chord string
chori- skin, membrane
chrom- color
chy- juice
chyt- fluid
-cide kill
cipit- head
circ- ring, around
cirrh- orange-colored
cleido- clavicle
clon- violent motion
co- with
coagul- drive together
coarct- pressed together
cochl- snail
coel- hollow
collat- brought together
condyl- knuckle, knob
coni- cone
contigu- adjoining
contra- against
copul- bond, link
corn- horny
corp- body
corpusc- little body
cost- rib
counter- opposite
cox- hip
crani- skull
crib- sieve
cric- circle
crypt- hidden
cubit- elbow
-culus(m) little
cuspi- point
cut- skin
cyan- blue
cyst- bladder, bag
cyt- cell
dactyl- finger or toe
de- from, out
debil- weak

deca- ten
decid- falling
decuss- a crossing
dendro- tree
den- tooth
derm- skin
desm- a bond
dext- right-side
di- two, separate
diastol- standing apart
didym- double, twin
dilat- expand
dimin- lessen
dipl- two, double
diurn- daytime, daily
dors- back
dur- hard
dya- two
e- without
ect- outer
-ectomy cut out
ectop- displaced
ef- away from
embol- inserted
emet- vomit
-emia blood
encephal- brain
end(o)- within
ent- within
epi- beside, upon
epithe- covered
erythr- red
eso- inward
esth- feel
etio- cause
ex- out
exacerb- violent
excit- arouse
excret- throw out
expir- breathe out
expuls- drive out
extern- outer

exud- sweat
falx, falc- sickle
febr- fever
fenestr- window
ferro- iron
fibr- fiber
fili- thread, son or daughter
fimbri- fringe
fiss- cleft
fistul- tube
flacc- flabby
flagell- whip
follicul- little bag
foram- opening
foss(a) trench
fove(a) pit
gala- milk
gangli- knot, swelling
gast- stomach, belly
gera- (geri-) old age
gingiv- gums
glauc- gray
glen(o)- socket
gli(a)- glue
glom- ball
glott- tongue
glut- swallow
glyc- sweet
goni- seed
gracil- slender
grav- heavy
gyn- woman
haust- draw up
hem(a)- blood
hepa- liver
hiat- opening
hist- tissue
hol(o)- whole
homeo- alike
homo- same, human
humer- shoulder
humor fluid

hy- y-shaped
hyal- glassy
hydat- watery
hydr- water
hyg- health
hyp(o)- under
hyper- over, above
iatro- of a physician
-icle little
icter- jaundice
ideo- one's own
il- not, into
ilia flank
ilio- intestine
im- not, into
in- into, not
inan- empty
infarct filled in
infer- (infra-) under
infundibul- funnel
inguin- groin
inter- between
intercal- insert
intim- innermost
intrins- contained within
ipsi- same
is(o)- same, equal
ischi- hip
isthm- narrow passage
-ites having to do with
-itis inflammation
-ium small
jejun- hunger
kera- horn
kilo- thousand
kine- move
kym(o)- wave
kypho- bent
labi- lip
lac- milk
lacer- torn
lachr- tears

HUMAN ANATOMY AND PHYSIOLOGY

JOAN G. CREAGER
Marymount College of Virginia

Wadsworth Publishing Company
A Division of Wadsworth, Inc.
Belmont, California

Biology Editor: Jack C. Carey

Art Director: Detta Penna

Art Editor: Wendy C. Calmenson

Copy Editor: Susan Weisberg

Illustrators: Catherine Brandel, Darwen Hennings, Vally Hennings, Joel Ito, Patricia Johnson, Nelva Richardson, Victor Royer, Evanell Towne.

Cover Designer: Stephen Rapley

Photographs by Elliott Varner Smith copyright © 1983.

Cover illustration: Ken Finch

Cover photography: Dow, Clement & Simison

Printed in the United States of America
1 2 3 4 5 6 7 8 9 10—87 86 85 84 83

Library of Congress Cataloging in Publication Data

Creager, Joan G.
   Human anatomy and physiology.

   Bibliography: p.
   Includes index.
   1. Human physiology.   2. Anatomy, Human.   I. Title.
QP34.5.C73   1983   612   612   82-8377
ISBN 0-534-01033-4   AACR2

ISBN 0-534-01033-4

PREFACE

The more students understand what they read (as opposed to memorizing by rote), the greater the rewards they will find in their study of human anatomy and physiology, and the longer they will remember what they have studied. This text helps students to understand and remember what they read. The details of human anatomy and physiology are organized around unifying themes and concepts, such as homeostasis. Introductory sections in most chapters include background on embryological development to provide a context for understanding the material. Optional clinical applications also provide another context for understanding. A complete system of pedagogical features greatly facilitates learning.

An emphasis on unifying concepts such as homeostasis   This text emphasizes homeostasis as the major organizing concept in understanding the structure and function of the body. This important basic biological concept, which operates in living organisms at many levels, is considered in this text at the chemical level, at the cellular level, and at the system level. Unit IV, Homeostatic Systems, which includes chapters in circulation, respiration, digestion, metabolism, kidney function, and electrolyte and acid-base balance, emphasizes the roles of these various systems in maintaining relatively stable internal conditions within the living human body. Even in the consideration of the continuity of life in Unit V, the concept of homeostasis helps to integrate ideas about the physiology of pregnancy and various stages of life from conception to death.

This text also emphasizes complementarity of structure and function and the hierarchical levels of complexity that contribute to the organization of the body as a whole. These and other themes introduced in Chapter 1 will help students incorporate detailed information into meaningful concepts and avoid memorizing without understanding. These themes provide a way to "see the forest" instead of getting bogged down in the details of the "trees."

Accuracy and readability, checked by more than eighty reviewers   The text was carefully and thoroughly reviewed by research specialists and professors of anatomy and physiology to help insure accuracy, currency, and clarity of presentation.

Developmental context provided   Most chapters open with introductory sections on development to provide background for understanding the structure and function of the mature form. The last chapter describes stages of life from prenatal development to aging and death. It explains how structure and function at various stages differ from adult structure and function. Because most health-science curricula do not require a separate course in embryology, students may not acquire an understanding of development unless the topic is included in the anatomy and physiology course. A knowledge of the way congenital defects affect the structure and function of the body will be helpful to students in clinical settings.

Optional clinical applications   To motivate students and to help maintain their interest, optional clinical applications are included in three forms:

1. *Boxed inserts* (of one or two paragraphs) give brief glimpses into applications relevant to the main text. These inserts appear at various points throughout the text.
2. *End-of-chapter sections on major disorders* and a self-pronouncing list of *clinical terms* are included in nearly every chapter. The sections on disturbances in structure and function help to explain how an understanding of normal structure and function can be applied to treating diseases and injuries.
3. *Boxed essays* in nearly every chapter treat high-interest topics, dealing with current and sometimes controversial ideas about application of anatomy and physiology to health and behavioral sciences. Essay topics include radioactivity, rheumatoid arthritis, biofeedback, interferon, cancer, and natural childbirth.

An entire chapter is devoted to nutrition, another to genetics, and significant portions of other chapters are devoted to the effects of stress.

A complete system of pedagogical features   Each chapter begins with a *chapter outline* that provides an overview of the content of the chapter, and the *introduction to the chapter* describes the general organization and major functions of the system to be described. *Objectives*, or statements of what students are expected to accomplish, are listed *at the beginning of each major section* within the chapter and are repeated in the *chapter summary*. This arrangement will help students keep the objectives in mind as they study the sections of each chapter and as they review what they have studied. The detailed *chapter summary* at the end of each chapter includes objectives and emphasizes major concepts. An extensive review section following the chapter summary includes a *list of important terms*, specific *questions* numbered to correspond to the objectives within the chapter, and *problems* that require application of information in the chapter or additional research. *References and readings* acknowledge the sources used in writing the chapter and provide easily accessible sources of further information about topics considered in the chapter. The extensive *glossary* and *index* also add to the pedagogical value of the text.

Acknowledgments. No book is ever solely the product of the efforts of its authors, and more than one hundred people have contributed to this one. Many of my colleagues in colleges and universities have conscientiously reviewed this book in manuscript form and contributed many constructive criticisms. Marymount College of Virginia provided copying service for several drafts of the manuscript.

Illustrating a book of this size requires the talents and assistance of many people. The artists include Joel Ito, Patricia Johnson, Nelva Richardson, Darwen Hennings, Vally Hennings, Judy McCarty and the staff at Innographics, Catherine Brandel, Victor Royer, Evanell Towne, Lisa Palacio, Alan Noyes, Joan Carol, photographer Elliott Varner Smith, and models Eilleen Kimball and Mark deLuna. Others who contributed to the illustrations include Joyce R. Isbel and her staff at Alexandria Hospital, who provided all X rays; technicians at Arlington Hospital who provided electroencephalograms and electrocardiograms; Lucia Young and others at Sharpe Health School, and staff members at Childrens Hospital National Medical Center, who arranged for me to take a number of photographs; staff members at Northern Virginia Community College—Alexandria Campus and at George Mason University, who provided slides and photomicrographic equipment; Herbert Wilson and his staff at the Armed Forces Institute of Pathology, who provided many illustrations; and the many individuals who gave permissions and provided photographs of their own work.

Manuscript and illustrations do not by themselves make a book; many talented people helped to put this book together. They include editors Jody Larson, Mary Arbogast, and Susan Weisberg, proofreader Kathy Lee, and especially Wendy Calmenson, who coordinated all of the artwork and prepared page layouts for all of the many pages of this text. Diane Moser prepared the discussion of how to use study aids. Leland Moss and the staff at Dharma Press served as compositors and provided the most error-free typesetting I have ever seen. Detta Penna, a lady with a flair for design and a dedication to meeting deadlines, coordinated all aspects of production with the able assistance of the staff at Wadsworth.

Biology editor, Jack Carey, with the assistance of Shirley Taylor, has worked unstintingly from the time he saw promise in the first sample chapters through many long months of reviews and revisions and more months of production to see this book published.

Finally, my husband, John, has proofread every page at every stage, and in spite of enduring such tedium and numerous inconveniences, has remained steadfast in his encouragement and support.

Thanks, everybody! Though I take responsibility for any errors that may remain, I am exceedingly grateful to all who have helped to make this book a current consideration of the important concepts of anatomy and physiology.

Joan G. Creager

REVIEWERS

This text was carefully reviewed by more than eighty specialists and professors of anatomy and physiology (many of whom are listed below) and reflects the author's consistent concern for accuracy, currency, and clear explanations.

David Bohr, The University of Michigan Medical School
William J. Brett, Indiana State University
Thomas E. Brown, Atlantic Community College
Robert H. Catlett, University of Colorado
Arthur K. Champlin, Colby College
Robert R. Chilcote, University of Chicago
Paul Churchill, Wayne State University Medical School
Nancy Corbett, Thomas Jefferson University
Monroe Cravats, Work College of the City of New York
Paul Desha, Tarrant County Junior College
Winifred B. Dickinson, University of Steubenville
Robert L. DePew, Pasadena City College
Peggy Dobry
Jessie Dolson, Delta College
Jon R. Fortman, Mississippi University for Women
Susan A. Foster, Mount Hood Community College
Ira Fowler, University of Kentucky
Walter Freeman, University of California, Berkeley
John Frehn, Illinois State University
Norman Goldstein, California State University, Hayward
Esta Grossman, Washetenaw Community College
Aslam Hassan, Lipid Research Center,
    Cincinnati General Hospital
Harlo N. Hadow, Coe College
John P. Harley, Eastern Kentucky University
Terrance L. Higgins, Wesley College
Theodore M. Hollis, Pennsylvania State University
Kathleen A. Koshelnyk, University of Colorado
Gerald L. Lllewellyn, Virginia Commonwealth University
Alexander Lucas, University of California, Berkeley

Robert W. Maitlen, The Defiance College
Donald H. Mansfield, Idaho State University
Ivonna McCabe, Tacoma Community College
Erwin D. Mickelberg, Augsburg College
Alar Mirka, University of Oregon Health Sciences,
    School of Medicine
Fred D. Morgan, Warner Southern College
James M. Moulton, Bowdoin College
Robert Nabors, Tarrant County Junior College
Jonathan C. Oldham, Metropolitan State College
Ingrith D. Olsen, University of Washington
Richard G. Pflanzer, Indiana University
L. Jack Pierce, Mountain View College
E. M. Turner Radtke, NCEA
Harry Reasor, Miami Dade Community College
Louis Renaud, Prince George's Community College
Robert J. Robbins, Michigan State University
Robert D. Rubin, Santa Rosa Junior College
Charles L. Rutherford, Virginia Polytechnic Institute
    and State University
Judith Shea, North Shore Community College
David Smith, San Antonio District Junior College
Paul M. Spannbauer, Hudson Valley Community College
Lawrence Stark, University of California, Berkeley
Aubery Taylor, University of South Alabama
Pauline Tepe, Phoenix College
Judith A. Theile, Hudson Valley Community College
Paula Timiras, University of California, Berkeley
Martha Van Bolt, Charles Stewart Mott Community College
Karen VanWinkle-Swift, San Diego State University
Donna M. Van Wynsberghe, University of Wisconsin
Rose Leigh Vines, California State University, Sacramento
C. Thomas Wiltshire, Culver-Stockton College
Donald L. Wise, College of Wooster
Mary Wise, Northern Virginia Community College
Stephen L. Wolfe, University of California, Davis
Richard D. Worthington, University of Texas, El Paso

HOW TO USE THE STUDY AIDS
IN THIS BOOK

In each chapter of this book you will find several carefully designed study aids. They will help you to focus on the most significant information and to master the important concepts.

An introduction to each unit provides the overall context for the chapters to follow.

A Chapter Outline begins each chapter. As you start to study a chapter, look over the chapter outline to preview the overall contents, note the main topics to be considered, and get a sense of the flow of ideas within the chapter.

One or more Study Objectives begins each chapter section. The objectives divide the chapter into manageable sections, so that you can keep each one clearly in mind as you read. Before you begin to study each chapter section, take a moment to fix in your mind the objective(s) for that section. Then, after you complete each section, go back to the beginning to review the objective. Can you do what the objective requires?

Important Terms are introduced in **bold-faced** type. As you glance over the section you just read, can you define all the **bold-faced** terms?

A detailed Summary outline concludes each chapter. Each section of the outline begins with a restatement of an objective. The major points under each objective are the essential points you should know to achieve the objective. Look over the points under each objective. If any points remain unclear, now is the time to go back to that numbered objective and the following chapter section for another review.

A list of Important Terms at the end of each chapter focuses on vocabulary you need to know from that chapter. Is there any term here you can't define? Look back in the chapter to review where it first appears in **bold-faced** type.

A Glossary of terms, with phonetic pronunciation, at the back of the book provides an additional source of definitions for key terms.

Review Questions at the end of the chapter are also numbered to correspond with the chapter section objectives. First try to answer them without looking back in the book. Then compare your answer with the appropriate section in your text, and relate your answer to the primary objective.

Problems at the end of each chapter provide more challenging questions.

References and Readings for further study are provided at the end of each chapter.

Clinical Applications are included in the book to relate human anatomy and physiology to interesting applications that are relevant to your field of study. These applications are presented in four ways:

1. *Boxed inserts* of one or two paragraphs appear within the body of the text.
2. *The last section of each chapter* (or the last part of some subsections of chapters) discusses clinical applications.
3. *A list of clinical terms* appears at the end of nearly every chapter.
4. *Boxed essays* discuss high-interest applications in detail.

BRIEF CONTENTS

CONTENTS

*To my
husband,
John*

UNIT ONE

LEVELS OF ORGANIZATION

The human body is a magnificent thing. Its many systems and components perform highly complex functions in a carefully regulated and often very subtle way. Because so many of these processes seem automatic, people sometimes tend to take the body's functioning for granted.

For example, you might be used to thinking of your stomach as only a bag that receives the food you eat, but it's much more complex than that. When food enters the stomach, its presence stimulates nerves, sending signals to centers in the brain. The brain responds with signals that cause contraction of muscles in the walls of the stomach, mixing and propelling the food; the same nerve impulses stimulate secretion of substances to start the chemical breakdown, or digestion, of proteins. The stomach produces these substances in such a way that normally only the proteins in the food are digested, and not the proteins in the cells of the stomach itself. The stomach cells are stimulated by the products of digestion, and they release a regulatory chemical into the blood. This regulatory chemical travels back through the circulatory system to the stomach and stimulates further secretion of digestive substances.

The process that takes place in the stomach is but one example of the complicated functions taking place in the human body. The more we learn about these processes, the more marvelous the body seems.

If you wanted to study an automobile, you might begin by determining what its major components are and how they are arranged to make the automobile run. You might then study the materials used to make the various parts of the car. Finally, you might make a detailed study of the different components—body, engine, fuel system, electrical system, and so on—to see how their structure is related to their function and how regulation is accomplished.

Likewise, in studying the processes of the human body, we must first understand how the parts of the body are organized. We will begin with a study of the body as a whole—its major components and how they are arranged to carry out basic life processes (Chapter 1). We will then study the fundamental units of the body at the chemical level (Chapter 2), the cellular level (Chapter 3), and the tissue level (Chapter 4). In subsequent chapters we will consider the structure and function of the various systems and the ways in which these systems are regulated.

1

THE BODY AS A WHOLE

DEFINITION OF THE SUBJECT

Objective 1. Define anatomy and physiology and summarize briefly the historical development of these subjects.

Anatomy is the study of structure. **Physiology** is the study of function. Long before these terms came into formal use, people were fascinated by the structure and function of their own bodies. Some of the important landmarks in the development of anatomy and physiology are considered in this section, providing a historical perspective for the study of the current state of these sciences.

Though the ancient Chinese acupuncturists made some efforts to relate body structure and function, Aristotle was the first known student of both anatomy and physiology in Western culture. His observations in the fourth century B.C. were extended by Galen in the second century A.D. In spite of the fact that Galen's observations were based on studies of dogs and other nonhuman animals, his writings remained the established authority for 1300 years. Then, Vesalius, an Italian physician, turned the study of anatomy into an experimental science. Not content with animal studies, he insisted on making direct observations from human cadavers. At the time this was a shocking notion, and it brought him into conflict with both state and religious authorities. Even his colleagues opposed his ideas. Despondent over such opposition, Vesalius destroyed many of his manuscripts and gave up teaching to become a court physician. Nevertheless, some records of his observations on human cadavers remained, and they served to correct some faulty ideas about the human body that were based on studies of other animals.

If we call Vesalius the founder of modern anatomy, we

might call William Harvey the founder of modern physiology. Harvey, born in England in 1597 and trained as a physician in Italy, is best known for demonstrating that blood circulates through the body. By observing the heartbeat of a frog or other animal, Harvey calculated that a volume of blood equivalent to all that is in the body leaves the heart in only a minute or two. He also tied off vessels and observed how the blood backed up in them. From these and other observations, he deduced that blood must circulate through a continuous system of vessels. As microscopes had not yet been developed, Harvey could not observe the tiny capillaries where blood moved from arteries to veins to complete the circuit. Nevertheless, Harvey's experimental methods and his interpretation of the results were of great benefit to the medical profession. Today, we take the circulation of blood so much for granted we find it hard to imagine that it was once not known.

Another giant in the science of physiology, Johannes Müller (1801-1858), combined a talent for accurate observation with a talent for applying the findings of physics, chemistry, and psychology to the study of the human body. His main contribution to physiology was to make it a comparative science, emphasizing similarities and differences among species of animals. His talent and enthusiasm for teaching fostered the development of many other outstanding physiologists. After Müller physiology grew in two directions—physical and chemical. The physicist-physiologists devised ingenious methods for recording and quantifying blood pressure, muscle contraction, and nerve impulses. The chemist-physiologists studied chemical changes that take place in the body. Some followed the changes in food as it was digested and particles were transported to the cells of the body; others studied chemical changes in the blood during respiration.

On the foundations laid by pioneers such as Aristotle, Galen, Vesalius, Harvey, and Müller, hundreds of researchers have built a sound understanding of human anatomy and physiology. But the task is not finished; new discoveries are being made every day. And physicians, nurses, technicians, and therapists apply these findings to create today's complex health technology.

Among the many concepts that scientists have developed over the centuries, five important ones help to unify and organize the large body of knowledge that has accumulated: (1) complementarity of structure and function—the idea that structure and function are closely related; (2) the constancy of the human body plan, with only small variations among individuals and over many generations; (3) the organization of functions into a set of basic life processes necessary for survival; (4) the idea that the body has hierarchical levels of complexity; and (5) the most powerful concept of all, homeostasis—the idea that the body's internal environment, though always changing, remains nearly constant. These concepts will be discussed in the following sections of this chapter.

COMPLEMENTARITY OF STRUCTURE AND FUNCTION

Objective 2. Define complementarity of structure and function and explain how it can be used to organize information about the human body.

Look at the back of your hand. Watch the stringlike tendons that move your fingers as you clench and relax your fist. Those tendons are connected to muscles in your arm. If, instead, these muscles were in your fingers, each finger would be so bulky that you would have far less freedom of movement. Touch the tip of your thumb and the tip of your index finger together. If you could not do that, you could not pick up small objects, write, or do many other things you do every day. Humans and a few other animals are the only organisms that can perform that movement. They are said to have *apposable* thumbs. The evolution of apposable thumbs allowed for the development of many human abilities.

As evidenced by the above examples, anatomical structures and their physiological functions are always closely related—structure and function are complementary. The anatomy (shape, size, and form) of nearly every structure in your body is well-suited for carrying out its function. The functions required for survival also help to determine what structures will be passed along from one generation to the next. Thus, structure influences function, and function influences structure—this **complementarity of structure and function** is a concept that will help you to organize the information you are learning.

BODY PLAN

Objective 3. Describe the general plan of the human body using accepted terminology.

Terminology is not an end in itself; it is simply a necessary means of communication about a complex subject. To talk about mathematics, we use such terms as sum, integer, zero, infinity, and equality. To talk about grammar we define such terms as noun, phrase, comma, and subject–verb agreement. Likewise, to talk about the structure and function of the body, we need to use the language of

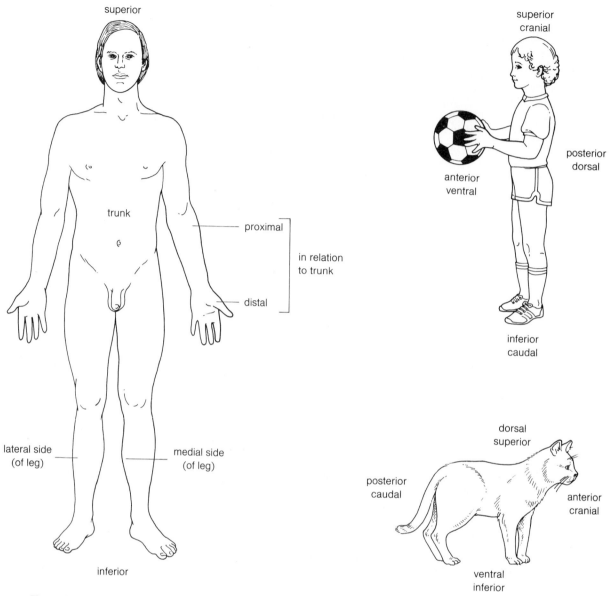

Figure 1.1 Anatomical terms of position.

anatomists and physiologists. Without such terminology we might find ourselves talking about the "whatcha-ma-call-it" on the "far side" of the "thing-a-ma-jig." Those terms are too vague to communicate as precisely as we need to. As you learn the language of anatomy and physiology, you will be acquiring a large new vocabulary; you may find it easier to remember and use this vocabulary if you think of it as a tool for understanding the major concepts.

Terms of Position

Terms used to describe the position of a structure or locate one structure in relation to another always assume that the body is in a specific position, known as the **anatomical position**: standing erect with face forward (that is, facing the viewer), hands at the sides with palms forward (Figure 1.1). The terms of position are listed and defined in Table 1.1.

Terms for Planes or Sections

In studying anatomy it is often helpful to imagine planes passing through the body (Figure 1.2). When such planes are passed through the body, they are called sections. A **sagittal section** divides the body into left and right portions. When this section lies along the midline of the body, dividing the body into equal left and right halves, it is called a **mid-sagittal section**. A **transverse** or **cross section** divides the body into superior and inferior portions. A **frontal section** or **coronal section** divides the body into anterior and posterior portions. These terms also can be used to describe sections through structures within the body.

Terms for Body Divisions and Body Cavities

The two major divisions of the body are the axial portion and the appendicular portion. The **axial** portion includes the head, neck, and trunk; the **appendicular** includes the appendages or arms, legs, shoulders, and hips. The main organs or viscera are located within the body cavities in the axial portion of the body (Figure 1.3). The **dorsal cavity** is composed of the **cranial cavity**, which contains the brain, and the **spinal cavity**, which contains the spinal cord. The **ventral cavity** is composed of the **thoracic cavity** and the **abdominopelvic cavity**. These ventral cavities are separated by a broad muscle called the **diaphragm**.

The left and right lateral portions of the thoracic cavity, called the **pleural cavities**, contain the lungs. The medial portion of the thoracic cavity, called the **mediastinum**, contains the heart, the thymus gland, and a part of the esophagus. The heart is further enclosed in the **pericardial cavity**. Together, these organs comprise the thoracic viscera.

The abdominopelvic cavity includes the **abdominal cavity** and the **pelvic cavity**. An imaginary plane extending from the anterior pubic bone to the posterior sacrum divides these cavities. (These bones of the pelvic area are described in Chapter 6.) The viscera of the abdominal cavity include the stomach, small intestine, most of the large intestine, liver, spleen, pancreas, and kidneys. The viscera of the pelvic cavity include the internal reproductive organs, the inferior portion of the large intestine, and the urinary bladder.

The abdominal cavity is divided into regions as shown in Figure 1.4. The central region, which surrounds the umbilicus, or navel, is called the **umbilical region**. Superior to the umbilical region is the **epigastric region**, and inferior to it is the **hypogastric region**. Lateral to the midline regions on both the left and right sides of the abdomen are three pairs of

regions. The most superior are the **hypochondriac regions**; next are the **lumbar regions** and, most inferior, the **iliac regions**. These regions are often used to describe the location of internal organs and the location of symptoms reported by individuals seeking medical attention.

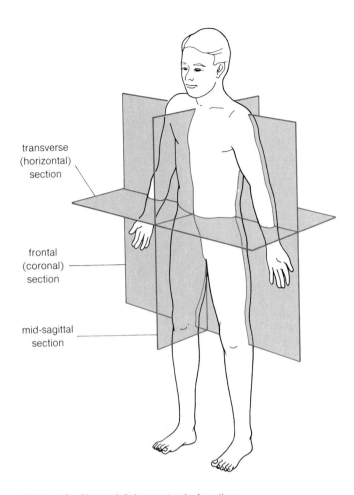

transverse (horizontal) section

frontal (coronal) section

mid-sagittal section

Figure 1.2 Planes defining anatomical sections.

Embodied in the term *hypochondriac* is a bit of medical and human history. Literally, the word means under the cartilage (of the ribs). Its use to describe a person with imaginary ailments comes from the outdated idea that symptoms often arose from these regions of the body. Thus, someone who constantly complained of symptoms became known as a hypochondriac.

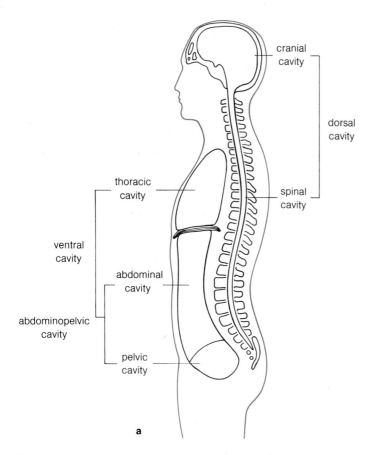

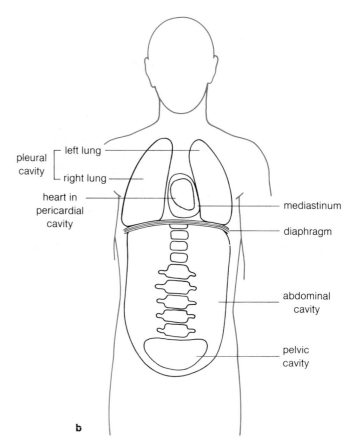

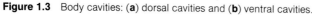

Figure 1.3 Body cavities: (**a**) dorsal cavities and (**b**) ventral cavities.

BASIC LIFE PROCESSES

Objective 4. List the basic life processes. Describe the ways each contributes to maintaining life and name the system(s) involved in carrying out the process.

Your body, like that of other living organisms, must carry out basic life processes to stay alive and to maintain the species. These processes include **movement, support, excitability, ingestion, digestion, metabolism, excretion, transport, respiration, integration, growth and repair, protection,** and **reproduction**. Some of these basic processes, such as metabolism, occur in all cells in all systems. Others, such as digestion, are accomplished by specialized systems. We can get an overview of the systems of the body by looking briefly at the processes each of them carries out.

The skin, or **integumentary system,** protects internal systems from damage. It also contains special structures that can detect changes in the environment such as temperature.

Beneath the skin are the muscles, or the **muscular system**. The muscles are attached to the bones of the **skeletal system**. The muscular and skeletal systems together make movement possible. The skeletal system supports the body and protects some of its internal organs. The major organs of these three systems are shown in Figure 1.5.

The **nervous system** receives information from special sensory receptors such as the eyes, ears, and skin receptors. It also transmits information from the receptors to the brain or spinal cord, and returns messages that cause responses such as movement. It can do these things because its cells are electrically **excitable**. The nervous system also helps to coordinate or integrate the functions of the other systems. The **endocrine system** produces chemicals called hormones, which also help to integrate the functions of other systems. The major organs of these two systems are shown in Figure 1.6.

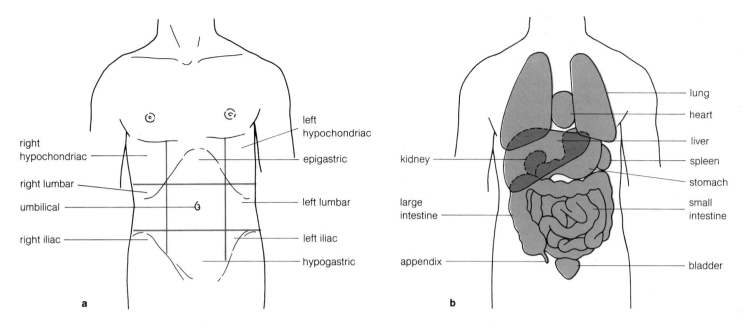

Figure 1.4 (**a**) abdominal regions and (**b**) internal organs.

Table 1.1	Terms of Position	
Term	Definition	Example
Anterior (*ante* = before)	Toward the belly or front side in humans; toward the head in other animals	The abdominal skin is anterior to the abdominal organs. A cat's head is anterior to its neck.
Ventral (*vent* = underside)	Toward the belly	The belly is ventral to the back.
Posterior (*post* = hindmost)	Toward the back in humans; toward the tail in other animals	The skin on the back is posterior to the lungs within the chest. A dog's hind legs are posterior to its front legs.
Dorsal (*dors* = back)	Toward the back	The back is dorsal to the belly.
Superior (*super* = above)	Toward the head	The head is superior to the chest.
Inferior (*infer* = below)	Toward the tail	The abdomen is inferior to the chest.
Medial (*medi* = middle)	Toward the midline	The mouth is medial to the cheeks.
Lateral (*later* = side)	Toward the side	The eyes are lateral to the nose.
Proximal (*proxim* = nearest)	Nearest the trunk	The ankle is proximal to the foot.
Distal (*dist* = distant)	Farthest from the trunk	The fingers are distal to the wrist.
Superficial	Near the surface	Skin is superficial to muscles.
Deep	Beneath the surface	The deep muscles lie beneath the superficial muscles.

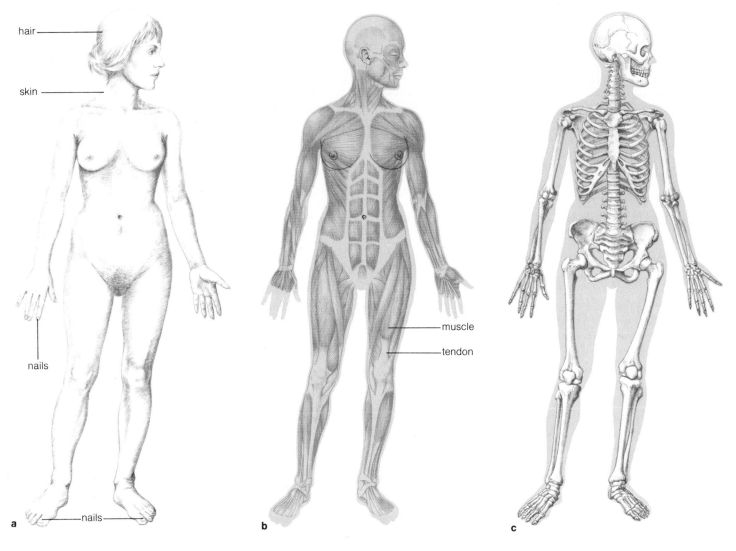

hair

skin

nails

nails

muscle

tendon

a

b

c

Figure 1.5 Organs of the (**a**) integumentary, (**b**) muscular, and (**c**) skeletal systems.

The **circulatory** and **lymphatic systems** are primarily responsible for transporting substances throughout the body. They also contain the cells that produce immunity and protect the body against infections. The **respiratory system** is closely related to the transport systems because it delivers oxygen to the blood and removes carbon dioxide from it. This process of gas exchange is called external respiration. The movement of oxygen from the blood into the cells and of carbon dioxide out of them is called internal respiration. These three systems are illustrated in Figure 1.7.

The **digestive system** is responsible solely for the ingestion of food and its digestion or breakdown into particles that can be transported throughout the body. The digestive system also excretes the waste materials from the digestive process. **Metabolism** occurs in all body cells, as food is used for energy, growth, and repair. Waste products of metabolism enter the blood and are excreted primarily by the **urinary system**. These systems are illustrated in Figure 1.8.

The body of an individual can exist for a lifetime without reproducing. However, a species can exist for only one generation unless some of its members reproduce. The human **male and female reproductive systems** carry out the process of reproduction, including, in the female, protecting and nourishing the developing individual until it is ready for independent existence (Figure 1.9).

As you study the following chapters, keep the basic

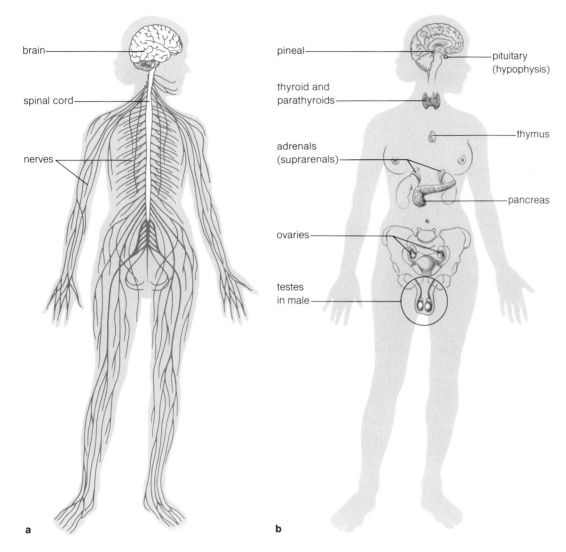

Figure 1.6 Organs of the (**a**) nervous and (**b**) endocrine systems.

life processes in mind. Try to classify every physiological function as an example of one of these processes. Table 1.2 lists the organs of each system and summarizes the processes they carry out.

LEVELS OF COMPLEXITY

Objective 5. List and describe briefly the levels of complexity of the human body from particles within cells to the whole body.

The human body functions as an entity, each of its parts contributing to the overall function. To begin to understand overall function, it is often useful to study components separately.

Like all other matter, living things are composed of particles called **atoms**, **molecules**, and **ions** (charged particles); these particles will be discussed in Chapter 2. Unlike nonliving matter, however, living things are able to rearrange these particles to maintain themselves and to reproduce. The smallest unit of living material capable of doing this is the **cell**. Cells contain specialized structures called **organelles**—the cell nucleus, for example. Whether a bacterial cell or a human muscle cell, each cell can perform most of the basic life processes. It is because of what hap-

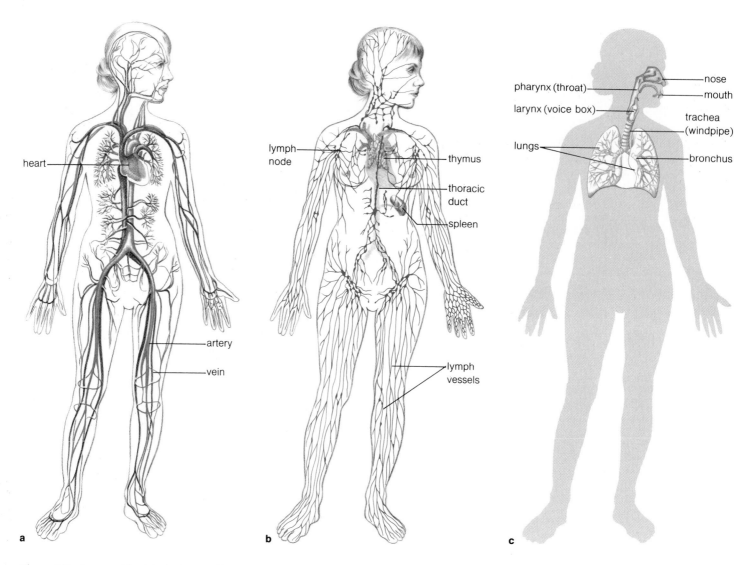

Figure 1.7   Organs of the (**a**) circulatory, (**b**) lymphatic, and (**c**) respiratory systems.

pens inside individual human cells that muscles contract, nerves conduct impulses, or glands secrete their products. The specifics of cellular function will be discussed in Chapter 3.

Cells are organized into tissues. A **tissue** is a group of similar cells specialized to carry out a particular function. For example, muscle cells are different from nerve cells, and they carry out different functions. All of the cells in muscle tissue work together to produce a muscle contraction. Likewise, the cells of any tissue work together to perform their particular function.

Tissues combine to form organs. An **organ** is a structured group of tissues working together to carry out a more general function. For example, the stomach is an organ. It is lined with a sheet of epithelial tissue containing glands that secrete digestive juices. Its wall contains muscle tissue, which contracts to mix foods inside the stomach; nerve tissue, which integrates the action of the muscles and glands; and connective tissue, which supports the organ.

Organs, in turn, form systems. A **system** is a group of related organs working in concert to perform related functions. Systems must be integrated structurally and functionally to produce a whole organism. In summary, the **levels of complexity** from simple to complex are: atoms and ions, molecules, organelles, cells, tissues, organs, systems, and the whole organism (Figure 1.10).

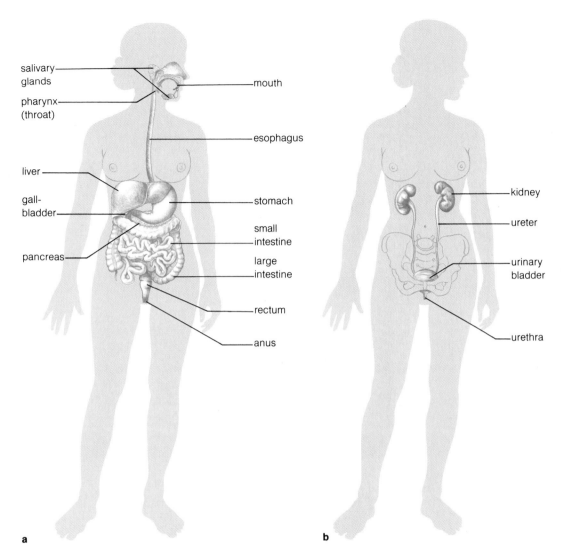

salivary glands

mouth

pharynx (throat)

esophagus

liver

stomach

gall-bladder

small intestine

pancreas

large intestine

rectum

anus

kidney

ureter

urinary bladder

urethra

a

b

Figure 1.8 Organs of the (**a**) digestive and (**b**) urinary systems.

HOMEOSTASIS

Objective 6. Define homeostasis and explain why it is an important unifying concept.

The concepts we have considered so far contribute to our understanding of the single most powerful concept in all of anatomy and physiology—homeostasis. **Homeostasis**, from the roots *homeo*, meaning alike, and *stasis*, meaning to stand, is *the stable internal environment within an organism that is essential for life.* Homeostatic mechanisms regulate the functioning of body components so that the body's physiological conditions are kept nearly constant. In health and in a resting state your body's homeostatic mechanisms keep your breathing rate at about fourteen to eighteen breaths per minute, your heart beating around seventy times per minute, and your body temperature close to 37°C (98.6°F). These are the optimum conditions for a well-running human machine.

Self regulation is a fundamental property of all homeostatic mechanisms. To be self-regulating, a homeostatic mechanism must have at least three components: a **sensor**, an **effector**, and a **control center**, each of which is a specific anatomical structure. The sensor detects changes in the internal environment and sends information, or **input**, to the control center. The control center causes certain events to occur, which we will call **output**. Output con-

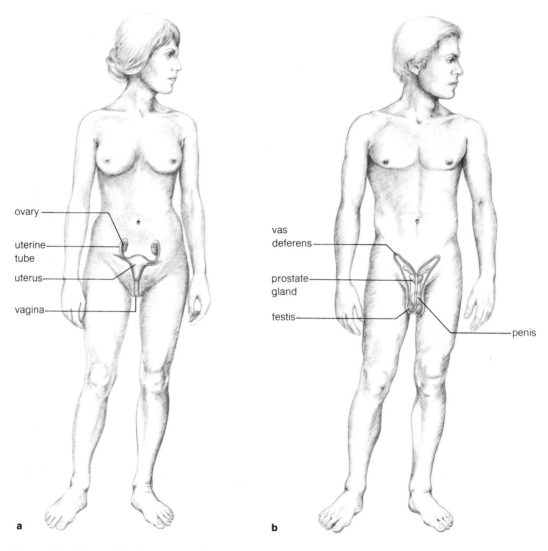

Figure 1.9 Organs of the female and male reproductive systems.

ovary

uterine tube

uterus

vagina

a

vas deferens

prostate gland

testis

penis

b

sists of signals that cause a change in a physiological condition—an increase or decrease in blood pressure, body temperature, or heart rate, for example. Effectors—muscles and glands—act to cause the change. Information about a change in the output is then relayed to the sensor. This is called **feedback**. The sensor detects the change, and the whole process begins again. *A sensor, an effector, a control center, and the processes of input, output, and feedback are essential for the operation of a homeostatic mechanism.*

The thermostatic control of a home heating system is an example of a mechanical homeostatic mechanism (Figure 1.11). Suppose the thermostat is set at a normal room temperature. When the air temperature drops below the

temperature at which the thermostat is set, this information is relayed to the sensor by feedback. The sensor relays this information (input) to the control center, where it causes the heating unit to switch on (output). Heat generated from the system causes the temperature of the room air to rise. When the air temperature rises above the set temperature, the sensor detects the change (feedback), and the switch turns the heating unit off. It stays off until the air temperature again drops below the thermostat setting (new input). The self-regulating action of this system maintains the air temperature within a narrow range near the thermostat setting.

Human body temperature is regulated by a similar

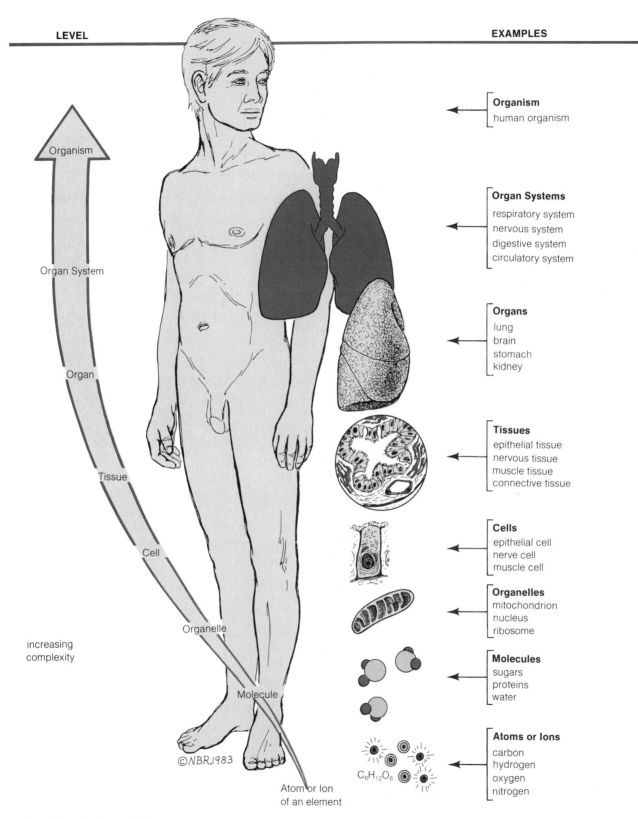

Organism

Organ System

Organ

Tissue

Cell

Organelle

increasing
complexity

Molecule

©NBR,1983

Atom or Ion
of an element

Organism
human organism

Organ Systems
respiratory system
nervous system
digestive system
circulatory system

Organs
lung
brain
stomach
kidney

Tissues
epithelial tissue
nervous tissue
muscle tissue
connective tissue

Cells
epithelial cell
nerve cell
muscle cell

Organelles
mitochondrion
nucleus
ribosome

Molecules
sugars
proteins
water

Atoms or Ions
carbon
hydrogen
oxygen
nitrogen

$C_6H_{12}O_6$

Figure 1.10 Levels of complexity.

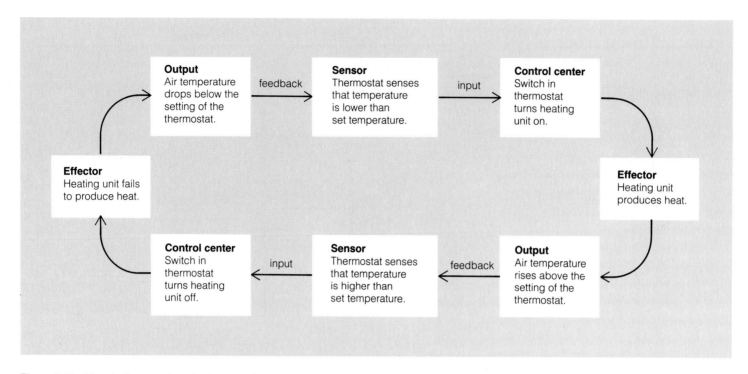

Figure 1.11 Steps in the operation of a thermostatically controlled heating unit, showing input, sensor, output, and feedback in a self-regulating mechanical homeostatic mechanism.

Table 1.2 The Systems of the Body		
System	Major Organs of the System	Basic Life Processes Carried Out
Integumentary	Skin	Protection
Muscular	Muscles	Movement
Skeletal	Bones and joints	Movement, protection, support
Nervous and sensory	Sense organs, nerves, brain, and spinal cord	Excitability, integration
Endocrine	Glands such as pituitary, thyroid, parathyroid, and adrenal	Integration
Circulatory and lymphatic	Heart, blood and lymph vessels, and blood	Transport, protection
Respiratory	Trachea, bronchi, and air passages of lungs	External respiration
Digestive	Mouth, stomach, intestines, liver, and pancreas	Ingestion, digestion, excretion
Urinary	Kidneys, passageways, and bladder	Excretion
Reproductive	Sex glands and passageways; uterus in female	Reproduction
All systems	Individual cells	Metabolism, growth and repair, and some degree of excitability

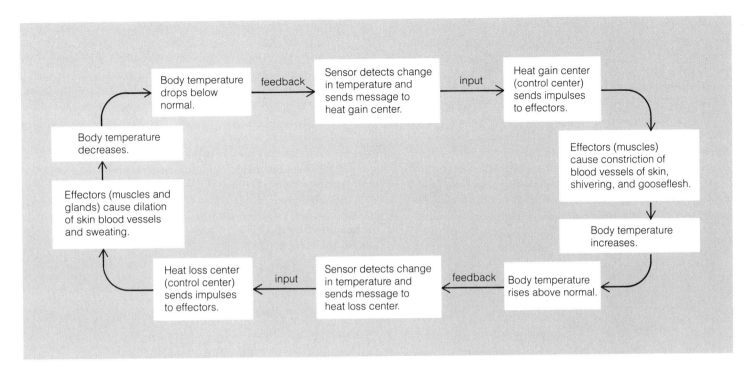

Figure 1.12 The regulation of body temperature.

mechanism (Figure 1.12). When body temperature changes, sensors in the base of the brain detect the change as blood passes through the vessels near them. If the temperature is lower than normal, the sensors relay signals to the **heat gain center**. The control center then sends signals that lead to physiological changes such as constriction or narrowing of the blood vessels so less heat is lost, shivering so muscles produce more heat by contracting, and "goose flesh," which would keep us warmer if we had more hair. These changes cause an increase in body temperature, including the temperature of the blood. Feedback is accomplished when the warmer blood passes by the sensors.

"Goose flesh" is caused by the contraction of tiny muscles attached to the base of individual hairs. In mammals with heavy fur these contractions cause hair to stand out and trap warm air around the body. Human goose flesh probably means that at one time humans were furry.

When you have been exercising, you feel hot and sweaty, and maybe short of breath. Even before you experience these things, the temperature of your blood increases slightly as heat is given off from contracting muscles. Sensors in the brain detect the temperature increase and send messages to the **heat loss center**. These messages cause output such as dilation or widening of blood vessels in the skin and release of sweat from the sweat glands. Both of these physiological effects tend to lower the body temperature. Sweat is mostly water, and, as it evaporates, it causes cooling of the skin and of the blood in dilated vessels near the surface. As the temperature of the blood drops, the change is fed back to the sensors as the blood passes by them.

Many other homeostatic mechanisms exist in the body. All have three anatomical components: sensor, effector, and control center. All have two physiological effects: output, or changes in the physiological conditions in the body, and feedback of the changes to the sensors. Because of the feedback component homeostatic mechanisms are self-regulating.

Feedback in self-regulating systems is always **negative feedback**. When the output increases to a certain point, sensors relay signals to the control center, which decreases the output. When the output decreases to a certain point, sensors again relay signals to the control center, which increases the output. In other words, negative feedback reverses the direction of the physiological change. Ultimately, an increase in temperature causes a decrease in heat production, and a decrease in temperature causes an increase in heat production. Thus, negative feedback maintains stable internal conditions.

In contrast, **positive feedback** accelerates a process; the information fed back causes an increase in the rate of the events detected by the sensor. For example, during the clotting of blood following an injury, the release of clotting factors in the later steps in the process stimulates the production of more of the factors that initiated the clotting process, resulting in faster clotting. The increase in the intensity of uterine contractions during labor is another example of positive feedback at work. Positive feedback, then, serves to hasten some physiological changes. Once these changes are accomplished, homeostatic mechanisms act to re-create stable conditions.

Homeostasis is an important unifying concept in anatomy and physiology because it emphasizes how structure and function interact to keep basic life processes operating at optimum rates and in a coordinated manner. Homeostasis must be maintained if the organism is to stay alive.

CLINICAL APPLICATIONS

Objective 7. Explain how the concept of homeostasis applies to health.

Homeostatic mechanisms are so important to maintaining normal physiological conditions that health may be thought of as meaning homeostasis. Most illnesses and injuries upset homeostasis in some way. Thus, they may be thought of as a loss of homeostasis. For example, a fractured bone or an injured joint disturbs the normal anatomical relationships of the body's parts. A loss of blood changes the total blood volume, reducing the blood pressure and the heart's pumping efficiency. Invasion of the body by an infectious agent triggers several events: White blood cells try to destroy some of the invaders directly; the immune system produces chemicals called antibodies that inactivate the invaders; and the whole body responds with symptoms such as pain, nausea, and fever. Knowing how the human body maintains homeostasis will help you to see how health can be maintained and how therapy can correct malfunctions and restore homeostasis.

The body's natural reaction to disturbances is to attempt to restore homeostasis. Most medical treatment is intended to help this process. Whether or not it is effective depends to a large extent on how well the would-be healers understand normal physiological processes and their regulation.

Clinical Terms

etiology (e-te-ol'o-je)   the study of the causes of diseases

pathology (path-ol'o-je)   the study of disorders of structure or function

pathophysiology (path''o-fiz-e-ol'o-je)   the study of the functional disorders produced by diseases

sign   observable evidence of a disease

symptom (simp'tum)   evidence of a disease reported by the affected individual

syndrome (sin'drōm)   a set of signs and symptoms that occur together

Essay: Human Characteristics and Human Dilemmas

We humans have many characteristics in common with other animals. Like most other animals, we can move; like other vertebrates, we have a spinal cord and vertebral column; like other mammals, we have hair and mammary glands; and like other primates, we have a large brain. With the anthropoid apes we share our apposable thumbs; and with the hominids we share our land-living habitat, our bipedal (two-footed) gait, and our large cerebrum, or higher brain, which carries out our thought processes.

Though we are like other animals in many ways, we are distinctly different from any other animal in important ways. We share curiosity, imitation, attention, and memory with some of the other animals, but we display these characteristics to a higher degree and with greater flexibility. We use our reasoning ability to adapt to and modify our environment. We make and use tools and create mental abstractions to a greater degree than any other animal. We are self-conscious—we wonder about our own existence. We are social, as are many other animals, but we develop social traditions and codes of behavior.

One characteristic that seems uniquely human is *altruism*, concern for the welfare of others beyond one's own interest. René Dubos, in the book *Beast or Angel?*, claims that altruism has been recognized among humans for thousands of years. Dubos cites as evidence the discovery of the remains of a man who died an estimated 50,000 years ago, at about fifty years of age. His bones showed that he had suffered from extensive arthritis. Since he undoubtedly had lived for many years after he was no longer able to gather food or hunt game, other members of his clan must have cared for him, possibly at the risk of their own survival.

This human desire to preserve human life and well-being is reflected in our use of tools and technology in medical science. We have created eyeglasses to correct vision, discovered the use of insulin and other therapies to control diabetes, and devised special diets to prevent mental retardation in individuals with hereditary metabolic diseases. With the aid of inventions such as pacemakers for the heart and artificial kidney machines, we can prolong the lives of people who otherwise would have died much sooner. Through special techniques we can determine whether or not an unborn child has certain genetic abnormalities. In the future, it may be possible to supply a normal gene to a person who has a defective one.

Altruism as part of our biological past helped make possible the survival of groups; however, Dubos says, "the really human aspect of altruism is not its biological origin or its evolutionary advantages, but rather the fact that humankind has now made it a virtue regardless of practical advantages or disadvantages." The advantages our technology has given us are not without their price. Our therapeutic intervention has already altered the composition of the human population. A greater number of people live to reach old age. More people with genetic defects survive to reproduce, and they may pass these defects on to their children. A higher proportion of the population are people who might have died from injury or illness but were saved to exist as invalids or partially disabled individuals. Fewer infants die, further increasing the size of the population. All these changes put a greater burden on society's resources. In spite of these disadvantages, our altruism still makes us feel that preserving life is good.

For better or for worse, the *human species is the first species capable of conscious participation in its own evolution*. Our big brains have given us this capability, yet with it comes very difficult questions: Are our brains "big enough" to know what is best for human evolution? Can anyone really tell with certainty the long-term effects of a genetic variation? Is it a good idea to let parents choose the sex of their children? Does anyone have the right to decide whether or not another person should be allowed to reproduce? If an individual chooses not to reproduce, does anyone else have the right to decide the opposite?

For these, and for many other questions, there are no easy answers. Our big brains have allowed us to create many human dilemmas.

CHAPTER SUMMARY

(Chapter summary points and review questions are numbered to correspond to the numbered objectives in the text of each chapter.)

Definition of the Subject

1. Define anatomy and physiology and summarize briefly the historical development of these subjects.
   a. Anatomy is the study of the structure of the body.
   b. Physiology is the study of its function.
   c. Important people in the development of anatomy and physiology as sciences include the anatomist Vesalius and the physiologists Harvey and Müller.

Complementarity of Structure and Function

2. Define complementarity of structure and function and explain how it can be used to organize information about the human body.
   a. Complementarity of structure and function means that the nature of a structure in the body influences how that structure will function, and, analogously, the functions a structure performs can over many generations influence the nature of the structure.
   b. Perceiving close relationships between structure and function is useful in organizing information about anatomy and physiology.

Body Plan

3. Describe the general plan of the human body using accepted terminology.
   a. Anatomical position of the body is the position of standing erect with hands at sides and palms forward.
   b. Terms of position are defined in Table 1.1.
   c. Planes or sections are shown in Figure 1.2.
   d. The body consists of the axial and appendicular portions.
   e. Cavities of the axial portion are shown in Figure 1.3.
   f. Abdominal regions are shown in Figure 1.4.

Basic Life Processes

4. List the basic life processes. Describe the ways each contributes to maintaining life and name the system(s) involved in carrying out the process.
   a. Basic life processes include movement, support, excitability, ingestion, digestion, metabolism, excretion, transport, respiration, integration, growth and repair, protection, and reproduction.
   b. The body systems and the processes they carry out are listed in Table 1.2.

Levels of Complexity

5. List and describe briefly the levels of complexity of the human body from particles within cells to the whole body.
   a. The human body functions as an entity, each of its parts contributing to the overall function.
   b. The cell is the fundamental unit of living organisms. It contains ions, atoms, molecules, and organelles, each of which has a particular function.
   c. Cells are organized into tissues; tissues into organs; organs into systems; and systems together make up the whole body.

Homeostasis

6. Define homeostasis and explain why it is an important unifying concept.
   a. Homeostasis is the stable, though constantly changing, internal environment.
   b. Homeostatic mechanisms regulate the functioning of all components of the body so that physiological conditions are kept nearly constant.
   c. Homeostatic mechanisms are self-regulating and involve a sensor, an effector, a control center, and the processes of input, output, and feedback.
   d. Homeostasis is an important unifying concept because it integrates structure–function relationships and the regulation of the functions of the structures.

Clinical Applications

7. Explain how the concept of homeostasis applies to health.
   a. Homeostasis and health might be equated.
   b. When homeostasis is disturbed by injury or disease,
      (1) the body's homeostatic mechanisms attempt to restore homeostasis.
      (2) the aim of medical treatment is intended to help restore homeostasis.

REVIEW

Important Terms

anatomical position	levels of complexity
anatomy	metabolism
anterior	organ
appendicular	organelle
axial	physiology
cell	posterior
complementarity of structure and function	respiration
	sagittal
cranial	spinal
dorsal	system
excitability	thoracic
feedback	tissue
frontal	transverse
homeostasis	ventral
integration	

Questions

1. **a.** What is the difference between anatomy and physiology?
   b. Who are some of the pioneers of anatomy and physiology, and what were their contributions?

2. What are some examples of complementarity of structure and function you can demonstrate on your own body?

3. Make a list of all the boldface terms pertaining to body plan and use them to describe the human body plan.

4. **a.** What are the basic life processes that occur in the human body?
   b. Which of these processes are carried out by each of the systems of the body?

5. Arrange the levels of complexity in the body from the whole organism down to the atom.

6. **a.** What is homeostasis?
   b. Suppose you are working with a patient who has a fever. How could you explain to the patient how her body normally maintains a temperature of about 37°C?

7. Discuss the statement that homeostasis is synonymous with health.

Problems

In each of the following problems, (a) identify the major concept to which the problem relates, and (b) find the flaw (if any) in the statements.

1. The nervous system controls and integrates the functioning of other systems of the body. The digestive system delivers food to the cells of the body. The reproductive system helps to maintain continuity from one generation to the next.

2. The human hand is constructed so that humans can do things many other animals cannot do. The stomach is well designed to serve its function as a food storage bag.

3. Tissues are composed of several different organs, which in turn are composed of cells, organelles, and molecules.

4. The internal conditions of the body are maintained in a nearly constant state. This state is maintained by positive feedback in which a process that has started constantly accelerates itself.

REFERENCES AND READINGS

Asimov, I. 1964. *A short history of biology.* Garden City, N.Y.: Natural History Press.

Borror, D. J. 1960. *Dictionary of word roots and combining forms.* Palo Alto, Calif.: Mayfield.

Dubos, R. 1974. *Beast or angel?* New York: Scribner's.

Eiseley, L. 1957. *Immense journey.* New York: Random House.

Kormondy, E. J., Sherman, T. F., Salisbury, F. B., Spratt, N. T. Jr., and McCain, G. 1977. *Biology.* Belmont, Calif.: Wadsworth.

Lovejoy, C. O. 1981. The origin of man. *Science* 211:341 (January 23).

Simpson, G. G. 1966. *Biology and man.* New York: Harcourt Brace Jovanovich.

Starr, C., and Taggart, R. 1981. *Biology: The unity and diversity of life* (2nd ed.). Belmont, Calif.: Wadsworth.

2

THE CHEMICAL LEVEL OF LIFE

WHY STUDY CHEMISTRY?

Objective 1. Explain why a study of basic chemistry is necessary to understand human physiology.

Chemistry is that branch of science concerned with matter—its properties and its interactions. Matter is anything that occupies space and has mass. This definition includes both nonliving things such as air, water, and rocks, and living things such as plants, animals, and human beings. Thus, many of the things that our bodies do can be described in terms of what matter does—that is, in chemical terms.

One of the best ways of explaining what matter is and how it behaves is to describe it as being composed of basic chemical "building blocks." Just as the twenty-six-letter English alphabet can be used to make thousands of words, the chemical building blocks can be used to make thousands of different substances. However, the complexity of chemical substances greatly exceeds the complexity of words. Very few English words contain more than twenty letters; complex chemical substances, by contrast, can contain as many as 20,000 building blocks!

Different chemical substances are capable of undergoing change and of interacting with one another. Most functions of the body are the result of such reactions. Metabolism, the breakdown of food to release energy and the making of the substance of the body, consists of many different chemical reactions. The conduction of nerve impulses, the contraction of muscles, and the regulatory action of hormones all involve function at the chemical level.

> By studying the chemistry of living things and the substances they produce, chemists have learned to manufacture complex molecules such as vitamins, antibiotics, hormones, and even fibers for clothing. One such molecule is vitamin C, also known as ascorbic acid. Our bodies cannot make vitamin C internally, but chemists can now make it fairly easily in the laboratory.
>
> Some proponents of healthy eating habits feel that vitamin C synthesized by chemists in test tubes is somehow inferior to vitamin C from natural sources, that is, synthesized by plants. However, vitamin C is a specific organic molecule. Whether it comes from an orange, a rose, or a laboratory, vitamin C has the same chemical structure and serves the same functions in our bodies.

Even homeostasis, the maintenance of near-constant internal conditions within an organism, is possible only when each of a large variety of chemical processes is occurring at the right time, in the right place, and at the proper rate. In many cases, homeostasis means *chemical* homeostasis. A major goal of the study of physiology is to understand how homeostasis is maintained. Reaching an understanding of the basic principles of chemistry can help achieve this goal.

THE CHEMICAL BUILDING BLOCKS

Objective 2. Define the terms atom, element, molecule, and compound; list the most common elements (and their symbols) found in the human body.

Objective 3. Describe the structure of an atom in terms of protons, neutrons, and electrons; explain the structure of ions and isotopes.

Chemical building blocks consist of particles too small to be seen even with a good microscope. However, over the years, chemists have been able to describe these particles by observing matter and deducing the characteristics of the particles from their observations.

Definitions

The smallest unit of matter is the **atom**. Atoms are not all the same; over a hundred different kinds of atoms are known. A substance composed of one kind of atom is called an **element**; each element has specific properties and is known by a unique name. For example, carbon is an element; a pure sample of carbon is composed of a vast number of carbon atoms.

Atoms can combine with other atoms in various ways. Sometimes the atoms of a single element can bond with each other. Carbon is such an element. A diamond is an arrangement of carbon atoms linked in a specific way; carbon atoms linked in a different way result in graphite, a soft black substance used in pencils. In writing the conventional way to designate elements is to use one- or two-letter symbols, with subscript numbers to indicate how many atoms are involved in various combinations. For instance, the elements oxygen and nitrogen, common gases in the atmosphere of the earth, usually occur as paired atoms: oxygen as O_2 (two atoms of oxygen combined) and nitrogen as N_2.

Atoms of one element can also combine with atoms of other elements. For example, CO_2—carbon dioxide—is one atom of carbon combined with two atoms of oxygen. H_2O—water—is made up of two hydrogen atoms bonded to an oxygen atom. These combined forms, called molecules, almost always have physical and chemical characteristics very different from the elemental atoms that compose them.

A **compound** is a substance that can be broken into two or more other substances by chemical means—that is, by undergoing a chemical reaction. The molecules of a compound always contain atoms of two or more elements. Thus, CO_2 and H_2O are compounds, but N_2 and O_2 are not.

A **molecule** is the smallest particle into which an element or compound can be divided without altering its chemical characteristics. O_2 and N_2 are examples of molecules, as are CO_2 and H_2O. Even individual atoms of some elements, such as carbon, are molecules because they can exist uncombined with other atoms.

> Sodium (Na) is a soft, metallic element that bursts into flame if exposed to oxygen. A 1 gram sample of sodium contains billions upon billions of sodium atoms. Chlorine (Cl) in pure form exists as Cl_2 molecules; it is a highly poisonous gas. When these two elements are combined, the result is the compound sodium chloride (NaCl), a white, crystalline solid commonly known as table salt. Countless numbers of NaCl molecules make up every grain of salt.

Table 2.1   Some Important Elements in Living Organisms

Element	Symbol	Atomic number	Electrons in outer shell	Percent by weight in human body	Biological occurrence
Oxygen	O	8	6	65	Component of most biological molecules; final electron acceptor in many energy-yielding reactions
Carbon	C	6	4	18	Basic atom of all organic compounds
Hydrogen	H	1	1	10	Component of most biological molecules; H^+ ion important component of solutions
Nitrogen	N	7	5	3	Component of proteins, nucleic acids, and many other biological molecules
Calcium	Ca	20	2	1.5	Found in bones and teeth; important in muscle contraction; controls many cellular processes
Phosphorus	P	15	5	1	Component of nucleic acids and molecules such as ATP carrying chemical energy; found in many lipid molecules
Sulfur	S	16	6	<1	Component of many proteins and other important biological molecules
Iron	Fe	26	2	<1	Important in energy-yielding reactions; component of oxygen carriers in blood
Potassium	K	19	1	<1	Important in conduction of nerve impulses
Sodium	Na	11	1	<1	Ion in solution in living matter; important in conduction of nerve impulses and transport of substances into cells
Chlorine	Cl	17	7	<1	Ion in solution in living matter
Magnesium	Mg	12	2	<1	Part of molecules important in photosynthesis; important in many enzyme-catalyzed reactions
Copper	Cu	29	1	Trace	Important in photosynthesis and energy-yielding reactions
Iodine	I	53	7	Trace	Component of hormones produced by thyroid gland
Fluorine	F	9	7	Trace	
Manganese	Mn	25	2	Trace	
Zinc	Zn	30	2	Trace	Found in enzymes or involved in activating enzymes
Selenium	Se	34	6	Trace	
Molybdenum	Mo	42	1	Trace	

< = less than

Over 95 percent of the human body consists of atoms of only four elements: carbon, hydrogen, oxygen, and nitrogen. Some of the elements found in living things, along with their symbols and properties, are summarized in Table 2.1. The compounds that make up the human body, however, can be highly complex arrangements of atoms. Using the "alphabet" in which CO_2 is a "word" (molecule) made up of three "letters" (atoms), a very simple sugar molecule contains twenty-four letters, $C_6H_{12}O_6$. Proteins, carbohydrates, fats, and other molecules of living organisms are compounds made up of thousands of letters.

Much of our study of the chemical level of life will concern complex compounds and the ways they are arranged to form the structure of the body. Some of our study will also concern the function of specific molecules in chemical reactions. As we will see, structure and function are related even at the chemical level.

Structure of Atoms

The atom is the smallest unit of any element that retains the properties of the element, yet atoms do contain smaller particles that together account for those properties. We will study only the particles called **protons**, **neutrons**, and **electrons**, though physicists study even smaller particles. Two important properties of these particles are mass and electrical charge. Mass is the amount of matter or substance present. Chemists arbitrarily designate the mass of a proton or a neutron as equal to one unit. In comparison to these particles electrons have a very small mass. With respect to electrical charge, electrons are negatively charged, protons are positively charged, and neutrons are neutral; that is, they have no charge. A third property of these particles—their location within the atom—will be discussed later (see Table 2.2). Atoms always have an equal number of protons and electrons, so they are electrically neutral.

The atoms of a particular element always have the same number of protons. The number of protons in an atom of a particular element is the **atomic number** of that element. The atomic numbers of elements range from 1 for hydrogen to 102 for nobelium.

Though all atoms of the same element have the same atomic number, they may not have the same atomic weight. The **atomic weight** is the sum of the number of protons and neutrons in an atom. Many elements consist of atoms with differing atomic weights. For example, carbon usually has six protons and six neutrons, giving it an atomic weight of 12. Some naturally occurring carbon atoms have one or two extra neutrons, giving them an atomic weight of 13 or 14. Laboratory techniques are available to create carbon atoms

Table 2.2	Properties of Atomic Particles		
Particle	Relative Mass	Charge	Location
Proton	1	Positive	Nucleus
Electron	1/1836	Negative	Around the nucleus
Neutron	1	Neutral	Nucleus

with two extra neutrons and an atomic weight of 14. Atoms with more or fewer than the usual number of neutrons are called **isotopes**.

Some isotopes are stable and others are not. Unstable, or radioactive, isotopes tend to break apart, emitting particles and radiation. The radiation can be detected by radiation counters, and so such isotopes are useful in following various kinds of chemical processes in living things. However, radiation also can be harmful to living systems, as will be discussed in the essay on radioactivity at the end of this chapter.

The particles within atoms are always arranged in a particular way. The protons and neutrons are always aggregated in the center, or nucleus, of the atom. Electrons are constantly in motion and form what is called an electron cloud around the nucleus. Because some electrons appear to have more energy than others, chemists use a model with concentric circles to suggest different energy levels. Electrons with the least energy are located nearest the nucleus, and those with greater amounts of energy are farther from the nucleus. Each energy level corresponds to one of the concentric circles or electron shells shown in Figure 2.1.

An atom of hydrogen has only one electron, which is located in the innermost shell. Helium has two electrons in this shell. The innermost electron shell can never contain more than two electrons. Larger atoms with more than two electrons always have two electrons in the inner shell and up to eight additional electrons in the second shell. The inner shell is filled before electrons are found in the second shell, the second shell is filled before the third, and so on. Very large atoms may have several more electron shells, but the outer shell is usually said to be filled if it contains eight electrons.

An important property of atoms whose outer electron shells are nearly full (they contain six or seven electrons) or nearly empty (they contain one or two electrons) is their tendency to form **ions**. Ions are charged particles produced when atoms gain or lose electrons. As shown in Figure 2.2, an atom of sodium with one electron in its outer shell may lose this electron and become a positively charged ion called a **cation**. It now has one more proton than it has electrons. Likewise, an atom of chlorine has seven electrons in its outer shell. It fills the shell by gaining an electron and thus becomes a negatively charged ion called an **anion**. Ions of elements such as sodium and chlorine are chemically more stable than their atoms because, as ions, their outer shell of electrons is full. Many of the elements listed in Table 2.1 are found in the human body in the form of ions. Those that have one or two electrons in their outer shell tend to lose the electrons to form ions with charges of +1 or +2, respectively; those that have seven electrons in their outer shell tend to gain an electron to form ions with charges of −1. In some instances atoms can gain or lose as many as three electrons. Ions commonly found in the body include Na^+, K^+, Ca^{2+}, and Cl^-.

CHEMICAL BONDS AND CHEMICAL REACTIONS

Objective 4. Distinguish among ionic, covalent, and hydrogen bonds and show how they are involved in holding atoms together.

Objective 5. Describe in general what happens in a chemical reaction.

Chemical bonds and chemical reactions have to do with energy, and energy is essential for life. When your body begins to run out of energy, you feel hungry and eat, thus replenishing your energy supply. However, many chemical reactions take place between the time you eat some food and the time the energy from that food can be used by your body. Let us see what happens to energy in chemical bonds and chemical reactions.

Chemical Bonds

Chemical bonds form between atoms through interactions of electrons in their outer shells. As we saw, in many cases these interactions result in the outer shells becoming filled with electrons. An atom with a full outer shell is more stable than one with a partially filled outer shell. Energy associated with those electron shells holds the atoms together. Three kinds of chemical bonds are found in living organisms: ionic, covalent, and hydrogen bonds.

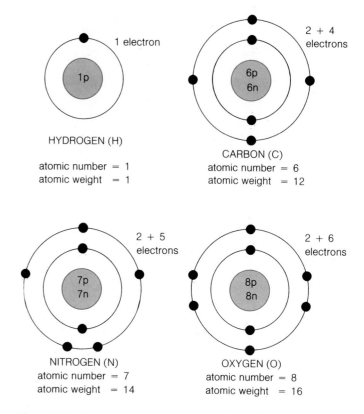

Figure 2.1 The structure of some atoms commonly found in the human body.

Ionic bonds result when ions having opposite charges combine to form molecules. Ions with positive charges (such as Na^+) and negative charges (such as Cl^-) attract each other, as already shown in Figure 2.2. Potassium iodide (KI) is another example of an ionically bonded compound.

Many compounds, especially those that contain carbon, are held together by **covalent bonds**. Instead of gaining or losing electrons, carbon atoms, which have four electrons in their outer shell, share electrons, as shown in Figure 2.3. One carbon atom can share an electron with each of four hydrogen atoms. Each hydrogen atom, likewise, shares an electron with the carbon atom. By the mutual sharing of electrons, the single shell of hydrogen is filled and made stable with two electrons, and the outer shell of carbon is filled and made stable with eight electrons. Sometimes a carbon atom shares two electrons with another atom; the other atom also shares two electrons with the carbon atom. When two pairs of electrons are shared, a double bond is formed. Chemists use a single line to represent a single pair of shared electrons and a double line to represent two pairs

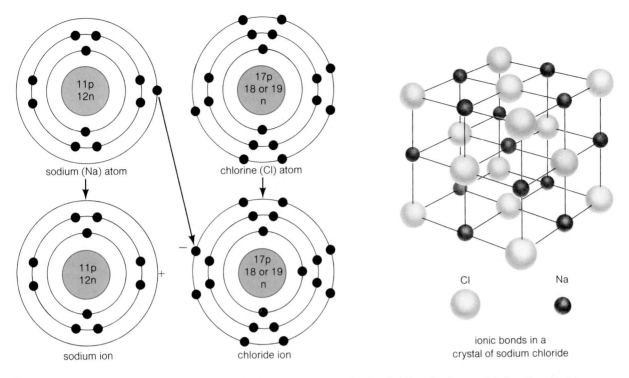

sodium (Na) atom

chlorine (Cl) atom

sodium ion

chloride ion

Cl

Na

ionic bonds in a
crystal of sodium chloride

Figure 2.2 The formation of sodium and chloride ions and the way these ions are held together in a crystal of sodium chloride.

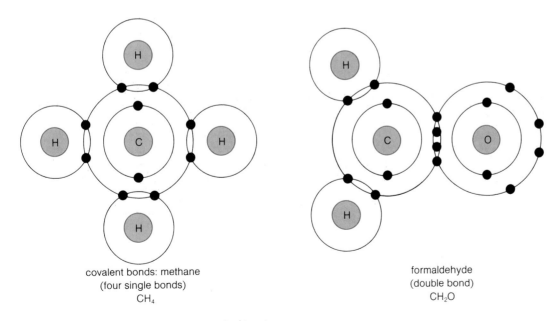

covalent bonds: methane
(four single bonds)
CH_4

formaldehyde
(double bond)
CH_2O

Figure 2.3 The sharing of electrons in covalent bonds.

of shared electrons. For example, methane is written

$$
\begin{array}{c}
\quad\quad H \\
\quad\quad | \\
H - C - H \\
\quad\quad | \\
\quad\quad H
\end{array}
$$

and formaldehyde is written

$$
\begin{array}{c}
\quad\quad H \\
\quad\quad | \\
H - C = O .
\end{array}
$$

A third type of chemical bond, the **hydrogen bond**, is much weaker than ionic or covalent bonds. Hydrogen bonds are important, however, in the chemical structure of living things. Oxygen and nitrogen nuclei attract electrons strongly; when linked with hydrogen, they share electrons unevenly—the electrons stay closer to the oxygen or nitrogen than to the hydrogen. Hydrogen bonds in biologically important molecules usually involve the placement of hydrogen between oxygen atoms, between nitrogen atoms, or between oxygen and nitrogen. Using ⋯ to represent a hydrogen bond, the combinations are as follows:

$$-O-H \cdots N-$$

$$-O-H \cdots O-$$

$$-N-H \cdots N-$$

$$-N-H \cdots O-$$

Water molecules hold on to each other with hydrogen bonds. Because the oxygen atom is much larger than the hydrogen atom, the electrons stay closer to the oxygen nucleus. In addition, the hydrogen nuclei are located on the same side rather than on opposite sides of the molecule (see Figure 2.4). The result is that water is a **polar compound**: Although electrically neutral, it has a positive side (the hydrogen side) and a negative side (the oxygen side). These weak charges allow the hydrogen part of one water molecule to form an association with the oxygen part of another water molecule. Because the hydrogen bond involves interaction of electrical charges, it is similar to an ionic bond, although it contains much less energy. Any compound whose hydrogen atoms have a weak charge because of unequal electron sharing may form hydrogen bonds.

Hydrogen bonds are responsible to some extent for the structure of large molecules including proteins and nucleic

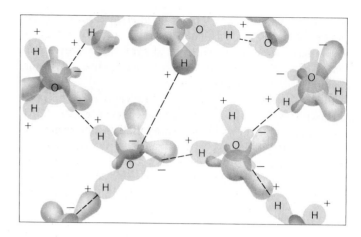

Figure 2.4 Hydrogen bonding, illustrated by water molecules.

acids (such as those shown in Figure 2.20). Both these types of molecules form long chains. These chains are coiled or otherwise wound about each other, and the coils are held together by hydrogen bonds. The functions of these molecules depend on their structure and on their ability to change shape—both of which involve making or breaking hydrogen bonds. Later we will study these molecules in more detail.

Chemical Reactions

Chemical reactions involve the breaking and reforming of chemical bonds. Associated with the breaking or forming of a bond is an energy change. Chemical bonds represent a way of storing chemical energy. Many of the chemical reactions that occur in living things involve the storage or release of energy.

Energy is often released when bonds are broken; that energy can be used in metabolic reactions. For example, the food we eat consists of molecules having chemical bonds that contain stored energy. During **catabolism**—the breakdown of substances—food is degraded, and energy is released. A catabolic reaction can be symbolized $XY \rightarrow X + Y + energy$, where XY represents a food molecule and where the energy released was originally stored in the bond between X and Y. Burning is a similar kind of reaction; it releases energy in the form of heat.

In contrast, energy can be used to form chemical bonds in the synthesis of new compounds. In **anabolism**—the build-up or synthesis of substances—energy is used to create bonds. An anabolic reaction can be symbolized

$X + Y + energy \rightarrow XY$, where the energy is stored in the new substance XY. Reactions like this occur in the body when small molecules are used to synthesize larger molecules. Hence, we can store energy for later use, or we can make needed new molecules.

Energy is always involved in chemical reactions. Those reactions that release energy are called **exothermic**; those that require energy to take place are called **endothermic**. For example, the breakdown of glucose to carbon dioxide and water with the release of energy is an exothermic reaction. The synthesis of proteins for body structure or the connecting of a number of glucose molecules to form glycogen (both of which require energy) are examples of endothermic reactions.

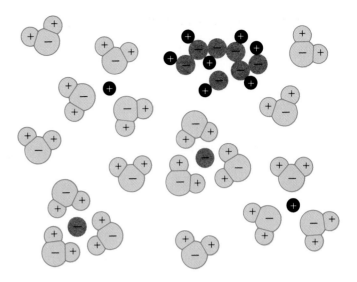

Figure 2.5 Water molecules surround positive and negative ions and help to hold those particles in solution.

WATER

Objective 6. Describe the properties of water that are important to its function in living things.

Water is so essential to life that you could live only a few days without it. It comprises about 60 percent of the total human body weight—more in infants and less in the elderly. Its concentration varies greatly from one part of the body to another. For example, bones and fatty tissue contain very little water, whereas brain tissue may contain as much as 75 percent water. Water is the medium in which many of the chemical reactions in the body take place. Let us consider some of the properties of water that make it so important to normal body function.

The fact that water is a polar compound—that is, it has positive and negative regions—accounts for many of its properties. This polarity not only makes it possible for water to form hydrogen bonds, it also accounts for water's ability to be an excellent solvent and for its ability to form a thin layer on membrane surfaces.

Water acts as a solvent for ions because the polar water molecules become oriented around ions. The positive area of water molecules is attracted to negative ions, and the negative area of water to positive ions. The result is that ions become dissolved and evenly distributed through the water medium (Figure 2.5). Water soluble substances—those that will dissolve in water—can be transported through the body by the blood and distributed through the watery fluids within and around cells.

Because of their polarity, water molecules tend to stick together and also to form thin layers. The ability to form layers makes water important in keeping the surfaces of membranes moist. The membrane surfaces within the

lungs, for example, must be kept moist for the diffusion of gases to take place during respiration.

Furthermore, water has a high specific heat; that is, it holds large quantities of heat energy and releases large quantities of heat energy when it evaporates. Because of these properties, water is important in the homeostatic regulation of body temperature. Through the evaporation of sweat, the body can get rid of excess heat. By conserving water, the body can retain heat. The slowness with which water gains or loses heat and the large amounts of water in the body together contribute significantly to the stabilization of body temperature.

Finally, water not only serves as a medium for chemical reactions, it also participates in many reactions. In dehydration synthesis, the elements of water are removed from reactants (substances that enter the reaction) to form a larger product molecule: $A—H + HO—B \rightarrow A—B + H_2O$. Examples of such reactions to be considered later in this chapter include the linking of monosaccharides (simple sugars) to form disaccharides (Figure 2.10), the linking of fatty acids to glycerol to make fats (Figure 2.11), and the linking together of amino acids to synthesize protein (Figure 2.15). Conversely, in degradation hydrolysis, water is often added to a reactant to form simpler product molecules: $A—B + H_2O \rightarrow A—H + HO—B$. Examples of such reactions include the reverse of the above reactions—the breaking down of larger molecules to release simple sugars, fatty acids, and amino acids.

The properties of water are summarized in Table 2.3.

Table 2.3 Properties of Water
1. Good solvent ability helps to dissolve substances for transport.
2. Ability to form layers helps to keep membranes moist.
3. Ability to store or release large quantities of heat helps to maintain body temperature.
4. Distribution throughout the body provides a medium for chemical reactions.
5. Chemical reactivity allows elements (H^+ and OH^-) to participate in many chemical reactions.

SOLUTIONS AND COLLOIDAL DISPERSIONS

Objective 7. Describe the properties of solutions and colloidal dispersions that are important to their function in living things.

Solutions and colloidal dispersions are examples of mixtures. Unlike a chemical compound that consists of molecules whose atoms are present in specific proportions, a **mixture** consists of two or more substances mixed in any proportion. Each of the substances in a mixture contributes to the properties of the mixture. For example, a mixture of sugar and salt could be made using any proportion of sugar and salt. The degree of sweetness and saltiness of the mixture would depend on the relative amounts of each substance present, but both sweetness and saltiness would be detectable.

A **solution** is a mixture of two or more substances in which the molecules of the substances are evenly distributed and will not separate out even upon standing. One substance is the **solvent**, the medium in which the other substances are dissolved. A dissolved substance, the **solute**, may consist of atoms, ions, or molecules. In the body water is the solvent in nearly all solutions. Typical solutes include the sugar glucose, the gases carbon dioxide and oxygen, and many different kinds of ions. A few proteins can also act as solutes in true solutions. Solutions used for intravenous feedings, saline (salt water) solution, and many liquid medications are examples of solutions used in therapeutic situations.

Colloids are particles too large to form true solutions, but they may form **colloidal dispersions**. Gelatin dessert is an example of a colloidal dispersion. Much of the substance surrounding the organelles of living cells is a very complex colloidal system. Colloids in the human body are usually formed from large protein molecules dispersed in water.

Colloidal dispersions are exemplified by proteins in blood or in the substance of cells. In colloidal dispersions large molecules are held in suspension by opposing electrical charges, layers of water molecules surrounding the particles, and other forces. Some colloidal systems have the ability to change from a semisolid state, like gelatin that has "set," to a more fluid state, like gelatin that has melted. Large colloidal molecules are important in creating osmotic pressure in cells and body fluids and can be involved in the function of cell membranes, as will be discussed in Chapter 3.

Though it was once thought that the properties of colloids helped to explain the behavior of the contents of cells that display amoeboid movement, it is now known that such movement is much more complex and involves processes similar to muscle contraction.

ACIDS, BASES, AND pH

Objective 8. Define acid, base, and pH; explain how these terms are useful in physiology.

Most living things exist in an environment that is neither very acidic nor very alkaline, or basic. The environment is said to be nearly chemically neutral. Likewise, with a few exceptions, the internal environment of living things is maintained in a range very near chemical neutrality. In the human body changes in the concentration of acids and bases can be life threatening.

Acids and bases readily form ions when placed in water solutions. Acids form hydrogen ions, H^+, and bases generally form hydroxyl ions, OH^-, or remove H^+ from solution. In a solution the greater the concentration of H^+, the stronger the acid, and the greater the concentration of OH^-, the stronger the base, or alkali. Thus, an **acid** is a hydrogen ion donor or a proton donor. (A hydrogen ion is a proton.) An acid "donates" H^+ to the solution. A **base** is a hydroxyl ion donor, sometimes also called a proton acceptor. A base "donates" OH^- to the solution; it can also accept H^+.

The presence of an excess of H^+ results in acid conditions, and the presence of an excess of OH^- results in alkaline or basic conditions. In living organisms H^+ often are released by carboxyl groups,

$$-\!\!\overset{\displaystyle O}{\underset{\displaystyle}{C}}\!\!-OH \longrightarrow -\!\!\overset{\displaystyle O}{\underset{\displaystyle}{C}}\!\!-O^- + H^+.$$

Carboxyl groups are found in organic acids, which will be discussed later.

Chemists have devised a scale, called the **pH scale**, to express the concentrations of acids and bases. This scale, shown in Table 2.4, is a logarithmic scale; that is, the concentration of hydrogen ions changes by a factor of 10 for each unit of the scale (each line of the table). As shown in the table, the pH is the exponent (without the minus sign) of the actual hydrogen ion concentration.

A solution at pH 7 is neutral—neither acidic nor basic. At this pH the concentrations of H^+ and OH^- are equal. Such is the case in pure, distilled water. Because huge numbers of ions are involved in any solution, we need a simple way to compare concentrations. To do this, chemists devised the concept of a **mole**, or **gram molecular weight**. The gram molecular weight of a compound is a weight in grams equal to the combined atomic weights of each atom in the compound. For example, the gram molecular weight of H_2O is 18—1 for each hydrogen and 16 for oxygen. So 1 mole of water is 18 grams of water.

Chemists determined that in pure water at 25°C, 0.0000001 part of each mole of water exists as H^+ and OH^- ions. This amount is conveniently expressed in scientific notation as 10^{-7} moles. The number 7 then becomes the 7 in pH 7, the pH of pure water and any other neutral substance.

At pH 2 the concentration of hydrogen ions is 10^{-2} (0.01) moles per liter; at pH 3 the concentration of hydrogen ions is 10^{-3} (0.001) moles per liter. Thus, the concentration of hydrogen ions at pH 3 is only one-tenth that at pH 2. Table 2.5 shows the pH of some body fluids and some other substances. As you can see in the table, the range of pH of blood is quite small—7.35–7.45. Variations outside this normal range create life-threatening conditions, as will be explained in Chapter 26.

COMPLEX MOLECULES

Objective 9. Define organic chemistry and identify the major functional groups of organic molecules.

Objective 10. List the four classes of physiologically important compounds.

The above discussion of the basic principles of general chemistry has paved the way for a discussion of **organic chemistry**, the study of compounds that contain carbon. Such compounds occur naturally in living things and in the products or remains of living things. The ability of carbon atoms to form long chains bonded together by covalent bonds makes possible the formation of an almost infinite number of chemical compounds.

Table 2.4 Hydrogen Ion (Proton) Concentration and pH			
Proton Concentration in Moles of Hydrogen per Liter of Water	Proton Concentration Written as an Exponent	pH Value	
1.0	10^0	0	Extremely acid
0.1	10^{-1}	1	
0.01	10^{-2}	2	
0.001	10^{-3}	3	Moderately acid
0.0001	10^{-4}	4	
0.00001	10^{-5}	5	Weakly acid
0.000001	10^{-6}	6	
0.0000001	10^{-7}	7	Neutral
0.00000001	10^{-8}	8	
0.000000001	10^{-9}	9	Weakly basic
0.0000000001	10^{-10}	10	
0.00000000001	10^{-11}	11	Moderately basic
0.000000000001	10^{-12}	12	
0.0000000000001	10^{-13}	13	
0.00000000000001	10^{-14}	14	Extremely basic

The simplest carbon compounds are the hydrocarbons—chains of carbon atoms with their associated hydrogen atoms. Methane (shown in Figure 2.3) is the simplest hydrocarbon. Octane,

$$
\begin{array}{c}
\ \ \ \ \text{H} \ \ \ \ \text{H} \ \ \ \ \text{H} \ \ \ \ \text{H} \ \ \ \ \text{H} \ \ \ \ \text{H} \ \ \ \ \text{H} \ \ \ \ \text{H} \\
\ \ \ \ | \ \ \ \ \ | \ \ \ \ \ | \ \ \ \ \ | \ \ \ \ \ | \ \ \ \ \ | \ \ \ \ \ | \ \ \ \ \ | \\
\text{H}-\text{C}-\text{C}-\text{C}-\text{C}-\text{C}-\text{C}-\text{C}-\text{C}-\text{H} \\
\ \ \ \ | \ \ \ \ \ | \ \ \ \ \ | \ \ \ \ \ | \ \ \ \ \ | \ \ \ \ \ | \ \ \ \ \ | \ \ \ \ \ | \\
\ \ \ \ \text{H} \ \ \ \ \text{H} \ \ \ \ \text{H} \ \ \ \ \text{H} \ \ \ \ \text{H} \ \ \ \ \text{H} \ \ \ \ \text{H} \ \ \ \ \text{H}
\end{array}
$$

is another hydrocarbon. Hydrocarbons include gasoline and other petroleum products, all of which are derived from the remains of living organisms.

In addition to hydrogen, other atoms such as oxygen and nitrogen can be attached to carbon chains. The atoms often form functional groups. A **functional group** is the part

Table 2.5 The pH of Various Substances	
Substance	pH
Hydrochloric acid	0.0
Stomach acid	1.0
Gastric juice	1.0–3.0
Lemon juice	2.5
Vinegar, beer, wine	3.0
Orange juice	3.5
Tomatoes, grapes	4.0
Coffee	5.0
Urine	5.0–7.0
Milk	6.5
Saliva	6.3–7.3
Pure water	7.0
Blood	7.35–7.45
Eggs	7.5
Ocean water	7.8–8.2
Household bleach	9.5
Milk of magnesia	10.5
Household ammonia	10.5–11.8
Oven cleaner	13.5
Sodium hydroxide	14.0

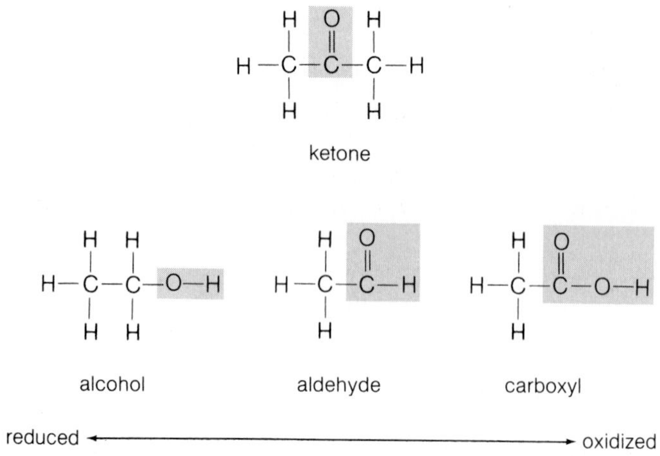

Figure 2.6   Oxygen-containing functional groups of organic molecules. The shaded portion of the molecule is the functional group.

ketone groups appear in the middle of chains, and alcohol groups appear anywhere along chains. Another example of a functional group is the amino group, —NH_2. Amino groups account for much of the nitrogen found in protein molecules of living organisms.

The relative amounts of oxygen in functional groups is significant. Groups with little oxygen, such as alcohol groups, are said to be **reduced**; groups with relatively more oxygen, such as carboxyl groups, are said to be **oxidized**. In general, the more reduced a molecule, the more energy it contains. (Hydrocarbons, having no oxygen, represent the extreme in reduced molecules; they contain large amounts of energy.) Conversely, the more oxidized a molecule, the less energy it contains. Oxidation releases energy from molecules. We shall discuss oxidation in detail in Chapter 23.

Organic molecules of physiological interest can be grouped in four major classes: carbohydrates, lipids, proteins, and nucleic acids. Enzymes, a particular group of proteins, are of sufficient importance to warrant special consideration. These classes of compounds will be discussed in the next sections of this chapter.

of a molecule that frequently participates in chemical reactions and that gives the molecule some of its chemical properties. Even at the chemical level, then, structure and function are related: The reactions a molecule may undergo depend upon which atoms are present and how they are put together.

Four important functional groups contain oxygen—alcohol, aldehyde, ketone, and carboxyl groups. Figure 2.6 shows their structure and how they link to carbon chains. Aldehyde and carboxyl groups appear at the ends of chains,

CARBOHYDRATES

Objective 11. Describe the general structure and chemical properties of carbohydrates and explain their role in the body.

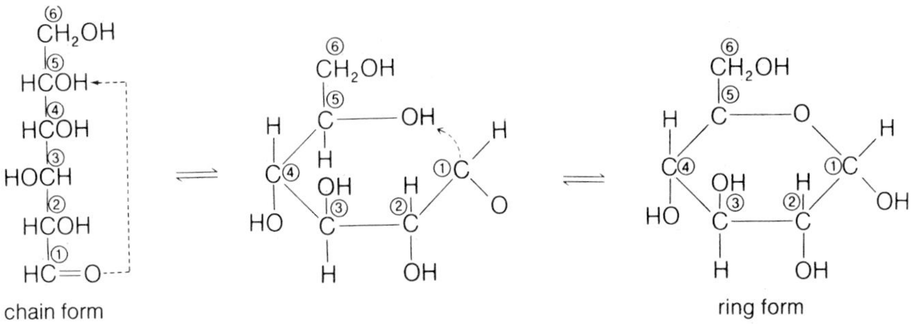

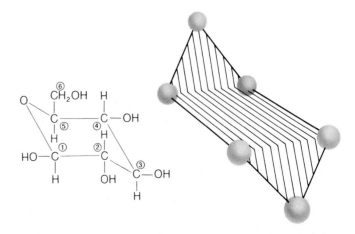

Figure 2.7 Structure of a glucose molecule. Dotted arrows show rearrangement of molecule to form ring structure.

chain form

ring form

Bread, potatoes, and honey are examples of foods that contain carbohydrates. **Carbohydrates** serve as the main source of energy for most living things, and the human body is no exception. Plants make carbohydrates, including structural carbohydrates such as cellulose and energy-storage carbohydrates such as starch. Other carbohydrates are located on the surface of cells, where they act as markers that make a cell chemically recognizable as a particular kind of cell. A small carbohydrate molecule, the sugar ribose, is found in nucleic acids.

All carbohydrates contain the elements carbon, hydrogen, and oxygen, generally in the proportion of two hydrogen atoms for each carbon and oxygen atom (CH_2O). The simplest carbohydrates are **monosaccharides**. They consist of a carbon chain with several organic alcohol groups (—OH) and either an aldehyde group

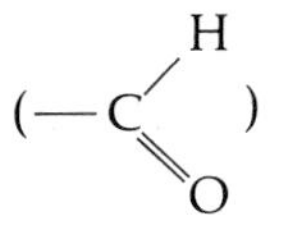

$$\left(-\overset{\displaystyle H}{\underset{\displaystyle O}{C}}\right)$$

or a ketone group

$$\left(-\overset{\displaystyle O}{\overset{\displaystyle \|}{C}}-\right).$$

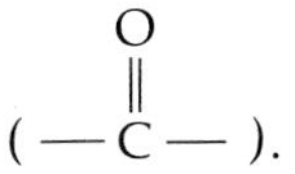

Most monosaccharides in the human body contain five or six carbons. **Glucose**, the most abundant monosaccharide, contains six carbons (see Figure 2.7). The straight chain configuration clearly shows the aldehyde group on carbon-1 and the alcohol groups on the other carbons. The ring structure is shown in the figure because it is the more likely configuration of glucose in solution. In glucose it is the aldehyde group that participates in most chemical reactions. Other monosaccharides, fructose and galactose, have the same number of atoms of carbon, hydrogen, and oxygen as glucose, but the atoms are arranged differently (see Figure 2.8). Fructose has a ketone group on carbon-2, and galactose has the alcohol groups arranged in a different

configuration from that of glucose. Ribose is a five-carbon monosaccharide.

Whenever diagrams or structural formulas are given for biochemical molecules, it is important to try to imagine each molecule as a three-dimensional object. The structural formula drawn out on a flat piece of paper only suggests the general relationship between the atoms in a molecule. Figure 2.9 indicates the three-dimensional shape of a glucose molecule. Though flat two-dimensional structural formulas

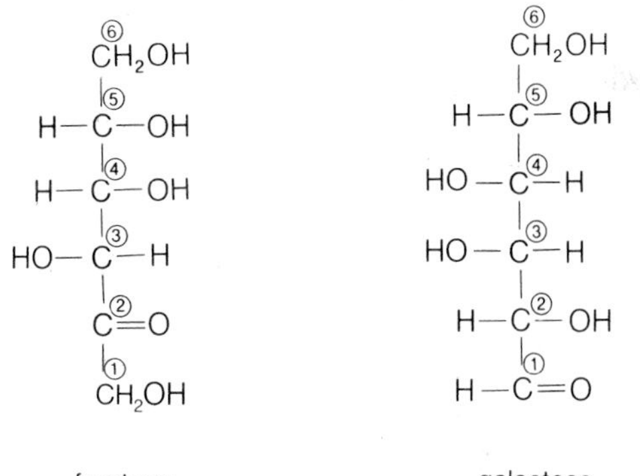

fructose

galactose

Figure 2.8 Structure of fructose and galactose molecules.

Figure 2.9 Three-dimensional representation of a glucose molecule.

will be used throughout this book, it should be emphasized that real molecules are three-dimensional.

Monosaccharides, or simple sugars, are the building blocks of more complex carbohydrates. Double sugars, or **disaccharides**, contain two units of a simple sugar, and **polysaccharides** contain many units of a simple sugar (Figure 2.10). Ordinary table sugar, sucrose, is a disaccharide composed of glucose and fructose. Other disaccharides of importance in the human body are lactose, or milk sugar, composed of glucose and galactose; and maltose, or malt sugar, composed of two molecules of glucose. Polysaccharides of importance in the human body include starch, glycogen, and cellulose. These polysaccharides are polymers (long, connected chains) of glucose. Starch is found in potatoes, rice, and cereals. Glycogen is stored in the liver of animals and to some extent in their muscles. Cellulose is found in most fruits and vegetables. The human body cannot digest cellulose as it lacks the enzymes necessary to break the particular bonds between its glucose units. Thus, cellulose passes through the digestive tract undigested and provides bulk or roughage in the diet. The properties of the carbohydrates described here are summarized in Table 2.6.

LIPIDS

Objective 12. Describe the general structure and chemical properties of simple lipids, compound lipids, and steroids; explain the roles of each in the body.

You are familiar with lipids from the fats in your diet such as butter or cooking oil. You are also undoubtedly

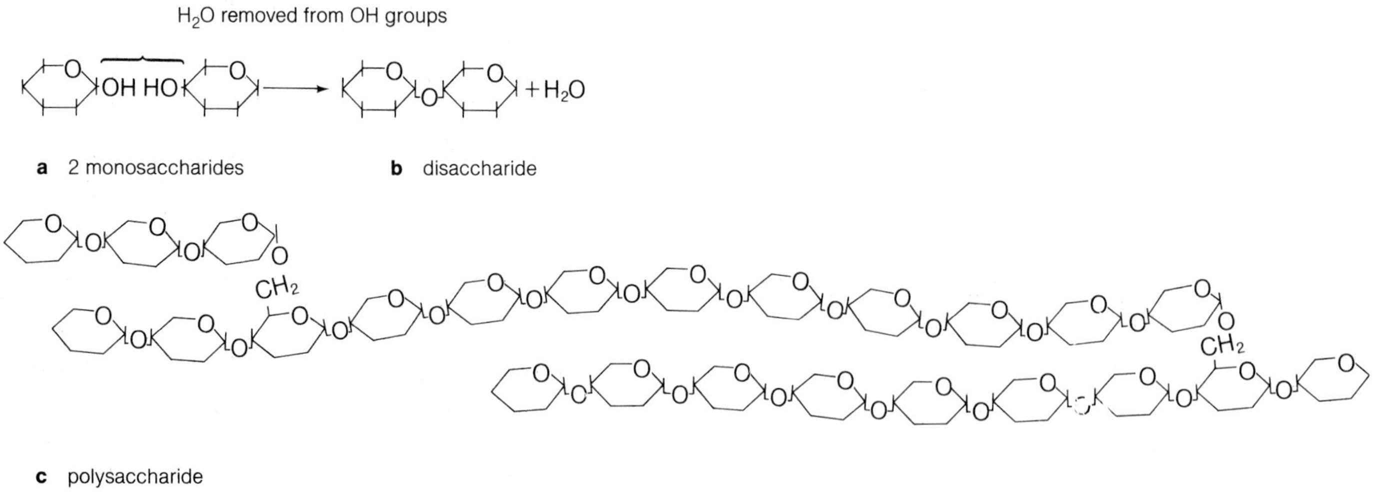

Table 2.6   Properties of Carbohydrates

Class of Carbohydrates	Examples	Description
Monosaccharides	Glucose	Six carbons, aldehyde functional group
	Fructose	Six carbons, ketone functional group
	Galactose	Six carbons, aldehyde functional group, alcohol groups arranged differently than in glucose
	Ribose	Five carbons, aldehyde functional group
Disaccharides	Sucrose	Contains glucose and fructose
	Lactose	Contains glucose and galactose
	Maltose	Contains two glucose units
Polysaccharides	Starch	Polymer of glucose found in plants, digestible by humans
	Glycogen	Polymer of glucose stored in the liver and muscles
	Cellulose	Polymer of glucose found in plants, not digestible by humans

H_2O removed from OH groups

a   2 monosaccharides   **b**   disaccharide

c   polysaccharide

Figure 2.10   The structure of (**a**) a monosaccharide, (**b**) a disaccharide, and (**c**) the polysaccharide starch. Most of the H and OH groups have been omitted from these diagrams.

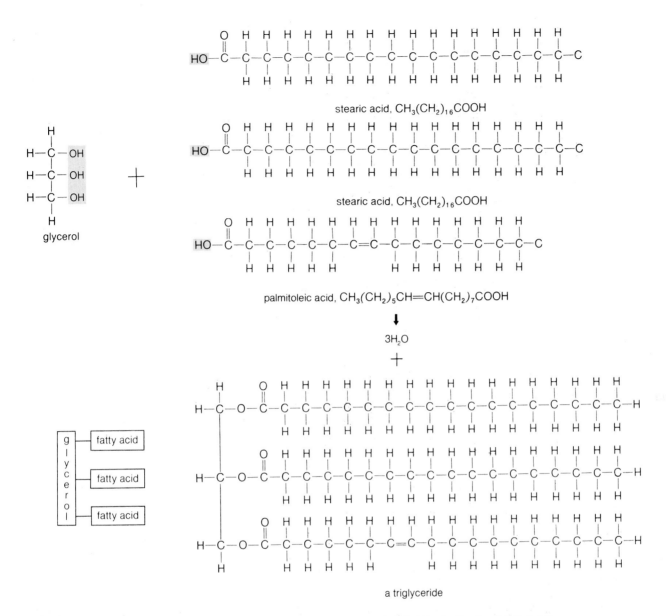

Figure 2.11 Glycerol and fatty acids, either saturated or unsaturated, are the building blocks of a simple lipid. A molecule of water is removed as each fatty acid is attached to glycerol.

aware of the controversy over cholesterol in the human diet and over the use of birth control pills that contain steroids. Dietary fats, cholesterol, and various steroids are all classified as **lipids**, substances insoluble in water but soluble in nonpolar substances such as ether or benzene.

Lipids serve three functions in the body. Some are incorporated into the structure of cells, especially into membranes; others are used for energy; and still others, like the steroid hormones from the adrenal and sex glands, regulate various processes in the body. Generally, lipids contain relatively more hydrogen and less oxygen than carbohydrates. The greater the proportion of hydrogen in a molecule, the more energy is stored in it. Thus, lipids contain even more energy than carbohydrates. As will be explained in Chapter 23, large amounts of energy are liberated when hydrogen atoms combine with oxygen; lipids provide large numbers of hydrogen atoms.

Simple lipids, or fats, consist of one molecule of glycerol, a three-carbon alcohol, and three molecules of fatty acids (Figure 2.11). A fatty acid consists of a long chain of

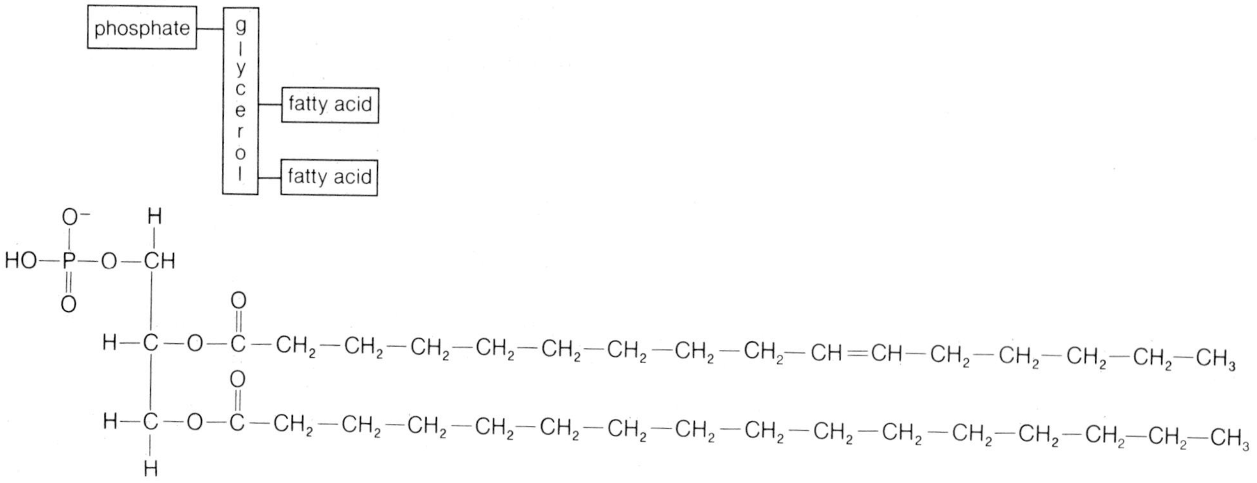

Figure 2.12 The structure of a phospholipid. The phosphate portion of the molecule is polar, and the fatty acid portion is nonpolar.

carbon atoms with their associated hydrogen atoms and a carboxyl (acid) group on the end of the chain. The synthesis of a fat from these building blocks involves the removal of the elements of a water molecule each time the carboxyl group of a fatty acid is connected to glycerol. A **triglyceride** is formed when three fatty acids are attached to glycerol; a **mono-** or **diglyceride** is formed when one or two fatty acids are attached.

Fatty acids may be saturated or unsaturated. A **saturated fatty acid** contains all of the hydrogen it can have; it is saturated with hydrogen. Some fatty acids contain double bonds between one or more pairs of carbon atoms. These fatty acids are said to be **unsaturated**, which means that they are not completely saturated with hydrogen. For example, palmitoleic acid (Figure 2.11) is unsaturated. Evidence exists that a diet high in saturated fats (a consequence of large amounts of animal fat) increases the likelihood of diseased arteries or heart attack.

Compound lipids are similar to simple lipids except that they contain some other components in addition to lipid. Of the compound lipids **phospholipids** are by far the most widely distributed in the body—they are found in the membranes of all cells. The structure of a phospholipid differs from a simple lipid by the substitution of a phosphate group,

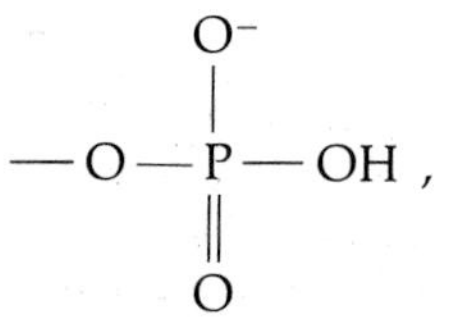

$$-O-P-OH \; ,$$

(with O^- above and O below the P)

for one of the fatty acids (Figure 2.12). The addition of the phosphate at the glycerol end of the molecule causes that end to be polar (charged); the fatty acid end of the molecule remains nonpolar (uncharged). Some phospholipids have other molecules attached to them. As will be discussed in Chapter 3, phospholipids are important in determining the characteristics of cell membranes.

Steroids are complex structures with a characteristic configuration of four connected ring structures (Figure 2.13). They include cholesterol, vitamin D, and a number of hormones from the sex glands and the cortex of the adrenal gland. Like phospholipids, cholesterol is found in the membranes of cells and may be deposited in the walls of blood vessels, where it contributes to atherosclerosis, the condition commonly called hardening of the arteries. The major characteristics of lipids are summarized in Table 2.7.

PROTEINS

Objective 13. Describe the general structure and chemical properties of amino acids as building blocks of protein; distinguish between structural proteins and enzymes.

Proteins are essential in the human diet for growth and maintenance of the body. Adequate protein seems to be especially important for normal development of the brain. Young children deprived of protein are stunted in their growth and mentally retarded.

Proteins are composed of building blocks called **amino**

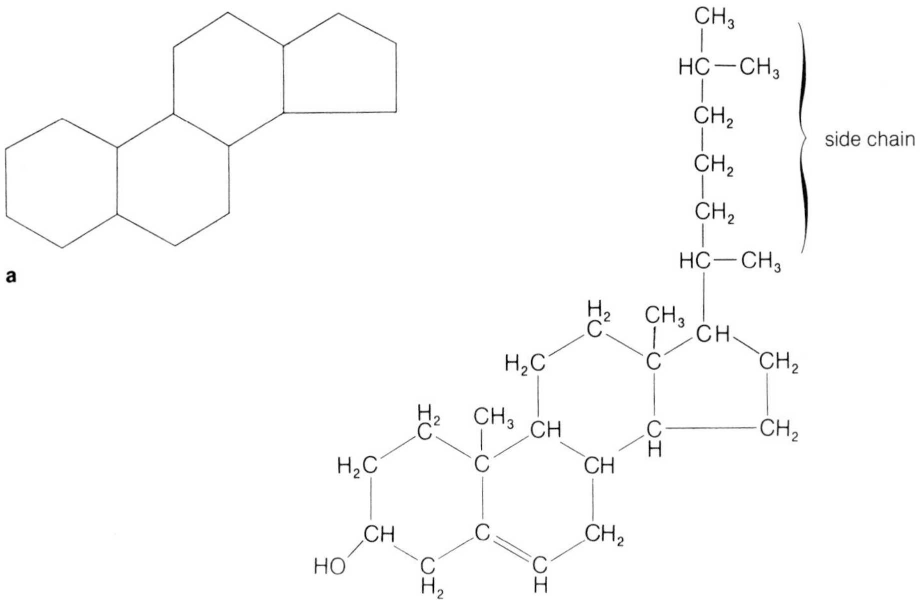

Figure 2.13 Structure of a steroid: (**a**) the typical arrangement of carbon rings and (**b**) cholesterol, with its long nonpolar side chain.

Table 2.7 Characteristics of Lipids

Class of Lipid	Characteristics
Simple lipid (fat)	Glycerol and three fatty acids form a triglyceride; mono- and diglycerides contain one and two fatty acids respectively; fatty acids may be saturated (contain all the hydrogen they can contain) or unsaturated (have double bonds in the carbon chain).
Compound lipids	Contain other components in addition to lipid; phospholipids contain phosphoric acid instead of one or more of the fatty acids; found in the membranes of cells.
Steroids	Contain a characteristic four-ring structure; include cholesterol, vitamin D, hormones from the adrenal and sex glands, and bile salts.
Other	A variety of substances having some properties of lipids; include porphyrins (a component of hemoglobin), vitamins A, E, and K, and prostaglandins (important regulatory molecules in cells).

acids. In addition to the elements carbon, hydrogen, and oxygen, amino acids contain nitrogen, and some also contain sulfur. The name for amino acids is derived from the fact that each has at least one amino group,—NH_2, and at least one acid (carboxyl) group,

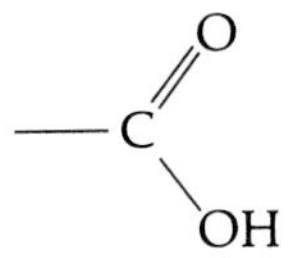

The structures of some of the twenty amino acids found in proteins are shown in Figure 2.14. The human body can make most amino acids, but some must be supplied in food because the body cannot make them. The latter are called **essential amino acids**. The quality of proteins in the diet is determined mostly by whether they provide adequate supplies of the essential amino acids. More will be said about amino acids in Chapters 23 and 24.

Amino acids are attached to one another by special linkages called **peptide bonds** to form long chains. A pep-

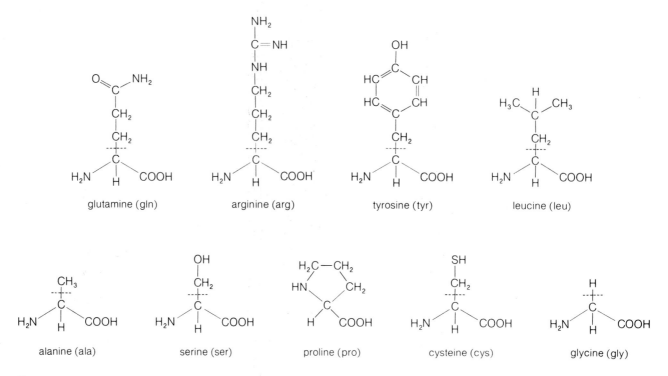

Figure 2.14 Some common amino acids. The carboxyl and amino groups are shown below the dashed lines, except for proline, which has the N-containing group in a ring structure.

tide bond is formed between an amino group of one amino acid and a carboxyl group of another amino acid (Figure 2.15). In addition to the amino and carboxyl groups, some amino acids have other functional groups, such as the sulfhydryl (—SH) group. This group is important in forming cross-linkages between chains of amino acids and in holding them in a three-dimensional configuration. In such a linkage two SH groups lose H and form a disulfide (—S—S—) linkage.

Proteins have several levels of structure. The primary structure of a protein consists of a chain of amino acids, usually one hundred or more in length, arranged in a specific sequence. Chains are then folded or coiled into a particular pattern, often a spiral or helix, which is held together by disulfide linkages, hydrogen bonds, and other forces. This constitutes the secondary structure. These molecules are further folded into globular (spherical) shapes or twisted into fibrous (threadlike) strands, forming the tertiary structure. Tertiary structure is maintained by the same relatively weak forces that maintain secondary structure. Some proteins can change back and forth between globular and fibrous shapes as weak bonds are disrupted and reformed. Certain very large proteins, like the globin of he-

moglobin, are aggregates of several globular components or subunits. Such aggregates form the quaternary structure of proteins.

Several factors can affect the hydrogen bonds that maintain protein structure. Highly acid or basic conditions, with a few exceptions, lead to destruction or disorganization of these bonds. Temperatures above 50°C also destroy such bonds. The disorganization of bonds that maintain the normal configuration of proteins is called **denaturation**. Methods of sterilization and disinfection often make use of heat or chemicals that kill microorganisms by denaturing their proteins. The cooking of meat tenderizes it by denaturing proteins.

One of the reasons that the temperature and pH of the body must be maintained within a narrow range is that extremes of temperature or pH alter proteins. Although a high fever is sometimes said to help the body to fight infection by interfering with the growth of microorganisms, it probably poses a greater threat to the body's own proteins than to those of the microorganisms.

Most proteins can be classified by their major roles in the body as structural proteins, motile proteins, enzymes, or regulatory proteins. Structural proteins include portions of

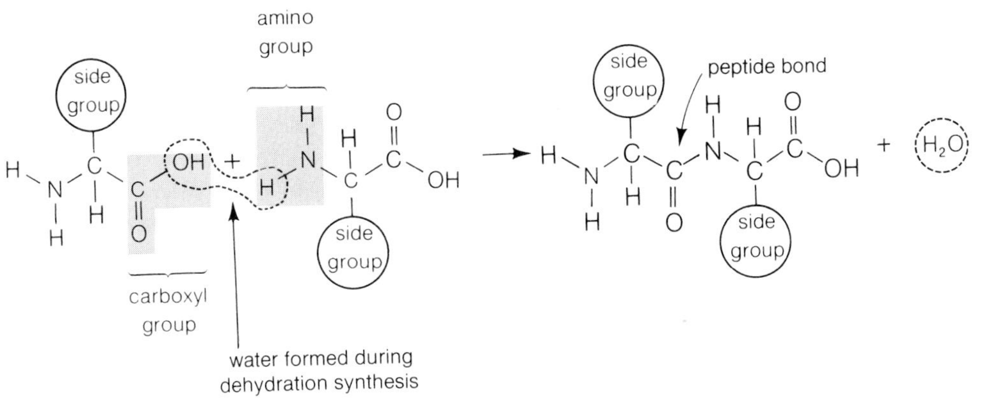

Figure 2.15 Amino acids can be attached to one another by the formation of a peptide bond.

cell membranes and the membranes of organelles; the keratin of skin, hair, and nails; and the collagen in cartilage and tendons. Keratin and collagen form long, strong fibers and are thus called fibrous proteins. Motile proteins include muscle proteins involved in muscle contraction and proteins of microtubules that provide a kind of internal skeleton within cells. Enzymes are proteins that control the rate of chemical reactions in the body; they are often globular and able to change shape as they control a reaction. Some proteins both contribute to the structure of cells and function as enzymes. Regulatory proteins act as hormones or form receptor sites on cell membranes, helping to determine what effects other chemicals will have on cells. Other proteins not so easily classified include antibodies that protect against infection, proteins that transport substances in the blood, and albumins that help to maintain blood osmotic pressure. Protein classification is summarized in Table 2.8.

Table 2.8 Classification of Proteins	
Type of Protein	Characteristics
Structural	Form the structure of cell parts or cell products, including portions of cell membranes; keratin of skin, hair, and nails; collagen in cartilage and tendons
Motile	Involved in muscle contraction and found in microtubules
Enzymes	Catalyze chemical reactions in cells
Regulatory	Form receptor sites on cell membranes; act as hormones
Other	Antibodies that protect against infection; proteins that transport substances in blood; albumins that help to maintain blood osmotic pressure

ENZYMES

Objective 14. Describe the characteristics of enzymes and explain how these characteristics contribute to the function of enzymes.

A fire in a fireplace on a cold winter's evening releases great amounts of heat energy. Usually we are not concerned about having precise control over the rate at which such energy is released. However, if energy were released in your body as it is from a fire, your body would not be able to use that energy because the rate of its release would not be under control. **Enzymes** control the rate of chemical reactions in living organisms so energy release can be controlled and the energy can be used by cells.

Chemical reactions in the body and even in nonliving substances are spontaneous; that is, given enough time, they would occur by themselves. However, many of these reactions do not regularly occur at any significant rate because they lack the energy necessary to start the reaction. For example, glucose is not spontaneously oxidized to H_2O and CO_2 at any significant rate. The energy required to start such a reaction is called the **activation energy** of the reaction. Activation energy can be thought of as a barrier over which molecules must be raised for a reaction to occur (Figure 2.16a). This condition is analogous to a rock resting in a depression at the top of a hill (Figure 2.16b). The rock would easily roll down the hill if it were pushed out of the depression. Activation energy is the effort required to lift the rock over the lip of the depression. Enzymes act as catalysts by lowering the activation energy necessary to

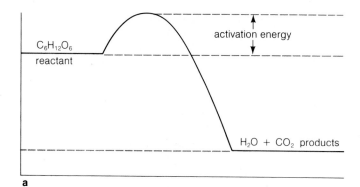

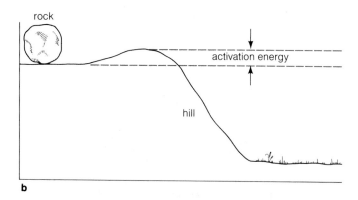

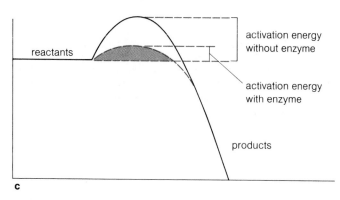

Figure 2.16 (**a**) The energy of activation for the oxidation of glucose, an energy "barrier" over which glucose molecules must be raised before they can be oxidized to H_2O and CO_2. (**b**) An analogous physical situation in which a rock is poised on a depression at the top of a hill. The rock will not move downward unless enough "activating energy" is added to raise it over the lip of the depression. (**c**) Enzymes increase the rate of a spontaneous reaction by reducing the activation energy. This reduction allows biological reactions to proceed rapidly at temperatures that can be tolerated by living organisms.

initiate a reaction (Figure 2.16c). In this way enzymes increase the rate of a reaction so that it can occur at temperatures living organisms can tolerate. (Another way to reduce activation energy might be to increase the temperature of the molecules, but the effective temperature increase would be greater than a living organism could tolerate.) In most cases in living organisms, enzymes increase the rate of a reaction from an unmeasurable low rate to a rate sufficiently high to keep the organism alive and functioning.

Enzymes are not used up in the reactions they initiate. Though enzyme molecules eventually "wear out," they can be used over and over again to catalyze a reaction. Like a catalyst in an inorganic chemical reaction, an enzyme increases the rate of a reaction without itself being permanently affected by the reaction. Enzymes are biological catalysts.

In addition to reducing activation energy, enzymes provide a surface on which the reactions take place. A certain area on the surface of an enzyme, the **active site**, is the site at which the enzyme forms a loose association with its substrate. The **substrate** is the substance the enzyme acts upon—the reactant. After forming a complex with the enzyme, the substrate undergoes chemical change, and the product or products of the reaction are formed (Figure 2.17). Sometimes a molecule similar in structure to the substrate becomes bound to the active site but is unable to undergo the reaction. This nonsubstrate ties up the active site and acts as a **competitive inhibitor** of the reaction; it competes with the substrate for the site, preventing the reaction from taking place whenever it occupies the active site.

Competitive inhibition is an important phenomenon. Some antibiotics kill microorganisms by competitively inhibiting one of their enzymes. Certain chemotherapeutic agents used to treat cancer inhibit enzymes in rapidly dividing cells and thus usually do more damage to those cells than to normal cells. Finally, some poisons kill people by competitive inhibition of essential enzymes.

Enzymes are usually named for the substrate they act upon by adding the suffix -*ase* to the name of the substrate. For example, the enzyme sucrase breaks down the sugar sucrose; lipase breaks down lipids, peptidase breaks peptide bonds, and phosphorylase acts on phosphate bonds.

Another very important characteristic of enzymes is their **specificity**. Cells contain hundreds of enzymes, each of which catalyzes one specific reaction. Their particular three-dimensional protein structure, especially the characteristic shapes of their active sites, account for this specificity. From a functional point of view, the specificity of enzyme reactions makes sure that only certain appropriate chemical reactions will take place at any given time. As will be explained in the consideration of protein synthesis, cells have control mechanisms determining which enzymes will be available in accordance with the cell's needs.

Factors that affect the rate of enzyme reactions include temperature; pH; and concentrations of substrate, product, and enzyme. Because enzymes are proteins, they are subject to denaturation by heat and extremes of pH just as other proteins are. In fact, most enzymes in the human body have an optimum temperature near normal body temperature and an optimum pH near neutral. The very acidic optimum pH of pepsin, a peptidase that breaks down proteins in the stomach, is an exception. An enzyme works most rapidly at its optimum temperature and pH.

Most enzymes will catalyze a reaction in either direction. That is, a substrate can react to make products (AB → C + D), or the reverse (C + D → AB). The concentrations of the substrates and products determine the direction and rate of the reaction. A high concentration of substrate drives the reaction toward the formation of product. If the product is removed as it is formed, as often occurs when the product of one reaction immediately becomes the substrate for another reaction, the reaction continues in the direction of forming more product (AB → C + D). However, if the product accumulates, the reaction is slowed considerably and may be driven in the opposite direction (C + D → AB). Finally, other things being equal, the rate of the reaction is affected by the amount of enzyme present. The more enzyme and thus the more active sites there are, the faster the reaction proceeds.

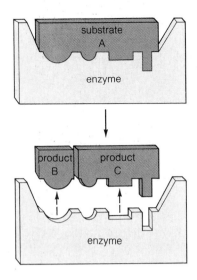

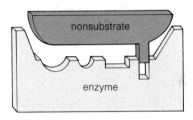

Figure 2.17 The surface of an enzyme has an active site on which its normal substrate fits. The reactants that fit there are converted to the products of the specific reaction catalyzed by the enzyme. If another molecule fits the active site well enough to attach and prevent the substrate molecules from occupying the site, this nonsubstrate molecule may inhibit the action of the enzyme.

NUCLEOTIDES AND NUCLEIC ACIDS

Objective 15. Describe the components of a nucleotide and compare the nucleotides of high-energy compounds, deoxyribonucleic acid (DNA), and ribonucleic acid (RNA). List the general functions of high-energy nucleotides and nucleic acids.

Nucleotides, so-named because they are the building blocks of nucleic acids, are also found in certain high-energy compounds and coenzymes. (Coenzymes are substances that work with enzymes; their properties will be discussed in Chapter 23.) A nucleotide consists of three parts: a nitrogen-containing base (so-called because it has basic, or alkaline, properties), a five-carbon sugar, and one or more phosphate groups (Figure 2.18).

The nucleotide adenosine triphosphate (ATP) is the main "energy currency" molecule of the cell (Figure 2.19). ATP is called an energy currency molecule because it is able to capture energy from the metabolism of food, transfer it from one part of a cell to another, and release it in a way the cell can use it. Other molecules that can store and release energy include guanidine triphosphate (GTP) and uridine triphosphate (UTP). In all these nucleotides the bonds between the phosphates contain far more energy than most chemical bonds; thus they are called high-energy bonds. When such a bond is formed, energy is stored; when it is broken, energy is released. Enzymes control the breaking and forming of these bonds so that energy is captured and delivered to appropriate sites in the cells when needed.

When the enzyme adenylate cyclase is present, ATP

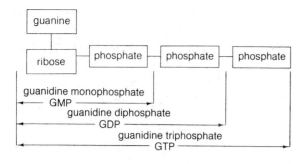

guanidine monophosphate
GMP
guanidine diphosphate
GDP
guanidine triphosphate
GTP

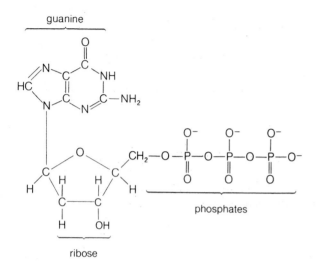

Figure 2.18   The structure of a nucleotide.

can be converted to cyclic adenosine monophosphate (cAMP) by the removal of two phosphate groups and rearrangement of the molecule into a ring form. Cyclic AMP and several other cyclic nucleotides are important in initiating specific activities within cells, as will be explained in later chapters.

Nucleic acids are very complex compounds found in all living organisms. They consist of long chains of nucleotides linked together. Ribonucleic acid (RNA) is a single chain of nucleotides; deoxyribonucleic acid (DNA) is a double chain of nucleotides arranged in the form of a double helix, or spiral. In both nucleic acids the phosphate and sugar molecules form the "backbone" of the strand. The nitrogen-containing bases attach to the sugar (Figure 2.20). A more detailed diagram of nucleic acids is provided in Figure 3.19, Chapter 3. The two nucleotide chains of DNA are held together by hydrogen bonds between the bases and by other forces. In DNA molecules adenine in one chain always pairs with thymine in the other chain, and cytosine always pairs with guanine.

The building blocks of the nucleotides of the two nucleic acids are somewhat different. RNA contains the five-carbon sugar ribose, and DNA contains a five-carbon sugar having one less oxygen atom, deoxyribose. Three of the nitrogen-containing bases are found in both DNA and RNA: cytosine, adenine, and guanine. In addition, DNA contains thymine, and RNA contains uracil (see Figure 2.21 and Table 2.9). Any particular DNA or RNA chain contains several hundred nucleotides with the bases arranged in a

a   ATP

adenylate cyclase

+ two phosphates

b   cyclic AMP

Figure 2.19   The structures of (**a**) ATP and (**b**) cyclic AMP.

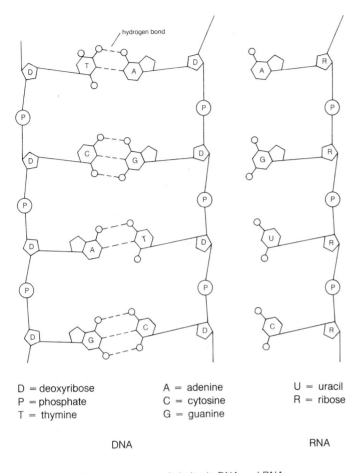

D = deoxyribose   A = adenine   U = uracil
P = phosphate   C = cytosine   R = ribose
T = thymine   G = guanine

DNA   RNA

Figure 2.20 The arrangement of chains in DNA and RNA.

particular sequence. The nearly infinite variety of possible sequences of bases makes it possible for DNA and RNA to contain a great many different pieces of information. The sequence of nucleotides, like the sequence of letters in words and sentences, conveys information about the proteins an organism will have. Like changing a letter in a word, changing a single nucleotide in the sequence may change the information it carries.

The roles of DNA and RNA in the body are related to their ability to convey information. DNA, the nucleic acid that is transmitted from one generation to the next, determines the characteristics of the new individual by supplying the information for the proteins the cells will contain. RNA, on the other hand, carries information from the DNA to the sites where protein is manufactured in cells and directs the actual assembly of proteins there. More will be said about these important molecules in Chapter 3.

Table 2.9 Components of DNA and RNA		
Component	Found in DNA	Found in RNA
Phosphoric acid	X	X
Ribose		X
Deoxyribose	X	
Adenine	X	X
Guanine	X	X
Cytosine	X	X
Thymine	X	
Uracil		X

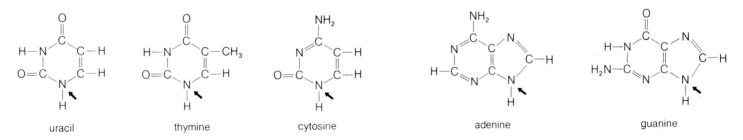

Figure 2.21 The nitrogen-containing bases of nucleic acids. The arrows indicate where the bases link to the sugars in the formation of nucleotides.

Essay: Radioactivity

Radioactivity, the ability of certain isotopes of some elements to emit radiation, is a two-edged sword. We can utilize radioactive elements to produce tremendous amounts of energy. Cancers and some other diseases can be treated successfully with radiation. On the other hand, excessive or prolonged exposure to radiation is a physiological disaster for essentially all life forms.

Radioactivity was first discovered in 1896, when photographic plates that had lain beneath a piece of uranium ore were developed and found to be mysteriously clouded. Investigators concluded that the uranium had given off a radiation that was similar to light but invisible and capable of penetrating material light could not penetrate. This ability of uranium (and many other elements) to give off radiation was called radioactivity. It was not until early in the twentieth century that a theory to describe the process of radioactivity was developed. At that time the arrangement of particles in atoms was unknown. The work with radioactive materials led to the now-accepted model of particle arrangement in an atom and to the recognition of isotopes, as described earlier in this chapter.

In the study of radioactivity investigators detected three kinds of emissions from the nuclei of atoms of radioactive elements: **alpha particles**, **beta particles**, and **gamma rays**. By measuring the mass and charge of the emissions, they identified alpha particles as helium nuclei (now known to consist of two protons, two neutrons, and no electrons), beta particles as electrons from the disintegration of a neutron into a proton and an electron, and gamma rays as electromagnetic radiation having wavelengths too short to be visible.

Radioactive emissions occur because of unbalanced energy relationships within the nuclei of radioactive atoms, causing some particles in their nuclei to fly apart, and the atoms to become different elements. Further studies showed that the emission of particles from radioactive substances continues at a constant rate regardless of temperature, pressure, or other conditions. The rates of emission for different elements are expressed as half-lives. The **half-life** of a radioactive element is the amount of time for half the original number of atoms in a sample to emit particles and undergo disintegration to form different elements. Half-lives can be expressed for emitters of alpha and beta particles. Emissions of gamma rays do not result in the formation of different elements.

Radioactive emissions affect living organisms by bombarding atoms within the cells, causing them to lose electrons and form ions. Thus, such emissions are often called **ionizing radiations**. The emissions also may break chemical bonds and form reactive products. When water molecules are bombarded by ionizing radiation, many eventually split into H^+ and OH^- ions. The OH groups may combine to form hydrogen peroxide, H_2O_2, an unstable product that releases oxygen. The oxygen is extremely reactive and interferes with the normal function of cells.

Our bodies are constantly bombarded with small amounts of radiation from outer space, although the earth's atmosphere protects us from part of that radiation. These emissions are thought to cause some cell mutations. If egg or sperm cells are affected, the mutations will appear in offspring and be transmitted from generation to generation. Emissions may cause any cell to become cancerous or to die.

Different emissions have different effects on the body. Alpha particles, though large and potentially capable of doing damage, are relatively harmless because they do not penetrate the skin. Most beta particles can penetrate only a few millimeters into tissues. Thus, the risk of tissue damage from beta particles is relatively small unless they happen to collide with matter inside a cell; they can then often cause damage. Gamma rays, emissions similar to X rays, can readily penetrate tissues and are the most likely to do damage. Substances that emit both beta particles and gamma rays may be particularly harmful.

The half-life of radioactive elements is another factor to be considered in assessing the likelihood of their doing damage. Some radioactive elements have long half-lives. If they enter the body through food or by other means and become incorporated into the tissues, they emit radiations into those tissues over a long period of time. Radioactive strontium, which is sometimes found in milk and becomes concentrated in the bones, has a half-life of 28 years. Radioactive iodine, on the other hand, has a half-life of 8.1 days.

The same properties of radioactive substances that cause inadvertent damage and death of cells can be used to destroy malignant or cancerous cells. For instance, cancer is often treated by placing radium or radioactive cobalt close to the cancerous tissue. Because cancerous cells are dividing and metabolizing more rapidly, they are more susceptible to damage than less active normal cells. The dosage of radiation must be carefully controlled. X rays, a penetrating radiation similar to gamma rays, can also be used to destroy malignant cells. The ability of certain tissues to accumulate particular elements can be used therapeutically. For example, as developing red blood cells and other rapidly dividing cells take up phosphorus, disorders in which excessive numbers of cells are produced can be treated by the introduction of radioactive phosphorus.

The ability of certain tissues to concentrate particular elements also can be used to diagnose abnormal conditions. Giving an individual a drink of fluid containing a small, known amount of radioactive iodine and measuring the radioactivity of the thyroid gland with a radiation counter makes it possible to determine whether the gland is making too much or too little of its hormones. Some controversy exists regarding the safety of this technique.

The use of X rays to penetrate soft tissue and highlight the location of bones is a well-established application of radiation in diagnosis of skeletal problems. Other diagnostic uses of X rays include chest X rays and the tracing of X-ray opaque substances through the intestine, kidneys, and blood vessels.

Whenever radioactive substances are used in diagnosis or treatment, the benefit of their use must be weighed against the risk of creating new pathology that may be more serious than the existing condition. Individuals subjected to radioactive substances and medical personnel who administer them must be protected against cumulative effects of radiation. Even the urine, feces, sweat, and vomited material of individuals receiving high doses of radioactive substances must be disposed of with care to avoid exposing others to the residual radioactivity.

The effects of radiation on the body may be cumulative throughout life. Small doses of radiation over a period of years could have the same probability of causing damage as a single dose equal to the sum of the small doses. Years of exposure to small amounts of radiation could amount to as much radiation as exposure to an atomic explosion! Even when no specific effects of radiation can be detected, the radiation may be accelerating the aging process.

Understanding the properties of radioactive materials, then, is important to the study of physiology for at least three reasons. First, it explains the cause of some mutations and other cell damage. Second, it can be applied to the selective destruction of malignant cells. And finally, it can be applied to an ever-increasing variety of diagnostic procedures. For each of radioactivity's potential benefits, though, there seems to be a potential risk. Radiation can kill cancers—or cause them. It can destroy individuals—or, over time, produce new species. It may be used to produce electrical power, or to produce the awesome destruction of nuclear war. Whether our understanding of radioactivity will lead us to use it responsibly remains to be seen.

CHAPTER SUMMARY

(Chapter summary points and review questions are numbered to correspond to the numbered objectives in the text of each chapter.)

Why Study Chemistry

1. Explain why a study of basic chemistry is necessary to understand human physiology.
   a. Functions at all levels of organization of the body involve functions at the chemical level.
   b. The maintenance of homeostasis likewise involves functions at the chemical level.

Chemical Building Blocks

2. Define the terms atom, element, molecule, and compound; list the most common elements (and their symbols) found in the human body.
   a. The above terms are defined as follows:
      (1) An atom is the smallest chemical unit of matter.
      (2) An element is a substance composed of one kind of matter.
      (3) A molecule is the smallest particle of a substance that retains the chemical characteristics of the substance; it usually consists of two or more atoms chemically combined.
      (4) A compound consists of atoms of two or more different elements chemically combined.
   b. The most common elements found in the body are carbon (C), hydrogen (H), oxygen (O), and nitrogen (N).

3. Describe the structure of an atom in terms of protons, neutrons, and electrons; explain the structure of ions and isotopes.
   a. The structural components of an atom are:
      (1) Positively charged protons found in the nucleus of the atom, each having one unit of mass
      (2) Uncharged neutrons found in the nucleus of the atom, each having one unit of mass
      (3) Negatively charged electrons found in the electron space of the atom, each having a mass of much less than one unit
   b. The number of protons in an atom determines its atomic number. The number of protons and neutrons in an atom determines its atomic weight.

c. Ions are atoms that have gained or lost one or more electrons.
 (1) Cations are positively charged ions.
 (2) Anions are negatively charged ions.
d. Isotopes are atoms of the same element that contain the same number of protons but different numbers of neutrons.

Chemical Bonds and Chemical Reactions

4. Distinguish among ionic, covalent, and hydrogen bonds and show how they are involved in holding atoms together.
 a. All chemical bonds contain energy that holds atoms together.
 b. The different kinds of bonds are as follows:
  (1) Ionic bonds involve the attraction of oppositely charged ions.
  (2) Covalent bonds involve the sharing of electrons between two atoms.
  (3) Hydrogen bonds involve weak attractions between a hydrogen nucleus and oxygen or nitrogen nuclei within or between molecules.
5. Describe in general what happens in a chemical reaction.
 a. Chemical reactions involve the breaking and forming of chemical bonds.
 b. Energy changes are associated with chemical reactions.
  (1) Catabolic reactions are said to be exothermic because they release energy.
  (2) Anabolic reactions are said to be endothermic because they require an input of energy in order to occur.

Water

6. Describe the properties of water that are important to its function in living things.
 a. The properties of water are summarized in Table 2.3.

Solutions and Colloidal Dispersions

7. Describe the properties of solutions and colloidal dispersions that are important to their function in living things.
 a. Solutions consist of a mixture in which one or more solutes are evenly distributed.
 b. Colloidal dispersions consist of particles too large to form true solutions distributed in a medium and held in suspension by electrical charges, layers of water molecules, and other forces.

Acids, Bases, and pH

8. Define acid, base, and pH; explain how these terms are useful in physiology.
 a. Acids release hydrogen ions (H^+); bases release hydroxyl ions (OH^-).
 b. The pH of a solution is a measure of its acidity or alkalinity, in which 7 is neutral, below 7 is acidic, and above 7 is alkaline, or basic.

Complex Molecules

9. Define organic chemistry and identify the major functional groups of organic molecules.
 a. Organic chemistry is a study of carbon-containing compounds.
 b. The functional groups of interest to physiologists are alcohols, aldehydes, ketones, carboxyl groups, and amino groups.
10. List the four classes of physiologically important compounds.
 a. The four classes of complex molecules are carbohydrates, lipids, proteins (including enzymes), and nucleic acids.

Carbohydrates

11. Describe the general structure and chemical properties of carbohydrates and explain their role in the body.
 a. Carbohydrates consist of chains of carbon atoms, usually having two hydrogen atoms and one oxygen atom associated with each carbon.
 b. The basic unit of a carbohydrate is a monosaccharide; disaccharides contain two units, and polysaccharides contain many units.
 c. Most carbohydrates are used by the body for energy.

Lipids

12. Describe the general structure and chemical properties of simple lipids, compound lipids, and steroids; explain the role of each in the body.
 a. Simple lipids or fats consist of one molecule of glycerol and three molecules of fatty acids, each of which may be saturated or unsaturated (contain double bonds in the carbon chain).
 b. Compound lipids contain some substance in addition to glycerol and fatty acids; phospholipids contain a molecule of phosphoric acid in place of one of the fatty acids.
 c. Steroids have a complex structure with a characteristic configuration of four connected ring structures; cholesterol, vitamin D, and hormones from the sex glands and adrenal glands are examples of steroids.
 d. Simple lipids serve to store energy in the body, compound lipids form part of the structure of the membranes of cells and organelles, and steroids usually act as chemical regulators (hormones).

Proteins

13. Describe the general structure and chemical properties of

amino acids as building blocks of proteins; distinguish between structural proteins and enzymes.

    a. Proteins are formed from amino acids, which have amino and carboxyl functional groups and are held together by peptide bonds.

    b. The chains of amino acids in proteins are coiled and folded into large complex shapes held together mostly by hydrogen bonds and disulfide linkages.

    c. Proteins may be classified according to function as:

        (1) Structural proteins, which form part of the structure of cells

        (2) Enzymes, which control the rate of chemical reactions

        (3) Other proteins, which serve certain transport and regulatory functions

Enzymes

14. Describe the characteristics of enzymes and explain how these characteristics contribute to the function of enzymes.

    a. Enzymes have the following properties:

        (1) They serve as biological catalysts by lowering the activation energy necessary to initiate a reaction.

        (2) They have active sites to which substrates can attach (and to which inhibitors can sometimes attach and block a reaction).

        (3) They are affected by temperature, pH, concentration of substrates and products, and concentration of the enzyme itself.

        (4) They demonstrate specificity by catalyzing only one type of reaction.

    b. These characteristics contribute to the function of enzymes by determining what reactions will occur and the rate at which they will occur.

Nucleotides and Nucleic Acids

15. Describe the components of a nucleotide and compare the nucleotides of high-energy compounds, deoxyribonucleic acid (DNA), and ribonucleic acid (RNA). List the general functions of high-energy nucleotides and nucleic acids.

    a. Nucleotides contain:

        (1) A nitrogen-containing base

        (2) A five-carbon sugar

        (3) One or more phosphate groups

    b. High-energy compounds include adenosine triphosphate (ATP), guanidine triphosphate (GTP), and uridine triphosphate (UTP).

    c. The components of DNA and RNA are summarized in Table 2.9.

    d. General functions:

        (1) High-energy nucleotides transfer and store energy.

        (2) Nucleic acids store and transmit information to direct the activities of cells.

REVIEW

Important Terms

acid	ion
active site	ionic bond
amino acid	isotope
anabolism	lipid
atom	mixture
atomic number	molecule
atomic weight	monosaccharide
base	neutron
carbohydrate	nucleic acid
catabolism	nucleotide
colloid	peptide bond
competitive inhibitor	phospholipid
compound	polar compound
compound lipid	polysaccharide
covalent bond	protein
denaturation	proton
disaccharide	radioactivity
electron	solute
element	solution
enzyme	solvent
essential amino acid	steroid
glucose	substrate
hydrogen bond	

Questions

1. Why study chemistry?

2. Tell what kind of chemical building block is indicated by each of the following symbols or formulas: C, O_2, CO_2, N, N_2, NH_2, H_2O.

3. a. Draw models of carbon, hydrogen, oxygen, nitrogen, and sodium atoms.

    b. Modify your drawings to show the formation of a sodium ion, a hydrogen ion, and the isotopes C^{14} and H^3.

4. Make a diagram to explain how each of the following is held together: a crystal of sodium chloride, a molecule of carbon dioxide, a molecule of carbon tetrachloride (one atom of carbon and four atoms of chlorine).

5. Using general information about chemical reactions, complete the equations for the following chemical reactions:

    a. $O_2 + C \rightarrow ?$

    b. $H^+ + OH^- \rightarrow ?$

    c. $NaOH + HCl \rightarrow H_2O + ?$
    d. $H_2CO_3 \rightarrow CO_2 + ?$

6. Explain how the following properties of water contribute to the normal functioning of living things: polarity, capacity as a solvent, high surface tension, ability to hold heat, ability to lose heat through evaporation, ability to participate in chemical reactions.

7. Determine which of the following are true solutions and which are colloidal dispersions: sugar syrup, saline, blood. Explain your answers.

8. Find the pH of each of the following solutions: pure water, a solution of H_2CO_3 that has an H^+ concentration of 10^{-5} moles per liter, a solution of HCl that has an H^+ concentration of 10^{-6} moles per liter. Which of the solutions is most acidic and by how much?

9. a. What is organic chemistry?
    b. What are the important functional groups found in organic compounds?

10. Name the four classes of complex molecules.

11. For carbohydrates: name the elements present, describe the functional groups, name the basic unit and its multiples, and discuss their function in the body.

12. a. Describe the building blocks of a simple lipid (fat) and distinguish between saturated and unsaturated fats.
    b. Describe how phospholipids and steroids differ in structure from simple lipids.
    c. List the major functions of each group of lipids.

13. a. Name the elements found in an amino acid, describe its functional groups, and explain how these groups form peptide bonds.
    b. Discuss the arrangement of amino acids in fibrous and globular proteins.
    c. Describe the major functions of proteins.

14. Describe the characteristics of enzymes that allow them to carry out their functions and list factors that affect the action of enzymes.

15. Describe the basic unit of a nucleic acid and explain how DNA and RNA differ in structure and function.

Problems

1. Given the following chemical reaction:
$$CO_2 + H_2O \rightleftharpoons H_2CO_3 \rightleftharpoons H^+ + HCO_3^-$$
and the information that the equilibrium of the reaction shifts as substances are added or removed, answer the following questions:
    a. What happens when an excess of CO_2 and H_2O are produced? (This would occur when metabolism is speeded up.)
    b. What happens when CO_2 and H_2O are removed?
    c. How do (a) and (b) affect the pH of the medium in which the reaction occurs?

2. Some antibiotics act by attaching to certain enzymes in microorganisms and acting as competitive inhibitors of the enzyme.

How might the antibiotic affect the chemical reaction controlled by the enzyme? What might happen to the microorganism? To the person taking the antibiotic?

REFERENCES AND READINGS

Anderson, P. D. 1976. *Clinical anatomy and physiology for allied health sciences.* Philadelphia: W. B. Saunders.

Arehart-Treichel, J. 1979. Chemical carcinogens: Part of the problem. *Science News* 115:411 (June 23).

Baum, S. J., and Scaife, C. W. 1975. *Chemistry: A life science approach.* New York: Macmillan.

Fuller, E. C. 1974. *Chemistry and man's environment.* Boston: Houghton Mifflin.

Sharon, N. 1974. Glycoproteins. *Scientific American* 230(5):78 (May).

Sharon, N. 1974. Carbohydrates. *Scientific American* 243(5):90 (November).

Wolfe, S. L. 1977. *Biology: the foundations.* Belmont, Calif.: Wadsworth.

3

THE CELLULAR LEVEL OF LIFE

ORGANIZATION AND GENERAL FUNCTION OF CELLS

Objective 1. Explain why the cell is considered the basic functional unit of living organisms.

Before the invention of the microscope it was difficult for those who tried to study the human body to understand much about how it worked. They were seriously hampered by the inability to see that the human body, and the bodies of other living things, were made up of cells. As we now know, cells are the smallest functional unit of living things. Many of the physiological processes that occur in the body occur at the cellular level.

As early as the seventeenth century, microscopic studies of specimens of living things showed they were divided into many similar units. Subsequent observations in the 1830s led to the **cell theory**: *All living things are composed of cells.* The units, or cells, were seen to contain a heavy, dense body—the nucleus—and a less dense granular substance—the cytoplasm. Since these early studies a great variety of types of cells have been described, and they have been found to contain many highly specialized structures besides the nucleus. These structures, the organelles, will be described later.

Cells are considered to be the functional units of living things not only because they appear as structural units, but also because they carry out most of the basic life processes. In general, the processes described in Chapter 1 that occur in whole organisms also occur at the cellular level. For example, movement occurs within cells; the membranes of cells, especially those of nerve and muscle cells, are excitable (respond to stimuli); cells ingest substances, metabolize them, and eliminate wastes; and finally, cells reproduce themselves.

Complex organisms such as humans have many different kinds of cells (Figure 3.1). Epithelial cells form sheets to line cavities or to cover organs. They absorb substances, produce secretions, or offer protection, depending on their location. Muscle cells form long fibers that shorten during contraction. Nerve cells (neurons) have a cell body with several long thin extensions (processes) that conduct nerve impulses. Several types of cells surround themselves with extracellular substances: Bone cells produce a hard substance; cartilage cells produce a less hard but still solid substance. As cells become highly specialized to carry out one particular function, they frequently become less able to carry out other functions. For example, highly specialized nerve cells have lost the ability to reproduce.

In this chapter we will consider the general structure of cells, their membranes, and their organelles, or "little organs." We will also consider how materials move into and out of cells, how cells make proteins, and how cells divide during growth and repair. Some processes that take place at the cellular level will be considered in later chapters. The contractility of muscle cells will be considered in Chapter 8, the excitability of membranes in Chapter 10, and energy production in cells in Chapter 23. Meiosis, the process of nuclear division by which eggs and sperm are produced, and genetics, the study of how characteristics are passed from one generation to the next, will be considered in Chapter 27.

CELL MEMBRANES

Objective 2. Describe the chemical and physical properties of cell membranes and explain how membranes contribute to the functioning of the cell.

Even with a good light microscope, you will have difficulty finding out very much about the membranes of a cell. Because these membranes can be seen only with the aid of an electron microscope, many of the properties of membranes have been determined by chemical analyses of cell functions rather than by visual observation.

What is now known about the membranes and organelles of cells is based on the results of many experiments, each of which required the use of highly specialized equipment and techniques. Although it is beyond the scope of this book to explain how these experiments were conducted, you should keep in mind that the information given here is based on carefully acquired experimental evidence.

The **plasma membrane** (often called the cell mem-

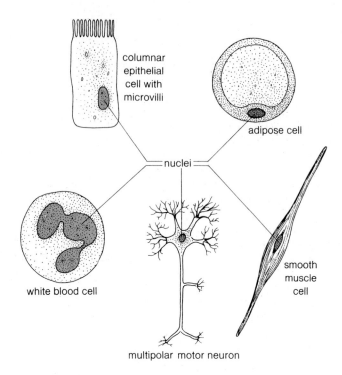

Figure 3.1 Some different types of cells.

brane) defines the boundaries of a cell; its structure is shown diagramatically in Figure 3.2. Similar membranes form the boundaries of organelles within cells. All membranes are composed of the same structural components. The plasma membrane consists of **phospholipids** arranged in two layers. The polar (charged) phosphate ends of the molecules are oriented toward the inner and outer surfaces, while nonpolar (fatty acid) ends point toward each other in the interior of the membrane.

Interspersed among the phospholipids are protein molecules that may extend partially or all the way through the lipid layers. Such embedded protein molecules are called **integral proteins**. Other protein molecules, the **peripheral proteins**, are loosely attached to the outer or inner surface of the membrane. Recent research has shown that, for the plasma membrane, most of the peripheral proteins project into the cytoplasm rather than toward the outer surface.

Carbohydrates are also associated with plasma membranes—sugars combine with proteins to form glycoproteins or with lipids to form glycolipids. These kinds of molecules cover about 7 percent of the outer surface of the membrane. Some carbohydrates serve as recognition sites that allow cells to recognize other cells in cell-to-cell interactions. Proteins and glycoproteins called antigens are also

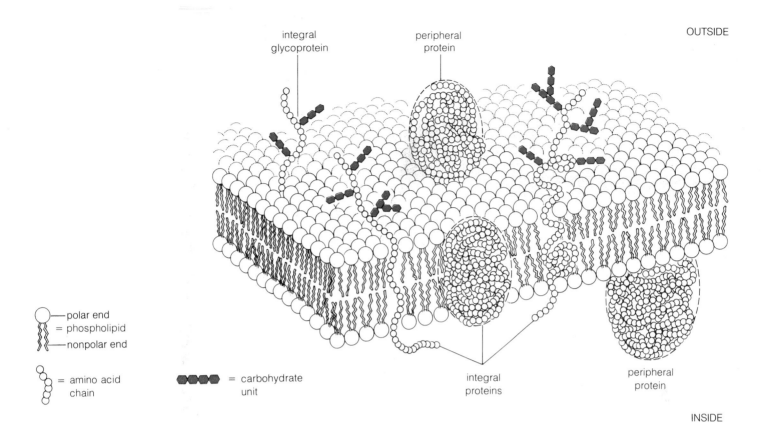

integral
glycoprotein

peripheral
protein

OUTSIDE

—polar end

= phospholipid

—nonpolar end

= amino acid
chain

= carbohydrate
unit

integral
proteins

peripheral
protein

INSIDE

Figure 3.2 A model of a cell membrane.

found on the surface of plasma membranes, where they are important in cell-to-cell interactions.

Good evidence exists that tiny pores in the cell membrane allow water molecules and some ions to cross the membrane. These pores probably are made of proteins that extend through the membrane.

The primary function of the plasma membrane is to regulate the internal environment of the cell and thus maintain homeostasis by controlling the passage of substances into and out of the cell. How these controls are exerted is discussed later in this chapter. Cell membranes also play a part in transmitting information. Chemical messengers, such as some of the hormones we will discuss in Chapter 15, attach to receptors on cell membranes. The presence of such messengers activates a second messenger, a substance that relays information. One such second messenger system involves an enzyme, adenylate cyclase, found in the membrane. This enzyme converts ATP inside the cell into cyclic AMP, a second messenger molecule. Cyclic AMP then acts as a specific signal molecule within the cell, stimulating the cell to carry out a particular function such as

speeding up a chemical reaction. Figure 3.3 illustrates this mechanism.

ORGANELLES

Objective 3. Describe the general structure and function of each of the organelles in the cell.

Your stomach, lungs, and heart are examples of organs of your body. Just as they are functional units of your body, **organelles** are functional units of a cell. Each cell has several different kinds of these little organs. Few of them can be seen with a light microscope; they are illustrated in Figure 3.4 as they might appear in an electron micrograph.

Endoplasmic Reticulum

The **endoplasmic reticulum** is an extensive network of interconnected vesicles, or sacs, and tubules bound by membranes. In some micrographs the endoplasmic reticulum (ER) appears to be continuous with the plasma membrane

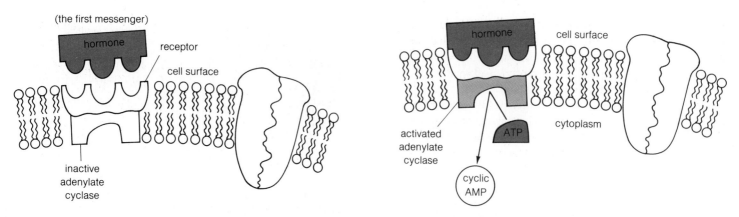

Figure 3.3 One mechanism by which cell membranes transmit information. A messenger such as a hormone binds to a receptor on the cell membrane. Its presence activates the enzyme adenylate cyclase to convert a molecule of ATP to cyclic AMP. The cyclic AMP acts as a specific signal within the cytoplasm of the cell. (M. Pines, *Inside the Cell*, DHEW Publication.)

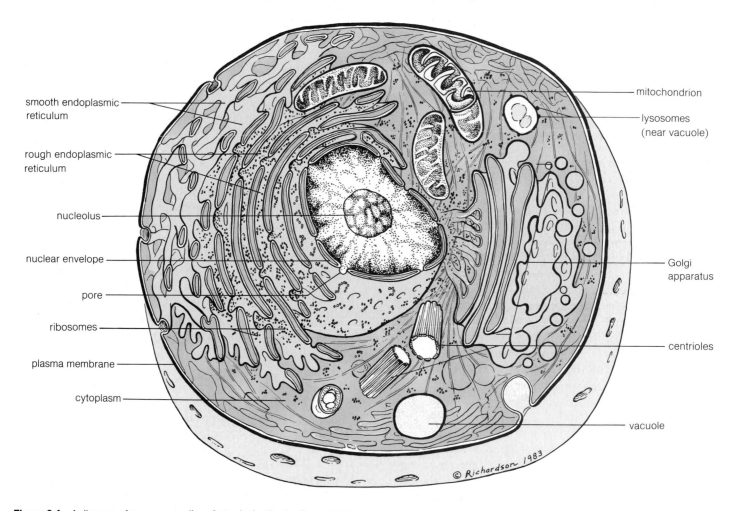

Figure 3.4 A diagram of some organelles of a typical animal cell, as might be seen in an electron micrograph. Some of the smaller organelles are shown larger than they actually are in relation to the rest of the cell.

and with the membrane system that surrounds the nucleus, the control organelle of the cell. It is now thought that the tubules of the ER serve as a transport system for proteins and possibly other large molecules synthesized by the cell.

Some parts of the ER are rough because of the presence of small structures called ribosomes; the rest is smooth (see Figure 3.5). Smooth ER is thought to be the site of synthesis of lipids such as cholesterol and also the site of breakdown of fats into smaller molecules that can be used for energy.

Ribosomes

Ribosomes, small bodies that lack membranes, are found on the surface of rough ER and also free in the cytoplasm. They serve as sites for protein synthesis, a process that will be described in more detail later. Cells that synthesize proteins for use outside the cell tend to have a greater proportion of their ribosomes attached to ER. Researchers believe that, as proteins are synthesized at the site of the ER-attached ribosomes, the proteins are transported to the lumen (inner cavity) of the ER and, through it, to the outside of the cell. Chemically, ribosomes consist of ribonucleic acid (RNA) and protein.

Golgi Apparatus

The **Golgi apparatus** usually appears as a stack of vesicles, or sacs, whose membranes have the same general structure as other membranes of the cell. Vesicles of the Golgi apparatus arise from the pinching off of other vesicles from the ER and the migration of these free vesicles through the cytoplasm to the Golgi apparatus. Vesicles of the Golgi apparatus contain proteins, which are processed by the Golgi apparatus. The proteins may be wrapped in membranous envelopes, converted to glycoproteins by the addition of a carbohydrate component, or changed from an inactive to an active form by the removal of a segment of the protein molecule. Products of the Golgi apparatus are usually extruded from the cell when a vesicle of the Golgi apparatus fuses with the plasma membrane. The Golgi apparatus also may be responsible for packaging certain enzymes into organelles called lysosomes.

Lysosomes

When cells engulf particles, as white blood cells do when they are destroying infectious organisms or debris from an injury, the particles are digested by enzymes from the **lysosomes**. Lysosomes, which contain many different digestive enzymes, generally average about 0.4 μm in diameter. (The abbreviation μm stands for micrometer. One microm-

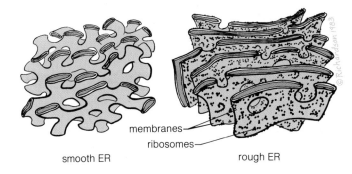

membranes
ribosomes

smooth ER   rough ER

Figure 3.5 Endoplasmic reticulum: tubular sacs of smooth ER and layers of rough ER in section.

eter is one-thousandth of a millimeter, or one millionth of a meter.) In some instances lysosomes fuse with vacuoles (sacs) containing foreign substances engulfed by the cell. The lysosomal enzymes then digest the foreign substances. Integrity of the lysosomal membranes prevents the enzymes from digesting the cell itself. However, when a cell is damaged or dies, its lysosomes rupture, and the enzymes digest the remains of the cell.

Mitochondria

Frequently called the "powerhouses" of the cell, **mitochondria** (Figure 3.6) are the sites of the oxidative reactions that produce energy for the cell. Structurally, the mitochondrion is composed of an outer smooth membrane and an inner folded membrane; the inner membrane folds are called **cristae**. Cells contain from hundreds to thousands of these small rod-shaped organelles that range in size from 0.5 to 1.0 μm in diameter and from 3 to 4 μm in length. Metabolically active cells contain large numbers of mitochondria. The cristae contain the enzymes and other molecules that carry out the energy-producing reactions of the cell. The matrix in the center of the mitochondrion contains some DNA and some ribosomes that are similar to those found in microorganisms.

Some biologists speculate that mitochondria were once free-living primitive organisms that became established as organelles of more complex cells. Whatever the source of mitochondria, the fact that they contain DNA and ribosomes indicates that they are capable of synthesizing some protein subunits without receiving instructions from the cell nucleus.

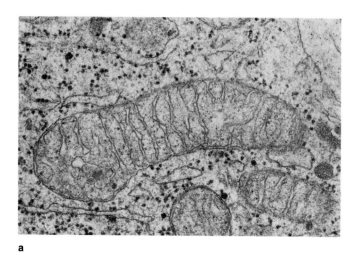

a

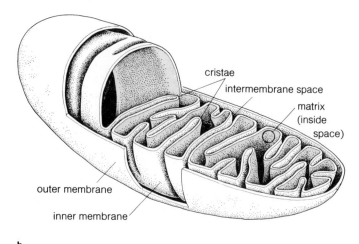

b

Figure 3.6 A mitochondrion: (**a**) from the intestinal epithelium of a chick, × 55,000 (courtesy J. J. Mais); and (**b**) in diagram to show the typical arrangement of inner membranes.

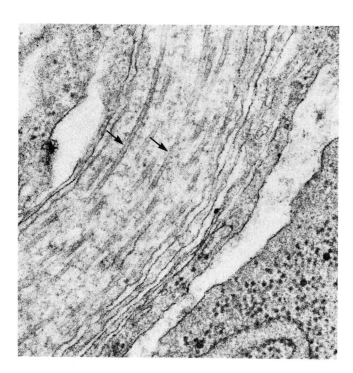

Figure 3.7 Microtubules (shown by arrows) as seen in longitudinal section through a cell, × 65,000. (Courtesy of M. P. Daniels, *Annals of The New York Academy of Sciences*, vol. 253, p. 535.)

Microtubules and Microfilaments

The internal structures that give rigidity to the cytoplasm and help to produce movement are the microtubules and microfilaments. Both consist of proteins devoid of any membrane covering. **Microtubules** are small, apparently hollow fibers composed of the protein tubulin. Visible only with powerful electron microscopes (see Figure 3.7), they form the spindle along which chromosomes move as they separate during cell division. **Microfilaments** are even smaller, solid structures, consisting of the protein actin, a protein also found in muscles. Microfilaments (Figure 3.8) account for amoeboid movement in cells and are particularly important in muscle contraction and in the movement of microvilli, which project from the surface of cells lining the small intestine. The movement of microvilli increases the rate at which digested food particles are absorbed into the blood and lymph.

Centrioles, Cilia, and Flagella

Each of these structures consists of sets of microtubules. The **centrioles** (Figure 3.9) are paired structures found in animal cells. Centrioles are always oriented at right angles to each other. Their internal structure consists of nine sets of three microtubules. They divide and move to the opposite ends of the cell during cell division.

Centrioles give rise to flagella and cilia. **Cilia** are short, hairlike cytoplasmic projections found on the surface of some cells, such as those that line the respiratory tract; they

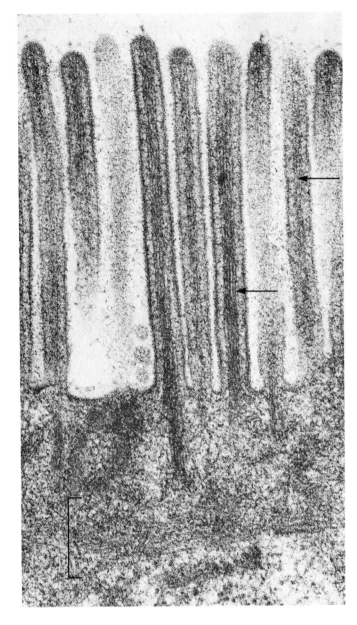

Figure 3.8 Microfilaments (arrows) in microvilli of the intestine of a chick and in the cytoplasm beneath the microvilli (bracket), × 80,000. Microfilaments are believed to provide the force for the movement of microvilli. (Courtesy of C. Chambers.)

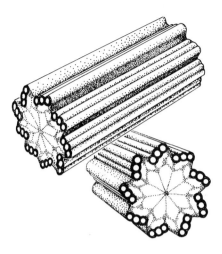

Figure 3.9 A diagram of a pair of centrioles, oriented at right angles as they usually are in the cell and containing nine sets of three microtubules.

pairs of tubules (doublets) around their periphery and a single pair (singlet) in their center (Figure 3.10).

Nucleus

As the control center of the cell, the **nucleus** (Figure 3.11) is essential for the long-term survival of a cell. (Human red blood cells, which normally have no nucleus at maturity, live only about four months.) The nucleus is surrounded by a **nuclear envelope** that consists of a double layer of membrane. The outer membrane is probably continuous at scattered points with the endoplasmic reticulum. Many large pores extend through this envelope, but they are closed by a protein-containing substance and do not allow materials to pass in and out freely.

The details of the control of passage of materials are unknown. Inside the nucleus, within the inner **nucleoplasm**, are the **chromosomes** and **nucleolus**. (Some cells have several nucleoli.) The nucleolus consists mainly of RNA, is irregularly shaped, and subject to change as the cell goes through stages of growth and division. Changes are related to the rate of synthesis of ribosomal RNA, as we shall see later. The nucleolus is not separated from the rest of the nucleus by a membrane.

The chromosomes (Figure 3.12), condensed into short rods during cell division, exist as more diffuse, elongated fibers at other times. Chromosomes are known to consist of DNA wrapped around a protein core; sometimes they are surrounded by protein as well. If the DNA of the forty-six chromosomes found in human cells were arranged end to

are also composed of sets of microtubules. Cilia often beat in waves and move materials such as mucus along the surface of cells. **Flagella**, also cytoplasmic projections, are generally longer than cilia but otherwise similar in structure. A flagellum causes movement of an entire cell—a human sperm, for example. Both cilia and flagella have nine

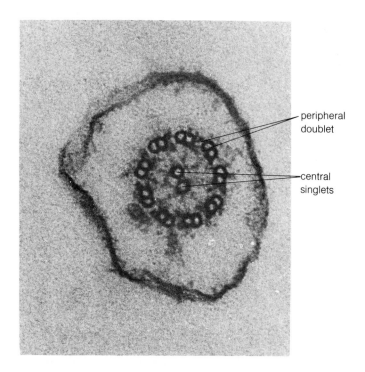

Figure 3.10 A cross-section through a flagellum, showing the arrangement of microtubules. (Courtesy of K. Fujiwara and The Rockefeller University Press.)

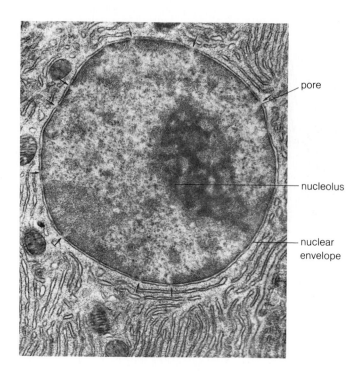

Figure 3.11 The nucleus of a bat pancreas cell, showing the nuclear envelope, pores, and nucleolus, × 13,000. (From W. Bloom and D. Fawcett, Textbooks of Histology, W. B. Saunders Co., 1975, with permission.)

end, the strand would be about 1½ meters long. To pack this amount of DNA into the confines of the nucleus, a body about 10 to 15 μm in diameter, requires that it be arranged compactly, as in fact it is. First the DNA helix is coiled, and then the coils are folded upon themselves. Because of the compact "supercoiled" arrangement, determining the exact sequence of information stored in DNA molecules still poses challenging research problems.

The chromosomes are important in two cellular processes. First, they dictate the nature of proteins that a cell can synthesize; they thereby control the function of the cell. Second, they transmit information for cellular control from one generation to the next. The chromosomes and their functions will be discussed further later in this chapter.

Cellular Inclusions and Extracellular Materials

In addition to the structured organelles, cells may contain vacuoles of ingested substances, stored fats, and granules of glycogen or other substances. Some cells also manufacture and secrete substances that become extracellular materials. These materials include mucus; the matrix of bone, carti-

lage, and connective tissue; and the basement membrane that underlies epithelial tissues.

Integration of Function

Organelles and other cellular structures work together to carry out the functions of cells. Together their activities help to maintain homeostasis within each cell. Their characteristics are summarized in Table 3.1.

PASSAGE OF MATERIALS ACROSS MEMBRANES

Objective 4. Describe the following passive processes and explain their importance in cell function: diffusion, facilitated diffusion, osmosis, filtration, and bulk flow.

Objective 5. Describe the process of active transport and explain (a) how it differs from passive processes, and (b) why it is important in cell function.

Objective 6. Distinguish between pinocytosis and

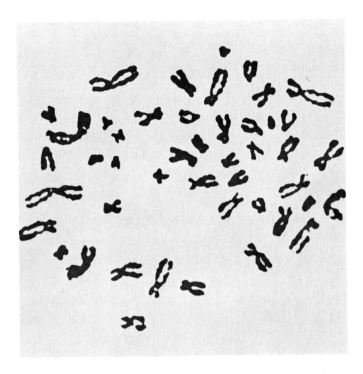

Figure 3.12 Chromosomes of a normal human cell, × 2300. This is the historic photograph by which Drs. Joe Hin Tjio and Albert Levan demonstrated that human cells contain forty-six chromosomes. (Courtesy of Dr. Tjio and the National Institute of General Medical Studies, National Institutes of Health.)

phagocytosis and describe the role of each in cell function.

A living cell is a dynamic entity, with substances constantly moving into and out of it. Understanding how these movements occur is essential to understanding how a cell functions. As described earlier, the plasma membrane consists of a mosaic of protein molecules imbedded in a lipid bilayer, with numerous tiny pores extending through the membrane. Some substances diffuse into and out of membranes through the pores, though electrical charges on the pores exert some control over such diffusion. Lipid-soluble substances dissolve in the lipid and diffuse through it. Still other substances are moved across the membrane by carrier molecules. Thus, the movement of an ion or molecule across a membrane is determined by a combination of factors: particle size, electrical charge, lipid solubility, and the availability of carrier substances in the membrane.

In considering the mechanisms by which substances move into and out of cells, we will first consider passive processes. **Passive transport** involves movement of a substance along a gradient—from higher to lower concentration or from higher to lower pressure. The cell expends no energy to move substances along a gradient; thus the substances are said to move passively. Passive transport processes include diffusion, facilitated diffusion, osmosis, filtration, and bulk flow.

Diffusion

Molecules and ions are in constant motion, resulting in their constant redistribution. Such motion can occur with or without the presence of a membrane. Though movement occurs in all directions, most movement occurs along the gradient. Thus, **diffusion** is the *net* movement of similar molecules from their area of higher concentration to their area of lower concentration. For example, if you drop a lump of sugar into a cup of hot coffee, the sugar molecules will eventually become evenly distributed throughout the coffee, even without stirring. At the beginning of the diffusion process the sugar molecules are present in highest concentration at the lump and in lowest concentration at the points in the coffee farthest from the lump. Thus, a **concentration gradient** is created—a range of concentrations starting with the high concentration at the sugar lump and becoming successively lower as the distance from the lump increases. Diffusion occurs as long as a concentration gradient exists because more sugar molecules move from high to low concentration than move in the other direction. The *net* movement is along the gradient.

Movement of sugar molecules continues once the concentration has become equal in all parts of the cup, but it is equal in all directions. A **dynamic equilibrium** has been reached—dynamic because molecules continue to move, equilibrium because there is no net change in concentration. Had we chosen to put salt in the coffee, equilibrium would have been reached more rapidly because the particles (ions) of salt are smaller than those of sugar, and they diffuse more rapidly. Had the coffee been cold rather than hot, any particles would have moved more slowly as the rate of molecular movement is directly proportional to temperature.

Substances that diffuse through membranes do so by dissolving in the lipids of the membrane or by passing through the pores of the membrane. Lipid-soluble substances will diffuse through the lipid layer at greater rates than they will diffuse through the protein parts of the membrane. However, diffusion through the lipid layer is affected by the solubility of the substance in lipid, temperature, and concentration gradient.

Other diffusion through the membrane probably occurs at points where integral protein molecules create a polar area, resulting in a pore. Again, substances move from higher to lower concentrations, but their movement is af-

Table 3.1 Characteristics of Organelles

Organelle	Characteristics
Endoplasmic reticulum	Network of interconnected vesicles and tubules bound by membranes; serves as transport system for proteins and possibly other large molecules synthesized by the cell; rough ER has ribosomes on the surface and acts as the site of protein synthesis; smooth ER lacks ribosomes and acts as the site of lipid synthesis.
Ribosomes	Small round bodies lacking membranes found on ER; consist of RNA and protein; function in protein synthesis.
Golgi apparatus	Large membrane-bound structure having the shape of a stack of vesicles; serves as a storage and processing organ for proteins and other products of a cell; may add carbohydrate to protein, wrap a protein in a membrane, or remove a segment from a protein before extruding the product from the cell.
Lysosomes	Membrane-bound bodies containing digestive enzymes; their enzymes are released into vacuoles or extruded into dead cells.
Mitochondria	Rod-shaped or spherical bodies having a smooth outer membrane and a folded inner membrane; contain enzymes that carry out the energy-producing reactions of the cell.
Microtubules	Hollow fibers composed of the protein tubulin; provide motility and internal support for the cell.
Microfilaments	Very small solid structures composed of the protein actin; account for motility and contractility of cells.
Centrioles	Paired structures that give rise to flagella and cilia; consist of nine sets of three microtubules.
Cilia	Short hairlike projections from the surface of certain cells; axis consists of a single pair of microtubules centrally located and nine pairs peripherally located.
Flagella	Relatively long projections from the surface of certain cells; axis consists of a single pair of microtubules centrally located and nine pairs peripherally located.
Nucleus	Large body surrounded by a nuclear envelope consisting of a double membrane with large pores; contains nucleoplasm, chromosomes, and one or more nucleoli; functions as the control center of the cell.
Chromosomes	Long, strandlike bodies consisting of DNA and protein; contain genetic information that controls the activities of the cell.
Nucleolus	Irregularly shaped body found in the nucleus; site of ribosome synthesis.

fected by electrical charges along the surface of the pore, the size of the pore, and the specific nature of the pore. Studies of the movement of small particles suggest that these pores are less than 0.8 nanometers (nm) in diameter. (A nanometer is one-billionth of a meter.) Only water molecules and other small molecules and ions can pass through these pores; for this reason the plasma membrane is said to be **selectively permeable**.

Different kinds of pores may exist for different kinds of ions, and charges on both pores and ions may affect passage of the ions through the pores. Calcium ions affect the permeability of membranes—the degree to which certain materials pass through the pores. For example, an increase in the concentration of calcium ions in the fluids around cells can decrease the permeability of the membrane. This effect is especially important in understanding nerve impulses and muscle contractions, which will be discussed in later chapters.

Facilitated Diffusion

Glucose and other sugar molecules too large to pass through the pores and not sufficiently soluble in the membrane lipids to diffuse through them are transported by facilitated diffusion or by active transport. (Active transport will be discussed later.) In **facilitated diffusion** the sugar molecule combines with a carrier substance (a protein molecule) that is imbedded in the membrane. A small portion of the protein molecule moves across the membrane with the sugar molecule. When the sugar is released into the cytoplasm, the carrier is available to facilitate, or aid in, the diffusion of another sugar molecule. Except for the carrier's ability to help the sugar molecule move across the membrane, this kind of diffusion is like any other kind of diffusion: It moves substances from an area of higher concentration to one of lower concentration. However, it does so at a faster rate than that of simple diffusion. When the sugar concentration is particularly high, the rate of movement is limited by the number of carrier molecules available. Certain other molecules also can move by facilitated diffusion, and movement can be in either direction across the membrane, depending on the concentration gradient.

Osmosis

Water passes through pores in cell membranes rapidly in both directions. If a concentration gradient exists, water will move from its own area of higher concentration to its own area of lower concentration at a greater rate than it moves in the opposite direction. This *net* movement of water across a selectively permeable membrane is **osmosis**. Osmosis occurs when nondiffusible solutes are more concentrated on one side of a membrane than on the other side, particularly if the membrane is permeable only to water molecules, as demonstrated in Figure 3.13. The presence of nondiffusible solutes on one side of the membrane creates a concentration gradient. As shown in Figure 3.14, water moves by osmosis through the selectively permeable membrane into the thistle tube in a greater amount than it moves in the opposite direction. The net movement of water into the tube reduces the concentration gradient and increases the volume of solution in the tube. Simply stated, **osmotic pressure** is the force under which water moves from an area of low solute concentration to an area of high solute concentration.

Cells normally are in osmotic balance with the fluids in their environment; that is, water is moving in and out of the cells at the same rate so that no *net* movement occurs. Both the cells and the fluids around them contain proteins and other molecules and ions that exert osmotic pressure. If a concentration gradient develops between a cell and its en-

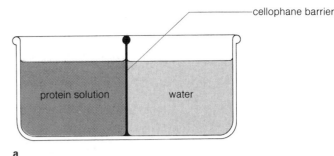

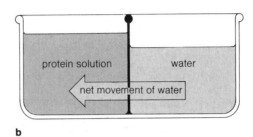

Figure 3.13 A laboratory demonstration of osmosis: (**a**) at beginning of experiment and (**b**) after osmosis has occurred. Water molecules move by osmosis from their area of higher concentration to their area of lower concentration in much greater numbers than they move in the opposite direction. The membrane in the diagram, like a living membrane, is permeable to water but not to protein molecules.

vironment, the net movement of water will be toward the area of higher concentration of solutes (lower concentration of water) until osmotic balance is restored.

Osmotic pressure can be stated in millimeters of fluid the pressure will support in a laboratory apparatus such as the one shown in Figure 3.14. In cells in a living organism physiologists often describe differences in solutions in terms of osmolarity rather than osmotic pressure. **Osmolarity** is expressed in osmols of solutes in a given volume of solution—osmols per liter, for example. **Osmols** express the number of particles (molecules and ions) in a solution. For nonionized substances such as glucose one osmol is the equivalent of one gram molecular weight, or one mole. (The gram molecular weight of a substance is the sum of the atomic weights of the atoms in the molecule expressed in grams.) For example, the molecular weight of glucose is 180, and a gram molecular weight of glucose is 180 grams. That amount of glucose dissolved in 1 liter of water would create a solution of 1 mole per liter, with an osmolarity of 1 osmol per liter. For ionized substances such as sodium chloride, in which each molecule produces two ions, or two particles, a gram molecular weight dissolved in 1 liter of water creates

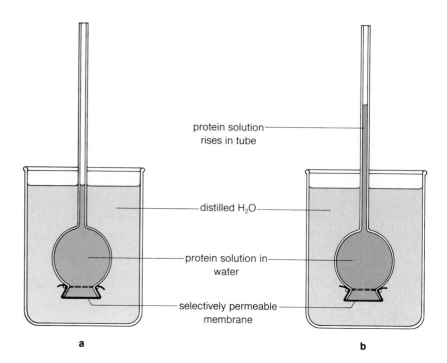

Figure 3.14 A laboratory apparatus to demonstrate the existence of osmotic pressure: (**a**) at the beginning of experiment and (**b**) after osmosis has occurred. The net flow of water is into the protein solution; the protein molecules cannot pass through the membrane.

protein solution rises in tube

distilled H$_2$O

protein solution in water

selectively permeable membrane

a

b

1 mole per liter, but two osmols of pressure, one for each kind of ion. The osmolarity of human body fluids, which is a great deal less than one osmol per liter, is usually expressed in milliosmols (1/1000 of an osmol) per liter. Normal osmolarity of fluids in and surrounding cells is about 300 milliosmols per liter.

Physiologists frequently have reason to refer to relationships between the osmolarity of solutions within cells and those of fluids surrounding them. The osmolarity of the contents of a cell is generally the basis for comparison. Solutions outside the cell are said to be **isosmotic** if they have the same osmolarity as the solution inside the cell, **hyperosmotic** if they have a higher osmolarity, and **hyposmotic** if they have a lower osmolarity than the cell.

In contrast to osmolarity, which is determined by the concentration of particles in a solution, **tonicity** is determined by whether or not water will move across a membrane separating two solutions. Again, the contents of a normal cell is used as a basis for comparison. Solutions outside the cell are said to be **isotonic** to those inside the cell if there is no net movement of water between the cell and the solution, that is, if there is no change in the volume of either the cell or the solution. A solution is **hypertonic** when it causes net movement of water out of the cell; that is, when the volume of the cell decreases and the volume of the solution increases. In such a situation cells shrivel and are said to be crenated. Conversely, a solution is **hypotonic**

when it causes net movement of water into the cell; that is, when the volume of the cell increases and the volume of the solution decreases. In such a situation cells burst and are said to be lysed (see Figure 3.15).

Vomiting, diarrhea, and a variety of other symptoms of illness can cause imbalances in the distribution of water between cells and their environment. Understanding what happens to cells when they contain too little or too much water is impŏrtant in treating individuals with such conditions. When cells are surrounded by isotonic fluids, fluid balance between the cells and their environment is maintained. If cells are surrounded by hypertonic fluids, the cells will lose water and become dehydrated. If, on the other hand, the cells are surrounded by hypotonic fluids, the cells will gain water, and their membranes may even burst.

Filtration

In some situations in the body substances are pushed through membranes by pressure, such as the pressure of flowing blood. This phenomenon, called **filtration**, is essentially the same as the movement of substances through filter paper in a funnel because those substances are pushed through the filter paper by the pressure of the solution standing in the funnel. This pressure is called **hydrostatic pressure**. Filtration occurs as blood flows through the capillaries, the smallest of blood vessels. Blood pressure

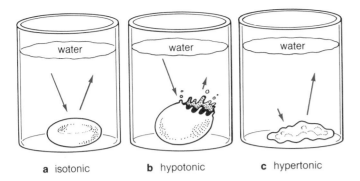

a isotonic   **b** hypotonic   **c** hypertonic

Figure 3.15 A cell placed in isotonic solution (**a**) will have no net movement of water; the same amount of water enters and leaves the cell. A cell placed in hypotonic solution (**b**) will gain more water than it loses; the cell will swell, and the membrane will eventually burst. This is called lysis. A cell placed in hypertonic solution (**c**) will lose more water than it gains; the cell will shrink, and the membrane will shrivel. This is called crenation.

pushing blood along the inside of capillaries also pushes nutrients and other substances through the walls of the capillaries out into the tissue fluids.

Bulk Flow

In the capillaries and in certain other locations in the body, water molecules move across membranes at more rapid rates than can be accounted for by diffusion. In all cases water is moving along a gradient created by osmotic pressure or hydrostatic (filtration) pressure. However, neither of these pressures accounts for the speed with which the water moves. The rapid movement of water appears to be due to a particular property of water molecules: Once moving in a given direction, water molecules tend to flow in streams through the pores of a membrane. This streaming property of water molecules is called **bulk flow**. Bulk flow is an important factor in the movement of fluids between the circulatory system and the cells of the body.

Active Transport

Each of the mechanisms of movement across membranes considered so far involves passive movement of substances from areas of higher concentration to areas of lower concentration. *These mechanisms do not require the cell to expend energy.* In contrast, **active transport** causes molecules to move against concentration gradients from areas of lower to areas of higher concentration. For example, sodium ions are pumped out of cells into extracellular fluids where the concentration of sodium is higher than inside the cells. This process, analogous to rolling something uphill, *does require energy from ATP.* Active transport begins much as facilitated diffusion does. The substance to be transported attaches to a carrier molecule that causes the substance to move across the cell membrane. An enzyme that is usually part of the carrier molecule releases energy from ATP. This energy is used to activate the carrier, to separate the substance being transported from the carrier, and to discharge the substance into or outside the cell. Energy is required because the substance is being moved against the concentration gradient.

The carrier molecule is a protein, sometime a glycoprotein, and it has on its surface a specific carrier site for the substance it transports. Attachment of a substance to a carrier molecule probably involves a change in the three-dimensional shape of the carrier molecule. Rates of movement by active transport depend primarily on the amount of carrier molecule-enzyme available to bring about the movement.

Actively transported substances include the following ions: Na^+, K^+, Ca^{2+}, Fe^{2+}, H^+, and I^-. Some sugars (crossing certain membranes), amino acids, and other organic substances are moved across membranes with the energy made available by the active transport of sodium in the same direction. The transport of sodium is so important in the function of cells that its active transport mechanism has been specifically named the **sodium pump**. It has been estimated that 40% of a cell's ATP is used for active transport of Na^+ and K^+ ions. This sodium pump is constantly transporting sodium ions out of cells against the concentration gradient; the gradient allows ions to diffuse back into cells. Potassium ions are actively transported into cells by the same carrier system (Figure 3.16). This might be called a coupled active transport system because two substances are transported by the same carrier.

Though glucose moves by facilitated diffusion where an appropriate concentration gradient exists, when movement is against the gradient, glucose is moved by active transport. In the intestine, where glucose is being absorbed from the digested food, the concentration of glucose in the blood vessels receiving it may be higher than in the intestinal tract. Thus, active transport is essential if glucose is to be absorbed.

In all cells that have been studied amino acids also cross membranes by active transport. It is thought that at least four different carrier systems exist to transport amino

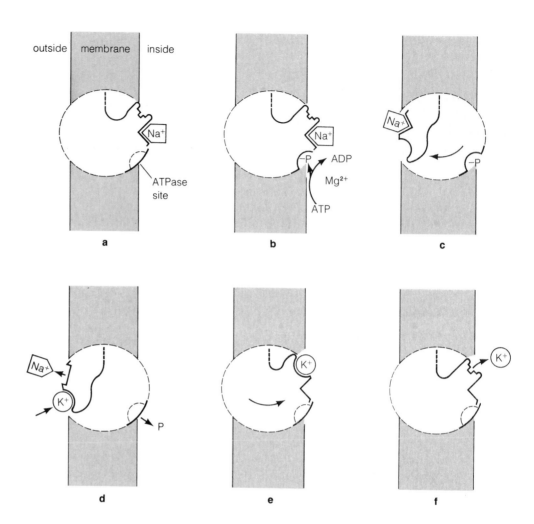

Figure 3.16 Active transport as illustrated by the sodium-potassium pump. In this diagram the carrier protein is represented by a large circle extending through the width of the cell membrane, with carrier sites for sodium and potassium and an ATPase site. (**a**) The carrier molecule binds Na^+ at the inside surface of the membrane. (**b**) The attachment of Na^+ activates ATPase; ATP is broken down to ADP and phosphate as energy is released. Mg^{2+} is required for this reaction. (**c**) The carrier molecule uses energy from ATP to move the Na^+ to the outside surface of the molecule. (**d**) K^+ attaches to its carrier site, causing Na^+ to be released from its carrier site. (**e**) The carrier molecule returns to its original position, moving K^+ across the membrane as it does so. (**f**) As the carrier molecule resumes its original position, it loses its affinity for K^+, and the K^+ is released to the inside of the cell.

acids. Each carrier transports a group of amino acids with similar chemical properties. For proper function some of these systems require a substance that contains vitamin B_6 (pyridoxine). Both amino acid transport and glucose transport are regulated by hormones, as we shall see in Chapter 23.

Active transport is essential to normal cell function because passive processes such as diffusion, osmosis, filtration, and bulk flow cannot increase the concentration of substances on either side of a membrane against a concentration gradient. Active transport *can* establish concentration gradients on which several other processes depend in one way or another. These processes include the initiation and transmission of nerve impulses, the contraction of muscles, the concentration of nutrients in cells, and the removal of wastes from them. It appears that, even within cells, for certain organelles such as mitochondria and the

endoplasmic reticulum, active transport (along with passive processes) is involved in the movement of substances across their membranes.

Pinocytosis and Phagocytosis

So far we have been concerned with the movements of particles of molecular size or smaller. Some cells also can take in large protein molecules or even large particles such as cellular debris from dead cells or microorganisms. The processes of pinocytosis and phagocytosis require energy and provide for the entry of these larger particles into cells. **Pinocytosis**, or "cell-drinking," is the taking in of small particles including water droplets. **Phagocytosis**, or "cell eating," is the taking in of larger particles. The difference between the two processes is primarily a matter of the size of the particles entering the cell. Protein molecules, water,

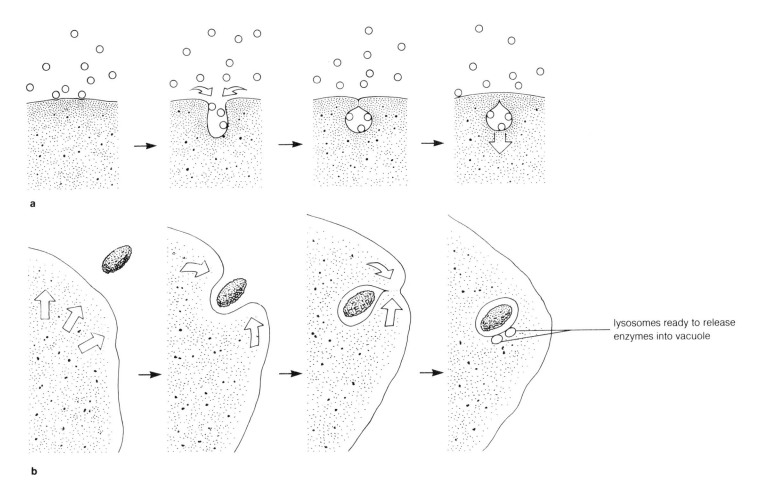

Figure 3.17 A diagrammatic representation of (**a**) pinocytosis and (**b**) phagocytosis.

lysosomes ready to release enzymes into vacuole

and ions can be taken in by pinocytosis; debris from dead cells and microorganisms are taken in by phagocytosis. Cells that have the ability to engage in phagocytosis are called **phagocytes**. By either process, once a particle is taken in, it becomes a vacuole (Figure 3.17). This vacuole may rupture, releasing the contents into the cytoplasm of the cell, or digestive enzymes from the lysosomes may be released into the vacuole and digestion take place there. In the latter case digested substances diffuse through the membrane of the vacuole into the cytoplasm. Eventually, the vacuoles themselves disintegrate. Undigestible substances are excreted.

Movement of Materials and Homeostasis

All the processes that result in the movement of materials into and out of cells contribute to maintaining the internal environment of cells in a constantly changing but relatively stable state and thus contribute to homeostasis. These processes are summarized in Table 3.2.

PROTEIN SYNTHESIS

Objective 7. Describe the cell parts and the steps involved in protein synthesis from DNA to the completed protein.

As you already know from Chapter 2, proteins are important as part of the structure of the body, as enzymes, and as molecules that control certain processes. They also act as carriers in the transport mechanisms described above. Proteins are essential for growth and repair of the body. How proteins are made within the cells of the body is a

Table 3.2	Mechanisms of Movement of Substances into and out of Cells
Process	Characteristics
Passive	Movement along a gradient; cell does not use energy to cause movement
Diffusion	Net movement of molecules from their higher to lower concentration with or without the presence of a membrane
Facilitated diffusion	Diffusion of molecules across a membrane with the assistance of a carrier molecule but without the expenditure of energy
Osmosis	Movement of water from higher to lower concentration (from lower to higher concentration of solutes); occurs across a selectively permeable membrane
Filtration	Movement of molecules along a pressure gradient; accounts for movement of nutrients and other substances from capillaries
Bulk flow	Rapid movement of water molecules along a gradient; caused by the streaming property of water molecules in motion
Active	Movement against a gradient; cell expends energy to cause movement
Active transport	Movement of a substance across a membrane against a gradient; requires expenditure of energy
Pinocytosis	Taking in of water droplets and other small particles; cell forms a vacuole around particle
Phagocytosis	Taking in of large particles such as debris from dead cells and microorganisms; cell forms a vacuole around particle

complex process that has been elucidated by painstaking research within the last few decades.

Cell Components Involved in Protein Synthesis

Earlier in this chapter the structure of the nucleus was discussed. The chromosomes within the nucleus were described as DNA molecules with associated proteins. Each chromosome may be thought of as a very long DNA molecule with thousands of nucleotides arranged in a double helix. The bases in the two chains of nucleotides in the helix are arranged so that hydrogen bonds and other forces hold the chains together by base pairing—adenine with thymine and cytosine with guanine, as explained in Chapter 2.

Chromosomes are now known to be divided into structural units of chromatin called nucleosomes (Figure 3.18). Each nucleosome consists of a coil of DNA containing 140 base pairs wrapped around a core. The core consists of a group of small basic proteins called histones. Other histones link the nucleosomes together. Additional protein molecules may also cover the surface of the DNA molecules; it is possible that these outer proteins play a role in determining which portions of the DNA direct a cell's activities at any given time.

The details of the molecular structure of DNA are shown in Figure 3.19. The width of the cylinder formed by the double helix is about 2 nanometers (nm), the base pairs are separated by a distance of 0.34 nm, and the helix makes one complete turn every 3.4 nm.

DNA contains the information necessary to direct the synthesis of all components of all cells in the body. With the exception of small amounts of DNA in mitochondria, all of the DNA of animal cells is found in the chromosomes. DNA includes information for the synthesis of structural proteins and enzymes, and enzymes control all chemical reactions, including those in which the lipids and carbohydrates of the cells are synthesized. DNA also contains information for the

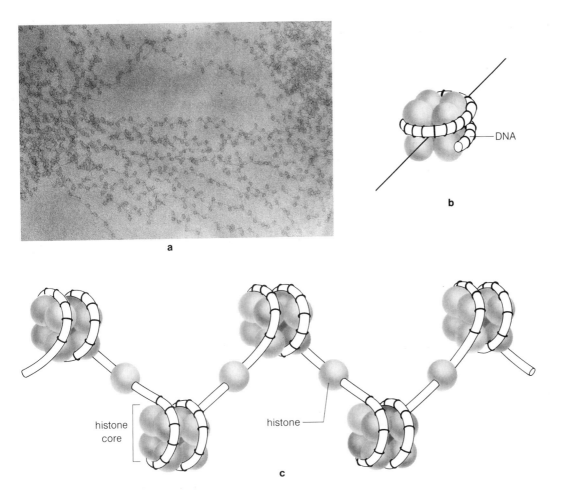

Figure 3.18 (a) Nucleosomes in chromatin isolated from a chicken erythrocyte nucleus, × 172,000. (Courtesy of A. L. Olins, from *The Molecular Biology of the Mammalian Genetic Apparatus*, ed. P. O. P. Ts'o. Elsevier/North Holland, 1977.) (b) A model for the structure of nucleosomes. Each of the distinct single or double coils is a nucleosome. The locations of the proteins called histones are shown. (From Olins and Olins, by permission of *American Scientist*.)

synthesis of RNA and for the synthesis of more DNA exactly like the existing DNA.

The Process of Protein Synthesis

To set the stage for protein synthesis, the hydrogen bonds between the paired chains of DNA are broken by enzymatically controlled reactions so the chains separate. Short sequences of unpaired DNA bases are thus made available to participate in **transcription** (Figure 3.20a), the process by which **RNA** is synthesized.

In the process of transcription RNA is synthesized according to information in the DNA template by base pairing. However, the bases in RNA differ from those in DNA, as noted in Chapter 2. Thus, in transcription cytosine and guanine pair with each other, but adenine in DNA pairs with uracil in RNA, and thymine in DNA pairs with adenine in RNA.

In transcription, the enzyme **RNA polymerase** binds to the exposed DNA that is to serve as the pattern, or template, for the synthesis of RNA (a). The building blocks of RNA, the nucleotides described in Chapter 2, must be present in

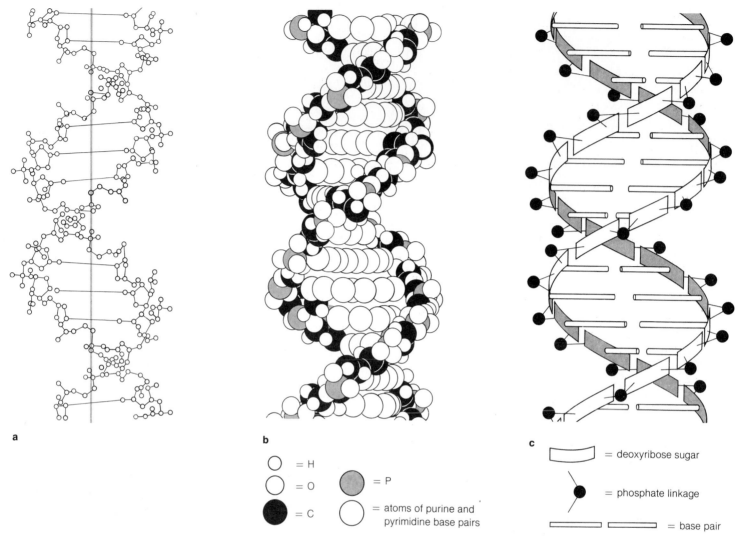

a

b

○ = H

○ = O

● = C

⬤ = P

○ = atoms of purine and pyrimidine base pairs

c

▭ = deoxyribose sugar

● = phosphate linkage

▭ ▭ = base pair

Figure 3.19 A diagrammatic representation of the structure of DNA: (**a**) the atoms of the backbone chains of DNA, (**b**) the packing of atoms into a double helix, (**c**) the relationships among deoxyribose sugars, phosphate linkages, and base pairs.

sufficient quantity in the nucleoplasm. These nucleotides are phosphorylated (coupled with phosphates containing high-energy bonds), thereby raising their energy content so they can participate in subsequent reactions. As shown in (b), after an enzyme binds to the first base in DNA (adenine in this case), the appropriate phosphorylated nucleotide (uridine triphosphate, U—PPP, in this case) joins the DNA base–enzyme complex. The base then attaches by base pairing to the base of DNA and two phosphate groups (PP) are released (c). The enzyme moves to the next base in DNA, and the appropriate phosphorylated nucleotide joins

the complex (d). The phosphate of the second nucleotide is linked to the ribose of the first nucleotide. This forms the first link in the "backbone" of a new molecule of RNA. Energy to form this link comes from the hydrolysis of ATP and the release of two more phosphate groups. The enzyme again moves to the next DNA base, and the process is repeated until the end of the DNA template is reached and the RNA molecule is completed.

At least three different kinds of RNA exist in animal cells—ribosomal RNA (rRNA), messenger RNA (mRNA), and transfer RNA (tRNA). Each consists of a single chain of

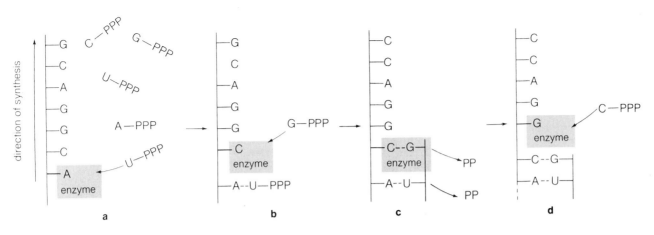

Figure 3.20 The transcription of RNA from template DNA. (See text for explanation.)

nucleotides, and each is formed by the process of transcription. To complete the story of protein synthesis, we will need more information about each of these kinds of RNA.

Ribosomal RNA is synthesized in the nucleolus. After the rRNA is synthesized, it is combined with protein to form ribosomal subunits. After passing through the pores in the nuclear envelope, the subunits come together in the cytoplasm to form **ribosomes**. Some ribosomes move to the endoplasmic reticulum, and others become distributed in clusters in the cytoplasm. Finished ribosomes consist of two subunits, one larger than the other. The smaller subunit serves as a binding site for transfer RNA, and the larger subunit contains the enzymes that control the formation of peptide bonds between amino acids during protein synthesis. The significance of these ribosomal functions will be clarified later.

Messenger RNA, like ribosomal RNA, is synthesized by transcription in accordance with a specific sequence of DNA bases. This sequence includes the exact amount of DNA necessary to make the exact amount of mRNA to convey the information for the synthesis of one chain of amino acids. Once synthesized, mRNA moves through nuclear pores and joins a ribosome.

On the ribosome the information coded in mRNA is used to direct the synthesis of a protein. This process of using information in mRNA to determine the sequence of amino acids in protein is called **translation**. In this process each sequence of three bases in mRNA specifies the location of one amino acid in the protein to be formed. These base triplets, called **codons**, can specify a particular amino acid, or they can act as a punctuation mark to indicate the termination of a protein molecule. In the **genetic code** shown

in Figure 3.21 at least one codon exists for each of the twenty amino acids found in proteins, and several different codons exist for some amino acids. Studies of the codons in the cells of many different organisms have shown this code to be the same (or nearly the same) in all cells, regardless of whether they are from an amoeba or a human being. This universality of the genetic code makes it possible to apply research on other organisms to our understanding of the transmission of information in human cells.

The use of the terms transcription and translation to describe protein synthesis is analogous to their use in ordinary language. For example, a stenographer *transcribes* shorthand notes into typewritten words—both are in the same language. Likewise, in protein synthesis the cell transcribes information in DNA to RNA—both in the "language" of nucleotides. A linguist *translates* one language to another—English to French or Spanish to English. Likewise, the cell translates information in RNA to protein structure—from the "language" of nucleotides to the "language" of proteins.

Many different kinds of **transfer RNA** (tRNA) have been isolated from the cytoplasm of cells. Like all other RNA, transfer RNA is synthesized by transcription from DNA in the nucleus and released into the cytoplasm. The function of tRNA is to carry amino acids to the ribosome for proper placement in a protein molecule. Generally,

		U		C		A		G		
U	UUU	phe	UCU	ser	UAU	tyr	UGU	cys	U	
	UUC		UCC		UAC		UGC		C	
	UUA	leu	UCA		UAA	*	UGA	*	A	
	UUG		UCG		UAG	*	UGG	try	G	
C	CUU	leu	CCU	pro	CAU	his	CGU	arg	U	
	CUC		CCC		CAC		CGC		C	
	CUA		CCA		CAA	gln	CGA		A	
	CUG		CCG		CAG		CGG		G	
A	AUU	ileu	ACU	thr	AAU	asn	AGU	ser	U	
	AUC		ACC		AAC		AGC		C	
	AUA		ACA		AAA	lys	AGA	arg	A	
	AUG	met	ACG		AAG		AGG		G	
G	GUU	val	GCU	ala	GAU	asp	GGU	gly	U	
	GUC		GCC		GAC		GGC		C	
	GUA		GCA		GAA	glu	GGA		A	
	GUG		GCG		GAG		GGG		G	

first base of codon · *third base of codon*

Figure 3.21 The genetic code consists of codons of messenger RNA. Most codons specify amino acids. The asterisks indicate terminator codons that specify the end of a message.

ala = alanine
arg = arginine
asn = asparagine
asp = aspartic acid
cys = cysteine
gln = glutamine
glu = glutamic acid
gly = glycine
his = histidine
ileu = isoleucine
leu = leucine
lys = lysine
met = methionine
phe = phenylalanine
pro = proline
ser = serine
thr = threonine
try = tryptophan
tyr = tyrosine
val = valine

tRNA consists of seventy-five to eighty nucleotides arranged in a cloverleaf configuration (Figure 3.22). Amino acids attach to the free end of the molecule shown at the top of the figure. Each tRNA has a particular sequence of three bases called the **anticodon**, shown at the bottom of the figure. The anticodon attaches by base pairing to the appropriate codon on the mRNA. As with the codons, at least one anticodon exists for each of the twenty amino acids, and several anticodons exist for some amino acids. Thus, a cell can have as many kinds of tRNA as there are anticodons.

At the time of synthesis of any protein (Figure 3.23), it can be assumed that all of the needed RNAs are available in sufficient quantities. These RNAs can be reused many times before they fail to function. Of the RNAs involved in protein synthesis mRNA is produced in the most precise quantities in accordance with the cell's needs for a particular enzyme or structural protein. Once the mRNA has joined a ribosome, the ribosome initiates protein synthesis and provides the site for the assembly of the protein molecule.

The detailed diagram (Figure 3.24) shows the mRNA aligned on the ribosome (a) and the arrival of the first tRNA (b). The smaller unit of the ribosome provides a site for binding the tRNA in a configuration such that its anticodon can be matched with the codon of the mRNA. This matching of codon and anticodon is the process by which the coded information acts to specify the sequence of amino

acids in the protein. After the arrival of the second amino acid (c) the formation of a peptide bond between the two amino acids is catalyzed by an enzyme built into the structure of the larger ribosomal unit (d). As the ribosome moves along the mRNA, a third amino acid arrives at the proper site, and the first tRNA is released into the cytoplasm (e). A second peptide bond is formed (f), and the process continues until a terminator codon is recognized by the ribosome. At this point the finished protein is released, and the mRNA is available to synthesize another molecule of the same protein. Likewise, the ribosome and the tRNAs are available to participate in the synthesis of the same or a different protein.

Control of Protein Synthesis

Within the nucleus of any cell there is a full complement of DNA that, if active, could direct the synthesis of any and all components of the body's cells. However, at any time only about 1 to 5% of the DNA is active. Regulation of DNA activity during transcription is one way that protein synthesis can be controlled. Much of what is known about the regulation of DNA activity has been determined from studies of bacterial cells; it is not yet clear how well these findings correlate with processes in human cells. However,

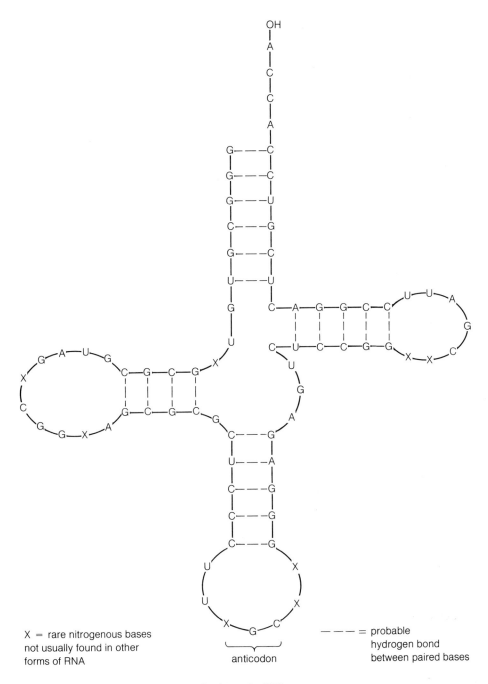

X = rare nitrogenous bases not usually found in other forms of RNA

anticodon

－－－＝ probable hydrogen bond between paired bases

Figure 3.22 The structure of a molecule of transfer RNA.

it can be said that certain proteins, associated with the DNA, control which segments of the DNA will engage in transcription. Regulation of gene action is the topic of many current research studies.

Mechanisms exist for regulating the amount of various proteins synthesized after the mRNA has reached the ribosomes. One such mechanism involves hormones that cause the release of cyclic AMP into the cell. Cyclic AMP, in turn, may regulate the activity of the mRNA. Though a detailed discussion of these mechanisms is beyond the scope of this book, the net result of such regulation is to help to maintain homeostasis within cells.

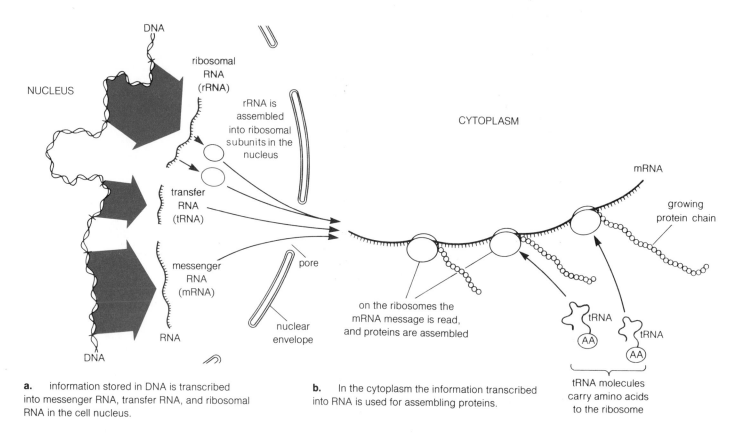

a. information stored in DNA is transcribed into messenger RNA, transfer RNA, and ribosomal RNA in the cell nucleus.

b. In the cytoplasm the information transcribed into RNA is used for assembling proteins.

Figure 3.23 An overview of protein synthesis.

CELL DIVISION: MITOSIS

Objective 8. Describe the process of DNA replication.

Objective 9. Describe the major stages in the process of mitotic cell division and explain its significance in normal body function.

The ability of cells to produce new cells is an essential property of living things. Without this ability even small cuts and scratches would not heal. The fertilized egg from which your body developed would never have progressed from the one-cell to the two-cell stage. Repair of injuries, growth, and development all involve the division of cells.

We will consider two processes concerned with cell division: (1) the **replication** (duplication) of DNA, and (2)

mitotic cell division, in which two new cells like the original cell are produced. Cells destined to produce eggs or sperm divide by a different process, called meiosis, which will be considered in Chapter 27.

Mutations or changes in the DNA of a cell occasionally occur during mitosis; they may be an important factor in the development of cancer. Mutations that occur during meiosis cause changes in the DNA of eggs or sperm; these changes can have significant effects on the offspring and on future generations.

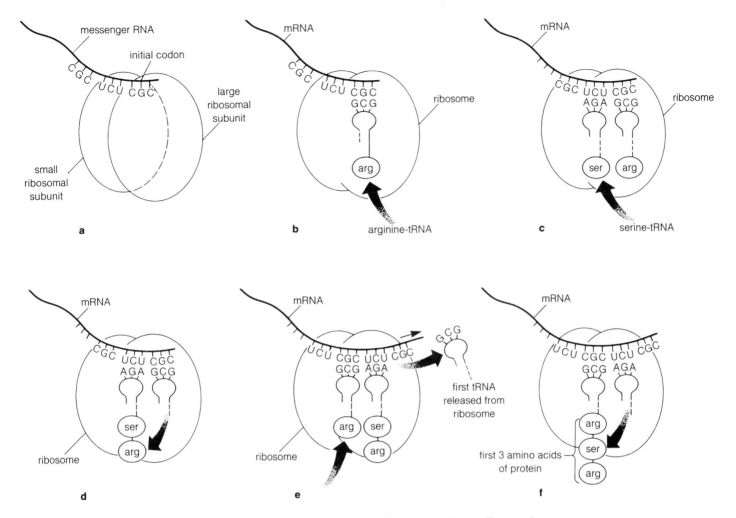

Figure 3.24 A detailed diagram of the role of ribosomes, mRNA, and tRNA in protein synthesis. (See text for explanation.)

DNA Replication

Just as **DNA** serves as a template for the synthesis of RNA in protein synthesis, it can also serve as a template for the synthesis of more DNA. In preparation for cell division segments of the nucleotide chains of a double helix of DNA separate, exposing chains of unpaired bases. The mechanism of DNA replication (Figure 3.25) is similar to RNA synthesis. Though each chain of double-stranded DNA is replicated separately, a small segment of DNA of the chain to be replicated must be present to start or prime the replication process. Each nucleotide chain of DNA serves as the template for the synthesis of a partner chain. A molecule of

the enzyme **DNA polymerase** binds to the site of the terminal base in the primer chain and to its paired base in the template (a). Phosphorylated nucleotides containing adenine, thymine, cytosine, or guanine are present in the surrounding nucleoplasm. A nucleotide that can pair with the exposed base joins the enzyme–primer–template complex (b). Energy from the breaking of bonds in the phosphates is used, and the enzyme catalyzes the joining of the nucleotide to the primer (c). The enzyme moves along the template (d); another nucleotide enters the complex and is added to the new strand of DNA. The process continues until a new molecule of DNA exactly like the original partner of the template chain is synthesized.

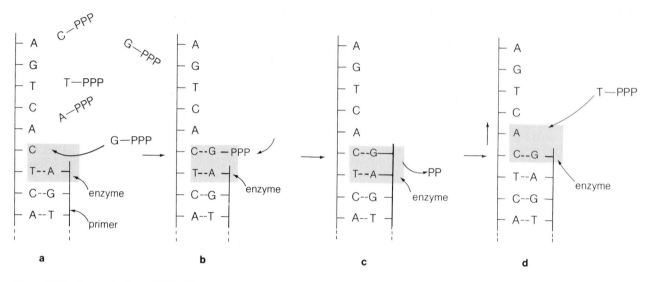

Figure 3.25 The replication of DNA. (See text for explanation.)

Each new chromosome consists of one old and one new chain of DNA (Figure 3.26). Evidence for this comes from experiments in which radioactively labeled nucleotides were provided to cells while they were replicating DNA. In such experiments half of the radioactive material appears in each chromosome, indicating that each chromosome contains half of the newly synthesized DNA.

Though DNA consists of a double helix, it is thought that the information that controls cellular processes may be stored on only one chain. For example, when RNA is being produced, only one chain of the DNA molecule serves as a template. The role of the second chain may be limited to serving as a template for the synthesis of new DNA. If we call the RNA synthesizing template the "information" molecule and the paired strand the "companion" molecule, then in DNA replication each information molecule serves as a template for the companion molecule, and the companion molecule serves as a template for the information molecule.

Mitosis

Cells capable of dividing go through a mitotic division cycle (Figure 3.27). Stage G_1 (gap or growth stage 1) is the stage in which cells are carrying on normal metabolic activity but not dividing or preparing to divide. G_1 can last from hours

to years. Highly specialized cells such as nerve and muscle cells in adults have lost their ability to divide, and they remain in stage G_1 for years. Cells in the deepest layers of the epidermis of the skin continue to divide throughout life.

Factors responsible for triggering division in cells that can divide are not well understood, but when a cell prepares to divide, it enters the S (synthesis) stage. In this stage DNA is replicated as described earlier, and the histones and other proteins of chromosomes are duplicated. After spending 6 to 8 hours in stage S, the cell enters stage G_2. G_2 is the stage between the completion of DNA replication and the beginning of mitotic division; it lasts from 2 to 5 hours. Together, stages G_1, S, and G_2 are called **interphase**. The G stages are periods during which no events related to DNA replication are known to occur—they may be thought of as "gaps" in the division process.

After G_2 the cell undergoes **mitosis**, the actual division of the nucleus. Mitosis is a *continuous* process, though biologists divide it into stages for convenience in studying it. The events to be described here and the stages in which they occur are a way of summarizing the process (see Figure 3.28). In **prophase**, the first stage of mitosis, the replicated chromosomes (which contain two times the normal amount of DNA) fold on themselves and become shorter and thicker (thus becoming visible with a light microscope). The nucleolus and nuclear envelope disintegrate, and their

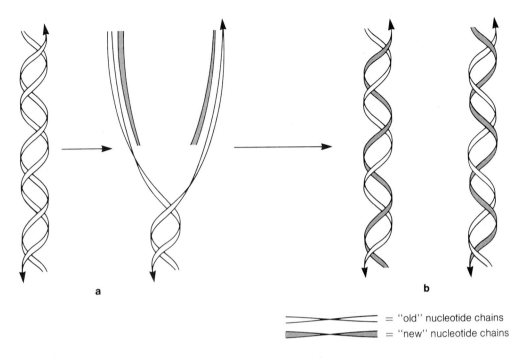

= "old" nucleotide chains
= "new" nucleotide chains

Figure 3.26 The arrangement of old and new chains of DNA in replication.

fragments are scattered in the cytoplasm. Centrioles separate and move to opposite sides of the cell, and spindle fibers form between the centrioles. In **metaphase** the double chromosomes, each half of which is called a chromatid, move to the center of the spindle. The chromatids of the double chromosomes each contain a kinetochore, which was replicated in the S phase along with the rest of the chromosome. The kinetochore of each chromatid attaches to a spindle fiber. In **anaphase** a force developed by the spindle fibers pulls on the kinetochores, and the chromatids separate and move to opposite ends of the spindle. In **telophase**, the chromatids, now called chromosomes, have arrived at opposite poles of the cell. The nucleolus and nuclear envelope reappear around each set of chromosomes, the spindle fibers disappear, and the chromosomes unfold (becoming too dispersed to be distinguished individually with a light microscope).

Following these stages that constitute mitosis or nuclear division—or concurrently with telophase—the cell undergoes **cytokinesis**, the division of the cytoplasm. In cytokinesis in animal cells the cytoplasm around the two new nuclei becomes furrowed, and the plasma membrane pinches in between the nuclei to complete the formation of two new cells. This pinching in is accomplished by contraction of a ring of microfilaments that forms at the furrow.

The chromosomes of the cells resulting from mitosis

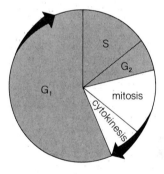

Figure 3.27 The cell cycle. Interphase includes G_1, S, and G_2 of the cycle. The time spent in phase G_1 is variable, but the other stages are of relatively constant length for a given type of cell.

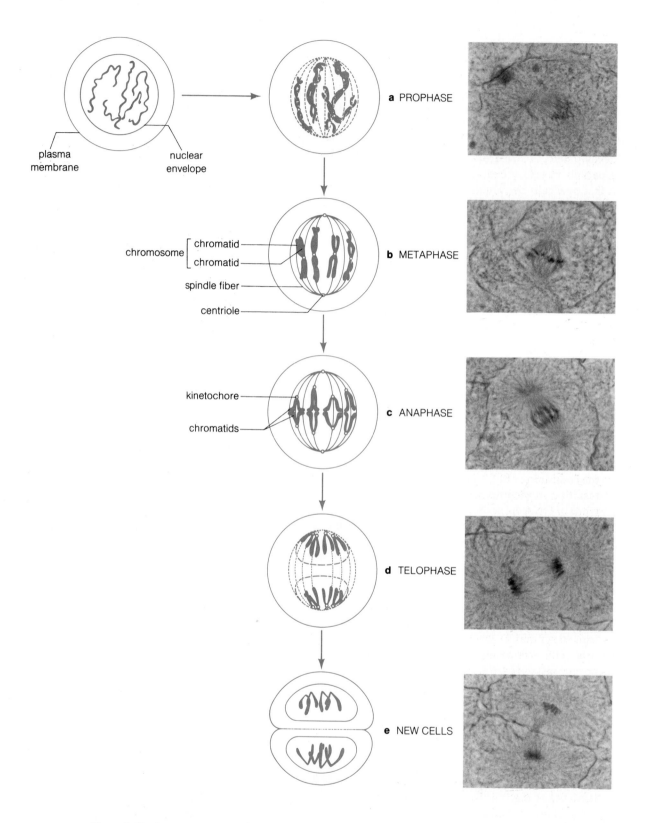

Figure 3.28 The major events in the process of mitosis. The process is shown diagramatically on the left and as it appears in the whitefish embryo on the right, × 1000. (Photographs by author.)

are identical to those of the original cell: Each cell has received one of each kind of chromosome that existed in the original cell. The cytoplasm is divided between the two cells in approximately equal quantities. Table 3.3 summarizes the events of DNA replication, mitosis, and cytokinesis.

Mitosis and cytokinesis occur during growth, during the repair of tissues after injury, and during embryonic development. They are accompanied by **differentiation**, especially in embryonic tissues. The result of differentiation is that new cells become increasingly specialized with each cell division. Differentiation leads to the formation of the different tissues and organs of the body. (Some additional details of the formation of tissues are provided in Chapter 4.) The process of differentiation is guided by factors present in adjacent cells and by genetic information the cells contain. The regulatory molecules that control protein synthesis also control differentiation.

Table 3.3	Events of DNA Replication, Mitosis, and Cytokinesis
Stage	**Events**
Interphase	
G_1	Metabolism, no known events related to cell division
S	Synthesis of DNA to replicate chromosomes Replication of kinetochore
G_2	No known events related to cell division
Prophase	Chromosomes fold on themselves and become shorter and thicker. Nucleolus and nuclear envelope disappear. Centrioles separate and move to opposite side of the cell. Spindle fibers form between centrioles.
Metaphase	Chromosomes move to center of spindle. Kinetochores of each chromatid attach to spindle fibers.
Anaphase	A force developed by spindle fibers pulls on kinetochores; the chromatids separate and move to opposite ends of spindle.
Telophase	One of each kind of chromosome arrives at each of the poles of the cell. Nucleolus and nuclear envelope reappear. Spindle fibers disappear. Chromosomes unfold and become longer and thinner.
Cytokinesis	Cytoplasm becomes furrowed between the two new nuclei. Plasma membrane completes the separation of the new cells.

Recombinant DNA

In recent years researchers have found ways to manipulate processes that occur during the replication of DNA in simple organisms. One technique involves the combining of DNA from two different organisms, resulting in **recombinant DNA**. For example, a segment of DNA from another organism can be inserted into the DNA of certain bacteria. The bacterial cell then has all of its own capabilities in addition to whatever new capabilities are acquired from the added DNA. If the DNA segment for directing the synthesis of insulin is added to the microorganism's DNA, that organism can then synthesize insulin. Such a technique has the potential for causing microorganisms to synthesize a number of useful chemical products. This technique also offers the possibility that normal genes might some day be inserted into human chromosomes to replace defective ones, though this has not yet been done successfully.

As discussed in the essay at the end of Chapter 1, the ability of human beings to participate in the evolution of their own species has already caused changes in the human population. Should it become possible to manipulate human genetic material, particularly at the level of the fertilized egg cell, we humans would find ourselves faced with some very difficult ethical issues.

CLINICAL TERMS

anaplasia (an-ap-lā′ze-ah)   reversion of cells to an undifferentiated form

atrophy (at′ro-fe)   a decrease in size, or wasting away, of a cell, tissue, or other part

biopsy (bi′op-se)   inspection of living tissue, usually by removal of a piece of the tissue for study

carcinoma (kar-sin-o′mah)   a malignant growth made up of epithelial cells

carcinoma-in-situ   a growth made up of epithelial cells lacking invasive properties

hyperplasia (hi-per-pla′ze-ah)   an abnormal increase in the number of cells in a tissue

hypertrophy (hi-per′trof-e)   an enlargement of a tissue due mainly to an increase in the size of the cells

metaplasia (met-ah-pla′ze-ah)   a change of one kind of cells into another kind of cells

necrosis (ne-kro′sis)   death of a portion of a tissue

sarcoma (sar-ko′mah)   a malignant growth made up of cells resembling embryonic connective tissue

Essay: Cancer

Throughout the world, over 2 million people die of cancer each year. In the United States the death rate from cancer is about 1.7 deaths per thousand, second only to the death rate of 4.3 per thousand from heart and circulatory diseases. Nearly half the deaths from cancer are caused by malignancies affecting the digestive organs, and another third are caused by lung cancer alone. The death rates do not tell the whole story, however; many of these deaths are preceded by long and expensive periods of illness. The incidence of cancer makes it an important area of human disease for massive research effort.

In normal tissues cell division proceeds in an orderly fashion. Regardless of whether the cell divisions are causing growth of the organism or repair of damaged tissues, regulatory factors prevent the division process from continuing beyond that needed for the tissue to reach normal size or the repair to be complete. One of these factors is called **contact inhibition**: When cells become packed together so that they are touching one another, the division process is halted. This phenomenon has been demonstrated in laboratory tissue cultures in which normal cells are allowed to form sheets over a piece of glass in a culture container. In normal cells the rate of cell division slows or stops when a complete sheet is formed; in cancer cells division continues, and cells pile on top of one another. Contact inhibition thus fails to occur in cancer cells, and the cells continue to divide uncontrollably.

Excessive cell division may also produce benign growth, in which the cells are contained within a single, encapsulated mass called a benign tumor. As long as the cells are confined to the tumor, they usually can do only limited damage to the body. **Malignant** growth, or cancer, on the other hand, is invasive. Malignant cells break out of the capsule (or even lack a capsule) and invade adjacent tissue. It is from this property of invasiveness that cancer gets its name. The word cancer means crab; it suggests that, like the claws of a crab, cells from a malignant growth spread out in all directions.

Malignant growth frequently metastasizes. In **metastasis** the cancer cells go beyond adjacent tissue, breaking away from the original growth and entering the blood or lymph. Once this happens, they migrate to many other sites in the body. There, the cancer cells continue to divide until the body is filled with many sites of malignant growth.

The causes of cancer are not fully understood. However, it is known that some chemicals are **carcinogenic**, or cancer causing. These include certain chemicals found in cigarette and other smoke, asbestos, nickel, and certain dyes, to mention only a few of the many substances implicated in the induction of cancer. Radiation, including ultraviolet rays and X rays, also can induce cancer. Evidence for the effect of ultraviolet rays is seen in the high incidence of skin cancers in people who live in very sunny climates and the appearance of cancers on the skin surfaces most frequently exposed to sunlight. Evidence for the effect of X rays is demonstrated by the incidence of leukemia (a cancer of the white blood cells) among radiologists—ten times as high as among other physicians. Japanese people exposed to radiation from World War II nuclear bombing show five times the incidence of leukemia seen in the rest of the population.

Food additives, atmospheric pollutants, and viruses have also been implicated in the induction of cancer. Certain viruses apparently invade susceptible cells and modify the cells' DNA. This process may not produce cancer for many years after exposure to the virus, so establishing viruses as causative agents of cancer is difficult.

Determining how various agents induce cancer is the goal of much current research effort. Part of the difficulty of determining how cancerous growth occurs lies in the fact that the mechanisms that start and stop the division of normal cells are not yet understood. The theories that seem most worth investigation are mutation and selective gene activation.

Evidence for the mutation theory is as follows: First, agents that are known to cause mutations (radiations and chemicals) also appear to cause cancer. Second, the incidence of cancer increases with age. As the number of body cell mutations also increases with age, it is possible that cumulative effects of mutations contribute to the initiation of malignancy. However, the mutation theory fails to explain occasional cases of spontaneous remission. **Remission** is the condition in which symptoms and evidence of the disease disappear.

A second theory, that of selective gene activation, does account for remissions. If certain genes that are not normally expressed suddenly become active, their expression could lead to uncontrolled cell division. A remission might occur when for some reason these genes cease to be expressed. Research into the mechanisms that control gene activation may provide insight into both the process of normal cell division and the aberrations in this process that lead to cancer.

It is possible that the mechanism of the induction of cancer is different from any of the hypotheses proposed here. It seems likely that more than one mechanism may be involved and that some combination of these hypotheses will contribute to an eventual understanding of the complex process of the regulation of cell division and how its disturbance causes cancer.

Immunological deficiences may explain why the body does not respond to kill the cancer cells. All cells have antigens on their plasma membranes, as discussed earlier in this chapter. If cancer cells have specific "cancer cell" antigens, the normal response of the body should be to develop antibodies (chemical substances that inactivate antigens) to the "cancer cell" antigens. Several mechanisms have been suggested for how cancer cells might escape recognition by the body's immunological defense system and avoid being attacked by antibodies. First, the cancer cells might not be detected in their early stages; by the time they are detected, too many cancer cells would exist to be destroyed by the available antibodies. Second, cancer cells may mask their surface antigens in some way to prevent detection. Finally, cancer cells may reproduce so rapidly that they flood the body with antigens and over-whelm the antibody-producing capability.

One of the best ways to prevent death from cancer is early diagnosis and treatment before the malignancy has metastasized. Early diagnosis can be facilitated by self-examination of breasts or testes; "Pap smears" to detect cervical cancer; and medical attention for cancer's warning signals: nagging cough, changes in a wart or mole, a sore that does not heal, changes in bowel or bladder habits, difficulty in swallowing, or any unusual bleeding or discharge. Lung cancer is now clearly associated with smoking. As early detection is difficult, the best prevention is never to smoke or to stop smoking.

Some research efforts are going into developing new techniques for early detection of cancer. One test can now be used to detect liver cancer. This test is based on the presence of alpha-fetoprotein, a substance found in the blood of many animals during fetal life but not normally in any significant quantity after birth. However, its concentration increases in the presence of liver cancer, and thus it can be used diagnostically.

Three general methods of treatment for cancer are currently available: surgical removal, radiation, and chemotherapy. Surgical removal is the treatment of choice when it is likely that all the malignant cells can be removed. Radiation works by causing sufficient damage to malignant cells that they are rendered incapable of dividing. Chemotherapy generally involves giving drugs that are similar to the building blocks of DNA. The nitrogenous bases in such drugs can combine with template DNA but fail to allow the cell to function normally after division. Other drugs interfere with the action of certain vitamins that are essential to the action of some enzymes required for cell division. Both radiation and chemicals affect rapidly dividing malignant cells more than normal cells. Though they are able to derange the metabolism of cancer cells they often have serious side effects on normal cells and thus on the affected individuals. The three treatment methods are often used in combination. For example, after surgical removal of a malignant growth radiation or chemotherapy may be used to destroy any malignant cells that might have escaped removal.

In the future immunotherapy may be a significant form of cancer treatment. If it becomes possible to create specific agents that could recognize and destroy cancer cells without affecting normal cells, such treatment would have obvious advantages over those that produce undesirable side effects. The fact that remissions of malignancies sometimes occur after bacterial infections suggests that stimulating the body's own immunological mechanisms can possibly cause immunological reactions against cancer cells. For example, tuberculosis vaccine has been used effectively in some instances to bring about remission. Finally, it might be possible to produce vaccines against common forms of cancer based on the specific antigens found on the surface membranes of such cells.

CHAPTER SUMMARY

(Chapter summary points and review questions are numbered to correspond to the numbered objectives in the text of each chapter.)

Organization and General Function of Cells

1. Explain why the cell is considered the basic functional unit of living organisms.
   a. Cells are considered the basic functional unit of living organisms because most of the basic life processes are carried out at the cellular level.
   b. The human body contains many different kinds of cells, each of which has a characteristic shape and size and a particular function to perform.

Cell Membranes

2. Describe the chemical and physical properties of cell membranes and explain how membranes contribute to the functioning of the cell.
   a. The cell (plasma) membrane consists of two layers of phospholipids through which protein molecules are interspersed as integral parts of the membrane or as peripherally attached molecules. Glycolipids and glycoproteins are associated with portions of the outer surface of the membrane.
   b. The cell (plasma) membrane regulates the passage of substances into and out of the cell and also transmits information to the inside of the cell.

Organelles

3. Describe the general structure and function of each of the organelles in the cell.
   a. The endoplasmic reticulum (ER) is an extensive network of interconnected membrane-bound vesicles that transports proteins and possibly other substances synthesized by the cell. The surface of smooth ER is thought to be the site of lipid synthesis and the rough ER (with its ribosomes) the site of protein synthesis.
   b. Ribosomes, small bodies that lack membranes, are found on the rough ER and in the cytoplasm. They serve as sites for protein synthesis.
   c. The Golgi apparatus consists of a stack of membrane-bound vesicles. It processes proteins synthesized by the cell.
   d. Lysosomes contain digestive enzymes that are released when a cell engulfs particles, is injured, or dies.
   e. Mitochondria consist of an outer smooth membrane and an inner folded membrane, which surrounds the matrix. Mitochondria contain the enzymes that carry out oxidative energy-producing reactions.
   f. Microtubules and microfilaments give rigidity to the cytoplasm and produce movement. Microtubules are hollow fibers composed of tubulin; microfilaments are solid fibers composed of actin.
   g. Centrioles, cilia, and flagella each consist of a set of microtubules. Centrioles give rise to cilia and flagella; cilia and flagella are capable of wavelike movements that propel cells or substances around them.
   h. The nucleus is the control center of the cell. It is surrounded by a nuclear envelope and contains chromosomes and one or more nucleoli.
   i. Cell inclusions are not true organelles, but rather consist of ingested substances such as fat or glycogen.
   j. Extracellular materials are substances, such as mucus and the matrix of bone and cartilage, that are secreted from cells.

Passage of Materials across Membranes

4. Describe the following passive processes and explain their importance in cell function: diffusion, facilitated diffusion, osmosis, filtration, and bulk flow.
   a. All of the above processes are passive; that is, they do not require cells to expend energy.
   b. In diffusion molecules move from their area of higher concentration to their area of lower concentration.
   c. In facilitated diffusion a second molecule enhances the rate of diffusion along a concentration gradient.
   d. Osmosis is a special case of diffusion of water molecules.
   e. In filtration pressure such as that from flowing blood pushes substances through membranes.
   f. In bulk flow the streaming property of water molecules causes them to flow more rapidly than can be explained by diffusion alone.

5. Describe the process of active transport and explain (a) how it differs from passive processes, and (b) why it is important in cell function.
   a. Active transport involves a carrier molecule and energy from ATP to move substances against a concentration gradient.
   b. It differs from passive processes because it requires energy and because it can produce movement against a concentration gradient.
   c. It is important to normal cell function because it makes possible the concentrating of substances on one side or the other of a membrane where such concentrations are needed for proper function.

6. Distinguish between pinocytosis and phagocytosis and describe the role of each in cell function.
   a. Both pinocytosis and phagocytosis involve the movement of particles into cells by engulfment. In pinocytosis the particles are small and dissolved; in phagocytosis the particles are large.
   b. Pinocytosis allows cells to take in water, ions, and protein molecules; phagocytosis allows cells called phagocytes to engulf microorganisms and debris.

Protein Synthesis

7. Describe the cell parts and the steps involved in protein synthesis from DNA to the completed protein.
   a. To initiate protein synthesis, the DNA of a segment of a chromosome directs the synthesis of messenger RNA. (Ribosomal and transfer RNAs are synthesized in a similar process.)
   b. Messenger RNA moves to the ribosomes or cytoplasm, where its codons direct the placement of anticodons of transfer RNA.
   c. Transfer RNA carries specific amino acids to the site of synthesis.
   d. The amino acids specified by the codon–anticodon matching are then linked together by enzymes that cause peptide bonds to form between the amino acids.
   e. Protein synthesis is controlled by information in DNA and through the action of regulatory substances.

Cell Division: Mitosis

8. Describe the process of DNA replication.
   a. In DNA replication the two nucleotide chains of DNA separate, and each chain serves as a template for the synthesis of its partner chain.
   b. Phosphorylated nucleotides, available in the nucleus, bind by base pairing to the template DNA.
   c. Energy from the breaking of bonds in the phosphates is used to join the nucleotide to the primer.
   d. Subsequent nucleotides are added to the growing DNA molecule by repetitions of (b) and (c) above.

9. Describe the major stages in the process of mitotic cell division and explain its significance in normal body function.
   a. Mitotic cell division is a process whereby replicated DNA in chromosomes is separated into two new nuclei and ultimately by cytokinesis into two complete new cells exactly like the parent cell.
   b. In the S stage of interphase, when the cell shows no signs of undergoing mitosis, the chromosomes are duplicated, but the duplicates remain attached.
   c. The continuous process of mitosis is arbitrarily divided into stages:
      (1) In prophase, the first stage of mitosis, when chromosomes become visible through a light microscope, the nuclear envelope and nucleoli disappear, and the spindle apparatus forms.
      (2) In metaphase the chromosomes line up in the center of the spindle.
      (3) In anaphase the chromatids of the replicated chromosomes separate and move toward the poles of the spindle apparatus.
      (4) In telophase the new nuclear membranes and nucleoli reappear, and cytokinesis (the division of the cytoplasm that accompanies mitosis) occurs.

REVIEW

Important Terms

active transport	metastasis
anticodon	microfilament
bulk flow	microtubule
carcinogenic	mitochondrion
centriole	mitosis
chromosome	nucleolus
cilia	nucleus
codon	organelle
diffusion	osmosis
DNA	passive transport
endoplasmic reticulum	phagocytosis
facilitated diffusion	pinocytosis
filtration	plasma membrane
flagellum	replication
genetic code	ribosomal RNA
Golgi apparatus	ribosome
hyperosmotic	RNA
hyposmotic	sodium pump
isosmotic	transcription
lysosome	transfer RNA
messenger RNA	translation

Questions

1. List several reasons for calling the cell the unit of structure and function of a living organism.

2. Describe the arrangement of phospholipids, proteins, glycolipids, and glycoproteins in the plasma membrane and explain how the chemical and physical properties of these substances contribute to the functions of the membrane.

3. Describe the structure and function of each of the organelles of a typical cell.

4. Suppose certain cells in the body have the following contents in their cytoplasm: 200 milliosmols of K^+, 10 milliosmols of Na^+, water, 10 milliosmols of glucose, and a large quantity of protein molecules and Cl^-. They are suspended in extracellular fluid that contains 10 milliosmols of K^+, 200 milliosmols of Na^+, water, 15 milliosmols of glucose, and only a few molecules of protein. Assume that only passive processes are affecting the movement of materials across the membranes. Describe the movement of each substance.

5. Assume that the cells in the above situation have come to equilibrium. Explain how active transport could restore the original concentration of Na^+ and K^+.

6. List the similarities and differences between pinocytosis and phagocytosis.

7. a. Describe the synthesis of ribosomal, messenger, and transfer RNA.

    b. List the steps in protein synthesis in sequence from the formation of messenger RNA to the release of a protein molecule from the ribosome.

    c. Given the following sequence of bases on a DNA molecule—AAAGAATAACAAAGAGGATGA—determine the corresponding codons, anticodons, and amino acid sequence in the portion of protein that would be produced.

8. List the steps in the process of DNA replication.

9. List the main events that occur in each stage of mitosis and explain the circumstances under which mitosis occurs.

Problems

1. Apply your knowledge of cells to determine the effects of the following hypothetical situations:

    a. A cell has no nucleus.

    b. A cell lacks mitochondria.

    c. A cell lacks ribosomes.

    d. A cell has an especially large Golgi apparatus.

    e. The cell membrane is deficient in phospholipids.

2. Determine at least one possible sequence of transfer RNA, messenger RNA, and DNA that would produce the following protein segment: alanine-glutamic acid-serine-valine-arginine-leucine-tryptophan.

REFERENCES AND READINGS

Arehart-Treichel, J. 1980. Emphasis on cancer prevention. *Science News* 118:123 (August 23).

Croce, C. M., and Kpropwski, H. 1978. The genetics of human cancer. *Scientific American* 238(2):117 (February).

Dustin, P. 1980. Microtubules. *Scientific American* 243(2):67 (August).

Goldman, R. D., Milstead, A., Schloss, J. A., Starger, J., and Yerna, M. 1979. Cytoplasmic fibers in mammalian cells: Cytoskeletal and contractile elements. *Annual Review of Physiology* 41:703.

Grobstein, C. 1977. The recombinant-DNA debate. *Scientific American* 237(1):22 (July).

Gunn, R. B. 1980. Co- and counter-transport mechanisms in cell membranes. *Annual Review of Physiology* 42:249.

Guyton, A. C. 1981. *Textbook of medical physiology* (6th ed.). Philadelphia: W. B. Saunders.

Kornberg, R. D., and Klug, A. 1981. The nucleosome. *Scientific American* 244(2):52 (February).

Kupfermann, I. 1980. Role of cyclic nucleotides in excitable cells. *Annual Review of Physiology* 42:629.

Levin, D. L., Devesa, S. S., Godwin, J. D., II, and Silverman, D. T. 1974. *Cancer rates and risks.* Washington, D.C.: U.S. Department of Health, Education and Welfare (DHEW Publication No. NIH 79–691).

Lodish, H. F., and Rothman, J. E. 1979. The assembly of cell membranes. *Scientific American* 240(1):48 (January).

Marx, J. L. 1980. Calmodulin: A protein for all seasons. *Science* 208:728 (April 18).

Old, L. J. 1977. Cancer immunology. *Scientific American* 236(5):62 (May).

Olins, D. E., and Olins, A. L. 1978. Nucleosomes: The structural quantum in chromosomes. *American Scientist* 66:704 (November–December).

Pederson, T. 1981. Messenger RNA biosynthesis and nuclear structure. *American Scientist* 69:76 (January–February).

Pines, M. 1978. *Inside the cell.* Washington, D.C.: Department of Health, Education and Welfare, The National Institute of General Medical Sciences (DHEW Publication No. NIH 78–1051).

Rich, A., and Kim, S. H. 1978. The three-dimensional structure of transfer RNA. *Scientific American* 238(1):52 (January).

Rubenstein, E. 1980. Diseases caused by impaired communication among cells. *Scientific American* 242(3):102 (March).

Sloboda, R. D. The role of microtubules in cell structure and cell division. *American Scientist* 68:290 (May–June).

Wetzel, R. 1980. Applications of recombinant DNA technology. *American Scientist* 68:664 (November–December).

Wolfe, S. L. 1977. *Biology: The foundations.* Belmont, Calif.: Wadsworth.

Wolfe, S. L. 1981. *Biology of the cell* (2nd ed.). Belmont, Calif.: Wadsworth.

4

TISSUES

DEFINITION AND CLASSIFICATION OF TISSUES

Objective 1. Define the term tissue and list the four categories of tissues and their major functions.

As discussed in the last chapter, the cell is the basic unit of structure and function of the body. However, the cells of a multicellular organism are specialized in function, and they do not work independently.

Imagine that the body is similar to a large organization, such as a modern hospital. A hospital provides a number of different services, and no single hospital employee performs every one of them. For example, as a member of a surgical team, you would be responsible for performing certain tasks in surgery. You would not also be expected to provide meals for hospitalized people or to sweep the halls, though you might be capable of doing these things. Similarly, each cell in an organism has a particular set of functions, a "specialty," even though all cells in an organism contain the same genetic information.

To carry the analogy further, you would not be the only hospital worker performing your kind of job. You would be one of a group of staff members who have roughly the same duties—groups such as nurses, laboratory technicians, surgeons, housekeepers, and kitchen workers. Likewise, organisms have different types of tissues, each type containing large numbers of cells with similar structures and functions.

Groups of cells that have the same structural characteristics and perform the same functions are called **tissues**. In this chapter we will consider the structure and location of different kinds of tissues and see how their structures and functions are related.

The many kinds of tissue are grouped into four general categories: (1) epithelial tissue, (2) connective tissue, (3) muscle tissue, and (4) nervous tissue.

Epithelial tissues cover surfaces, line cavities, and form the major portion of many glands. They protect the surfaces they cover against abrasion and against the entry of harmful agents. Some epithelial surfaces secrete certain beneficial products; others allow for the absorption of nutrients.

Connective tissues comprise a diverse group of tissues, each member of which consists of cells surrounded by matrix. **Matrix** consists of cell products and tissue fluids. Matrix fills the spaces between the cells; its composition differs depending on the type of connective tissue. For example, in bone the matrix is hard, in cartilage the matrix is semisolid, and in most other forms of connective tissue it is soft and jellylike. Blood with its fluid matrix is usually classified with connective tissues. Connective tissues support and protect the body and assist in the transport of substances.

Muscle tissues, which have the ability to contract, are involved in many kinds of movement—movement of food through the digestive tract, pumping of blood, and movement of body parts or the whole body. The functions of muscle tissue are explained in Chapter 8.

Nerve (or nervous) **tissues** have the ability to receive stimuli, carry signals, and coordinate conscious and unconscious activities. The functions of nervous tissue are presented in Chapter 10.

DEVELOPMENT OF TISSUES

Objective 2. Describe how the three germ layers form from a fertilized egg and name the tissues derived from each layer.

All of the cells, tissues, organs, and systems of the human body develop from a single cell—the fertilized egg. Included within the nucleus of that egg is all the information necessary to initiate the growth and development of all body parts.

This fertilized egg cell (Figure 4.1a) divides by mitosis, first becoming two cells, then four, eight, sixteen cells, and so on. It soon becomes a solid ball of cells called a **morula** (b). By the end of the first week of development, some of these rapidly dividing cells rearrange, forming a hollow ball, the **blastocyst** (c). The blastocyst has an outer cell layer and an inner cell mass. The outer layer of cells goes on, along with tissues from the mother, to form the placenta. During the second week of development the inner cell mass forms a plate of cells called the embryonic disc (d). Some cells on either side of the embryonic disc divide and rearrange to

create two new cavities, the **amniotic cavity** and the yolk sac. The yolk sac later becomes the **gut cavity**.

The cells of the embryonic disc are the only ones that will eventually become the new individual; most of the others contribute to the placenta or membranes that surround the embryo. Disc cells are now arranged in two layers, each of which is a **primary germ layer**. The layer nearest the amniotic cavity is the **ectoderm** (*ecto* = outer); the one nearest the gut cavity is the **endoderm** (*endo* = inner). During the third week of development the embryonic disc cells become oriented into a head end and a tail end. Ectoderm cells near the tail end proliferate and grow forward between the two existing layers. This third layer becomes the **mesoderm** (*meso* = middle), the last of the embryonic germ layers.

What we have seen so far are the early steps in cell **differentiation**—that is, as these embryonic cells divide they are becoming *different* from one another. Each primary germ layer develops into tissues and organs with specialized structures and functions. The tissues arising from the primary germ layers are summarized in Table 4.1. Note in the table that nervous tissue is derived from ectoderm, and that muscle and connective tissues develop from mesoderm. In contrast, some epithelial tissues arise from each of the germ layers.

More information about the development of body systems will be given at the beginning of most of the remaining chapters.

EPITHELIAL TISSUES

Objective 3. Identify the characteristics of epithelial tissues and explain how these characteristics are related to the location and function of the tissues.

Objective 4. Distinguish between mucous membranes and serous membranes in terms of structure, function, and location.

Objective 5. Distinguish between exocrine and endocrine glands and describe the structure, function, and location of the various exocrine glands.

Characteristics of Epithelial Tissues

Of all the tissues of your body epithelial tissue is the easiest to observe. The surface of skin, which covers your entire body, consists of epithelial tissue, or **epithelium**. Your mouth, nose, ears, and other body openings are lined with epithelium. Less apparent are the internal epithelial tissues.

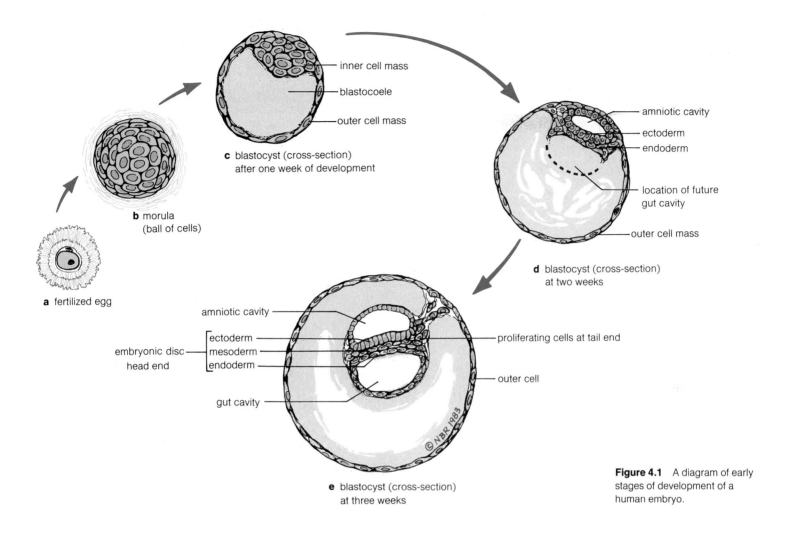

c blastocyst (cross-section)
after one week of development

inner cell mass
blastocoele
outer cell mass

b morula
(ball of cells)

a fertilized egg

amniotic cavity
ectoderm
endoderm
location of future
gut cavity
outer cell mass

d blastocyst (cross-section)
at two weeks

amniotic cavity

embryonic disc
head end
ectoderm
mesoderm
endoderm

gut cavity

proliferating cells at tail end

outer cell

e blastocyst (cross-section)
at three weeks

Figure 4.1 A diagram of early stages of development of a human embryo.

Table 4.1 Tissues and Organs Derived from Each of the Embryonic Germ Layers

Ectoderm	Mesoderm	Endoderm
Epithelium of skin and its derivatives	Bones, cartilage, and other connective tissues, including blood	Epithelium of digestive and respiratory systems, except mouth and anus
Nervous system	Muscles	Epithelium of thyroid, para-thyroid, thymus, liver, and pancreas
Pituitary gland	Organs of urinary and reproduc-tive systems, except linings of cavities	Epithelial lining of part of bladder and urethra
Adrenal medulla		
Epithelial parts of most sense organs	Epithelial coverings of organs and linings of body cavities and blood vessels	
Lining of mouth and anus		
Pineal gland	Adrenal cortex	

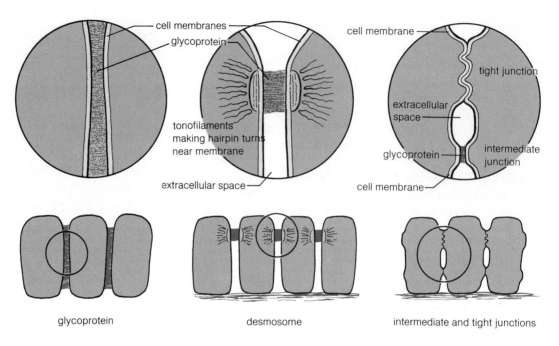

cell membranes
glycoprotein

cell membrane

cell membrane

tight junction

extracellular
space

tonofilaments
making hairpin turns
near membrane

glycoprotein

intermediate
junction

extracellular space

cell membrane

glycoprotein

desmosome

intermediate and tight junctions

Figure 4.2 How epithelial cells are held together: (**a**) glycoprotein deposits, (**b**) desmosomes, and (**c**) intermediate and tight junctions.

Many of the organs of the digestive, respiratory, urinary, and reproductive systems are lined with epithelium; all blood vessels are lined with epithelium. Finally, much of the tissue of glands consists of epithelial cells that secrete the products of the glands.

Several characteristics are common to all epithelial tissues. First, the cells of epithelia are capable of dividing by mitosis. In multilayered epithelial tissue cell division is usually limited to the bottom layer of cells, with cells moving upward toward the surface as division occurs, and changing shape as they move. The epithelium of the skin grows in this manner, as will be described in Chapter 5.

Second, epithelial tissues are attached to the underlying connective tissue by a noncellular **basement membrane**. The basement membrane consists of glycoprotein from the epithelial cells and a meshwork of reticular and collagen fibers from the connective tissue. (These fibers will be described in the discussion of connective tissue.)

Third, the cells of epithelial tissues are tightly packed together and held to each other by one of several mechanisms: (1) glycoprotein deposits, (2) desmosomes, (3) intermediate junctions, and (4) tight junctions (Figure 4.2). **Glycoprotein deposits** consist of a combination of polysac-charides and protein. They are secreted from the epithelial cells and actually stick the cells together, much in the same way that they help to hold epithelial cells to the basement membrane (a). **Desmosomes** (b) consist of large numbers of fibers called tonofilaments arranged in hairpin turns along the inside of the cell membrane, and of glycoprotein deposits in the intercellular space. Tight and intermediate junctions are found together (c) where there is a very tight seal between the cells. In a **tight junction** the cell membranes of the adjacent cells come into contact with each other near the surface ends of the cells. Where the membrane of one cell curves in, the other curves out (like the pieces of a jigsaw puzzle), and the outer portions of the membranes actually fuse together. In an **intermediate junction**, which is usually found below the tight junction, the cell membranes are held together by glycoprotein. Here the glycoprotein is present in smaller quantity than in a desmosome, and tonofilaments are entirely lacking.

Finally, epithelial tissues lack blood vessels. However, the underlying connective tissues are generally well supplied with blood vessels. Nutrients enter epithelial tissues by diffusing through the basement membrane and on through each layer of epithelial cells.

Structure, Location, and Function of Epithelial Tissues

Epithelial cells come in three basic shapes: **squamous**, or flat, cells; **cuboidal**, or cube-shaped, cells; and **columnar**, or cylindrical, column-shaped cells.

Since the cells are tightly packed together, epithelial tissues usually occur in "sheets." If the sheet consists of a single layer of cells, the tissue is called **simple** epithelium. If it is made up of two or more layers of cells, it is called **stratified** epithelium. Stratified epithelia are further classified by the shape of the cells in their outermost layer. A third type of epithelium is called **pseudostratified** epithelium (*pseudo* = false) because it appears to have more than one cell layer. On closer examination, however, it turns out to be a single sheet of cells having different heights, all of which touch the basement membrane. A final type of epithelium is **transitional** epithelium, in which the cells are capable of changing shape in response to stress.

Combining different cell shapes with the various types of layering gives us the several different structural classes of epithelial tissues discussed below. Figure 4.3 summarizes these structural types. Locations and functions of each class are given in Table 4.2.

Simple squamous epithelium **Simple squamous epithelium** (Figure 4.4) consists of a single layer of flat, many-sided cells with a central nucleus. Because the cells are extremely thin, the nucleus causes a bulge in the surface of each cell. This tissue is widely distributed throughout the body. It lines parts of the urinary, gastrointestinal, and male reproductive systems. As **endothelium**, it lines the heart and all of the blood and lymph vessels. As **mesothelium**, it lines the abdominal, pleural, and pericardial cavities and covers the surfaces of the organs within these cavities.

In most locations the function of simple squamous epithelium is to protect the underlying tissues. However, in the smaller blood and lymph vessels this thin tissue allows many substances to pass through it.

Simple cuboidal epithelium **Simple cuboidal epithelium** (Figure 4.5) consists of a single layer of cube-shaped cells with centrally placed nuclei. It is found in parts of the kidney and in the secretory portions and excretory ducts of many glands. In the ducts its function is to protect, and in the secretory portions of glands its function is to secrete.

Simple columnar epithelium **Simple columnar epithelium** (Figure 4.6) consists of a single layer of tall, cylindrical cells with nuclei placed near the base of the cell. Most of the simple columnar epithelium is found lining the gastrointestinal tract from the stomach to the anus and in the ex-

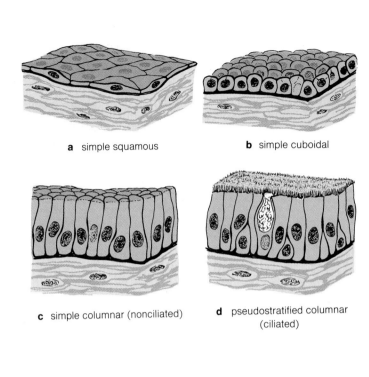

a simple squamous   **b** simple cuboidal

c simple columnar (nonciliated)   **d** pseudostratified columnar (ciliated)

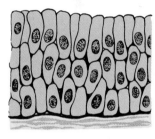

e stratified squamous

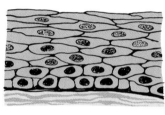

f stratified columnar

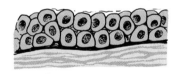

g stratified cuboidal

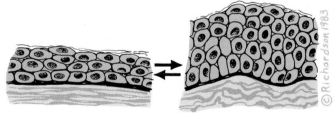

h transitional (distended)   **i** transitional (undistended)

Figure 4.3 Classification of epithelial tissues.

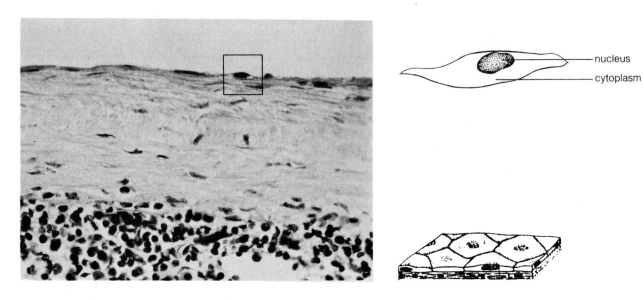

nucleus

cytoplasm

Figure 4.4 Simple squamous epithelium from the human spleen, × 374. (Armed Forces Institute of Pathology, negative number 71–9194.)

Table 4.2	Structure, Locations, and Functions of Epithelial Tissue	
Structure	Locations	Functions
Simple squamous	Lining of blood vessels, lining of body cavities, some parts of kidney tubules	Protection, absorption
Simple cuboidal	Secretory portion and ducts of some glands, part of kidney tubules	Secretion, protection
Simple columnar	Lining of gastrointestinal tract, excretory ducts of some glands	Absorption, protection, secretion
Pseudostratified columnar	Lining of trachea and parts of male reproductive system	Protection, secretion
Stratified squamous	Epidermis, lining of vagina, mouth, and esophagus	Protection, secretion, limited absorption
Stratified cuboidal	Ducts of sweat glands (a rare tissue)	Protection
Stratified columnar	Male urethra (a rare tissue)	Protection
Transitional	Lining of ureter and urinary bladder	Protection

cretory portions of many glands. The primary function of this tissue is secretory, and **secretory granules** can be seen in some of these cells. However, the tissue also protects the organs it lines and allows for the absorption of nutrients in the gastrointestinal tract.

The simple columnar epithelium of the upper respiratory tract and the uterine tubes is ciliated. The cilia help to move fluids along the passageways. (Cilia were described in Chapter 3.) In the respiratory tract the cilia help to push debris out of the lungs or nasal cavity toward the pharynx, where it can be ejected or swallowed. In the uterine tubes the cilia help to move an egg, or ovum, from the ovary to the uterus. These tissues also contain goblet cells, single-celled glands that secrete mucus, to be described in more detail later. Mucus secreted by these cells helps to lubricate the surfaces of passageways and entraps debris that might enter the passageways so it can be removed by the cilia.

Pseudostratified columnar epithelium **Pseudostratified columnar epithelium** (Figure 4.7) appears to have more than one layer of cells because the nuclei are not all at the same level when the tissue is studied in sagittal section. However, *all* of the cells rest on the basement membrane, and some grow longer than others. The unequal lengths of the cells give the single layer of cells the appearance of being more than one layer. Found in the respiratory and male reproductive tract, this kind of tissue is usually ciliated and contains goblet cells. It too is capable of undergoing cell division to rapidly repair itself whenever it is damaged. The functions of this

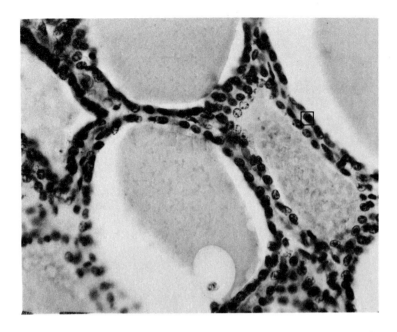

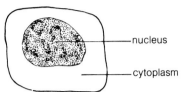

nucleus

cytoplasm

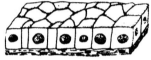

Figure 4.5 Simple cuboidal epithelium from the thyroid gland, × 374. (Armed Forces Institute of Pathology, negative number 71–9196.)

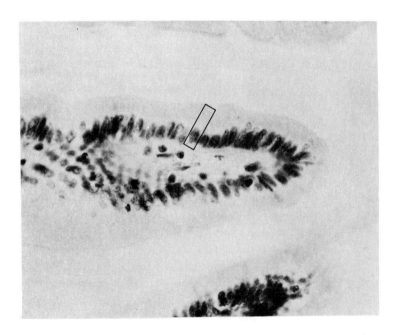

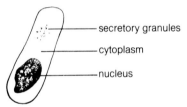

secretory granules

cytoplasm

nucleus

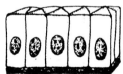

Figure 4.6 Simple columnar epithelium, from the small intestine, × 488. (Armed Forces Institute of Pathology, negative number 71–9197.)

tissue are to protect the passageways it lines and to secrete mucus, which lubricates the surface and entraps debris.

Stratified squamous epithelium **Stratified squamous epithelium**, illustrated in Figure 4.8, contains many layers of cells, but the outer layer is always made up of flattened (squamous) cells. The **epidermis** of the skin is an example of stratified squamous epithelium. As will be discussed in more detail in Chapter 5, keratin forms a waterproof layer on the exposed surface of skin tissue. Other stratified squamous epithelia are found in the esophagus and vagina; these tissues do not have the keratin layer. The function of all stratified squamous epithelia is primarily protection, although the epidermis has a modest ability to absorb some

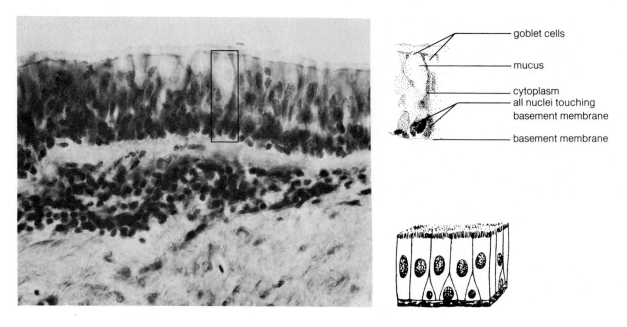

Figure 4.7 Pseudostratified columnar epithelium with goblet cells, × 259. (Armed Forces Institute of Pathology, negative number 71–9198.)

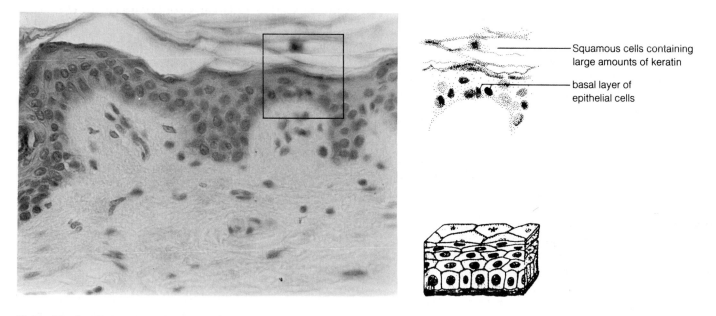

Figure 4.8 Stratified squamous epithelium from human skin, × 340. (Photograph by author.)

substances. Glands within some of these tissues produce secretions, as will be discussed later in this chapter.

Stratified cuboidal and columnar epithelia Stratified cuboidal and columnar epithelia are rare in the human body. **Stratified cuboidal epithelium** consists of at least two layers of cells, the surface layers being cube-shaped. It lines the ducts

of the larger sweat glands. **Stratified columnar epithelium** also consists of at least two layers of cells, the surface layer being cylindrical in shape. It lines parts of the epiglottis and parts of the male urethra. These tissues protect the organs they line.

Transitional epithelium **Transitional epithelium** (Figure 4.9)

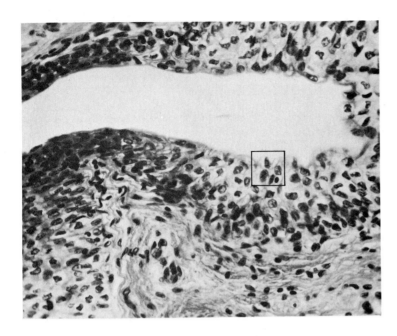

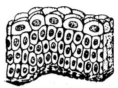
nucleus
cytoplasm

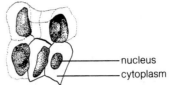

Figure 4.9 Transitional epithelium from the ureter, × 259. (Armed Forces Institute of Pathology, negative number 71–9203.)

is characterized by the presence of several layers of cells that can change shape when the tissue is stretched. Found in the ureters and the urinary bladder, the cells of this tissue become flattened when they are under tension (as when the bladder is full) and rounded when they are not under tension (as when the bladder is empty).

Membranes

In several sites in the body a sheet of epithelium and its underlying connective tissue together constitute a **membrane**. These multilayered membranes are of two major types—serous membranes and mucous membranes. **Serous membranes** line the closed internal body cavities and cover the surfaces of the organs in these cavities, which include the abdominal, pleural, and pericardial cavities mentioned earlier. The squamous epithelium and underlying connective tissue in Figure 4.4 is a serous membrane. Serous membranes are lubricated by a clear fluid similar to intercellular fluid (the fluid that bathes the cells of most tissues). Because of this lubrication organs can move during respiration and digestion without causing significant friction between surfaces.

Mucous membranes line the internal surfaces of organ systems where passageways lead to the outside of the body. These systems include the digestive, respiratory, urinary, and reproductive systems. All epithelial tissues previously described as able to secrete mucus, along with the connec-

tive tissue that underlies them, are examples of mucous membranes. These membranes protect the organs they line; their mucous secretions moisten and lubricate the membrane.

Glands

In addition to forming sheets of cells, epithelial tissues also contribute to the formation of glands, structures that produce secretions. Glands may be unicellular or multicellular. Unicellular glands consist of single, modified epithelial cells; multicellular glands are more complex. In the development of multicellular glands the epithelium forms pouches that grow inward from the surface of the epithelium. Toward the end of development some glands lose their connection with the surface epithelium (such as the lining of the digestive tract) and become ductless, or **endocrine**, glands. Others retain their connection with the epithelium through ducts and become ducted, or **exocrine**, glands.

Exocrine glands can be unicellular or multicellular. Unicellular glands, though ductless, release their secretions directly into the lumen (inner cavity) of the organ in which they are found. Only one type of unicellular gland is of significance in humans—the **goblet cell**, which produces mucus (see Figure 4.6). Goblet cells are interspersed among the other epithelial cells in mucous membranes and are so named because of their goblet or wine-glass shape when they are filled with secretion.

Multicellular exocrine glands (Figure 4.10) are classified as **simple** if they have a single duct and **compound** if they have branched ducts. These glands are also classified according to the shape of the secretory portion of the gland. Some glands have **tubular** (tubelike) secretory portions; others have **acinar** or **alveolar** (saclike) secretory portions. Tubular glands may have branching or coiled tubes; acinar glands may have branches that form many alveoli or acini within the secretory portion of the gland.

Exocrine glands also vary in the manner in which they produce secretions; the glands and their secretions are classified accordingly as merocrine, apocrine, or holocrine. The cells of some glands synthesize substances and simply discharge them without any part of the cell being released. Such glands and their secretions are said to be **merocrine**. The cells of certain other glands collect their products in the apical end (the end nearest the surface). The apical end breaks away from the cell and is released with the secretion. Such glands and their secretions are termed **apocrine**. Cells in still other glands accumulate secretory products, and eventually the whole cell and its accumulated product separates from the tissue. Such glands and their secretions are termed **holocrine**.

A variety of exocrine glands are present in the body. The major glands, their structure, location, manner of secretion, and an example of a secretion are listed in Table 4.3.

> Endocrine glands, such as the pituitary and thyroid, release their secretions into the intercellular fluids. These secretions then diffuse to and enter blood vessels, through which they are transported to other parts of the body. The secretions of endocrine glands are called **hormones**. These glands and their hormones will be discussed in Chapter 15.

CONNECTIVE TISSUES

Objective 6. List the four classes of connective tissues and describe their major characteristics.

Objective 7. Distinguish among the types of connective tissue proper in terms of structure, function, and location.

Objective 8. Distinguish among the types of cartilage in terms of structure, function, and location.

Objective 9. Distinguish among the types of bone in terms of structure, function, and location.

Classes of Connective Tissue

Connective tissue is aptly named—in general, it connects body parts together. It forms the bones that make up the framework of the body; it holds the bones together, holds the muscles to the bones, and holds the skin to the muscles. Though connecting things is the major function of connective tissues, they do perform some other functions as well.

In the embryo some of the mesoderm develops into a tissue called **mesenchyme**, which gives rise to all adult connective tissues. Connective tissues consist of cells surrounded by an extracellular matrix of varying consistency. These tissues can be grouped into four general classes on the basis of the characteristics of the matrix: (1) blood, (2) connective tissue proper, (3) cartilage, and (4) bone. **Blood** is a connective tissue in which various blood cells are dispersed in a fluid matrix. Because of its special properties, blood will be discussed separately in Chapter 16. **Connective tissue proper** connects many parts of the body to each other and serves as "packing" material. Its matrix consists of various types of fibers imbedded in a relatively fluid ground substance. **Cartilage** has its cells imbedded in a fairly solid but flexible matrix, and **bone** has its cells imbedded in a solid matrix.

Connective Tissue Proper

Connective tissue proper includes several different kinds of tissue, each of which has its own characteristic types and arrangement of fibers. These tissues include (1) loose, or areolar, connective tissue, with its loosely packed, irregularly arranged extracellular fibers; (2) dense connective tissue, with its more abundant fibers, often arranged in bundles; (3) reticular connective tissue, in which the fibers form a network (reticulum) that supports the other structures in an organ; (4) adipose tissue, in which fat globules inside cells rather than fibers give the tissue its definitive appearance; and (5) pigmented connective tissue, which is found in the iris and choroid coat of the eye and has cells containing granules of pigment, usually melanin.

Loose or areolar connective tissue **Loose connective tissue** (Figure 4.11) is found at sites where there is usually little tension on the tissues—between the skin and the skeletal muscles and beneath most epithelial linings of organs. This abundant tissue contains a variety of cell types and their products as well as several different kinds of fibers.

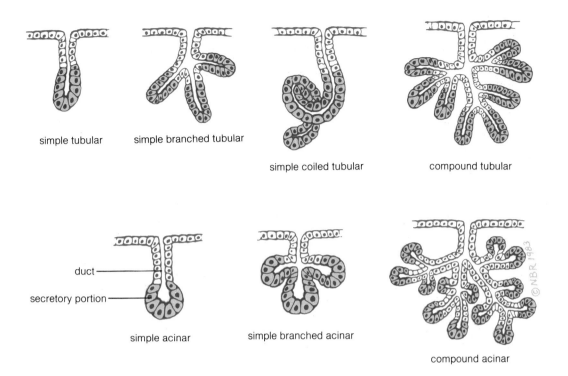

simple tubular

simple branched tubular

simple coiled tubular

compound tubular

duct

secretory portion

simple acinar

simple branched acinar

compound acinar

Figure 4.10 Types of multicellular exocrine glands. Notice that simple glands have no branches in the ducts, although they may have branches in their secretory portions. Compound glands always have branches in the ducts. Glands may have tubular or acinar secretory portions.

Table 4.3 Structure, Location, Manner of Secretion, and Examples of Secretions of Exocrine Glands				
Gland	Structure	Location	Manner of secretion	Example of secretion
Goblet cell	Unicellular	Mucous membranes	Merocrine	Mucus
Intestinal glands	Simple tubular	Small intestine	Merocrine	Enzymes
Sweat glands	Simple coiled tubular	Skin	Merocrine and apocrine	Sweat
Sebaceous glands	Simple alveolar or simple branched alveolar	Skin	Holocrine	Oil and wax
Liver	Compound tubular, but very complex	Abdominal cavity	Merocrine	Bile
Pancreas	Compound alveolar	Abdominal cavity	Merocrine	Enzymes
Mammary glands	Compound alveolar	Chest area	Apocrine	Milk
Salivary glands	Compound alveolar and compound tubulo-alveolar	Jaw area	Merocrine	Saliva

Fibroblasts, the most numerous of the cells in loose connective tissue, synthesize and secrete proteins that make up the fibers of all connective tissues; they also synthesize and secrete glycoproteins (polysaccharides combined with proteins). These substances comprise the **ground substance** of the matrix. Much of the ground substance of loose connective tissue consists of **hyaluronic acid**, which gives the ground substance its jellylike consistency. The basement membrane between epithelial and connective tissue also contains glycoproteins.

The enzyme hyaluronidase destroys hyaluronic acid in tissues, reducing their viscosity and thereby permitting easier movement of substances in tissue spaces. Some microorganisms produce hyaluronidase; the action of the enzyme helps the organisms to invade tissues.

Other cell types in loose connective tissues include histiocytes, mast cells, lymphocytes, and other white blood cells. **Histiocytes**, also called tissue macrophages, are phagocytic cells native to connective tissues. **Mast cells** produce and release several substances, including histamine, serotonin, and heparin. Histamine, released at the time of cell injury, is important in initiating the inflammatory reaction, as will be explained in the essay at the end of this chapter. The exact functions of serotonin and heparin in connective tissue are not well understood, though in other parts of the body serotonin is a transmitter of neural impulses and heparin prevents blood clotting. **Lymphocytes** and other **white blood cells** migrate into loose connective tissue in large numbers following tissue injury. The lymphocytes are involved in the development of immunity (as described in Chapter 20), and the other white blood cells are primarily involved in phagocytizing foreign substances that have entered the tissue.

The three kinds of fibers found in connective tissues are (1) collagenous, (2) elastic, and (3) reticular fibers. Collagenous fibers, the strongest of all the connective tissue fibers, consist of parallel, coiled molecules of the whitish protein **collagen**. These molecules are arranged in parallel and overlapping strands in the fiber. Thus, collagenous fibers have high tensile strength and flexibility, much like a rope. Collagenous fibers do not branch, and they do not stretch. Elastic fibers consist of thinner molecules of a fibrous, yellowish protein, **elastin**. The elastin molecules branch to form an interconnected network of fibers capable of stretching and snapping back to their original length. Elastic fibers in the connective tissue of the walls of arteries and in the skin beneath the epidermis account for the resiliency of these tissues. **Reticular fibers** consist of thin, delicate fibers whose molecules branch like elastin and overlap like collagen. They may be immature collagenous fibers whose development has been arrested.

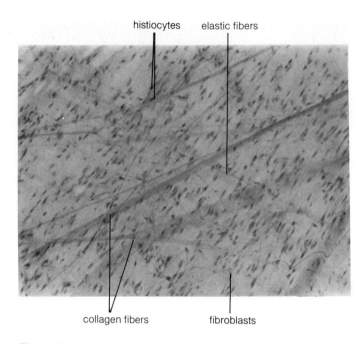

Figure 4.11 Cells and fibers of loose connective tissue, × 75. (Photograph by author.)

Gelatin, the protein found in gelatin desserts, is made from collagen (by boiling it with water or acid). Gelatin is easily digestible and is thus a good source of protein in the diet. However, gelatin contains no tryptophan and only small amounts of tyrosine and cystine; thus it must be supplemented with other proteins that contain these amino acids to provide an adequate diet.

Dense connective tissue **Dense connective tissue** is characterized by the close packing of its fibers; however, there are many gradations of dense connective tissues. Two categories of dense connective tissues are distinguished according to the arrangement of fibers in their matrix. **Dense, irregularly arranged connective tissues** consist of all types of fibers, with collagenous fibers predominating. These fibers are arranged irregularly in a tough feltwork. Fibroblasts are the most common cell. This kind of tissue is found in the dermis of the skin and in the membranes that cover bones and cartilage. **Dense, regularly arranged connective tissue** usually has a matrix consisting primarily of collagen fibers arranged in large, parallel bundles. Typically, a few fibroblasts are the only cells present. This tissue is found in fascia, tendons, aponeuroses, and ligaments. **Fascia** is a

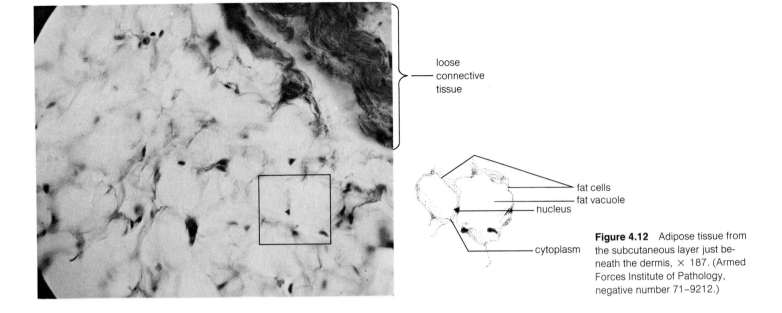

loose connective tissue

fat cells
fat vacuole
nucleus
cytoplasm

Figure 4.12 Adipose tissue from the subcutaneous layer just beneath the dermis, × 187. (Armed Forces Institute of Pathology, negative number 71–9212.)

glistening white sheet of tissue that covers muscles; **tendons** are bands of tissue that connect bones and muscles; **aponeuroses** are essentially sheetlike tendons that attach muscles to bones or to other muscles; **ligaments** attach one bone to another. Structurally, ligaments are similar to tendons, except that some ligaments contain large numbers of elastic fibers and are thus known as yellow ligaments.

Reticular connective tissue   **Reticular connective tissue** consists of a network (reticulum) of fibers formed by special cells called **reticular cells**. These fibers are not distinguishable from the reticular fibers made by fibroblasts in loose connective tissue, although they are formed in a different way. Reticular connective tissue forms the framework of the liver, spleen, and lymph nodes.

Adipose tissue   **Adipose**, or fat, tissue lacks a matrix and contains a few of all types of fibers and large numbers of fat cells (Figure 4.12). A **fat cell** contains a large, central, fat-filled vacuole; its nucleus and cytoplasm have been pushed to the perimeter of the cell. These cells are often called **signet ring cells** because they resemble a signet ring when seen in cross section. Fat cells are scattered through loose connective tissue and are also found aggregated into separate tissues in several locations, including the fat layers beneath the skin, around the kidneys and heart, around the joints as padding, and in the marrow cavities of long bones. In addition to functioning as protective padding, adipose tissue also insulates the body against heat loss and serves as

a storage depot for fat that can be metabolized to produce energy. Adipose tissue is a metabolically active tissue. How fat is stored and later mobilized is discussed in Chapter 23.

Pigmented connective tissue   Though limited to only a few places in the body, such as certain structures in the eye (the choroid, ciliary body, and the iris), **pigmented connective tissue** constitutes a distinctive type of tissue. The cells are irregular in shape and contain granules of pigment, usually melanin. Some evidence suggests that these cells are derived from the neural crests, some cells that develop near the neural tube (see Chapter 10) of the embryo. All other pigmented cells are epithelial cells of the skin. They will be discussed in the next chapter.

The characteristics of connective tissue proper are summarized in Table 4.4.

Cartilage

Like other connective tissues, cartilage consists of cells, fibers, and ground substance. The cells of developing cartilage are called **chondroblasts** (*chondro* = cartilage). These cells produce the fibers and ground substance of the matrix, eventually becoming entrapped in their own products. The cells are then called **chondrocytes**, and the cavities they occupy are called **lacunae**. Often more than one cell occupies a lacuna; these cells are the progeny of the chondroblast that first occupied the space. The ground substance

Table 4.4	Characteristics of Connective Tissue Proper	
Tissue Type	Characteristics	Location
Loose (areolar)	Fibroblasts and many other kinds of cells; all three kinds of fibers in a loose network	Between skin and skeletal muscles and beneath most epithelial linings
Dense		
Irregular	Feltwork of mostly collagenous fibers; fibroblasts are the pre-dominant cell	Dermis of the skin and membranes that cover bones and cartilage
Regular	Large bundles of mostly col-lagenous fibers; few cells, mostly fibroblasts; yellow ligaments contain elastic fibers	Fascia, tendons, aponeuroses, and ligaments
Reticular	Network of reticular fibers	Framework of liver, spleen, and lymph nodes
Adipose	Large numbers of fat cells each with a fat-filled vacuole; a few fibers of each type; an actively metabolic tissue	Scattered through loose connective tissue, and as a distinct tissue beneath the skin, around heart and kidneys, around joints, and in bone marrow
Pigmented	Irregularly shaped cells con-taining pigment granules	A rare tissue, found in the iris and choroid coat of the eye

of cartilage consists of chondroitin sulfate, a complex polysaccharide. Cartilage has no blood supply, and the chondrocytes are nourished by nutrients that diffuse through the ground substance.

Because cartilage is nourished by diffusion of nutrients, its thickness is limited by the distance nutrients can diffuse rapidly enough to maintain the cells. This means of nourishment also accounts for the slow healing of cartilage following an injury.

The nature and arrangement of fibers varies among different types of cartilage. On the basis of the predominant fibers three types of cartilage are recognized: (1) hyaline, (2) elastic, and (3) fibrous.

Hyaline cartilage **Hyaline cartilage** (Figure 4.13) has a bluish-white color in fresh preparations. Chondrocytes in lacunae are clearly visible with a microscope, but special microscopic techniques are needed to distinguish ground

substance and the thin collagenous fibers. Hyaline cartilage is the most widely distributed of the three types. It forms the costal cartilages of the ribs and the cartilages of the nose, larynx, trachea, and bronchi. Because of the weakness of the fibers in hyaline cartilage, it is the weakest type of cartilage. It is usually not found in areas where stresses are great.

Elastic cartilage **Elastic cartilage** (Figure 4.14) is slightly yellowish in color because of the presence of interlacing elastic fibers. Like other cartilage, it contains chondrocytes. This type of cartilage is resilient, and, when deformed, it springs back to its original shape. Elastic cartilage is found in the external ear, the epiglottis, the eustachian tube, and in some places in the laryngeal cartilages.

Fibrous cartilage **Fibrous cartilage**, the strongest type of cartilage, contains many dense collagenous fibers, chondrocytes, and a limited amount of ground substance. It is found in the intervertebral discs, the pubic symphysis (the joint between the pubic bones), and the articular cartilages (cartilages that cover the surfaces of bones where they form a joint with another bone). Though the articular cartilages are often classified as hyaline cartilage, they have more

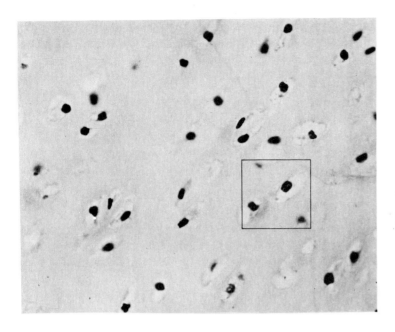

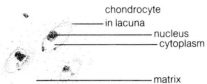

Figure 4.13 Hyaline cartilage from the trachea, × 412. (Armed Forces Institute of Pathology, negative number 71–9215.)

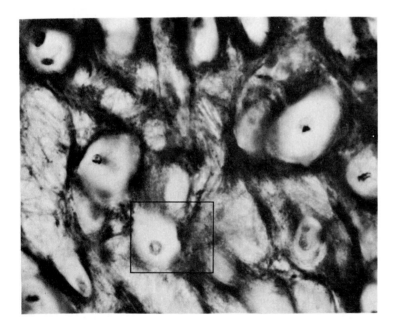

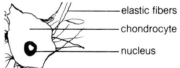

Figure 4.14 Elastic cartilage from the larynx, × 412. (Armed Forces Institute of Pathology, negative number 71–9216.)

and stronger collagenous fibers than are typical of hyaline cartilage.

Bone

Of all the connective tissues, bone has the hardest intercellular matrix. Its cells, the **osteocytes** (*osteo* = bone), lie in lacunae. The matrix of bone consists of about one-third organic substances and two-thirds inorganic substances. The organic part is made up of collagen and chondroitin sulfate. The inorganic part is made up mostly of the minerals calcium carbonate and calcium phosphate, which give bone its hardness. Bone is a highly vascular tissue; that is, it has many blood vessels running through it. The arrange-

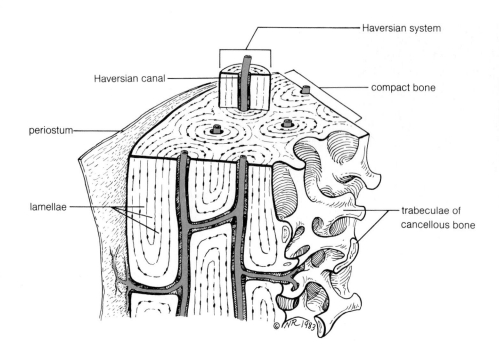

a

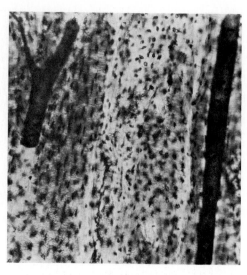

b

Figure 4.15 A section through a long bone showing the Haversian systems of compact bone and the trabeculae of cancellous bone: (**a**) diagram and (**b**) photomicrograph, × 75. (Photograph by author.)

ment of blood vessels and other structures makes it possible to distinguish two types of bone: (1) compact bone and (2) cancellous, or spongy, bone (Figure 4.15).

Compact bone **Compact bone** (Figure 4.16) contains **Haversian systems**, also called **osteons**. A Haversian system consists of a **Haversian canal** containing blood vessels and nerves, concentric layers of bone matrix (**lamellae**), and osteocytes (bone cells) in **lacunae**, which lie mostly between the lamellae. Cytoplasmic processes extend from the osteocytes into the **canaliculi**, tiny crevices in the matrix. Nutrients reach the osteocytes by diffusing from the blood vessel in the Haversian canal through the canaliculi; wastes move in the opposite direction.

For the most part, the Haversian systems are arranged parallel to the long axis of a bone, though there are connections between adjacent systems. Blood is supplied to the Haversian systems by **nutrient arteries**, which usually pass obliquely through the surface of a bone in a **nutrient canal**.

Compact bone is found on the outer surface of most bones. Between the compact bone and the marrow cavity in many bones is an area of cancellous or spongy bone.

Cancellous bone **Cancellous**, or spongy, bone contains osteocytes in lacunae and a matrix of organic and inorganic

substances like that of compact bone. However, the matrix is arranged in an irregular meshlike structure without Haversian systems. Thin plates of bone called **trabeculae**, common in cancellous bone, often extend into the marrow cavity. Because of the irregular spacing of the trabeculae, spongy bone is weaker and lighter than compact bone.

Bone development and bone shaping The complex processes of bone development and bone shaping are described in some detail in Chapter 6. For now it is sufficient to note two things. First, bone is laid down by cells called **osteoblasts** either in a membrane (membranous bone formation) or in cartilage (endochondral bone formation). Second, bone is continuously reshaped throughout life by the osteoblasts laying down small amounts of new bone and by the **osteoclasts**, bone-dissolving cells, removing small amounts of bone at other sites.

MUSCLE TISSUES

Objective 10. Distinguish among the three types of muscle tissues in terms of structure, function, and location.

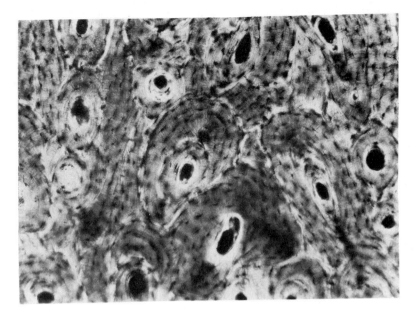

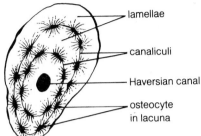

Figure 4.16 A cross-section from the shaft of a long bone, showing the components of a Haversian system, × 85. (Photograph by author.)

All muscle tissue has the ability to contract. This ability is what makes movement possible. The process of contraction occurs at the molecular level; it will be discussed in detail in Chapter 8. Here we are concerned with the characteristics of the three different types of muscle: (1) skeletal, (2) smooth, and (3) cardiac. These characteristics are summarized in Table 4.5.

Skeletal muscle **Skeletal muscle** (Figure 4.17) forms the muscles of the body that are usually attached to the bones. Its action is **voluntary**; that is, it may be consciously controlled by the individual and requires stimulation by a nerve before it contracts.

Each muscle consists of many individual, unbranched muscle **fibers**, arranged in bundles. Each fiber of a muscle is a single cell; it extends the entire length of the muscle. Each cell contains many nuclei, all located at the periphery of the cell. The **sarcoplasm**, or cytoplasm of skeletal muscle, is highly organized. The striations, or "stripes," seen with a light microscope that are one of the distinguishing characteristics of skeletal, or striated, muscle are formed by the orderly arrangement of the protein molecules involved in the contractile process.

Smooth muscle **Smooth muscle** (Figure 4.18) is found in the walls of the digestive tract, uterus, urinary bladder, blood vessels, and respiratory passages. Its action is generally **involuntary**; that is, cells do not require nerve stimulation to contract.

Smooth muscle cells are smaller than skeletal muscle

Table 4.5	Characteristics of Muscle Tissues	
Skeletal	Smooth	Cardiac
Voluntary	Involuntary	Involuntary
Fibers contain many nuclei	Fibers contain one nucleus	Fibers contain many cells connected by intercalated discs
Striated	Nonstriated, smooth sheets or bands	Striated (lightly)
Unbranched fibers found attached to bones	Unbranched fibers found in internal organs	Branched fibers found in heart

cells. They are spindle shaped, round in the middle and tapered at the ends.

Though smooth muscle cells contain the same kinds of contractile proteins as skeletal muscle cells, the arrangement of these molecules is less orderly, and thus no striations are apparent in smooth muscle. Smooth muscle is usually arranged in bands or sheets within the walls of an organ. It contracts more slowly and is able to sustain contraction longer than skeletal muscle.

Cardiac muscle **Cardiac muscle** (Figure 4.19) is found only in the heart and in the walls of the large blood vessels near their connection to the heart. It is involuntary like smooth

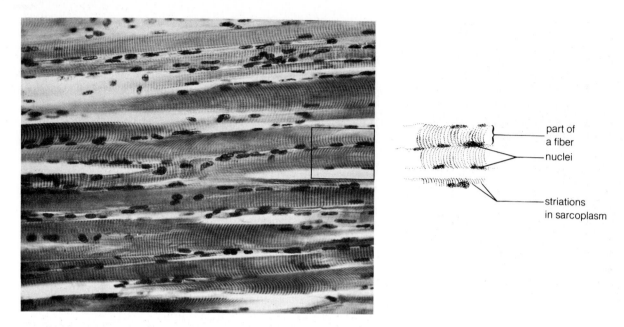

part of
a fiber
nuclei

striations
in sarcoplasm

Figure 4.17 Skeletal muscle, × 225. (Armed Forces Institute of Pathology, negative number 72–13786.)

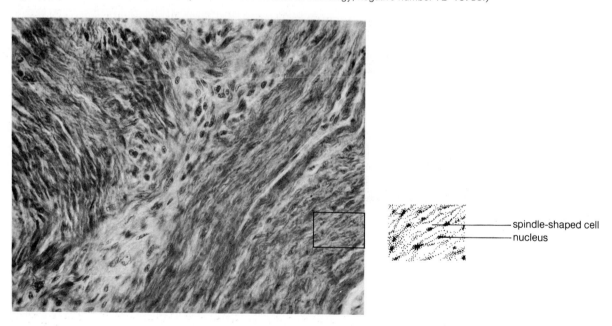

spindle-shaped cell
nucleus

Figure 4.18 Smooth muscle, × 225. (Armed Forces Institute of Pathology, negative number 71–9163.)

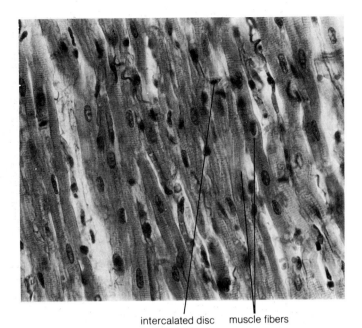

Figure 4.19 Cardiac muscle, × 340. (Photograph by author.)

intercalated disc   muscle fibers

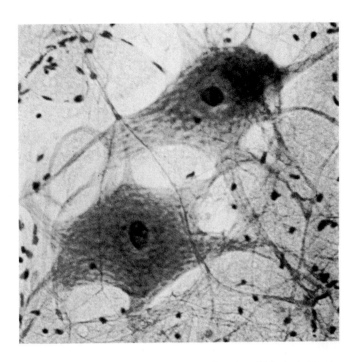

Figure 4.20 Neurons and neuroglia. (Carolina Biological Supply Company.)

muscle and striated like skeletal muscle. However, the striations are lighter and less definite than in skeletal muscle. Cardiac muscle has branching fibers and specialized cell junctions called **intercalated discs**. The other specialized properties that enable cardiac muscle to contract regularly throughout life will be discussed in Chapter 17.

NERVOUS TISSUE

Objective 11. Distinguish between neurons and neuroglial cells in terms of structure, function, and location.

Nervous, or nerve, tissue consists of two types of cells; the neurons, which conduct impulses, and the neuroglial cells, which perform other functions (Figure 4.20). Their main common property is that both are found only in nervous tissue.

Neurons **Neurons** consist of a **cell body** (soma), an **axon**, and usually several **dendrites**. In general, the axon conducts impulses away from the cell body; the dendrites conduct impulses toward the cell body. An individual nerve fiber is composed of a bundle of axons (or sometimes dendrites), as we shall see in Chapter 10. Neurons make up the impulse-conducting portion of the brain, spinal cord, and nerves.

Neuroglial cells **Neuroglia**, also called glial cells, are literally the "glue" of the nervous system (*glia* = glue). As shown in Figure 4.20, some of the glial cells provide a supporting network for neurons. They may also help to nourish the neurons. Most neuroglia are found within the central nervous system, but one kind, the **Schwann cell**, is associated with neurons outside the central nervous system. This kind of cell produces a fatty substance called myelin that insulates many axons. Glial cells will be discussed in more detail in Chapter 10.

Essay: Inflammation

One evening after a hard day you are slicing some delicious-looking fresh vegetables for your dinner. Suddenly the knife takes a wrong turn in a carrot—you've cut your hand. Luckily, the cut isn't too bad. The bleeding soon subsides, and you put on a bandage and continue fixing your meal.

Shortly after this the area around the cut starts to swell, turn red, and grow hot. The area is tender to the touch and may throb with pain. The cut has become inflamed.

Inflammation is the term used for these visible effects—redness, swelling, heat, and pain or itching—and other less visible effects as well. Inflammation, the body's response to tissue damage from injury or infection, is the initial step in the healing process. Yet inflammation, particularly the resulting pain, is often uncomfortable. In severe or abnormal cases inflammation itself can be harmful.

What happens in the inflammatory process, and why? Let's follow the process on the cellular and tissue levels and briefly look at the effects. Figure 4.21 shows the steps in the process diagrammatically.

When cells are damaged, **histamine** is released into the surrounding tissue fluids and diffuses into nearby capillaries (the smallest blood vessels) and venules (the smaller veins). It causes the blood vessels to become more permeable, allowing fluids to leave the blood and accumulate around the injured cells, so swelling occurs. It also causes the blood vessels to dilate, or increase in size, so more blood flows into the area. This increase in the amount of blood just beneath the epidermis causes the skin to become red and hot to the touch. The increased blood supply brings blood clotting factors, nutrients, and other important substances to the injured area and removes wastes and excess fluids. Though histamine has some unpleasant effects, it has beneficial effects as well.

Infections such as the common cold, insect bites, and allergies like hay fever, also cause tissue injury and the release of histamine. The red, watery eyes and runny nose of hay fever and the itching of an insect bite are caused by the release of histamine. The drugs called **antihistamines** alleviate the above symptoms by reducing the permeability and diameter of blood vessels. Unfortunately, antihistamines also have unpleasant side effects, such as sleepiness, dizziness, disturbed coordination, digestive disturbances, and thickening of mucous secretions.

To return to the inflamed cut—the fluid that enters the injured tissue also carries the chemical components of the blood-clotting mechanism (see Chapter 16). If the injury has caused bleeding, the bleeding is stopped by the formation of a blood clot in the opening of the skin. The dried clot is called a scab. Clotting also takes place in the intercellular fluids around the injury, where it greatly reduces the movement of fluids around the damaged cells, effectively walling off the injured area from the rest of the body. This walling off inhibits the spread of infectious organisms or toxic substances that might have entered the injured area.

Pain associated with injury is thought to be due to the release of a chemical such as **bradykinin**, a molecule consisting of nine amino acids. An injection of bradykinin (given to a consenting volunteer) causes much more pain than a similar injection of saline. How bradykinin stimulates pain receptors in the skin is unknown. Pain is a valuable sensation because it causes us to protect an injured area and prevent further injury. But pain sometimes lasts longer or is more severe than is needed to warn us; then drugs such as aspirin may be given to alleviate it. It is likely that these drugs interfere in some way with the pain signals reaching the brain rather than with the bradykinin directly.

Inflamed tissues also appear to release another chemical called **leukocytosis-promoting** (LP) **factor**. In leukocytosis leukocytes (white blood cells) increase in numbers in the blood, probably by being released from the organs that form them. The LP factor makes more leukocytes available, and many of them find their way to the wounded area. Some of these cells squeeze through the walls of the blood vessels in a process called **diapedesis** and enter the intercellular fluid around the wound.

Most of the leukocytes are phagocytic. They are attracted to microorganisms, which have entered the tissue from the air or the object that caused the wound, and to debris that remains from dead cells. This attraction is called **chemotaxis**. In the battle between the microorganisms and the phagocytes, many of the phagocytes die while carrying out their clean-up operation. The accumulation of dead phagocytic cells and the material they have ingested forms the white or yellow fluid we call **pus**. Pus continues to form until the infection has been brought under control and the microorganisms have been prevented from spreading.

Though the LP factor, and the phagocytes thereby made available, usually prevent the infection from spreading or getting worse, sometimes these natural defenses are overwhelmed. The infection may enter the blood and spread throughout the body. **Antibiotics**, drugs that inhibit the growth of certain microorganisms, are often used to minimize the chances of infection spreading from the site of serious injuries.

In addition to some blood cells acting as phagocytes, other blood cells produce **immune reactions** destined to help overcome the initial infection and to recognize the organism and prevent future infections by the same organism. These immune reactions are discussed in Chapter 20.

During the entire inflammatory reaction, the healing process is also underway. Once the inflammatory reaction has subsided and most of the debris has been cleared away, healing accelerates. Epithelial cells in the basal layer of the epidermis proliferate, and new epidermis replaces the part that was destroyed. In the digestive tract and other organs that are lined with epithelium, an injured lining can be similarly replaced.

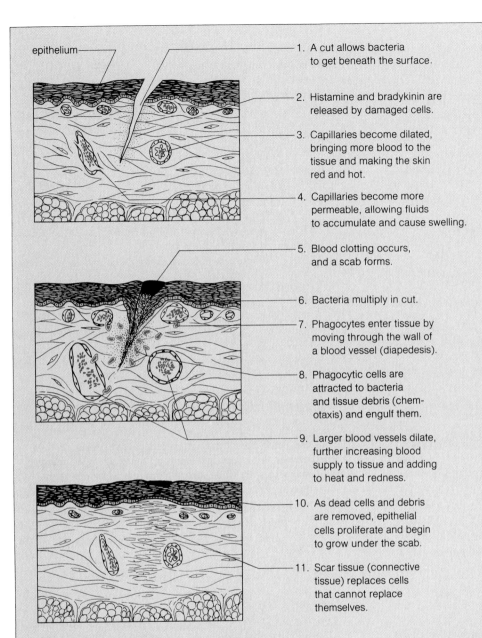

epithelium

1. A cut allows bacteria to get beneath the surface.

2. Histamine and bradykinin are released by damaged cells.

3. Capillaries become dilated, bringing more blood to the tissue and making the skin red and hot.

4. Capillaries become more permeable, allowing fluids to accumulate and cause swelling.

5. Blood clotting occurs, and a scab forms.

6. Bacteria multiply in cut.

7. Phagocytes enter tissue by moving through the wall of a blood vessel (diapedesis).

8. Phagocytic cells are attracted to bacteria and tissue debris (chemotaxis) and engulf them.

9. Larger blood vessels dilate, further increasing blood supply to tissue and adding to heat and redness.

10. As dead cells and debris are removed, epithelial cells proliferate and begin to grow under the scab.

11. Scar tissue (connective tissue) replaces cells that cannot replace themselves.

Figure 4.21 Steps in the processes of inflammation and healing.

Beneath the epidermis fibroblasts proliferate and produce fibers, thereby forming new connective tissue called **scar tissue**. Scar tissue replaces damaged muscle and nerve cells, which themselves cannot divide. Though scar tissue is not able to contract (like muscle cells) or carry signals (like nerve cells), it does provide a strong, durable "patch" that allows the remaining normal tissue to function. Deep cuts are often sutured (stitched together) to minimize the amount of scar tissue and prevent disfigurement.

Several factors affect the healing process. The tissues of young people heal more rapidly than those of older people. Their cells divide more quickly, their bodies are generally in a better nutritional state, and their blood circulation is more efficient. As you might guess from the many contributions of blood to healing, good circulation is extremely important. Certain vitamins are also important in the healing process. Vitamin A is essential for the division of epithelial cells, vitamin C is essential for the production of collagen and other components of connective tissue, and vitamin K is required for blood clotting. Vitamin E also may promote healing and reduce the amount of scar tissue formed.

And so, after several days, if everything has gone well, the cut you suffered while slicing vegetables has healed. It's no longer painful, red, or swollen. All that's left of the cut is a very thin scar where your skin has repaired itself—and, hopefully, a reminder to be more careful when using a kitchen knife.

CHAPTER SUMMARY

(Chapter summary points and review questions are numbered to correspond to the numbered objectives in the text of each chapter.)

Definition and Classification of Tissues

1. Define the term tissue and list the four categories of tissues and their major functions.
   a. A tissue is a group of similar cells that work together to perform a particular function.
   b. The four categories of tissues and their major functions are:
      (1) Epithelial tissues, which perform the functions of protection, absorption, and secretion
      (2) Connective tissues, which connect parts of the body and provide support and protection
      (3) Muscle tissues, which contract and make movement possible
      (4) Nervous tissues, which receive and carry signals and provide for responsiveness and communication

Development of Tissues

2. Describe how the three germ layers form from a fertilized egg and name the tissues derived from each layer.
   a. Development proceeds from the fertilized egg to the morula, blastocyst, and embryonic disc.
   b. By the end of the third week of human development, the following three germ layers have become established:
      (1) Ectoderm gives rise to the epithelium of the skin and the nervous system.
      (2) Mesoderm gives rise to connective tissues, muscles, and parts of various internal organs.
      (3) Endoderm gives rise to epithelium that lines various organs and to several glands associated with the digestive tract.

Epithelial Tissues

3. Identify the characteristics of epithelial tissues and explain how these characteristics are related to the location and function of the tissues.
   a. Epithelial tissues:
      (1) form sheets of cells that cover or line organs.
      (2) are capable of mitosis.
      (3) are attached to the underlying connective tissue by a basement membrane.
      (4) are tightly packed together and held to each other by glycoprotein deposits, desmosomes, or tight and intermediate junctions.
      (5) lack blood vessels and so receive nutrients by diffusion.
   b. Epithelial tissues are classified by cell shape and the number of layers of cells.
      (1) Simple epithelia consist of one layer of cells and may be squamous (flattened), cuboidal (cube shaped), or columnar (cylindrical).
      (2) Stratified epithelia consist of more than one layer of cells and are named according to the shape of the outermost layer of cells, which may be squamous, cuboidal, or columnar.
      (3) Pseudostratified epithelia consist of one layer of cells of differing heights.
      (4) Transitional epithelium consists of cells that can change shape.
   c. The structures, locations, and functions of epithelial tissues are summarized in Table 4.2.

4. Distinguish between mucous membranes and serous membranes in terms of structure, function, and location.
   a. Membranes consist of a sheet of epithelium and the underlying connective tissue.
   b. Serous membranes are lubricated by a clear fluid that reduces friction between the surfaces of the internal organs they cover.
   c. Mucous membranes produce mucus and protect the internal surfaces of cavities in the organs of the digestive, reproductive, respiratory, and urinary systems.

5. Distinguish between exocrine and endocrine glands and describe the structure, function, and location of the various exocrine glands.
   a. Glands, structures that produce secretions, include:
      (1) Endocrine glands, which lack ducts and release their secretions into the intercellular fluids.
      (2) Exocrine glands, which have ducts and release their secretions through the ducts to the surface of the organ to which they are attached.
   b. The structure, location, manner of secretion, and examples of secretions for exocrine glands are summarized in Table 4.3.

Connective Tissues

6. List the four classes of connective tissues and describe their major characteristics.
   a. The four classes of connective tissues are blood, connective tissue proper, cartilage, and bone. All consist of cells surrounded by extracellular matrix, which usually contains fibers.
   b. The major characteristics of each class are as follows:
      (1) Blood consists of various types of blood cells in a fluid matrix.
      (2) Connective tissue consists of cells surrounded by a relatively fluid matrix containing several types of fibers.
      (3) Cartilage consists of cells imbedded in a fairly solid but flexible matrix with varying kinds and numbers of fibers.
      (4) Bone consists of cells imbedded in a solid fibrous matrix.

7. Distinguish among the types of connective tissue proper in terms of structure, function, and location.

    a. The characteristics of the types of connective tissue proper are summarized in Table 4.4.

8. Distinguish among the types of cartilage in terms of structure, function, and location.

    a. Cartilage consists of chondrocytes in cavities called lacunae and a matrix of chondroitin sulfate ground substance interspersed with fibers.

    b. The structure, function, and location of various types of cartilage are as follows:

        (1) Hyaline cartilage has thin collagenous fibers and is found in low-stress areas such as the ribs, nose, and respiratory system.

        (2) Elastic cartilage has elastic fibers and is found in the external ear and parts of the respiratory system.

        (3) Fibrous cartilage contains many dense collagenous fibers and is found in high-stress areas such as between vertebrae and on the joint surfaces of bones.

9. Distinguish among the types of bone in terms of structure, function, and location.

    a. Bone consists of osteocytes imbedded in a matrix of organic and inorganic substances.

    b. The structure, function, and location of the two types of bone are as follows:

        (1) Compact bone contains Haversian systems, which carry blood vessels and nerves, lamellae, and canaliculi; it is found on the outer surface of most bones, where it contributes to the strength of the bone.

        (2) Cancellous (spongy) bone is arranged in an irregular meshwork and has trabeculae extending into the marrow cavity; it contributes to the support function of bone while minimizing its weight.

Muscle Tissues

10. Distinguish among the three types of muscle tissues in terms of structure, function, and location.

    a. Skeletal muscle is voluntary, has multinucleated fibers, is striated, and is attached to bones.

    b. Smooth muscle is involuntary, has fibers with one nucleus, is nonstriated, and is found in internal organs.

    c. Cardiac muscle is involuntary, has multinucleated fibers, is striated, and is found only in the heart.

Nervous Tissue

11. Distinguish between neurons and neuroglial cells in terms of structure, function, and location.

    a. Neurons consist of a cell body, an axon, and several dendrites; they carry signals through the nervous system.

    b. Neuroglial cells are of several types; they support, insulate, and maybe help to nourish the neurons.

REVIEW

Important Terms

adipose	histiocyte
blastocyst	lacuna
canaliculi	lamella
cartilage	matrix
chondrocyte	membrane
collagen	mesoderm
columnar	muscle
connective	nerve
cuboidal	neuroglia
ectoderm	neuron
elastin	osteocyte
endocrine	osteon
endoderm	pseudostratified
epithelium	squamous
exocrine	tissue
fibroblast	transitional
goblet cell	

Questions

1. a. Define the term tissue.

    b. List the distinguishing characteristics of each of the four major tissues.

2. Describe the development of the human embryo through the establishment of the three germ layers and list the tissues derived from each layer.

3. a. How are epithelial tissues classified?

    b. Name one example of each type of epithelial tissue and give its function and location.

    c. How are epithelial cells held together?

4. Describe the structure, function, and location of:

    a. Serous membranes

    b. Mucous membranes

5. a. How do endocrine and exocrine glands differ?

    b. How are exocrine glands classified?

    c. Give an example of each type of exocrine gland and describe its structure, location, and secretion.

6. What are the distinguishing characteristics of the four classes of connective tissues?

7. Give an example of each type of connective tissue proper and describe its structure, function, and location.

8. Give an example of each type of cartilage and describe its structure, function, and location.

9. Describe the distinguishing characteristics of compact and of cancellous bone.

10. Describe the structure, function, and location of the three types of muscle tissue.

11. Describe the distinguishing characteristics of neurons and of neuroglial cells.

Problems

1. The absence of any one of the three primary germ layers in an embryo would lead to the death of the embryo. Determine which organs and tissues would be missing if an embryo lacked (a) ectoderm, (b) mesoderm, or (c) endoderm.

2. Design an experiment to determine whether the secretion of a gland is holocrine, apocrine, or merocrine.

3. Use your knowledge of the inflammatory process to explain to a nonscientist the possible effects of taking antihistamines.

REFERENCES AND READINGS

Bloom, W., and Fawcett, D. W. 1975. *Textbook of histology.* Philadelphia: W. B. Saunders.

Copenhaver, W. M., Kelly, D. E., and Wood, R. L. 1978. *Bailey's textbook of histology* (17th ed.). Baltimore, Md.: Williams and Wilkins.

Eyre, D. R. 1980. Collagen: Molecular diversity in the body's protein scaffold. *Science* 207:1315 (March 21).

Hertzberg, E. L., Lawrence, T. S., and Gilula, N. B. 1981. Gap junctional communication. *Annual Review of Physiology* 43:479.

Kuehl, F. A., and Egan, R. W. 1980. Prostaglandins, arachidonic acid, and inflammation. *Science* 210:978 (November 28).

Satir, B. 1975. The final steps in secretion. *Scientific American* 233(4):29 (October).

Staehelin, L. A., and Hull, B. E. 1978. Junctions between living cells. *Scientific American* 238(5):141 (May).

UNIT TWO

PROTECTION, MOVEMENT, AND SUPPORT

Now that you are familiar with the levels of organization in the body from the chemical level to the tissue level, you are ready to study the organ systems of the body. This unit will deal with the skin or integumentary system, the skeletal system, including the joints, and the muscular system. Each of these systems is involved in performing one or more of the functions of protection, movement, and support: The skin protects; the skeletal system offers both protection and support; and the muscular system, with its connections to the skeletal system, provides movement. The discussions of these systems will emphasize the relationship between structure and function and show how each system contributes to the maintenance of homeostasis.

5

THE SKIN

ORGANIZATION AND GENERAL FUNCTIONS

Objective 1. Describe the organization and general functions of the skin.

The integumentary system consists of a single organ—the skin, and the skin derivatives—hair, skin glands, and nails. Your skin separates you from the rest of the world. It covers the entire body and is the largest organ in the body, accounting for about 15 percent of total body weight. In an adult the skin has a surface area of about 1.8 square meters and varies in thickness from 0.5 millimeters on the eyelids to 5 millimeters on the back between the scapulae (shoulder blades).

The skin has two main parts, the outer **epidermis** and the inner **dermis**. These layers are tightly fastened together, and the dermis is bound to underlying muscles by the subcutaneous layer of connective tissue. (The word roots *derm* and *cut* refer to the skin. Thus, the term subcutaneous means beneath the skin.) The dermis is usually much thicker than the epidermis, but where heavy calluses have formed in response to pressure or rubbing, the epidermis is thicker than the dermis.

The skin protects underlying structures against abrasion and dehydration, and its glands allow fluid loss during sweating. By regulating the amount of sweating and the amount of blood flowing through the dermal blood vessels, the skin also helps to regulate body temperature and maintain homeostasis. The pigment melanin in the skin helps to protect against ultraviolet radiation. The millions of sensory receptors in the skin contribute to homeostasis by receiving stimuli from the environment, to which the body makes appropriate responses. (These sensory receptors will be described in Chapter 14.) Finally, the skin is instrumental in synthesizing vitamin D and other compounds and may play a role in absorbing substances from the environment.

DEVELOPMENT

Objective 2. Describe the development of the ectodermal and the mesodermal components of the skin.

In Chapter 4 the embryonic germ layers ectoderm, mesoderm, and endoderm were described. The outer, or ectodermal, layer of the embryo gives rise to the epidermis of the skin. During the first seven weeks of development the epidermis consists of a single layer of cells; at birth it has become many layers. All of the derivatives of skin—hair, nails, and glands—come from ectoderm. Though they lie in the dermis, the sensory receptors too are derived from the neural portion of the ectodermal layer.

The middle, or mesodermal, layer of the embryo gives rise to the dermis. Early in embryonic development blocks of mesoderm called **somites** develop between the ectoderm and endoderm. From each somite three kinds of tissues differentiate. One of these, the dermatome, gives rise to the dermis of the skin. The other two, the myotome and the sclerotome, give rise to the muscles and bones, respectively (Figure 5.1). Though the dermis first appears as isolated blocks of tissue, these blocks grow together to form a complete layer of tissue beneath the epidermis.

TISSUES

Objective 3. Describe the structure of the epidermis and the dermis.

Objective 4. Distinguish between thick skin and thin skin.

The epidermis and the dermis fit together in a wavy configuration similar to the middle layer of a piece of corrugated cardboard. Figure 5.2 provides an overview of the structure of skin. Labeled structures will be discussed later in this chapter. The border between the dermis and the underlying subcutaneous tissue is less distinct than that between the epidermis and the dermis. The subcutaneous tissue consists of loose connective tissue containing adipose (fat) cells and is not considered part of the skin. Though hair follicles and glands extend into the dermis, they are derived from epidermis.

Epidermis

As mentioned in Chapter 4, epidermis is composed of stratified squamous epithelium. It contains four, or in thick skin five, different strata as explained below (Figure 5.3). The deepest cells that lie next to the dermis—termed the **stratum basale**—divide throughout life, pushing the cells above

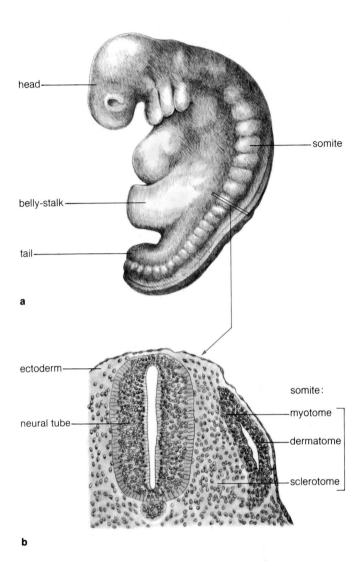

Figure 5.1 (**a**) Development of somites, shown in a whole mount of a four-week-old human embryo, × 20, (**b**) the components of somites, shown in transverse section, × 100.

them toward the surface. The cells moving toward the surface take on the characteristics of each successive stratum, eventually being sloughed off at the same rate that new cells grow. Complete renewal of the epidermis takes from fifteen to thirty days, depending on the area of the body and the age of the individual. (The rate of renewal decreases with age.)

The cells of the stratum basale lie on a basement membrane immediately next to the top portion of the dermis. Interspersed among these cells are **melanocytes**, cells capable of synthesizing the pigment **melanin**. (The formation and function of pigment will be discussed later.)

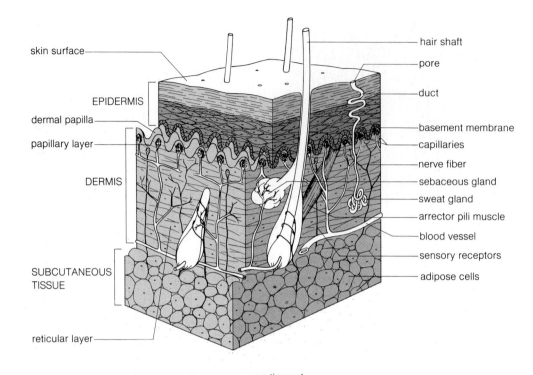

skin surface

hair shaft

pore

EPIDERMIS

duct

dermal papilla

basement membrane

papillary layer

capillaries

nerve fiber

DERMIS

sebaceous gland

sweat gland

arrector pili muscle

blood vessel

sensory receptors

SUBCUTANEOUS
TISSUE

adipose cells

reticular layer

a

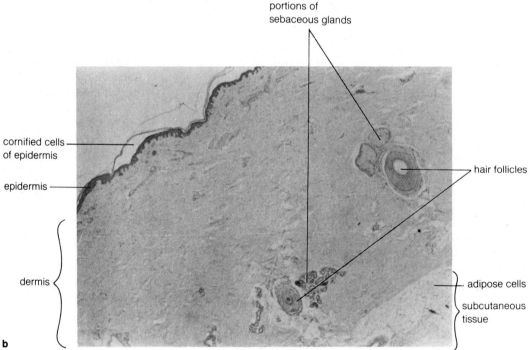

portions of
sebaceous glands

cornified cells
of epidermis

epidermis

hair follicles

dermis

adipose cells

subcutaneous
tissue

b

Figure 5.2 Structures found in thin skin: (**a**) diagrammatically represented, × 10, (**b**) photomicrograph × 21. (Photograph by author.)

The **stratum spinosum** contains many-sided cells arranged in eight to ten layers. The name spinosum derives from the fact that these cells shrink and take on a spiny appearance as they are prepared for microscopic observation. Spinosum cells have oval nuclei, and their cytoplasm contains small fibers of a protein destined eventually to become the waterproofing protein **keratin**. Though most cell division takes place in the stratum basale, some cell division occurs in the stratum spinosum. Thus, these two layers are sometimes referred to collectively as the **stratum germinativum**.

The two or three layers of cells in the **stratum granulo-**

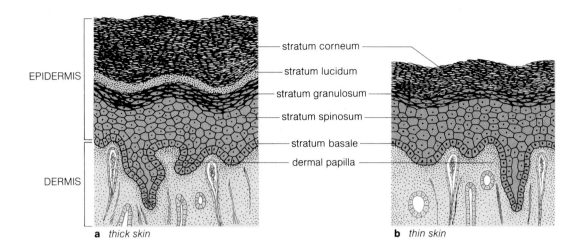

stratum corneum
stratum lucidum
stratum granulosum
stratum spinosum
stratum basale
dermal papilla

DERMIS

a *thick skin*

b *thin skin*

Figure 5.3 A comparison of (**a**) thick skin and (**b**) thin skin.

sum are somewhat flattened. They contain darkly staining granules of **keratohyaline** derived from the protein in the lower layer.

The **stratum lucidum**, composed of flattened nonnucleated cells, is apparent only in thick skin such as that found on the palms of the hands and the soles of the feet. This layer gives such skin its translucent appearance because of the presence within it of **eleidin**, another intermediate substance produced in the development of keratin.

The **stratum corneum** consists of twenty-five or more layers of dry, squamous cells. Dead cells in the upper layers are constantly being shed from the surface; those that remain have lost their nuclei and are filled with keratin. The loss of the nucleus leads to the death of the cells; the presence of large amounts of keratin provides a barrier against water entering or leaving the body. These cells also provide a mechanical barrier against light waves, bacteria, and other substances entering the body.

The epidermis contains no blood vessels and few nerve endings (sensory receptors). Cells are nourished by nutrients diffusing from blood vessels in the dermis; as nutrients can diffuse only short distances, the uppermost cells literally may starve to death. Accumulation of keratin in these cells may also contribute to their death, though the reason for this is not clear. Because most nerve endings are imbedded in the dermis, stimuli from the environment such as pressure, heat, and cold must pass through the epidermis. A few nerve endings that respond to touch and pain extend into the epidermis and so are more easily stimulated.

The terms **thin skin** and **thick skin** refer primarily to the number of layers and relative thickness of the epidermis. Hair follicles are present only in thin skin. The stratum lucidum is apparent only in thick skin, though some histologists believe that with proper microscopic techniques thin

skin may eventually be shown to have a thin layer of lucidum. The stratum granulosum may also be reduced in thin skin, and the stratum corneum may be quite delicate. Most of the body is covered with thin skin; only the palms of the hands and the soles of the feet are covered with thick skin. Skin technically classified as thin skin may in fact be thicker than skin classified as thick skin. This occurs when thin skin contains an unusually thick layer of dermis, as is found in the skin of the back. Any thin skin subjected to pressure or abrasion can take on the characteristics of thick skin as the rate of mitosis in the basal layer increases. Such areas are called calluses.

Dermis

The dermis lies in close association with the epidermis. Being a connective tissue, the dermis has an intercellular matrix. Some of this matrix forms part of the **basement membrane** that helps hold the epidermis and dermis together. The epidermis also secretes a portion of the basement membrane. Dermal papillae, shown in Figure 5.2, project into folds in the epidermis in a tongue-and-groove arrangement that helps to hold the dermis and epidermis together. The dermal papillae also create the ridges that constitute fingerprints and footprints. In the tanning of leather the epidermis is removed from the dermis, leaving the toughened dermis that constitutes leather.

The dermis is divided into two layers, the **papillary layer** and the **reticular layer** (see Figure 5.2). In addition to the papillae the papillary layer contains capillaries and nerve endings (sensory receptors). Extending into the reticular layer are sebaceous (oil) glands, sweat glands, hair follicles, and many blood vessels and nerve endings. Both the papillary and reticular layers consist of dense connective

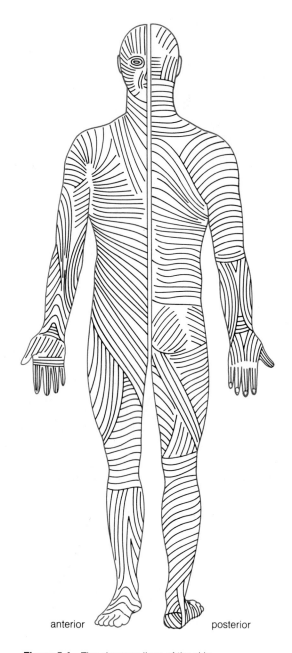

anterior   posterior

Figure 5.4 The cleavage lines of the skin.

tissue in which the collagen and elastic fibers run in all directions. The reticular layer is thicker and contains more fibers than the papillary layer. In addition to the fibers running in different directions, some of the collagen fibers in the reticular layer are organized into bundles of fibers running in the same direction. Separations between these bundles form cleavage lines in the skin (Figure 5.4). Surgeons generally make incisions along these lines because

such incisions are less likely to gape and therefore will heal more rapidly.

The reticular layer varies in thickness according to the amount of fat it contains. No clear line of demarcation exists between the reticular layer of the dermis and the subcutaneous connective tissue beneath it. Both have adipose tissue interspersed within them, and the amount of fat in the tissue increases with depth beneath the surface. Because the **fatty subcutaneous** tissue is loosely packed, it allows for the injection of fluids containing medications.

Both stretching and aging affect the dermis. During pregnancy or a period of excessive weight gain, the dermis stretches and can be ruptured. The rupture of the dermis leaves thin lines visible through the epidermis, often referred to as stretch marks. During aging the number of elastic fibers in the dermis decreases, causing the ratio of collagen to elastic fibers to increase and the elasticity of the skin to decrease. Reduced elasticity leads to sagging of the skin and formation of wrinkles. The degree of elasticity can be observed by pinching the back of the hand and observing the time required for the skin to return to its normal position.

PHYSIOLOGY

Objective 5. Explain the role of the skin in each of the following functions: protection, pigment formation, temperature regulation, absorption, synthesis, and sensory reception.

Your skin is subjected to the influences of a host of factors in the external environment—microorganisms, toxic substances, and other objects that touch, abrade, and tear it; sunlight, heat, cold, wind, rain; even radiation from outer space. The skin performs a variety of functions that prevent these factors from upsetting the homeostatic balance inside the body. It acts as a barrier to most substances in the environment, but it can selectively absorb a few substances. It receives stimuli interpreted in the brain as touch, pressure, hot, cold, and pain. The body's responses to these stimuli help to regulate body temperature and to avoid injury. Should an injury occur, the skin undergoes an inflammatory reaction (described in Chapter 4) and repairs the damage done to it. The skin even makes use of sunlight to synthesize vitamin D.

Protection

The skin provides at least three barriers to invasion of the body. Though the surface of the skin is teeming with microorganisms that tend to feed upon the skin's secretions, intact skin prevents these organisms and other foreign substances in the environment from entering the body. Some of the secretions consumed by the microorganisms are poisonous to them and have a bacteriocidal effect. Thus, the surface of the skin serves as a barrier both mechanically and chemically. The waterproof layer of keratin in the outer cells provides a second barrier. Finally, the basement membrane, a combination of protein-polysaccharide secretions of epithelial cells and matrix of dermal connective tissue, provides yet another barrier against substances entering the body.

Pigment Formation and Skin Color

As mentioned earlier, the pigment melanin is produced by melanocytes found in the stratum basale. Though blood circulating in the blood vessels of the dermis contributes to the color of the skin, the amount and distribution of melanin is a significant factor in skin color. As melanocytes produce melanin, some of it is released and phagocytized by epithelial cells.

To some extent sunlight stimulates melanin production. Ultraviolet radiation can damage cells, as you know if you have ever had a painful sunburn. Melanin absorbs some of this radiation, as well as visible light, so increased melanin production in the epidermis protects underlying tissues.

Genetic factors contribute significantly to the natural color of the skin. The number of melanocytes in the skin is the same for all races, but the amount of melanin produced by those cells varies. Greater amounts of melanin result in darker skin, and the amount of melanin produced is determined by several genes. Albinos lack one of the genes necessary for the manufacture of melanin, so their bodies lack this pigment altogether. In most races melanin is found only in the strata basale, spinosum, and granulosum; in blacks epithelial cells carry melanin to all strata. Another pigment, **carotene**, found in the upper layers of the epidermis, is responsible for yellow skin tones.

Blood circulating in the dermis accounts for the pinkness of the skin most visible in lighter skinned people. When blood vessels are dilated and more blood passes through the dermis, the skin reddens appreciably. Blood vessels in the skin dilate under at least two conditions: If you have been exercising strenuously, your body temperature increases, and blood vessels dilate as a part of the reaction that lowers your body temperature. If you have become embarrassed, your body's emotional response causes the blood vessels of your face to dilate, and you are said to be blushing.

Exposure to the sun may produce a deep tan in light-skinned individuals, but it also dries the skin and increases the risk of skin cancer. In addition, ultraviolet rays increase the rate at which elastic fibers are lost and hence accelerate the aging of the skin. Each summer tan brings closer the day of dry skin and wrinkles.

Temperature Regulation

Skin plays an important role in the regulation of body temperature (Figure 5.5). As we have seen, the maintenance of human body temperature near 37°C is an example of a homeostatic mechanism; such maintenance requires that the amount of heat produced by the body be balanced by the same amount of heat loss.

Body heat comes from cellular metabolism, particularly that of muscle cells. When the cells are very active, they give off great quantities of heat. Consider, for example, what happens when you run a mile or two. Your leg muscles are working hard and producing a large amount of heat. The temperature of your blood rises, and the rise is detected by temperature sensors in your brain. Your brain signals your skin to change in two ways. First, the blood vessels near the skin surface dilate. Warm blood passing through these dilated vessels conducts heat to the epidermis. The heat then radiates into the cooler environment like heat from an automobile radiator, and the blood cools, just like the water in the radiator. Second, your skin releases large amounts of sweat. The sweat lying on the surface of the skin evaporates, drawing large quantities of heat from the body. In fact, sweating is the main mechanism for heat loss. All the while, your skin surface gives off heat to passing air currents by a process called convection. In summary, then, the excess heat produced by running is lost in four ways: conduction and radiation from the dilated blood vessels, evaporation of sweat, and convection of heat from the skin surface to air currents. These functions of the skin prevent your body from overheating when you run or perform other strenuous exercise.

When you stop running, of course, less heat is produced because your cells slow down their metabolic rate. Your brain sensors detect the falling temperature of the blood and signal a decrease in the diameter of the skin blood vessels and a cessation of sweating.

Heat loss may go too far. Suppose you have finished running and are covered with sweat, but you fail to put on a jacket. Soon, because sweat continues to evaporate on your

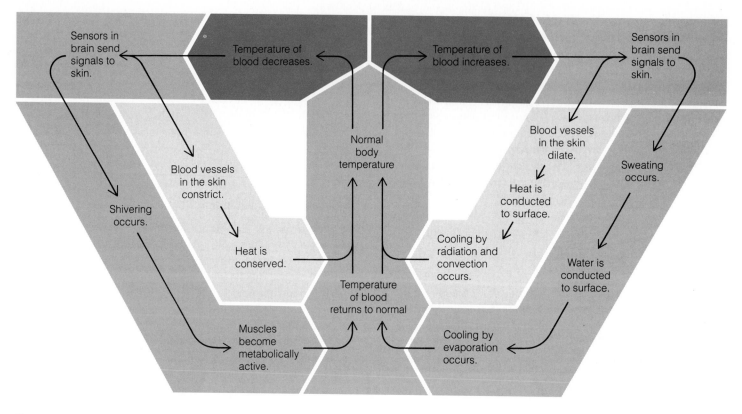

Figure 5.5 Regulation of body temperature.

skin, you will begin to feel chilled. As your blood cools, other brain sensors come into play. They send two signals: One constricts the blood vessels in your skin—in effect, shutting off the radiator. The other starts the muscles shivering—increasing cellular metabolism and raising body heat. Small involuntary, smooth muscles attached to the hair follicles, the **arrector pili**, erect the hairs away from the surface of the skin, making goose flesh (see box on p. 16).

Absorption

Though absorption of materials through the human skin is limited by the protective barriers already described, small quantities of a few substances do manage to enter the blood stream by cutaneous (through the skin) absorption. Small molecules of gases such as oxygen and carbon dioxide can diffuse through the normal barriers, as can fat-soluble vitamins (A, D, E, and K) and certain steroid hormones (cortisol). Absorption of fat-soluble substances is possible because they dissolve in the fatty materials in the skin, particularly in the secretions of the sebaceous glands (discussed

in a later section). It may be that absorption is almost entirely through these glands. Some toxic substances, such as insecticides, can be absorbed through the skin. However, absorption through the skin is not a significant avenue of entry into the body for most substances.

Synthesis

The skin synthesizes a number of substances that remain in the skin—keratin, melanin, and carotene. In addition, skin contains a substance—dehydrocholesterol—from which it synthesizes vitamin D in the presence of ultraviolet light. (Small amounts of ultraviolet light—far short of that required for a sunburn—are sufficient.) Once synthesized, vitamin D enters the blood and helps to regulate calcium and phosphorus metabolism; thus it is essential for the development of strong bones. Children who are exposed to adequate amounts of sunshine require smaller amounts of vitamin D in their diets than those who aren't exposed to the sun. Those who receive vitamin D neither in their diets nor

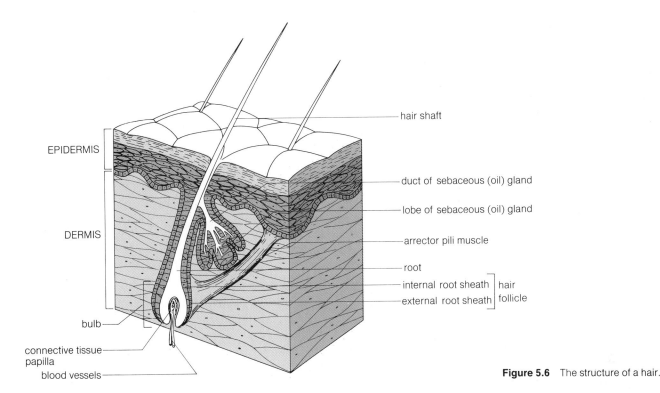

EPIDERMIS

DERMIS

bulb

connective tissue papilla

blood vessels

hair shaft

duct of sebaceous (oil) gland

lobe of sebaceous (oil) gland

arrector pili muscle

root

internal root sheath ⎤ hair
external root sheath ⎦ follicle

Figure 5.6   The structure of a hair.

through exposure to sunlight develop a vitamin deficiency disease called rickets. This disease is discussed in the next chapter.

Sensory Reception

Large numbers of various sensory receptors are located in the skin, where they play an important role in detecting changes in the environment. They are discussed in Chapter 14.

DERIVATIVES OF THE SKIN

Objective 6. Describe the structure and function of the following derivatives of the skin: hair, nails, sebaceous glands, and sweat glands.

Though the skin is a single large organ, it has within it or on its surface several different structures—hair, fingernails, toenails, sweat glands, and sebaceous, or oil, glands. Even the mammary glands are highly specialized sweat glands. (They will be considered in Chapter 28.) We call these structures skin derivatives because they develop from the epidermis of the skin.

Hair

In humans hair is largely a vestigial structure; that is, it remains from an earlier evolutionary state but serves little or no function. Though your entire body is covered with **hairs**, or **pili**, except for the palms of your hands and the soles of your feet, most of that hair is not functional. Scalp hair does protect the scalp from overexposure to the sun's rays, and eyelashes and tiny hairs inside the nose and ear canals help to prevent foreign particles from entering those organs.

Each hair (Figure 5.6) consists of a **hair shaft** that extends beyond the skin surface and a **hair root** that lies within the hair follicle. The **hair follicle** itself consists of epidermis that has grown down into the dermis to surround a connective tissue papilla. This epithelial tissue is arranged in two layers, the internal and external sheaths. A sebaceous gland and a small arrector pili muscle are associated with each hair follicle. The function of the muscle was explained in the discussion of temperature regulation; the function of the sebaceous gland will be discussed later.

Cells of the stratum basale in the hair bulb divide to produce new hair cells, and the hair is pushed up through the follicle by the basal growth. Growth normally occurs at an average rate of 0.3 millimeters per day. Blood vessels at the base of the hair bulb provide nourishment for the hair cells. Nutrients diffuse upward through the follicle but never reach the ends of a long hair. Therefore, the shaft of hair consists of dead cells, and loss of hair occurs by breaking of the shaft. (All of the rinses and conditioners we use on our scalp hair are applied to dead tissues.) As many as a hundred hairs are lost from the scalp per day, but those hairs are continuously replaced by regrowth of hair in the follicles. When hair fails to grow from follicles in certain areas of the scalp, baldness results. Baldness may be caused by genetic factors, hormonal imbalances, scalp injuries and diseases, and dietary deficiencies.

Straight hairs are symmetrically round, while curly hairs are somewhat flattened. The shape of hair is genetically determined.

Hair color is determined by the amount of pigment (melanin) deposited in the shaft of the hair. In cross-section a hair appears as a hollow tube with pigment deposited in the walls and spaces. Dark hair has a large amount of melanin, blond hair has a small amount, and red hair has an intermediate amount. Hair appears white because the cells in the hair bulb fail to produce pigment. In the absence of pigment the light is reflected from the air spaces within the hair. Hair appears gray because of a mixture of pigmented and white hairs.

Because hair contains concentrations of trace elements as great as ten times that found in blood or urine, hair is a potentially useful material for diagnostic tests. Heavy metals such as lead, arsenic, cadmium, and mercury are concentrated in the hair of individuals exposed to these toxic substances. Various pathological (disease-producing) conditions lead to abnormal concentrations of substances in the hair—for example, an excess of sodium and a deficiency of calcium in children with cystic fibrosis, a deficiency of magnesium and calcium in those with phenylketonuria, and a deficiency of zinc in malnourished individuals. (These conditions are discussed in Chapter 24.)

Nails

A **nail** (Figure 5.7) consists of a **nail plate** attached to a **nail bed** and partially covered at its proximal end by **cuticle**. Adjacent to the cuticle is the **lunula** (little moon), a thick white part of the nail. The lunula appears white and the remainder of the nail pink because the thickness of the lunula obscures the blood in the vessels of the underlying connective tissue while the remainder of the nail allows the blood to show through. Nails consist of modified, highly

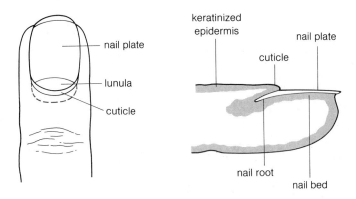

Figure 5.7 The structure of a nail: (**a**) top external view, (**b**) side internal view.

keratinized cells of the stratum corneum. Nail growth occurs by division of cells beneath the cuticle at the base of the nail. As a nail grows, cells are transformed into true nail cells, and the existing nail is pushed distally at a rate of about 2 millimeters per month. Nails help to protect the fingers and toes, and humans sometimes use nails for such functions as picking up small objects.

Sebaceous Glands

Most **sebaceous glands** are associated with hair follicles (see Figure 5.6); they are found all over the body surface wherever there is hair. They are simple, branched alveolar glands that produce an oily, holocrine secretion called **sebum**. Sebum, which consists mainly of lipids, helps to keep hairs soft, pliable, and waterproof. Regular brushing of hair helps to spread the sebum to the ends of the hairs, giving them a natural sheen.

Sweat Glands

Sweat glands are of two types, merocrine and apocrine. The merocrine, or excretory, sweat glands are widely distributed over the surface of the body. They produce a watery, merocrine secretion that is important in temperature regulation. Apocrine sweat glands are found mainly in the armpits and groin area. They produce a white, cloudy, apocrine secretion, which contains organic substances that give rise to odor. Emotional stimuli lead to the release of apocrine sweat. All sweat glands are simple, coiled tubular, exocrine glands like the one shown in Figure 5.2. Sweat from merocrine glands is conducted to the surface by way of a duct and emptied through a pore in the skin; sweat from apocrine glands is released into a hair follicle.

CLINICAL APPLICATIONS

Objective 7. Describe how the physiology of the skin is altered by acne and other lesions.

Acne

Acne affects over 80 percent of teenagers sometime between puberty and early adulthood; it sometimes affects older adults as well. It is caused by the action of male sex hormones on sebaceous glands. These hormones are produced by the adrenal glands as well as the testes, so both males and females can be affected. During adolescence higher hormone concentrations cause the sebaceous glands to increase in size and to produce more sebum. When sebum accumulates in excess, microorganisms feed upon the secretions. The duct of the gland or the surrounding skin surface becomes infected and inflamed.

Acne occurs in varying degrees of severity (Figure 5.8). The least severe is a "blackhead," in which the hair follicle and associated sebaceous gland become plugged with keratin and excessive secretions. The plugged duct may rupture, releasing the secretions into the surrounding tissues, causing a break in the skin and initiating an inflammatory reaction. Bacteria infect the area and cause more inflammation. If the condition increases in severity, more tissue destruction and scarring occur. Finally, in the most severe cases, lesions extend over many parts of the body, and some of the lesions become encysted in connective tissue.

Treatment includes frequent cleansing of the skin and the use of topical medications to reduce the risk of infection. Sometimes individuals affected by acne are advised to avoid fatty foods, but the connection between diet and sebum production is not at all well established. Dermatologists often prescribe topical antibiotics or low dosages of oral antibiotics in an attempt to reduce the likelihood of bacterial infections. Continuous use of an oral antibiotic over a long period of time depletes natural intestinal flora; continuous use of any antibiotic may lead to the development of antibiotic-resistant strains of bacteria. A new experimental chemical, *cis*-retinoic acid, has been tested on small groups of individuals suffering from severe and persistent acne with good results. The chemical seems to work by inhibiting sebum production, and its effects seem to last for several months after treatment has been terminated.

In most cases acne disappears or decreases in severity as the body adjusts to the hormonal changes of puberty, and homeostasis is reestablished in the functioning of the sebaceous glands.

Other Skin Lesions

Skin lesions (breaks in the continuity of the skin) can result from infections, irritations, or impaired circulation of the blood to the skin, as well as being symptoms of certain diseases. Some common types of skin lesions are described below.

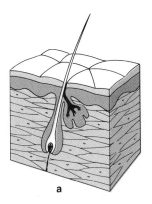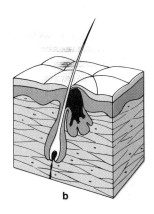

a   b

Figure 5.8 Acne begins with (**a**) a "blackhead," in which the duct of a sebaceous gland is plugged with excessive secretions. (**b**) Some blackheads become infected with microorganisms, inflamed, and filled with pus.

Impetigo is a bacterial infection of the skin, usually caused by streptococcus or staphylococcus. The body's inflammatory reaction produces pus-filled bumps, or pustules, on the skin's surface. Impetigo, which is easily spread if the pustules are scratched, is treated with antibiotics.

Measles and **chickenpox** are viral infections involving the whole body. Measles produces a dry rash, and chickenpox causes pustule formation; both diseases also have other effects on the body. No cure exists for these diseases. Measles vaccine is given to many young children, and if its use becomes worldwide, the disease might be eradicated.

Eczema lesions are patches of reddened, raw, watery skin. Irritation is thought to be one of the causes, but it is likely that eczema is a sign of another disorder, such as hypersensitivity to some substance, rather than a disease in itself.

Decubitus ulcers (bedsores) are caused by a combination of irritation and lack of blood circulation. Without sufficient blood flow in the dermis, the epidermis starts to die of starvation, resulting in open sores. Bedridden individuals are particularly susceptible to these lesions; their occurrence and severity can be reduced by frequent changes of position and massage to stimulate increased blood flow to affected areas.

Dermatitis, meaning skin inflammation, is a symptom of a variety of allergies and other diseases, including pellagra and other vitamin-deficiency diseases. Treatment is generally directed at identifying and correcting the problem that caused the dermatitis.

Clinical Terms

abrasion (ab-ra'zhun)   rubbing or scraping off of skin or mucous membrane

athlete's foot   a superficial fungus infection of the skin of the foot

bulla (bul'ah)   a large blister or fluid-filled vesicle

carbuncle (kar'bun-kl)   an inflammation of subcutaneous tissue that eventually discharges pus

contusion (kon-tu'zhun)   a bruise

crust   a layer of solid matter formed by dried secretions

cyst (sist)   a sac filled with liquid or semisolid material

dermatology (der-mat-ol'o-je)   the study of diseases of the skin

erythema (er-ith-e'mah)   redness of the skin due to inflammation and engorgement of capillaries

excoriation (ex-ko-re-a'shun)   loss of superficial skin, often by scratching

fissure (fish'ūr)   a groove or cleft; a crack in the skin

keloid (ke'loid)   a growth of dense tissue often appearing during the healing of an injury to the skin

keratolytic (ker"at-o-lit'ik)   pertaining to a substance that dissolves keratin

macule (mak'ūl)   a discolored spot on the skin

nevus (ne'vus)   a new growth of skin of congenital origin; a birthmark

nodule (nod'ūl)   a small swelling or protruberance

papule (pap'ūl)   a small, solid elevation on the skin

petechia (pe-te'ke-ah)   a small red spot formed by the effusion of blood into the skin

pruritis (pru-ri'tis)   intense itching

psoriasis (so-ri'as-is)   a skin disorder consisting of scaly red patches

pustule (pus'tūl)   a small, pus-filled elevation

vesicle (ves'ik-l)   a small, fluid-filled sac, a small blister

wart   a nonmalignant epithelial growth caused by a virus

Essay: Burns

Do you remember the last time you accidentally touched a hot object or stayed too long in the sun? Your life probably was not endangered, but you did suffer severe pain. Serious burns can be life threatening, and the treatment of burns is a complex medical problem. Each year in the United States approximately 75,000 people are hospitalized for severe burns involving 30 percent or more of the body surface. Of these, 30,000 require hospital stays in intensive care units. Even with intensive care over 10,000 people die of burns annually, making burns the third leading cause of accidental death. One-third of these victims are children under the age of fifteen.

Burns may be caused by exposing the skin to heat, or to chemicals, electricity, or radiation. All these agents destroy proteins and cause cells to die. Heat causes damage by denaturing (rearranging the structure of) proteins. Chemicals react with molecules in the skin and damage the tissue. Electricity and radiation introduce energy into complex molecules and cause damage by rearranging those molecules. Radiation is particularly dangerous because it can cause a burn without a sensation of pain. This is one reason people can become sunburned so severely: It doesn't hurt while it's happening—only later on as the body responds to the damage.

The severity of a burn is determined by the degree of destruction of epithelial cells, although the terminology of "degrees" is now obsolete. In **partial-thickness burns**, some of the stratum basale remains. Its cells divide and replace the epidermis that was lost. In **full-thickness burns** the stratum basale is completely destroyed. Because no epithelial cells capable of dividing remain, skin grafts are necessary to repair the damage of the burn.

For convenience the extent of burns is estimated by the "rule of nines" (Figure 5.9), in which the surface area of the body is divided into areas that each account for about 9 percent of the area (or a multiple of 9 percent). Together these areas account for 100 percent of the body surface. Being able to estimate the percent of surface area damaged is important in determining how much fluid a burned person needs to replace that lost from damaged tissues.

In addition to the local effects of burns, systemic effects (effects to the body as a whole) also occur in severe burns. Because the body's protective covering is destroyed, large amounts of fluid seep out, as noted above. Because blood vessels are damaged, proteins as well as fluid are lost from the blood, thereby reducing the blood volume and eventually leading to shock. (Shock is a condition in which adequate amounts of blood fail to circulate to the tissues.) Urine production decreases, and wastes may accumulate in the tissues. Moreover, the risk of infection is very high because the natural barrier to infection, the skin, has been destroyed.

One problem in burn treatment has been the removal of

eschar, the dead skin that covers a severely burned area. Until recently this tissue was allowed to separate from the burned area spontaneously over a period of several weeks. Now it is possible to remove it surgically and to replace it with skin grafts within a few days of the injury. Use of a laser scalpel reduces blood loss from the surgical removal of eschar because it cauterizes blood vessels as the incision is made.

In areas where tissue destruction includes or goes beyond the stratum basale of the epidermis, new skin cannot grow back. In skin grafting thin sheets of healthy epidermis from an uninjured region of the body are moved to the burned area, where they can proliferate and protect the underlying tissues. In addition, skin grafts can be a temporary means of preventing fluid loss and infection. For this short-term purpose sheets of skin from other mammals as well as from other humans can be used.

In some cases where burning has destroyed large areas of skin, it's not possible to use the burn victim's own epidermis for grafts. However, the body's immune system recognizes and rejects skin from donors as foreign. Researchers have developed a synthetic, or artificial, skin made from carbohydrates and protein fibers from cattle that does not seem to be recognized as foreign by the immune systems of recipients. As a result, the artificial skin can be used to prevent fluid loss and can serve as a base for the recipient's fibroblasts to grow into, forming a new protective layer of scar tissue to replace the destroyed skin.

It has long been known that burn victims often suffer from malnutrition. They are under great stress as their bodies maintain a hypermetabolic state (a higher than normal metabolic rate) and their skin cells undergo rapid division. Current research is directed toward increasing the calories consumed by burn victims. A by-product of that research is a greater understanding of the regulation of metabolism.

A variety of other research efforts are directed toward controlling infection, preventing rejection of skin grafts, and regulating blood volume and cardiac output. For example, a burned person can be placed inside a plastic isolation tent to prevent exposure to airborne bacteria. Proper temperature and humidity can be maintained in the filtered air that passes through the tent. Controlling air temperature helps to regulate body temperature, and controlling humidity helps to prevent fluid loss. Thus, the individual is protected from three of the hazards that contribute to mortality in burn patients—infection, failure of the body's temperature-regulating mechanism, and excessive fluid loss.

Much research is directed toward improving care for burn victims and increasing our understanding of the biological processes of wound healing. Although mortality from deep and extensive burns is still fairly high (two out of fifteen), burn treatment centers around the nation report a 33 to 50 percent improvement in survival over the past two decades.

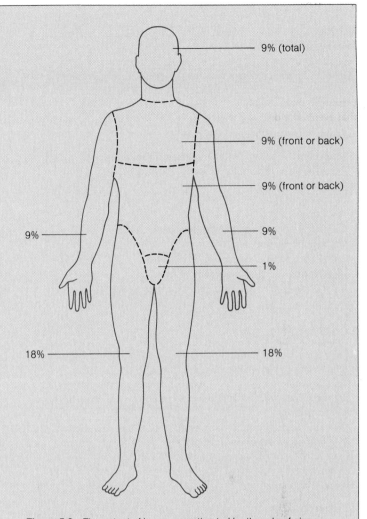

Figure 5.9   The extent of burns, as estimated by the rule of nines.

CHAPTER SUMMARY

(Chapter summary points and review questions are numbered to correspond to the numbered objectives in the text of each chapter.)

Organization and General Functions

1. Describe the organization and general functions of the skin.
  a. The skin, or integumentary system, consists of two main parts:
    (1) epidermis
    (2) dermis
  b. The primary functions of the skin include:
    (1) protection
    (2) prevention of excessive fluid loss
    (3) regulation of body temperature
    (4) reception of stimuli from the environment

Development

2. Describe the development of the ectodermal and the mesodermal components of the skin.
  a. The epidermis of the skin, skin derivatives (hair, nails, and glands), and the sensory receptors are derived from ectoderm.
  b. The dermis of the skin is derived from the dermatome portion of the mesoderm.

Tissues

3. Describe the structure of the epidermis and the dermis.
  a. The epidermis consists of many layers of cells.
    (1) The innermost layer, the stratum basale, continuously undergoes mitosis.
    (2) Cells move outward and are transformed as they become part of each of the outer layers.
    (3) The outermost layer, the stratum corneum, consists of dead cells filled with the waterproof substance keratin.
  b. The dermis lies beneath the epidermis and consists of:
    (1) The papillary layer, where the dermal papillae project into folds in the epidermis
    (2) The reticular layer, where fibers and fat cells are found
    (3) The blood vessels and nerves, which are distributed within the dermis

4. Distinguish between thick skin and thin skin.
  Thin skin differs from thick skin in that the former has no stratum lucidum, the stratum granulosum is reduced in thickness, and hair follicles are present.

Physiology

5. Explain the role of the skin in each of the following functions: protection, pigment formation, temperature regulation, absorption, synthesis, and sensory reception.
  a. The skin protects the body with:
    (1) antiseptic secretions
    (2) a waterproof outer layer
    (3) a basement membrane between the epidermis and the dermis
  b. Pigments protect the skin from excessive radiation from the sun and also determine the color of the skin and hair.
  c. The skin is involved in temperature regulation as follows:
    (1) Excess heat is removed by conduction of heat from the blood vessels to the surface, where it is lost by radiation and convection, and by the production of sweat, which cools the skin as it evaporates.
    (2) Heat is conserved when the above processes are prevented from occurring.
  d. The skin also allows for:
    (1) the absorption of a few substances
    (2) the synthesis of keratin, melanin, and vitamin D
    (3) the reception of sensations

Derivatives of the Skin

6. Describe the structure and function of the following derivatives of the skin: hair, nails, sebaceous glands, and sweat glands.
  a. Hair grows in epidermal follicles and protects the body from radiation and from the entry of foreign objects into sense organs.
  b. Nails consist of modified stratum corneum. They are of limited function in humans.
  c. Sebaceous glands are associated with hair follicles and produce an oily secretion called sebum.
  d. Sweat glands are of two types:
    (1) Merocrine sweat glands, found all over the body, produce watery, merocrine secretions and assist in temperature regulation.
    (2) Apocrine sweat glands, found in the armpits and groin, produce apocrine secretions.

Clinical Applications

7. Describe how the physiology of the skin is altered by acne and other lesions.
  a. Acne is a skin lesion affecting 80 percent of teenagers. It is caused by male sex hormones stimulating the activity of sebaceous glands and subsequent infections in these glands and the surrounding tissues.
  b. Other lesions result from infections, irritations, or reduced blood flow. They include eczema, impetigo, decubitus ulcers (bedsores), and dermatitis.

REVIEW

Important Terms

acne

arrector pili

basale

carotene

corneum

cuticle

dermal papilla

dermis

eleidin

epidermis

germinativum

granulosum

hair follicle

hair root

hair shaft

keratin

lucidum

lunula

melanin

melanocyte

nail

papillary layer

recticular layer

sebaceous gland

sebum

somite

spinosum

subcutaneous

sweat gland

Questions

1. **a.** List the two main parts of the skin.
   b. List the main functions of the skin.

2. List the structures in the skin that are derived from ectoderm and the structures that are derived from mesoderm.

3. **a.** Name the five layers of the epidermis in order from the lower layer outward and describe the structure of each layer.
   b. Name the two layers of the dermis and describe the structure of each layer.

4. How does thin skin differ from thick skin?

5. **a.** Describe the three barriers in the skin that protect the body from microbial invasion.
   b. Explain how skin color is produced and how pigment protects the body.
   c. Describe the role of the skin in decreasing and increasing body temperature and explain why this process is called a homeostatic mechanism.
   d. What kinds of materials can be absorbed through the skin, and how do they escape the natural barriers?
   e. Name four substances synthesized in the skin.

6. **a.** Describe the structure and function of hair.
   b. Describe the structure of a nail.
   c. Describe the structure of sebaceous glands and the nature of their secretions.
   d. Describe the structure of the two types of sweat glands and the nature of their secretions.

7. **a.** Discuss the cause, effects, and treatment of acne.
   b. List three other types of skin lesions and the symptoms they produce.

Problems

1. If the skin is broken and microbes penetrate the stratum corneum, what remaining skin barriers and other defense mechanisms might prevent a generalized infection? (Use information from all chapters you have studied so far.) What are some of the limitations of the use of various topical ointments and solutions?

2. Design an experiment to demonstrate the effects of the body's temperature-regulating mechanism.

3. One severely burned person is placed in a plastic isolation tent maintained at 30°C and high humidity and receives a high-protein diet. Eschar is removed by laser surgery, and grafts of synthetic skin are placed over the larger burned areas. Another similarly burned person is placed in a typical hospital room and receives a standard diet. Eschar is allowed to separate spontaneously, and pig skin grafts are used to cover the larger burned areas. Explain how each different treatment might affect the recovery of the individuals.

REFERENCES AND READINGS

Anonymous. 1979. Clear advances in acne therapy. *Science News* 115:118 (February 24).

Anonymous. 1979. Drug therapy without peaks and valleys. *Science News* 115:102 (February 17).

Copenhaver, W. M., Kelly, D. E., and Wood, R. L. 1978. *Bailey's textbook of histology* (17th ed.). Baltimore, Md.: Williams and Wilkins.

Guyton, A. C. 1981. *Textbook of medical physiology* (6th ed.). Philadelphia: W. B. Saunders.

Maugh, T. H. 1978. Hair: a diagnostic tool to complement blood serum and urine. *Science* 202:1271 (December 22).

Office of Information, National Institutes of Health. 1978. Burn care research. *News and Features from NIH.* Bethesda, Md.: U.S. Department of Health, Education and Welfare (November).

Pihl, R. O., and Parkes, M. 1977. Hair element content in learning disabled children. *Science* 198:204 (October 14).

6

SKELETAL SYSTEM

ORGANIZATION AND GENERAL FUNCTIONS

Objective 1. Describe the basic plan of the skeletal system and list its major functions.

The skeletal system consists of all 206 bones of the body; the joints between these bones; the ligaments that hold bones together; and the cartilage of the nose, outer ear, larynx, and ends of bones. It performs several functions. Some of the bones protect internal organs. For example, your skull forms a hard cover for your brain, and your ribs and sternum (breastbone) form a protective cage around your heart and lungs. Other bones make a rigid framework that supports the rest of your body. In addition to supporting and protecting your body, the bones provide surfaces for the attachment of muscles. Whenever you move, muscles contract, usually causing joints to bend. You can move your whole body, as when you run or swim; you can move a part, as when you write or talk. All of your movements are possible because of muscles pulling on bones. Even when you are not making any conscious movements, muscles attached to your ribs help you to breathe.

Bone tissue performs still other functions. It provides a reservoir of calcium and other minerals and is actively involved in maintaining calcium balance in the body. Red bone marrow, a tissue inside certain bones, produces blood cells. This process, hemopoiesis, will be discussed in Chapter 16.

In summary, the skeletal system supports, protects, provides a reservoir of calcium and other minerals, makes blood cells, and, with the muscular system, provides for movement. Bones also provide useful anatomical landmarks for describing the location of other organs. Thus, many of the terms used in describing the skeletal system will appear again and again as you study other systems.

Though it really functions as a whole, the skeleton (Figure 6.1) is usually divided into two parts for study. These parts are the **axial** skeleton, which supports the trunk and head, and the **appendicular** skeleton, which supports the appendages (arms and legs) and connects them to the axial skeleton. The axial skeleton includes the skull, vertebrae, ribs, sternum, and hyoid bone. The appendicular skeleton includes the pectoral girdle and the bones of the upper appendages and the pelvic girdle and the bones of the lower appendages. The bones of each upper appendage are the humerus, radius, ulna, carpals, metacarpals, and phalanges; the bones of each lower appendage are the femur, tibia, fibula, tarsals, metatarsals, and phalanges. All of the bones of the appendicular skeleton are paired—one on the left and one on the right side of the body.

Each appendage is connected to the axial skeleton by a group of bones called a **girdle**. The **pectoral** girdle, which holds the arms to the trunk, includes the scapulae and the clavicles—one of each on each side of the body. The **pelvic** girdle, which attaches the legs to the trunk, consists of two coxal bones, each of which includes an ilium, ischium, and pubis. Because the sacrum and coccyx are intimately associated with the coxal bones, they give stability to the pelvic girdle although they are part of the vertebral column. The bones of the appendicular skeleton are summarized in Table 6.1.

DEVELOPMENT OF THE SKELETAL SYSTEM

Objective 2. Describe the ossification and remodeling of (a) a membranous bone, and (b) an endochondral bone.

Bone, as noted in Chapter 4, is a type of connective tissue whose matrix contains mineral deposits. This hard matrix gives bones the properties that are important in their supporting and protecting functions.

In Chapter 5 it was mentioned that **sclerotomes**, portions of embryonic mesodermal somites, give rise to some bones; such bones include the vertebrae, ribs, and scapulae. Though some somitic tissue migrates to the head, many bones of the head develop from unsegmented (nonsomitic) mesoderm. Bones of the limbs develop from somites but not from the sclerotome portion. They are first laid down as cartilage models; the cartilage later is replaced by bone in the process called **endochondral** (within cartilage) **ossification** (bone formation). In contrast, some bones, especially those derived from unsegmented mesoderm, are laid down di-

rectly as bone within a connective tissue membrane. This process is called **membranous ossification**. Though the processes of endochondral and membranous ossification differ in ways to be described presently, the process of bone deposition and the bone that results is the same in both cases.

Most of the bones of the appendicular skeleton are endochondral; the flat bones of the skull are membranous; and the bones of the face, base of the skull, and other parts of the axial skeleton are partly endochondral and partly membranous.

Though each bone has its own developmental schedule, a few have begun to ossify by the eighth week of development and many more by the twelfth week. All bones continue to grow after birth. Ossification is not complete in all bones until about age 25.

Membranous Bones

Before the formation of a membranous bone begins, a sheet of connective tissue membrane develops in the area where the bone will be laid down. Numerous small blood vessels grow into the area of the membrane, and undifferentiated embryonic cells proliferate in the membrane. Some of these cells differentiate into **osteoblasts**, or bone-forming cells, which begin to deposit the bone matrix within the membrane. As the bone becomes more dense, the osteoblasts are trapped in the matrix and can no longer divide. Now they are called **osteocytes**, the metabolically active cells of mature bone. The peripheral portion of the membrane that remains unossified is now called the **periosteum**, an appropriate term because it literally means around bone. As membranous bones are developing in the skull of an embryo, the brain grows too. The bones constantly grow and change shape to accommodate a larger brain. Untrapped osteoblasts on the surface continue to form bone as inner cells become trapped. New bone is deposited on the outer surfaces of the skull bones, and completed bone is absorbed on the inner surfaces. Bone absorption is accomplished by **osteoclasts**, another kind of cell that differentiates from the embryonic cells.

Endochondral Bones

Before the formation of an endochondral bone, a mass of hyaline cartilage having the general shape of the future bone is laid down (Figure 6.2). This cartilage model is covered by a membrane, the **perichondrium** (Figure 6.2a). Because many of the bones that develop endochondrally are long bones (see the section on types of bones for definition of long

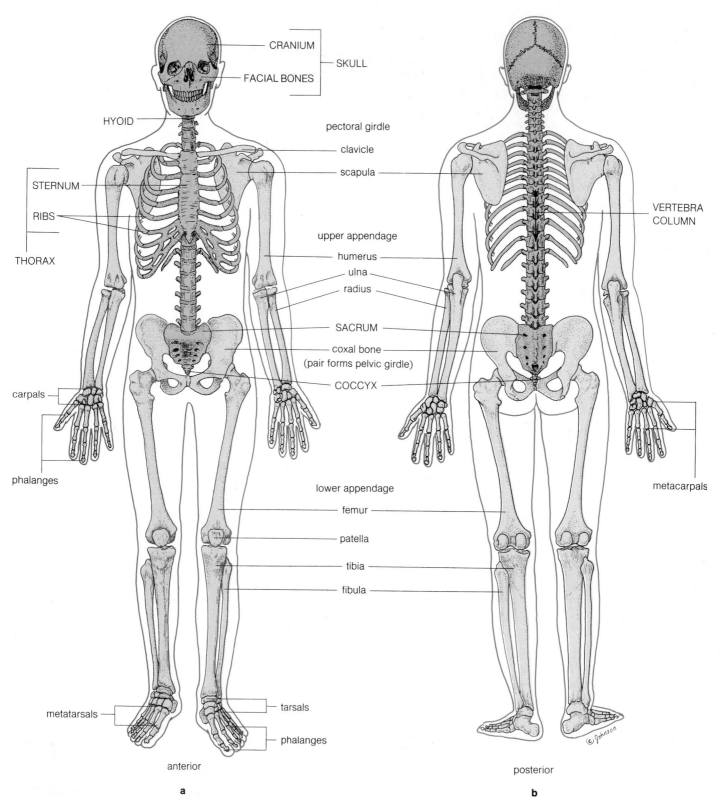

CRANIUM

SKULL

FACIAL BONES

HYOID

pectoral girdle

clavicle

scapula

STERNUM

RIBS

THORAX

VERTEBRA COLUMN

upper appendage

humerus

ulna

radius

SACRUM

coxal bone
(pair forms pelvic girdle)

COCCYX

carpals

phalanges

metacarpals

lower appendage

femur

patella

tibia

fibula

metatarsals

tarsals

phalanges

anterior

posterior

a

b

Figure 6.1 The human skeleton: (**a**) anterior view, (**b**) posterior view. The bones of the axial skeleton are shown in gray and labeled in capital letters; those of the appendicular skeleton are shown in color and labeled in lowercase letters.

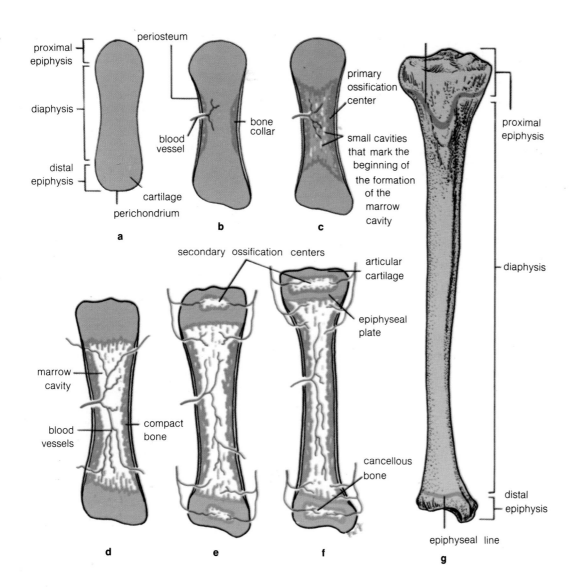

Figure 6.2 The formation of endochondral bone: (**a**) a cartilage model, (**b**) formation of collar, (**c**) beginning of primary ossification, (**d**) formation of marrow cavity and entry of blood vessels into it, (**e**) formation of secondary ossification centers, (**f**) cartilage remaining at articular surfaces and epiphyseal plates, (**g**) fully formed bone with remaining epiphyseal lines.

bone), we will follow the process in a long bone such as the femur. Because different events take place in different regions of the bone, we will use the terms **diaphysis** and **epiphysis** to refer to the middle and the end of the bone, respectively.

The first evidence of endochondral ossification appears in the middle of the diaphysis at the **primary ossification center**, where cartilage cells proliferate and increase the mass of the cartilage. The matrix of the cartilage becomes

reduced in amount, and what remains becomes calcified (hardened by mineral deposits). The calcification of cartilage is different from the mineralization of bone and is *not* to be confused with it. Once cartilage becomes calcified, nutrients can no longer diffuse into it, and the cartilage cells die. Shortly after these changes in the cartilage become established, embryonic cells in the perichondrium differentiate into osteoblasts; the osteoblasts deposit a perforated collar of compact bone around the calcified cartilage. The peri-

Table 6.1	Bones of the Appendicular Skeleton			
	Upper Appendage		Lower Appendage	
Component	Anatomical Name	Common Name	Anatomical Name	Common Name
Girdle	Pectoral	Shoulder	Pelvic	Hip
Proximal segment	Humerus	Upper arm	Femur	Thigh
Middle segment	Radius, ulna	Forearm	Tibia, fibula	Leg
Distal segment	Carpals, metacarpals, phalanges	Hand	Tarsals, metatarsals, phalanges	Foot

chondrium in the area of the bony collar is now called periosteum because it covers bone (Figure 6.2b). Blood vessels grow through the perforations in the bony collar and extend into the area of calcified cartilage.

Along with the blood vessels embryonic cells capable of becoming osteoblasts also enter the area of calcified cartilage at a time when the calcified cartilage is disintegrating and a primitive **marrow** or **medullary cavity** begins to form (Figure 6.2c). The embryonic cells align themselves on the surfaces of remnants of calcified cartilage and differentiate into osteoblasts. The osteoblasts secrete collagen and create a matrix around themselves where minerals are deposited. Bone laid down in this manner enlarges and expands the collar and forms a network of cancellous bone within the marrow cavity. Eventually, some of this bone is reabsorbed by osteoclasts, and the marrow cavity is enlarged. Many blood vessels grow into the marrow cavity (Figure 6.2d).

The above processes occur in long bones starting as early as the eighth week of embryonic development and continuing far into childhood, with each bone having its own developmental schedule. The ossification process begins at the middle of the diaphysis of each bone and spreads in both directions toward the epiphyses at a rate characteristic of each bone.

About the time of birth **secondary ossification centers** are established in the epiphyses of the long bones (Figure 6.2e). Calcification and disintegration of cartilage, proliferation of blood vessels and osteoblasts, and deposition of collagen and minerals occur in the same way as in primary ossification centers. The secondary centers are separated from the primary center by what remains of the cartilage

model, the **epiphyseal plates** (Figure 6.2f). Each epiphysis also has a sheet of articular cartilage covering the end of the bone where it will articulate (come in contact) with another bone in a joint.

Have you ever wondered how bones can be strong enough to support a child's body and at the same time continue to grow? We can answer that question by studying the events that take place in the secondary ossification centers and in the epiphyseal plates. During growth cartilage cells in the epiphyseal plates divide by mitosis and increase the length of the bone; thus the epiphyseal plates move further apart. Ossification continues at both ends of the primary center, and, at the same time, ossification in the secondary centers provides rigidity at the ends of the bones where they form joints with other bones. Large quantities of collagen give the bone tensile strength, and minerals give it rigidity. Growing cartilage is protected by the rigidity of both the epiphyses and the diaphysis. At puberty sex hormones suppress the division of cartilage cells, thus contributing to the narrowing of the epiphyseal plates. When growth is completed at about age seventeen, the cartilage cells cease to divide, but ossification continues until about age twenty-five. At this time the diaphysis unites with the epiphyses, leaving only the **epiphyseal line** at the site at which longitudinal growth once occurred (Figure 6.2g). Bones also grow in diameter by the action of osteoblasts just beneath the periosteum. At the same time, osteoclasts dissolve minerals from bone and enlarge the marrow cavity. Consequently, the thickness of the bones remains nearly constant.

You might think that, once growth is completed, bones become unchanging structures. However, this is not the case. Bones are well supplied with blood vessels and are metabolically active tissues in which minerals are constantly being removed and redeposited. They require nutrients, vitamins, and minerals, not only for development but also for maintenance, once they are formed. Vitamins A and C are essential for proper mineralization, and vitamin D increases the absorption of calcium and phosphorus from the food, thereby assuring a sufficient supply of minerals for calcification of bone. Parathyroid hormone from the parathyroid gland and the hormone calcitonin from the thyroid gland are also essential in bone metabolism; their roles will be discussed in Chapter 15.

In addition to being metabolically active, bones are constantly being remodeled—a little bone tissue added along one surface and a little reabsorbed along another. Debris from damaged bone cells is reabsorbed by osteoclasts and replaced by osteoblasts depositing new bone. Certain areas of bones are thickened or reinforced in response to stresses placed on them by physical activity.

The processes of bone formation and reabsorption occur throughout life. In childhood and adolescence more bone is formed than is destroyed; such bone has a high content of collagen. In adulthood up to about age forty the processes are in equilibrium; after forty more bone is destroyed than is formed. In old age the marrow cavity enlarges, and minerals and collagen are lost from the matrix, causing the bones to become brittle and subject to fracture.

CHARACTERISTICS OF BONES

Objective 3. List the types of bones found in the body, describe the structure of a long bone, and identify the markings found on bones.

Bones come in a variety of shapes and sizes, but they share many characteristics. All bones have collagen-containing matrix and mineral deposits that make them sturdy supporting structures; their shapes help them to provide appropriate kinds of support and protection. All bones have a blood supply that carries nutrients to their cells and removes wastes from them. At the same time, each bone has certain definitive characteristics. A person familiar with these characteristics could assemble a human skeleton from a box of bones, placing each bone in its proper anatomical position.

Types of Bones

Bones can be classified by their shape as long, short, flat, or irregular (Figure 6.3). **Long bones** have a long diaphysis, or shaft, and two epiphyses. Most are slightly curved, and this curvature increases the ability of the bones to absorb shocks and distribute stresses. Long bones have a large central marrow cavity extending over most of the length of the diaphysis. Examples of long bones are the humerus, radius, ulna, metacarpals, femur, tibia, fibula, and metatarsals. **Short bones** are often approximately cube shaped and are composed of peripheral compact bone and central spongy or cancellous bone. (Refer back to Chapter 4 for a discussion of these tissue types.) Short bones have very small marrow spaces. The carpals, tarsals, and phalanges are examples of short bones. **Flat bones** have a sandwichlike structure where the "bread" is compact bone and the "filling" is spongy bone called **diploe**. Within the spongy bone are many small marrow spaces. The bones of the cranium, sternum, and ribs are examples of flat bones. **Irregular bones** are bones that do not fit in any of the above categories. They include the vertebrae, the hyoid bone, and some of the facial bones. Irregular bones usually have peripheral compact bone and central spongy bone with mar-

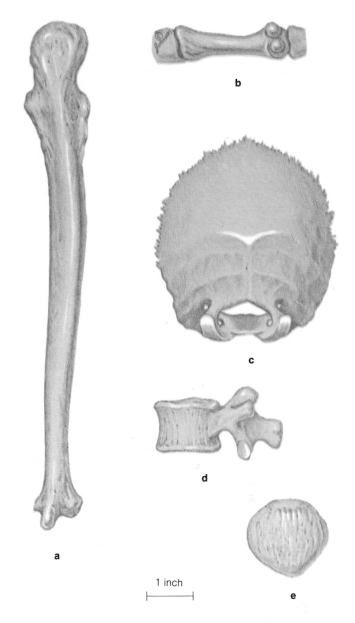

Figure 6.3 Types of bones: (**a**) long bone, (**b**) short bone, (**c**) flat bone, (**d**) irregular bone, (**e**) sesamoid bone.

1 inch

row spaces, but the relative amounts of each type of bone tissue varies.

Two other types of bones are defined by their location. **Sesamoid bones** are imbedded in tendons where excessive pressure exists. The patella, or kneecap, is an example of a sesamoid bone. Though the patellas are the only sesamoid bones regularly present in humans, some individuals have additional sesamoid bones (in tendons of the shoulder, for example). **Wormian bones** or **sutural bones** are found between the **sutures** (joints) of the skull (Figure 6.4). Such bones develop from isolated ossification centers between the larger bones. Some skulls have no Wormian bones, and others have many. Both Wormian bones and extra sesamoid bones develop from extra ossification centers that somehow form during embryological development.

Structure of a Long Bone

Many of the parts of a long bone were mentioned in the discussion of endochondral bone development. As shown in Figure 6.5, the diaphysis consists primarily of compact bone, and the epiphyses consist of outer compact bone and inner spongy bone. Marrow is found within the spongy bone and within the medullary or marrow cavity. The medullary cavity is lined with a membrane called the **endosteum**, which is similar in function to the periosteum, though it lies on the inner surface instead of the outer surface.

Bone marrow is of two types: red and yellow. **Red bone marrow** is a hemopoietic tissue; that is, it is capable of producing blood cells. It is found in many of the bones of infants and young children; in adults it is located primarily in the ribs, sternum, vertebrae, and the coxal bones—areas having the highest body core temperature. **Yellow bone marrow** gradually replaces much of the red bone marrow as a child matures. Under normal circumstances the yellow bone marrow (which consists mostly of fat cells) cannot produce blood cells, but when great need for blood cells exists (following blood loss) some yellow marrow can become red again as it begins to produce blood cells. Yellow marrow is found primarily in the shafts of the long bones of adults.

Bones have an extensive blood supply. Figure 6.5 shows how blood is circulated through bones. A blood vessel enters a bone through a **nutrient foramen** (a **foramen** is a hole in the bone) and passes through to the marrow cavity. Branches of this vessel pass obliquely through the matrix of compact bone in channels called **Volkmann's canals**. Smaller branches enter the **Haversian canals**, which pass through the center of the Haversian systems, or osteons (see Chapter 4). The nutrient artery is but one source of blood entering the bones. Numerous small epiphyseal vessels enter the long bones near their ends, and their smaller branches supply osteons. Furthermore, the periosteum has a rich blood supply.

Bone Markings

Bones have surface markings that are characteristic of some of their functions. The ends of some bones have **depres-**

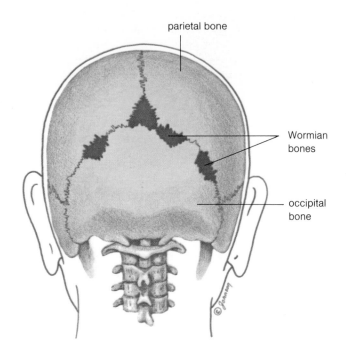

Figure 6.4 Wormian bones in one of the typical locations. They may also be found between other skull bones.

sions, while the ends of other bones have rounded **processes** that fit into the depressions, forming joint surfaces. Bones also have protrusions for the attachment of muscles and tendons, and **fissures**, grooves, or openings for the passage of blood and lymph vessels and nerves. The general characteristics of bone markings are summarized in Table 6.2. The markings of specific bones are summarized in Tables 6.4, 6.5, and 6.7. Refer to drawings of appropriate bones to identify each kind of marking.

AXIAL SKELETON I: BONES OF THE HEAD

Objective 4. Locate and identify the bones of the axial skeleton found in the head and describe their structural characteristics.

The axial skeleton (Table 6.3), as its name implies, forms an axis down the midline of the body. The main part of this axis is the **vertebral column**. Lateral to the vertebral column are the bones of the **thorax**, the **ribs** and the **sternum**, which form a sturdy cagelike structure that protects

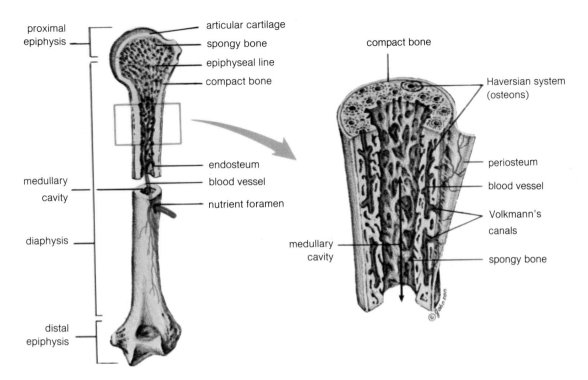

Figure 6.5 The structure of a long bone.

the heart and lungs. These are discussed in the following section.

Superior to the vertebral column is the skull, also a part of the axial skeleton, which includes the **cranial bones** and the **facial bones**. The cranial bones support and protect the brain, and the facial bones give structure to the face. Minor variations in the shape of the facial bones contribute to the individuality of each human face. Other bones considered to be part of the axial skeleton include the **hyoid bone** and the **middle ear bones**.

The skull consists of twenty-two bones, eight of which form the cranium and fourteen of which form the face. These bones are labeled in Figures 6.6, 6.7, and 6.8, each of which shows most of the bones from one of several perspectives.

Bones of the cranium   The bones of the **cranium** enclose the brain. The frontal bone forms the forehead, the paired parietal bones form the crown of the head, and the occipital bone forms the back of the head and the base of the skull. It is the occipital bone that articulates with the vertebral column. The paired temporal bones form the sides of the

cranium, and the ethmoid and sphenoid form much of the floor of the cranium. Locate these bones in the figures before you move on to the consideration of each individual bone.

The **frontal** bone consists of a large curved plate. At the *supraorbital margin* it curves under sharply to form the roof of the orbits (sockets) for the eyes. Above each orbit is a *supraorbital foramen*, through which blood vessels and nerves pass to supply the tissues of the forehead.

The parietal bones are located on each side of the cranium just posterior to the frontal bone. Together they form the roof and bulging sides of the cranium.

The **occipital** bone joins the parietals and forms the base of the cranium. It has a large hole in it, the *foramen magnum*. The brainstem becomes the spinal cord as it passes through the foramen. Blood vessels also pass through the foramen magnum. On either side of the foramen magnum are the *occipital condyles*, processes with convex surfaces that articulate with the first cervical vertebra. Superior to each condyle are the *hypoglossal canals*, through which the hypoglossal cranial nerves leave the cranium. (The cranial nerves will be considered with the nervous system.) Lateral to each condyle is a *condyloid canal*, through which

Table 6.2 Bone Markings

Openings	
Fissure	A slit between two bones through which nerves or blood vessels pass, such as the superior orbital fissure of the sphenoid bone
Foramen	A hole within a bone through which nerves or blood vessels pass, such as the foramen magnum of the skull
Meatus	A tubelike passageway within a bone, such as the auditory meatus of the temporal bone
Sinus	A cavity within a bone, such as the frontal sinus of the frontal bone

Depressions	
Fossa	A simple depression or hollowing in or on a bone, such as the mandibular fossa of the temporal bones
Sulcus	A groove that may contain a blood vessel, nerve, or tendon, such as the malleolar sulcus of the tibia

Joint Processes	
Condyle	A large convex protrusion at the end of a bone, such as the medial or lateral condyles of the femur
Head	A round protrusion separated from the rest of a bone by a neck, such as the head of the humerus or femur
Facet	A flat smooth surface, such as the facets of the ribs

Processes for the Attachment of Ligaments, Tendons, and Muscles	
Crest	A prominent ridge on a bone, such as the iliac crest of the coxal bone
Epicondyle	A second protrusion above a condyle, such as the medial or lateral epicondyles of the femur
Line	A less prominent ridge on a bone, such as the linea aspera of the femur
Tubercle	A small round protrusion, such as the greater tubercle of the humerus
Tuberosity	A large, round, and usually roughened protrusion, such as the ischial tuberosity of the coxal bone
Trochanter	A large protrusion found only on the femur

Table 6.3 Bones of the Axial Skeleton

Skull		22 bones
Cranial bones	*8 bones*	
Frontal	1	
Parietal	2	
Temporal	2	
Occipital	1	
Sphenoid	1	
Ethmoid	1	
Facial bones	*14 bones*	
Maxilla	2	
Palatine	2	
Nasal	2	
Lacrimal	2	
Inferior nasal conchae	2	
Zygomatic	2	
Vomer	1	
Mandible	1	
Middle ear bones		6 bones
Hyoid		1 bone
Vertebral Column		26 bones
Cervical vertebrae	7	
Thoracic vertebrae	12	
Lumbar vertebrae	5	
Sacrum	1	
Coccyx	1	
Thorax		25 bones
Ribs	24	
Sternum	1	
Total bones of axial skeleton		80 bones

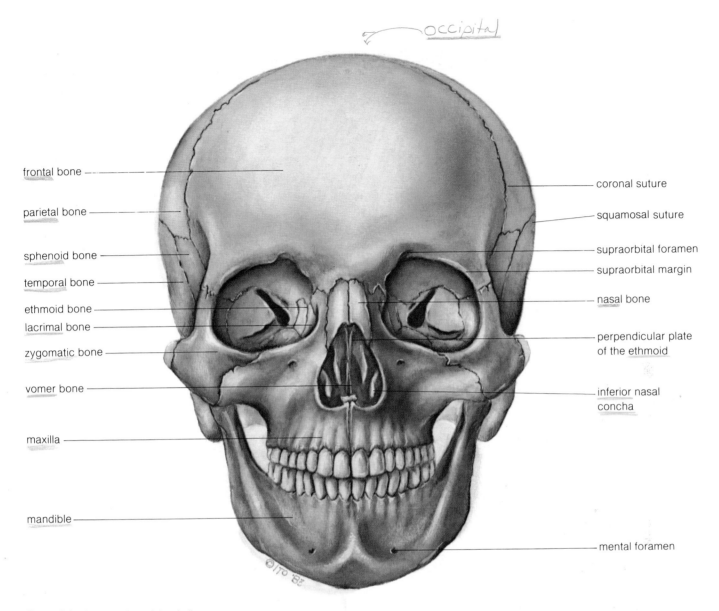

occipital

frontal bone

parietal bone

sphenoid bone

temporal bone

ethmoid bone

lacrimal bone

zygomatic bone

vomer bone

maxilla

mandible

coronal suture

squamosal suture

supraorbital foramen

supraorbital margin

nasal bone

perpendicular plate of the ethmoid

inferior nasal concha

mental foramen

Figure 6.6 Anterior view of the skull.

a vein carrying blood from the brain passes. Rough ridges on the occipital bone mark the location of the attachments of neck muscles.

The **temporal bones** (Figure 6.9) join the parietal bones and extend downward to form the sides and part of the base of the cranium. The *zygomatic process*, extending from the *squamosal portion*, joins the zygomatic bone to form the zygomatic arch (cheek bone). The *mandibular fossa* forms part of the joint by which the mandible (lower jaw) is attached to the cranium. (These structures will be discussed in more detail with the discussion of the facial bones.) The *external auditory meatus* is the opening for the ear canal. It leads into

the middle ear where the **malleus, incus,** and **stapes** are located. The *cochlea* and *semicircular canals* are surrounded by the *petrous portion* of the temporal bone.

The *mastoid process*, which extends from the *mastoid portion* of the temporal bone, serves as the point of attachment of several neck muscles. The mastoid portion itself contains air spaces that drain into the middle ear cavity; infection of these air spaces is called mastoiditis. The *styloid process* provides a point of attachment for muscles and ligaments of the hyoid bone, neck, and tongue. The *internal auditory meatus* (see Figure 6.8) is an opening in the petrous portion; the cranial nerve from the cochlea and semicircular

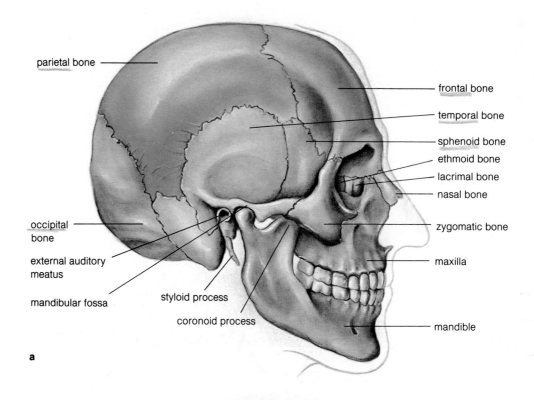

parietal bone

frontal bone

temporal bone

sphenoid bone

ethmoid bone

lacrimal bone

nasal bone

occipital bone

zygomatic bone

external auditory meatus

maxilla

mandibular fossa

styloid process

coronoid process

mandible

a

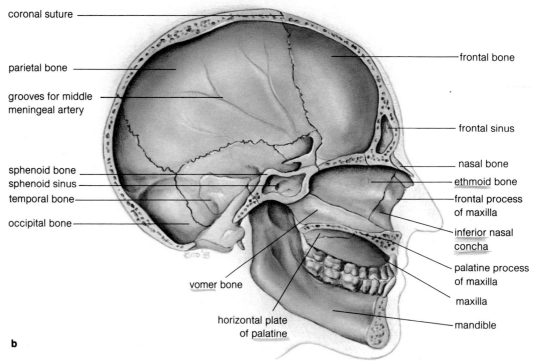

coronal suture

frontal bone

parietal bone

grooves for middle meningeal artery

frontal sinus

nasal bone

ethmoid bone

sphenoid bone

sphenoid sinus

frontal process of maxilla

temporal bone

occipital bone

inferior nasal concha

palatine process of maxilla

vomer bone

maxilla

horizontal plate of palatine

mandible

b

Figure 6.7   Lateral views of the skull: (**a**) external surface of the left side of the skull, (**b**) internal surface of the right side of the skull, after a midsagittal section, (**c**) next page, top left, an elderly man who has lost all of his teeth, and (**d**) next page, top right a child with two sets of teeth apparent. (X rays courtesy of Alexandria Hospital, Alexandria, Virginia, Joyce R. Isbel, R.T.)

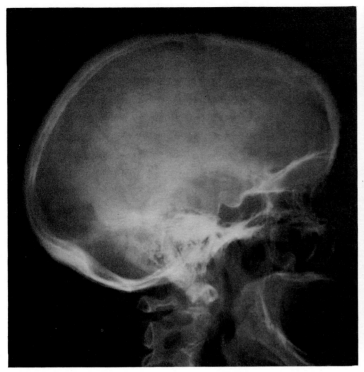

c

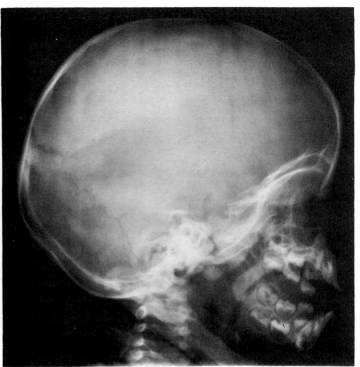

d

canals passes through this meatus to the brain; the facial cranial nerve also passes through this meatus.

The **ethmoid bone** (Figures 6.6 and 6.10) is an irregularly shaped bone that forms part of the anterior portion of the cranial floor. It also extends downward to form part of the nasal septum, the midline division of the nose. The cranial portion contains the *cribriform* ("sieve") *plate*, through which sensory nerve fibers from the nasal epithelium pass to the brain, and the *crista galli* ("cock's comb"), a triangular process to which the membranes that cover the brain are attached. The portion of the ethmoid that extends inferiorly from the cranium consists of the *perpendicular plate*, which forms a large portion of the nasal septum, and the *lateral masses*, which lie between the nasal cavity and the orbits of the eyes. Each lateral mass contains two scroll-shaped, membrane-covered bones, the *superior nasal concha* and the *middle nasal concha*. Inside the lateral mass are small sacs called sinuses. The conchae increase the surface area inside the nasal cavity; their surface membranes contain receptors for the sense of smell.

The **sphenoid** bone (Figures 6.8 and 6.11) is a large, relatively flat bone with wing-shaped projections. Both the *greater* and the *lesser wings* of the sphenoid form part of the cranial floor. The *pterygoid processes* extend downward to form part of the lateral wall of the nasal cavity. Because the borders of the sphenoid touch on each of the other cranial bones, the sphenoid acts as a keystone holding the cranium together. The medial portion of the bone is hollow and contains the large *sphenoidal sinus* (Figure 6.7). Its superior surface has a depression, the *sella turcica* ("Turkish saddle"), in which the pituitary gland lies. Just anterior to the sella turcica is another, shallower depression where some fibers of the optic nerves from the eyes pass to the opposite side of the brain. These nerves pass through the *optic foramina* of the lesser wing. Two other pairs of foramina are visible in the superior view. On each side is a *foramen rotundum*, through which a branch of the trigeminal nerve passes, and a *foramen ovale*, through which another branch of that nerve passes.

Sutures The joints of the skull are all classified as **sutures**, with the exception of the joints that attach the mandible to the skull. Sutures are immovable points between the skull bones. The cranial sutures (Figure 6.7a) are as follows: The *coronal suture* lies between the frontal and parietal bones. The *squamosal sutures* lie between the parietal and temporal bones on either side of the head. The *lambdoidal suture* lies

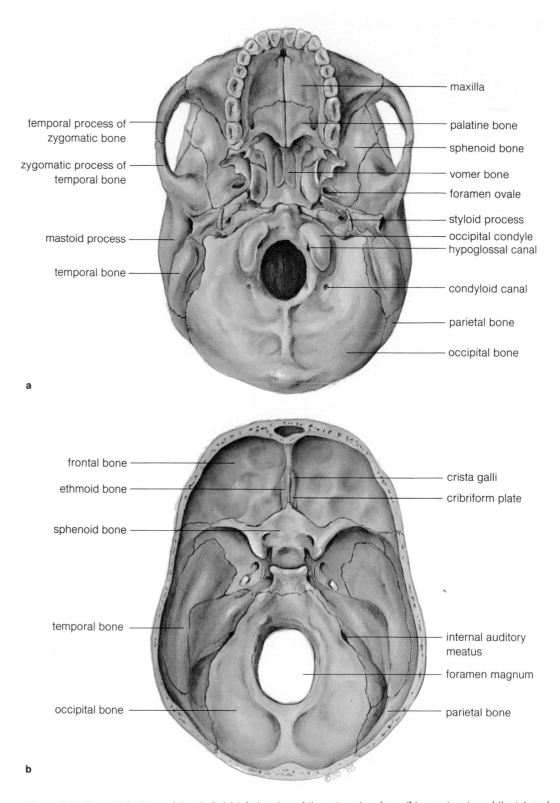

maxilla

temporal process of
zygomatic bone

palatine bone

sphenoid bone

zygomatic process of
temporal bone

vomer bone

foramen ovale

styloid process

occipital condyle

mastoid process

hypoglossal canal

temporal bone

condyloid canal

parietal bone

occipital bone

a

frontal bone

crista galli

ethmoid bone

cribriform plate

sphenoid bone

temporal bone

internal auditory
meatus

foramen magnum

occipital bone

parietal bone

b

Figure 6.8 Views of the base of the skull: (**a**) inferior view of the external surface, (**b**) superior view of the internal surface, after removal of the upper part of the cranium.

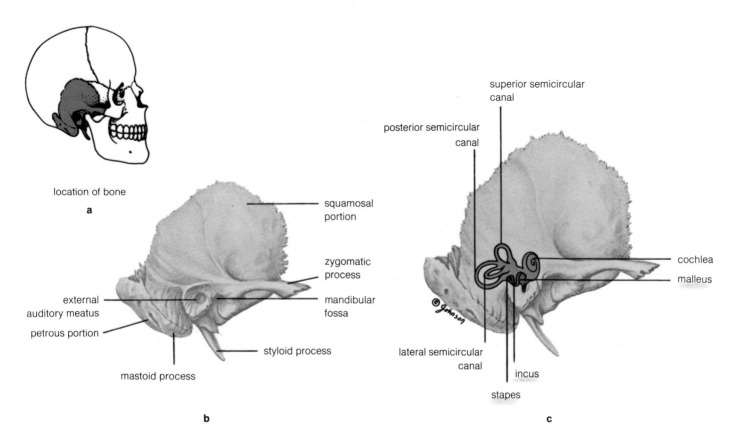

Figure 6.9 The temporal bone: (**a**) location of bone in skull, (**b**) lateral view of the external surface of the right temporal bone, (**c**) lateral view of the temporal bone, after removal of some of the petrous portion to expose the middle ear bones, cochlea, and semicircular canals.

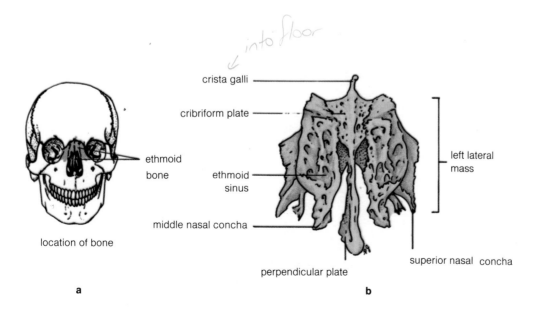

Figure 6.10 The ethmoid bone: (**a**) anterior view of the skull, showing the location of the ethmoid bone, (**b**) enlarged, anterior view of the ethmoid bone.

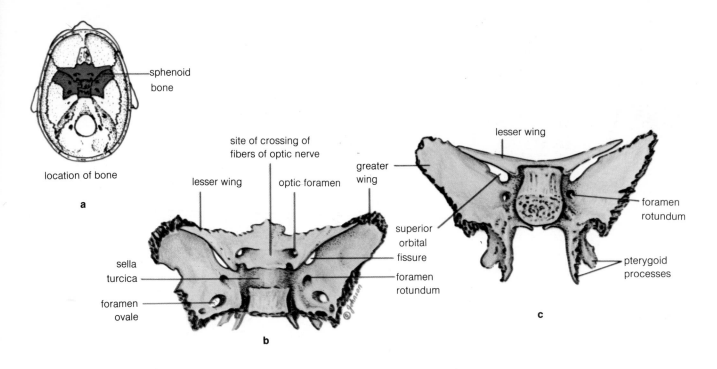

location of bone

a

sphenoid
bone

site of crossing of
fibers of optic nerve

lesser wing

optic foramen

greater
wing

lesser wing

superior
orbital
fissure

foramen
rotundum

sella
turcica

foramen
ovale

foramen
rotundum

pterygoid
processes

b

c

Figure 6.11 The sphenoid bone: (**a**) superior view of the internal floor of the skull, showing the location of the sphenoid bone, (**b**) enlarged, superior view of the sphenoid bone, (**c**) an enlarged posterior view of the sphenoid bone.

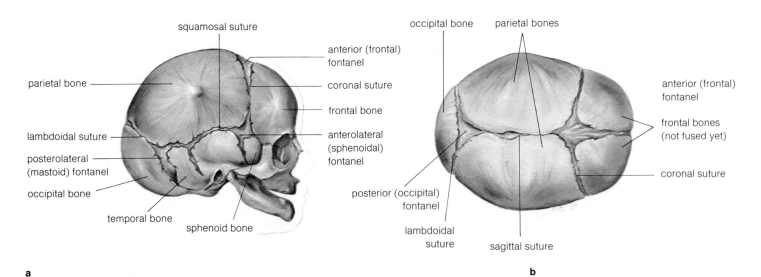

squamosal suture

anterior (frontal)
fontanel

coronal suture

frontal bone

anterolateral
(sphenoidal)
fontanel

parietal bone

lambdoidal suture

posterolateral
(mastoid) fontanel

occipital bone

temporal bone

sphenoid bone

occipital bone

parietal bones

anterior (frontal)
fontanel

frontal bones
(not fused yet)

coronal suture

posterior (occipital)
fontanel

lambdoidal
suture

sagittal suture

a

b

Figure 6.12 Fontanels of a newborn infant: (**a**) superior view, (**b**) lateral view.

between the occipital and parietal bones. The *sagittal suture* (best seen in Figure 6.12) is located between the parietal bones in the midline of the skull.

Fontanels   In the human infant at birth the sutures of the skull are not completely immovable. Bone is still developing within the tough membrane that extends across the suture sites. **Fontanels** (Figure 6.12), or "soft spots," are membranes in which bone has not yet been laid down. They are found where a junction of two or more sutures will eventually form. Two fontanels lie in the midline on the superior surface of the skull; two additional pairs lie near the temporal bone. Fontanels are said to close when bone is laid down in the membrane and the edges meet and fuse, forming sutures. The *anterior*, or *frontal, fontanel* is the largest of the fontanels and the last to close at eighteen to twenty-four months of age. The *posterior*, or *occipital, fontanel*, a smaller fontanel, is usually closed at two months of age. The small, irregularly shaped *anterolateral*, or *sphenoidal, fontanels* are usually closed by three months of age, and the large, irregularly shaped *posterolateral*, or *mastoidal, fontanels* are usually closed by twelve months of age.

Fontanels allow the head to be slightly compressed and sometimes distorted during the birth process, thereby easing the delivery. Distortions disappear shortly after birth as the plates of bone move back to their normal positions. The fontanels also allow for bone growth and increase in the size of the cranium before the sutures close.

Facial bones   The **facial bones**, as listed in Table 6.3, include six paired bones, the maxilla, palatine, nasal, lacrimal, inferior nasal conchae, and zygomatic, and two unpaired bones, the vomer and mandible. These bones can be located on Figures 6.6, 6.7, and 6.8.

The pair of **maxillae** (Figure 6.13) are fused by a midline suture. Together, they articulate with every other facial bone except the mandible. Each maxilla forms a lateral surface of the nose and the inferior part of an eye orbit, and each contains an air sac called a *maxillary sinus*. The *zygomatic process* forms a portion of the cheek bone, and the *palatine process* forms part of the *hard palate*. The maxillae also contain *alveoli*, the bony sockets for the upper teeth (see Figure 6.7). The *infraorbital foramen* provides a passageway from the orbit of the eye for a nerve and an artery.

A pair of **nasal** bones (Figure 6.13) forms the bridge of the nose. These small bones, each about the size of a fingernail, are joined by sutures to the maxillae, the frontal bones, and each other.

The **lacrimal** bones (Figure 6.13), which are about the same size as the nasal bones, form part of the lateral wall of the nasal cavity and part of the medial surface of each orbit.

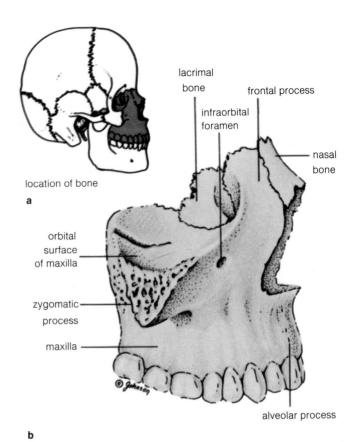

Figure 6.13   (**a**) Shaded area of skull shows location of maxilla, lacrimal, and nasal bones. (**b**) Lateral view of these bones.

Each of these bones has a foramen through which the lacrimal duct carries tears to the nasal cavity.

The **palatine** bones (Figure 6.14) articulate with the palatine processes of the maxillae to complete the hard palate.

The **inferior nasal conchae** (Figure 6.14), one concha on either side of the nose, are scroll-shaped bones. They are similar to the other conchae that are part of the ethmoid bone. The inferior conchae articulate with the maxillae. Together, the conchae provide a large surface area, which is covered by a highly vascular membrane that helps to warm and moisten air as it is inhaled.

The **vomer**, a single shovel-shaped bone, forms the inferior portion of the nasal septum between the ethmoid and the maxillae. It is best seen in Figure 6.7b.

The paired **zygomatic** bones (Figures 6.6 and 6.7a) articulate with the zygomatic processes of both the maxillae and the temporal bones. The zygomatic bones in combination with these processes form the cheek bones.

The **mandible**, or jaw bone (Figure 6.15), consists of a body and two rami. (A ramus, singular of rami, is a projecting part.) It contains alveoli, or sockets, for the lower teeth. Two pairs of foramina are found in the mandible; each serves as a passageway for nerves and blood vessels. A *mental foramen* is located on each side of the mandible below and between the sockets of the bicuspids. A *mandibular foramen* is located on the medial surface of each ramus. The mandible articulates with the squamosal portion of the temporal bone (Figure 6.7a) at a depression called the *mandibular fossa*. The *mandibular condyle* fits into this fossa to form a sliding hinge joint—the only movable joint in the skull. The *coronoid process* is the point of attachment of the temporal muscle, a muscle that is important in movements of the mandible.

Sinuses A number of hollow air sacs called **sinuses** (Figure 6.16) are found within the bones of the face and cranium. The frontal bone contains a pair of sinuses, the sphenoid bone and the maxillae each contain a single sinus, and the ethmoid bone contains many small sinuses. Each of these sinuses is lined with a mucous membrane and has a small opening through which mucus can drain into the nasal cavity. The sinuses have no essential function, though they give resonance to the voice and make the skull lighter than it would be if composed of solid bone.

> Though mucus can drain out of the sinuses, infectious organisms and irritants in the nasal cavity can move into the sinuses. The resulting inflammation, **sinusitis**, frequently accompanies a cold or an allergy. If the membranes swell enough to block drainage from the sinuses into the nasal cavity, fluid pressure builds up in the sinuses, and a sinus headache results.

Special Bones

Strictly speaking, the bones of the middle ear and the hyoid bone are not part of the cranium or the face, but, because they are located in the head area, they are considered here. The middle ear bones, or **auditory ossicles**, are located in a chamber within the petrous portion of the temporal bone.

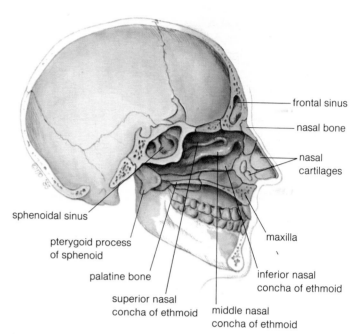

Figure 6.14 Sagittal section showing the bones that form the lateral wall of the nasal cavity.

(labels: frontal sinus; nasal bone; nasal cartilages; maxilla; inferior nasal concha of ethmoid; middle nasal concha of ethmoid; superior nasal concha of ethmoid; palatine bone; pterygoid process of sphenoid; sphenoidal sinus)

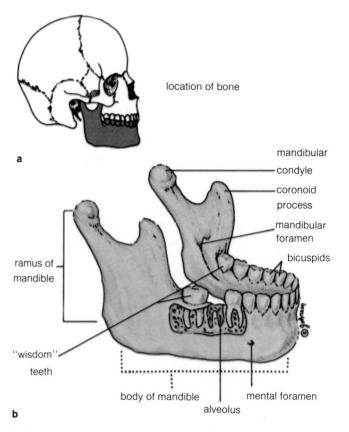

location of bone

a

b

(labels: mandibular condyle; coronoid process; mandibular foramen; bicuspids; mental foramen; alveolus; body of mandible; "wisdom" teeth; ramus of mandible)

Figure 6.15 (**a**) Location of the mandible, (**b**) Lateral view of the mandible.

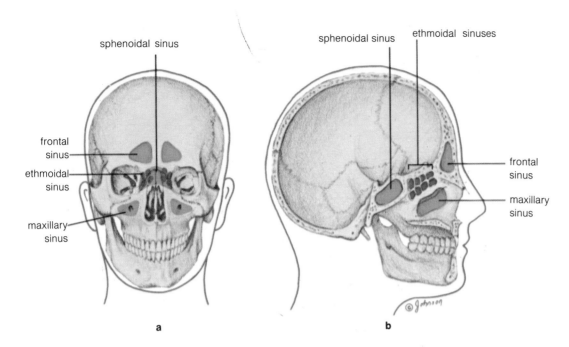

Figure 6.16 The sinuses: (**a**) anterior view, (**b**) lateral view of sagittal section.

Together, the three bones transfer vibrations from the tympanic membrane, or ear drum, to the oval window, which leads ultimately to the cochlea, the organ of hearing. The ossicles (Figure 6.17) are the **malleus**, attached to the tympanic membrane, the **incus**, and the **stapes**, attached to the oval window. More will be said about the role these bones play in hearing in Chapter 14.

The **hyoid bone** (Figure 6.18) is a U-shaped bone located in the neck just below the angle of the mandible. It is attached by ligaments to the styloid processes of the temporal bones. The hyoid has a *body* and two pairs of hornlike projections, the *greater cornua* and the *lesser cornua*. Each projection is a *cornu*. Both the body and the horns serve as points of attachment for muscles of the neck and tongue. The hyoid does not articulate (form a joint) with another bone.

Table 6.4 summarizes the characteristic markings of the bones of the axial skeleton located in the head.

AXIAL SKELETON II: BONES OF THE TRUNK

Objective 5. Locate and identify the bones of the axial skeleton found in the trunk and describe their structural characteristics.

The bones of the axial skeleton found in the trunk include the bones of the vertebral column and the bones of the thorax.

Vertebral Column

The *vertebral column* (Figure 6.19) consists of twenty-four vertebrae plus the sacrum and coccyx. These bones, along with the *ribs* and *sternum,* make up the skeleton of the trunk.

The vertebral column has five regions: from top to bottom, the cervical, thoracic, lumbar, sacral, and coccygeal. Of the twenty-four vertebrae seven are found in the cervical region, twelve in the thoracic region, and five in the lumbar region. The sacral and coccygeal regions each consist of a single bone, the sacrum and the coccyx, respectively. Four of the regions have a natural curvature. In lateral view the curvature is convex (bulging anteriorly) in the cervical and lumbar regions and concave (bulging posteriorly) in the thoracic and sacral regions. These curvatures of the spine (vertebral column) increase its strength and weight-bearing ability and its shock-absorbing capacity. Because infants have not yet developed the convex cervical and lumbar spinal curvatures, they have a continuous anterior concave curvature. As they become able to hold the head erect, sit, and stand, the convex curvatures appear.

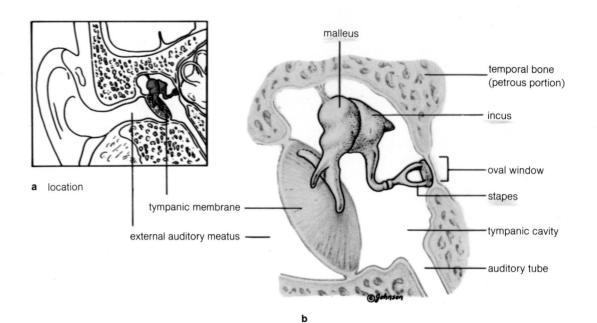

Figure 6.17 Auditory ossicles; (**a**) location, (**b**) detailed view of ossicles.

Bone	Marking
Table 6.4 Markings of the Major Bones of the Head	
Frontal (Figure 6.6)	Supraorbital margin—an arched ridge inferior to eyebrow
	Supraorbital foramen—an opening through which blood vessels and nerves pass
Occipital (Figures 6.7, 6.8)	Foramen magnum—an opening at the base of the skull
	Occipital condyle—convex process that forms a joint with the first cervical vertebra
	Condyloid canal—opening through which a vein passes from the brain
Temporal (Figure 6.9)	*Squamosal portion* Zygomatic process—projection that joins the zygomatic bone
	Mandibular fossa—depression that forms a joint with the mandible
	Petrous portion Middle ear bones and cochlea imbedded in petrous portion
	Mastoid portion Mastoid process—protruberance behind ear to which muscles attach
	Styloid process—spikelike process in front of mastoid process to which muscles attach
	External auditory meatus—opening through which the auditory tube passes
	Internal auditory meatus—opening on inside of skull through which cranial nerves pass
Ethmoid (Figure 6.10)	Cribriform plate—plate of bone containing many small holes through which branches of the olfactory nerve pass
	Crista galli—projection to which meninges attach
	Perpendicular plate—vertical portion that forms part of nasal septum
	Lateral mass—lateral portion of bone filled with air spaces
	Superior nasal concha—part of lateral wall of nasal cavity
	Middle nasal concha—also part of lateral wall of nasal cavity

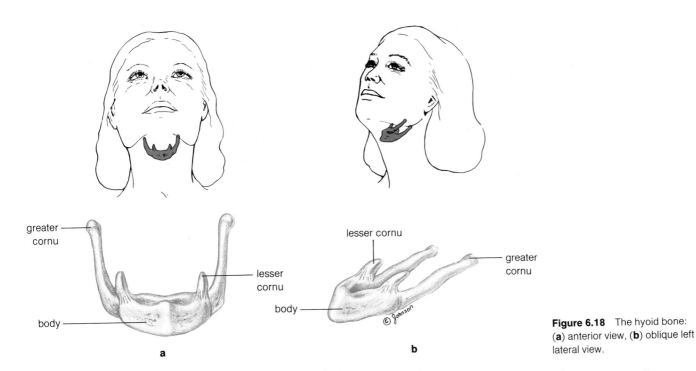

greater
cornu

lesser
cornu

body

a

lesser cornu

greater
cornu

body

b

Figure 6.18 The hyoid bone: (**a**) anterior view, (**b**) oblique left lateral view.

Table 6.4	Markings of the Major Bones of the Head (continued)
Bone	**Marking**
Sphenoid (Figure 6.11)	Ethmoid sinus—air space lined with mucous membrane, found in lateral mass
	Greater wing—lateral projection that forms part of eye orbit
	Lesser wing—thin superior projection that also forms part of orbit
	Pterygoid process—inferior projection that forms part of lateral nasal wall
	Sphenoidal sinus—one of several mucous membrane–lined spaces within body of sphenoid
	Sella turcica—saddle-shaped depression in which pituitary gland lies
	Optic foramen—opening in orbit through which optic nerve passes
	Foramen rotundum—opening through which a portion of the trigeminal nerve passes
	Foramen ovale—opening through which another portion of the trigeminal nerve passes
Maxilla (Figures 6.13, 6.14)	Zygomatic process—lateral portion that forms part of the orbit
	Palatine process—posterior portion that forms part of the hard palate
	Alveolar process—portion that contains the alveoli or tooth sockets
	Infraorbital foramen—opening just below orbit through which nerves and blood vessels pass
Mandible (Figure 6.15)	Ramus—portion projecting upward from body to form joint with temporal bone
	Mental foramen—opening on outer surface between bicuspids through which nerves and blood vessels pass
	Mandibular foramen—opening on inner surface through which nerves and blood vessels are distributed to teeth
	Mandibular condyle—end of ramus that forms joint with mandibular fossa of temporal bone
	Coronoid process—a more anterior projection of the ramus to which the temporal muscle attaches

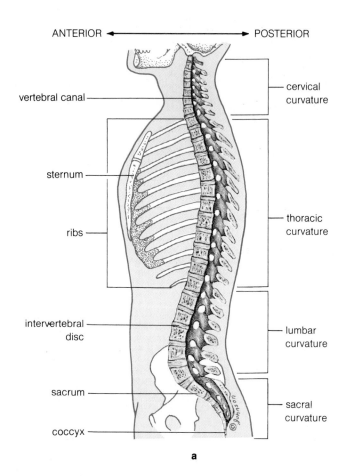

ANTERIOR ←——————→ POSTERIOR

vertebral canal

cervical curvature

sternum

ribs

thoracic curvature

intervertebral disc

lumbar curvature

sacrum

sacral curvature

coccyx

a

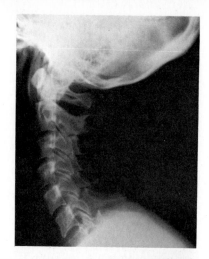

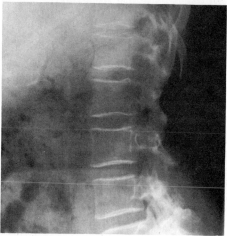

b

Figure 6.19 The ribs, sternum, and vertebral column: (**a**) lateral view showing individual bones and natural curvature of the vertebral column, (**b**) lateral X-ray view of cervical (top) and lumbar (bottom) vertebrae. (X rays courtesy of Alexandria Hospital, Alexandria, Virginia, Joyce R. Isbel, R.T.)

Extreme curvatures of the spine are not uncommon. An exaggerated convex curvature of the lumbar region is called **lordosis**, or swayback; lateral, or side-to-side, curvatures are called **scoliosis**; and an exaggerated concave curvature of the thoracic region is called **kyphosis**, or hunchback.

A typical **vertebra** (Figure 6.20) has an anterior *body* (centrum) and several posterior structures that form a bony covering for the spinal cord. The *vertebral foramen* through which the spinal cord passes is surrounded by the vertebral body, the *pedicles* (the paired anterior parts of the arch), the *laminae* (the paired posterior parts of the arch that fuse in the midline), and the *spinous process*. The vertebral foramina of

all twenty-four vertebrae form the *vertebral canal*. Extending laterally from the pedicles on either side of the vertebra are the paired *transverse processes*. Between adjacent vertebrae is an *intervertebral foramen*, formed from notches in each vertebra, through which a spinal nerve passes from the spinal cord.

Joints are found in the vertebral column between the bodies of adjacent vertebrae and between the articulating processes. Each vertebra has a pair of *superior articulating processes* and a pair of *inferior articulating processes*. The articulating processes of one vertebra join the processes of adjacent vertebrae somewhat like the overlapping shingles on a roof (Figure 6.20b). Other joint surfaces called *facets*, located on the bodies and transverse processes of vertebrae in the thoracic region, articulate with the ribs.

In addition to these general characteristics the vertebrae of each region have specialized characteristics (Figure 6.21).

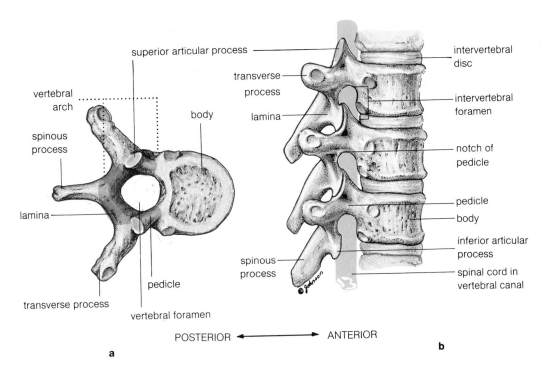

Figure 6.20 A typical vertebra: (**a**) superior view, (**b**) right lateral view.

The superiormost **atlas** has facets that articulate with the occipital condyles; it lacks a centrum or body. The second cervical vertebra, the **axis**, has a *dens*, or *odontoid process*, that extends into the vertebral foramen of the atlas. Embryologically the dens starts out being the centrum of the atlas; as development proceeds, it separates from the atlas and becomes attached to the axis.

All seven of the **cervical vertebrae** have short transverse processes, each process having a *transverse foramen* through which blood vessels and nerves pass. Except for the atlas, all cervical vertebrae have a bifid, or two-pronged, spinous process. Muscles attached to these processes contribute to movement of the neck.

Each of the twelve **thoracic vertebrae** is characterized by the presence of long spinous processes and thick, stubby transverse processes. Both the transverse processes and the bodies of these vertebrae have facets that articulate with the ribs. Muscles attached to the spinous processes contribute to movement of the back.

The five **lumbar vertebrae** have relatively short spinous processes and relatively long transverse processes. The largest and "chunkiest" of the vertebrae, they have large superior and inferior articulating processes, whose artic-

ular surfaces are directed laterally. The articulations form strong, slightly movable joints, which bend forward or backward when muscles attached to the spinous processes contract.

The **sacrum** and **coccyx** (Figure 6.22) are formed from the fusion of nine separate embryonic vertebrae, five forming the sacrum and four forming the coccyx. The union of vertebrae in the sacrum is represented by *transverse lines* visible on its anterior surface. Four pairs of *pelvic foramina* on the anterior (ventral) surface communicate with four pairs of *dorsal foramina* on the posterior (dorsal) surface. Nerves and blood vessels pass through these foramina. In the posterior dorsal midline is the *median sacral crest*, a remnant of the spinous processes of the fused vertebrae. Also apparent are the *lateral sacral crests*, to which various muscles are attached.

Between the anterior and posterior surfaces of the sacrum in the midline is the *sacral canal*, a continuation of the vertebral canal. During embryonic development the spinal cord extends into this canal, but in adults the spinal cord extends only to the first or second lumbar vertebra. Thus, in adults the lower vertebral canal and the sacral canal contain spinal nerve roots that have branched from the spinal cord.

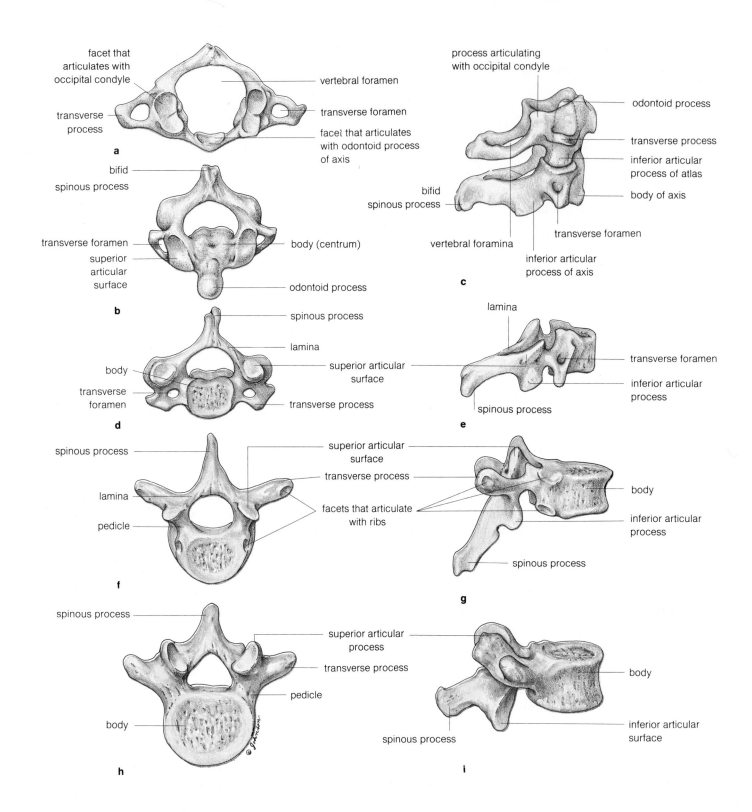

Figure 6.21 Characteristics of certain vertebrae: (**a**) atlas, (**b**) axis, (**c**) articulation of atlas and axis, (**d**) superior view of cervical vertebra, (**e**) lateral view of cervical vertebra, (**f**) superior view of thoracic vertebra, (**g**) lateral view of thoracic vertebra, (**h**) superior view of lumbar vertebra, (**i**) lateral view of lumbar vertebra.

The *sacral hiatus,* an area in which the spinous processes generally do not fuse, is covered with fibrous connective tissue.

An anesthetic can be administered through the fibrous tissue of the sacral hiatus to block pain sensations in the pelvic area. Such anesthesia (called a caudal block or spinal block) is often used during childbirth because, as little enters the mother's bloodstream, it has minimal effects on the fetus.

The **coccyx,** a triangular bone that represents the vestige (remnant) of a tail, is attached by ligaments to the sacrum. It serves as a point of attachment for important pelvic muscles, and it also may act as a shock absorber when a person sits down. Falls or blows to the coccyx often result in fractures or dislocations.

Thorax

The *thorax,* or chest, which contains within its cavity the heart and lungs, is a bony cage formed by the ribs and sternum along with the thoracic vertebrae described above (Figure 6.23).

The **sternum,** or breastbone, is located in the anterior midline of the thorax. It is about 15 centimeters long and consists of three parts—the *manubrium,* the *body,* or *gladiolus* ("little sword" because of its shape), and the *xiphoid process.* The lateral edges of the sternum articulate with the ribs. The first two ribs articulate with the manubrium, and the next eight articulate directly or indirectly with the gladiolus. The xiphoid process has no ribs attached to it; rather, it serves as an attachment point for some of the abdominal muscles.

Twelve pairs of **ribs** are normally present in the thorax, one pair extending from each thoracic vertebra. Of these, the first seven pairs are called **true ribs** because they articulate directly with the sternum by means of small pieces of hyaline cartilage, the *costal cartilages.* Ribs eight through twelve are called **false ribs.** The superior three of these articulate by cartilage with the costal cartilage of the seventh rib and thus are attached indirectly to the sternum. The inferior two are called **floating ribs** because their anterior ends are not attached to either the sternum or the cartilage of another rib. Of course, these ribs are not literally floating because they are attached to the muscles of the body wall and to the thoracic vertebrae.

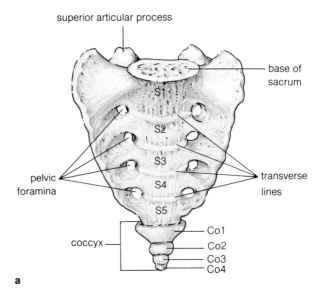

a

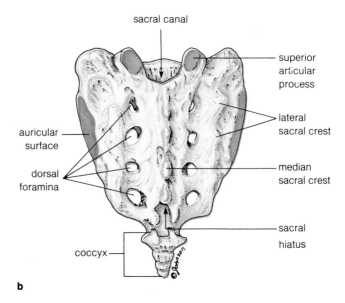

b

Figure 6.22 The sacrum and coccyx: (**a**) anterior view, (**b**) posterior view.

Each individual rib (Figure 6.24) has a *head,* a *neck,* and a *shaft.* The heads of ribs two through nine have two *facets,* which articulate with the body (centrum) of the corresponding thoracic vertebrae; the heads of the first rib and of the last three ribs have only one facet. The *tubercle* of each of the first nine ribs has a facet that articulates with the trans-

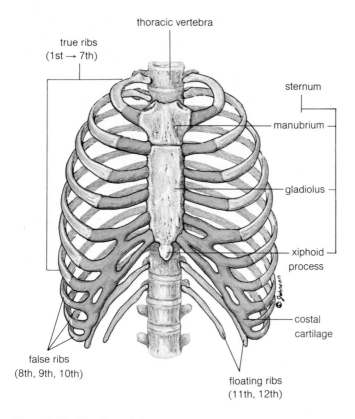

Figure 6.23 The ribs and sternum.

Labels on figure: thoracic vertebra; true ribs (1st → 7th); sternum; manubrium; gladiolus; xiphoid process; costal cartilage; false ribs (8th, 9th, 10th); floating ribs (11th, 12th)

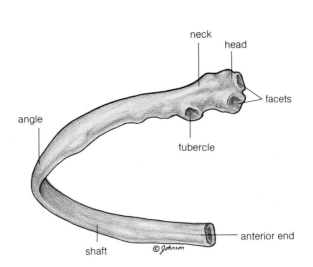

Figure 6.24 A detailed view of a rib.

Labels on figure: neck; head; facets; angle; tubercle; shaft; anterior end

verse process of a thoracic vertebra; the last three have no such facets. The anterior end of the shaft joins the costal cartilage, except in the case of floating ribs.

The markings of the bones of the trunk are summarized in Table 6.5.

APPENDICULAR SKELETON

Objective 6. For each of the following parts of the appendicular skeleton, locate the bones and identify their structural characteristics: (a) pectoral girdle, (b) upper appendage, (c) pelvic girdle, and (d) lower appendage.

The above consideration of the axial skeleton makes it apparent that its functions in supporting the body and protecting internal organs are more significant than its function in movement. In contrast, the appendicular skeleton is more important in movement.

The bones of the appendicular skeleton, listed in Table 6.6, comprise four groups—the **pectoral girdle**, the **upper appendage**, the **pelvic girdle**, and the **lower appendage**. Each girdle attaches an appendage to the axial skeleton. Notice that all the bones of the appendicular skeleton are paired—one of each lies on the left and on the right sides of the body. Therefore, in the following discussion when a single bone is described, you should remember that one is present on each side of the body.

Pectoral Girdle

The **pectoral girdle** (Figure 6.25) consists of two paired bones, a scapula and a clavicle. These bones and the muscles associated with them form the shoulders. It is not a complete girdle because the scapulae do not articulate posteriorly.

The **clavicle** is a slightly curved, rod-shaped bone, sometimes called the collar bone. It extends from the manubrium of the sternum to the acromion process of the scapula.

The **scapula** is a large, flat bone with many processes and projections. On the anterior surface of the scapula is the *subscapular fossa*, where a large muscle attaches. Medial to this fossa is the *vertebral border*, which extends from the *superior angle* to the *inferior angle*. These angles provide convenient anatomical landmarks on the scapula, as do the borders and other markings labeled in Figure 6.25.

The lateral portion of the bone comprises the *glenoid fossa*, the *acromion process*, and the *coracoid process*. The acromion process articulates directly with the clavicle; the cor-

Table 6.5 Markings of the Bones of the Trunk

Bone	Marking
Vertebra (Figure 6.20)	Body (centrum)–anterior, flat, round mass that is the weight-bearing structure
	Vertebral foramen—hole in center of vertebra formed by the body, pedicles, and laminae; passageway for spinal cord
	Pedicles—projections extending posteriorly from body
	Laminae—posterior parts of vertebra from which spinous process projects
	Intervertebral foramen—opening between vertebrae through which spinal nerves pass
	Superior articulating processes—processes that project upward (superiorly) from laminae
	Inferior articulating processes—processes that project downward (inferiorly) from laminae
	Transverse processes—processes projecting laterally from laminae
Atlas (Figure 6.21)	Facets—indentations that articulate with occipital condyles
Axis (Figure 6.21)	Odontoid process—peglike projection around which the atlas rotates
Cervical vertebrae (Figure 6.21)	Transverse foramina—holes in the transverse processes through which an artery, vein, and some nerves pass
Thoracic vertebrae (Figure 6.21)	Facets—smooth surfaces with which the ribs articulate
Sacrum (Figure 6.22)	Pelvic foramina—pairs of openings on the anterior surface through which nerves and blood vessels pass
	Dorsal foramina—pairs of openings on the posterior surface through which blood vessels and nerves pass
	Median sacral crest—a structure in the dorsal midline formed from the fusion of spinous processes
	Sacral canal—a continuation of the vertebral canal within the sacrum
	Sacral hiatus—an area covered by fibrous connective tissue where spinous processes failed to fuse
Sternum (Figure 6.23)	Manubrium—superiormost portion of the sternum
	Gladiolus—large middle portion of the sternum
	Xiphoid process—inferiormost portion of the sternum
Ribs (Figure 6.24)	Head—projection from posterior portion that articulates with body of thoracic vertebrae
	Neck—narrow portion just below the head
	Shaft—main part of rib
	Facets—smooth surfaces on head that articulate with thoracic vertebrae
	Tubercle—process just below neck that articulates with transverse process of thoracic vertebra

Table 6.6 Bones of the Appendicular Skeleton	
Pectoral girdle	4 bones
Scapula	2
Clavicle	2
Upper appendage	60 bones
Humerus	2
Radius	2
Ulna	2
Carpals	16
Metacarpals	10
Phalanges	28
Pelvic girdle	2 bones
Coxal bones	2
Lower appendage	60 bones
Femur	2
Tibia	2
Fibula	2
Patella	2
Tarsals	14
Metatarsals	10
Phalanges	28
Total bones of the appendicular skeleton	126 bones

acoid process attaches to the clavicle by strong ligaments that stabilize the pectoral girdle. The glenoid fossa is a depression into which the head of the humerus fits.

On the posterior surface of the scapula is a large *spine* that terminates laterally in the acromion process. Both the *supraspinous fossa* and the *infraspinous fossa* are sites of attachment of large muscles that move the humerus at the shoulder joint. Other muscles extend from the spine and the vertebral border of the scapula to the vertebral column.

These muscles play an important role in attaching the pectoral girdle to the axial skeleton; they are, in fact, the *only* attachment between the scapula and the vertebral column because no joint exists between these bones.

Upper Appendage

The bones of the **upper appendage** include the humerus in the upper arm, the radius and ulna in the forearm, and the carpals, metacarpals, and phalanges in the wrist and hand. (Refer back to Figure 6.1.)

The **humerus** (Figure 6.26) is a long, relatively thick bone with a large smooth head at the proximal end and a number of projections at the distal end. The *head* of the humerus articulates with the glenoid fossa of the scapula; it is separated from the *shaft* by the *anatomical neck*, a slight narrowing in the diameter of the bone. The *surgical neck*, slightly distal to the anatomical neck, designates the location of a common fracture of the humerus. Lateral to the head are the *greater tubercle* and the *lesser tubercle*, which serve as points of attachment for the ligaments of the shoulder joint. The *intertubercular groove* is a depression in which rests the tendon of the long head of the biceps brachii muscle. (As noted in Chapter 4, ligaments join bones to one another, and tendons join muscles to bones.) Other markings on the shaft of the humerus include the *deltoid tuberosity*, where the deltoid muscle attaches, and the *radial groove*, which marks the course of the radial nerve.

The distal end of the humerus has a *medial epicondyle* and a *lateral epicondyle*, where muscles that move the forearm attach; the other structural characteristics of the distal humerus form parts of the elbow joint (Figure 6.27). The *capitulum* ("little head") articulates with the radius, and the *trochlea* articulates with the *trochlear notch* of the ulna. The *coronoid fossa* is a depression on the anterior surface into which the coronoid process of the ulna fits. On the posterior surface of the distal humerus is the *olecranon fossa*, which articulates with the olecranon process of the ulna.

The **radius** and the **ulna** (Figure 6.27) are the bones of the forearm. The *head* of the radius is located proximally, where it articulates with the capitulum of the humerus. At the distal end of the radius the *styloid process* extends along the lateral surface of one of the carpals; it can be felt through the skin as a bump on the thumb side of the wrist.

The *head* of the ulna is located distally. It also has a *styloid process*, which can be felt as a bump on the little finger side of the wrist. The proximal end of the ulna has a long projection, the *olecranon*, which articulates with the humerus and can be felt through the skin as the "crazy bone." Bumping the crazy bone causes pain because the ulnar nerve is stimulated.

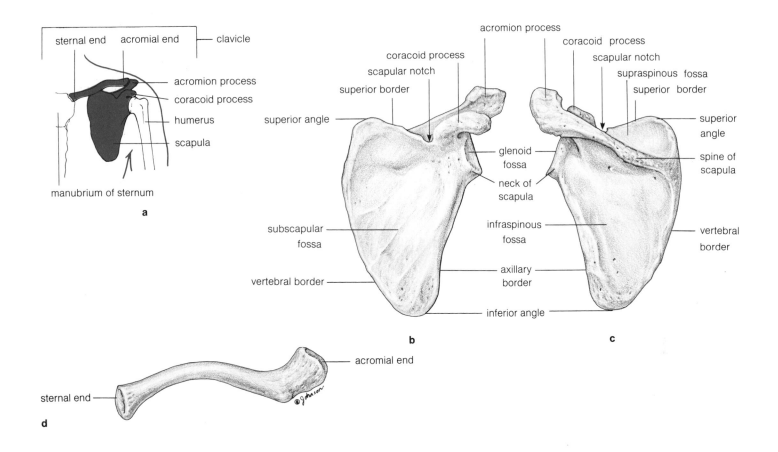

Figure 6.25 The pectoral girdle: (**a**) anterior view of the left part of the girdle (ribs have been removed), (**b**) anterior view of the scapula, (**c**) posterior view of the scapula, (**d**) inferior view of the clavicle.

In addition to their articulations with the humerus, the radius and ulna articulate with each other. The head of the radius fits into the *radial notch* of the ulna. The ability of the radius to rotate around the ulna is possible in part because of this joint. No matter how the radius is rotated, it always lies on the thumb side of the forearm.

Other markings on these bones include the radial tuberosity and the nutrient foramina. The *radial tuberosity* serves as a point of attachment for the biceps brachii muscle. The *nutrient foramina* of both the radius and the ulna mark the point at which blood vessels enter the tissue of the bones.

The bones of the wrist and hand include eight **carpals**, five **metacarpals**, and fourteen **phalanges** (Figure 6.28). The carpals, named in the figure, form the wrist. The most proximal scaphoid and lunate bones form joints with the

radius and ulna, respectively. Several of the carpals articulate with other carpals, and the more distal ones articulate with the metacarpals. The metacarpals form the bony structure of the hand and the proximal portion of the thumb. The phalanges are named according to their position in the fingers or digits—proximal, middle, and distal. However, the first digit, or thumb, has only two phalanges.

Pelvic Girdle

The **pelvic girdle** consists of the two **coxal bones** (Figure 6.29). Each is formed from the fusion of three bones during embryonic development: the ilium, ischium, and pubis. The **ilium** constitutes the superior and lateral por-

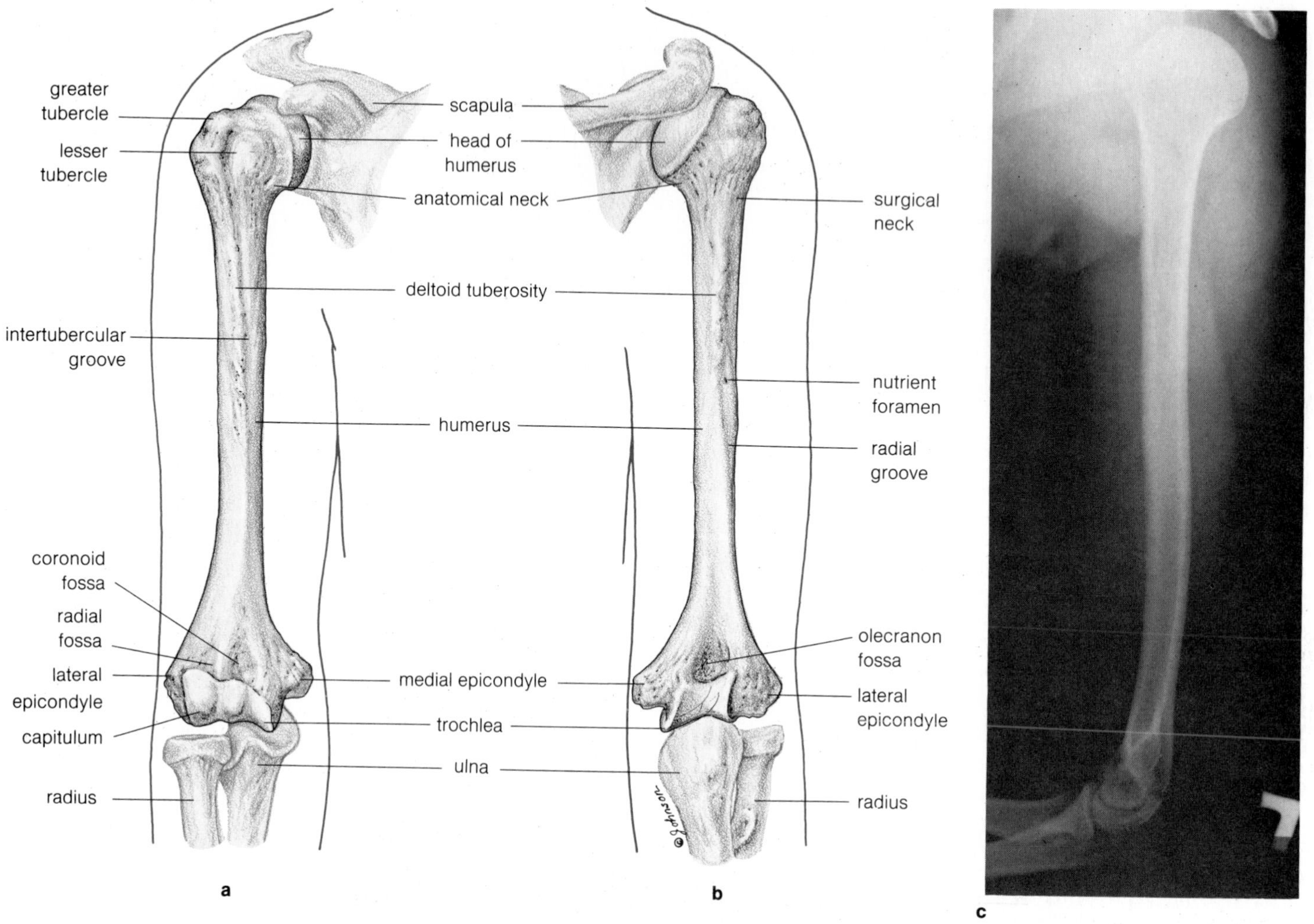
greater tubercle
lesser tubercle
scapula
head of humerus
anatomical neck
surgical neck
deltoid tuberosity
intertubercular groove
nutrient foramen
humerus
radial groove
coronoid fossa
radial fossa
olecranon fossa
lateral epicondyle
medial epicondyle
lateral epicondyle
capitulum
trochlea
ulna
radius
radius
a
b
c

Figure 6.26 The right humerus: (**a**) anterior view, (**b**) posterior view, (**c**) X ray of left posterior view (rotated), showing articulation with radius and ulna (X ray courtesy of Alexandria Hospital, Alexandria, Virginia, Joyce R. Isbel, R.T.)

tion of each coxal bone; its superior edge can be felt as a ridge of bone when you place your hands on your hips. The **ischium** is the portion of the coxal bone you sit on, and the **pubis** is the anterior portion. The *spines, crests, fossae,* and *lines* on the coxal bone represent the points of attachment of muscles of the abdomen, hip, and thigh. They are identified in Figure 6.29. The *greater sciatic notch* is closed by a ligament to form a foramen through which part of the sciatic nerve passes.

On the internal surface of the coxal bone two articulating surfaces are seen. The left pubis articulates with the right pubis to form the *pubic symphysis.* This joint is immovable except during late pregnancy and delivery (see Chapter 7). The articular surface of the ilium joins with the sacrum to form the *sacroiliac joint,* also a relatively immovable joint. The large, membrane-covered opening formed by the union of the inferior ramus of the pubis and the ramus of the ischium, through which blood vessels and the obturator nerve pass, is called the *obturator foramen.*

On the lateral surface of the coxal bone is the *acetabulum,* the socket of the ball-and-socket joint of the hip. Within the acetabulum parts of the three bones that form the coxal bone fuse. Outgrowth of these bones and their cartilage extensions form the rims of the acetabulum.

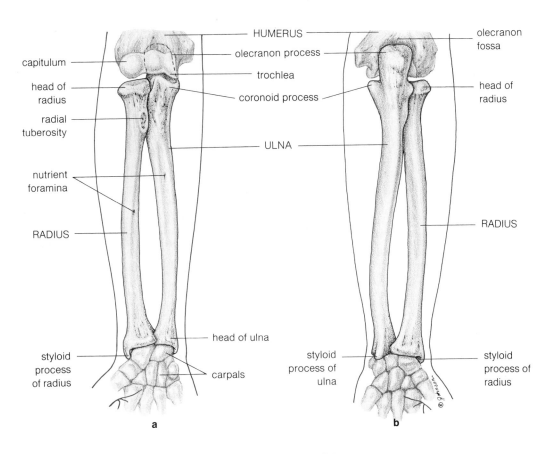

capitulum

head of radius

radial tuberosity

nutrient foramina

RADIUS

styloid process of radius

HUMERUS

olecranon process

trochlea

coronoid process

ULNA

head of ulna

carpals

a

olecranon fossa

head of radius

RADIUS

styloid process of ulna

styloid process of radius

b

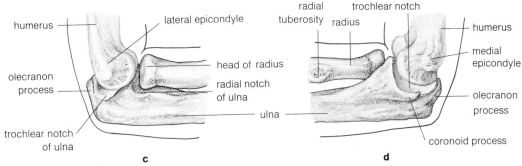

humerus

olecranon process

trochlear notch of ulna

lateral epicondyle

head of radius

radial notch of ulna

ulna

c

radial tuberosity

radius

trochlear notch

humerus

medial epicondyle

olecranon process

coronoid process

d

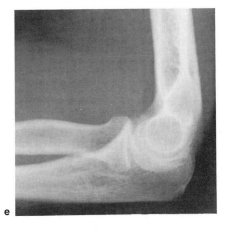

e

Figure 6.27 The right radius and ulna: (**a**) anterior view, (**b**) posterior view, (**c**) lateral view of articulation with the humerus, (**d**) medial view of articulation with the humerus, (**e**) X ray of medial view. (X ray courtesy of Alexandria Hospital, Alexandria, Virginia, Joyce R. Isbel, R.T.)

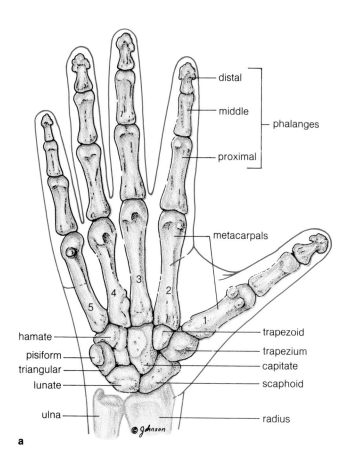

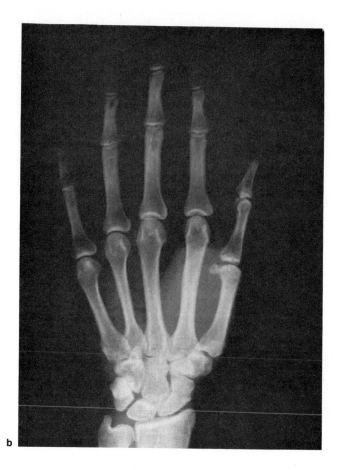

Figure 6.28 Carpals, metacarpals, and phalanges of right hand, palmar view: (**a**) diagram, (**b**) X ray. (X ray courtesy of Alexandria Hospital, Alexandria, Virginia, Joyce R. Isbel, R.T.)

Lower Appendage

The bones of the *lower appendage*, shown in Figure 6.1, are the femur, tibia, fibula, patella, tarsals, metatarsals, and phalanges.

The **femur**, or thigh bone (Figure 6.30), has a *head*, a *neck*, and a *shaft*. The head fits into the acetabulum of the coxal bone, and the anatomical neck is the site of attachment of capsular ligaments that hold the head in the joint socket. The *fovea capitis* is the site of attachment of an intraarticular ligament—a ligament found within the joint capsule. (Joint capsules will be explained in Chapter 7.) At the proximal end of the shaft are the *greater trochanter* and the *lesser trochanter*, sites for the attachment of thigh muscles. The *intertrochanteric line* on the anterior surface is another site of ligament attachment. The *intertrochanteric crest* serves a similar purpose on the posterior surface. Also on the poste-

rior surface are the *nutrient foramen*, the *linea aspera*, and the *popliteal surface*, sites at which muscles attach to the femur.

At the distal end of the femur the *medial condyle* and the *lateral condyle* form part of the knee joint surface. *Epicondyles*, located proximal to each condyle, serve as points of muscle attachment. The *patellar surface* and the *posterior intercondylar fossa* are also found on the distal end of the femur.

The **patella**, a sesamoid bone, is imbedded in the tendon of the quadriceps femoris muscle. It will be discussed in more detail with the discussion of the knee joint in Chapter 7.

The tibia and fibula (Figure 6.31) form the bony structure of the leg. The **tibia**, the heavier of the two bones, is the weight-bearing bone. At its proximal end *lateral* and *medial tibial condyles* articulate with the femur. At its distal end a *medial malleolus* extends around a portion of the medial surface of the talus.

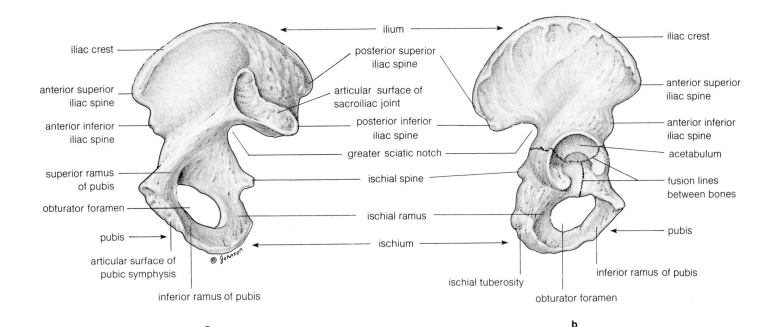

iliac crest

ilium

posterior superior
iliac spine

iliac crest

anterior superior
iliac spine

articular surface of
sacroiliac joint

anterior superior
iliac spine

anterior inferior
iliac spine

posterior inferior
iliac spine

anterior inferior
iliac spine

greater sciatic notch

acetabulum

superior ramus
of pubis

ischial spine

fusion lines
between bones

obturator foramen

ischial ramus

pubis

pubis

ischium

inferior ramus of pubis

articular surface of
pubic symphysis

© Johnson

ischial tuberosity

inferior ramus of pubis

obturator foramen

a

b

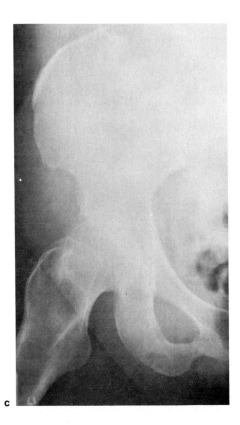

c

Figure 6.29 The coxal bone: (**a**) view of the internal surface, (**b**) view of the external surface, (**c**) X ray view, left, below, showing head of femur in acetabulum. (X ray courtesy of Alexandria Hospital, Alexandria, Virginia, Joyce R. Isbel, R.T.)

The **fibula**, a much thinner bone than the tibia, lies lateral to the tibia and articulates with it at both its proximal and distal ends. The fibula has a *lateral malleolus* that extends over part of the lateral surface of the talus. The malleoli show through the skin as bony projections on either side of the ankle. In many ankle fractures one or the other of the malleoli breaks off. Several other features of these bones are labeled in Figure 6.31.

The bones of the ankle and foot include the seven **tarsals**, five **metatarsals**, and fourteen **phalanges** (Figure 6.32). Of the tarsals the **talus** is the main bone in the articulation of the leg bones with the foot, and the **calcaneus** is the heel bone. Other tarsals are labeled in the figure. The distal tarsals articulate with the metatarsals about midway along the length of the foot. The metatarsals articulate with the proximal phalanges at the point where the toes join the rest of the foot. Notice that, like the thumb, the first, or great, toe has only two phalanges.

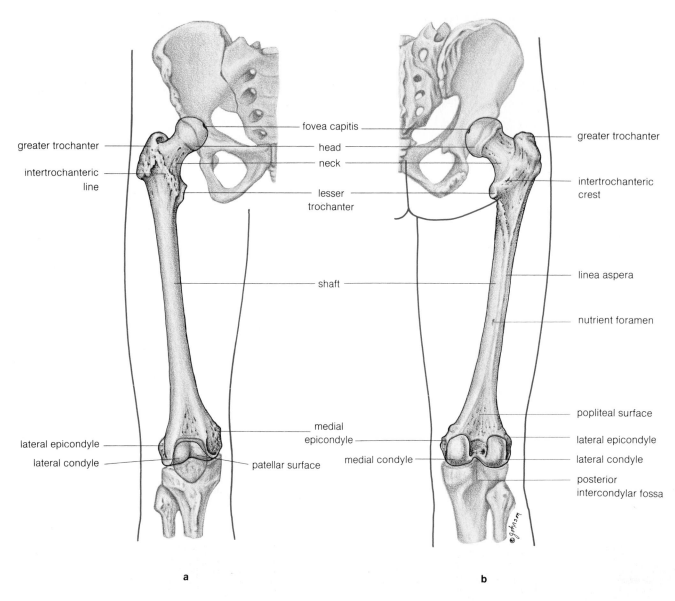

greater trochanter

intertrochanteric
line

fovea capitis

head

neck

lesser
trochanter

shaft

greater trochanter

intertrochanteric
crest

linea aspera

nutrient foramen

lateral epicondyle

lateral condyle

medial
epicondyle

patellar surface

popliteal surface

lateral epicondyle

lateral condyle

posterior
intercondylar fossa

medial condyle

a

b

Figure 6.30 The right femur: (**a**) anterior view, (**b**) posterior view.

The arches of the foot (Figure 6.33) include two longitudinal arches and one transverse arch. The *medial longitudinal arch* is formed by the calcaneus (heel bone), talus, navicular, cuneiforms, and three metatarsals. The *lateral longitudinal arch* is formed by the calcaneus, the cuboid, and the two lateral metatarsals. The *transverse arch* is formed by the cuboid and cuneiforms and the proximal ends of the metatarsals. Tendons of certain leg muscles and strong ligaments of the foot itself normally hold the bones of the foot in these characteristic arched positions. The arches support the body's weight and act as shock absorbers during walking and running.

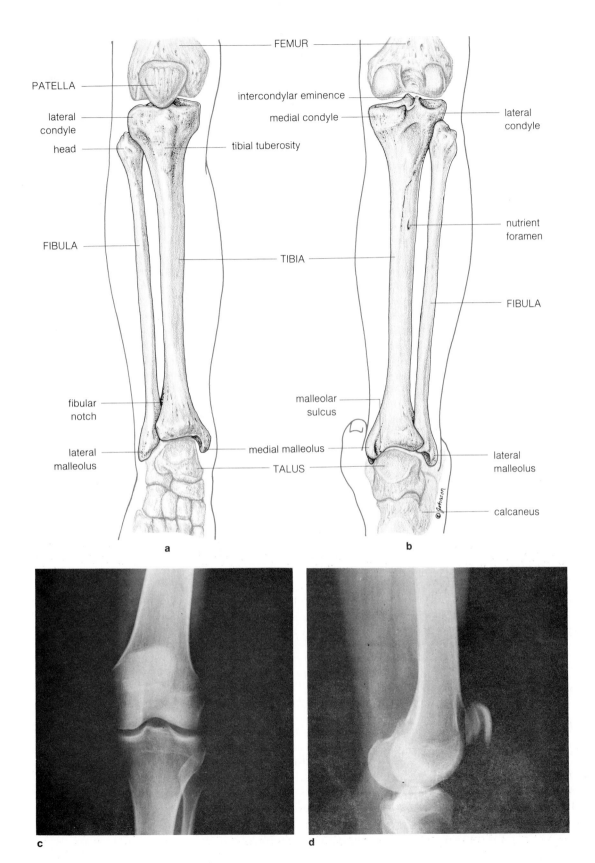

FEMUR

PATELLA

lateral condyle

head

FIBULA

intercondylar eminence

medial condyle

tibial tuberosity

TIBIA

lateral condyle

lateral condyle

nutrient foramen

FIBULA

fibular notch

lateral malleolus

malleolar sulcus

medial malleolus

TALUS

lateral malleolus

calcaneus

a

b

c

d

Figure 6.31 The right tibia and fibula: (**a**) anterior view, (**b**) posterior view, (**c**) X ray of posterior view, (**d**) X ray of lateral view (note patella to right and above joint), (X rays courtesy of Alexandria Hospital, Alexandria, Virginia, Joyce R. Isbel, R.T.)

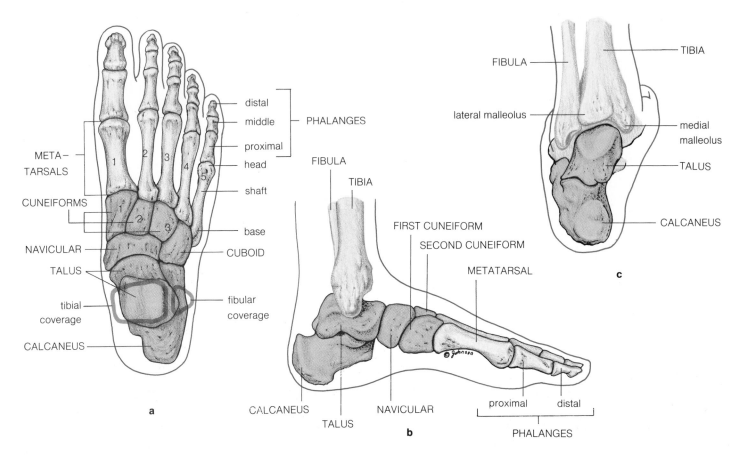

Figure 6.32 The foot: (**a**) superior view of right foot, (**b**) medial view of left foot, (**c**) posterior view of articulation of right foot with leg bones.

Markings on bones of the appendicular skeleton are summarized in Table 6.7.

Your arches can be easily damaged. If your body weight is excessive, your arches weaken from supporting the weight, and eventually you may have flat feet. If you wear poorly fitted shoes for jogging or other sports, you will place unnecessary stress on your arches. If you wear high-heeled shoes, you throw the weight of your body on the distal ends of the metatarsals. Not only does this place stress on the metatarsals and the arches, it also makes it much more difficult to maintain your balance and puts additional stress on your lower back.

SKELETAL DIFFERENCES DUE TO AGE AND SEX

Objective 7. Describe variations in the structure of bones due to age and sex.

Differences Due to Age

We have already studied the fontanels of an infant and how they close during the first months of life, but other age differences are also apparent in bones and joints. That these differences exist should not be surprising because bone is a metabolically active tissue and because bones are subjected to various stresses throughout life.

During the period of skeletal growth striking changes in the proportions of various bones occur. At birth an in-

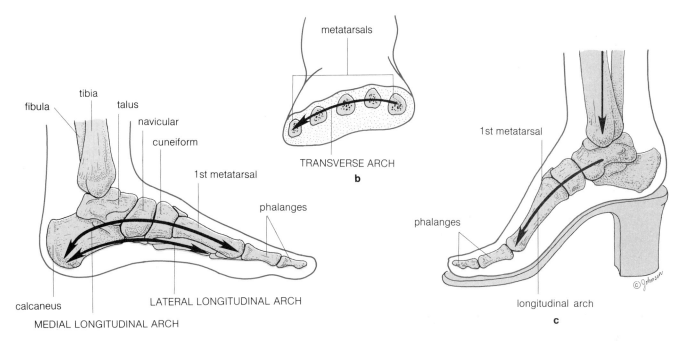

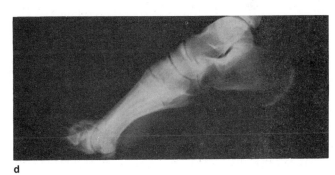

Figure 6.33 Arches of the foot: (**a**) longitudinal arches of the left foot, (**b**) transverse arch of the right foot (with toes removed), (**c**) alteration of weight distribution during the wearing of high-heeled shoes, (**d**) X ray at right shows medial view of right foot.

fant's head accounts for about one-fourth of its height, but in an adult the length of the head accounts for only about one-eighth of the total height. This is because bones of the trunk, as well as the appendages, grow faster than the skull. Curvatures of the vertebral column change from the anterior concavity of the infant to the alternating convex–concave curvatures described earlier for the adult skeleton. Changes in the bones of the face also occur, as clearly evidenced by the larger and sharper features of an adult face compared with an infant face. As already noted, the epiphyseal plates of the growing bones disappear, leaving only the epiphyseal lines as evidence of growth sites.

Even after growth is complete, the skeleton continues to change. Bone deposition occurs on the outer surfaces of bones, particularly near the joints, and absorption occurs on the inner surfaces. Marrow cavities thus become larger, and external processes more pronounced. As aging occurs, the growth of external processes often takes place in such a way as to limit mobility of the joints, and this increasingly limits various movements of the body. When bone is deposited near the articular cartilages, it severely limits joint movement. Such bone deposits, along with deterioration of articular cartilages, are manifestations of **osteoarthritis**, a common joint disease of the elderly (see Chapter 7).

Table 6.7 Markings on Bones of the Appendicular Skeleton	
Bone	Marking
Scapula (Figure 6.25)	Subscapular fossa—hollow anterior surface
	Vertebral border—edge nearest vertebrae
	Superior angle—point at which superior and vertebral borders meet
	Inferior angle—point at which axillary and vertebral borders meet
	Glenoid fossa—depression that articulates with humerus
	Acromion process—projection at lateral end of spine that articulates with the clavicle
	Coracoid process—anterior projection from superior border
	Spine—sharp ridge running across posterior surface
	Supraspinous fossa—depression superior to spine
	Infraspinous fossa—depression inferior to spine
Humerus (Figure 6.26)	Head—smooth, spherical projection on proximal end
	Anatomical neck—groove just below head
	Surgical neck—region below anatomical neck, so named because it is frequently the site of a fracture
	Greater tubercle—anteriolateral projection near head
	Lesser tubercle—anterior projection just below anatomical neck
	Intertubercular groove—long depression between tubercles where a tendon of the biceps brachii muscle lies
	Deltoid tuberosity—rough area near the middle of the shaft where the deltoid muscle attaches
	Radial groove—depression in deltoid tuberosity through which radial nerve passes
	Medial epicondyle—medial projection on distal end
	Lateral epicondyle—lateral projection on distal end
	Capitulum—rounded knob between the condyles that articulates with the radius
	Trochlea—projection on distal end that articulates with ulna
	Coronoid fossa—depression above trochlea that articulates with coronoid process of ulna
	Olecranon fossa—depression above and posterior to trochlea that articulates with the olecranon process of ulna
Radius (Figure 6.27)	Head—process at proximal end that articulates with the capitulum of the humerus and the radial notch of the ulna
	Styloid process—projection on lateral surface of distal end
	Radial tuberosity—roughened surface near head on which biceps brachii muscle inserts
Ulna (Figure 6.27)	Head—rounded process at distal end
	Styloid process—projection at distal end (toward little finger side of hand)
	Olecranon process—proximal projection that forms elbow
	Radial notch—concavity into which head of humerus fits

Table 6.7 Markings on Bones of the Appendicular Skeleton (continued)

Bone	Marking
Coxal bone (Figure 6.29)	Iliac crest—superior boundary of ilium
	Iliac fossa—concave anterior surface of ilium
	Anterior superior iliac spine—projection at anterior end of iliac crest
	Posterior superior iliac spine—projection at posterior end of iliac crest
	Anterior inferior iliac spine—projection below anterior superior spine
	Posterior inferior iliac spine—projection below posterior superior spine
	Ischial spine—projection above ischial tuberosity
	Ischial tuberosity—large inferior process that bears weight in sitting position
	Obturator foramen—opening surrounded by pubis and ischium
	Greater sciatic notch—notch on posterior surface of ilium
	Acetabulum—depression formed by fusion of ilium, ischium, and pubis; articulates with head of femur
Femur (Figure 6.30)	Head—rounded proximal projection that articulates with acetabulum
	Neck—constriction just below head
	Fovea capitis—indentation on head where a ligament attaches
	Greater trochanter—inferiolateral projection near head
	Lesser trochanter—small projection inferior and medial to greater trochanter
	Intertrochanteric line—anterior line between trochanters to which a ligament attaches
	Intertrochanteric crest—posterior rough area between trochanters to which a ligament attaches
	Linea aspera—lengthwise ridge on posterior surface to which muscles attach
	Popliteal surface—rough area on posterior surface to which muscles attach
	Medial condyle—medial projection at distal end
	Lateral condyle—lateral projection at distal end
	Medial epicondyle—small projection proximal to medial condyle
	Lateral epicondyle—small projection proximal to lateral condyle
	Patellar surface—depression between condyles beneath patella
	Posterior intercondylar fossa—posterior depression between condyles
Tibia (Figure 6.31)	Lateral tibial condyle—depression on proximal end that articulates with lateral condyle of the femur
	Medial tibial condyle—depression on proximal end that articulates with medial condyle of the femur
	Medial malleolus—medial projection at distal end of tibia
Fibula (Figure 6.31)	Lateral malleolus—lateral projection at distal end of fibula

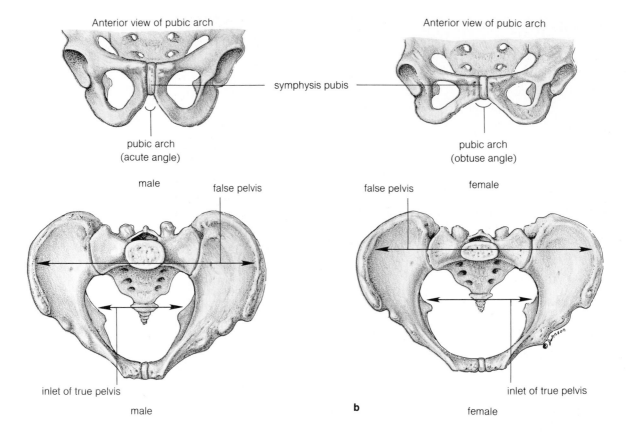

Anterior view of pubic arch

Anterior view of pubic arch

symphysis pubis

pubic arch
(acute angle)

pubic arch
(obtuse angle)

male

false pelvis

false pelvis

female

inlet of true pelvis

inlet of true pelvis

a

male

b

female

Figure 6.34 The differences in the structure of the pelvis related to sex: (**a**) anterior view of a male pubic arch, and superior view of male pelvic girdle, (**b**) anterior view of a female pelvic arch and superior view of female pelvic girdle, (**c**) X ray, next page, top. Is this a male or female pelvis? (X ray courtesy of Alexandria Hospital, Alexandria, Virginia, Joyce R. Isbel, R.T.)

Differences Due to Sex

The most marked differences between the skeletons of males and females are found in the pelvis. As shown in Figure 6.34, the male pelvis is narrow and deep, whereas the female pelvis is wide and shallow. The *inlet of the true pelvis* is somewhat heart-shaped in the male and much wider in diameter and nearly round in the female. The *false pelvis* is much wider in females than in males. Finally the *pubic arch* is narrow in males and wide in females. The characteristics of the female pelvis provide a wide basinlike pelvic area for a developing fetus and also allow for the passage of the fetus through the true pelvic inlet and on through the birth canal. These and other sexual differences in the skeleton are summarized in Table 6.8.

Table 6.8	Sexual Differences of Skeletons
Part	Difference
Skull	The female skull is lighter in weight, and the muscle attachments are less pronounced than in the male skull. In the female the facial area is more rounded and the jaw is usually proportionately smaller than in the male.
Sacrum	The female sacrum is wider, and the sacral curvature bends more sharply posteriorly than in the male sacrum.
Coccyx	The female coccyx is more movable than the male coccyx.
Pelvis	The female coxal bones are thinner and lighter in weight, and the muscle attachments are less pronounced than in the male coxal bones. The female ischia are more flared, and the acetabula are farther apart and smaller than in the male.
Pelvic cavity	The female pelvic cavity is shorter and wider in diameter than the male pelvic cavity.

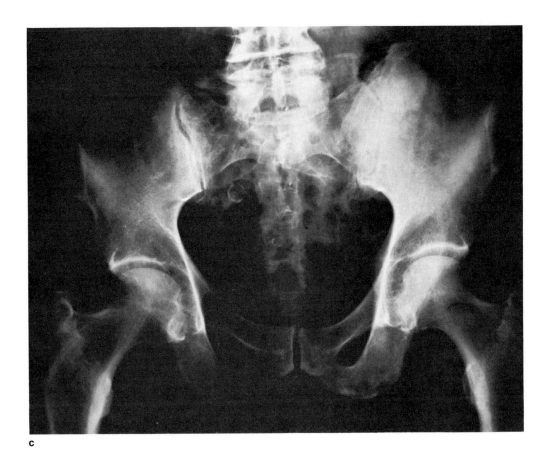

c

CLINICAL APPLICATIONS

Objective 8. Discuss the alterations of the structure and function of bones in the following clinical conditions: (a) fractures and the ways they heal, (b) osteomalacia and rickets, and (c) osteoporosis.

Bones are subject to a number of structural problems that lead to inadequate support or impaired movement of the body. These conditions may be caused by injury or disease.

Fractures

Fractures, one of the most common problems affecting bones, are more often due to twisting or excess lateral tension on bones than to compression. Though we may think of a fracture as primarily involving a bone, the tissues around the bone are also affected. Skin and muscles may be bruised or lacerated, and blood vessels and nerves may be damaged.

Fractures are classified according to whether the bone protrudes through the skin. In a **closed,** or **simple, fracture** the skin is not broken. However, in an **open,** or **compound, fracture,** an end of a broken bone tears through the skin and muscles, and the person is at serious risk of infection. Fractures may also be classified as **complete,** when the bone is broken into two parts, or **incomplete** (greenstick) when the bone is cracked without being broken apart. Greenstick fractures are common in children because the bones contain more collagen fibers and less mineral than adult bones. In a **comminuted fracture** the bone is broken into several fragments. These and some other types of fractures are illustrated in Figure 6.35.

Pain and swelling accompany fractures as they do many other kinds of injuries. Consequently, it is difficult to diagnose a fracture without using X ray unless a protruding bone or a clear deformity of the part is visible or can be felt through the skin.

Even when it is known without X ray that a fracture is present, X-ray photographs are usually taken to determine the position of the fractured bone, whether other fractures are present, and whether there are fragments of bone or periosteum that might interfere with healing.

The healing of a fracture is a relatively long and complex

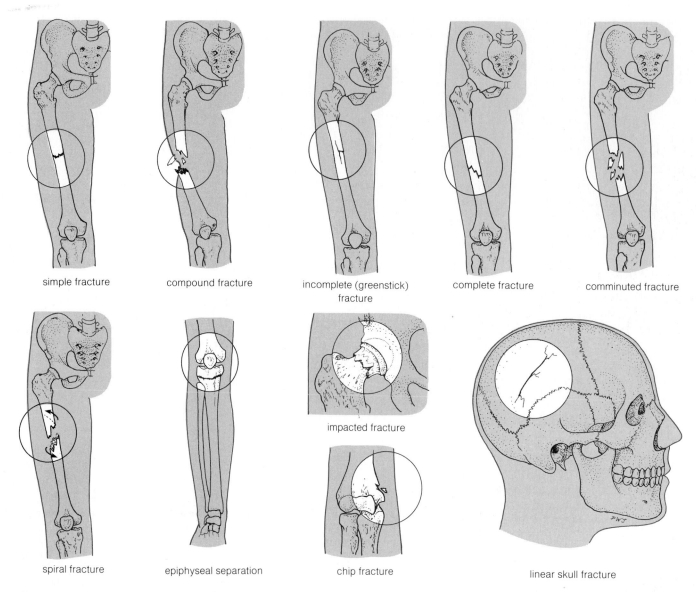

simple fracture

compound fracture

incomplete (greenstick) fracture

complete fracture

comminuted fracture

spiral fracture

epiphyseal separation

impacted fracture

chip fracture

linear skull fracture

Figure 6.35 Some different kinds of fractures.

process. Unlike most other injuries in which connective tissue scars form, a fracture heals by the growth of bone around the broken ends. To prevent deformity and to maintain function, the ends of a broken bone must be lined up in their original position before healing begins. This is called **reduction**, or setting, of a fracture. **Closed reduction** is done by manipulating the ends of the bone beneath the skin. **Open reduction** makes use of surgical procedures to place the parts of the bone in proper position and often also involves the use of rods inside the bone or plates and screws along the surface of the bone (Figure 6.36).

During the healing process (Figure 6.37) a blood clot forms, and phagocytic cells clean up the tissue debris surrounding the fracture. Then cells of the endosteum and periosteum differentiate into chondroblasts and osteoblasts and invade the clot. New cartilage and bone tissue in the shape of a collar forms around the ends of the broken bone on the inner and outer surfaces. This growth is called a **callus**. New spongy bone grows across the fracture line, and finally it is converted to compact bone. Bone remodeling continues until only a slightly thickened area around the fracture is apparent in an X ray.

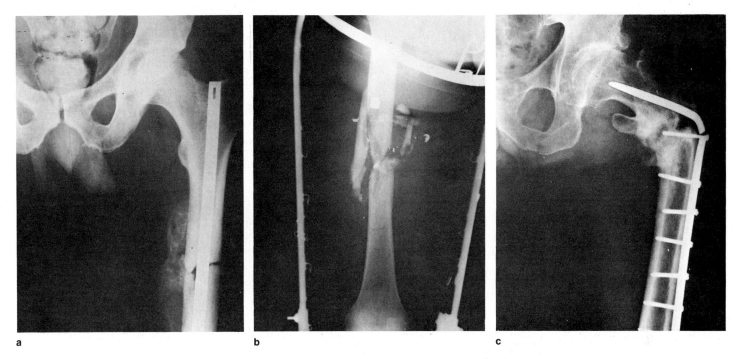

Figure 6.36 The open reduction of fractures: (**a**) reduction of a fracture using a rod inserted in the marrow cavity, (**b**) a comminuted fracture before reduction, (**c**) reduction of the comminuted fracture. (Armed Forces Institute of Pathology negative numbers (**a**) 53–11950, (**b**) 219506–19102, and (**c**) 219506–19103.)

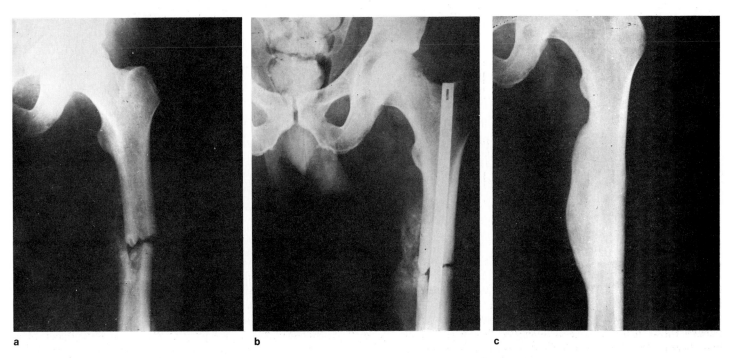

Figure 6.37 The healing of a fracture: (**a**) the fracture at the time of injury, (**b**) the open reduction of the fracture, (**c**) the healed fracture, showing the rod removed and the callus that has formed around the fracture site. (Armed Forces Institute of Pathology negative numbers (**a**) 219506–22034–0, (**b**) 219506–22034–W, and (**c**) 219506–22034–X.)

The length of time required for a fracture to heal depends on the quality of the reduction and immobilization and on the adequacy of the blood supply to the fracture area. If blood vessels were damaged at the time of the fracture, the circulation to the area of the fracture may be diminished and the healing process slowed down. Individuals are encouraged to place weight on a fractured limb as soon as the limb can withstand it so that healing along usual stress lines is promoted. Early weight-bearing improves the blood circulation and accelerates healing.

The plaster cast has been the traditional method of immobilizing a fracture in spite of the fact that it is hot, heavy, itchy, and impossible to keep clean. Fiberglass is now being used as material for forming casts. It is three times as strong as plaster and weighs only half as much. Because it is porous and waterproof, air can reach the skin beneath, so itching is reduced, and the cast itself can be washed. Walking casts made of fiberglass make it easier for people with leg fractures to move about. Furthermore, they make it possible for some weight to be placed on the fracture. This creates stress in the bone and stimulates bone growth as well as increasing the circulation of blood.

Osteomalacia and Rickets

Osteomalacia, called **rickets** when it occurs in childhood, is a disease in which the bones contain insufficient amounts of calcium and phosphorus. Three causes are discussed here: kidney disease, vitamin D deficiency, and an inherited defect. Certain kinds of kidney disease allow excess excretion of calcium; because the concentration of calcium in the blood is maintained at a nearly constant level, calcium is removed from the bones to replace that lost from the blood. Vitamin D deficiency leads to inadequate absorption of calcium from the food, the blood calcium concentration drops, and again calcium is removed from the bones. In the inherited condition vitamin D–resistant rickets, the kidneys do not respond to vitamin D and excrete excessive amounts of phosphate, preventing it from being incorporated into the bones. This inherited condition is difficult to treat; administration of vitamin D does not alleviate the condition because increasing calcium absorption is of no use unless phosphate is available to combine with the calcium.

Osteoporosis

Osteoporosis is a disease in which bone loses minerals and protein fibers from its matrix. Individuals taking hydrocortisone for arthritis, allergies, or other disorders are especially prone to bone loss. Hydrocortisone blocks the formation of new bone and decreases the absorption of calcium so that normal bone maintenance is impaired and some existing bone is lost. Diabetic individuals are also subject to bone loss; those taking oral hypoglycemic medica-

tions are more prone to bone loss than those receiving insulin injections. Even without receiving hydrocortisone, many elderly people suffer from osteoporosis. For unknown reasons white women are particularly susceptible to the condition, both white and black men somewhat susceptible to it, and black women are particularly resistant to it. The spine and other parts of the skeleton undergo degeneration, and the person becomes hunched and especially susceptible to fractures. Sometimes in elderly persons, a bone breaks and causes a fall, rather than a fall causing a fracture.

A bone scan (Figure 6.38) is frequently done on an individual who has had a malignancy and who is suspected of having metastasis to the bones. In a bone scan a radioactive substance is given the individual, and radiographs are taken over the next few minutes. During that time the radioactive substance is incorporated into the bone marrow and is seen as "black dots" on the developed film. Malignant tissue takes up the radioactive substance more rapidly than other tissue and thus can be detected as an intensely dark area.

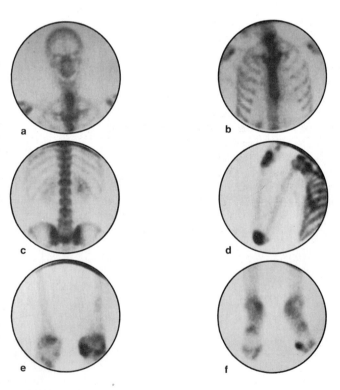

Figure 6.38 A bone scan showing the incorporation of a radioactive substance in the bone marrow: (**a**) head and neck, (**b**) thorax, (**c**) lumbrosacral area, (**d**) arm, (**e**) thighs and knees, (**f**) ankles and feet. (Courtesy of Alexandria Hospital, Alexandria, Virginia, Joyce R. Isbel, R.T.)

Clinical Terms

achondroplasia (ah-kon-dro-pla′ze-ah)   a genetic defect leading to dwarfism

acromegaly (ak-ro-meg′al-e)   enlargement of the bones of the face, hands, and feet due to excess growth hormone in adult life

Colles' fracture   a fracture of the lower end of the radius in which the bone fragment is displaced posteriorly

craniotomy (kra-ne-ot′o-me)   any surgical procedure that involves severing bones of the cranium

flat foot   the loss of curvature of one or more of the arches of the foot

orthopedic (or-tho-pe′dik)   pertaining to the treatment of bone and joint disorders and the correction of deformities

osteitis deformans (os-te-i′tis de-for′manz)   an inflammation of bone in which some skeletal parts become thickened and others thinned; Paget's disease

osteoblastoma (os″te-o-blas-to′mah)   a tumor produced from bone-forming cells

osteogenesis imperfecta (os″te-o-jen′e-sis im-per-fek′tah)   a disorder caused by a genetic defect that leads to improper synthesis of collagen and thus to defects in skin, cartilage, tendons, and bones

osteomyelitis (os″te-o-mi-el-i′tis)   an inflammation of the marrow cavity and usually the surrounding bone tissue

osteosarcoma (os″te-o-sar-ko′mah)   a malignant growth of bone tissue

Pott's fracture   a fracture of the lower part of the fibula accompanied by injury to the articulation of the fibula with the tarsals

---

CHAPTER SUMMARY

(Chapter summary points and review questions are numbered to correspond to the numbered objectives in the text of each chapter.)

Organization and General Functions

1. Describe the basic plan of the skeletal system and list its major functions.
   a. The skeletal system consists of all of the bones and cartilages of the body. It includes:
      (1) the axial skeleton, which supports the head and trunk
      (2) the appendicular skeleton, which supports the appendages
   b. The general functions of the skeletal system are:
      (1) support
      (2) protection
      (3) storage of calcium and phosphorus
      (4) provision of surfaces for the attachment of muscles
      (5) formation of blood cells

Development of the Skeletal System

2. Describe the ossification and remodeling of (a) a membranous bone, and (b) an endochondral bone.
   a. In the formation of a membranous bone osteoblasts deposit bone in connective tissue membranes.
   b. In the formation of an endochondral bone:
      (1) a cartilage model of the bone is laid down

   (2) blood vessels grow into the perichondrium of the primary ossification center, and cells become differentiated into osteoblasts
   (3) bone is laid down in a collarlike structure around the future shaft of the bone
   (4) the cartilage disintegrates and is replaced by bone
   (5) similar processes occur at the ends of the bones in the secondary ossification centers until skeletal growth is completed

Characteristics of Bones

3. List the types of bones found in the body, describe the structure of a long bone, and identify the markings found on bones.
   a. Bones are classified by shape as long, short, flat, or irregular.
   b. Bones are classified by location or manner of development as:
      (1) sesamoid bones, which develop in a tendon
      (2) Wormian bones, which develop from independent centers of ossification between the larger skull bones
   c. A long bone consists of:
      (1) two epiphyses and a diaphysis
      (2) a medullary cavity lined with endosteum
      (3) an outer membrane called the periosteum
   d. Bone markings are summarized in Table 6.2.

Axial Skeleton I: Bones of the Head

4. Locate and identify the bones of the axial skeleton found in the head and describe their structural characteristics.

 a. The axial skeleton consists of the bones of the skull, the vertebral column, ribs, sternum, hyoid, and middle ear bones (see Table 6.3).

 b. Structural characteristics of the bones of the head are related to their functions as follows:

  (1) Most bones of the cranium are shaped to protect the brain.

  (2) Some bones have processes and depressions where muscles attach.

  (3) Most bones have openings through which nerves and blood vessels pass.

  (4) Special structures associated with bones of the head include sutures, fontanels, meati (plural of meatus), and sinuses.

Axial Skeleton II: Bones of the Trunk

5. Locate and identify the bones of the axial skeleton found in the trunk and describe their structural characteristics.

 a. The vertebral column is a major supporting structure of the trunk.

 b. The ribs and sternum, with the vertebral column, provide a protective "cage" around the heart and lungs.

 c. Bones of the trunk have processes and depressions where muscles attach, and some have openings through which nerves and blood vessels pass.

Appendicular Skeleton

6. For each of the following parts of the appendicular skeleton, locate the bones and identify their structural characteristics: (a) pectoral girdle, (b) upper appendage, (c) pelvic girdle, and (d) lower appendage.

 a. The appendicular skeleton consists of the pectoral girdle, the pelvic girdle, and the bones of the upper and lower appendages, as listed in Table 6.6.

 b. Structural characteristics of these bones are related to their functions as follows:

  (1) These bones have processes and/or depressions where muscles attach.

  (2) Some have openings through which nerves and blood vessels pass.

  (3) These bones have articular surfaces where they form joints with other bones.

  (4) The girdles attach the appendages to the axial skeleton.

  (5) The appendicular skeleton serves many of the same functions as the axial skeleton but is more important in movement than the axial skeleton.

  (6) The markings on bones of the appendicular skeleton are listed in Table 6.7.

Skeletal Differences Due to Age and Sex

7. Describe variations in the structure of bones due to age and sex.

 a. The structure of the skeleton changes with age.

  (1) After birth the trunk and appendages grow at a more rapid rate than the skull.

  (2) After growth is complete, bones continue to be reshaped and remodeled, and some degeneration occurs.

 b. The male and female skeletons differ in size and shape.

  (1) The female pelvic girdle is larger, shallower, and more bowl shaped than the male skeleton.

  (2) Other differences are summarized in Table 6.8.

Clinical Applications

8. Discuss the alterations of the structure and function of the bones in the following clinical conditions: (a) fractures and the ways they heal, (b) osteomalacia and rickets, and (c) osteoporosis.

 a. Fractures:

  (1) are classified as simple (closed) or compound (open), and as complete, incomplete, or comminuted

  (2) are set by open or closed reduction

  (3) heal by forming a callus around the fracture site

 b. Osteomalacia in adults and rickets in children are diseases in which bones are lacking in minerals because of an inadequate supply of calcium or vitamin D, or because of inherited vitamin D resistance.

 c. Osteoporosis is a disease in which bone mass is lost, and remaining bone is less dense.

REVIEW

Important Terms

appendicular	fissure
axial	fontanel
callus	foramen
closed reduction	fossa
cranium	fracture
crest	Haversian canal
depression	marrow
diaphysis	meatus
endochondral	medullary cavity
endosteum	membranous
epiphyseal line	nutrient foramen
epiphyseal plate	open reduction
epiphysis	ossification

osteoblast

osteoclast

osteocyte

osteomalacia

osteoporosis

pectoral

pelvic

perichondrium

periosteum

primary ossification center

process

rickets

secondary ossification center

sesamoid bone

sinus

sulcus

suture

trochanter

tubercle

tuberosity

Volkmann's canal

Wormian bone

Note: The names of individual bones are found in boldface type and the names of their markings are found in italics in the text.

Questions

1. **a.** What are the functions of the skeletal system?
   b. What are the main divisions of the skeletal system, and how are they related to each other?

2. **a.** How does the development of a membranous bone differ from the development of an endochondral bone?
   b. What occurs during the remodeling of a bone?

3. **a.** How are bones classified by shape?
   b. What is the difference between a sesamoid bone and a Wormian bone?

4. **a.** Name the bones of the axial skeleton.
   b. Cite five examples of complementarity of structure and function in the bones of the head.
   c. What is a suture?
   d. What is a fontanel, and where are fontanels found?
   e. What is a sinus, and where are sinuses found?

5. **a.** Compare the structures of the different types of vertebrae.
   b. Compare the structures of the different types of ribs.
   c. How do the ribs connect the vertebrae with the sternum?

6. **a.** Name the bones of the appendicular skeleton.
   b. Which bones are part of the pectoral girdle? the pelvic girdle? the upper appendage? the lower appendage?
   c. Classify the structural characteristics of the major bones of the appendicular skeleton as openings, depressions, articular surfaces, or surfaces for the attachment of other structures.
   d. From what bones are the arches of the foot formed, and what is the function of arches?

7. **a.** How is the skeleton of an adult different from the skeleton of an infant?
   b. How is the structure of a male skeleton different from a female skeleton?

   c. What is the significance of the specialized structure of the female pelvis?

8. **a.** List five different kinds of fractures and describe their characteristics.
   b. How does a fracture heal?
   c. What are the advantages of early weight-bearing on a fractured bone?
   d. How are the diseases of osteomalacia and osteoporosis similar, and how are they different?

Problems

1. X rays of the bones of the hand are sometimes used to estimate the rate at which epiphyseal plates are closing in the distal forearm and wrist of a growing child. Research this topic and determine how the technique could be used to determine whether a child's growth rate is abnormal.

2. Two individuals have similar leg fractures. One received a walking cast and the other a regular cast and crutches. Which person's fracture would heal faster and why?

3. Devise a new method of immobilizing a fracture in an ambulatory person that would be equally effective but less cumbersome than a plaster or fiberglass cast.

REFERENCES AND READINGS

Anonymous. 1979. New therapies, new forms of an old vitamin. *Science News* 115:181 (March 24).

Copenhaver, W. M., Kelly, D. E., and Wood, R. L. 1978. *Bailey's textbook of histology* (17th ed.). Baltimore, Md.: Williams and Wilkins.

Christakos, S., and Norman, A. W. 1978. Vitamin D_3-induced calcium binding protein in bone tissue. *Science* 202:70 (October 6).

Evans, F. G. 1957. *Atlas of human anatomy.* Totowa, N.J.: Rowman and Littlefield.

Gray, H. 1973. *Anatomy of the human body* (29th American ed.). C. M. Goss, ed. Philadelphia: Lea and Febiger.

Russell, C. 1979. Chinese medicine: old and new. *Science News* 116:292 (October 27).

Schlossberg, L. 1977. *The Johns Hopkins atlas of human functional anatomy.* G. D. Zuidema, ed. Baltimore, Md.: Johns Hopkins Press.

Snell, R. S. 1978. *Atlas of clinical anatomy.* Boston: Little, Brown.

7

ARTICULATIONS

ORGANIZATION AND GENERAL FUNCTIONS

Objective 1. Relate articulations to the skeletal system and describe their general functions.

Articulations, also called **joints** or **arthroses**, are the points at which bones are joined to each other or at which a bone is joined to cartilage. (It is from the word arthrosis that we get arthritis, meaning joint inflammation.) Though the joints constitute part of the skeletal system, they are considered separately because of their importance in the movements of the body and its parts.

Some joints help to support parts of the skeletal system, but most provide for movement. Some joints provide both movement and support. Most joints are movable, though some are not. Immovable joints fasten bones together to form rigid supporting structures such as the skull. Movable joints allow one bone to move in relation to another. For example, a pivot joint between the first and second cervical vertebrae allows turning of the head; a ball-and-socket joint at the shoulder or hip allows a wide range of movements of a limb. Several other kinds of joints are present in the body. Together, they allow us to perform many kinds of activities from the heavy work of the dockside stevedore to the intricate movements of an eye surgeon.

CHARACTERISTICS OF JOINTS

Objective 2. List the general characteristics of the three types of joints.

Objective 3. Describe the structure, function, and location of fibrous joints.

Objective 4. Describe the structure, function, and location of cartilaginous joints.

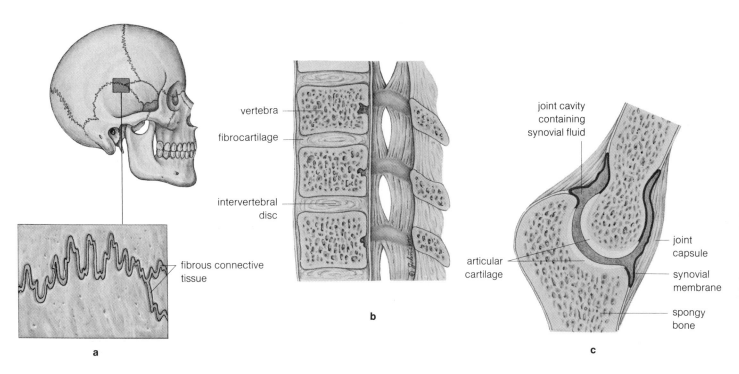

Figure 7.1 Types of joints: (**a**) a synarthrosis, an immovable fibrous joint, (**b**) an amphiarthrosis, a slightly movable cartilaginous joint, (**c**) a diarthrosis, a freely movable synovial joint with a joint cavity.

Objective 5. Describe the structure, function, and location of (a) synovial joints and (b) bursae and tendon sheaths; (c) describe the properties and function of synovial fluid.

Objective 6. List and define the kinds of movement that occur at synovial joints.

Joints are classified according to their structure and the degree of movement they allow. On this basis three types of joints are recognized (Figure 7.1):

1. synarthroses—immovable or slightly movable fibrous joints

2. amphiarthroses—slightly movable cartilaginous joints

3. diarthroses or synovial joints—freely movable joints that have a synovial cavity, or joint cavity.

The characteristics of these joints are summarized in Table 7.1.

Synarthroses (Fibrous Joints)

In a **synarthrosis** (Figure 7.1a) the bones are held together by fibers of connective tissue; thus a synarthrosis is also called a **fibrous joint**. The fibers extend from one bone to the other and hold the two bones together tightly. There is little or no movement at such a joint. The **sutures** of the skull are examples of one kind of synarthrosis. Another kind of synarthrosis, called a **syndesmosis**, is located between the distal ends of the tibia and fibula, just above the ankle, and between the radius and ulna near the wrist. Again, fibers of connective tissue extend between these bones and bind them together, but in this instance the bones do not fit together as tightly as in a suture, and a slight amount of movement is possible.

> Trauma from athletic injuries and automobile accidents often causes excessive movement at a synarthrosis. If the joint does not return to its normal position, the person experiences chronic pain until the bones are manipulated back to their normal positions.

Amphiarthroses (Cartilaginous Joints)

In an **amphiarthrosis** (Figure 7.1b) bones are held together by a piece of cartilage interposed between them and fas-

Table 7.1   Characteristics of Types of Joints

Type of Joint	Properties	Mobility	Examples
Synarthrosis (fibrous joint) (Figure 7.1)	Bones held together by fibers; no joint cavity present	Immovable or slightly movable	
Suture	Fibers hold bones tightly together	Immovable	Coronal, sagittal, and lambdoidal sutures
Syndesmosis	Fibers bind bones but not as tightly as above	Slightly movable	Tibiofibular and radioulnar joints
Amphiarthrosis (cartilaginous joint) (Figures 7.1, 7.2)	Cartilage interposed between bones of the joint; fibers hold bone and cartilage together; no joint cavity present	Slightly movable	
Symphysis	Fibrous cartilage between bones; fibers and ligaments stabilize joint	Slightly movable	Intervertebral joints and pubic symphysis
Synchrondrosis	Hyaline cartilage interposed between bones	Slightly movable	Joint between first costal cartilage and sternum; joint between bone and epiphyseal cartilage during bone growth
Diarthrosis (synovial joint) (Figures 7.1, 7.4)	Has joint cavity, joint capsule, synovial membrane, and synovial fluid; ligaments stabilize joint and muscles extend across joint; bone ends within joint covered with hyaline articular cartilage	Freely movable	
Gliding	Flat or slightly curved articular surfaces	Side-to-side and back-and-forth movements	Joints between carpals and between tarsals
Hinge	Convex and concave articulating surfaces	Movement in only one plane	Elbow and knee joints
Pivot	Rounded bone fits in depression in another bone	Rotation	Joint between radius and ulna, and between atlas and axis
Ellipsoid (condyloid)	Oval condyle fits into an elliptical depression in another bone	Back-and-forth and side-to-side movements	Joints between metacarpals and phalanges of fingers
Saddle	Projection of one bone fits in saddle-shaped depression in another bone	Same as ellipsoid, but freer movements	Joint between metacarpal and phalanx of thumb
Ball-and-socket	Ball-like projection of one bone fits into socketlike depression in another bone	Most freely movable of all joints; allows movement in three planes and rotation of bone on its own axis	Shoulder and hip joints

tened tightly to both; thus an amphiarthrosis is also called a **cartilaginous joint**. Such joints are further classified as symphyses or synchrondroses.

A **symphysis** is a slightly movable joint in which the articular surfaces of the bones are covered with hyaline cartilage, and a piece of fibrous cartilage is interposed between them. Collagen fibers from the fibrous cartilage attach to the bones and bind them together. Ligaments also connect the bones to each other and reinforce the union.

Symphyses are found between the vertebrae, where they provide strong support for the vertebral column and allow slight movement. By twisting and bending your back, you can demonstrate to yourself that these joints are slightly movable. The fibrous cartilage in an intervertebral joint has special characteristics that provide for weight-bearing and allow it to act as a shock absorber (Figure 7.2). This cartilage (also sometimes referred to as a **disc**) consists of an inner gelatinous pulp, the **nucleus pulposus**, and an outer set of

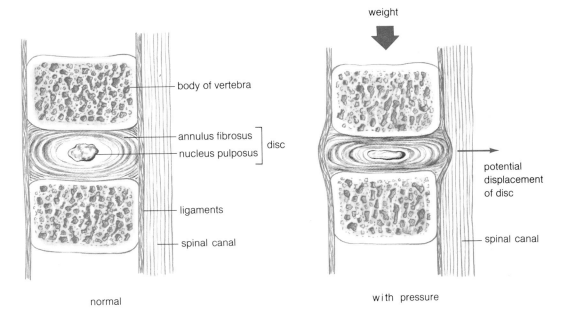

weight

body of vertebra

annulus fibrosus ⎤
nucleus pulposus ⎦ disc

ligaments

spinal canal

normal

potential
displacement
of disc

spinal canal

with pressure

Figure 7.2   An intervertebral joint, an example of a symphysis.

concentric rings of fibers, the **annulus fibrosus**. When you stand erect, the disc is slightly compressed and flattened; as you walk, the pulpy portion acts as a shock absorber.

A similar joint, the **pubic symphysis**, joins the coxal bones anteriorly. This joint is movable only during late pregnancy and delivery, when the fibers that connect the cartilages of the bones have become stretched. Movement of this joint during delivery eases the passage of the infant through the birth canal.

Another type of amphiarthrosis, the **synchondrosis**, is a slightly movable joint in which hyaline cartilage is interposed between the bones. The union of the first costal cartilage to the sternum is an example of such a joint. Other synchondroses exist as temporary joints during the growth of bones. These joints occur between the bone of the diaphysis and epiphyseal cartilage of a growing bone and disappear when growth is complete.

Diarthroses (Freely Movable Synovial Joints)

The majority of joints in the body are diarthroses. These freely movable joints are located in all of the places one normally thinks of as movable joints—shoulder, hip, elbow, knee, wrist, ankle, and many places in the hands and feet.

A **diarthrosis** is also called a **synovial joint** because it has a joint cavity that contains synovial fluid, which lubricates the joint (Figure 7.1c). A synovial joint is surrounded

If an intervertebral disc is subjected to severe pressure, it may rupture (herniate), and the nucleus pulposus may push into the body of the vertebra or out to the side of the joint, where it can create painful pressure on adjacent spinal nerves. Pain is felt in the area of the body supplied by the affected nerves.

by a fibrous **joint capsule**, which helps to maintain the alignment of the bones of the joint. Ligaments outside the capsule also help to stabilize the joint. Muscles attach to the bones of a given joint and extend over the joint; contraction of the muscles causes movement at the joint. Inside the capsule are the ends of the bones, extending into the joint cavity. The articular surfaces of the bones are covered with **articular cartilage**, a smooth hyaline cartilage that reduces friction when the ends of the bones move against each other. Friction is further reduced by the lubricating action of the synovial fluid.

Synovial fluid is secreted by the **synovial membrane**, a membrane that lines joint cavities, bursae and tendon sheaths. Synovial fluid consists of interstitial fluid (fluid found between cells of a tissue) that has a high concentration of hyaluronic acid, the primary lubricant.

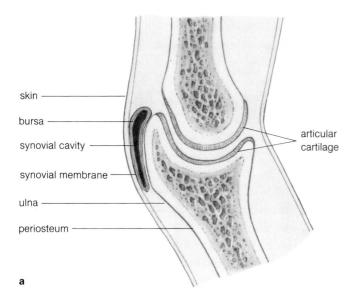

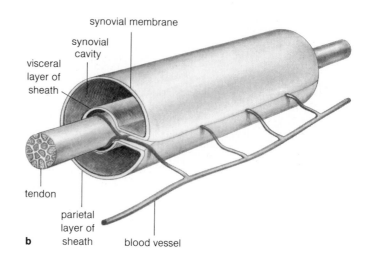

Figure 7.3 (**a**) A bursa, (**b**) a tendon sheath.

Bursae and Tendon Sheaths

Bursae and **tendon sheaths** are saclike structures made of connective tissue, lined with synovial membrane and filled with synovial fluid (Figure 7.3). They are similar to joint cavities and are usually located near a joint at a point of excessive friction. Bursae may be subcutaneous, lying between the skin and an underlying bone, or they may lie between a tendon and a bone. Their main function is to reduce friction, permitting easy movement of one part on another. A few of the more prominent bursae include the prepatellar bursa between the skin and the patella, the olecranon bursa in the elbow, and the subscapular bursa beneath the scapula. Bursae also are found in the hips, heels, and other sites. **Tendon sheaths** are tube-shaped structures, similar to bursae, that surround tendons subjected to great pressure. Tendons possessing such sheaths may be observed on the back of the hand when the fingers are held straight out and spread apart. They also are found along the anterior surface of the foot.

Synovial Joints and Their Movements

Though we will discuss movements of specific major joints in detail later in this chapter, we can now consider the various types of synovial joints and the nature of the movements each allows. All joint movements are described in terms of the body being in anatomical position. The six types of synovial joints, according to their shapes and the movements they allow, are: (1) gliding, (2) hinge, (3) pivot, (4) ellipsoid, (5) saddle, and (6) ball-and-socket (Figure 7.4).

A **gliding joint** (Figure 7.4a) is the simplest of the synovial joints. The articular surfaces of a gliding joint are flat or slightly curved, permitting only back-and-forth or side-to-side movements. No rotation or twisting is possible because the bones are packed closely together or held in place by ligaments. Gliding joints are found between the carpal bones, between the tarsal bones, and between the articulating processes of the vertebrae.

A **hinge joint** (Figure 7.4b) allows movement primarily in one plane. In a hinge joint the convex surface of one bone fits into the concave surface of another bone. The elbow and the knee are examples of hinge joints. You can demonstrate to yourself the movements of a hinge joint. Bend your elbow so your hand moves toward your shoulder. This movement is called **flexion** because it decreases the angle between the bones that make up the joint. Now straighten your arm. This movement is called **extension** because it increases the angle between the bones of the joint. Notice that flexion and extension are opposite movements, and that the movement is limited to one plane.

A **pivot joint** (Figure 7.4c) also allows movement in only one plane. In a pivot joint a rounded or pointed bone fits into a depression in another bone. The joints between the atlas and axis and between the radius and ulna just below the elbow are examples of pivot joints. The primary movement at a pivot joint is **rotation**. You can demonstrate rotation by extending your arm in front of you with the

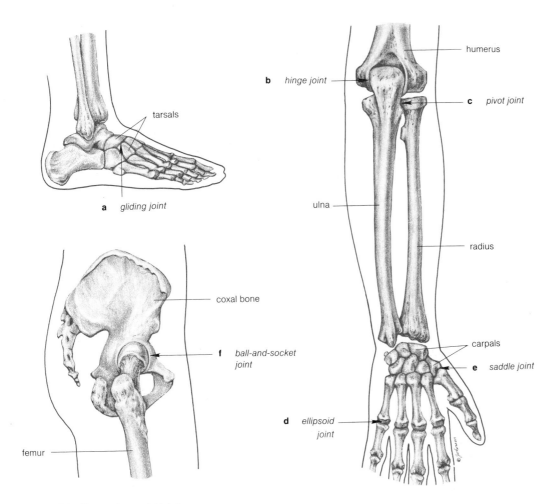

Figure 7.4 Types of synovial joints.

palm up. Then move your forearm so that your hand is palm down and notice that the radius (the bone that goes from your elbow to your thumb) rotates over the ulna (the other bone in your forearm). You can also rotate or turn your head from side to side because of the pivot joint between the two most superior vertebrae.

An **ellipsoid**, or **condyloid**, **joint** (Figure 7.4d) allows movement in two planes, back-and-forth and side-to-side. In an ellipsoid joint an oval (egg-shaped) condyle of one bone fits into an elliptical depression in another bone. The joints between the bones in the palm of your hand and the bones of your fingers are examples of ellipsoid joints. To demonstrate the side-to-side movement, spread your fingers apart and move them back together again. The spreading apart movement is called **abduction** because the

fingers are moving away from the midline of the hand—an imaginary line extending down the middle finger. (To abduct literally means to carry away; in the movement of body parts abducting them is carrying them away from a midline.) Moving your fingers back together again is called **adduction** because the fingers are moving back toward the midline. Abduction and adduction are opposite movements within one plane. The other plane of movement at the ellipsoid joints is the back-and-forth movement. You can demonstrate this by bending a finger toward the palm of your hand and straightening it again. The bending is flexion, and the straightening is extension. In these particular joints **hyperextension** is also possible, as you can demonstrate by bending your finger backward toward the back of your hand.

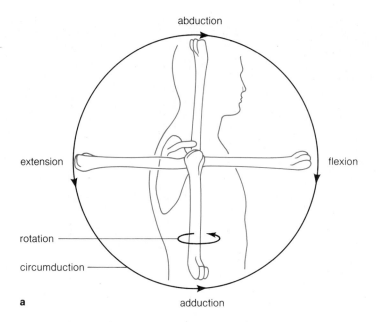

abduction

extension

flexion

rotation

circumduction

a

adduction

Figure 7.5 Movements of a ball-and-socket joint: (**a**) diagrammed, (**b**) flexion and extension, (**c**) circumduction. (Photographs by Elliott Varner Smith.)

Individuals who have an unusual amount of flexibility in the joints between the carpals and metacarpals are sometimes said to be "double jointed." However, the joints are not really double; they have exactly the same structural components as other synovial joints. The joints simply have greater flexibility.

A **saddle joint** (Figure 7.4e) allows the same movements as an ellipsoid joint, but the movements are freer. The joint between the metacarpal of the thumb and the carpals of the hand is an example of a saddle joint. Compare the freedom of movement of your thumb with that of your other fingers to demonstrate to yourself that movement is freer at a saddle joint than at an ellipsoid joint.

A **ball-and-socket joint** (Figures 7.4f and 7.5) is the most freely movable of all joints. In a ball-and-socket joint,

as the name suggests, a ball-like structure on one bone fits into a socketlike structure in another bone. Three kinds of movement are possible at a ball-and-socket joint. First, the bone with the ball-shaped articulation can rotate in the socket. You can demonstrate this by holding your arm out in front of you with the elbow extended and rotating your whole arm back and forth on its own axis. (Its axis is an imaginary line that goes straight down the midline of the arm from shoulder to fingertip.) This movement is **rotation**. Be sure you distinguish between the rotation of the humerus in the ball-and-socket joint and the rotation at the pivot joint in the forearm. The second kind of movement at a ball-and-socket joint is abduction-adduction. When you raise your arm up and away from your side, you abduct it; when you bring your arm close to your side you adduct it. The third kind of movement is flexion-extension. The natural swing of your arm when you walk is an example of flexion and extension—the forward swing is flexion, and the backward swing is extension. Yet another kind of move-

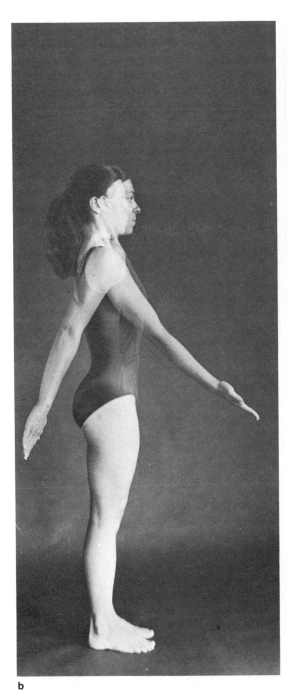

b

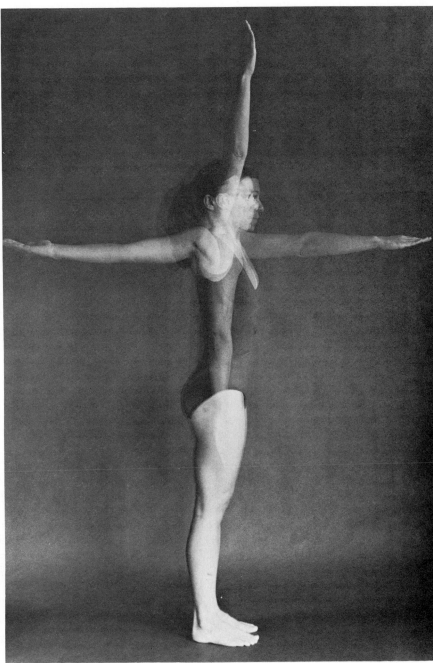

c

ment, **circumduction**, is the combination of flexion, extension, abduction, and adduction. You can demonstrate circumduction by swinging your arm so that your fingertips describe a circle with its center at the shoulder joint. These movements are illustrated in Figure 7.5.

Special Movements

In addition to the movements described for each of the types of joints, special kinds of movements occur at only certain joints (Figure 7.6). At the ankle joint **inversion** is the

Figure 7.6 Special kinds of movements. (Photographs by Elliott Varner Smith.)

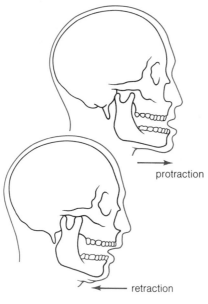

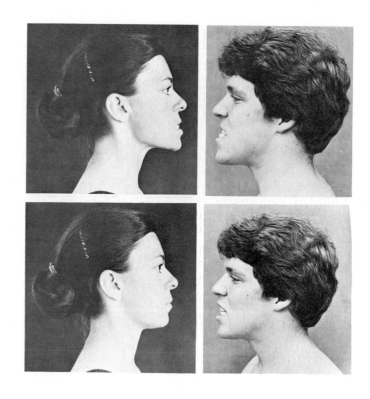

a protraction–retraction

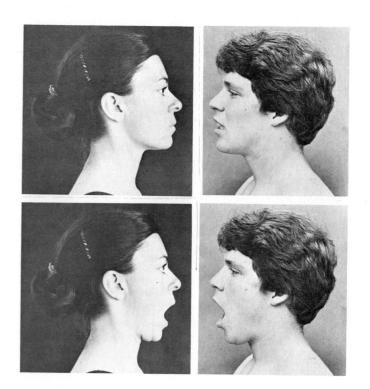

b elevation–depression

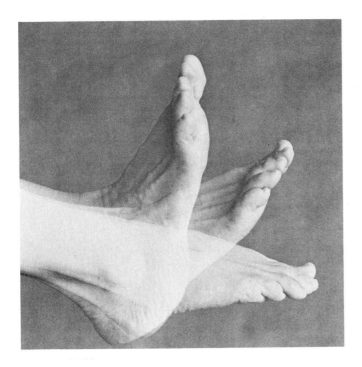

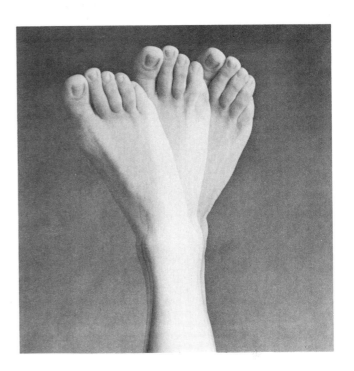

c dorsiflexion–plantarflexion

d inversion–eversion

rotation of the sole of the foot inward, and **eversion** is the rotation of the sole of the foot outward. Also at the ankle joint **flexion** or **dorsiflexion** is the drawing of the foot toward the shin and **plantarflexion** is the extension of the toes away from the shin. Standing on tiptoes requires plantarflexion of the foot; walking on the heels requires dorsiflexion.

The rotation of the forearm at the pivot joint of the radius and ulna results in **supination** or **pronation** of the palm of the hand. To demonstrate pronation, rotate the radius until the palm of the hand is posterior. To demonstrate supination, rotate the radius back again until the palm of the hand is anterior. Recall from Chapter 1 that, when the body is in anatomical position, the palms of the hands are parallel with the anterior surface of the body; that is, they are in *supine* position.

Movements of the lower jaw or mandible illustrate two other kinds of movement: **elevation-depression** and **protraction-retraction**. Your mandible is elevated when your mouth is closed and depressed when your mouth is open; it is protracted when you thrust your lower jaw outward so your lower teeth extend beyond your upper teeth and retracted when you pull your lower jaw back to its normal position.

The various kinds of joint movements are summarized in Table 7.2.

JOINTS OF THE AXIAL SKELETON

Objective 7. Describe the characteristics and movements of the joints of the axial skeleton.

Joints of the axial skeleton function primarily to support the body; a few of these joints are also movable. Axial skeleton joints include the sutures of the skull and facial bones; the synovial joints that attach the mandible to the skull; and the cartilaginous and synovial joints of the vertebral column, ribs, and sternum.

As noted earlier, the sutures of the skull are immovable fibrous joints. The joints between the facial bones are also sutures.

The only movable joints in the skull are the synovial joints of the mandible. The condylar process of the mandible articulates with the mandibular fossa of the temporal bone. The types of movement possible at this joint are elevation-depression, protraction-retraction, and a small amount of side-to-side movement such as occurs when food is being ground between the molars.

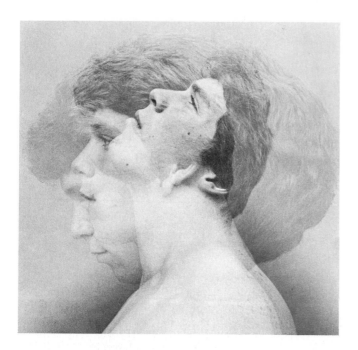

Figure 7.7 Nodding the head.

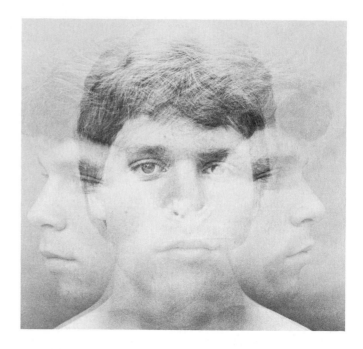

Figure 7.8 Rotation of the head. (Photographs by Elliott Varner Smith.)

The joints of the vertebral column include the articulation of the atlas (first cervical vertebra) with the occipital condyles, the articulation of the atlas and axis, the intervertebral joints between the remaining vertebrae, the joints of the sacrum, and the articulations of the ribs with the thoracic vertebrae. At the articulation of the atlas with the skull the occipital condyles fit into depressions in the atlas, forming ellipsoid joints, and allow a rocking motion such as occurs in nodding the head "yes." At the articulation of the atlas and axis the dens of the axis projects into the vertebral foramen of the atlas, forming a pivot joint. Rotation of the head from side to side, such as in shaking the head "no," occurs at this joint. These movements are illustrated in Figure 7.7 and Figure 7.8. Both of the articulations of the atlas are synovial joints, as are the joints between the articulating processes of the remainder of the vertebrae. Symphyses are found between the bodies of all vertebrae. The synovial joints in the cervical region provide for rotation, flexion, and hyperextension of the neck, while the symphyses provide support for the vertebral column. In addition to the symphyses and synovial joints between the thoracic vertebrae, synovial joints also exist between the facets of the vertebrae and the ribs. These joints allow a small amount of movement of the ribs such as occurs during breathing. In the lumbar region symphyses between the vertebral bodies and synovial joints between the articulating processes allow for only slight movements of flexion, extension, and rotation.

The joints of the sacrum include the articulation with the fifth lumbar vertebra superiorly and the articulation with the coccyx inferiorly, both of which are symphyses. Two other joints, the **sacroiliac joints**, are found between the lateral edges of the sacrum and the posterior edges of each ilium, a portion of a coxal bone. These joints are a combination of a fibrous and a synovial gliding joint; they have limited movement through early adulthood and become almost entirely fused by midlife. During the later months of pregnancy and during delivery these joints temporarily become slightly movable in response to hormonal stimulation.

In addition to their articulations with the vertebrae, most of the ribs also articulate with the sternum. The first seven ribs articulate directly with the sternum by way of small costal cartilages; the next three articulate with the costal cartilage of the seventh rib. These joints are variable in structure; some are cartilaginous, and some have small synovial sacs at their articulation with the sternum. Movement at these joints is limited and occurs during breathing.

Like the sacroiliac joint that attaches the pelvic girdle to the axial skeleton, the sternoclavicular joint attaches the pectoral girdle to the axial skeleton. This synovial, gliding joint lies between the clavicle and the manubrium of the sternum. Movement at this joint can be detected by placing the fingers of the right hand over the sternal end of the left clavicle and shrugging the shoulders.

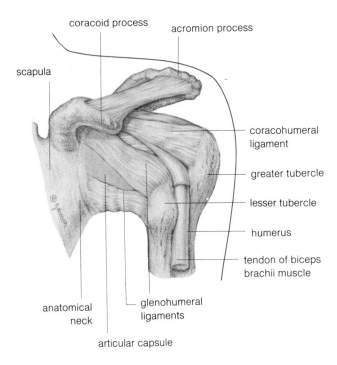

Figure 7.9   The shoulder joint.

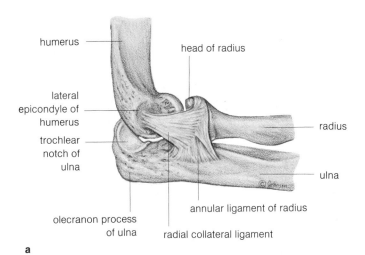

a

b

Figure 7.10   The elbow joint: (**a**) articulation of humerus and forearm bones, (**b**) X ray. (X ray courtesy of Alexandria Hospital, Alexandria, Virginia, Joyce R. Isbel, R.T.)

JOINTS OF THE APPENDICULAR SKELETON

Objective 8. Describe the characteristics and movements of the joints of the appendicular skeleton.

In contrast to the joints of the axial skeleton, which have limited movement and are mostly supporting structures, the joints of the appendicular skeleton are generally freely movable joints. Grouped by location, these joints include the joints of the pectoral girdle and upper appendage and the joints of the pelvic girdle and lower appendage. All are paired structures, one on the left and one on the right side of the body (except for the pubic symphysis).

Joints of the Pectoral Girdle

The joints of the pectoral girdle include the sternoclavicular joint described above and the joint between the clavicle and the acromion process of the sternum. This acromioclavicular joint is a gliding joint that allows elevation, depression, protraction, and retraction of the shoulder.

Joints of the Upper Appendage

The **shoulder joint** (Figure 7.9) is encased in an articular capsule partially surrounded by ligaments. Though the lig-

aments and the more superficial muscles of this joint provide both protection and excellent mobility, the bones are easily dislocated, or moved out of alignment, a very painful event. As a ball-and-socket joint, this joint allows flexion, extension, abduction, adduction, circumduction, and medial and lateral rotation.

The **elbow** joint (Figure 7.10) contains within one joint capsule three articulations—radius and ulna each with the humerus and radius and ulna with each other. The articulations of the forearm bones with the humerus form a hinge joint that limits movement to a single plane; flexion and extension occur here. The articulation between the radius and ulna allows rotation of the radius about the ulna.

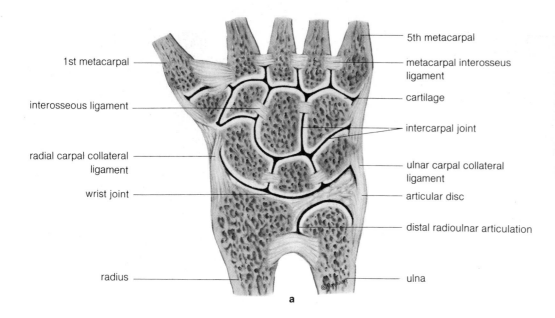

1st metacarpal

interosseous ligament

radial carpal collateral ligament

wrist joint

radius

5th metacarpal

metacarpal interosseus ligament

cartilage

intercarpal joint

ulnar carpal collateral ligament

articular disc

distal radioulnar articulation

ulna

a

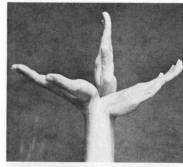

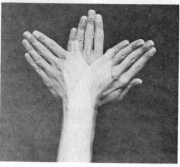

b

Figure 7.11   Joints of the wrist and hand: (**a**), shown in a section through the hand, (**b**) movements of the wrist. (Photographs by Elliot Varner Smith.)

At the **wrist** the distal ends of the radius and ulna again articulate. The radius also articulates directly with some of the carpals, and the ulna articulates with carpals indirectly through an intervening cartilage disc. These joints and some of the joints of the hand are shown in Figure 7.11. The radiocarpal and ulnocarpal joints allow flexion, extension, abduction, adduction, and circumduction of the wrist. The free movement at the carpometacarpal joint of the thumb makes the thumb apposable; the carpometacarpal joints of the other four digits provide somewhat less freedom of movement. It will help you to remember these movements if you try each of them with your own wrist and hand.

Joints of the Pelvic Girdle

The joints of the pelvic girdle include the sacroiliac joint and the pubic symphysis, an unpaired, midline joint. These relatively immovable joints have been described previously.

Joints of the Lower Appendage

The **hip joint** (Figure 7.12) is formed by the articulation of the head of the femur and the acetabulum of the coxal bone. Its outer surface is covered by ligaments, as shown in the figure. Beneath the ligaments is the articular capsule, and within the joint cavity itself is the **ligamentum teres**, which runs from the fovea capitis to the capsule and helps to hold the femur in the socket. This ball-and-socket joint is capable of the same movements as the shoulder joint: flexion (drawing the knee toward the abdomen), extension (thrusting the thigh out behind the body), abduction (moving the thigh away from the body), adduction (moving the thighs close together), circumduction (the combination of these movements to describe a large circle with the entire leg), and rotation of the femur on its own axis. In medial rotation the knee is moved from its anterior position to a medial position, and in lateral rotation the knee is moved to a lateral position. Try each of these movements with your own thigh to understand how they occur.

The **knee joint** (Figure 7.13) is an unstable and complex joint. Externally it is encased in ligaments between bones and tendons of muscles of the thigh and leg. The large **patellar ligament** and the **patella**, enclosed within the tendon of the quadriceps femoris muscle, are prominent on the anterior surface. Beneath these structures the condyles of the femur provide relatively flat surfaces for articulation. No deep depressions are present in this joint, so it is relatively easy for the tibia to slip out of the normal articulating position. The **medial** and **lateral menisci** (singular, menis-

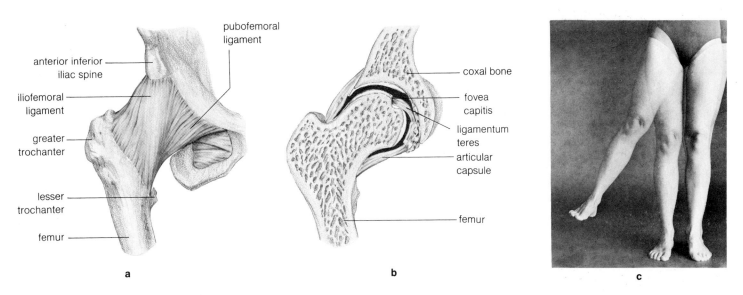

Figure 7.12 The right hip joint: (**a**) view of the anterior surface of the joint, showing ligaments, (**b**) section through the joint, showing the joint capsule and the structures within it, (**c**) lateral movement. (Photograph by Elliott Varner Smith.)

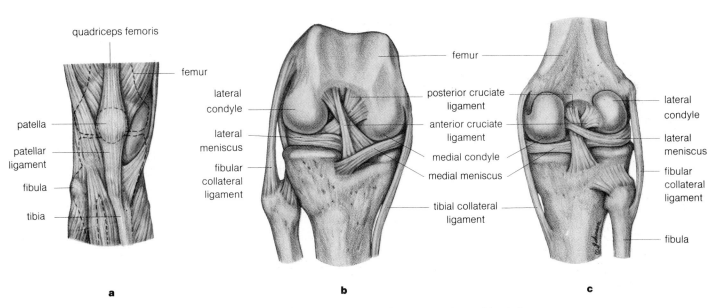

Figure 7.13 The right knee joint: (**a**) anterior superficial view with muscles, tendons, and ligaments intact, (**b**) anterior view of the knee joint flexed with the joint cavity exposed, (**c**) posterior view of the knee joint extended with the joint cavity exposed.

Table 7.2 Movements and Their Definitions

Pairs of Antagonistic Movements

Flexion—the decreasing of the angle between two bones	Extension—the increasing of the angle between two bones
Abduction—the movement of a limb away from the midline of the body	Adduction—the movement of a limb toward the midline of the body
Medial rotation—the turning of a bone on its own axis toward the midline of the body	Lateral rotation—the turning of a bone on its own axis from the midline of the body
Inversion—the rotation of the sole of the foot inward	Eversion—the rotation of the sole of the foot outward
Supination—the placing of the palm of the hand in anatomical position	Pronation—the rotation of the palm of the hand away from anatomical position
Elevation—the raising of a body part	Depression—the lowering of a body part
Protraction—the thrusting forward of a body part	Retraction—the withdrawal of a body part
Dorsiflexion—the bending of the foot toward the shin (tibia)	Plantarflexion—the bending of the foot away from the shin (tibia)

Unpaired Movements

Hyperextension—the excessive extending of a body part in the opposite direction of flexion

Circumduction—movement describing a circle

cus), concave discs of fibrous cartilage, lie between the articulations of the condyles. Their thick outer edges help to prevent dislocation of the tibia. **Collateral ligaments** around the lateral surfaces of the joint capsule also serve to stabilize the joint. **Cruciate**, or crossing, **ligaments** resist twisting and turning movements and anterior displacement of the tibia. As shown in the posterior view of the knee joint (Figure 7.13c), additional ligaments are present on the posterior surfaces of the joint.

The synovial cavity of the knee joint is extensive and irregular in shape. It extends proximally from the patella beneath the quadriceps femoris muscle to form a large bursa called the suprapatellar bursa. Other bursae, not connected to the joint cavity, include the infrapatellar bursa located distal to the patella, and the prepatellar bursa beneath the skin anterior to the patella.

The movements of the knee joint generally are limited to flexion (moving the leg toward the back of the thigh) and extension (straightening the leg). When the knee is flexed, the tension on the collateral ligaments is reduced, and a slight amount of rotation and circumduction is possible at the joint.

Two joints are found between the tibia and the fibula—the **superior tibiofibular joint**, just below the knee, and the **inferior tibiofibular joint** near the ankle. The **interosseous membrane** lies between these joints and holds the two bones together. Neither of these joints is movable to any extent. Their main function is to stabilize the fibula in relation to the tibia and to allow the fibula to accommodate movements of the ankle.

Quick pivot turns, such as are required in football, basketball, and other sports, place a strain on the knee joint and often result in injuries to the ligaments. Dislocation of the knee joint because of torn ligaments is also a frequent occurrence. Finally, damage may be done to the menisci in severe injuries.

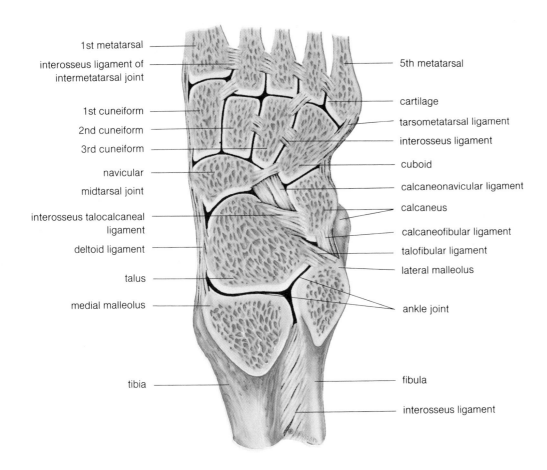

1st metatarsal
interosseus ligament of intermetatarsal joint
1st cuneiform
2nd cuneiform
3rd cuneiform
navicular
midtarsal joint
interosseus talocalcaneal ligament
deltoid ligament
talus
medial malleolus
tibia

5th metatarsal
cartilage
tarsometatarsal ligament
interosseus ligament
cuboid
calcaneonavicular ligament
calcaneus
calcaneofibular ligament
talofibular ligament
lateral malleolus
ankle joint
fibula
interosseus ligament

Figure 7.14 Synovial joints of the right ankle and foot, shown in a section through the ankle and foot.

Joints of the **ankle** and **foot** are shown in Figure 7.14. The ankle joint, formed by articulations of the malleoli of the tibia and fibula with the talus, allows dorsiflexion, plantarflexion, and limited circumduction. Articulations of the talus with other tarsals allow inversion and eversion of the foot. The tarsometatarsal joints are more limited in movement than the comparable joints in the hand; the great toe is especially limited in movement compared to the thumb.

The major joints of the body and their movements are summarized in Table 7.3.

Immobility or lack of movement may lead to impaired function of joints. Tendons and ligaments lose some of their elasticity, and joints become less mobile. These effects are seen in individuals confined to bed because of injury or illness and even in healthy individuals, such as those confined to a space capsule. Impairment of function can be mimimized by range of motion exercises—moving each joint through its complete arc of movement in each plane in which it moves. Passive exercises can be done for a bedridden person by someone else moving each limb through its range of motion.

Table 7.3 Summary of Major Joints and Their Movements

Joint	Type	Movement
Most skull joints	Sutures	Immovable
Temperomandibular	Hinge	Elevation, depression, protraction, retraction
Atlantooccipital	Ellipsoid	Back-and-forth and side-to-side movements
Atlantoaxial	Pivot	Rotation
Intervertebral		
Bodies	Symphyses	Slight movement
Arches	Gliding	Rotation, flexion, hyperextension
Sacroiliac	Synarthrosis	Slight movement
Costovertebral	Gliding	Slight movement during breathing
Sternocostal	Gliding and synchrondoses	Slight movement during breathing
Sternoclavicular	Gliding	Slight movement when shrugging shoulders
Acromioclavicular	Gliding	Elevation, depression, protraction, retraction
Shoulder	Ball-and-socket	Flexion, extension, adduction, abduction, circumduction, medial and lateral rotation
Elbow	Hinge	Flexion, extension
Radioulnar	Pivot	Rotation of radius about ulna
Wrist	Ellipsoid	Flexion, extension, abduction, adduction, circumduction
Carpometacarpals		
Fingers	Ellipsoid	Back-and-forth and side-to-side movements
Thumb	Saddle	Freer back-and-forth and side-to-side movements
Hip	Ball-and-socket	Flexion, extension, adduction, abduction, circumduction, medial and lateral rotation
Knee	Hinge	Flexion, extension; when flexed, some circumduction and rotation
Superior tibiofibular	Gliding	Stabilizes fibula; almost no movement
Inferior tibiofibular	Syndesmosis	Stabilizes fibula; almost no movement
Ankle	Hinge	Dorsoflexion, plantarflexion, limited circumduction
Intertarsals	Gliding	Inversion, eversion
Tarsometatarsals	Gliding	Back-and-forth and side-to-side movement, but much more limited than similar joints in hands; form arches of foot

CLINICAL APPLICATIONS

Objective 9. Discuss the alterations of the structure and function of joints in the following conditions: (a) osteoarthritis, (b) dislocations, (c) sprains, (d) strains, and (e) bursitis.

Osteoarthritis

Osteoarthritis, the most common form of arthritis, is a degenerative disease of the joints. The articular cartilages degenerate (Figure 7.15), and new bone grows in the form of spurs in the joint cavity. Though these spurs interfere with movement of the joint, inflammation is not as severe as in rheumatoid arthritis (see essay below). The incidence of osteoarthritis increases with age. It is rarely seen before the age of forty but affects over 85 percent of people over 70. As the disease progresses, affected joints become less mobile, more enlarged, and often more painful. Osteoarthritis is not generally a crippling disease unless it affects weight-bearing joints.

Dislocation

A **dislocation** is a displacement of the articular surfaces of a joint; it usually involves damage to the ligaments surrounding the joint.

Most dislocations result from falls, blows, or extreme exertion and are most often seen in the joints of the thumb, fingers, knee, or shoulder. Picking up a small child by one arm is a dangerous practice because it often dislocates the child's shoulder. Symptoms of dislocation include swelling, pain, and loss of motion. Treatment consists of returning the bones to their normal positions and immobilizing the joint while healing takes place.

Occasionally, a child is born with dislocated hips because the rim of the acetabulum is not deep enough to retain the head of the femur in its proper position. In such instances the child may be placed in traction (Figure 7.16) to allow the acetabulum to develop further and become stronger before it is allowed to bear weight.

Sprains and Strains

A **sprain** is a twisting of a joint without dislocating it. Such an injury causes damage to ligaments and also often damages tendons, muscles, blood vessels, and nerves. Severe sprains are quite painful and require immobilization during the healing process.

In contrast to a sprain a **strain** is a less severe stretching or twisting of a joint. Muscles and tendons may be stretched and become somewhat painful, but only minor damage is done to the tissues of the joint.

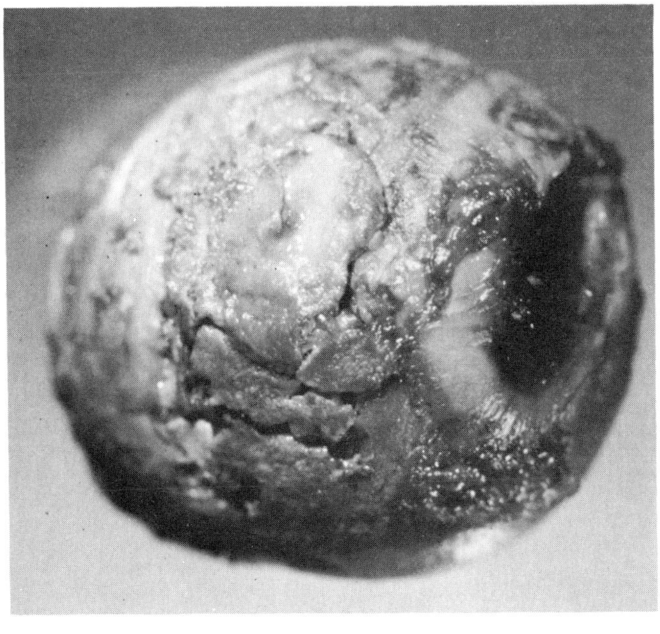

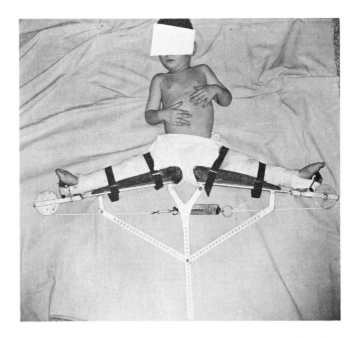

Figure 7.15 The head of the femur removed during the surgical replacement of a hip joint in the treatment of osteoarthritis. Notice the eroded surface of the bone where the articular cartilage is missing. (Armed Forces Institute of Pathology negative number 53–11950.)

Figure 7.16 A child in traction for the treatment of congenital hip dislocation. (Armed Forces Institute of Pathology negative number 58–10063.)

Bursitis

Bursitis is an inflammation of a bursa. It can occur in any bursa, but it is most common in the subscapular bursa near the shoulder, the olecranon bursa at the elbow, and the prepatellar bursa of the knee. Bursitis can result from injury or infection, or occur as a complication of rheumatoid arthritis. Once bursitis has occurred in a bursa, excessive use of the nearby joint often precipitates another painful episode. In chronic bursitis calcium deposits build up in the bursa, causing extreme pain and restriction of movement. Treatment includes rest and analgesics following an acute attack, with later physical therapy to prevent loss of function. Hydrocortisone injections are sometimes used to reduce the inflammation of bursitis, and in seriously immobilized joints forceful manipulation under anesthesia may be used to restore movement.

Clinical Terms

ankylosis (ang-kil-o'sis) abnormal immobility of a joint

arthralgia (ar-thral'je-ah) pain in a joint

bunion (bun'yon) swelling of a bursa in the great toe

contracture (kon-trakt'yur) a reduction in the movement of a joint, often due to shortening of muscles acting on the joint

foot drop the hanging of the foot in a plantar-flexed position, often due to prolonged immobility

spondylitis (spon-dil-i'tis) an inflammation of a vertebra

spondylosis (spon-dil-o'sis) ankylosis or immobility of a vertebral joint

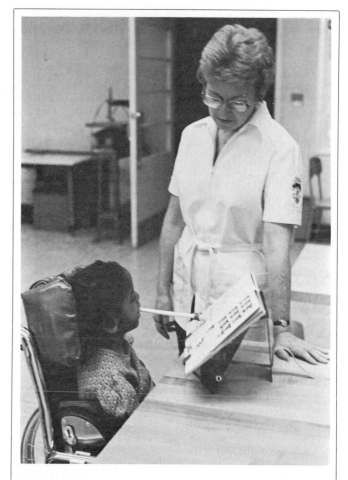

Figure 7.17 This child suffering from arthrogryposis is developing communication skills by learning to turn pages with a mouth stick. Arthrogryposis is a congenital generalized fibrous ankylosis (immobility) of the joints, in this case severe enough to prevent movement of the upper extremities. With encouragement from the therapist, she succeeds in turning the pages as the therapist reads to her. (Photograph by author. Used with permission of the D.C. Public Schools, Department of Special Education, Sharpe Health School Administration, and the Department of Human Services of the District of Columbia.)

Essay: Rheumatoid Arthritis

Among the several forms of arthritis **rheumatoid arthritis** is most likely to lead to crippling disabilities. In contrast to the forms of arthritis that afflict the elderly, this form can strike at any age and frequently affects individuals between the ages of thirty and forty. Because of the early onset and severe effects, rheumatoid arthritis can cause many years of suffering for its victims.

Rheumatoid arthritis affects all organs and tissues of the skeletal system, but its most obvious effects are seen in the joints of the hands and feet. The disease may be acute or chronic, with relatively symptom-free periods interspersed with painful attacks. One of the primary symptoms of rheumatoid arthritis is early morning joint stiffness, which is seen in nearly all individuals having the disease. Initially, it may affect only one or a few joints, but as the disease progresses, additional joints are affected, usually bilaterally—the same joints on the left and right sides of the body. Joints become deformed, and their functions impaired (Figure 7.18). In some cases joints fuse and become immovable. In addition to affecting the joints, rheumatoid arthritis also can cause inflammation of tendons, subcutaneous tissue, skin, and even blood vessels.

Rheumatoid arthritis is sometimes classed as an autoimmune disease. In such a disease, the body produces autoantibodies against its own proteins and attacks them in the same way it would foreign substances (antigens) (see Chapter 20). The autoimmune response is complex, but it appears to involve "mistaken identity." In rheumatoid arthritis autoantibodies attack the synovial membranes in joints, causing inflammation and destruction.

Autoantibody complexes can be detected in the blood as **rheumatoid factor**. Rheumatoid factor also can be detected in the synovial fluid of rheumatoid joints and in subcutaneous nodules (lumps) that often develop in individuals with this disease. The factor sometimes appears in the blood plasma of relatives of individuals affected by rheumatoid arthritis, suggesting that its presence is genetically determined. However, for unknown reasons some individuals who have the rheumatoid factor (and thus a gene that leads to its formation) fail to develop the disease.

No definitive answer exists to the question of what causes rheumatoid arthritis. Nevertheless, it is clear that some antigenic substance initiates the disease. It may be that no single agent is responsible in all cases. In some individuals the disease may be initiated by a virus, in others by a bacterial agent, and in still others by some unknown factor. Recent studies of rheumatoid synovial cells in tissue culture have demonstrated that some of these cells produce an enzyme, collagenase, that digests collagen. The relationship of this enzyme (and the resorption of cartilage that it causes) to the autoimmune disease process in rheumatoid arthritis is not yet known, and the problem is still under study.

No cure exists for rheumatoid arthritis; although some treatments are effective for some individuals, no treatment works in all cases. Most therapy involves treating symptoms to allow victims of the disease to pursue nearly normal lives. Hydrocortisone and other steroid derivatives lessen inflammation and thereby reduce joint damage; however, long-term hydrocortisone therapy weakens bone structure (as discussed in Chapter 6) and has other undesirable side effects. Large doses of aspirin, which decrease inflammation and reduce pain, are very effective therapy because aspirin combats the most incapacitating effects of the disease. Finally, physical therapy is used to keep joints movable, increasing the individual's ability to function normally.

When rheumatoid arthritis, other forms of arthritis, or injuries and stresses lead to crippling degeneration of a joint, it is often possible to replace the natural joint with a prosthetic device (a device to replace a missing part). This is done most frequently in weight-bearing joints to enable the patient to walk again, but it also can be done on finger joints to restore finger dexterity. Both hip and knee joints can be replaced now, and work is underway to develop a technique for replacing ankle joints. As the art of joint replacement becomes more advanced, more and more victims of rheumatoid arthritis and other crippling conditions will benefit.

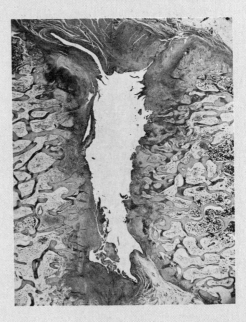

Figure 7.18 A microscopic view of the sternoclavicular joint from an individual who suffered from rheumatoid arthritis, × 9. The clear area is the joint cavity. Notice the roughened surfaces of the bones extending into the cavity. Though the joints of the hands and feet are most likely to be affected by rheumatoid arthritis, this photomicrograph illustrates that other joints can be affected. (Armed Forces Institute of Pathology negative number 71–2627.)

CHAPTER SUMMARY

(Chapter summary points and review questions are numbered to correspond to the numbered objectives in the text of each chapter.)

Organization and General Functions

1. Relate articulations to the skeletal system and describe their general functions.
    a. Articulations, also called joints or arthroses, are the points at which bones are joined or come in close proximity to each other, or at which a bone is joined to cartilage.
    b. Joints help to support the parts of the skeletal system, and many also make it possible for one bone to move in relation to another.

Characteristics of Joints

2. List the general characteristics of the three types of joints.
    a. Synarthroses are immovable or slightly movable fibrous joints.
    b. Amphiarthroses are slightly movable cartilaginous joints.
    c. Diarthroses, or synovial joints, are freely movable joints that have a synovial cavity (see Table 7.1).
3. Describe the structure, function, and location of fibrous joints.
    a. Fibrous joints are held together by fibers of connective tissue that extend from one bone to another; little or no movement occurs at a fibrous joint.
    b. Fibrous joints include:
        (1) sutures of the skull
        (2) syndesmoses between the radius and ulna and between the tibia and fibula
4. Describe the structure, function, and location of cartilaginous joints.
    a. Cartilaginous joints are held together by a piece of cartilage interposed between the bones; such joints are slightly movable.
    b. Cartilaginous joints include:
        (1) symphyses between vertebrae and between pubic bones
        (2) synchondroses between some of the ribs and the sternum, and at the epiphyseal plates of growing bones
5. Describe the structure, function, and location of (a) synovial joints and (b) bursae and tendon sheaths; (c) describe the properties and function of synovial fluid.
    a. Synovial joints are:
        (1) surrounded by a joint capsule, have a joint cavity lined with synovial membrane and filled with synovial fluid, and have the cartilage-covered articular surfaces of the bones extending into the cavity
        (2) highly movable joints found at all sites in the body where more than slight movement is possible
    b. Bursae and tendon sheaths are:
        (1) connective tissue sacs closely resembling synovial cavities

        (2) found at points of excessive friction
    c. Synovial fluid is secreted by the synovial membrane and serves to lubricate the surfaces inside a synovial cavity, bursa, or tendon sheath.
6. List and define the kinds of movement that occur at synovial joints.
    a. The types of synovial joints are:
        (1) gliding joints, which allow back-and-forth and side-to-side movements
        (2) hinge joints, which allow bending in a single plane
        (3) pivot joints, which allow rotation of one bone in relation to another
        (4) ellipsoid, or condyloid, joints, which allow back-and-forth and side-to-side movements
        (5) saddle joints, which allow movements that are similar to but freer than an ellipsoid joint
        (6) ball-and-socket joints, which allow very free movements, including abduction, adduction, flexion, extension, and circumduction
    b. Specific kinds of movement are defined in Table 7.2.

Joints of the Axial Skeleton

7. Describe the characteristics and movements of the joints of the axial skeleton.
    a. Immovable or slightly movable joints of the axial skeleton include sutures of the skull and facial bones, cartilaginous joints of the vertebral column and ribs, and a variety of joints of the sacrum.
    b. Freely movable joints of the axial skeleton include the hinge joints of the mandibles, the pivot and condyloid joints that allow movement of the head, and some of the joints between the ribs and the vertebral column.

Joints of the Appendicular Skeleton

8. Describe the characteristics and movements of the joints of the appendicular skeleton.
    a. Joints of the pectoral girdle include the sternoclavicular joint and the joint between the clavicle and the acromion process of the scapula; they allow limited movement.
    b. Joints of the upper appendage include:
        (1) the ball-and-socket joint of the shoulder, which allows a wide range of movements
        (2) the hinge joint of the elbow
        (3) a variety of joints in the wrist and hand
    c. Joints of the pelvic girdle include the sacroiliac joint and the pubic symphysis, both of which are relatively immovable.
    d. Joints of the lower appendage include:
        (1) the ball-and-socket joint of the hip, which allows a wide range of movements
        (2) the hinge joint of the knee
        (3) a variety of joints in the ankle and foot

Clinical Applications

9. Discuss the alterations of the structure and function of joints in the following conditions: (a) osteoarthritis, (b) dislocations, (c) sprains, (d) strains, and (e) bursitis.

    a. Osteoarthritis is a degenerative disease in which the articular cartilages of joints disintegrate, and bony spurs develop in joint cavities; these changes cause painful and limited movement of affected joints.

    b. A dislocation is the displacement of the articular surfaces of a joint with damage to ligaments.

    c. A sprain involves damage to joint structures and soft tissues without displacement of the articular surfaces.

    d. A strain involves stretching of muscles or tendons without major damage to the joint.

    e. Bursitis is an inflammation of a bursa from infection or injury, or as a complication of rheumatoid arthritis.

REVIEW

Important Terms

abduction	hyperextension
adduction	inversion
amphiarthrosis	osteoarthritis
arthrosis	pivot joint
articular cartilage	plantarflexion
ball-and-socket joint	pronation
bursa	protraction
circumduction	retraction
depression	rheumatoid arthritis
diarthrosis	rotation
dorsiflexion	saddle joint
elevation	sprain
ellipsoid (condyloid) joint	strain
eversion	supination
extension	suture
flexion	symphysis
gliding joint	synarthrosis
hinge joint	synovial
	tendon sheath

Questions

1. a. What is a joint?
    b. What are the major functions of joints?

2. What are the three types of joints found in the body?

3. What are the characteristics of fibrous joints, and where are such joints found?

4. a. How do cartilaginous joints differ in structure and function from fibrous joints?
    b. Where are cartilaginous joints found?

5. a. What is a synovial joint?
    b. What are its functional characteristics?
    c. Where are synovial joints found?
    d. How does a bursa differ from a synovial joint cavity?
    e. What is synovial fluid, and what is its function?

6. List the six types of synovial joints and describe the types of movement that are possible in each type.

7. a. Classify the joints of the axial skeleton as synarthroses, amphiarthroses, or diarthroses.
    b. What are the functions of the joints of the axial skeleton?

8. a. Describe the structure and function of the shoulder and hip joints and explain how they are alike and how they are different.
    b. Describe the structure and function of the elbow and knee joints and explain how they are alike and how they are different.

9. a. What are the effects of osteoarthritis?
    b. How can the degree of damage to a joint be used to distinguish between dislocations, sprains, and strains?
    c. What is bursitis?

Problems

1. Devise exercises you can do to demonstrate the kinds of movement that can occur in the neck, vertebral column, shoulder, elbow, wrist, hip, knee, and ankle.

2. Several surgical techniques for replacing injured or degenerated joints have been developed. Do some library research on joint replacement.

REFERENCES AND READINGS

Copenhaver, W. M., Kelly, D. E., and Wood, R. L. 1978. *Bailey's textbook of histology* (17th ed.). Baltimore, Md.: Williams and Wilkins.

Evans, F. G. 1957. *Atlas of human anatomy.* Totowa, N.J.: Rowman and Littlefield.

Glynn, L. E. 1977. Recent concepts on the pathogenesis of rheumatoid arthritis. *La Ricerca Clinical Laboratory* 7:299.

Gray, H. 1973. *Anatomy of the human body* (29th American ed.). C. M. Goss, ed. Philadelphia: Lea and Febiger.

Schlossberg, L. 1977. *The Johns Hopkins atlas of human functional anatomy.* G. D. Zuidema, ed. Baltimore, Md.: Johns Hopkins Press.

Sonstegard, D. A., Matthews, L. S., and Kaufer, H. 1978. The surgical replacement of the human knee joint. *Scientific American* 238(1):44 (January).

Trotter, R. J. 1979. Preventing the curve. *Science News* 115:298 (May 5).

Woolley, D. E., Harris, E. J., Jr., Mainardi, C. L., and Brinckerhoff, C. E. 1978. Collagenase immunolocalization in cultures of rheumatoid synovial cells. *Science* 200:773 (May 19).

8

MUSCULAR SYSTEM: CHARACTERISTICS AND PHYSIOLOGY

ORGANIZATION AND GENERAL FUNCTIONS

Objective 1. Describe the organization of skeletal muscles in relation to the skeletal system and state the main functions of the skeletal muscular system.

We saw in the last two chapters how the structure of bones and joints, particularly in the appendicular skeleton, allow for movement. Movement would be impossible, however, without an organ system capable of exerting force or effort on the skeletal framework. The skeletal muscular system is the organ system that accomplishes this.

In addition to skeletal muscle the body also contains smooth muscle and cardiac muscle. The general characteristics of these three types of muscle tissue were described briefly in Chapter 4. The physiology of smooth muscle will be discussed as a part of the physiology section in this chapter; that of cardiac muscle will be discussed in Chapter 17.

Muscles, the organs of the muscular system, have the ability to contract—that is, to exert a force when they are stimulated. Skeletal muscles are attached to bones, so they exert force across joints. (Many of the bone markings described in Chapter 6 are the sites of muscle attachment.) The bones and their joints provide a framework for the body; the rigid bones serve as levers and transmit the force exerted by the muscles.

The muscular system consists of over six hundred individual muscles. Some of the muscles of the human body are shown in Figures 8.1 and 8.2.

Muscles are usually described in groups according to their anatomical location. Muscles of the axial skeleton include scalp and facial muscles, neck muscles, and trunk muscles. Muscles of the appendicular skeleton include muscles that hold the pectoral and pelvic girdles in position

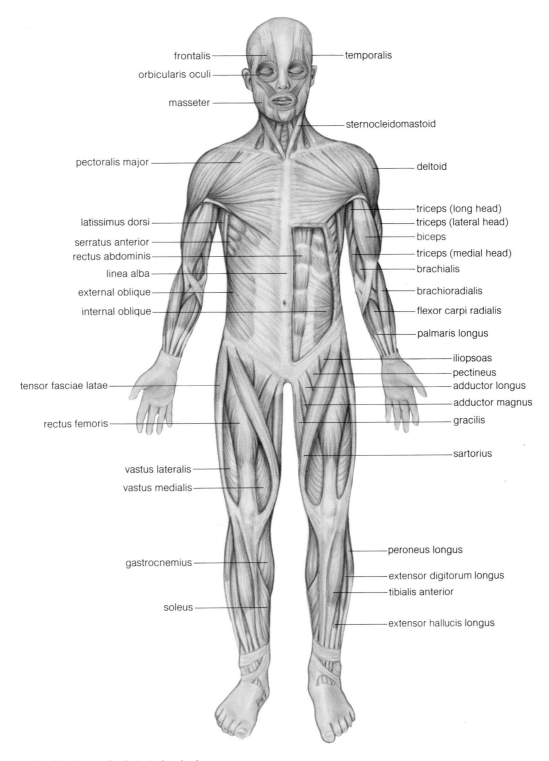

frontalis
temporalis
orbicularis oculi
masseter
sternocleidomastoid
pectoralis major
deltoid
triceps (long head)
latissimus dorsi
triceps (lateral head)
serratus anterior
biceps
rectus abdominis
triceps (medial head)
linea alba
brachialis
external oblique
brachioradialis
internal oblique
flexor carpi radialis
palmaris longus
iliopsoas
pectineus
tensor fasciae latae
adductor longus
adductor magnus
rectus femoris
gracilis
sartorius
vastus lateralis
vastus medialis
peroneus longus
gastrocnemius
extensor digitorum longus
tibialis anterior
soleus
extensor hallucis longus

Figure 8.1 Some muscles of the human body (anterior view).

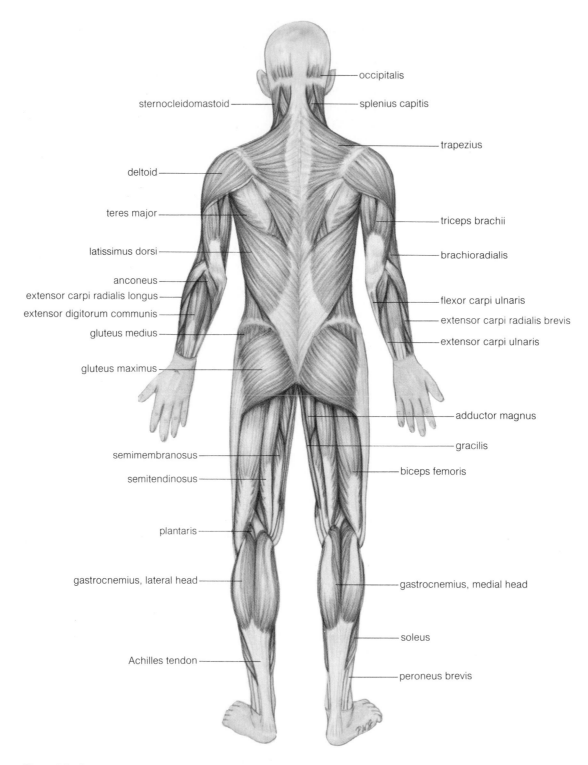

occipitalis

sternocleidomastoid

splenius capitis

trapezius

deltoid

teres major

triceps brachii

latissimus dorsi

brachioradialis

anconeus

extensor carpi radialis longus

flexor carpi ulnaris

extensor digitorum communis

extensor carpi radialis brevis

gluteus medius

extensor carpi ulnaris

gluteus maximus

adductor magnus

gracilis

semimembranosus

biceps femoris

semitendinosus

plantaris

gastrocnemius, lateral head

gastrocnemius, medial head

soleus

Achilles tendon

peroneus brevis

Figure 8.2   Some muscles of the human body (posterior view).

relative to the axial skeleton, muscles that move the limbs in relation to the girdles, and muscles that move each of the joints of the limbs. These groups of muscles will be considered in Chapter 9.

In addition to the property of **contractility** (the ability to exert a force), muscles have three other important properties: excitability, elasticity, and extensibility. **Excitability** is the ability to respond to stimuli. **Elasticity** is the ability of a muscle to return to its original shape after it has contracted or stretched. **Extensibility** is the ability of a muscle to undergo stretching.

By contracting, muscles perform three functions. The first, of course, is to move the body or its parts. The second is to maintain posture, and the third is to produce heat. How muscles move the body or its parts will be discussed in Chapter 9.

In maintaining posture, different groups of fibers (cells) of a muscle contract alternately. For example, back muscles hold the vertebral column in a vertical position when you stand or sit. Because some of the fibers of these muscles relax while others contract, they can maintain posture for a relatively long time.

Muscles produce heat when they contract and cause movement. The feeling of being hot following strenuous exercise is caused by the heat produced by skeletal muscles. Likewise, the ability to keep warm on a cold day by exercising or by shivering is also possible, in part, because muscles produce heat when they contract. Thus, heat from muscle metabolism helps to maintain body temperature, though it can lead to overheating during strenuous exercise. These functions of skeletal muscle—movement, maintenance of posture, and production of heat—all contribute to the maintenance of homeostasis.

DEVELOPMENT OF THE SKELETAL MUSCULAR SYSTEM

Objective 2. Describe the development of the skeletal muscular system.

The skeletal muscular system develops from **myotomes** (blocks of mesoderm in the embryonic trunk area, described in Chapter 5) and from less highly organized mesoderm in the head area. Muscle development begins about four weeks after conception. Each myotome gives rise to many muscle fibers, or muscle cells. Each fiber is a single, multinucleated cell derived from the fusion of several embryonic muscle cells called myoblasts. Although myoblasts are capable of dividing, adult skeletal muscle cells have lost the ability to divide.

As myotomes develop (Figure 8.3), they elongate and extend anteriorly, toward the midline of the body, or distally, into the limb buds. The orientation of developing muscles is influenced by the presence of cartilage models of bones. Each myotome is associated with a sclerotome; sclerotomes give rise to vertebrae. As will be explained in Chapter 10, spinal nerves branch from the spinal cord and exit between vertebrae. One spinal nerve grows into each developing myotome and innervates—that is, supplies both sensory and motor nerve branches to—the muscles that develop from that myotome. As development continues, muscle fibers migrate into complex patterns, which eventually result in adult muscles. The primary nerve of each myotome may also branch to adjacent myotomes in an overlapping pattern. Even after extensive migration of myotomes and branching of nerve fibers, the embryological origin of a muscle usually can be traced by determining the main spinal nerve that innervates it. A muscle, the nerve that stimulates it to contract, and the nerve that carries sensory information about its contractile state constitute an important functional unit arising early in development and persisting throughout life.

SKELETAL MUSCLE TISSUE

Objective 3. Describe the organization of a skeletal muscle from the whole muscle level to the molecular level.

Whole muscles consist of skeletal muscle tissue and connective tissue arranged in a highly organized pattern. The ends of some muscles attach by connective tissue fibers directly to the periosteum of a bone. Other muscle ends attach to bone by strong cordlike structures called **tendons**. Still other muscles attach to nearby structures by flat sheets of connective tissue called **aponeuroses**.

A whole muscle (Figure 8.4a) is covered by a connective tissue sheath, the **epimysium**. Beneath the epimysium each skeletal muscle consists of many muscle fibers arranged in bundles called **fasciculi**. Each bundle, or fasciculus, is surrounded by a connective tissue sheath, the **perimysium**, and each muscle fiber, or cell, is surrounded by a thin connective tissue sheath, the **endomysium**.

Just as the whole muscle consists of many fibers, each fiber (cell) consists of many small **myofibrils**, and each myofibril consists of many still smaller **myofilaments** (Figure 8.4b). The myofilaments are of two types: the thick myofilaments are made of molecules of the protein **myosin**, and the thin myofilaments are made of molecules of the proteins **actin**, **troponin**, and **tropomyosin**.

In addition to the myofibrils and myofilaments each

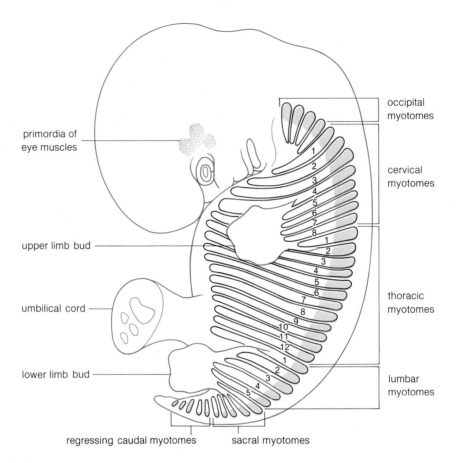

Labels on figure:
primordia of eye muscles
upper limb bud
umbilical cord
lower limb bud
occipital myotomes
cervical myotomes
thoracic myotomes
lumbar myotomes
sacral myotomes
regressing caudal myotomes

Figure 8.3 Diagram of embryonic myotomes at about four weeks development. Shaded areas show approximate size and location of myotomes, and unstippled areas indicate the area into which the myotome extends as it develops.

skeletal muscle cell has many nuclei and certain cytoplasmic structures enclosed within its plasma membrane. The plasma membrane of a muscle fiber with its surrounding connective tissue is called the **sarcolemma**, and the cytoplasm inside is called the **sarcoplasm**. Within the sarcoplasm is a highly organized system of vesicles, the **sarcoplasmic reticulum**, a structure similar to the endoplasmic reticulum of other cells (Figure 8.5).

The functional unit of a myofibril is a **sarcomere** (Figure 8.4c and d), a repeating arrangement of thick and thin myofilaments. When a muscle shortens, the sarcomeres decrease in length. Understanding the highly organized arrangement of myofilaments in sarcomeres assists in understanding the contractile process; it also explains the striations seen in microscopic views of skeletal (and cardiac) muscle fibers (shown in Chapter 4).

Under high magnification, several bands, zones, and lines can be seen associated with a sarcomere. A sarcomere extends from one Z-line to the next, a distance of about 2 μm in a resting sarcomere. In each sarcomere the thick myosin filaments are located entirely within the broad A-band. The thin filaments are anchored to the Z-line and extend from it toward the thick filaments in the A-band. Near the Z-line where only thin filaments are present, the sarcomere appears lighter under the microscope. This is the I-band (isotropic band, so named because of the way light passes through it). Both kinds of filaments are present in the A-band (anisotropic band), except in the H-zone in the middle of the A-band, where the filaments do not overlap in a resting sarcomere. In a contracted sarcomere, the thin filaments more completely overlap the thick ones, partially or completely obliterating the H-zone. The characteristic

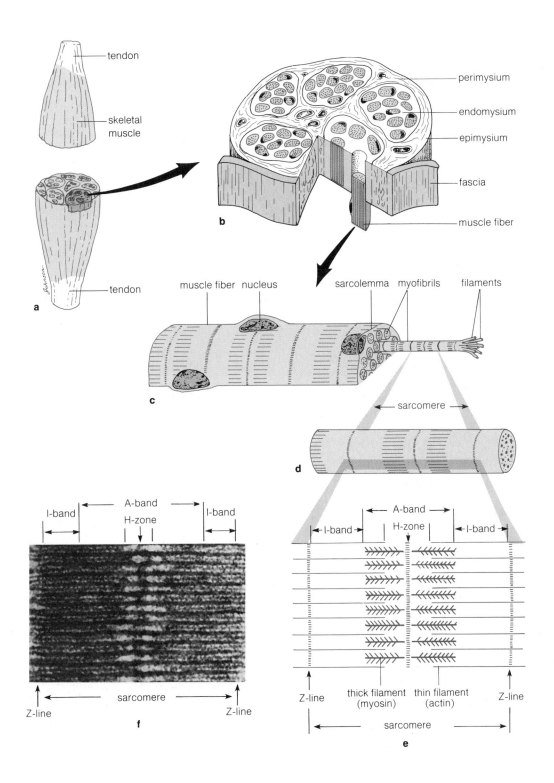

Figure 8.4 Structure of skeletal muscle: clockwise, (**a**) whole muscle cut through belly, × 10, (**b**) cross section through whole muscle, × 30, (**c**) portion of muscle fiber with myofibril projecting from it, × 90, (**d**) myofibril showing sarcomere, (**e**) diagram of a sarcomere, (**f**) photomicrograph of a sarcomere, × 16,200. (Photomicrograph courtesy of H. E. Huxley.)

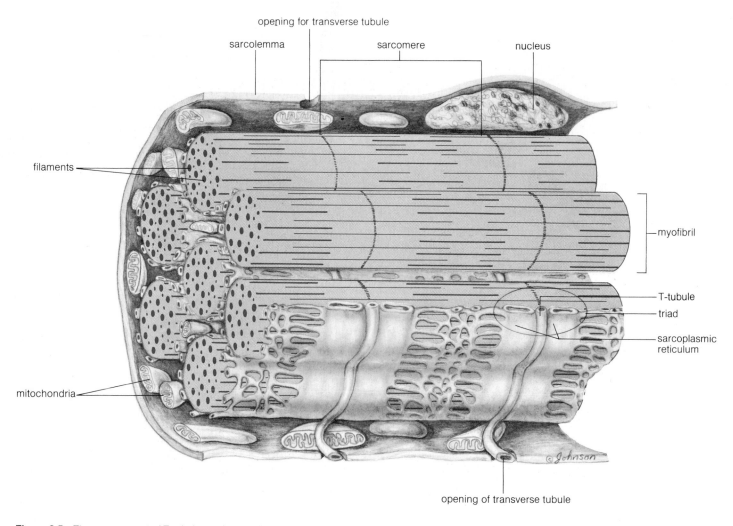

opening for transverse tubule

sarcolemma

sarcomere

nucleus

filaments

myofibril

T-tubule

triad

sarcoplasmic reticulum

mitochondria

opening of transverse tubule

Figure 8.5 The arrangement of T-tubules and sarcoplasmic reticulum around myofibrils in a muscle fiber, or cell.

striations seen under the microscope are created by the alternation of dark A-bands and light I-bands.

Another specialized structure found in skeletal and cardiac muscle is the system of **transverse tubules**, T-tubules (Figure 8.5). T-tubules are extensions of the plasma membrane that penetrate deeply into each muscle fiber. They are located at the junctions of A- and I-bands in mammalian skeletal muscle (two sets of tubules per sarcomere) and run perpendicular to both the myofibrils and the sarcoplasmic reticulum. The T-tubules are closely associated with two layers of sarcoplasmic reticulum. When a muscle fiber is stimulated, the T-tubules conduct action potentials (signals) along their membranes into the muscle fiber.

PHYSIOLOGY OF MUSCLE

Objective 4. Explain the steps in the processes of excitation, contraction, and relaxation.

Objective 5. Describe the role of the following in muscle physiology: (a) motor unit, (b) mechanics of muscle contraction, and (c) metabolism of muscle contraction.

Objective 6. Compare the properties of smooth muscle to those of skeletal muscle.

The physiology of muscle action is a complex process, which includes excitation, contraction, and relaxation. First, these cellular processes will be discussed. Then the cellular processes will be related to motor units—the functional units, each of which includes a nerve fiber and all the muscle fibers it innervates. Next, cellular processes and motor unit activities will be related to body movments as we consider the mechanics of muscle contraction. Some characteristics of metabolism related to muscle contraction will be discussed. Finally, the physiology of smooth muscle will be compared to that of skeletal muscle. (Cardiac muscle physiology will be considered in Chapter 17.)

Excitation of Muscle Cells

Skeletal muscle is stimulated to contract by nerve impulses traveling at a rate of about 100 meters per second. When a stimulus reaches the membrane of a muscle cell, the permeability of the membrane to sodium and potassium ions is altered. The result is a change in the balance of electrical charges, creating an electrical potential, or **action potential**. The details of how this change comes about will be discussed shortly. For now, it's important to know that the action potential moves along the muscle cell membrane, spreading down into the T-tubules. When the action potential passes the region of the sarcoplasmic reticulum, it causes the sarcoplasmic reticulum to release calcium ions (Ca^{2+}) into the sarcoplasm. It takes roughly a millisecond (1/1000 second) for this to occur. Calcium ions act as mediators between excitation, an electrical event, and contraction, a mechanical event.

The Contraction Process

The **sliding filament theory** of contraction, proposed in the 1950s by H. E. Huxley and based on electron microscopic studies, is now generally accepted. According to this theory, muscle shortening occurs when the thin filaments of a sarcomere slide over the thick filaments so that greater overlap exists between them (Figure 8.6).

Actin and **myosin** are protein molecules that bring about the generation of force in the contraction process. Actin is a globular protein; actin molecules are arranged like two strings of beads wound in a spiral to form an actin filament. Myosin is a much larger molecule with a globular head and a long tail piece (Figure 8.6b). The heads of myosin molecules project laterally from a thick filament toward the surrounding actin filaments. These heads are called **cross-bridges** (Figure 8.6c). The head of each myosin molecule contains an enzyme capable of releasing energy from **ATP**. Magnesium ions are required for this enzyme to function.

The proteins **troponin** and **tropomyosin**, which are closely associated with actin, also are important in regulating the attachment of actin to the cross-bridges. Calcium ions can bind to troponin, causing a change in its molecular configuration. This in turn alters the configuration of tropomyosin, to which troponin binds. As the structure of this troponin-tropomyosin complex changes, the complex shifts position on the surface of the actin filaments. This shift exposes previously covered areas called **active sites** on the surfaces of the actin molecules. Myosin cross-bridges are then able to bind to these active sites.

The steps in the contraction process shown in Figure 8.7 are as follows: In a relaxed muscle (a) ATP is bound to the head of a myosin molecule. Though energy is available for contraction, no contraction occurs because the troponin–tropomyosin complex on the thin filaments blocks the myosin binding sites on the actin. Following excitation, calcium ions released into the sarcoplasm cause the troponin–tropomyosin complex to withdraw into a "groove" between the chains of actin molecules (b). An enzyme in the myosin head splits ATP to ADP and phosphate, energizing the cross-bridge, and cross-bridges bind to actin (c). The energized cross-bridges swivel, causing the myofilaments to slide along one another (d). Each time a cross-bridge completes a swiveling movement, a new molecule of ATP replaces the ADP. The formation of a new ATP-myosin bond breaks the existing cross-bridge attachment and allows a new one to form (Figure 8.7e). If calcium ions remain available in sufficient quantity, steps c, d, and e occur over and over again at the rate of 50 to 100 times per second. These repetitive steps constitute the **contraction cycle**.

It is important to note that, in the contraction process, no shortening of either the actin or the myosin filaments occurs. The sarcomere shortens because of the sliding of the actin filaments produced by cross-bridge movements. The H-zones and I-bands shorten, but the width of the A-band remains constant. (Refer back to Figure 8.6a.) The most significant event in this process is the cyclic change in the position of the myosin heads and the resultant movement of the filaments in relation to each other. This movement is a little like the movement of the oars of a boat. Rowing with oars pushes a boat across the water—or the water along the sides of the boat—in somewhat the same way that myosin and actin filaments slide along one another.

The Relaxation Process

It may come as a surprise to you that the relaxation of a muscle fiber that has contracted is *not* a passive process. Like contraction, relaxation also requires ATP. When a muscle is stimulated, the sarcoplasmic reticulum releases calcium ions for only a few milliseconds; repetitive stimuli are required for calcium to continue to be released. As soon as stimulation ceases, calcium begins to be returned to the

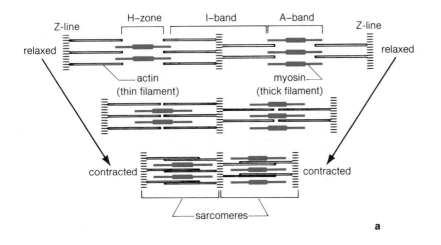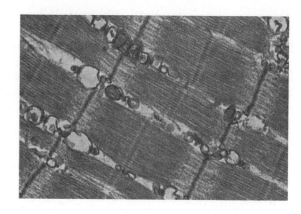

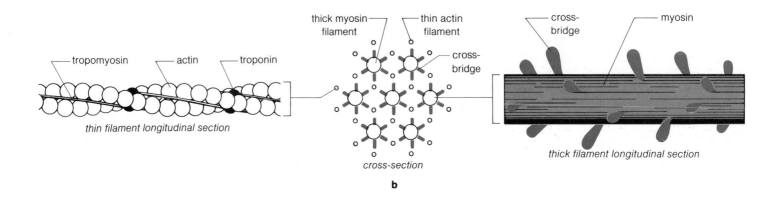

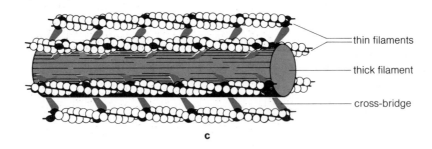

Figure 8.6 The arrangement of filaments in a sarcomere: (**a**) a diagram of the change in the arrangement of filaments from the relaxed to the contracted state, and a photomicrograph of filaments, (**b**) the structure and arrangement of filaments, (**c**) interrelation of actin and myosin. (Photomicrograph courtesy of Patricia Schulz.)

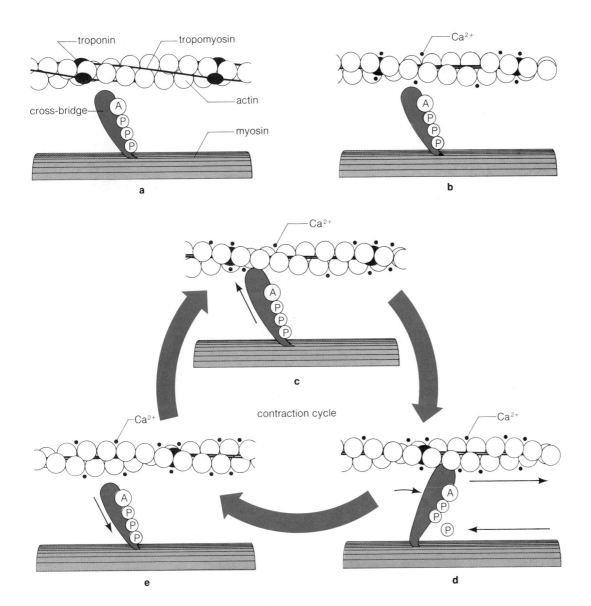

Figure 8.7 Steps in the contraction process: (**a**) ATP attaches to myosin. (**b**) Calcium ions cause the troponin-tropomyosin complex to move away from the reactive sites on actin. (**c**) Energized cross-bridge binds to actin. (**d**) The energized myosin head swivels, causing the filaments to slide past one another. (**e**) New ATP attaches to myosin, and the head returns to its earlier shape, ready to form another cross-bridge. Steps c, d, and e constitute the contraction cycle. These steps occur over and over again at the rate of 50 to 100 times per second as long as calcium ions are available in adequate concentration.

sarcoplasmic reticulum by active transport, a process that requires ATP. However, contraction continues to occur for several hundred milliseconds, or until enough calcium is removed from the troponin–tropomyosin complex to allow these molecules to block reactive sites on actin. When myosin cannot attach to actin, the muscle relaxes. However, the actin filaments slide back to their relaxed position, and the sarcomeres lengthen only when an external force (load) is exerted on the muscle. The role of calcium in the contraction and relaxation processes is summarized in Figure 8.8.

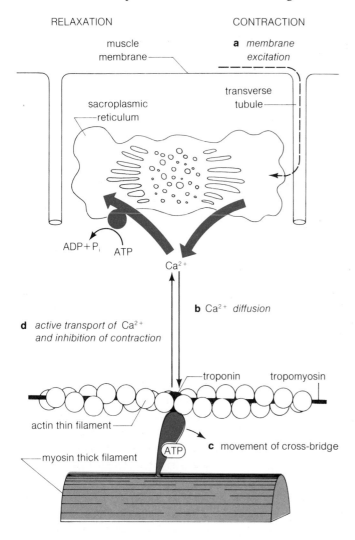

Figure 8.8 The role of calcium ions in the contraction and relaxation processes: (**a**) Excitation of the membrane causes calcium ions to be released from the sarcoplasmic reticulum. (**b**) Calcium ions diffuse through sarcoplasm, and some bind to troponin-tropomyosin, causing it to move away from the active sites of actin. (**c**) Contraction occurs. (**d**) Calcium ions are actively transported back to the sarcoplasmic reticulum, and the troponin-tropomyosin complex again covers the active sites of actin, restoring its inhibition of contraction.

Starting verse:	The SR releases the—calcium.
(Sing each line a half note higher)	The calcium connects to the—troponin.
	Troponin moves tropo—myosin.
	Tropomyosin releases the—actin.
	The actin connects to the—myosin.
	The myosin breaks the—ATP.
	The ATP releases the—energy.
	The energy causes con—traction.
	And that's how the muscle works.
Chorus:	These proteins going to—move around
	These muscles going to—jump around.
	These bones soon going to—leap around.
	When the actin and myosin react.
Finishing verse:	The ATP connects to the—myosin.
(Sing each line a half note lower)	The myosin releases the—actin.
	The actin connects to new—myosin.
	And this results in—contraction.
	Till the SR absorbs the—calcium.
	The calcium releases the—troponin.
	Troponin returns tropo—myosin.
	Tropomyosin protects the—actin.
	And the muscle is now relaxed.

"The Muscle Song" sung to the tune of "Dry Bones." Reprinted with permission from *Journal of College Science Teaching* 8(4):228 and with the permission of the author, Nancy Ann Dahl.

Contraction and relaxation can be used to explain the development of **rigor mortis**, the rigidity of muscles that occurs several hours after death. When an organism dies, cellular metabolism slowly comes to a halt. When ATP is no longer available, cross-bridges between actin and myosin cannot be broken, and calcium ions cannot be returned to the sarcoplasmic reticulum. Consequently, cross-bridges remain, making the muscle rigid until actions of enzymes from ruptured lysosomes degrade actin and myosin proteins. If bacteria are present, their enzymes also degrade proteins. Rigor mortis disappears some fifteen to twenty-five hours after death as proteins are degraded.

The Motor Unit

Having considered the processes that occur at the cellular level in muscles, we are ready to consider the role of the motor unit in controlling muscle contraction. A **motor unit** consists of a single motor neuron (nerve cell) and the muscle fibers it innervates (Figure 8.9). (The structure of neurons is explained in Chapter 10.) Motor units controlling precise movements such as those in the fingers have three to six muscle fibers per motor neuron; those controlling gross movements such as those in the back have several hundred fibers per motor neuron. Some leg muscles such as the calf muscle (gastrocnemius) have as many as 1900 muscle fibers per motor neuron.

The branch of an axon that serves a particular muscle fiber has many small terminal branches that lie in grooves in the muscle cell membrane. The portion of the muscle plasma membrane that lies beneath these nerve endings is called the **motor end plate**. The terminal ends of the axon and the motor end plate together constitute the **myoneural** (muscle-nerve) **junction**.

As a nerve impulse reaches the terminal end of the axon, small sacs called **synaptic vesicles** fuse with the axon membrane and release a chemical transmitter, **acetylcholine**. Acetylcholine diffuses across the **synaptic cleft**, the space between the axon membrane and the motor end plate. In this area the muscle cell membrane is folded into **subneural clefts** and has acetylcholine receptor sites on its surface (Figure 8.10c). When a sufficient number of these sites are stimulated by acetylcholine, the motor end plate becomes depolarized.

To understand depolarization, it is important to realize that a resting muscle cell membrane is polarized; that is, it has a small positive charge at the outer surface and a small negative charge at the inner surface. This polarized state is maintained by the transport of sodium ions and potassium ions across the membrane. Acetylcholine acts to depolarize the muscle cell membrane by causing it to become suddenly more permeable to sodium ions. The positive sodium ions entering the cell reduce the electrical charge across the membrane; the membrane is then said to be depolarized. When depolarization of the motor end plate reaches a certain level, it creates an action potential. This action potential is propagated along the T-tubules and causes the sarcoplasmic reticulum to release calcium ions. (See Chapter 10 for a more detailed discussion of depolarization and action potentials.)

Along with receptor sites for acetylcholine the motor end plate also contains an enzyme, **cholinesterase**, that breaks down acetylcholine. About 5 milliseconds after the release of acetylcholine, cholinesterase has broken acetyl-

choline down into its component parts, acetate and choline. The effect of cholinesterase is to prevent continuous stimulation of a muscle fiber after the release of acetylcholine. A portion of the choline diffuses back to the axon and is reused to synthesize more acetylcholine for transmission of subsequent impulses.

Events at the myoneural junction can be interfered with by a variety of chemicals and by certain diseases. The chemical d-tubocurarine (curare) used as a poison on arrowheads by some South American Indians and also during surgery to prevent muscle contractions, causes paralysis by binding to the acetylcholine receptor sites on the motor end plate. The drug is not destroyed by cholinesterase and binds very tightly to the receptor sites, blocking the action of acetylcholine. Although curare paralyzes all skeletal muscles, death results because the muscles involved in respiration are paralyzed. Some nerve gases and certain pesticides inactivate cholinesterase. This allows acetylcholine to maintain the muscle fiber in a depolarized state, and new stimuli have no effect. Again, the end result is paralysis.

The sequence of events in muscle contraction from nerve stimulation to relaxation are summarized in Table 8.1.

Mechanics of Whole Muscle Contraction

Much of what is known about the mechanics of muscle contraction has been learned through laboratory experiments performed either on isolated muscles or on bundles of muscle fibers. The force produced by a whole muscle when it contracts is called muscle **tension**, and the force exerted on a muscle by a weight is called the **load**. For example, when you pick up a book, the book is the load and the force produced by the muscles in your arm is the tension. Thus, load and tension are opposing forces.

When the tension in a muscle is sufficient to lift a load, the contraction is said to be **isotonic** (same tension). Any time a muscle in your body moves a part of your body or participates in moving your whole body, it is engaging in an isotonic contraction. In such a contraction the force or tension in the muscle remains equal to the load, and the muscle shortens. In contrast, when the tension in a muscle is used to support a load (a book you are carrying, for exam-

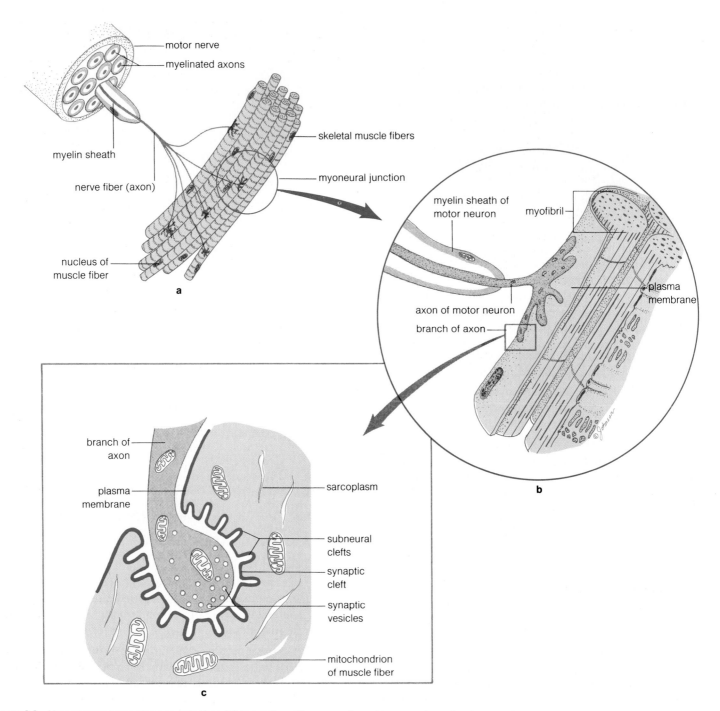

Figure 8.9 How an axon innervates a muscle fiber: (**a**) In a motor unit an axon of a motor neuron branches to several muscle fibers. (**b**) Each branch of the axon forms a myoneural junction. (**c**) The branch of the axon rests in a groove in the muscle fiber, the motor end plate. (**d**) Photomicrograph of a myoneural junction. (The myelin sheath insulates the axon except at the junction, as explained in Chapter 10.) (Photomicrograph courtesy of J. E. Heuser.)

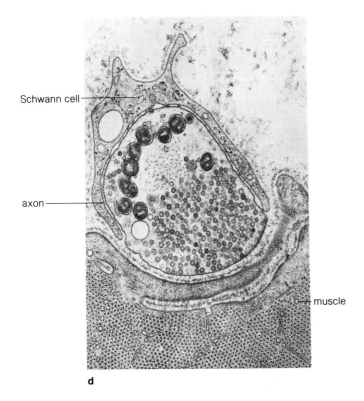

Schwann cell

axon

muscle

d

Table 8.1	Sequence of Events in Muscle Contraction from Nerve Stimulation to Relaxation

1. An action potential travels along the axon of a motor neuron and initiates the release of acetylcholine from synaptic vesicles in its axon terminals.

2. Acetylcholine diffuses across the synaptic cleft and binds to receptor sites of the motor end plate, bringing about depolarization, after which it is destroyed by cholinesterase.

3. An action potential passes from the motor end plate over the muscle plasma membrane and into the T-tubules, where it stimulates release of calcium ions from the sarcoplasmic reticulum into the sarcoplasm.

4. Calcium ions bind to troponin-tropomyosin and prevent these proteins from inhibiting contraction.

5. Energy from ATP causes energized myosin cross-bridges to bind to actin.

6. Energized cross-bridges move, causing actin filaments to slide along the myosin filaments.

7. ATP binds to myosin, releasing the cross-bridges from actin.

8. Steps 5, 6, and 7 are repeated many times as long as calcium remains to inhibit troponin-tropomyosin.

9. Unless stimuli continue to affect the sarcoplasmic reticulum, calcium is pumped back into it by active transport, using ATP for energy.

10. When sufficient calcium has been removed, troponin and tropomyosin inhibit the binding of cross-bridges to actin; when force is exerted on the muscle, it returns to its original length.

ple) or to push against an immovable object, the contraction is said to be **isometric** (same length). In an isometric contraction the muscle maintains the same length but develops tension during the period of the contraction.

A **twitch** is the response of a muscle to a single action potential in its membrane. Both isotonic and isometric twitches can be produced, depending on whether the muscle is allowed to shorten and lift a load (isotonic) or is placed at a fixed length and allowed to develop tension (isometric) as shown in Figure 8.10.

Three phases of a twitch can be distinguished: the latent period, the period of contraction, and the period of relaxation. The **latent period** is the time between the stimulus and the beginning of the contraction. During this period the nerve action potential is conducted to the axon terminals, acetylcholine is released and binds to the motor end plate, the action potential passes over the membrane, and calcium inhibits the action of troponin and tropomyosin. As is demonstrated by the longer latent period in an isotonic twitch, some of this time is spent developing enough tension to overcome the load imposed before shortening can begin to occur. In an isometric twitch force is measured as soon as it begins to be exerted. In the graph of the isometric twitch tension is recorded in grams; in the graph of the isotonic twitch the distance the muscle shortens is recorded

in millimeters (mm). The total length of the **contraction period** (the time the line on the graph is rising) is the time during which tension is rising or shortening is occurring. The **relaxation period** in the isotonic twitch is considerably shorter than in the isometric twitch because, as tension exerted by the muscle declines in the isotonic twitch, the load pulls the muscle back to its original length.

Muscles respond differently to different strengths of stimuli. With regard to single muscle fibers, each fiber in a motor unit has its own threshold for responding to a stimulus. A **threshold stimulus** is a stimulus just strong enough to create an action potential in the muscle fiber. A **subthreshold stimulus** is a stimulus not sufficiently strong to create an action potential. The fiber being stimulated contracts when it receives a threshold stimulus, but fails to

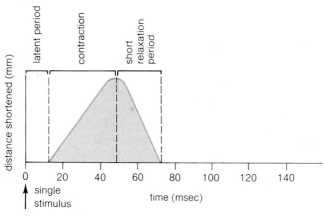

a *isotonic twitch*

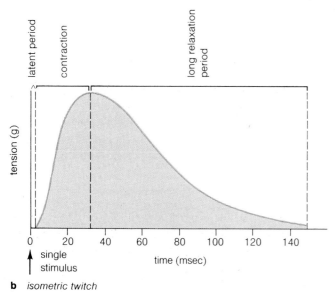

b *isometric twitch*

Figure 8.10 A graphic representation of the phases of a muscle twitch.

When stimuli above the threshold level are given at intervals sufficiently long to allow relaxation between them (Figure 8.11), a series of twitches is produced. The muscle responds to each stimulus in the same way. If, however, a second stimulus is given before complete relaxation of the muscle's response to the first stimulus, the force produced by the second contraction will be stronger than the first; similarly, the third will be stronger than the second. This phenomenon is called **summation**. When stimuli are applied at a fairly rapid rate (twenty to thirty stimuli per second in frog muscle, for example), **incomplete tetanus** occurs; the muscle barely begins to relax when the next stimulus arrives. When stimuli are applied at an even more rapid rate (forty to fifty stimuli per second in frog muscle), **complete tenanus** occurs; the muscle cannot begin to relax before the next stimulus arrives. If, when doing work, we maintain our muscles at maximum levels of contraction, we are maintaining them in tetanic contraction because the muscle fibers are being stimulated at a high frequency.

> The use of the word tetanus to describe normal processes in muscles should not be confused with the use of the word tetanus to describe an infection caused by the bacterium *Clostridium tetani*. Toxin produced by this organism leads to severe, painful spasms and rigidity of voluntary muscles. When these spasms affect the muscles of the jaw, "lockjaw" is the result; when the spasms affect the respiratory muscles, death usually ensues unless a respirator is used.

Most of the work we do involves short-term tetanic contractions of one set of muscles followed by short-term tetanic contractions of other sets of muscles. For example, in running, the muscles of one leg contract, and then the muscles of the other leg contract. The small amount of time between the muscle contractions of the same leg allows those muscles to relax and become ready to contract again. As a result, such muscles can work for long periods.

When a series of maximal stimuli are delivered to a resting muscle at intervals long enough to allow relaxation (Figure 8.12), the phenomenon of **treppe** is observed. Under this condition each of the first few contractions produces more tension than the preceding one, creating a staircase effect on a graph. Athletes make use of this effect in their warming-up exercises. They do, in fact, increase the strength of their maximal contractions, provided the warming-up is not carried to the extreme of fatiguing the muscles.

contract when it receives a subthreshold stimulus. According to the "all-or-none" law, when a fiber contracts, it contracts maximally. With regard to whole muscles the degree of contraction (amount of tension or amount of shortening produced) is determined by two factors: (1) how many motor units are stimulated, and (2) how frequently the fibers in the muscle are being stimulated. Thus, the response of a whole muscle is the sum of the responses of the individual fibers. When a large number of fibers are caused to contract, the degree of tension or the degree of shortening is greater than if a small number of fibers are caused to contract. Similarly, when the frequency of stimulation increases, the force of the contraction increases up to the maximum possible for the fibers being stimulated.

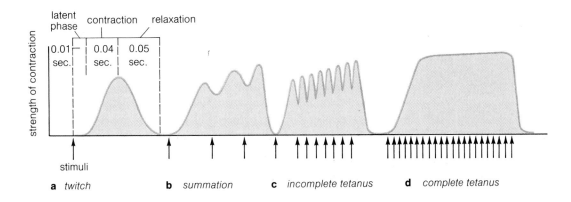

Figure 8.11 Effect of varying the frequency of stimuli: (**a**) twitch, (**b**) summation, (**c**) incomplete tetanus, (**d**) complete tetanus. Note the approximate time of the latent phase, contraction, and relaxation in each situation.

Fatigue occurs when a muscle has been repeatedly stimulated, and the tension the muscle can produce decreases.

Muscle tone is a low level of tension maintained by the contraction of skeletal muscles in response to stimuli initiated by specialized sensory structures within the muscles called stretch receptors. (Stretch receptors are discussed in Chapter 10.) Such tonic contractions are responsible for maintaining posture. Because individual motor units contract alternately, posture usually is maintained without fatigue. However, when a particular posture is held for a long period of time, fatigue may occur. We experience this as a stiff neck or other mild muscle ache.

Exercise can affect the size of muscles. When muscles are repeatedly and forcefully contracted over several weeks, either isotonically or isometrically, the muscle mass increases. The increase in mass is due to increases in the number of filaments in the sarcomeres, in the number of mitochondria, and in the amount of sarcoplasm; it does not involve the division of muscle cells to increase the number of cells. Increase in the size of muscle cells is called **hypertrophy**. Hypertrophy is accompanied by increase in strength because the amount of force a muscle can exert depends on the number of filaments it contains.

In contrast, muscle cells can also undergo **atrophy**, a reduction in the size of individual cells. In atrophy the numbers of filaments and mitochondria and the amount of sarcoplasmic reticulum are reduced. A lack of exercise or immobilization of muscles (in a cast, for example) lead to atrophy. An injury to a nerve that supplies a muscle can also lead to atrophy because the muscle will receive no stimuli to contract. In diseases or injuries that involve damage to nerves that supply muscles, atrophy may be prevented or retarded by frequent mild electrical stimulation of the muscles.

Muscle Metabolism

Energy from ATP is necessary for muscle contraction, as described earlier. Glucose or other nutrients and oxygen are required to make large quantities of ATP, and carbon dioxide is given off in this process. During extreme exertion the supply of ATP may become depleted, and the muscles will fatigue. However, muscles resist fatigue by storing the compounds phosphocreatine, glycogen, and myoglobin,

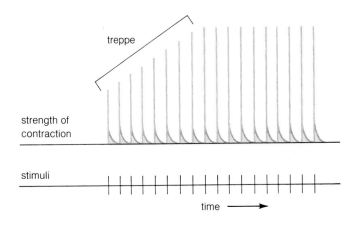

Figure 8.12 The phenomenon of treppe.

and by generating small amounts of ATP without using oxygen.

In a resting muscle some of the ATP produced reacts with creatine, forming **phosphocreatine** and ADP. Energy from ATP is stored in a high-energy bond in phosphocreatine. When a muscle is active, some of the energy from phosphocreatine is transferred back to ATP, where the energy can be used to power contraction.

$$\text{ATP} + \text{creatine} \xrightleftharpoons[\text{active muscle}]{\text{resting muscle}} \text{phosphocreatine} + \text{ADP}$$

Phosphocreatine serves as an energy source for the few seconds necessary for metabolic processes in the muscle cells to begin to produce greater quantities of ATP.

Resting muscle cells store considerable amounts of **glycogen**, a carbohydrate molecule consisting of many glucose units. When a muscle is active, the glycogen can be broken down and the glucose metabolized for energy. However, the metabolism of glucose produces large quantities of energy only when adequate amounts of oxygen are available. Oxygen enters muscle cells from the blood; an oxygen-carrying pigment in muscle cells called **myoglobin** increases the rate at which oxygen enters muscle cells. Even so, the amount of oxygen entering the muscle cells may not be enough to allow the cells to metabolize glucose aerobically (with oxygen). When the oxygen delivery to a muscle is not sufficient to produce the needed energy, glucose can be metabolized anaerobically (without oxygen). Large quantities of glucose are used to produce only small quantities of energy, and a large quantity of a substance called **lactic acid** is produced, creating a condition referred to as **oxygen debt**. The oxygen debt is the amount of oxygen that must be consumed over and above the resting level after exercise has ceased to restore the metabolic state that existed before exercise.

After strenuous exercise has ceased, the oxygen debt is "paid" as oxygen is used to metabolize lactic acid, and the stores of phosphocreatine and glycogen are replenished. These activities are accomplished as oxygen and glucose are metabolized in muscle (and also liver) cells in greater quantities than they are used for energy when exercise is not occurring.

The main steps in muscle metabolism are summarized in Figure 8.13. (These metabolic processes are considered in more detail in Chapter 23.)

Fast and Slow Skeletal Muscle Fibers

Most muscles contain a mixture of different kinds of muscle fibers, which can be categorized as slow or fast. In slow fibers the release of energy from ATP occurs relatively slowly, and thus the speed of contraction is slow. These fibers are relatively resistant to fatigue. In fast fibers the release of energy from ATP occurs relatively rapidly, so contraction is also rapid. Some, but not all, fast fibers fatigue easily. In large limb muscles, where both types of fibers are present, the slow fibers are the first to be stimulated in most movements. Only when more forceful movements are required are the fast fibers also stimulated.

Muscles that contain many fast fibers are called fast muscles; because of their paleness they are also called white muscles. Conversely, muscles that contain many slow fibers are called slow muscles; because of their redness they are also called red muscles. Redness is due to the presence of myoglobin and to the large number of blood-filled capillaries found in such muscles. For example, the posture-maintaining muscles of the back are mainly red muscles, and the muscles of the hands that are capable of skilled movements are mainly white muscles.

Different kinds of exercise cause different kinds of responses in certain skeletal muscle fibers. For example, strenuous (muscle-strengthening) exercises such as push-ups and weight-lifting apparently cause an increase in the size of slow fibers, thereby increasing the strength and mass of those fibers, as noted earlier. On the other hand, endurance exercises such as swimming and jogging apparently cause slow fibers to be transformed into fast fibers, thereby increasing the rate at which energy can be supplied for contraction without significantly increasing the size of the fibers.

Smooth Muscle

Smooth muscle is found in the walls of internal organs rather than attached to bones. In contrast to the voluntary control of skeletal muscle, smooth muscle is generally involuntary; that is, it responds to physiological events in our bodies without our having conscious control over it, though we may be aware of its actions. For example, we might be aware of partially digested food moving through the intestine or changes in the size of the pupils of our eyes, but we cannot consciously control these processes. Contractions of smooth muscles are usually less precise than those of skel-

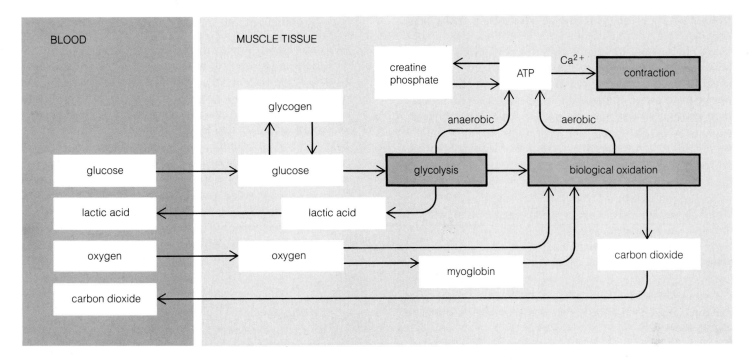

Figure 8.13 Main steps in muscle metabolism.

etal muscles, but they can be sustained over longer periods of time.

Each smooth muscle fiber consists of a single spindle-shaped cell bounded by a plasma membrane and containing a single nucleus. Within these cells the thin filaments are more numerous and the thick filaments are less numerous than in skeletal muscle fibers. Furthermore, the fibers are arranged in a somewhat random pattern. As a result, smooth muscle lacks sarcomere organization and therefore lacks the striations seen in skeletal muscle. Actin and myosin filaments do overlap each other and presumably slide along one another during contraction, though the details of the mechanism are not well understood. Tropomyosin serves the same function as in skeletal muscles, but the sarcoplasmic reticulum and the T-tubules are very poorly developed. Calcium is required for smooth muscle to contract; it diffuses into the muscle cell from extracellular fluids or is released from the sarcoplasmic reticulum when the cell is stimulated and is actively transported back to the sarcoplasmic reticulum or out of the cell, producing relaxation.

Smooth muscle is innervated by both sympathetic and parasympathetic neurons; the effects of stimulation of smooth muscle by such neurons will be discussed in Chapter 13. The mechanism of stimulation in smooth muscle dif-

fers from that in skeletal muscle in that smooth muscle has no discrete neuromuscular junctions. Swollen areas on an axon simply release their transmitter into extracellular fluids, and it diffuses to receptor sites on the membranes of several adjacent smooth muscle cells. Thus, smooth muscle responds more slowly to nerve stimuli and is less precise in its action than is skeletal muscle. In contrast to skeletal muscle, which can be stimulated only by neural stimuli, smooth muscle can be either excited or inhibited by various neural and hormonal stimuli, such as acetylcholine and norepinephrine, as will also be explained in Chapter 13.

Smooth muscle is classified according to its properties as **multiunit** or **visceral** (single-unit). However, some smooth muscle has some of the properties of both types, and all gradations from purely multiunit to purely visceral can be found in the body.

Visceral smooth muscle is found in sheets in the walls of hollow organs such as those of the digestive tract, the ureters of the urinary tract, and the uterus of the female reproductive system. In addition to responding to neural stimuli, visceral smooth muscle can contract spontaneously and rhythmically without being stimulated by neurotransmitters or hormones. The mechanism by which these cells spontaneously contract is not well understood, but it appears that they can generate an electrical activity that spreads from the membrane of one cell to that of adjacent cells. **Gap junctions** that link the cytoplasm of adjacent cells permit ions to flow from cell to cell, making a sheet of cells function together. Visceral smooth muscle responds to stretching by first increasing its tension and then gradually decreasing its tension when stretching is prolonged. This property, called **plasticity**, partly accounts for the ability of the smooth muscle of the bladder to reduce tension as it fills with urine.

Multiunit smooth muscle contracts in more discrete, smaller units than visceral muscle because electrical activity is not transferred from cell to cell as in visceral muscle. However, multiunit muscle is very sensitive to chemicals such as acetylcholine and norepinephrine from neurons. These chemicals tend to persist and cause repeated firing of the muscle cell rather than generating a single action potential, thus prolonging the duration of contraction. Multiunit smooth muscles are found in some large blood vessels and in the iris and the ciliary body of the eye.

CLINICAL APPLICATIONS

Objective 7. Discuss the alteration of muscle structure and function in muscular dystrophy; define spasm, cramp, fibrillation, and fasciculation.

Muscular Dystrophy

Muscular dystrophy refers to a group of serious diseases affecting skeletal muscle. Dystrophy means degeneration, and, as the name implies, muscle cells are reduced in size and eventually destroyed in the course of the disease. Several forms of muscular dystrophy are recognized; all are inherited. The most common is Duchenne muscular dystrophy, inherited as a sex-linked recessive characteristic (see Chapter 27) and usually diagnosed in young males between age two and ten (Figure 8.14). The degeneration of muscles usually begins in the pelvic girdle area and spreads to the legs, abdomen, and spine. The disease progresses relentlessly until the patient dies in early adulthood. Other less debilitating forms of the disease are usually diagnosed in adolescence or adulthood. These include limb-girdle dystrophy, which affects the muscles of shoulder, hip, and upper limbs; facioscapulohumeral dystrophy, which affects muscles of the face and shoulder; and myotonic or distal dystrophy, which affects the muscles of the hands, forearm, and foreleg.

Although the cause of muscular dystrophy is known to be a genetic defect, the mechanism of the cell degeneration is unknown, and research is currently focused on the biochemistry of muscle degeneration. It is suspected that one or more enzymes may be absent or defective. Abnormal constituents have been found in the urine of individuals having muscular dystrophy, and the membranes of cells other than muscle cells have been shown to have structural defects. For example, the membranes of red blood cells from persons with muscular dystrophy contain unusually small amounts of certain lipids. It is thought that this defect may be due to the absence of an enzyme, which may account for abnormalities in other cells, including muscle cells. Whatever the cause, microscopic examination clearly indicates that dystrophic

muscle tissue degenerates and is replaced by fat and connective tissue (Figure 8.15).

No effective treatment exists for muscular dystrophy other than physical therapy and the use of braces to overcome some of the disabilities caused by the wasting of muscles. Experiments with animals have recently shown that the chemicals leupeptin and pepstatin can delay the degeneration of muscle tissue; these chemicals inhibit the action of enzymes that digest proteins. Genetically dystrophic chickens treated with these chemicals

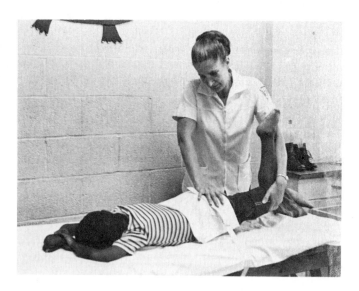

Figure 8.14 This child who has muscular dystrophy is placed in prone position while the therapist stretches his hip flexor muscles. The passive stretching exercise prevents increases in the contractures of the affected muscles. (A contracture is a shortening or distortion of a muscle.) (Photograph by author. Used with permission of the D.C. Public Schools, Department of Special Education, Sharpe Health School Administration, and the Department of Human Services of the District of Columbia.)

show far less degeneration of muscle tissue than those untreated. Similar treatment for humans afflicted by muscular dystrophy may be available in the future.

Some biochemical abnormalities found in individuals with muscular dystrophy are also found in individuals who are unaffected but who carry a recessive gene for the disease. One such abnormality involves the amounts of certain lipids in erythrocyte cell membranes. The ability to use biochemical tests to determine whether a person carries a defective gene for muscular dystrophy would make it possible for concerned individuals to know whether they might transmit such a gene to their offspring before they decide to have a child. Such tests are presently available in a few medical centers and research is underway to improve the tests' reliability.

Spasm, Cramp, Fibrillation, and Fasciculation

Various kinds of involuntary contractions sometimes occur in skeletal muscles. These include spasms, cramps, fibrillations, and fasciculations.

In a muscle **spasm** fibers of the muscle contract in a twitch-like contraction. Such contractions may be forceful and painful. Causes include toxins (poisons) and chemical imbalances in body fluids; massage may alleviate the pain by increasing the circulation of blood to the affected muscle and thus removing accumulations of damaging substances.

Muscle **cramps** involve tetanic contractions of muscle fibers. One explanation for such contractions is that exercise causes an increase in sensory stimuli from the muscles back to the spinal cord. These stimuli cause the cord to send additional motor stimuli to the muscle in a kind of feedback loop until involuntary tetanic contraction is produced. Voluntary contraction of opposing muscles (on the opposite side of a limb) will often alleviate the pain of a muscle cramp by breaking the "vicious cycle" of stimuli passing between the cramped muscle and the spinal cord.

Fasciculation is an uncoordinated contraction of a fasciculus, or bundle of fibers in a muscle; it can be seen through the skin. In contrast, a **fibrillation** is an uncoordinated contraction of various individual muscle fibers within a muscle; it cannot be observed with the naked eye. Persistent occurrence of either fasciculation or fibrillation usually indicates nerve damage.

Clinical Terms

myalgia (mi-al'je-ah)   pain in one or more muscles

myopathy (mi-op'ath-e)   any disease of a muscle

myositis (mi-o-si'tis)   inflammation of a skeletal muscle

myotonia (mi-o-to'ne-ah)   increased irritability and contractility of a muscle accompanied by decreased ability to relax

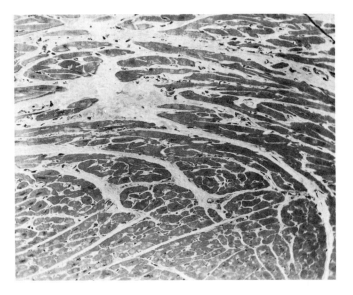

a

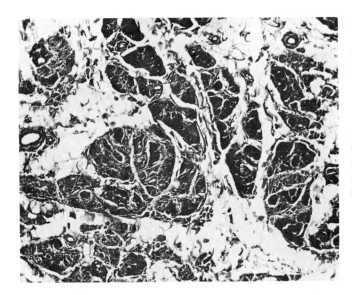

b

Figure 8.15   Muscle tissue (**a**) from a normal individual, × 145; (**b**) from an individual with muscular dystrophy, × 90. (Armed Forces Institute of Pathology negative numbers (**a**) 67–11316, and (**b**) 65–2050.)

Essay: Myasthenia Gravis

Myasthenia gravis is a disease characterized by easily fatigued muscles, particularly those of the limb girdles and those involved in eye movements, speech, and swallowing. The disease can begin at any age, with a peak age of onset between twenty and thirty, and its course is highly variable and unpredictable. Some patients experience only modest muscle impairment and live otherwise normal lives. Others experience a sudden onset of the disease with increasingly severe loss of muscle function, terminating in respiratory failure and death after only three or four months. Most patients experience a waxing and waning degree of impairment between these extremes.

The disease is an uncommon and puzzling one. Its incidence is only 3 or 4 per 100,000, and it affects women twice as often as men. Although it was recognized in 1672, it is not yet fully understood. In spite of its low incidence, it is worthy of discussion here because of recent advances in our knowledge of its causes.

It is now well established that in many affected individuals the direct cause of the symptoms of myasthenia gravis is a reduction in the number of functional acetylcholine receptors on the motor end plates of skeletal muscles. The receptors are probably destroyed by circulating antibodies that react with them. Thus, the disease is classified as an autoimmune disease, in some respects similar to rheumatoid arthritis (see the essay on rheumatoid arthritis in Chapter 7).

Part of the evidence for the reduction in acetylcholine receptor sites in myasthenia gravis patients comes from research with bungarotoxin, a small protein molecule found in cobra venom (and the component of the venom that causes paralysis). In experimental animals bungarotoxin has been shown to bind irreversibly to acetylcholine receptors. The toxin can be used in the laboratory to estimate relative numbers of receptors in a sample of muscle tissue. Such estimates have shown that biopsy muscle tissue from individuals with myasthenia gravis has only about 30 percent of the normal number of receptor sites. It has also been shown that a certain protein found in the blood of myasthenia gravis patients blocks the binding of bungarotoxin to acetylcholine receptors. Presumably, this protein binds to the receptors itself and may account for the impaired muscle function.

The disease has been produced experimentally in several animals including baboons, where it closely resembles the human disease. When serum (fluid from clotted blood) from an animal with myasthenia gravis is injected into a normal animal, symptoms of myasthenia gravis are produced. Thus, a circulating antibody that attaches to acetylcholine receptors seems to be the direct cause of the symptoms of the disease.

The problem of how the autoimmune process is initiated in myasthenia gravis is the subject of much current research. The thymus gland is implicated in two ways: (1) It is the source of tissue-destroying T-cells (see Chapter 20), and (2) it is a source of some embryonic muscle cells that have acetylcholine receptors on their surfaces. (Why muscle cells should be present in the thymus is not known.) It is thought that these muscle cells in some way stimulate the formation of antibodies to the acetylcholine receptors and that the antibodies then may attack skeletal muscle cells and cause myasthenia gravis. An explanation has been offered as to why this autoimmune reaction occurs only in a few individuals who have myasthenia gravis. It has been suggested that the ability to produce antibodies to embryonic muscle cells from the thymus is normally suppressed early in development, but in myasthenia gravis victims the ability reappears to some degree later in life. What triggers this antibody formation remains a mystery. Although not fully accepted, this explanation is consistent with the high variability in the severity of the disease and in the age of onset (from childhood to middle age).

The nature of thymus gland involvement remains puzzling. The gland is enlarged in about two-thirds of affected persons and contains a tumor in about one-tenth of them. Removal of the thymus has proved beneficial in some cases. However, a few individuals without myasthenia gravis who have had thymic tumors surgically removed have subsequently developed the disease. The effects of radiation therapy on thymic tumors, with or without surgery, is also unpredictable in individuals with myasthenia gravis. In some it alleviates the disease and in others it makes it worse.

At the present time treatment of this disease involves the use of drugs that inhibit cholinesterase, thereby allowing the available receptors to be stimulated by acetylcholine in higher concentration and over a longer period of time. This treatment must be continued throughout the life of an affected person. It compensates somewhat for the defect but does not cure it. As more is learned about the nature of the antibody and how it is produced, it may be possible to prevent antibody formation or reverse its action and free the receptor sites.

CHAPTER SUMMARY

(Chapter summary points and review questions are numbered to correspond to the numbered objectives in the text of each chapter.)

Organization and General Functions

1. Describe the organization of skeletal muscles in relation to the skeletal system and state the main functions of the skeletal muscular system.
   a. Muscles of the skeletal muscular system are attached to the bones of the skeleton.
   b. The main functions of the skeletal muscular system are:
   (1) movement
   (2) maintenance of posture
   (3) heat production

Development of the Skeletal Muscular System

2. Describe the development of the skeletal muscular system.
   a. The muscular system develops from myotomes and from less highly organized mesoderm in the head area.
   b. Each myotome has one main nerve associated with it, though later branching of nerves creates overlap in innervation of the myotomes.

Skeletal Muscle Tissue

3. Describe the organization of a skeletal muscle from the whole muscle level to the molecular level.
   a. Whole muscles are covered by epimysium and are attached to bones or other structures by tendons or aponeuroses.
   b. Muscles are made up of bundles of fibers covered with perimysium.
   c. Individual fibers are covered with endomysium.
   d. A muscle fiber is the cell of a muscle tissue and has sarcolemma, T-tubules, and a sarcoplasmic reticulum.
   e. Each fiber contains myofibrils that are made up of:
   (1) thick myofilaments of myosin
   (2) thin myofilaments of actin, troponin, and tropomyosin
   f. The functional unit of a myofibril is the sarcomere, which shortens during contraction as the actin and myosin filaments slide over one another.

Physiology of Muscle

4. Explain the steps in the processes of excitation, contraction, and relaxation.
   a. In excitation:
   (1) the plasma membrane becomes depolarized

   (2) the wave of depolarization passes along the T-tubules and stimulates the sarcoplasmic reticulum to release calcium ions
   (3) the calcium ions diffuse into the sarcoplasm and some bind with troponin, causing the troponin-tropomyosin complex to shift position and expose the active sites on the actin filaments
   b. In contraction:
   (1) energy from ATP energizes the myosin cross-bridges, causing them to bind to actin
   (2) energy is released, and the heads of the myosin molecules swivel, causing the actin and myosin filaments to slide over one another so that the sarcomere shortens
   (3) this cycle repeats as long as Ca^{2+} and ATP are present
   c. In relaxation:
   (1) calcium is pumped back to the sarcoplasmic reticulum in a process that uses ATP
   (2) the troponin-tropomyosin complex shifts position, covering the reactive sites of actin
   (3) the actin filaments slide back to their original positions, and the sarcomere returns to its original length, provided an external force acts in this direction

5. Describe the role of the following in muscle physiology: (a) motor unit, (b) mechanics of muscle contraction, and (c) metabolism of muscle contraction.
   a. A motor unit has the following properties:
   (1) It consists of all of the branches of an axon and the muscle fibers it innervates.
   (2) The portion of the muscle plasma membrane that lies beneath the nerve endings is the motor end plate.
   (3) The myoneural junction consists of the axon terminals and the motor end plate of the muscle cells innervated.
   b. When a nerve impulse reaches the axon terminals:
   (1) synaptic vesicles release acetylcholine
   (2) acetylcholine diffuses across the synaptic cleft and the subneural clefts and attaches to receptor sites on the membrane
   (3) the action of acetylcholine on the receptor sites depolarizes the membrane
   (4) acetylcholine is broken down by cholinesterase, and some choline is returned to the axon for reuse
   c. The mechanics of muscle contraction involve the following:
   (1) The force produced by a muscle is tension.
   (2) The opposing force is the load the muscle lifts.
   (3) Contractions are isotonic when the tension remains the same and the muscle shortens; they are isometric when the muscle remains the same length and the tension increases.
   (4) A twitch is the response of a muscle fiber to a single stimulus. It involves a latent period, a contraction period, and a relaxation period.

(5) Stimuli may be categorized as subthreshold or threshold, depending on whether they create an action potential.

(6) When stimuli are given in such rapid succession that the muscle never relaxes before the next stimulus, a tetanic contraction is produced.

(7) When a resting muscle receives a series of maximal stimuli at intervals long enough to allow relaxation between stimuli, treppe is produced.

(8) Muscle tone is a low level of tension maintained by contraction of some fibers of muscles.

(9) Muscles may become hypertrophic if forcefully exercised or atrophic if not used.

d. Some special properties of metabolism in muscles are that:
(1) muscle cells store energy in phosphocreatine
(2) muscle cells also contain glycogen, which can be broken down into glucose
(3) when muscles are rapidly using energy, glucose undergoes anaerobic glycolysis, lactic acid is produced, and an oxygen debt is created

6. Compare the properties of smooth muscle to those of skeletal muscle.

a. Smooth muscle shares the properties of excitability and contractility with skeletal muscle.

b. Smooth muscle is found in the walls of internal organs and blood vessels and has the following properties:
(1) spindle-shaped cells with a single nucleus
(2) involuntary control
(3) a lesser degree of organization of myofilaments than skeletal muscle

c. Smooth muscle is of two types:
(1) Visceral smooth muscle contracts spontaneously, and a wave of contraction can spread from cell to cell, but it may also respond to neural or hormonal stimulation.
(2) Multiunit smooth muscle responds to stimuli from the sympathetic and parasympathetic nervous systems and to hormones.

Clinical Applications

7. Discuss the alteration of muscle structure and function in muscular dystrophy; define spasm, cramp, fibrillation, and fasciculation.

a. Muscular dystrophy is a group of diseases caused by a genetic defect; it leads to degeneration of certain muscles, depending on the type of the disease. Affected muscles become less able to contract and are eventually paralyzed.

b. Common muscle disorders are defined as follows:
(1) A spasm is a painful contraction due to chemical imbalance in the muscle.
(2) A cramp is a tetanic contraction due to excessive motor stimuli, often following exercise.
(3) A fasciculation is an uncoordinated contraction of a bundle of muscle fibers.
(4) A fibrillation is an uncoordinated contraction of individual fibers within a muscle.

REVIEW

Important Terms

acetylcholine	myofilament
actin	myoglobin
"all-or-none" law	myoneural junction
aponeurosis	myosin
ATP	myotome
atrophy	perimysium
cholinesterase	phosphocreatine
contractility	plasticity
contraction cycle	relaxation period
contraction period	sarcolemma
cramp	sarcomere
elasticity	sarcoplasm
endomysium	sarcoplasmic reticulum
epimysium	sliding filament theory
excitability	smooth muscle
extensibility	spasm
fasciculation	subneural cleft
fatigue	subthreshold stimulus
fibrillation	summation
hypertrophy	synaptic cleft
isometric	tendon
isotonic	tetanus
latent period	threshold stimulus
motor end plate	transverse tubule
motor unit	treppe
multiunit smooth muscle	tropomyosin
muscular dystrophy	troponin
myasthenia gravis	twitch
myofibril	visceral smooth muscle

Questions

1. a. What are the properties of muscles that enable them to cause movement?
   b. What other functions besides movement do muscles perform?

2. What are myotomes, and what is their role in the development of muscles?

3. Create a model or diagram that describes the structure of skeletal muscle tissue. (Use pipe cleaners, rubber bands, or other objects to make your model.)

4. **a.** What chemical substances are involved in the processes of excitation, contraction, and relaxation of a muscle?
   b. How is each substance involved?
   c. Write a coherent paragraph describing the steps in these processes and showing where each chemical is involved.

5. **a.** What is a motor unit, and what is its role in muscle contraction?
   b. How are acetylcholine and cholinesterase involved in muscle contraction?
   c. What is the difference between an isotonic and an isometric contraction?
   d. How are the following types of contractions different? (1) twitch, (2) summation, (3) tetanic contraction, and (4) treppe?
   e. How are subthreshold and threshold stimuli different?
   f. What major chemical substances are involved in muscle metabolism?
   g. How is each of the substances involved in the production of energy for muscle contraction?
   h. How are fast muscle and slow muscle fibers different?

6. **a.** How does smooth muscle differ from skeletal muscle?
   b. How does the function of multiunit smooth muscle differ from visceral smooth muscle?

7. **a.** What is muscular dystrophy, and what are its effects?
   b. What are some limitations on the treatment and prevention of muscular dystrophy?
   c. Distinguish among spasms, cramps, fasciculations, and fibrillations.

Problems

1. Certain kinds of diseases of the muscles involve some kind of defect at the myoneural junction. Predict the effects of the following defects and identify the disease (if known) with which each defect is associated:
   a. Failure of axons to release acetylcholine
   b. Absence of the enzyme that destroys acetylcholine
   c. Deficiency of calcium ions in the sarcoplasmic reticulum

2. Design an experiment you can safely do on yourself to determine which of your muscles fatigues most easily.

REFERENCES AND READINGS

Anonymous. 1979. Target of the error in myasthenia. *Science News* 115:102 (February 17).

Astrand, P. O., and Rodahl, K. 1977. *Textbook of work physiology: Physiological basis of exercise* (2nd ed.). New York: McGraw-Hill.

Clausen, J. P. 1977. Effects of physical training on cardiovascular adjustments to exercise in man. *Physiological Reviews* 57(4):779.

Cohen, C. 1975. The protein switch of muscle contraction. *Scientific American* 223(5):36 (November).

Eisenberg, E., and Greene, L. E. 1980. The relation of muscle biochemistry to muscle physiology. *Annual Review of Physiology* 42:293.

Evans, F. G. 1957. *Atlas of human anatomy.* Totowa, N.J.: Rowman and Littlefield.

Ganong, W. F. 1981. *Review of medical physiology* (10th ed.). Los Altos, Calif.: Lange Medical Publications.

Guyton, A. C. 1981. *Textbook of medical physiology* (6th ed.). Philadelphia: W. B. Saunders.

Hartshorne, D. J., and Siemankowski, R. F. 1981. Regulation of smooth muscle actinomyosin. *Annual Review of Physiology* 43:519.

Howland, J. L., and Iyer, S. L. 1977. Erythrocyte lipids in heterozygous carriers of Duchenne muscular dystrophy. *Science* 198:309 (October 21).

Jolesz, F., and Sreter, F. A. 1981. Development, innervation, and activity-pattern induced changes in skeletal muscle. *Annual Review of Physiology* 43:531.

Kao, I., and Drachman, D. B. 1977. Thymic muscle cells bear acetylcholine receptors: Possible relation to myasthenia gravis. *Science* 195:74 (January 7).

Lester, H. A. 1977. The response to acetylcholine. *Scientific American* 236(2):107 (February).

Libby, P., and Goldberg, A. L. 1978. Leupeptin, a protease inhibitor, decreases protein degradation in normal and diseased muscles. *Science* 199:534 (February 3).

Lou, M. F. 1979. Human muscular dystrophy: Elevation of urinary dimethylarginines. *Science* 203:668 (February 16).

Murphy, R. A. 1979. Filament organization and contractile function in vertebrate smooth muscle. *Annual Review of Physiology* 41:737.

Plishker, G. A., Gitelman, H. J., and Appel, S. H. 1978. Myotonic muscular dystrophy: Altered calcium transport in erythrocytes. *Science* 200:323 (April 21).

Schlossberg, L. 1977. *The Johns Hopkins atlas of human functional anatomy.* G. D. Zuidema, ed. Baltimore, Md.: Johns Hopkins Press.

Stanley, E. F., and Drachman, D. B. 1978. Effect of myasthenia immunoglobulin on acetylcholine receptors of intact mammalian neuromuscular junctions. *Science* 200:1285 (June 16).

Stracher, A., McGowan, E. B., and Shafiq, S. A. 1978. Muscular dystrophy: Inhibition of degeneration in vivo with protease inhibitors. *Science* 200:50 (April 7).

Symposium on myasthenia gravis. 1978. *Thorax* 33(5):666 (October).

Tregear, R. T., and Marston, S. B. 1979. The crossbridge theory. *Annual Review of Physiology* 41:723.

9

MUSCULAR SYSTEM: MUSCLE ACTIONS

In Chapter 8 we considered the general characteristics and physiology of muscles; in this chapter we will study the specific actions of the major muscles of the body.

ACTIONS OF MUSCLES

Objective 1. Relate the properties of levers to muscle action.

Objective 2. Define the terms that describe muscle actions.

Levers

The bones and joints form a complex set of levers that produce skeletal movement when the muscles attached to the bones contract. We can apply the physical principles of the lever to understanding skeletal movement. A **lever** has three basic parts, the fulcrum, the point of effort, and the resistance, or load (Figure 9.1). The **fulcrum** is the point about which the lever moves. In the body the fulcrum is always a joint. The **point of effort** is the attachment of a muscle to a bone; it is where the force is exerted. The **resistance** (load) is the force to be overcome or the weight to be lifted.

Levers are divided into three classes, depending on the placement of the fulcrum, the resistance, and the effort. In a **first-class lever** the fulcrum is placed between the effort and the resistance. For example, the posterior neck muscles contract to produce the effort to overcome the weight of the anterior skull, rocking the head back (Figure 9.1a). In a **second-class lever** the resistance is between the fulcrum and the effort. The use of leg muscles to stand in a tip-toe position is a possible example of this kind of lever (Figure 9.1b), though some anatomists claim that no example of a second-class lever exists in the body. In a **third-class**

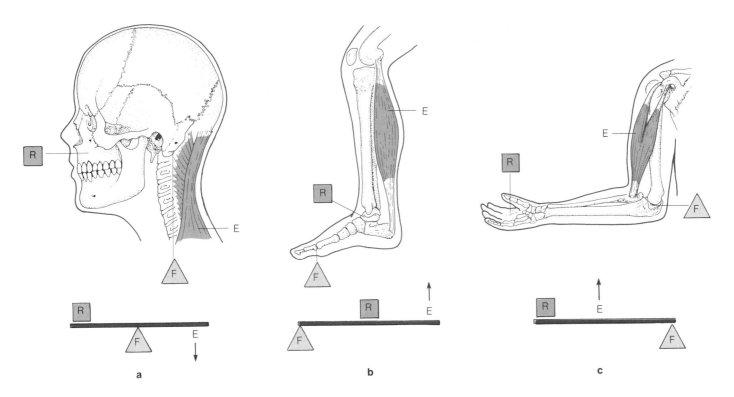

Figure 9.1 Classes of levers: (**a**) first-class lever, (**b**) second-class lever, (**c**) third-class lever. F = fulcrum, E = point of effort, R = resistance.

lever the effort is between the fulcrum and the resistance (Figure 9.1c). This arrangement is typical of many of the muscles and joints of the body. Though lever action is important in movement, many movements cannot be classified according to these classical lever types.

Two principles of lever action are important in understanding their role in body movement: (1) Levers amplify force and velocity of movement, and (2) the length of the lever arm between the point of effort and the resistance determines the amount of amplification of force and velocity. A playground teeter-totter illustrates these principles. Placing a heavy child on one end of the teeter-totter will cause a lighter child on the other end to go up as the heavy child goes down. The force applied by the heavy child is amplified as it is transferred to the other end of the board. The velocity of movement is also amplified; the greater the difference in the weights of the two children, the faster the lighter child will ride up on the board. It is a common practice to equalize the forces exerted by children of unequal weight by adjusting the position of the board at the fulcrum so that the lighter child is further from the fulcrum

than the heavier child. Because the total force applied is the product of the weight of the child times the distance between the fulcrum and the child, the forces exerted by the two children can be equalized. This illustrates the relationship between the forces and their effects on amplification of force and velocity.

If we apply these concepts to levers in the body, it is apparent from Figure 9.1 that, when effort is applied at some distance from the resistance, the force produced by that effort is amplified. Many of the muscles of the body are attached to the bones so as to amplify the force produced when the muscle contracts.

Muscle Terminology

Muscles are generally attached to bone or connective tissue at two points. The least movable attachment is the **origin** of the muscle; the most movable attachment is the **insertion**. In the appendages the origin is usually proximal to the insertion. The movement produced when the muscle contracts and pulls on the insertion is the **action** of the muscle. The different kinds of movements have already been described in Chapter 7 in the discussion of joints and their movements; they are summarized in Table 7.2.

Muscles often act together to create a certain movement. A muscle that causes a particular action is an **agonist**, or **prime mover**. Muscles that work with the agonist are **synergists**. For each movement there is usually an opposite movement—for example, flexion and extension are opposites. A muscle that performs the opposite action to that of an agonist is an **antagonist**. Among pairs of muscles each can be either the agonist or the antagonist, depending on the movement. For example, in flexing the elbow the flexor is the agonist, and the extensor is the antagonist; in extending the elbow the roles are reversed. Because a single muscle can exert a force in only one direction, an antagonistic muscle is required to cause movement in the opposite direction.

Muscles are named for a variety of characteristics: (1) movements they perform, (2) shapes, (3) origin and insertion, (4) multiple points of origin, (5) location, and (6) size. Muscles named for the movement they perform may be called flexors, extensors, abductors, adductors, or levators. (A levator is a muscle that elevates a part of the body.) Muscles named for their shapes include the trapezius (shaped like a trapezoid) and the rhomboideus (shaped like a rhomboid). The origin and insertion appear in the name of the sternohyoid muscle; its origin is on the sternum, and its insertion on the hyoid. Muscles having multiple origins (more than one proximal attachment) are said to have "ceps," or heads; a biceps has two heads, a triceps three heads, and a quadriceps four heads. The name may describe the location as in the tibialis anterior, located on the anterior surface of the tibia, or the tibialis posterior, located on the posterior surface of the tibia. The size of the muscle may be reflected in the name, as in the gluteus maximus, the large muscle that forms each buttock. Associating characteristics of muscles with their names is a help in remembering the names.

The **innervation** of a muscle—that is, what nerve supplies it with motor fibers that stimulate it to contract—reveals some information about its development as nerves become associated with myotomes early in development, and they migrate together (see Chapter 8). Though not derived from myotomes, facial muscles develop from a certain portion of the mesoderm that is largely under the control of the facial nerve (cranial nerve VII). Knowing the location of nerves in relation to muscles is important in surgical procedures either to prevent damage or to attempt to restore function after injury.

The names, locations, origin, insertions, actions, and innervations of the major muscles of the body are listed in Table 9.1 near the end of this chapter. (Actions were defined in Chapter 7.) Certain muscles have been selected for emphasis in the text to illustrate their actions in the movement of certain joints or because of other important functions. Muscles, regardless of whether they are associated with the axial or the appendicular skeleton, are paired—one on each side of the body.

MUSCLES OF THE AXIAL SKELETON

Objective 3. Locate and describe the action of the major muscles of (a) the head and neck, (b) the trunk, (c) the abdominal wall, and (d) the pelvic floor.

Muscles of the Head and Neck

Muscles of the head and neck can be divided into four groups according to their function. They are the muscles of facial expression, the muscles of mastication, the muscles that move the tongue and assist in swallowing, and the muscles that move the head.

The muscles of **facial expression** (Figure 9.2) lie beneath the skin of the scalp, face, and throat. You can determine the effects of several of these muscles by studying the figure and then attempting to contract each muscle as you look at yourself in a mirror. You raise your eyebrows and wrinkle your forehead by contracting the frontal part of the **occipitofrontalis**. You close your eyes or your mouth by contracting the appropriate **orbicularis** muscle. You use the **major** and **minor zygomatic** muscles to smile and the **depressor** muscles to create a sad or "down-in-the-mouth" expression. The **platysma** muscle lies just beneath the skin; it gives the neck a smooth appearance and also helps to pull the angle of the mouth downward, as in pouting. The deeper **buccinator** muscle is sometimes called the trumpeter's muscle because it aids in puckering the lips to blow air out of the mouth.

The muscles of **mastication**, or chewing (Figure 9.3), include the **temporalis**, **masseter**, **buccinator**, and the deeper **pterygoids**. The masseter is the primary muscle used in closing the mouth by elevating the jaw. The temporalis and medial pterygoid are synergists with the masseter in raising the mandible; they are antagonists in retracting and protracting the mandible. The lateral pterygoids open the jaws, protract the mandible, and cause the mandible to move from side to side. The coordinated action of these muscles makes possible the chewing of food. The buccinator, already mentioned as a muscle of facial expression, is also involved in mastication. It can produce a sucking motion and also helps to keep food between the teeth.

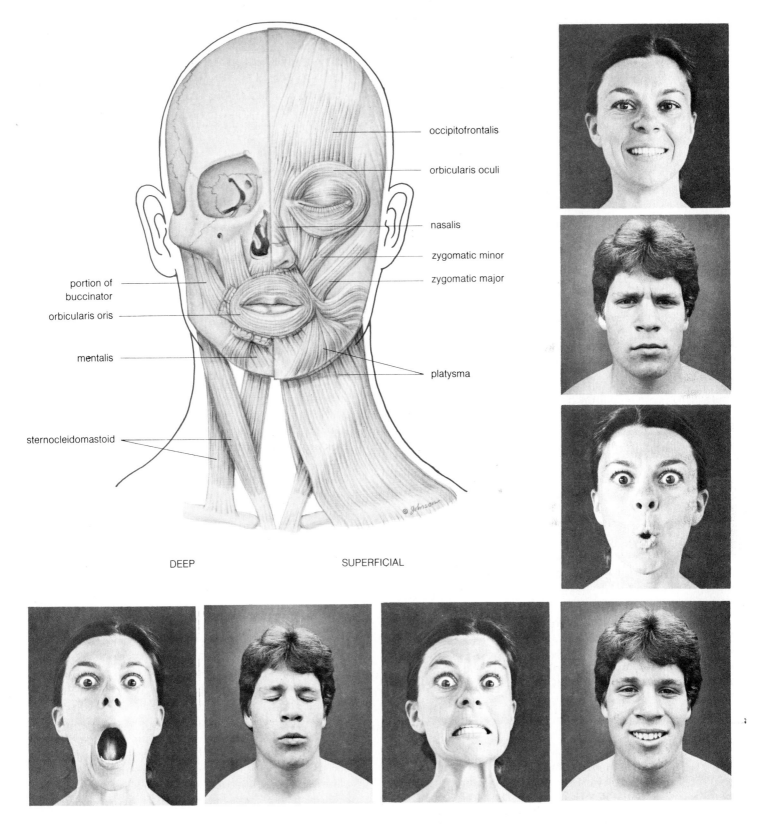

occipitofrontalis

orbicularis oculi

nasalis

zygomatic minor

zygomatic major

portion of buccinator

orbicularis oris

mentalis

platysma

sternocleidomastoid

DEEP

SUPERFICIAL

Figure 9.2 The muscles of facial expression. (Photographs by Elliott Varner Smith.)

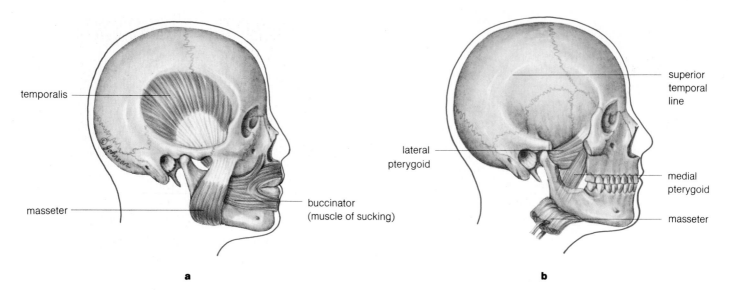

temporalis

masseter

buccinator
(muscle of sucking)

a

superior
temporal
line

lateral
pterygoid

medial
pterygoid

masseter

b

Figure 9.3 Muscles of mastication: (**a**) superficial muscles, (**b**) deep muscles.

In some individuals the eruption of a third molar ("wisdom tooth") may cause a spasm of the masseter and temporalis muscles. This condition, called trismus, may be so severe that the person cannot open his or her mouth.

The muscles associated with the **tongue** include the **genioglossus**, **stylohyoid**, **hyoglossus**, and **styloglossus** (Figure 9.4). The genioglossus extends from the chin (genio) to the tongue (glossus); it depresses the tongue and pulls it forward. The stylohyoid extends from the styloid process of the temporal bone to the hyoid bone; it elevates the hyoid, to which the hyoglossus is attached. The hyoglossus is also attached to the tongue, so together these muscles elevate the tongue. The styloglossus, which extends from the styloid process to the tongue, retracts the tongue. These and other muscles work together to move the tongue in mixing food and pushing it out of the mouth into the pharynx. They are also important in moving the tongue in the articulation of words.

Several **neck** muscles are involved in moving the head (Figure 9.4). The **sternocleidomastoid** extends from sternum (sterno) and clavicle (cleido) to the mastoid process of the temporal bone. When both the left and right sternocleidomastoid muscles contract, the neck is flexed so the chin is touching the chest. When only one of these muscles

contracts, the head is rotated to face the side toward the contracting muscle. A posterior muscle, the **splenius capitis**, is an antagonist of the sternocleidomastoid. When these muscles contract on both sides of the head at the same time, they extend the neck and tilt the head back. When only one contracts, it rotates the head to face the same direction as the contracting muscle. Two deeper muscles, the **semispinalis capitis** and the **longissimus capitis**, are shown in Figure 9.6 with the deep muscles of the back and trunk. Both of these muscles extend the neck (bend the head back). When one semispinalis capitis muscle contracts, it rotates the face toward the side of the contracting muscle; when one longissimus capitis muscle contracts, it extends the head toward the contracting muscle.

Muscles of the Trunk

Muscles of the trunk include those of the back (Figures 9.5 and 9.6) and the rib cage (Figure 9.7). The pectoral muscles, although located on the trunk, will be discussed with the pectoral girdle muscles because their actions are associated with the shoulder joint. Most of the superficial trunk muscles shown in Figure 9.5 are likewise associated with the pectoral or pelvic girdles and will be discussed later. When these muscles are removed, the deep muscles of the back are exposed. These are the muscles that move the trunk (Figure 9.6).

The major muscle of the **trunk** is the **sacrospinalis**. It is

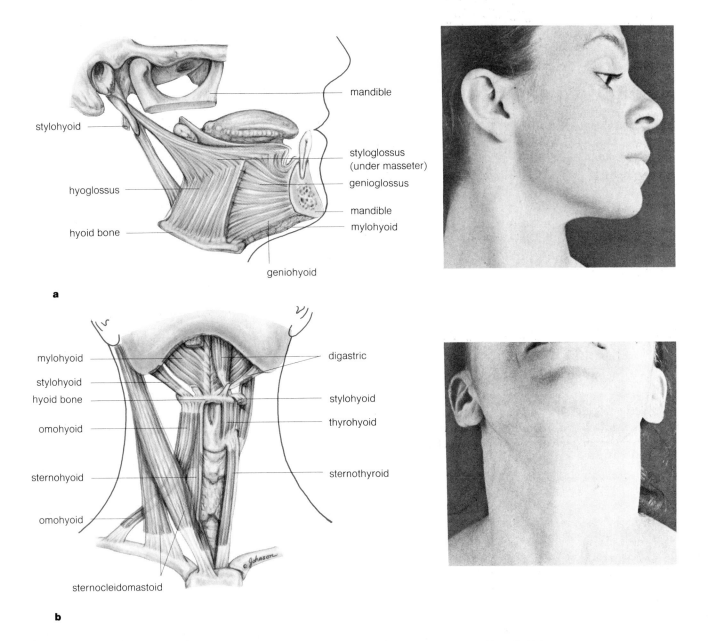

Figure 9.4 Muscles of the tongue and neck: (**a**) lateral view, (**b**) anterior view. (Photographs by Elliott Varner Smith.)

divided into the lateral **iliocostalis**, the intermediate **longissimus**, and the medial **spinalis**. The iliocostalis is further divided into three portions, the **lumborum**, the **thoracis**, and the **cervicis**, each named for the area of the vertebral column in which it is found. The longissimus is likewise divided into the **thoracis**, **cervicis**, and **capitis**. (The longissimus capitis has already been mentioned as a muscle that moves the head.) Together, all the parts of the sacrospinalis act as extensors of the spine. Portions of it act to rotate the spine or to bend it laterally from side to side. This lateral movement is called abduction because it moves the spine away from the midline of the body. Another major muscle of the trunk is the **quadratus lumborum**. It too extends, rotates, and abducts the spine.

The muscles of the **rib cage** (Figure 9.7) include the **external intercostals** and the **internal intercostals**. These are wide, short muscles that have their origins on a superior rib and their insertions on the next inferior rib. Another mus-

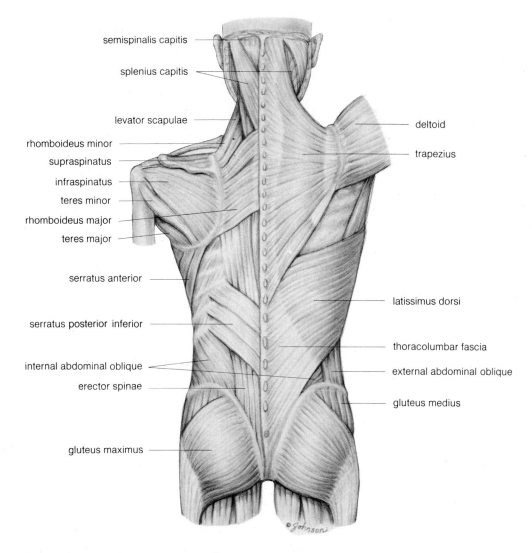

Figure 9.5 Superficial muscles of the back and trunk, with most superficial muscles shown on the right and the next deeper layer of muscles shown on the left.

semispinalis capitis

splenius capitis

levator scapulae

rhomboideus minor

supraspinatus

infraspinatus

teres minor

rhomboideus major

teres major

serratus anterior

serratus posterior inferior

internal abdominal oblique

erector spinae

gluteus maximus

deltoid

trapezius

latissimus dorsi

thoracolumbar fascia

external abdominal oblique

gluteus medius

cle, the **diaphragm**, lies within the body cavity and separates the thoracic and abdominal cavities. Together, these muscles are responsible for the movements in breathing, as will be explained in Chapter 21.

Muscles of the Abdominal Wall

The muscles of the abdominal wall (Figure 9.8) are the **rectus abdominis**, the **external** and **internal obliques**, and the **transverse abdominis**. The rectus abdominis muscles are a pair of long, flat muscles lying on either side of the midline connective tissue, the **linea alba**. Horizontal lines across this muscle, the **tendinous inscriptions**, represent the embryonic divisions between myotomes. The rectus abdominis muscles are flexors of the spine and act as antagonists to the sacrospinalis muscles. The other abdominal muscles form the lateral abdominal wall. Their arrangement in layers, like the layers of a three-ply automoble tire, increases the strength of the abdominal wall. The outermost muscle is the external oblique; its fibers run on a diagonal from the ribs

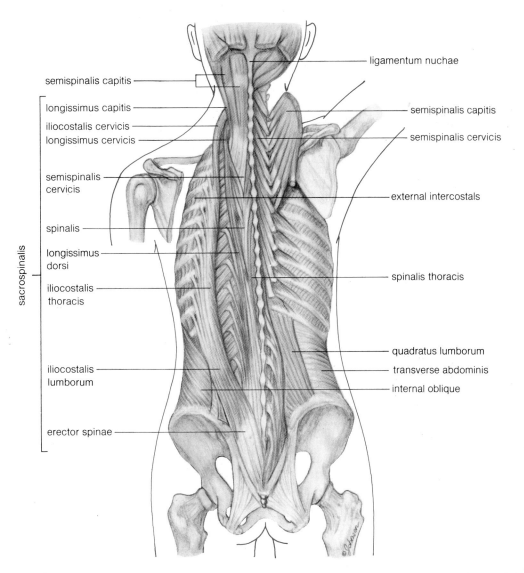

semispinalis capitis

longissimus capitis
iliocostalis cervicis
longissimus cervicis

semispinalis
cervicis

spinalis

longissimus
dorsi

iliocostalis
thoracis

iliocostalis
lumborum

erector spinae

sacrospinalis

ligamentum nuchae

semispinalis capitis

semispinalis cervicis

external intercostals

spinalis thoracis

quadratus lumborum
transverse abdominis
internal oblique

Figure 9.6 Some intermediate and deep muscles of the back and trunk, after removal of most of the muscles in Figure 9.5.

down and forward to the pelvic area. The fibers of the middle muscle, the internal oblique, run on a diagonal from the iliac crest up and forward to the ribs and xiphoid process. The fibers of the innermost layer, the transverse abdominis, run in a transverse direction from the iliac crest, lumbar fascia, and rib cartilages to the linea alba. These muscles compress the abdomen during such actions as defecation, coughing, and childbirth. They also play a role in the maintenance of posture and can contribute to twisting motions and forced expirations.

Sometimes a separation develops between the fibers of an abdominal muscle or the diaphragm, producing a **hernia**. In the area of herniation underlying tissues and organs protrude through the gap in the muscle fibers. Such separation often results from heavy lifting, obesity, or lack of exercise followed by weakening of the muscles. Some hernias are congenital—that is, present at birth; they result from muscle groups failing to fuse during development.

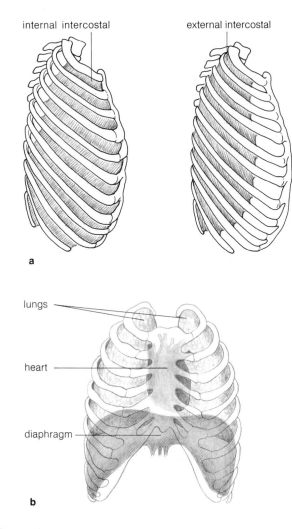

internal intercostal   external intercostal

a

lungs

heart

diaphragm

b

Figure 9.7 The muscles of breathing: (**a**) the external and internal inter-costals, (**b**) the diaphragm.

Muscles of the Pelvic Floor

The muscles of the pelvic floor are the **levator ani** and the **coccygeus**. Together, they form the pelvic diaphragm, which supports the pelvic organs and forms the floor of the pelvic area. When these muscles become weakened or lose their tone, organs can protrude through openings. Such protrusion is called **prolapse**. Uterine prolapse is not uncommon in women who have had numerous pregnancies or who have sustained unrepaired injuries during childbirth. The arrangement of these muscles in the female, as they appear from inside the pelvic cavity, is shown in Figure 9.9. The arrangement of the levator ani in relation to other structures in the male is shown in Figure 9.10. This figure

shows the perineal area (the area around the anus and uro-genital openings) as seen externally after removal of the skin and scrotum.

MUSCLES OF THE APPENDICULAR SKELETON

Objective 4. Locate and describe the action of the major muscles of (a) the pectoral girdle and shoulder joint, (b) the elbow, (c) the wrist and hand, (d) the pelvic girdle and hip joint, (e) the knee, and (f) the ankle and foot.

Muscles of the Pectoral Girdle and Shoulder Joint

Muscles that move the pectoral girdle and hold it to the trunk are closely associated with those that move the shoulder joint (Figures 9.5 and 9.11). Among the muscles that move the **pectoral girdle** is the **trapezius**. It is a large muscle shaped like a trapezoid, running from the thoracic vertebral column to the spine and acromion process of the scapula and to the distal clavicle. Because of its large size and several insertions, it has several actions. The whole muscle rotates the scapula and abducts the arm. The superior portion elevates the glenoid fossa, the middle portion adducts the vertebral border of the scapula, and the inferior portion depresses the vertebral border of the scapula.

Beneath the trapezius are the **levator scapulae**, the **rhomboideus major**, and the **rhomboideus minor**. As the name suggests, the levator scapulae elevates the scapula. Both the rhomboideus muscles adduct the scapula; the rhomboideus major also rotates it slightly upward.

The **serratus anterior**, which extends from the scapula laterally and anteriorly to the ribs, holds the scapula against the wall of the trunk. When the ribs are fixed, it pulls the scapula forward, such as in reaching or pushing movements; when the scapula is fixed, it elevates the ribs.

The **pectoralis minor**, an anteriorly located muscle, lies beneath the larger pectoralis major, whose action is discussed below. The pectoralis minor extends from the ribs to the coracoid process of the scapula. When the ribs are stationary, it depresses and anteriorly rotates the scapula; when the scapula is stationary, it assists in elevating the ribs during respiration.

The muscles that move the arm at the **shoulder joint** are closely associated with those that move the pectoral girdle (see Figures 9.5 and 9.11). The large chest muscle, the **pectoralis major**, extends from the clavicle, sternum, and ribs to the humerus. It flexes, adducts, and medially rotates

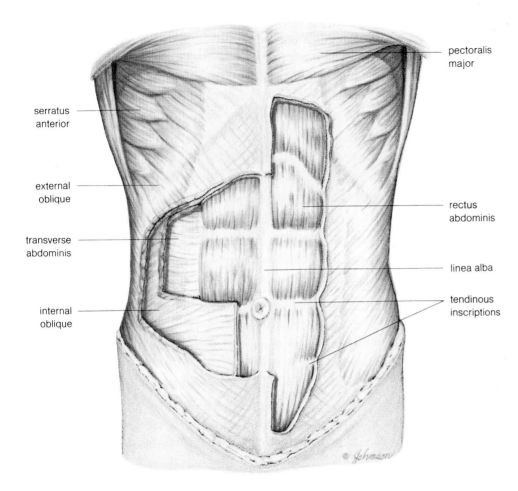

serratus anterior

external oblique

transverse abdominis

internal oblique

pectoralis major

rectus abdominis

linea alba

tendinous inscriptions

© Johnson

Figure 9.8 Muscles of the abdominal wall.

the arm. The **deltoid**, a triangular muscle that forms the fleshy part of the shoulder, extends from the clavicle and scapula to the humerus. Its action is to abduct the arm. The **latissimus dorsi**, a broad, flat, sheetlike muscle, extends from the lower thoracic and lumbar vertebrae, sacrum, and iliac crest to the humerus. It extends, adducts, and medially rotates the arm. Swinging the arm along the side of the body requires alternate contractions of the pectoralis major and the latissimus dorsi.

Beneath the deltoid muscle and attached to various surfaces of the scapula are four other muscles that assist with movements of the shoulder joint (see Figure 9.5). The **supraspinatus** lies superior to the spine of the scapula and assists the deltoid in abducting the arm. The **infraspinatus** lies inferior to the spine of the scapula and rotates the arm

laterally. The **teres minor** lies inferior to the infraspinatus and also rotates the arm laterally. The **teres major** originates from the inferior angle of the scapula, runs diagonally toward, and inserts distal to, the lesser tubercle of the humerus. It assists with extension, adduction, and medial rotation. These underlying muscles are important in maintaining stability of the shoulder joint.

The pectoralis major is frequently congenitally absent, either wholly or in part. It is also removed in the surgical procedure called radical mastectomy often done as a treatment for breast cancer.

Muscles of the Elbow Joint

Muscles of the **elbow joint** (Figure 9.12) generally have their origins on the scapula or humerus and their insertions on the radius or ulna. They cause flexion or extension at the elbow joint and movement of the forearm. The two-headed **biceps brachii** extends from the scapula to the radius and flexes and supinates the forearm. The **brachialis** has its origin beneath the biceps brachii on the anterior surface of the humerus and its insertion on the ulna. It is also a flexor of the forearm. The **brachioradialis** assists the biceps brachii in flexing and supinating the forearm. (Supination places the palm upward.). The **triceps brachii** is a three-headed muscle with origins on the scapula and humerus. It inserts by a tendon to the olecranon process of the ulna. Its action is to extend the forearm. Two small muscles, the **supinator** and the **pronator teres** run from the humerus and ulna to the radius. As their names imply, they supinate or pronate the forearm. (Pronation places the palm downward.)

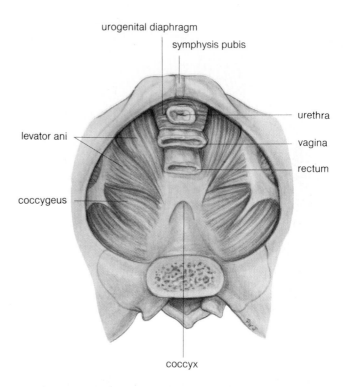

Figure 9.9 Muscles of the female pelvic floor, as seen from inside the pelvic cavity.

Figure 9.10 Muscles of the pelvic floor and perineum of the male, as seen in external view with skin removed.

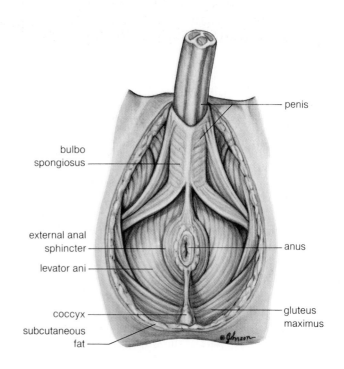

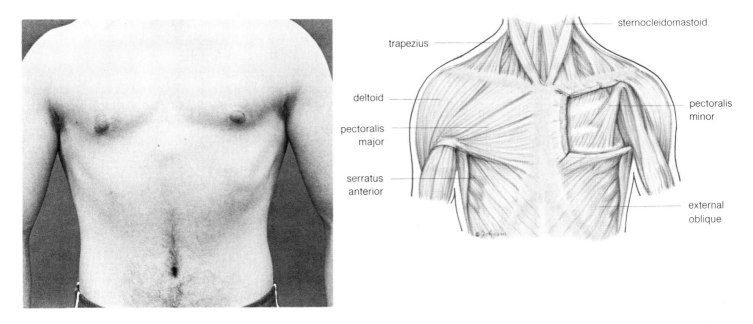

Figure 9.11 Muscles of the anterior chest. (Photograph by Elliott Varner Smith.)

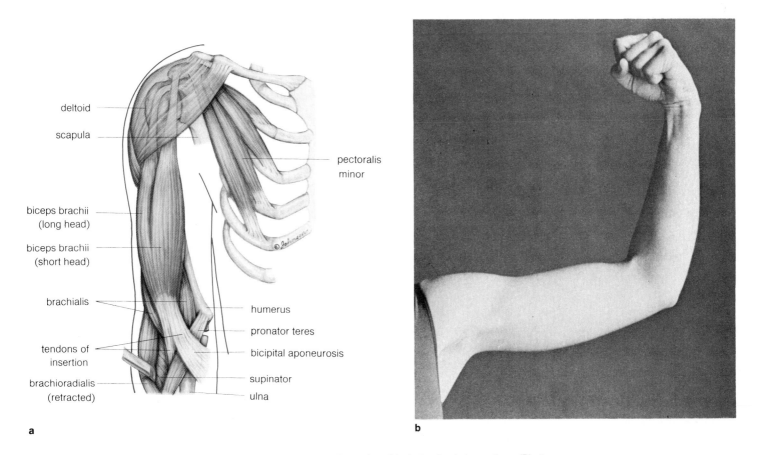

a

b

Figure 9.12 Muscles of the shoulder and elbow: (**a**) anterior view of muscles, (**b**) photo of anterior surface. (Photograph by Elliott Varner Smith.)

Muscles of the Wrist, Hand, and Fingers

The major muscles of the **wrist**, **hand**, and **fingers** are shown in Figure 9.13. Many more muscles are present than are shown in the figure; of those shown six are discussed here to illustrate the types of movement that occur. All of the muscles discussed have their origins on the humerus, though they have little action at the elbow.

Two major flexors on the anterior surface of the forearm are the lateral **flexor carpi radialis** and the more medial **flexor carpi ulnaris**. The names of these muscles indicate their action (flexing the carpi, or wrist) and the bone they most nearly parallel. Of these muscles the radialis is also an abductor of the hand, and the ulnaris is an adductor of the hand.

The extensors, antagonists of the flexors, are located on the posterior surface of the forearm. They are the **extensor carpi radialis longus** and the **extensor carpi ulnaris**. In addition to their extensor action, these muscles act synergistically with the above flexors in abduction and adduction; the extensor carpi radialis longus acts with the corresponding flexor in abduction, and the ulnar muscles work together in adduction.

Among the muscles acting on the hand and fingers, the **flexor digitorum profundus** flexes the wrist and phalanges, and the **extensor digitorum** extends the wrist and phalanges. Several other muscles intrinsic to (entirely within) the hand control flexion and extension of the joints between each of the phalanges and allow spreading the fingers and closing them together again. Muscles of the thumb allow a wide range of rotational movement.

> When a person has a broken bone in the forearm or wrist, the cast usually extends above the elbow. Casting above the elbow is necessary to immobilize the wrist muscles that extend above the elbow.

Muscles of the Pelvic Girdle and Hip

In our study of the deep muscles of the back and trunk (see Figure 9.6), we have already encountered some muscles that extend from the pelvic girdle upward along the vertebral column. These muscles support the trunk and help to maintain posture. They also help to keep the pelvic girdle firmly attached to the sacrum.

Many of the muscles that move the **thigh** (Figure 9.14) by bending the hip joint have their origins on either the ilium or the pubic bone and their insertions on the femur or tibia. The **iliopsoas**, sometimes considered to be two separate muscles, the **iliacus** and the **psoas major**, flexes the thigh. When the thigh is stationary, it flexes the trunk. This muscle is often stretched or torn in the activities of ballet dancers. The **rectus femoris** is also a flexor of the thigh. Because its insertion is on the tibia by way of the patellar tendon, it is also an extensor of the leg.

The **gluteus maximus**, the heaviest muscle in the body, which forms much of the buttock, is an extensor of the thigh. It also rotates the femur laterally. Anterior to and partially beneath the gluteus maximus are the other two muscles of the gluteal group, the **gluteus medius** and the **gluteus minimus**. Both help to stabilize the femur in the acetabulum, and both are abductors of the thigh. The **tensor fasciae latae** is a muscle imbedded in fascia that lies on the lateral surface of the hip. It is also an abductor of the thigh.

A group of three adductors occupy the medial aspect of the thigh. All originate on the pubis and pull the femur toward the midline. They are the superficial **adductor longus** and the deeper **adductor magnus** and **adductor brevis**. As the names indicate, these muscles adduct the thigh. A small, superficial, straplike muscle, the **gracilis**, adducts the thigh and also flexes the leg.

Muscles of the Knee Joint

We have already mentioned the rectus femoris and the gracilis as muscles that move the leg by causing extension of the **knee joint**. The **rectus femoris** is part of a group of four muscles, the **quadriceps femoris group**, that lie on the anterior surface of the thigh and extend the leg. The other muscles of this group are the **vastus lateralis**, **vastus intermedius**, and **vastus medialis** (Figure 9.14). The vastus intermedius is not visible in the figure because it lies beneath the rectus femoris muscle. Another muscle of the anterior thigh is the **sartorius**, a straplike muscle that flexes both the thigh and the leg. Its action is important in crossing one leg over the other or in assuming the cross-legged yoga or tailor's position.

The **hamstring group** occupy the posterior aspect of the thigh. The tendons of these muscles in the thigh of a pig are used to suspend a ham during curing, hence the name hamstring. The members of this group are the **biceps femoris**, **semitendinosus**, and **semimembranosus** (Figure 9.14). One head of the biceps has its origin on the ischium and the other on the femur. The biceps muscle also has two insertions, on the fibula and on the tibia. Its actions are to flex the knee joint and extend the thigh. The semitendinosus and the semimembranosus are both extensors of the thigh.

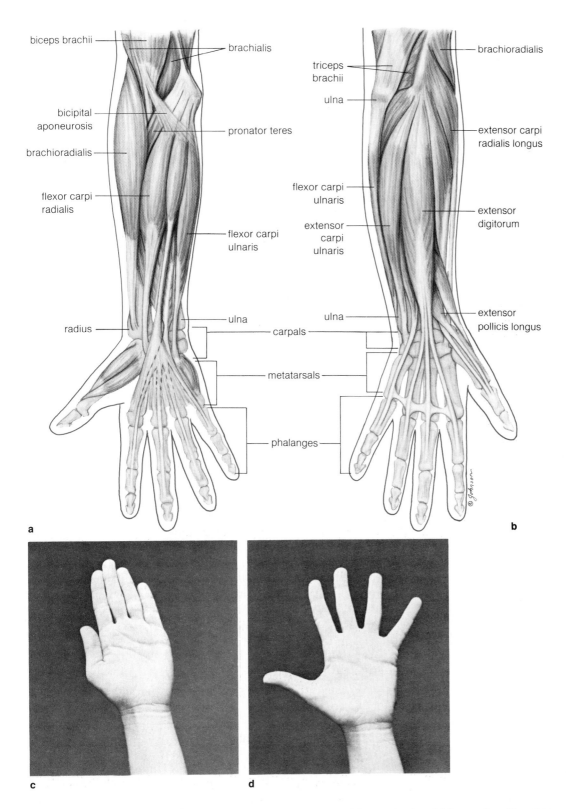

Figure 9.13 Muscles that move the wrist and hand: (**a**) anterior view, (**b**) posterior view, (**c**) fingers closed together, (**d**) fingers spread apart. (Photographs by Elliott Varner Smith.)

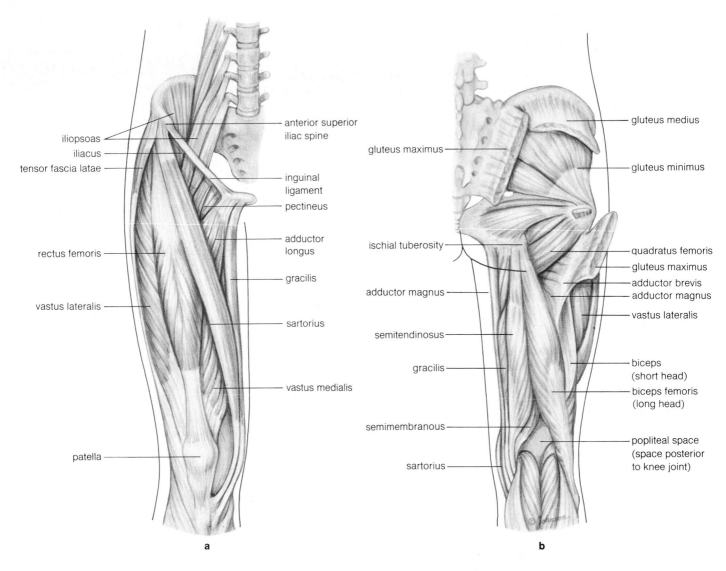

Figure 9.14 Muscles of the right pelvic girdle and thigh: (**a**) anterior view, (**b**) posterior view.

Muscles of the Lower Leg, Ankle, and Foot

As with the wrist and hand, only a few of the many muscles of the **ankle** and **foot** are considered here. The selected muscles and a few additional ones are shown in Figure 9.15. On the anterior surface of the leg, lateral to the tibia, is the **tibialis anterior**. It is a flexor of the foot and also acts to invert the foot. On the posterior surface of the leg in the area of the calf is the large **gastrocnemius** muscle. Its origins are on the condyles of the femur, and its insertion is on the calcaneus by way of the **Achilles tendon**. Its actions are to flex the leg by bending the knee joint and to extend or plantarflex the foot. Beneath the gastrocnemius is the **soleus**, also inserted by way of the Achilles tendon and also a plantarflexor of the foot. An even smaller muscle, the

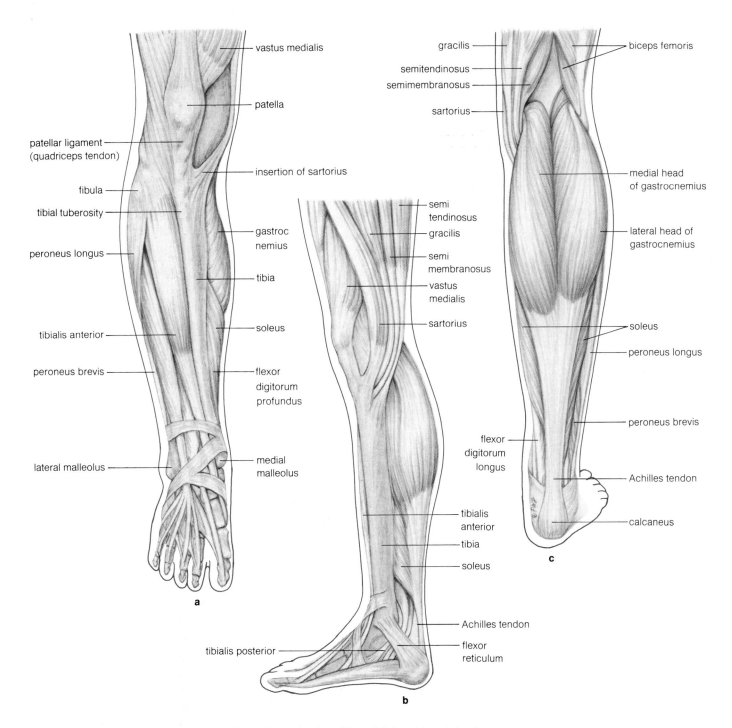

Figure 9.15 Muscles of the right leg, ankle, and foot: (a) anterior view, (b) medial view, (c) posterior view.

In figure (a):
vastus medialis
patella
patellar ligament (quadriceps tendon)
insertion of sartorius
fibula
tibial tuberosity
gastrocnemius
peroneus longus
tibia
tibialis anterior
soleus
peroneus brevis
flexor digitorum profundus
lateral malleolus
medial malleolus
a

In figure (b):
semi tendinosus
gracilis
semi membranosus
vastus medialis
sartorius
tibialis anterior
tibia
soleus
Achilles tendon
flexor reticulum
tibialis posterior
b

In figure (c):
gracilis
semitendinosus
semimembranosus
sartorius
biceps femoris
medial head of gastrocnemius
lateral head of gastrocnemius
soleus
peroneus longus
peroneus brevis
flexor digitorum longus
Achilles tendon
calcaneus
c

tibialis posterior, seen in the medial view in Figure 9.15, extends, plantarflexes, and inverts the foot. Two muscles on the lateral surface of the leg, the **peroneus longus** and the **peroneus brevis**, plantarflex and evert the foot.

The Achilles tendon is named after the mythical Greek hero Achilles. According to the legend, Achilles's mother dipped him in the river Styx when he was a baby, holding him only by the heel of one foot. This made him invulnerable except where the water had not touched the back of his heel. He was an invincible warrior until the battle of Troy, when he was pierced by an arrow in the one place he could be wounded.

Cutting the Achilles tendon results in a crippling injury even without mythical explanation: Without the support of the gastrocnemius muscle, one is unable to stand on the injured leg. The action of this muscle, through the lever of the foot (Figure 9.1b), is what keeps us from falling on our faces. A torn Achilles tendon is one of the most serious athletic injuries, particularly for runners.

TABLE OF MUSCLE ACTIONS

In Table 9.1 the major muscles are listed by region of the body. The information given for each muscle is: name, general location, origin, insertion, action, and innervation. When studying information about muscles, it is important to note what clues the name of the muscle gives about its origin, insertion, and action. It is also helpful to attempt to locate each muscle on your own body, to contract the muscle, and to compare what happens in your body with the action described in the table. Finally, it is helpful to group together muscles with similar actions and to compare them with the groups having antagonistic actions. For example, the flexors are usually on one surface of a limb and the extensors on the opposite surface. Abductors are usually located lateral to the joint they move, and adductors are usually medial to the joint they move.

Table 9.1   Muscle Characteristics and Actions

Muscle	Location	Origin	Insertion	Action	Innervation
Muscles of Facial Expression					
Occipitofrontalis	Forehead and scalp	Occipital bone	Muscles of eye orbit	Wrinkles forehead, raises eyebrows	Cranial nerve VII
Orbicularis oculi	Encircles eyelid	–	–	Closes eye	Cranial nerve VII
Orbicularis oris	Encircles mouth	–	–	Puckers lips	Cranial nerve VII
Platysma	Anterior neck	Fascia of deltoid and pectoralis major	Mandible	Draws corners of mouth down	Cranial nerve VII
Buccinator	Cheeks	Maxillae	Skin of sides of mouth	Smiling, sucking	Cranial nerve VII
Muscles of Mastication					
Masseter	Side of mandible	Zygomatic arch	Mandible	Closes jaw	Cranial nerve V
Temporal	Lateral skull	Temporal bone	Mandible	Closes jaw	Cranial nerve V
Pterygoids	Medial to ramus of mandible	Pterygoid process of sphenoid	Mandible	Protrudes jaw and moves it from side to side	Cranial nerve V

Table 9.1 Muscle Characteristics and Actions (continued)

Muscle	Location	Origin	Insertion	Action	Innervation
Muscles of the Tongue					
Genioglossus	Beneath tongue	Mandible	Tongue and hyoid bone	Depresses and protracts tongue	Cranial nerve XII
Styloglossus	Cheek	Styloid process of temporal	Tongue	Elevates and retracts tongue	Cranial nerve XII
Stylohyoid	Behind mandible	Styloid process of temporal	Hyoid bone	Elevates and retracts tongue	Cranial nerve VII
Hyoglossus	In and beneath tongue	Hyoid	Within tongue	Depresses tongue	Cranial nerve XII
Muscles of the Neck					
Sternocleidomastoid	Lateral neck	Sternum and clavicle	Mastoid process of temporal	Flexes and rotates head	Cranial nerve XI and cervical nerves 2, 3
Semispinalis capitis	Back of neck	Upper 6 thoracic and lower 4 cervical vertebrae	Occipital bone	Extends head and bends it laterally	Cervical nerves 1–5
Splenius capitis	Back of neck	Ligamentum nuchae	Mastoid process of temporal	Extends head	Cervical nerves 2–4
		Upper thoracic vertebrae	Occipital bone	Bends and rotates head	
Longissimus capitis	Lateral neck	Upper 6 thoracic and lower 4 cervical vertebrae	Mastoid process of temporal	Extends, bends, and rotates head	Middle and lower cervical nerves
Muscles of the Trunk					
Sacrospinalis	Posterior trunk			Extends spine, maintains posture	Cervical nerve 1 to lumbar nerve 5
Iliocostalis					
lumborum		Iliac crest and lumbar vertebrae	Lower 6 ribs		
thoracis		Lower 6 ribs	Upper 6 ribs		
cervicis		Upper 6 ribs	Cervical vertebrae 4 to 6		
Longissimus					
thoracis		Iliac crest and lumbar vertebrae	Thoracic vertebrae and ribs		
cervicis		Upper 6 thoracic vertebrae	Cervical vertebrae 2 to 6		
capitis		(See neck muscles.)			
Quadratus lumborum	Between ilium and last rib	Iliac crest	12th rib	Extends or abducts spine	Thoracic nerve 12 and lumbar nerves 1,2
Muscles of Breathing					
Diaphragm	Between abdominal and thoracic cavities	Lower circumference of thorax	Central tendon	Increases volume of thoracic cavity	Phrenic nerves

(continued)

Table 9.1 Muscle Characteristics and Actions (continued)

Muscle	Location	Origin	Insertion	Action	Innervation
Muscles of Breathing (cont.)					
External intercostals	Superficial, between ribs	Inferior border of rib	Superior border of inferior rib	Elevates ribs	Intercostal nerves
Internal intercostals	Deep, between ribs	Inner surface of rib	Superior border of inferior rib	Depresses ribs	Intercostal nerves
Muscles of the Abdominal Wall					
External oblique	Superficial, lateral abdomen	Lower 8 ribs	Iliac crest, linea alba, and pubis	Compresses abdomen	Intercostal nerves
Internal oblique	Middle layer, lateral abdomen	Iliac crest, fascia of back	Lower ribs, pubis, linea alba	Compresses abdomen	Intercostal nerves
Transverse abdominis	Inner layer, lateral abdomen	Lower ribs, iliac crest, fascia of back	Pubis and linea alba	Compresses abdomen	Intercostal nerves
Rectus abdominis	Medial abdomen	Pubis	Costal cartilage of ribs 5–7	Compresses abdomen and flexes trunk	Intercostal nerves
Muscles of the Pelvic Floor					
Levator ani	Pelvic floor	Pubis, ischium	Coccyx	Supports pelvic organs	Pudenal nerve
Coccygeus	Pelvic floor	Ischium	Coccyx, sacrum	Supports pelvic organs	Pudenal nerve
Muscles of the Pectoral Girdle					
Pectoralis minor	Deep, chest	Ribs 3–5	Coracoid process of scapula	Depresses scapula, rotates shoulder, elevates ribs	Pectoral nerve
Serratus anterior	Lateral thorax	Upper 8 ribs	Vertebral border of scapula	Rotates scapula, elevates ribs	Long thoracic nerve
Trapezius	Superficial, upper back	Occipital bone, ligamentum nuchae, vertebrae C7–T12	Spine of scapula, acromion process of clavicle	Elevates, adducts, or depresses scapula; elevates clavicle	Cranial nerve XI, cervical neryes 3 and 4
Levator scapulae	Posterior neck	Upper cervical vertebrae	Vertebral border of scapula	Elevates scapula	Cervical nerves
Rhomboideus major	Deep, upper back	Vertebrae T2–5	Vertebral border of scapula	Adducts and upwardly rotates scapula	Cervical nerves
Rhomboideus minor	Deep, upper back	C7 and T1 vertebrae	Superior angle of scapula	Adducts scapula	Cervical nerves
Muscles of the Shoulder Joint					
Pectoralis major	Superficial, chest	Clavicle, sternum, cartilage of ribs 2–6	Greater tubercle of humerus	Flexes, adducts, and medially rotates arm	Pectoral nerves
Latissimus dorsi	Superficial, lower back	Vertebrae T6–L5, lower ribs, iliac crest	Humerus	Extends, adducts, and medially rotates arm	Thoracodorsal nerve
Deltoid	Top of shoulder	Clavicle, acromion, and spine of scapula	Deltoid tuberosity of humerus	Abducts arm	Axillary nerve

Table 9.1   Muscle Characteristics and Actions (continued)

Muscle	Location	Origin	Insertion	Action	Innervation
Muscles of Shoulder Joint (cont.)					
Supraspinatus	Above spine of scapula	Supraspinous fossa	Greater tubercle of humerus	Abducts arm	Suprascapular nerves
Infraspinatus	Below spine of scapula	Infraspinous fossa	Greater tubercle of humerus	Laterally rotates arm	Suprascapular nerve
Teres major	Between scapula and humerus	Inferior angle of scapula	Lesser tubercle of humerus	Adducts, extends, and medially rotates arm	Lower subscapular nerves
Teres minor	Above teres major	Axillary border of scapula	Greater tubercle of humerus	Laterally rotates arm	Axillary nerve
Muscles of the Elbow Joint					
Biceps brachii	Anterior upper arm	Glenoid fossa and coracoid process	Radial tuberosity	Flexes and supinates forearm	Musculocutaneous nerve
Brachialis	Anterior upper arm	Lower anterior humerus	Coronoid process of ulna	Flexes pronated forearm	Musculocutaneous nerve
Brachioradialis	Lateral forearm	Upper lateral humerus	Styloid process of radius	Flexes forearm	Radial nerve
Triceps brachii	Posterior humerus	Scapula and humerus	Olecranon process of ulna	Extends lower arm	Radial nerve
Pronator teres	Anterior upper forearm	Medial epicondyle of humerus	Middle of radius	Pronates and flexes forearm	Median nerve
Supinator	Anterior upper forearm	Lateral epicondyle of humerus	Upper radius	Supinates forearm	Radial nerve
Muscles of the Knee Joint					
Sartorius	Anterior thigh	Anterior superior iliac spine	Medial head of tibia	Adducts thigh and flexes knee	Femoral nerve
Gracilis	Medial thigh	Pubic bone	Medial head of tibia	Adducts thigh and flexes knee	Obturator nerve
Quadriceps femoris group					
Rectus femoris	Superficial, anterior thigh	Anterior inferior iliac spine	Tibia via patellar tendon	Flexes thigh and extends lower leg	Femoral nerve
Vastus lateralis	Lateral thigh	Linea aspera of femur	Tibia via patellar tendon	Extends lower leg	Femoral nerve
Vastus intermedius	Deep, anterior thigh	Shaft of femur	Tibia via patellar tendon	Extends lower leg	Femoral nerve
Vastus medialis	Medial thigh	Linea aspera of femur	Tibia via patellar tendon	Extends lower leg	Femoral nerve
Hamstring group					
Biceps femoris	Posterior thigh	Ischial tuberosity and linea aspera	Lateral head of fibula	Extends thigh and flexes lower leg	Sciatic nerve
Semitendinosus	Posterior thigh	Ischial tuberosity	Medial shaft of tibia	Extends thigh and flexes lower leg	Sciatic nerve
Semimembranosus	Posterior thigh	Ischial tuberosity	Medial condyle of tibia	Extends thigh and flexes lower leg	Sciatic nerve

(continued)

Table 9.1   Muscle Characteristics and Actions (continued)

Muscle	Location	Origin	Insertion	Action	Innervation
Muscles of the Ankle and Foot					
Tibialis anterior	Anterolateral lower leg	Lateral condyle of tibia	Cuneiform and meta-tarsal 1	Flexes and inverts foot	Deep peroneal nerve
Gastrocnemius	Superficial, calf of leg	Posterior surface of con-dyles of femur	Calcaneus via Achilles tendon	Flexes lower leg and extends foot	Tibial nerve
Soleus	Deep, calf	Proximal tibia and head of fibula	Calcaneus via Achilles tendon	Extends (plantarflexes) foot	Tibial nerve
Peroneus longus	Lateral leg	Lateral condyle of tibia and head of fibula	Cuneiform and meta-tarsal 1	Plantarflexes and everts foot	Common peroneal nerve
Peroneus brevis	Lateral leg	Lower lateral shaft of fibula	Metatarsal 5	Plantarflexes and everts foot	Common peroneal nerve
Tibalis posterior	Posterior leg	Posterior surface of tibia and fibula	Tarsals	Extends (plantarflexes) and inverts foot	Tibial nerve
Muscles of the Wrist and Hand					
Flexor carpi radialis	Superficial anterior forearm	Medial epicondyle of humerus	Metacarpals 2 and 3	Flexes and abducts wrist	Median nerve
Flexor carpi ulnaris	Superficial anterior forearm	Medial epicondyle of humerus and distal ulna	Metacarpal 5 and carpals	Flexes and adducts wrist	Ulnar nerve
Extensor carpi radialis longus	Posterior forearm	Lateral epicondyle of humerus	Metacarpal 2	Extends and abducts wrist	Radial nerve
Extensor carpi ulnaris	Posterior forearm	Lateral epicondyle of humerus and ulna	Metacarpal 5	Extends and adducts wrist	Radial nerve
Flexor digitorum pro-fundus	Deep, anterior forearm	Proximal, anteromedial ulna	Base of distal phalanges	Flexes wrist and phalanges	Median and ulnar nerves
Extensor digitorum	Posterior forearm	Lateral epicondyle of humerus	Middle and distal phalanges	Extends wrist and phalanges	Deep radial nerve
Muscles of the Thigh					
Iliopsoas (Iliacus and psoas major)	Iliac fossa and poste-rior pelvic cavity	Iliac fossa and verte-brae T12 to L5	Lesser trochanter of femur	Flexes thigh (or trunk if femur is fixed)	Femoral nerve and lum-bar nerves 2–4
Gluteus maximus	Buttocks	Ilium, sacrum, and coccyx	Gluteal tuberosity of femur	Extends and laterally ro-tates thigh	Inferior gluteal nerve
Gluteus medius	Buttocks	Lateral surface of ilium	Greater trochanter of femur	Abducts and rotates thigh	Superior gluteal nerve
Gluteus minimus	Buttocks	Lateral surface of ilium	Greater trochanter of femur	Abducts and rotates thigh	Superior gluteal nerve
Tensor fasciae latae	Lateral hip	Anterior superior iliac spine	Fascia lata and tibia	Abducts thigh	Superior gluteal nerve
Adductor brevis	Medial thigh	Pubic bone	Upper linea aspera	Adducts thigh	Obturator nerve
Adductor longus	Medial thigh	Pubic bone	Middle linea aspera	Adducts thigh	Obturator nerve
Adductor magnus	Medial thigh	Pubic bone	Lower linea aspera	Adducts thigh	Obturator nerve
Gracilis	Medial thigh	Pubic bone	Medial head of tibia	Adducts thigh and flexes knee	Obturator nerve

CLINICAL TERMS

fibromyositis (fi″bro-mi-o-si′tis)   inflammation of muscle and its accompanying fibrous tissue

fibrosis (fi-bro′sis)   formation of fibrous tissue, often to replace degenerating muscle tissue

fibrositis (fi-bro-si′tis)   inflammation and hyperplasia of fibrous sheaths surrounding skeletal muscle, usually accompanied by stiffness and pain

shin splints   strain of the flexor digitorum longus muscle, which causes pain along the tibia; often seen in athletes

torticollis (tor-tik-ol′is)   a twisting of the neck caused by contraction of some cervical muscles; wryneck

---

Essay: Exercise and Fitness

Most of us accept the idea that exercise is essential for fitness. But what is fitness? Is it the same for everyone? How does lack of exercise reduce fitness, how does performing exercise contribute to it? Answers to these questions are important to individuals desiring to maintain their own fitness, as well as to health and athletic professionals.

What Is Fitness?

One definition of fitness is the ability to meet the demands of the environment. However, people face different environments today than their ancestors did even 200 years ago. If we live in or near a large city and do work that requires us to sit at a desk for long periods of time, then our environment demands far less of us physically than if we were professional athletes or manual laborers. People with desk jobs or others who have little physical activity are termed sedentary people—literally, sitters. However, some physiologists believe the human body functions better when muscles and joints are frequently used; sedentary individuals may not get enough exercise to keep their bodies functioning normally. Fitness, then, also means maintaining the body's ability to function normally.

Physiological Effects of Exercise

The most immediate effects of exercise involve the heart, blood vessels in the muscles, and the respiratory system. Exercise increases the heart rate, the stroke volume (volume of blood pumped each time the heart contracts), and the cardiac output (liters of blood pumped per minute). It also causes blood vessels in the working muscles to dilate, thereby increasing the blood supply to those muscles. The respiratory rate increases, thus supplying more oxygen to the blood and offsetting the increased oxygen consumption of the muscle cells.

Individuals who have been exercising regularly display some long-term changes in their hearts. Such trained individuals have a larger stroke volume and a slower heart rate at rest than untrained individuals. They also tend to have larger hearts and exhibit smaller increases in heart rate for a given amount of work than untrained persons. In other words, training allows the heart to meet the demands of exertion without as great an increase in the heart rate as in an untrained individual.

Exercise has other important effects on the body. One of these effects is psychological: People who exercise regularly report that they feel better. Regular exercise may also increase the likelihood of remaining active at a more advanced age than would be possible without regular exercise. Some evidence exists to show that regular exercise decreases the severity of myocardial infarctions (heart attacks). Finally, exercise may affect the appetite-regulating mechanism so that one has less tendency to overeat when exercising regularly than when leading a sedentary life.

Strength, Endurance, and Flexibility

An exercise program can be designed to increase the strength of muscles, cardiorespiratory and muscle endurance, or flexibility of the joints. Strength of muscles increases most rapidly when maximum tension is produced in the muscle, such as would be accomplished with weight-lifting or through isometric exercises.

Cardiorespiratory endurance is increased by endurance types of exercise, which elevate the heart rate to a specific level, the **training pulse**. The appropriate training pulse for a given individual is determined by the physical condition of the individual and especially by the amount of increase in heart rate caused by a given degree of exertion. This determination should be made by a physician, using results of a physical examination, an analysis of blood lipids, and a stress test. Muscle endurance—the duration of effective performance—increases when the rate at which energy can be supplied to the muscle fibers increases. Such endurance is largely dependent on the cardiorespiratory endurance.

Flexibility of joints may be increased by stretching exercises. Such exercises should gradually increase the range of motion of a joint, the maximum angle through which a body part can be moved.

What Kind of Exercise and How Much?

What kind of exercise and how much an individual needs to maintain fitness depends to a large degree on how fit that person is already and on the kind of lifestyle the person leads or plans to lead. A sudden effort to improve fitness by strenuous exercise after years of sedentary life may lead to serious problems. The body of a sedentary person has little reserve cardiac capacity to meet new demands placed on it if the person begins a strenuous exercise program too suddenly.

When a person goes from rest to maximal exercise, the increase in oxygen used in cellular metabolism increases as much as ten times in untrained individuals and as much as twenty-five times in trained individuals. The increased demand of the cells for oxygen is met by an increase in cardiac function as the heart rate and stroke volume both increase. Because heart rate is directly proportional to the amount of oxygen used, increase in an individual's heart rate during exercise can be used to measure the degree of exertion that person is experiencing. The resting heart rate for a healthy young adult is about 70 beats per minute and for a trained athlete somewhat less. The maximum heart rate during exercise for a healthy young adult is about 190 beats per minute; it decreases by about 1 beat per minute per year to a maximum of 160 beats per minute at age sixty-five.

Fitness programs usually make use of maximum heart rates to determine the kind and duration of exercise for participants. The training pulse is determined by the age of the exerciser and how much out of condition the person is; it is usually 65 to 85 percent of the maximum heart rate. At this pulse rate a safe overload is placed on the heart, one that causes the heart to increase in strength. At heart rates above the training pulse muscle metabolism becomes partly anaerobic, the heart is not further strengthened, and no additional training effect occurs.

Three factors to consider in designing an exercise program are intensity, frequency, and duration. The intensity is determined by the training pulse. Several studies have shown that the optimal frequency of training sessions is at least three times per week, on alternate days. The duration of the sessions varies from ten to forty minutes, depending on the program. Each session consists of three phases: a warm-up phase, a workout phase at the training pulse, and a cool-down phase. Many such programs have been published; each has some advantages and some disadvantages. An example of one program is summarized here. The summary illustrates the kinds of activities that might be included in a fitness program. Before you engage in a fitness program, study the reference (Morehouse and Gross, 1975) or another similar one.

Our bodies have not changed as much as our lifestyles in modern, technologically advanced societies. Thousands of years in the future human beings may have different physical structures and physiology than we have now—adapted in part to a less strenuous way of life. For the present, though, most of us are better off in terms of health and well-being if we pursue some regular program for maintaining fitness.

An Example of a Fitness Program. (Summarized from Morehouse and Gross (1975) with the permission of Dr. Morehouse)

Minimum fitness *prevents physical deterioration and requires meeting the following five requirements daily:*

---

1. Turning and twisting your body joints to near-maximum range of motion.

2. Standing for two hours a day.

3. Lifting something heavy for 5 seconds (half the maximum weight you can lift).

4. Getting your heart rate up to 120 beats/minute for 3 minutes.

5. Burning up 300 calories/day in physical activity. (see Table 23.1 for calories used in selected activities.)

General fitness *increases fitness above the minimum and creates a reserve to meet changing demands of the environment.*

The pulse test *determines whether you are fit enough to engage in moderate exercise. Symptoms such as profuse sweating, cramps, achy legs, a tremor or twitching in the legs, shortness of breath, difficult breathing, or a painful pounding of the heart indicate that you may not be able to tolerate an exercise program. Should you experience any of these symptoms after a mild exercise, stop your test and seek medical advice.*

The Test	Pulse Rates That Indicate Lack of Fitness to Continue
1. Take your resting pulse.	100 or more
2. Stand quietly for 1 minute and take pulse.	110 or 10 beats/minute higher than resting pulse
3. Step up and down a stairstep at 30 steps/minute for 1 minute. Immediately sit down and take pulse.	120 or more
4. Repeat step 3.	120 or more
5. Repeat step 3 again.	120 or more
6. Rest 1 minute and take pulse.	110 or more

The fitness program *is divided into three stages of eight weeks each and requires three 10-minute sessions on alternate days each week. The first stage develops muscle tissue, the second endurance, and the third strength. All develop flexibility. To begin the program, determine your training pulse (TP) from the following table:*

Age	Stage One TP	Stage Two TP	Stage Three TP	Maintenance TP
Under 30	120	140	150	150–160
30–44	110	130	140	140–150
45–60	100	120	130	130–140
Over 60	100	110	120	120–130

Stage One

Limbering (1 minute) (to be done leisurely)
1. Reach as high as you can above your head with one arm. *Stretch!* Repeat with the other arm.

2. Extend arms and *twist* trunk in each direction.

3. Lean over, bending knees slightly, and grasp arms around knees; gently pull shoulders toward knees.

4. Turn head to side and use hands to push head a little farther to each side.

Muscle Buildup (4 minutes)
1. Put hands against wall at height of shoulders. Place chest against wall and push back to starting position. Do fifteen to twenty times until exertion feels heavy. To increase exertion, stand farther from wall, push against a counter, or do push-ups from the floor.

2. Sit on the floor, bend knees, and hook feet under a piece of furniture. Place hands on abdomen and lean back until abdominal muscles begin to quiver after 20 seconds. Increase distance of lean-back to increase exertion.

3. Check pulse after each set of these two exercises to be sure training pulse has not been exceeded.

4. Repeat set of exercises for 4 minutes.

Endurance (5 minutes)
1. Engage in some activity to get pulse rate up to training pulse by the end of the second minute and keep it there until the end of 5 minutes. Running in place, jogging, or any exercise you enjoy will do.

2. Check pulse rate at 2 minutes and at 5 minutes. Keep walking around while you take your pulse.

3. Walk around slowly at the end of your workout.

Stage Two

Limbering (1 minute, optional) Repeat activities in Stage One.
Muscle Buildup (4 minutes)
1. Do twice as many push-aways as you did in Stage One and do them faster. Reduce the exertion so you can do them fast.

2. Do sit-back in position that causes abdominal muscles to quiver in 30 seconds.

3. Repeat above set of exercises, take pulse, and repeat twice again.

Endurance (6 minutes)
1. Do 30 seconds of activity at same rate you used in Stage One. In next 30 seconds speed up to new training pulse.

2. During next 30 seconds walk at a rate that keeps pulse no lower than old training rate.

3. For remainder of 6 minutes alternate between activities to maintain new training pulse for 30 seconds and old training pulse for 30 seconds.

4. Take pulse during lower activity periods.

5. Walk around slowly at the end of your workout.

Stage Three

Limbering (1 minute, optional) Repeat activities in Stage One.
Muscle Strength (2 minutes)
1. Make push-aways so difficult that you can do no more than five. Do push-ups on floor and elevate feet on a stairstep or a chair.

2. Make sit-back so difficult that you can hold position for only 5 seconds before your abdominal muscles begin to tremble. Place hands on chest or above head and lean very far back to do this.

3. Check pulse rate between each set and do three sets of exercises.

Endurance Sprint (8 minutes)
1. Do Stage Two activity for 15 seconds at Stage Two training pulse. In the next 15 seconds speed up until pulse reaches Stage Three training pulse.

2. Alternate periods of slow and fast activity in 15 second intervals as above for 8 minutes. Try to keep muscles relaxed as you do this activity. The agonist muscles can contract best when the antagonist muscles are relaxed.

Maintenance

To maintain the fitness gained by the program, meet the five requirements for minimum fitness daily. In each of the three weekly workouts do the activities of one stage (a different stage each day), but do them at your maintenance pulse rate.

CHAPTER SUMMARY

(Chapter summary points and review questions are numbered to correspond to the numbered objectives in the text of each chapter.)

Actions of Skeletal Muscles

1. Relate the properties of levers to muscle action.
   a. The bones and joints form a complex set of levers that are moved by the contraction of muscles attached to the bones.
   b. These various kinds of levers allow the body or its parts to move.
2. Define the terms that describe muscle actions.
   a. Each muscle has its origin at the proximal or least movable attachment, and its insertion at the distal or most movable attachment.
   b. Muscle actions describe the kind of movement a muscle causes. (These terms were defined in Chapter 7 and should be reviewed.)
   c. The main muscle in a movement is the prime mover, or agonist; muscles that work with the agonist are synergists.
   d. Muscles that perform opposite movements to the agonist are antagonists.

Muscles of the Axial Skeleton

3. Locate and describe the action of the major muscles of (a) the head and neck, (b) the trunk, (c) the abdominal wall, and (d) the pelvic floor.
   a. Muscles of the head and neck include:
      (1) muscles of facial expression
      (2) muscles of mastication
      (3) muscles that move the tongue and assist in swallowing
      (4) muscles that move the head
   b. Muscles of the trunk include:
      (1) the back muscles that move the back and maintain posture
      (2) the muscles of breathing
   c. The abdominal muscles compress the abdomen and flex the spine.
   d. The muscles of the pelvic floor support the pelvic organs.
   e. The properties of these muscles are listed in Table 9.1.

Muscles of the Appendicular Skeleton

4. Locate and describe the action of the major muscles of (a) the pectoral girdle and shoulder joint, (b) the elbow, (c) the wrist and hand, (d) the pelvic girdle and hip joint, (e) the knee, and (f) the ankle and foot.
   a. Muscles of the pectoral girdle move the girdle and hold it to the axial skeleton.
   b. Muscles of the shoulder joint cause the various movements that are possible at that joint—abduction, adduction, flexion, extension, and circumduction.
   c. Muscles of the elbow flex and extend that joint and rotate the forearm.
   d. Muscles of the wrist and hand are quite numerous; they cause various movements of the wrist joint and move the joints of the fingers and the apposable thumb.
   e. Muscles of the pelvic girdle hold the girdle firmly to the axial skeleton.
   f. Muscles of the hip joint cause abduction, adduction, flexion, extension, and circumduction.
   g. Muscles of the knee joint flex and extend the leg.
   h. Muscles of the ankle and foot flex and extend the foot and perform some rotational movements; they also cause limited movement of the toes.
   i. The properties of these muscles are described in Table 9.1.

REVIEW

Important Terms

action

agonist

antagonist

fulcrum

hernia

innervation

insertion

lever

origin

point of effort

resistance (load)

synergist

Review specific actions (flexion, extension, and so on) from the Important Terms list in Chapter 7.

Questions

1. How can the lever principle be used to explain muscle action?
2. Define the terms pertaining to muscle action.

3. a. List the main muscles of facial expression and give their location and action.

b. Use the names of muscles to explain how mastication occurs.

c. Which muscles assist in moving the tongue and pushing food to the back of the mouth for swallowing?

d. What neck muscles are involved in the following actions: (1) flexion, (2) extension, and (3) rotation?

e. Which muscles are involved in flexing, extending, and rotating the trunk?

f. Which muscles are involved in breathing?

g. How do the abdominal muscles function to flex the spine and compress the abdomen?

h. What is the function of the muscles of the pelvic floor?

4. a. Which muscles hold the pectoral girdle to the axial skeleton?

b. Which muscles hold the pelvic girdle to the axial skeleton?

c. Which muscles and muscle actions are involved in: (1) throwing a ball? (2) kicking a ball? (3) walking up a stairway? (4) opening a door? (5) writing? (6) standing on tiptoes? (7) getting out of bed? (8) jogging? (9) swimming?

Problems

1. Select a specific injury that is frequently sustained by people who engage in your favorite sport. Use your knowledge of the skeletomuscular system and the sport to suggest ways of minimizing the chance of such an injury occurring.

2. Use what you have learned about muscle actions and exercise to devise an exercise program that you feel would improve your physical condition and that you would get some satisfaction out of following.

REFERENCES AND READINGS

Astrand, P. O., and Rodahl, K. 1977. *Textbook of work physiology: Physiological basis of exercise* (2nd ed.). New York: McGraw-Hill.

Evans, F. G. 1957. *Atlas of human anatomy*. Totowa, N.J.: Rowman and Littlefield.

Gallistel, C. R. 1980. From muscles to motivation. *American Scientist* 68:398 (July–August).

Ganong, W. F. 1981. *Review of medical physiology* (10th ed.). Los Altos, Calif.: Lange Medical Publications

Gray, H. 1973. *Anatomy of the human body* (29th American ed.). C. M. Goss, ed. Philadelphia: Lea and Febiger.

Hinson, M. M. 1981. *Kinesiology* (2nd ed.). Dubuque, Iowa: Wm. C. Brown.

Holloszy, J. O. 1976. Adaptations of muscular tissue to training. *Progress in Cardiovascular Diseases* 18(6):445.

Merriman, J. E. 1978. Exercise prescription for apparently healthy individuals and for cardiac patients. In N. K. Wenger, ed., Exercise and the heart. *Cardiovascular Clinician* 9(3):81.

Morehouse, L. E., and Gross, L. 1975. *Total fitness in 30 minutes a week*. New York: Simon and Schuster.

Schlossberg, L. 1977. *The Johns Hopkins atlas of human functional anatomy*. G. D. Zuidema, ed. Baltimore, Md.: Johns Hopkins Press.

Selkirk, E. E. 1976. *Physiology* (4th ed.). Boston: Little, Brown.

UNIT THREE

CONTROL AND INTEGRATION

Having considered the levels of complexity of the human body in Unit I and its mechanisms for protection, support, and movement in Unit II, we will consider in Unit III how the basic life processes are controlled and integrated so that the body functions as a total organism. Two systems—the nervous system and the endocrine system—work together to control and integrate body function. We will now look at the roles of each of these systems, paying particular attention to the complex interactions of these systems with each other and with other systems of the body.

Chapter 10 provides an overview of the nervous system, explains the basic properties of neural function, and de-scribes the structure and functions of the spinal cord and spinal nerves. Chapter 11 focuses on the anatomy of the brain and its basic functions, Chapter 12 describes the more complex functions of the brain, and Chapter 13 concentrates specifically on the autonomic nervous system. Chapter 14 explains how sensory receptors provide input for the nervous system. Chapter 15, the final chapter of the unit, discusses the role of the endocrine glands in the control and integration of the body and the ways neural and endocrine functions interact. By studying the chapters of this Unit, we will see why it truly can be said of the human body that the whole is greater than the sum of its parts.

10

THE NERVOUS SYSTEM: PROPERTIES OF NERVE TISSUE AND SPINAL CORD

ORGANIZATION AND GENERAL FUNCTION

Objective 1. Describe the general organization of the nervous system.

Objective 2. Explain briefly how the nervous system functions to maintain homeostasis.

As you read this sentence, millions of neural signals are traveling through your body. Your intact nervous system allows you to read this sentence, process the symbols (words) to find meaning in it, and at the same time maintain your posture and carry out various internal body processes.

Though the nervous system functions as an integrated whole, we can divide it into parts for convenience in studying it. Furthermore, we can consider its parts from either a structural or a functional point of view.

Structurally, the two major parts of the nervous system are the **central nervous system** (CNS), which consists of the brain and spinal cord, and the **peripheral nervous system** (PNS), which consists of the **somatic nervous system** (serving the framework of the body) and the **autonomic nervous system** (serving the viscera). The somatic nervous system is further divided into the **cranial nerves** and the **spinal nerves**; the autonomic nervous system is divided into the **sympathetic division** and the **parasympathetic division** (Figure 10.1). In each part of the nervous system cells called neurons and their processes, called nerve fibers, are responsible for generating and carrying signals.

Functionally, the nervous system is a complex network of interconnected nerve fibers, something like a computer. Both the nervous system and a computer have input, processing, and output functions, but the human nervous system is far more intricate than the most advanced computer. If we use the computer analogy, the brain and spinal cord (CNS) constitute the processing unit. **Sensory nerve fibers** (part of the somatic nervous system) provide input by carrying signals from sense organs (**receptors**) to the brain and spinal cord. **Motor nerve fibers** provide output by carrying signals from the brain or spinal cord to muscles and other organs (**effectors**).

With this general overview of the structural and functional organization of the nervous system, we can now consider some of the parts of the peripheral nervous system in more detail.

The somatic nervous system consists of sensory nerve fibers and motor nerve fibers. Sensory nerve fibers carry signals *from* receptors in all parts of the body *to* the CNS. They convey information about heat, cold, pressure, pain, and touch from the skin; about body position from joints and muscles; and about sensations from the viscera or internal organs. Sensory fibers are also called **afferent** fibers because they carry signals *from* the sensory receptors *to* the CNS (*a*fferent = bring to). In contrast, motor nerve fibers carry signals *from* the CNS *to* the skeletal muscles, causing these muscles to contract, as described in Chapter 8. Motor fibers are also called **efferent fibers** because they carry signals *away from* the CNS (*e*fferent = carry outward). For example, when a painful stimulus is received, sensory fibers carry signals to the spinal cord. From the spinal cord motor fibers carry signals to muscles, causing them to contract and move the painful part away from the stimulus. This sort of interaction occurs when, for instance, you touch something hot.

The autonomic nervous system consists of motor nerves that serve the visceral or internal organs, stimulating smooth and cardiac muscles to contract and glands to secrete. Literally, autonomic means self-governing; thus, the autonomic nervous system usually functions without our being conscious of its activities. The two divisions of this system, the sympathetic and the parasympathetic, work together to regulate blood pressure, body temperature, digestion, urinary output, heart rate and force of heart muscle contraction, and many other physiological processes. In general, the sympathetic division helps the body to respond to stress—the "fight-or-flight" response—and the parasympathetic division returns the body to a nonstress level of function. These divisions continually respond to small

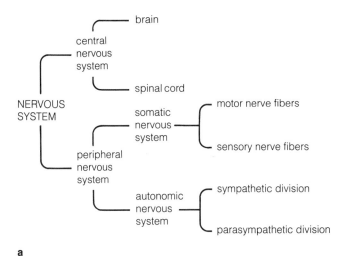

a

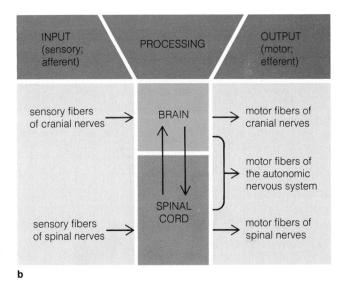

b

Figure 10.1 Organization of the nervous system: (**a**) structural organization, (**b**) functional organization.

changes and help to maintain nearly constant internal conditions (homeostasis).

Some textbooks classify specialized sensory nerves from the senses of the head (eyes, ears, and organs of taste and smell) as a separate system, but in this text we will treat them as particularly important parts of the somatic system. We will also consider the autonomic nervous system as a purely motor system, though some texts include the sensory fibers from internal organs as a part of the autonomic system. Sensory fibers that serve internal organs are anatomically and physiologically like those that serve the skin and muscles, so we will include them with the somatic sensory fibers. Our classification system in this text should help us to think about nervous system function in an orderly way; however, our main objective is to understand both structure and function, not simply to classify them.

In the broadest sense the functions of the nervous system are integration and coordination. It performs these functions by detecting changes in the external and internal environment, by processing the sensed information, and by sending out motor signals to effectors. The nervous system also interacts with the endocrine system, as will be explained in later chapters. Together, these systems maintain homeostasis—the endocrine system by initiating relatively slow changes and the nervous system by initiating relatively rapid ones. As we begin our detailed study of how the nervous system works, keep in mind this overall homeostatic function.

Failure of the neural tube to close throughout its length during development is a relatively common birth defect, appearing in 1 in 2000 births in the United States. If the defect involves the brain area of the neural tube, the fetus will have no brain or a poorly developed one. If the defect involves the spinal cord, the condition is called spina bifida. When the spinal cord and its meninges protrude from the body and form a kind of lump on the back, the condition is called myelomeningocele (Figure 10.3). Individuals affected by spina bifida or myelomeningocele have varying degrees of paralysis, depending on which of the spinal nerves are affected and how severely their distribution is disturbed.

DEVELOPMENT

Objective 3. Describe the general development of the nervous system.

As described in Chapter 4, the outer surface of the early embryo consists of the embryonic tissue ectoderm. Ectodermal cells of the neural place in the midline of the posterior surface form a neural groove and migrate below the surface to form a neural fold and finally a hollow **neural tube**. Some cells extend laterally to form the **neural crests** (Figure 10.2a). By the end of the first month of development, the neural tube extends from the head to the tail of the embryo and is completely closed. Its anterior end has begun to differentiate into regions of the brain, such as the cerebrum, cerebellum, and medulla. The long cavity enclosed by the neural tube becomes the central canal of the spinal cord and the ventricles of the brain. Different areas of the neural tube give rise to the brain and spinal cord, the motor portions of the cranial and spinal nerves, and the retina and optic nerves of each eye, as well as a portion of the pituitary gland (Figure 10.2b). The cells of the neural crest give rise to the sensory nerve fibers, the autonomic nervous system, and the medulla of the adrenal gland. Each of these structures will be discussed in more detail later. For now, in considering relationships between the nervous and endocrine systems, keep in mind that the adrenal medulla and a part of the pituitary gland are derived from the same embryonic tissue as the nervous system.

Early in development the neural ectoderm differentiates into two types of cells: Some are destined to form **neurons**, the impulse-conducting cells, and others are des-

tined to form most of the various **neuroglia**, which support, protect, and nourish the neurons. In contrast to most other body systems, very little mesodermal connective tissue is associated with the nervous system; rather, the ectodermal neuroglial cells perform most of the functions normally carried out by connective tissue. The **meninges**, the membranes that cover the external surfaces of the brain and spinal cord, are the primary examples of mesodermal connective tissue associated with the central nervous system. The sheaths around bundles of peripheral nerve fibers are also formed from connective tissue.

CELLS AND TISSUES

Objective 4. Distinguish between neurons and neuroglia, including Schwann cells; describe the structure, function, and location of neurons and of each type of neuroglia.

Objective 5. Describe the structure of nerves, tracts, ganglia, and nuclei.

Neurons

Neurons (nerve cells) carry neural signals called impulses or action potentials to other neurons and also to other cells of the body. They give rise to the nerve fibers that make up nerves, tracts of the spinal cord and brain, and information-processing parts of the brain. Several different types of neurons are shown in Figure 10.4; three types of them are

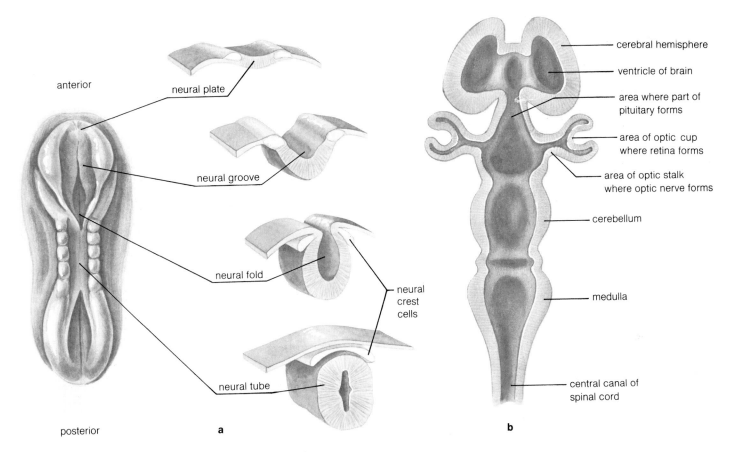

anterior

neural plate

neural groove

neural fold

neural crest cells

neural tube

posterior

a

cerebral hemisphere

ventricle of brain

area where part of pituitary forms

area of optic cup where retina forms

area of optic stalk where optic nerve forms

cerebellum

medulla

central canal of spinal cord

b

Figure 10.2 Development of the nervous system: diagrams of (**a**) transverse sections through an embryo during the first month of development, (**b**) coronal (frontal) sections at five weeks, showing how the retina and optic nerve begin to develop from the optic cup and optic stalk, respectively.

shown in more detail in Figure 10.5. Though neurons display many variations, they have many structures in common. Most have one axon and several dendrites extending from the **cell body**. Impulses always travel along a neuron from dendrite to axon end, as will be explained later.

The **cell body**, or **soma**, contains most of the cytoplasm and many of the organelles usually found in cells—mitochondria, Golgi apparatus, nucleus, and nucleolus. The cell body also contains **Nissl granules**, a complex of endoplasmic reticulum and ribosomes that serves as the site of protein synthesis for the neuron. **Neurofibrils** are found in the cell body near the **axon hillock**, where the axon joins the cell body.

The **axon** of a neuron is a long, thin process extending from the hillock. In most neurons it extends in only one direction from the cell body. However, in many sensory neurons the axon consists of two parts, the **peripheral process**,

which extends from the dendrites to the cell body, and the **central process**, which extends from the cell body to the **terminal branches** (Figure 10.5b). Sometimes the peripheral process is considered to be a dendrite because it carries the signal toward the cell body. Axons also may have **collateral branches**, making it possible for an impulse traveling along the axon to be distributed to several sets of terminal branches. Most axons are myelinated; that is, they are surrounded by an insulating substance called **myelin** in somewhat the same way as the coating on an electrical cord insulates the metal wires. An interneuron (Figure 10.5c) has many of these parts. Such neurons are found in the spinal cord.

Dendrites are shorter processes than axons in most neurons. They connect directly with the cell body, or with the peripheral process of the axons in the case of sensory neurons. Unlike axons, dendrites are not myelinated.

Schwann Cells

Schwann cells, sometimes considered a kind of neuroglial cell, are found wrapped around the axons of myelinated neurons of the peripheral nervous system (Figure 10.6). During embryonic development Schwann cells become associated with an axon, growing and wrapping around the axon. As this wrapping process occurs, several layers of Schwann cell membranes are placed around the axon, and the cytoplasm of the Schwann cell is squeezed out toward the outermost layer of this spiral. Thus, the myelin sheath consists of many layers of Schwann cell membrane. Peripheral to the myelin is the Schwann cell body, with its nucleus and various organelles. Many Schwann cells are required to produce a myelin sheath on a single axon. As shown in Figure 10.5, the myelin sheath has numerous small constrictions called **nodes of Ranvier**. These nodes represent minute spaces between adjacent Schwann cells. As will be explained later, impulses jump from one node to the next as they are conducted along a myelinated neuron. Schwann cells are also associated with unmyelinated neurons, but in that case the axons are only partially surrounded by Schwann cell membranes.

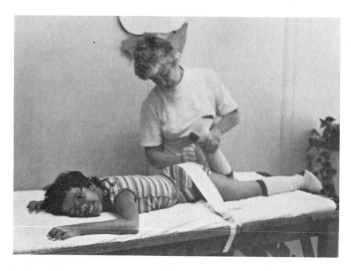

Figure 10.3 The child shown here has a myelomeningocele. The therapist is stretching a tight rectus femoris muscle. Such passive stretching of muscles helps to prevent contractures (shortening or distortion of muscles). (Photograph by author. Used with permission of the D.C. Public Schools, Department of Special Education, Sharpe Health School Administration, and the Department of Human Services of the District of Columbia.)

Neuroglia

In addition to the neurons and the nonconducting Schwann cells of the peripheral nervous system, four types of neuroglia are found primarily in the central nervous system: ependymal cells, astrocytes, oligodendrocytes, and microglia (Figure 10.7). The word neuroglia is derived from the word root *glia*, meaning glue. At the time these cells were named, it was thought that they were primarily concerned with holding, or "gluing," together the cells of the central nervous system. Since then other functions of these cells have been discovered.

Ependymal cells form a sheet that lines the ventricles of the brain and the central canal of the spinal cord. **Astrocytes**, named for their star shape, create a supporting network for neurons and blood vessels; they also may help to transport nutrients from blood to neurons. **Oligodendrocytes**—literally, sparsely branched cells—have only a few short dendrites and a short axon. These cells pro-central nervous system. Finally, **microglia**, the only glial cells of mesodermal origin (the others being derived from ectoderm), are thought to protect nerve cells against infection. These small phagocytic cells migrate to the site of an injury in the central nervous system and destroy microorganisms and cellular debris.

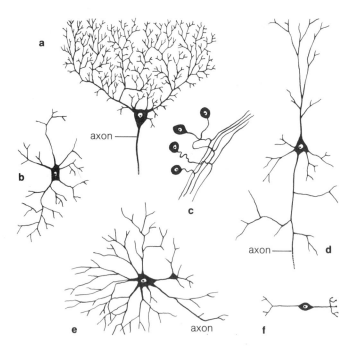

Figure 10.4 Some nerve cells: (**a**) Purkinje cell from cerebellum, (**b**) interneuron from spinal cord, (**c**) sensory cells from spinal ganglion, (**d**) pyramidal motor cell from cerebral cortex, (**e**) motor cell from spinal cord, (**f**) bipolar cell from retina of eye.

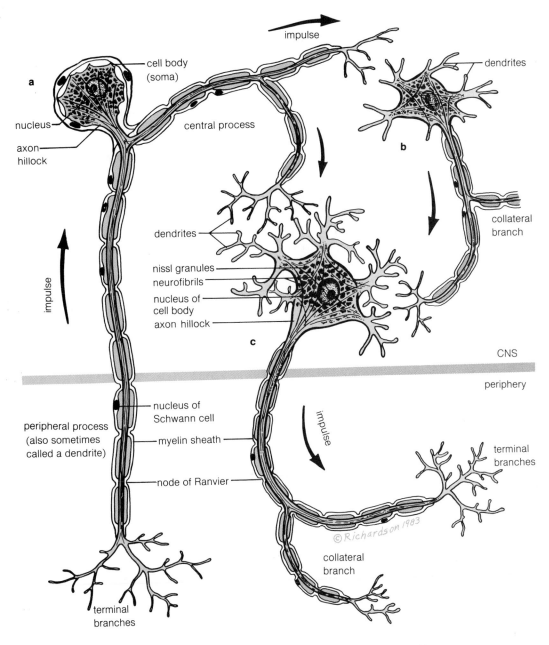

Labels in the figure:

cell body (soma)

a

nucleus

axon hillock

impulse

central process

dendrites

b

collateral branch

dendrites

nissl granules

neurofibrils

nucleus of cell body

axon hillock

c

CNS

periphery

nucleus of Schwann cell

peripheral process (also sometimes called a dendrite)

myelin sheath

impulse

node of Ranvier

terminal branches

©Richardson 1983

collateral branch

terminal branches

collateral branch

impulse

impulse

Figure 10.5 Detailed structure of typical neurons: (**a**) sensory neuron, (**b**) interneuron, (**c**) motor neuron.

Nerves and Tracts

Bundles of nerve fibers in the peripheral nervous system are called **nerves**; those in the central nervous system are called **tracts**. Nerves contain mostly myelinated and a few unmyelinated axons, surrounded by several connective tissue sheaths. Most nerves, except for some cranial nerves (nerves that branch directly from brain), contain both sensory and motor fibers. A connective tissue sheath, the **endoneurium**, surrounds each fiber. Another connective tissue sheath, the **perineurium**, binds groups of fibers together into **fascicles**. Yet another connective tissue sheath, the **epineurium**, covers the whole nerve, including its sev-

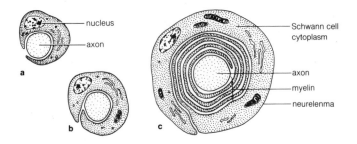

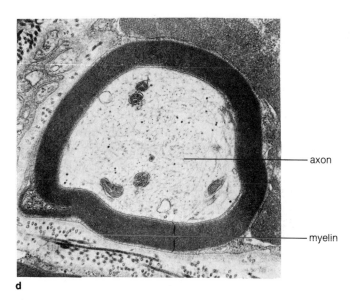

Figure 10.6 (a–c) a myelinated axon in cross section showing the myelin wrapping created by the Schwann cell as it develops, (d) photomicrograph of cross section of myelinated axon. (Photomicrograph from *Journal of Cell Biology* 52:719 (1972), courtesy of T. L. Lentz and The Rockefeller University Press.)

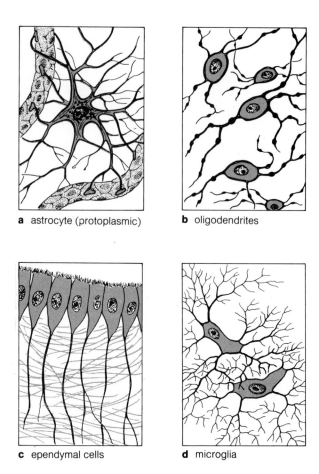

a astrocyte (protoplasmic)   b oligodendrites

c ependymal cells   d microglia

Figure 10.7 Neuroglia: (a) astrocytes, (b) astrocytes, (c) oliogodendrocytes, (d) ependymal cells and (d) microglia.

eral fascicles. Blood and lymph vessels are often located within the connective tissue between fascicles of large nerves and may form a sizable portion of the nerve (Figure 10.8).

Nerve fibers in tracts of the CNS are mostly myelinated; they acquire their myelin from the activities of oligodendrocytes rather than from Schwann cells. The myelin that surrounds the fibers of tracts gives the tracts a whitish color; thus they are recognized as **white matter** of the central nervous system. Cell bodies and dendrites lack myelin, and these areas are recognized as **gray matter**.

Ganglia and Nuclei

The cell bodies of the fibers of both nerves and tracts are usually aggregated in large groups to the side of the main pathway of the fibers. In the peripheral nervous system these aggregations are called **ganglia** (see Figure 10.28). Within the central nervous system they are called **nuclei** (see Figure 11.9, Chapter 11), but they are not to be confused with cellular nuclei. Each nucleus in the brain consists of many cell bodies, each having its own cellular nucleus. Terms pertaining to the nervous system are summarized in Table 10.1.

NERVE DEGENERATION AND REGENERATION

Objective 6. Describe the process by which injured neurons degenerate and the process by which they may regenerate.

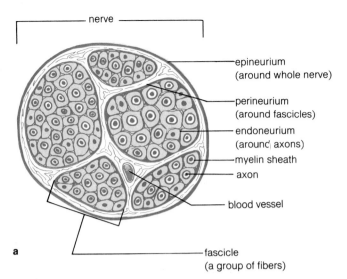

nerve

epineurium
(around whole nerve)

perineurium
(around fascicles)

endoneurium
(around axons)

myelin sheath

axon

blood vessel

a

fascicle
(a group of fibers)

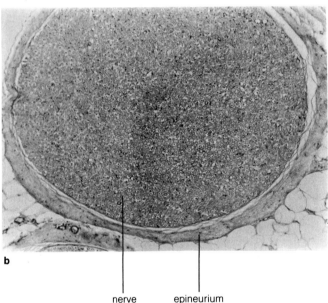

b

nerve   epineurium

Figure 10.8 (**a**) a diagram of a cross section of a nerve, (**b**) a photomicrograph of a nerve, × 73. (Photograph by author.)

Table 10.1	Selected Terms Pertaining to the Nervous System	
	PNS	CNS
Axons (white matter)	Aggregated into nerves	Aggregated into tracts
Cell bodies and dendrites (gray matter)	Collected into ganglia	Collected into nuclei
Myelin-producing cells	Schwann cells	Oligodendrocytes

injury. The portion of each axon and its sheath distal to the injury undergoes **Wallerian degeneration**; the axon first swells and then degenerates (disintegrates), then the myelin surrounding the axon also degenerates. Phagocytic cells destroy fragments of the degenerating tissue. At the time of injury the cell body itself swells, and the Nissl granules break into small fragments. These fragments synthesize proteins to repair the damaged axon. The living portion of the axon grows distally through a canal of endoneurium and remaining Schwann cells at 1 to 4 millimeters per day, as shown in Figure 10.9. Thus, injury to peripheral, myelinated axons may be repaired over a period of weeks to months. However, the distribution of the new axons may be less precise than the original innervation because no myelin sheath ever existed at their terminal ends and because all of the original channels may not still exist.

Until recently, neurons of the central nervous system were thought to have extremely limited regenerative ability. They lack the endoneurium channels found in the peripheral nervous system, and when injured their associated oligodendrocytes die, so their regrowth is haphazard in an area where precise connections are essential for normal function. Furthermore, astrocytes form a network of scar tissue that blocks much of the growth of injured axons. However, new grafting techniques are being developed to provide channels for axon growth. (See essay on page 270.)

Neurons, unlike many other cells, cannot divide. Shortly after birth human nerve cells lose the ability to reproduce. However, injured neurons in peripheral, myelinated nerves can regenerate axons if the cell body of the neuron is not damaged and if the endoneurium remains to provide a channel to guide the growth of the regenerating axon.

When a nerve is injured, as it might be in a deep wound, many axons are likely to be damaged, but their cell bodies, located in more proximal ganglia, may have escaped

INITIATION AND CONDUCTION OF NERVE IMPULSES

Objective 7. (a) Explain how the property of excitability contributes to the functioning of the nervous system; (b) describe the processes of initiation and conduction of an impulse along a neuron; (c) list and describe briefly the factors that affect the initiation and conduction of an impulse.

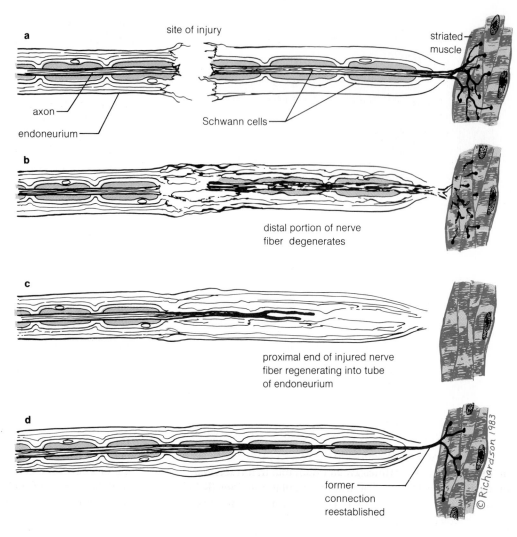

site of injury

striated muscle

axon

endoneurium

Schwann cells

distal portion of nerve fiber degenerates

proximal end of injured nerve fiber regenerating into tube of endoneurium

former connection reestablished

© Richardson 1983

Figure 10.9 Degeneration and regeneration of a peripheral axon: (**a**) site of injury in an axon, (**b**) degeneration of distal end of axon, (**c**) proximal end of axon regenerating and growing through the tube of endoneurium, (**d**) contact reestablishment with muscle cells.

Excitability

Though nearly all cells have an electric potential difference between the inside and the outside of the cell membrane, this potential difference is especially significant in neurons; because of it they display the property of **excitability**—the ability to respond to a stimulus and initiate and conduct an electrical impulse. To understand excitability, we need to explore some of the basic facts about electricity.

It is a fundamental property of matter that oppositely charged particles (+ and −) attract each other. The force of

this attraction increases as the particles come closer together or as the number of oppositely charged particles increases. When particles with unlike electrical charges are separated, a force is produced. This force is called a **potential difference** (PD), measured in volts. Because the PDs that exist across cell membranes are small, they are measured in thousandths of volts, or millivolts (mV).

In living cells potential differences are created by charged particles (ions) in and around the cells. Each cell contains intracellular fluid and is surrounded by extracel-

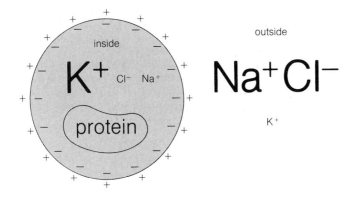

Figure 10.10 The large number of negatively charged protein molecules ⁻ P ⁻ within the cell and the large number of Na⁺ outside the cell are the major contributors to the potential difference between the inside and the outside of the membrane in a resting cell. The resting potential difference in most nerve cells is about −70 millivolts; that is, the inside is more negative than the outside by that amount.

lular fluid. Both of these fluids contain ions, but the concentrations of the various ions in each of the fluids differ. The concentration of sodium ions (Na⁺) in extracellular fluids is about twenty times greater than that in intracellular fluids; in contrast, the concentration of potassium ions (K⁺) in intracellular fluids is about twenty-five times greater than that in extracellular fluids. Intracellular fluids also contain large numbers of negatively charged protein molecules. Differences in the concentrations of charged particles create a potential difference across the cell membrane, and the cell is said to be **polarized**.

In resting, polarized neurons (those that have not been stimulated recently) the potential difference—about −70 mV—is called the **resting potential**. Thus, at the resting potential of −70 mV, the inside of the membrane is more negative than the outside by 70 mV (Figure 10.10).

In a resting cell potassium ions tend to diffuse out of the cell more easily than sodium ions diffuse in. The exact reasons for this difference are not well understood. Because large protein molecules and negatively charged ions cannot easily diffuse across the cell membrane, the inside of a cell tends to become more negative than the outside. These events create the negative potential difference. Furthermore, as sodium ions leak slowly into the cell, they are actively transported out again, and as potassium ions leak out of the cell, they are actively transported back into the cell by the

action of the **sodium-potassium pump** (see Chapter 3). This combination of active transport and passive diffusion of ions maintains the potential difference across the cell membrane.

When excitable cells are stimulated, the permeability of their membranes changes abruptly, altering the potential difference. More specifically, then, excitability refers to the ability of a cell to change its permeability to sodium and potassium ions when triggered by a stimulus. The fact that neurons and muscle cells are excitable is extremely important in the normal functioning of the body. Excitability is essential for the initiation and conduction of the impulses that transmit information, without which consciousness would cease and paralysis would occur.

Initiation and Conduction of Impulses

In much of the foregoing discussion we have used the general term **signal** to refer to the information being carried by the nervous system. The relaying of signals involves two processes: (1) the initiation and conduction of electrical impulses along individual neurons, and (2) the transmission of chemical messages from one neuron to the next across gaps or synapses between neurons.

Initiation of an impulse As previously noted, resting neurons have a potential difference, or resting potential, created by a difference in the concentration of ions between the inside and the outside of their membranes. To initiate an impulse, a neuron must be stimulated. Neurons normally receive stimuli in two ways: either from sensory receptors or from other neurons. When a neuron is stimulated, a rapid sequence of events occurs. The membrane's permeability to sodium ions suddenly increases at the point of stimulation, though the increase persists for only 1 millisecond (msec; 1/1000 second). Sodium ions rush into the cell for this brief time and create a positive potential difference of about +30 mV at the point of entry. Such a change in membrane potential is called **depolarization**; in this state the affected part of the membrane is less polarized than in the resting state.

As suddenly as the cell membrane became more permeable, it again becomes less permeable to sodium ions—all within 1 to 2 milliseconds—and the ions enter the cell at the lower resting rate. Meantime, the permeability to potassium increases, and potassium ions move out of the cell, again making the membrane negative on the inside. The process is called **repolarization**.

The rapid sequence of depolarization and repolarization is called the **action potential**, or **impulse**; the action potential (impulse) is the basic means of communication within the nervous system. After the impulse is completed, the sodium-potassium pump becomes active; sodium ions are pumped out of the cell, and potassium ions are pumped into the cell until the original resting state of ionic concentrations is achieved.

Conduction of an impulse   Once part of the membrane of a neuron is depolarized at the point where the stimulus was applied, adjacent portions of the membrane become depolarized, and a wave of depolarization spreads along the neuron (Figure 10.11). This is a little like throwing a pebble into still water and creating waves in all directions from the point at which the pebble hit. The **conduction** of an impulse is simply the passage of an action potential along a neuron. The impulse is the same regardless of what kind of stimulus—light, sound, heat, or touch—created it. At any point along a neuron the whole process of depolarization and repolarization takes only about 2 milliseconds (Figure 10.12).

Factors that Affect Initiation and Conduction of Impulses

Strength of stimulus   For an impulse to be initiated, the stimulus must be strong enough to depolarize the neuron beyond the **threshold level** of depolarization for that neuron (Figure 10.13a). This threshold determines the minimum strength of stimulus to which a neuron will respond with an action potential. It varies among neurons and according to different conditions affecting a particular neuron.

Summation   A stimulus too weak to initiate an impulse is called a **subthreshold**, or **subliminal**, **stimulus** (Figure 10.13b). If a series of these stimuli reach a neuron in rapid succession, their accumulated effects may succeed in initiating an impulse. This additive effect of several subthreshold stimuli is called **summation** (Figure 10.13c). One explanation of summation is that each subthreshold stimulus depolarizes the membrane slightly so that a subsequent subthreshold stimulus may add to the earlier stimuli and depolarize the membrane enough to reach the threshold. Various types of summation exist; they will be discussed later.

All-or-none principle   Once a neuron has received a stimulus above the threshold level, it conducts an impulse of constant maximum size throughout the length of the neuron. Thus, the **all-or-none principle** states that a neuron either conducts or does not conduct an impulse; if it conducts an

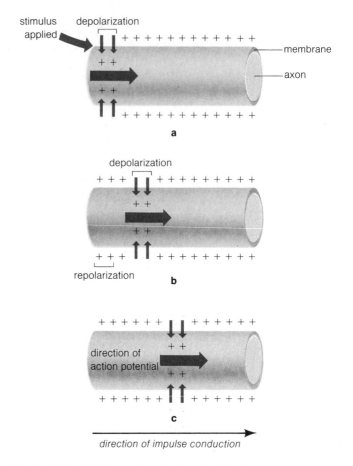

Figure 10.11   Initiation and conduction of an impulse.

impulse or action potential, that impulse is always of maximum size. Therefore, according to the all-or-none principle, a neuron can be thought of as being either "on" or "off." Increasing the strength of a stimulus beyond the threshold level will not increase the size of the impulse.

Refractoriness   For a brief period of time immediately after being stimulated, a time corresponding roughly to the duration of the action potential, a neuron cannot be restimulated by any stimulus, no matter how strong. This period is called the **absolute refractory period**. At a slightly later time an unusually strong stimulus may successfully initiate an impulse, even though a threshold level stimulus would not be able to do so. This occurs during what is called the **relative refractory period**.

Saltatory conduction   The properties of impulse conduction described so far apply to unmyelinated neurons. However,

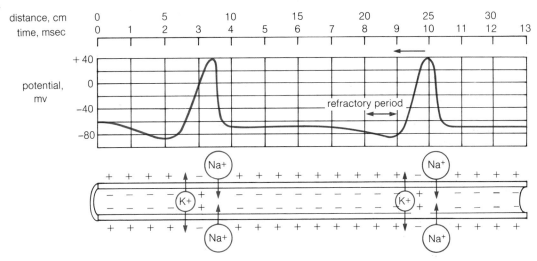

Figure 10.12   Two action potentials traveling along an axon.

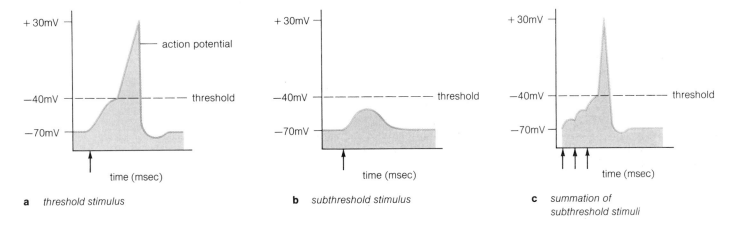

a   threshold stimulus

b   subthreshold stimulus

c   summation of subthreshold stimuli

Figure 10.13   (a) A threshold stimulus initiates an impulse, (b) but a subthreshold stimulus is too weak to initiate an impulse. (c) Summation of subthreshold stimuli can initiate an impulse. Arrows indicate times at which stimuli were applied.

the myelin sheath of many axons in the body insulates those axons except at the nodes of Ranvier (see Figure 10.5). When an impulse travels along a myelinated neuron, depolarization occurs only at the nodes; it leaps over the myelin from one node to the next. This process, **saltatory conduction**, gets its name from the root word *saltere*, which means to leap. Saltatory conduction accounts for the greater speed of an impulse traveling along a myelinated neuron than along an unmyelinated one; a great deal of time is saved by depolarizing the membrane only at the nodes instead of its entire length. Less energy is required for saltatory conduction than

for conduction along an unmyelinated neuron because smaller amounts of ATP are used to operate the sodium pump; when only small portions of the axon generate an action potential, less sodium enters the cell. In evolution saltatory conduction offered an advantage to those animals that had myelinated neurons, allowing them to respond more quickly and expend less energy in responding to stimuli from the environment.

Conduction velocity   The speed of an impulse is also affected by the diameter of the axon. Axons having a large diameter offer less internal resistance to the conduction of an impulse than those having a small diameter. Large myelinated fibers, such as some motor neurons that innervate skeletal muscles, may conduct impulses at speeds up to 100 meters per second due to saltatory conduction along large-diameter axons. In contrast, small unmyelinated fibers, such as those supplying visceral organs, conduct impulses at speeds of only 0.5 to 1 meter per second.

TRANSMISSION OF IMPULSES

Objective 8. Define synapse and neurotransmitter; distinguish between excitatory and inhibitory synapses.

Objective 9. Describe the physiological properties of the transmission of a signal across a synapse, including the effect of multiple synapses on the same neuron.

The Synapse

After a signal has traveled the length of a neuron, **transmission** of the signal to the next neuron in the neural pathway occurs. Such transmission takes place across a **synapse**, a specialized junction between the axon terminal of one neuron and the dendrite (or cell body or axon) of the next neuron (Figure 10.14). Transmission across a synapse is accomplished by a chemical substance called a **neurotransmitter**. The neuron whose axon releases the neurotransmitter is the **presynaptic neuron**; the neuron that receives the neurotransmitter is the **postsynaptic neuron**. The neuromuscular junction, already considered in Chapter 8, is a special kind of synapse where the signal is transmitted from a motor neuron to a muscle cell. In the nervous system the signal is transmitted from one neuron to another. As shown in Figure 10.14, a typical synapse consists of the **presynaptic knob** of an axon separated from the **postsynaptic region** of a dendrite or nerve cell body by the **synaptic cleft**.

Not all conduction paths are as simple as this one-axon-to-one-dendrite pattern. As shown in Figure 10.15, a single axon can form synapses with dendrites and cell bodies of several neurons, creating a **divergence** of the pathway. Alternatively, several axons can form synapses with dendrites and cell body of a single neuron, creating a **convergence** of pathways. In some cases axons form synapses with other axons. Regardless of the synaptic configuration, the process of chemical transmission is essentially the same.

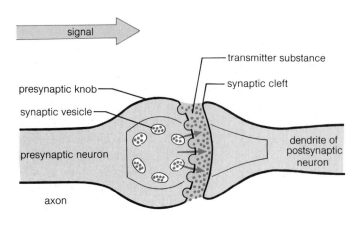

Figure 10.14   A synapse.

Mechanism of synaptic transmission   The neurotransmitter is synthesized in the axon terminals and stored in membrane-covered **vesicles**, which aggregate near the surface of the presynaptic knobs (see Figure 10.14). When an impulse arrives at a presynaptic knob, the permeability of the cell membrane changes, and calcium ions from the extracellular fluid enter the cytoplasm of the knob. The calcium ions cause some of the vesicles to move to the surface of the knob, where their membranes fuse with the cell membrane, releasing neurotransmitter into the synaptic cleft.

The transmitter quickly diffuses across the narrow synaptic cleft and binds with protein receptor molecules on the postsynaptic membrane. This binding action alters the membrane potential of the postsynaptic cell, opening channels in the membrane and allowing sodium ions to enter the cell. Finally, the neurotransmitter is inactivated, either by an enzyme on the postsynaptic membrane or by reuptake into the presynaptic knob. In the case of the neurotransmitter acetylcholine, the enzyme cholinesterase on the postsynaptic membrane breaks the transmitter into acetate and choline. Choline is then transported back to the presynaptic cell for reuse in the synthesis of acetylcholine. (New acetyl groups are produced by the presynaptic neuron.) In summary, transmission across a synapse involves synthesis, storage, release, reception, inactivation of the neurotransmitter, and sometimes reuptake, as shown in Figures 10.16 and 10.17.

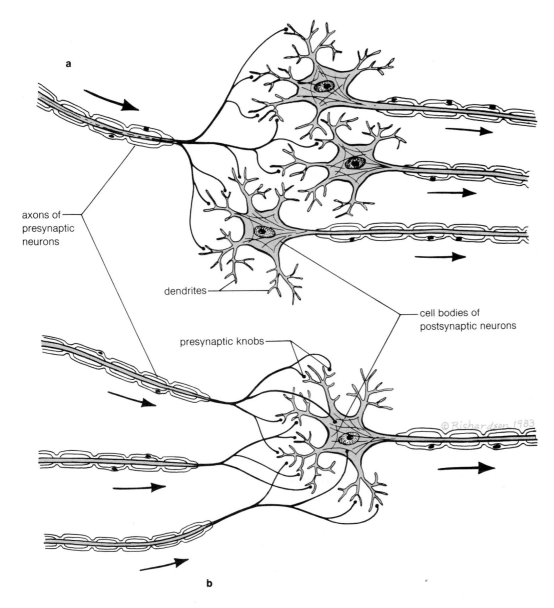

a

axons of presynaptic neurons

dendrites

cell bodies of postsynaptic neurons

presynaptic knobs

© Richardson 1983

b

Figure 10.15 Divergence and convergence of synapses: (**a**) divergence, (**b**) convergence.

Properties of synaptic transmission   When a neuron is stimulated, the wave of depolarization moves along the membrane in all directions from the point of stimulation like the ripples of water created by throwing a stone into a pond. However, signals are usually generated at the dendrite region because that is where most presynaptic knobs impinge on (come in close contact with) the cell. Thus, signals usually travel from dendrite to axon to axon terminals within a neuron and from presynaptic axon to postsynaptic dendrites across a synapse. Because only the axonal terminals can release a chemical transmitter, one-way signals are maintained throughout the nervous system. Thus, synaptic transmission causes all signals to obey the **principle of forward conduction**.

The effects of transmission across a synapse depend on the number of molecules of neurotransmitter reaching the

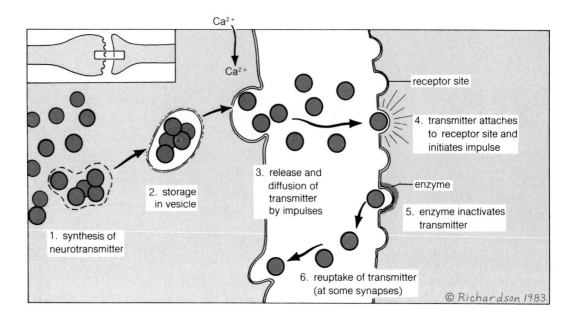

Ca²⁺

Ca²⁺

receptor site

4. transmitter attaches
to receptor site and
initiates impulse

enzyme

5. enzyme inactivates
transmitter

3. release and
diffusion of
transmitter
by impulses

2. storage
in vesicle

1. synthesis of
neurotransmitter

6. reuptake of transmitter
(at some synapses)

© Richardson 1983

Figure 10.16 Steps in the transmission of a signal across a synapse.

receptor sites on the postsynaptic membrane and on the interaction of the transmitter and receptor sites. This interaction can be excitatory or inhibitory.

An excitatory interaction alters the postsynaptic membrane and causes an influx of sodium ions, which depolarizes the cell. This creates an **excitatory postsynaptic potential (EPSP)**. Such transmission from a single presynaptic knob is unlikely to develop an action potential in the postsynaptic neuron; it does depolarize the membrane toward the threshold, making it easier for a subsequent transmission to create an action potential. This action of an EPSP is called **facilitation** (Figure 10.18a).

An inhibitory interaction between a transmitter and a receptor site alters the permeability of the postsynaptic membrane and allows either potassium ions to flow out or chloride ions to flow in. These ion movements change the membrane potential, causing it to be hyperpolarized (more polarized than in the resting state). This creates an **inhibitory postsynaptic potential (IPSP)**, as shown in Figure 10.18b. When a cell is hyperpolarized, the membrane potential is farther from the threshold than normal and therefore requires a stronger stimulus to reach threshold level. This action of an IPSP is called **inhibition**.

Several presynaptic knobs simultaneously releasing a chemical transmitter whose effect is excitatory can cause sufficient depolarization to initiate an action potential in the postsynaptic neuron, even though no single knob releases enough transmitter to exceed the threshold. This simulta-

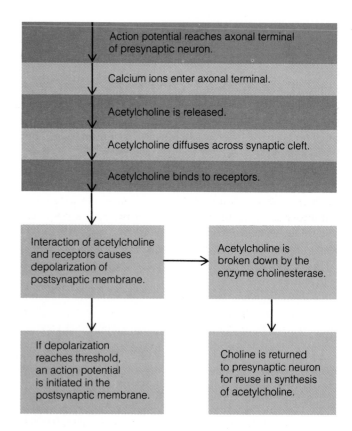

Action potential reaches axonal terminal of presynaptic neuron.

Calcium ions enter axonal terminal.

Acetylcholine is released.

Acetylcholine diffuses across synaptic cleft.

Acetylcholine binds to receptors.

Interaction of acetylcholine and receptors causes depolarization of postsynaptic membrane.

Acetylcholine is broken down by the enzyme cholinesterase.

If depolarization reaches threshold, an action potential is initiated in the postsynaptic membrane.

Choline is returned to presynaptic neuron for reuse in synthesis of acetylcholine.

Figure 10.17 A summary of events that occur in the transmission of a signal across a synapse.

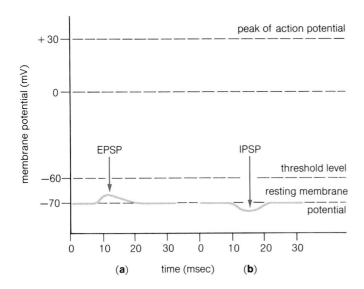

peak of action potential

EPSP

IPSP

threshold level

resting membrane potential

membrane potential (mV)

+30

0

−60

−70

0 10 20 30   0 10 20 30

(a)   time (msec)   **(b)**

Figure 10.18 Alteration of postsynaptic potentials: (**a**) An EPSP depolarizes the membrane and facilitates the initiation of an impulse. (**b**) An IPSP hyperpolarizes the membrane and makes the initiation of an impulse more difficult.

neous release of a chemical transmitter from several adjacent presynaptic knobs is called **spatial summation**. If a single presynaptic knob repetitively releases a chemical transmitter, the additive effects of the transmitter over a short period of time also can create a threshold stimulus. Such repetitive release is called **temporal summation**. These types of summation are illustrated in Figure 10.19.

At many neurons in the central nervous system both excitatory and inhibitory interactions can occur. Whether the total effect on the postsynaptic neuron is excitatory or inhibitory is determined by the net change in the membrane potential created by the combination of excitatory and inhibitory interactions. For example, if the excitatory interactions exceed the inhibitory interactions by an amount sufficient to create an action potential, the effect will be excitatory. Thus, the neurons of the central nervous system, and of the brain in particular, can be turned "on" or "off" by the net effect of these transmitter–receptor interactions. The overall effect of many such "on-off" events makes possible the coordination and integration of nervous system function.

Transmission across synapses is slower than impulse conduction along neurons because of the time required for the release, diffusion, and action of the transmitter. This **synaptic delay** may amount to about half a millisecond at each synapse at a body temperature of 37°C. Because of this

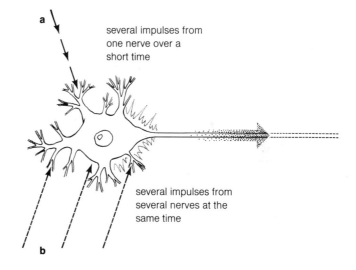

a

several impulses from one nerve over a short time

several impulses from several nerves at the same time

b

Figure 10.19 Summation: (**a**) temporal summation, (**b**) spatial summation.

synaptic delay the time a signal takes to travel from one point to another in the body can be used to estimate the number of synapses in the neural pathway. For example, at 100 meters per second (10 centimeters per millisecond), a signal can travel 5 centimeters along a neuron in the same amount of time it takes to cross a synapse. In the brain, where synapses are close together, traversing a 5 centimeter pathway with one synapse would take 1 millisecond; traversing the same distance over a pathway with three synapses would take 2 milliseconds—twice as long.

Repeated stimulation of the presynaptic knobs can lead to the depletion of the stored transmitter substance. When this occurs, the postsynaptic neuron cannot be stimulated by this pathway, and a condition called **synaptic fatigue** exists. This fatigue lasts for several seconds until the axonal terminals can synthesize a new supply of neurotransmitter. Synaptic fatigue is the only kind of fatigue that occurs in the nervous system; conduction along neurons is not subject to fatigue. Synaptic fatigue and inhibitory interactions are important factors in regulating neural function. They are also important in limiting the duration of seizures.

Neurotransmitters

As explained in the discussion of synapses, neurotransmitters are chemicals released from a presynaptic neuron that interact with specific receptor sites of a postsynaptic neuron. Early in their embryological development neurons have the potential to produce any one of several chemical transmitters, but as development proceeds, each neuron usually becomes limited to producing only one neurotransmitter. Recent research shows that some neurons contain two, or occasionally three, chemicals that can act as chemical messengers between cells. It is clear that transmitter–receptor interactions are much more complex when they involve cells that can produce more than one transmitter. It is beyond the scope of this book to discuss the various possibilities; suffice it to say that ongoing research efforts will undoubtedly lead to the discovery of many more kinds of neurons that contain more than one transmitter and to a more complete understanding of their roles in the function of the nervous system. At least thirty chemicals thought to have the capacity to act as neurotransmitters have been discovered, most of them in brain tissue, and more are likely to be found. Some of those neurotransmitters will be considered here.

Acetylcholine   The neurotransmitter **acetylcholine** is released at all neuromuscular junctions between motor neurons and skeletal muscle cells, at all synapses between preganglionic and postganglionic neurons in the autonomic nervous system (see Chapter 13), and at certain synapses between neurons in the central nervous system (see Chapter 11). As with all other neurotransmitters, the effect of acetylcholine depends on the nature of its interaction

Some flea collars for pets, pesticide strips, and other forms of insecticide contain a chemical that inhibits the action of cholinesterase in insects. Acetylcholine accumulates and binds to all receptor sites, blocking further excitation of the postsynaptic neurons. The fact that the absence of cholinesterase kills insects (and also humans) demonstrates the importance of this enzyme in neural function.

with its receptor. For example, at receptors in neuromuscular junctions, the effect is excitatory and, if it is sufficiently strong, will cause contraction of muscle fibers. At receptors in cardiac muscle the effect is inhibitory and will make the stimulation of contraction more difficult. At receptors on postsynaptic neurons the effect is usually excitatory. The enzyme **cholinesterase** is present on the membrane of the muscle cell or the postsynaptic neuron, where it breaks down acetylcholine into acetate and choline and terminates the action of the transmitter.

Norepinephrine   Another transmitter, **norepinephrine** (formerly called noradrenalin), is secreted by some neurons of the sympathetic nervous system and also by some neurons of the central nervous system. Norepinephrine is excitatory at some synapses and inhibitory at others, depending on the nature of the receptor to which it attaches. This transmitter is important in regulating the activity of visceral organs and in controlling certain brain functions. Norepinephrine is usually inactivated by reuptake into the presynaptic knob; it also can be inactivated by the action of **monoamine oxidase**, an enzyme that oxidizes the amino group of the neurotransmitter, rendering it ineffective.

Gamma aminobutyric acid   The interaction of **gamma aminobutyric acid** (GABA) with its receptor sites is usually inhibitory. GABA causes the membrane potential of the postsynaptic neuron to become more negative by increasing the membrane's permeability to potassium and chloride ions. Thus, the membrane becomes hyperpolarized.

Neuronal Pools

A **neuronal pool**, which might be thought of as an extremely complex set of synapses, consists of an area of thousands or millions of interconnected neurons. Such pools, found mainly in the central nervous system, particularly in the brain, regulate body functions and help to maintain homeostasis. Knobs of a presynaptic neuron may send signals to as many as a thousand postsynaptic neurons; likewise, a postsynaptic neuron may receive signals from as many as a thousand presynaptic neurons. Some presynaptic input leads to excitation, and some leads to inhibition. The number of knobs that discharge on a single postsynaptic neuron and whether the discharges lead to excitation or inhibition determine the nature of the effect.

The circuits in neuronal pools are extremely complex, but we can gain some understanding of their properties by studying the characteristics of four types: divergent, convergent, parallel after-discharge, and reverberating circuits. Refer to Figure 10.20 as you read about each kind of circuit.

In **divergent circuits** a single neuron can stimulate several other neurons, thereby amplifying the effect of the stimulus. For example, a single sensory neuron might form synapses with several other neurons and eventually send information to several parts of the brain.

In **convergent circuits** one postsynaptic neuron receives stimuli from several sources. For example, a motor

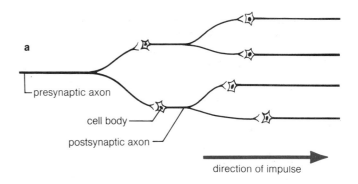

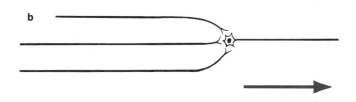

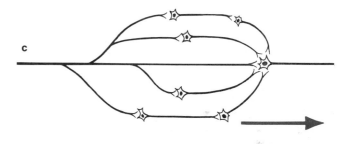

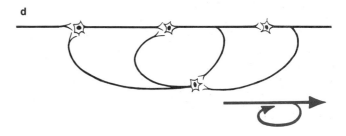

Figure 10.20 Circuits found in neuronal pools: (**a**) divergent, (**b**) convergent, (**c**) parallel after-discharge, (**d**) reverberating circuit.

In addition to the neurotransmitters discussed so far, which are endogenous (normally present in the body), certain exogenous chemicals (chemicals not normally present in the body) can affect the excitability of neurons. Though it is beyond the scope of this book to explain the effects of exogenous chemicals in detail, we will mention the effects of some of them here.

Chemicals in commonly used beverages—theobromine in cocoa, theophylline in tea, and caffeine in coffee—increase the excitability of neurons. Strychnine also increases excitability, but it does so by inhibiting the action of transmitters such as glycine in the spinal cord. When glycine interacts with its receptors, the postsynaptic neuron is inhibited; thus, strychnine appears to act by preventing inhibition. Some anesthetics increase the threshold for excitation. Lipid-soluble anesthetics such as ether dissolve in neuronal membranes and alter the permeability of the membrane. Certain other anesthetics block the release of transmitters or enhance the effects of inhibitory transmitter–receptor interactions. Local anesthetics such as those often used in dentistry appear to prevent depolarization by preventing sodium from being conducted across the membrane.

neuron might receive stimuli from several different neurons. Though regulation of the respiratory rate is more complex than can be accomplished by a single convergent circuit, such circuits contribute to its regulation. Stimuli from sensors of oxygen concentration in the blood, stimuli that are created by exertion, and stimuli associated with observation of an exciting event may converge to stimulate an increase in the respiratory rate.

In some circuits the output continues for several milliseconds after the initial stimulus has terminated. This phenomenon can be explained by the existence of **parallel after-discharge circuits**. In such circuits the initial stimulus comes directly from the presynaptic neuron. This same neuron stimulates other parallel circuits that have one or more synapses. Signals pass through these several circuits, each of which may have a different number of synapses. The combined delays of several synapses cause the postsynaptic neuron to receive a series of stimuli. This creates a burst of impulses, or an after-discharge, and causes the postsynaptic neuron to continue to respond for up to 15 milliseconds after receiving the first stimulus in the sequence. Such parallel circuits probably function in complex mental processes.

In **reverberating circuits** the postsynaptic, or output, neuron sends a branching collateral axon back to the presynaptic neuron, either directly or by way of one or more additional neurons. Each time a signal passes through the main pathway, collateral signals restimulate the input neuron and thus prolong neural activity. The strength of the collateral signal may be sufficient to excite the input neuron or only sufficient to facilitate it. Short-term memory, which is measured in minutes, may involve such circuits.

SPINAL CORD

Objective 10. Describe the structure of the spinal cord, including its major tracts.

Up to this point in the study of the nervous system, we have emphasized the cellular level of neurological function. However, no neurological function is accomplished by a single neuron, so it is essential that we consider higher functional levels—the spinal cord level, the lower brain level, and the higher brain (cerebral cortex) level. The spinal cord level, the subject of the remainder of this chapter, involves a variety of reflexes. The lower and higher brain levels, which involve subconscious and conscious activities of the brain, will be discussed in the next two chapters.

External Anatomy

The **spinal cord** is located inside the vertebral column and extends from the base of the brain, with which it is continuous, to the level of the second lumbar vertebra (Figure 10.21). In an adult the spinal cord is from 42 to 45 centimeters long; its diameter varies at different levels, being enlarged in the cervical and lumbar regions. The cord is also flattened so that its antero-posterior diameter is less than its left-to-right diameter. The **cervical enlargement** extends from the fourth cervical to the first thoracic vertebrae; it is the region from which nerves supplying the arms arise. The **lumbar enlargement** extends from the ninth to the twelfth thoracic vertebrae; it is the region from which the nerves supplying the legs arise.

It may seem strange that the lumbar enlargement should be in the thoracic region; this is the case because the spinal cord grows at a slower rate than the vertebral column. By adulthood the area within the vertebral column below the second lumbar vertebra contains spinal nerves that branched from the spinal cord at higher levels. These spinal nerves, labeled L2 through Co1 in Figure 10.21, are called, collectively, the **cauda equina**, or horse's tail.

The spinal cord terminates as the **conus medullaris**. Surrounding the conus medullaris is a fibrous connective tissue covering, the **filum terminale**, which anchors the spinal cord within the vertebral column. The filum terminale is an extension of the pia mater, one of the meninges, or coverings of the CNS, to be discussed later.

Though the divisions between segments of the spinal cord disappear during embryological development, the spinal cord can be considered to consist of thirty-one segments, each with an associated pair of spinal nerves.

Internal Anatomy

The internal anatomy of the spinal cord is best seen in cross section (Figure 10.22). In a cross section of the spinal cord we are looking at the cut ends of fibers that run longitudinally through the spinal cord, carrying impulses between the peripheral nervous system and the brain. Two indentations, the **posterior median sulcus** and the **anterior median fissure**, separate the spinal cord into left and right symmetrical halves. The inner butterfly-shaped area is the **gray matter** of the spinal cord. Gray matter is so named because it lacks myelin and therefore appears gray in an unstained preparation. Surrounding the gray matter are bundles of myelinated nerve fibers, called fasciculi or white columns, which together form the **white matter** of the spinal cord.

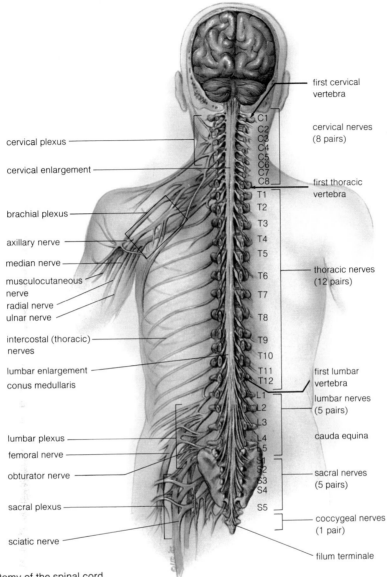

first cervical
vertebra

cervical nerves
(8 pairs)

first thoracic
vertebra

thoracic nerves
(12 pairs)

first lumbar
vertebra

lumbar nerves
(5 pairs)

cauda equina

sacral nerves
(5 pairs)

coccygeal nerves
(1 pair)

filum terminale

cervical plexus

cervical enlargement

brachial plexus

axillary nerve

median nerve

musculocutaneous
nerve

radial nerve

ulnar nerve

intercostal (thoracic)
nerves

lumbar enlargement

conus medullaris

lumbar plexus

femoral nerve

obturator nerve

sacral plexus

sciatic nerve

C1
C2
C3
C4
C5
C6
C7
C8
T1
T2
T3
T4
T5
T6
T7
T8
T9
T10
T11
T12
L1
L2
L3
L4
L5
S1
S2
S3
S4
S5

Figure 10.21 Gross anatomy of the spinal cord.

These fasciculi, which contain the spinal tracts, are white because of the myelin that is deposited around the nerve fibers within them.

In each segment of the spinal cord a spinal nerve arises from each side of the cord. Each spinal nerve connects with the cord through two nerve roots. The **dorsal nerve root** consists of a bundle of sensory axons (carrying incoming signals) whose cell bodies are located in the **dorsal root ganglion**. These axons extend into the **posterior horn** of the gray matter, where they often form synapses with other neurons, some of which are called interneurons. **Interneurons**, short neurons confined to the gray matter of the cord, form synapses with other interneurons and with the motor neurons whose cell bodies are located in the **anterior horn** of the gray matter. Aggregations of motor axons (carrying outgoing signals) from these cell bodies form the **ventral nerve roots**. The **lateral horns** lie between the anterior and posterior horns. The hollow **central canal** contains cerebrospinal fluid (to be discussed later). The meninges labeled in this figure will also be discussed later.

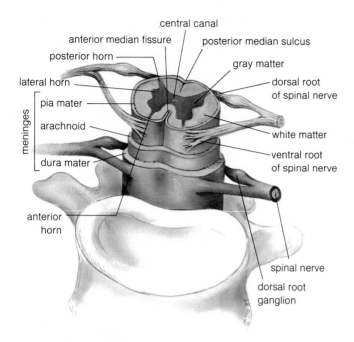

Figure 10.22 A cross section of the spinal cord, showing the internal anatomy of the cord with some surface of the cord visible to show meninges.

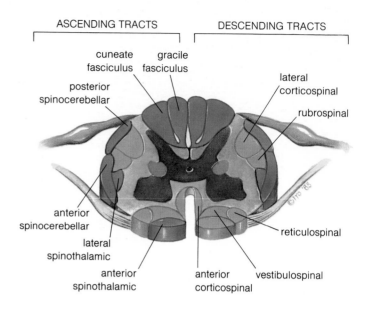

Figure 10.23 The tracts of the spinal cord. Ascending tracts are labeled on the left side of the diagram, and descending tracts are labeled on the right side of the diagram, though all are present on both sides of the cord.

Spinal Tracts

Within the white matter are two kinds of fasciculi, or bundles of axons: the **ascending tracts**, which carry sensory impulses to the brain, and the **descending tracts**, which carry motor impulses from the brain to the spinal nerves at various levels of the cord. Table 10.2 summarizes the major characteristics of those tracts. Note that many of the tracts are named by combining the names of their points of origin and termination. For example, the spinothalamic tract goes from the sensory axons of the posterior horn of the spinal cord to the thalamus, and the vestibulospinal tract goes from the vestibular nuclei of the medulla to the motor neurons of the anterior horn. (The parts of the brain mentioned here are described in more detail in the next chapter.)

Decussation, an important characteristic of some spinal tracts, is the crossing over of fibers from one side of the spinal cord to the other. Because of decussations movement and some sensations on one side of the body are controlled by a part of the brain on the opposite side of the body. For example, if a motor area of the left side of the brain is damaged, movement will be impaired on the right side of the body. Most decussations occur at the upper end

of the spinal cord or in the brain stem. Such tracts are said to be **contralateral**; that is, their origins and terminations are on opposite sides of the body from each other. Other tracts do not decussate and are said to be **ipsilateral**; their fibers run the length of the spinal cord and into the brain without crossing the midline of the cord.

MENINGES AND CEREBROSPINAL FLUID

Objective 11. Describe the location, structure, and function of the meninges.

Objective 12. Describe the location, composition, and function of cerebrospinal fluid.

Meninges

The connective tissue coverings of the central nervous system are the meninges: the outer dura mater, the middle arachnoid layer, and the inner pia mater (see Figures 10.22

Table 10.2 Major Spinal Tracts

Tract	A/D*	Origin	Termination	Characteristics
Gracile and cuneate fasciculi	A	Sensory axons in posterior horn	Medulla, and relayed to cerebral cortex	Convey information from one side of the body to the same side of the medulla. Information allows distinguishing closely adjacent touch stimuli; recognizing sizes, shapes, and textures; and sensing body position.
Posterior and anterior spino-cerebellar	A	Sensory axons in posterior horn	Cerebellum	Convey information for the control of muscle tone and posture to the same side of the cerebellum from which the stimuli came.
Lateral spino-thalamic	A	Sensory axons in posterior horn	Thalamus, and relayed to cerebral cortex	Conveys information about pain and temperature to the opposite side of the thalamus from which the stimuli came.
Anterior spino-thalamic	A	Sensory axons in posterior horn	Thalamus, and relayed to cerebral cortex	Conveys information about pressure and crude touch to the opposite side of the thalamus from which the stimuli came.
Lateral and anterior corticospinal	D	Motor area of cerebral cortex	Motor neurons of anterior horn	Convey information to stimulate voluntary muscle actions. Lateral tract crosses over in medulla; anterior tract crosses over in spinal cord.
Rubrospinal (rubro-red)	D	Red nucleus of brainstem	Motor neurons of anterior horn	Conveys information that controls muscle tone and posture. Crosses over in brain stem.
Reticulo-spinal	D	Reticular formation of brainstem	Motor neurons of anterior horn	Conveys information that increases muscle tone and motor activity. Cross over in brainstem.
Vestibulo-spinal	D	Vestibular nuclei of medulla	Motor neurons of anterior horn	Conveys information to the same side of the body to maintain equilibrium and balance.

*A = ascending, D = descending

and 10.24). All three layers of meninges surround the entire central nervous system and extend over the roots of the peripheral nerves as they leave the spinal cord. Here, they join the epineurium of each nerve.

The **dura mater**, literally "tough mother," lines the cranial cavity and forms a tube surrounding the spinal cord, terminating in a blind sac at the second sacral vertebra. Spinal nerves in the cauda equina pass through the sac. Between the dura mater and the vertebrae is the **epidural space**, which is filled with fat and connective tissue that serve to cushion and support the brain and spinal cord. When anesthesia in certain spinal nerves is desired, anesthetics can be injected into the epidural space and allowed to diffuse to the neural tissue. The dura mater itself consists of tough fibrous connective tissue. In certain places in the cranial cavity, the dura mater separates into two layers; the lower layer extends between lobes of the brain.

This arrangement of the dura helps to hold the brain in place in the cranial cavity. The space between the layers of dura mater is the **dural sinus**. As will be explained later, the dural sinus collects venous blood from the brain tissues to be returned to the heart.

The **arachnoid layer** is a thin, cobweblike membrane. It is separated from the dura mater by a small amount of serous fluid in the **subdural space**, and from the pia mater by the **subarachnoid space**. The subarachnoid space is filled with cerebrospinal fluid. Small folds in the arachnoid layer, the **arachnoid villi**, or **arachnoid granulations**, function as one-way passages and allow cerebrospinal fluid to diffuse from the subarachnoid space into the blood in the dural sinuses.

The **pia mater**, literally "soft mother," is a delicate membrane well supplied with blood vessels. It follows the contours of the brain and spinal cord.

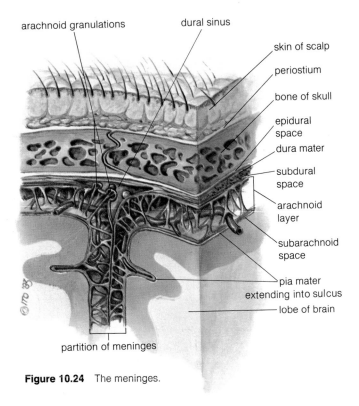

arachnoid granulations
dural sinus
skin of scalp
periostium
bone of skull
epidural space
dura mater
subdural space
arachnoid layer
subarachnoid space
pia mater extending into sulcus
lobe of brain
partition of meninges

Figure 10.24 The meninges.

Cerebrospinal Fluid

As mentioned in the discussion of the development of the nervous system, the cavity within the hollow neural tube becomes the central canal of the spinal cord and the ventricles of the brain. This continuous cavity is filled with **cerebrospinal fluid**, which is secreted by a special tissue in the roof of the ventricles. An opening from one of the ventricles allows the fluid to enter the subarachnoid space. Cerebrospinal fluid contains a relatively high concentration of sodium ions; because of sodium and other ions water is drawn into the fluid by osmosis. The result is that the pressure within the cavity containing cerebrospinal fluid can be regulated by the amount of sodium secreted. Therefore, in addition to acting as a shock absorber, the cerebrospinal fluid also can change in volume and regulate internal pressure within the cavity. The structure of the ventricles and the production and circulation of cerebrospinal fluid will be described with the discussion of the brain.

SPINAL NERVES

Objective 13. Describe the structure of spinal nerves, their distribution, and their arrangement into plexuses.

Structure

The **spinal nerves** are formed by the union of the dorsal and ventral roots shortly after they leave the spinal cord (Figure 10.25). Each spinal nerve has afferent (sensory) and efferent (motor) fibers; in general, efferents come from the ventral root, and afferents go into the dorsal root. Thus, all spinal nerves are **mixed nerves** because they carry both sensory and motor impulses.

After passing through the intervertebral foramen, each spinal nerve separates into posterior and anterior branches. The **posterior branch** innervates the muscles and skin of the posterior portion of the body. The **anterior branch** innervates the limbs and the lateral and anterior portions of the body. Spinal nerves in the thoracic and lumbar regions also have a **visceral branch**, which innervates internal organs. The **meningeal branch**, a small branch not shown in the figure, innervates the structures around the spinal cord—the vertebrae, ligaments, meninges, and blood vessels of the cord itself.

Distribution

The thirty-one pairs of spinal nerves are named and numbered according to the vertebrae with which they are associated. (Refer back to Figure 10.21.) They include eight pairs of cervical nerves, twelve pairs of thoracic nerves, five pairs of lumbar nerves, five pairs of sacral nerves, and one pair of coccygeal nerves. In the cervical region the first cervical nerve (C1) passes between the occipital condyles of the skull and the first cervical vertebra (atlas). Nerve C2 passes between the atlas and the axis. The fact that the atlas has a cervical nerve superior to it and another inferior to it accounts for the presence of eight cervical nerves even though there are only seven cervical vertebrae. In all other regions the spinal nerve passes inferiorly to the vertebra of the same number.

We mentioned earlier how motor nerves associate with embryonic myotomes, which later become muscles. The pattern of nerve supply to the skin (Figure 10.26) follows the developmental pattern of the dermatomes, other segmental blocks of tissue in the embryo that eventually form the dermis. (Nerve C1 does not supply a dermatome.) Even in the adult the segment of the skin supplied by a particular spinal nerve is called a dermatome, though separations no longer exist between them. Growth of the appendages and unequal growth in other areas result in adult dermatomes having unequal size and shape and varying degrees of overlap. Abnormalities in skin sensations in a dermatome can be used to detect damage to the spinal nerve that supplies the dermatome.

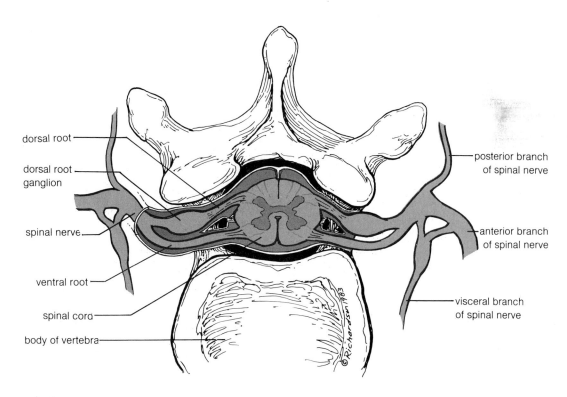

dorsal root

dorsal root
ganglion

spinal nerve

ventral root

spinal cord

body of vertebra

posterior branch
of spinal nerve

anterior branch
of spinal nerve

visceral branch
of spinal nerve

Figure 10.25 Spinal nerves branch from the spinal cord, as shown here.

Plexuses

A **plexus** is a branching, interconnected network of nerves. The anterior branch of each of the spinal nerves, except for thoracic nerves T2 through T12, enters a plexus from which fibers are redistributed to nerves supplying specific areas of the body. The four major plexuses are the cervical plexus, the brachial plexus, the lumbar plexus, and the sacral plexus (Figure 10.27).

The **cervical plexus**, formed from branches of nerves C1 through C4, lies beneath the sternocleidomastoid muscle of the neck (Figure 9.4, Chapter 9). Nerves branching from the cervical plexus supply the skin and muscles of the neck, scalp, and upper part of the shoulders. The **phrenic nerve** branches from the cervical plexus to innervate the diaphragm, a major muscle of the breathing mechanism. Damage to the spinal cord above the cervical plexus can impair or stop breathing because such damage affects the phrenic nerve. (The cervical plexus also contains fibers from two of the cranial nerves, the spinal accessory nerve and the hypoglossal nerve. Cranial nerves will be discussed in the next chapter.)

The **brachial plexus** includes branches of nerves C5 through T1, which form a network at the base of the neck near the clavicle. Nerves leading from the brachial plexus branch repeatedly to innervate the entire skin surface and muscles of the arm. Some of the major branches of the brachial plexus are the **radial nerve**, which supplies the posterior surface of the whole arm, the **musculocutaneous nerve**, which innervates the anterior upper arm, and the **median** and **ulnar nerves**, both of which supply the forearm. It is a branch of the ulnar nerve that is stimulated when you experience the sharp sensation of bumping your "crazy bone" or elbow.

The **lumbar plexus** is formed by nerves L1 through L4 (and in some individuals part of T12). It lies in the psoas major muscle, a deep muscle located between the lumbar vertebrae and the femur. The largest single branch of the lumbar plexus is the **femoral nerve**, which innervates the muscles and skin of the anterior thigh and leg. Other branches supply the lateral and medial thigh, the anterolateral abdominal wall, and portions of the pelvic organs.

Closely associated with the lumbar plexus is the **sacral plexus**, formed from branches of nerves L4 through S3 (and sometimes part of S4). Because of the overlapping branches

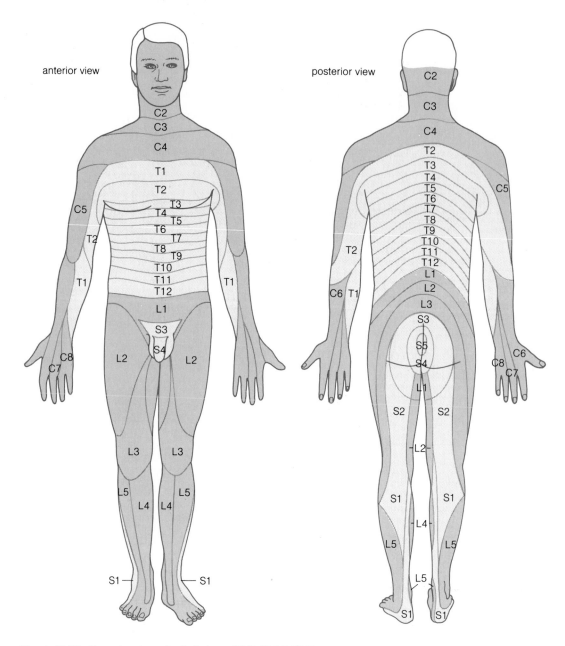

anterior view

posterior view

Figure 10.26 Dermatomes, and spinal nerve distribution to them.

and close proximity, the whole network of the lumbar and sacral plexuses is sometimes referred to collectively as the **lumbosacral plexus**. The major nerve of the sacral plexus is the **sciatic nerve**, the largest nerve in the body. It branches into the common peroneal and tibial nerves to supply the leg. Smaller nerves of the sacral plexus supply the gluteal muscles and portions of the pelvic organs. Intramuscular injections into the gluteus muscle should be given with care to avoid damage to the sciatic nerve and partial paralysis or loss of some sensation.

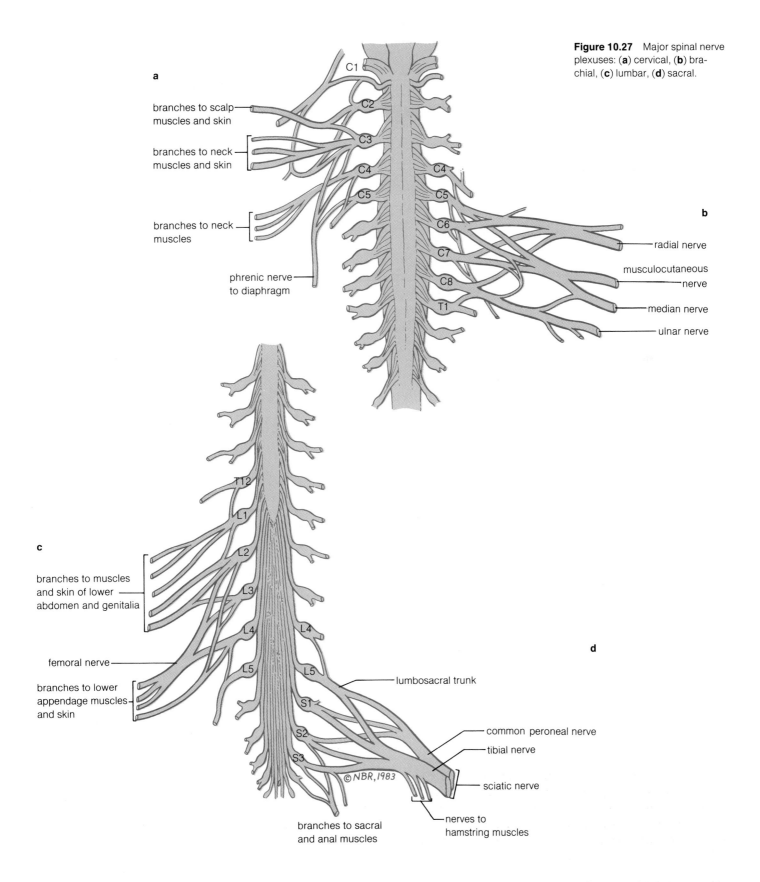

Figure 10.27 Major spinal nerve plexuses: (**a**) cervical, (**b**) brachial, (**c**) lumbar, (**d**) sacral.

a

branches to scalp muscles and skin

branches to neck muscles and skin

branches to neck muscles

phrenic nerve to diaphragm

C1
C2
C3
C4
C5

C4
C5
C6
C7
C8
T1

b

radial nerve

musculocutaneous nerve

median nerve

ulnar nerve

c

branches to muscles and skin of lower abdomen and genitalia

femoral nerve

branches to lower appendage muscles and skin

T12
L1
L2
L3
L4
L5

L4
L5
S1
S2
S3

d

lumbosacral trunk

common peroneal nerve

tibial nerve

sciatic nerve

nerves to hamstring muscles

branches to sacral and anal muscles

© NBR, 1983

REFLEXES

Objective 14. Describe the properties of a reflex arc.

Objective 15. Discuss briefly the withdrawal, crossed-extensor, and stretch reflexes, including the role of negative feedback in their function.

Reflex Arc

A **reflex** is a predictable, involuntary motor response to a specific stimulus. Many, though not all, reflexes function at the spinal cord level. This means that, though sensory impulses eventually may reach the brain, the response to the stimulus requires only the spinal cord and not the brain. Even reflexes that involve the brain may make use of only the brainstem; they are not normally consciously controllable. By the time sensory impulses reach the conscious part of the brain, the reflex has already occurred. Your eyes have blinked or your finger has been jerked away from a hot object before you become aware of what has happened.

The neural components of a typical spinal reflex are shown in cross section of the spinal cord in Figure 10.28. The conduction pathway of a **reflex arc** proceeds from a sensory receptor (in the skin, for example) through a sensory neuron to a synapse in the spinal cord. From this synapse the signals usually travel through one or more interneurons to a motor neuron, which connects to an effector (the motor end plate of a muscle, for example). One spinal reflex, the stretch reflex, involves only one synapse; when a muscle is stretched, the signal is transmitted from the sensory neuron directly to a motor neuron, causing the muscle to contract. No interneuron is involved. However, the vast majority of reflexes involve several interneurons.

Sensory receptors involved in a simple spinal reflex arc can be located in the skin, in a muscle or tendon, or in a visceral organ. They receive information about the external or internal environment. (More will be said about the properties of receptors in Chapter 14.) Information from sensory receptors is conducted along sensory neurons to synapses in the posterior horn of the spinal cord. A single long sensory neuron extends from each receptor to the spinal cord. Its cell body is in the dorsal root ganglion, and its axon consists of a central and a peripheral process. (Refer back to Figures 10.5 and 10.25.)

When present, the interneuron (sometimes called the association, or internuncial, neuron) relays information from the sensory neuron to the dendrite of a motor neuron. In Figure 10.28 the interneuron is confined to the left side of a single segment of the spinal cord. In some reflexes other interneurons conduct impulses to the other side of the

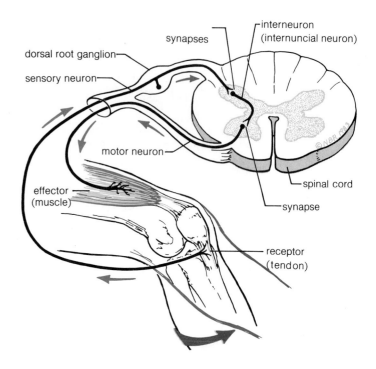

Figure 10.28 A reflex arc.

spinal cord and to adjacent segments of the spinal cord above or below the input level. Thus, signals can go to the same side (ipsilateral), the opposite side (contralateral), or both sides (bilateral) of the cord. They also may be relayed to several segments of the cord. Though not part of the reflex arc, other pathways can conduct the sensory information through nerve tracts in the spinal cord to the cerebral cortex, where conscious awareness of the reflex is elicited.

The motor neuron originates in the anterior horn of the spinal cord, where its short dendrites and cell body are located. A long motor axon carries efferent impulses to the motor end plates of many muscle fibers.

Examples of Reflexes

Withdrawal reflex The **withdrawal reflex**, sometimes referred to as the **flexor reflex**, occurs in response to a painful stimulus such as burning a finger or stepping on a tack. The reflex action is to contract muscles to flex joints in the injured limb and withdraw it from the source of the stimulus. It is clearly a protective reflex. Though the person is almost immediately conscious of the stimulus, the reflex has already caused withdrawal of the limb before conscious

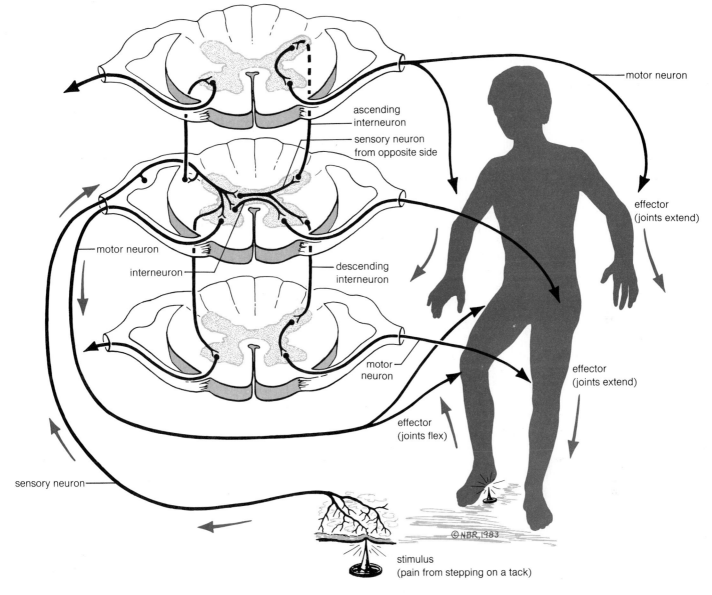

Figure 10.29 A crossed-extensor reflex involves association neurons that cross the spinal cord and that extend up and down the cord to adjacent segments.

awareness occurs. The reflex precedes conscious awareness because the reflex arc involves fewer synapses than the pathway to the cerebral cortex, where conscious awareness is created. This explanation involving the reflex arc is really only part of the story regarding the movements associated with withdrawal; divergent and parallel after-discharge circuits are also involved in integrating the complete response.

Crossed-extensor reflex The **crossed-extensor reflex**, also a response to a painful stimulus, occurs when the withdrawal reflex causes a movement that would throw the body off balance. It involves three kinds of interneurons (Figure 10.29). One interneuron carries signals from one side of the spinal cord to the other. An ascending interneuron carries signals upward, and a descending interneuron carries sig-

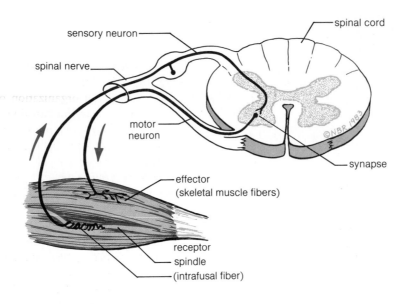

Figure 10.30 The stretch reflex. Note that there are no interneurons involved in this reflex.

nals downward to adjacent segments of the spinal cord. Interneurons carry the impulses to as many levels of the spinal cord as necessary to cause the appropriate muscles to contract or relax. The crossed-extensor reflex is so named because the sudden flexion of joints on one side of the body (jerking foot from a tack) requires extension of joints (extending arm) on the other side of the body to maintain balance.

Stretch reflex The **stretch reflex** functions in the motor control of skeletal muscles. Each skeletal muscle contains **muscle spindles**, which are a kind of stretch receptor that responds to stretching of muscle fibers (Figure 10.30). Likewise, each tendon contains **Golgi tendon organs**, which respond to changes in the tension on a tendon in a similar manner. The muscle spindle consists of small **intrafusal muscle fibers** attached to the sheaths of the regular (contractile) muscle fibers. The center of the intrafusal fibers lacks actin and myosin; instead, it is wrapped with a sensory nerve fiber. When a skeletal muscle is stretched, the spindle stretches and stimulates the nerve endings. Impulses travel along the sensory nerve fiber directly to the anterior horn of the spinal cord. Here, the sensory axon forms a synapse with

a motor neuron on the same side of the cord and without passing through an interneuron. The motor neuron stimulates the stretched muscle to contract. The signals from the spindles are stronger when the muscle is being increasingly stretched than when it is being maintained in a stretched position. Thus, variations in the strength of signals from the stretch receptors help to regulate contraction. The interactions between stretch receptors, Golgi tendon organs, and muscle contraction serve both to maintain posture and muscle tone and to control the degree of contraction during voluntary movement.

Reflexes and Negative Feedback

Reflexes, being direct responses to stimuli, help the body to react quickly to changes in the environment. Because the response minimizes the disturbing effect of the stimulus, the reflex can be viewed as a negative feedback mechanism (Figure 10.31). Recall from Chapter 1 that negative feedback suppresses the sensor when output is increasing. All self-regulatory systems involve negative feedback; such systems are essential in maintaining homeostasis.

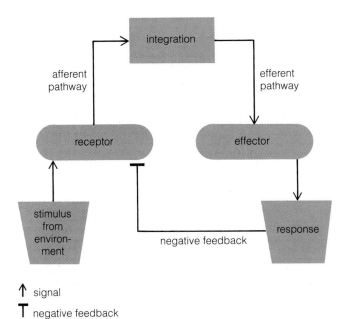

afferent pathway

efferent pathway

↑ signal

T negative feedback

Figure 10.31 A generalized reflex arc, illustrating negative feedback.

INTEGRATED FUNCTION OF THE NERVOUS SYSTEM

Objective 16. Explain how the functions of the nervous system studied in this chapter contribute to homeostasis.

The overall organization of the nervous system provides the capacity for carrying signals from sensory receptors throughout the body to effectors (muscles and glands) also distributed throughout the body. The excitability of neurons is the fundamental property that allows the body to detect and respond to changes, thereby helping to maintain homeostasis. The ability of neurons to regenerate new axons in the peripheral nervous system helps to assure continued function of nerves even after injury.

Reflex activity, the functional level of the nervous system emphasized in this chapter, contributes significantly to homeostasis. The withdrawal reflex minimizes injury; the crossed-extension reflex maintains balance and prevents further injury; the stretch receptors help to maintain muscle tone and posture and also regulate voluntary muscle activities. Together, such reflexes remove from conscious effort certain functions that must be carried on constantly.

The relationships of reflex-level functions with higher level functions will be developed in the next chapter. It is, as we shall see, the integration of all neural functions along with endocrine functions that ultimately maintains homeostasis.

CLINICAL APPLICATIONS

Objective 17. Explain briefly the clinical significance of each of the following reflexes: Babinski, plantar, patellar, and Achilles reflexes.

Objective 18. Discuss the nature of the malfunction in each of the following clinical conditions: (a) multiple sclerosis, (b) poliomyelitis, (c) neuritis, (d) neuralgia, (e) sciatica, and (f) meningitis.

Clinically Significant Reflexes

Neurologists use a variety of reflexes to assess neurological function. Because reflexes are under involuntary control, and because in a healthy individual a given stimulus produces a predictable response, reflexes are good diagnostic tools for studying the function of the spinal cord and the peripheral nervous system. When the spinal cord or nerves are damaged or diseased, the reflex response to a particular stimulus may be exaggerated, diminished, or obliterated. Deviations from the normal response in specific reflexes often indicate to a neurologist the location of a neurological defect. Only a few of the many clinically significant reflexes will be described here.

Babinski and plantar reflexes In the **Babinski reflex**, when the sole of the foot is stroked, the big toe is extended and the other toes may be spread in a fanlike configuration (Figure 10.32a). This reflex normally occurs only in children up to the age of 1½ years; neurologists attribute its presence to incomplete development of the corticospinal (pyramidal) tracts. In older children and adults this reflex is normally replaced by the **plantar reflex**. Elicited in the same way, the plantar reflex causes the toes to curl under (Figure 10.32b). The presence of this normal reflex indicates intact, mature corticospinal tracts. When the Babinski reflex is seen in individuals over 1½ years old, it indicates some kind of damage or disease in the corticospinal tracts. Thus, the presence of the Babinski reflex helps the neurologist to locate a defect,

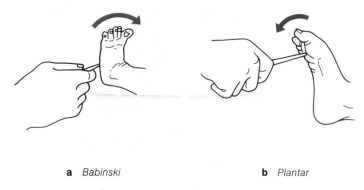

a *Babinski*   **b** *Plantar*

Figure 10.32 (**a**) Babinski reflex, (**b**) plantar reflex.

though it provides little information about what might have caused it.

Patellar reflex The **patellar**, or **knee-jerk**, **reflex** consists of the contraction of the quadriceps femoris muscle (on the anterior thigh) and the extension of the leg when the patellar tendon is stimulated. The degree of response following stimulation of the patellar tendon is a measure of the functioning of the stretch receptors and of the strength of facilitating and inhibiting inputs from the brain to the motor neurons in the spinal cord. When a patient shows a weak or absent patellar reflex, the peripheral nerves associated with the lumbar plexus may have been damaged, or inputs from higher centers via the spinal cord may be disrupted. When a patient shows an exaggerated knee jerk, the corticospinal tract may have been damaged and inhibition from the brain diminished. Evidence from autopsies often confirms the correlation between specific signs seen in live individuals and subsequently located defects, even when the defects cannot be identified in life.

Achilles reflex The **Achilles**, or **ankle-jerk**, **reflex** results in plantarflexion (extension of the foot) when the Achilles tendon is stimulated. Weakness or absence of this reflex may indicate damage to the peripheral nerves associated with the sacral plexus or to neurons within the spinal cord in the lumbosacral region. Exaggeration of the reflex usually occurs when the spinal cord tracts themselves have been damaged. The Achilles reflex is also important in diagnosing abnormalities in thyroid function. Though the contraction phase of the reflex is normal, the relaxation phase is disturbed in thyroid malfunction. In hypothyroidism (too little thyroid activity) the relaxation phase is slowed; in hyperthyroidism (overactive thyroid) it is accelerated.

Malfunctions of the Nervous System

Multiple sclerosis **Multiple sclerosis** is a progressive degenerative disease of the central nervous system, so named because of the many sites in which hardened (or sclerotic) scar tissue has replaced the normal myelin sheaths of neurons. The disintegration of myelin interferes with impulse conduction, and the formation of scar tissue, or **plaque**, exacerbates the condition. The cause of myelin degeneration is as yet unknown; researchers are studying the effects of immune reactions, viruses, and genetic factors. At the onset of the disease, which usually occurs between twenty and forty years of age, mild symptoms appear. An affected person may show one or more of the following symptoms: slight visual impairment, speech disturbances, uncoordinated handwriting, or impaired concentration.

The episodic and unpredictable nature of the disease may be one of the most dependable criteria for diagnosis. Symptoms often disappear for a period of weeks or months, only to be followed by new symptoms or a recurrence of previous symptoms in a more incapacitating form. The nature of the symptoms appears to depend on the location of the plaques. Because the symptoms vary greatly among individuals, and because each may be a symptom of another disease, the diagnosis of multiple sclerosis is rarely made until after several episodes of the disease have occurred. Death usually follows a period of ten to thirty years of gradually increasing disability. When death occurs, it is usually from a secondary infection associated with limited movement—bladder and kidney infection or pneumonia. In spite of efforts toward improved understanding of the disease, multiple sclerosis is still almost always fatal.

Poliomyelitis **Poliomyelitis** is an acute viral infection that destroys the cell bodies of motor neurons in the anterior horn of the spinal cord. Bulbar poliomyelitis affects motor neurons in the brainstem and may damage the respiratory centers in the medulla. Symptoms include stiff neck, muscle pain, headache, and fever. As the disease runs its course, the muscles served by the dying motor neurons become paralyzed. Because the disease affects only motor neurons, the individual retains sensory functions even in paralyzed limbs. Some motor neurons may remain undamaged so that, after recovering from the acute phase of the disease, individuals can sometimes regain partial or even total use of limbs through physical therapy. Effective immunization has been available for several decades, but parental complacency and some religious beliefs leave many children and adults unprotected from this seriously crippling disease.

Neuritis More a symptom than a specific disease, **neuritis** is a general term for disturbances of the peripheral nervous system. Either sensory or motor fibers or both may be damaged. Pain is nearly always present, and paralysis or unusual sensations such as tingling or coldness also may occur. Neuritis may be caused by trauma (blows, fractures), exposure to toxic substances (heavy metals and some drugs), or deficiencies of some B vitamins. Treatment is directed toward the cause when it is known. Aspirin or other drugs are given to relieve pain, and weakened muscles are massaged and stretched.

Neuralgia **Neuralgia** is pain in a circumscribed area innervated by a sensory nerve of the peripheral nervous system. It is often

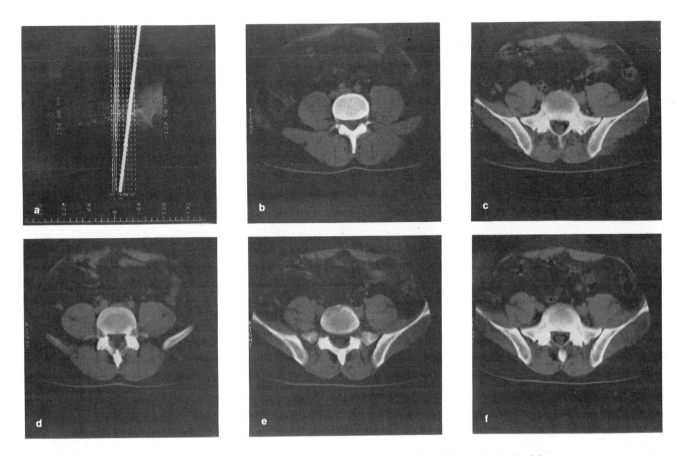

Figure 10.33 A CAT scan of the lumbar area in a thirty-three-year-old man complaining of lower back pain: (**a**) a longitudinal section of the vertebral region in which the dotted lines indicate the planes of the individual frames in the scan, (**b**) a frame showing a vertebra at the level of the intervertebral foramina, (**c**) a frame showing a vertebra at the level of the transverse processes, with white areas to the right showing sections through the ilia, (**d** through **f**) selected frames from the more inferior regions of the scan. (Courtesy of Alexandria Hospital, Alexandria, Virginia, Joyce R. Isbel, R.T.)

impossible to determine the cause of the pain and difficult to relieve it. In severe cases the sensory nerve supplying the painful area is surgically cut. The area becomes numb, but the pain is usually relieved.

Sciatica **Sciatica** is an irritation or neuritis of the sciatic nerve. The most common cause of sciatica is a "slipped," or herniated, intervertebral disc. A disc in the lumbar area herniates or protrudes from the vertebral column. The soft central part of the disc may be pushed out through the peripheral fibrous part, causing pressure to be placed on the sciatic nerve, or it may be pushed inward, causing pressure on nerve roots destined for the sciatic nerve. Treatment includes bed rest, exercises, muscle relaxants, physical therapy, pain medication, and sometimes surgery if the pressure on the nerve persists. Other causes of sciatica include osteoarthritis and pregnancy, if the weight and position of the fetus creates pressure on the sciatic nerve.

Computerized axial tomography (CAT scan) is a diagnostic technique in which a series of sections through the body can be observed and recorded on X-ray film. The technique is useful in diagnosing a variety of conditions; a diagnostic series for an individual with low back pain is shown in Figure 10.33. Abnormalities of the spinal cord, spinal nerves, vertebrae, and intervertebral discs could be observed if present.

Meningitis **Meningitis**, an inflammation of the meninges, is usually caused by an infectious organism. Several different kinds of bacteria and viruses can infect the meninges; antibiotics can be used to control bacterial infections, but no effective treatment exists for viral infections. In the latter case the person's symptoms are treated while the disease runs its course. Death or permanent brain damage may occur.

A spinal tap, or spinal puncture, may be used to diagnose the cause of meningitis. A sterile spinal needle is introduced into the subarachnoid space between the third and fourth lumbar vertebrae (below the inferior end of the spinal cord), and a sample of cerebrospinal fluid is withdrawn for laboratory study. In performing a spinal tap it is important to avoid damaging the nerves of the cauda equina. The spinal tap procedure can also be used to withdraw fluid and subsequently introduce an equal volume of anesthetic to induce spinal anesthesia or to measure pressure within the subarachnoid space.

Clinical Terms

analgesia (an-al-je'ze-ah)   absence of ability to sense pain

anesthesia (an-es-the'ze-ah)   loss of feeling or sensation

ataxia (ah-tax'e-ah)   inability to coordinate muscular activity

hypnosis (hip-no'sis)   artificially induced trancelike state

neurology (nu-rol'o-je)   the study of the nervous system

neuromata (nu-ro-mă'tah)   branches of neurons growing from the end of a nerve cut during an amputation

paresis (par'es-is)   slight or incomplete paralysis

sedation (se-da'shun)   the process of calming

shingles   an inflammatory disorder caused by the virus herpes zoster, which damages the cell bodies of dorsal root ganglia

whiplash   an injury caused by sudden hyperextension of the neck, which may lead to spinal nerve damage in the cervical area

Essay: Spinal Cord Injuries

Injuries to the spinal cord result from falls and blows, especially in conjunction with automobile and diving accidents. The extent of disability caused by a cord injury is determined by its location and its severity, which may be determined by studying a myelogram of the injured area. A myelogram is an X ray of the spinal cord after an opaque dye has been injected into the body so that it becomes concentrated in the cord. Figures 10.34 and 10.35 are examples of cervical and lumbar myelograms, respectively.

If the spinal cord is completely severed, all sensory and voluntary motor activity below the injury is permanently lost. Severing the cord in the upper lumbar region results in **paraplegia**—loss of sensation and motor function in those parts supplied by the spinal nerves distal to the injury, typically the legs. Severing the cord in the mid-cervical region results in **quadriplegia**—loss of sensation and voluntary motor function in all four limbs. If the cord is severed above spinal segment C3, respiratory arrest may occur as well.

The nature of the paralysis usually indicates whether the injury is in the cord or in the peripheral nerves. If the lesion is in the spinal cord, "spastic paralysis" often develops over a period of weeks or months, and the affected muscles are paralyzed in a contracted state. This is because the motor neurons

are no longer inhibited by impulses descending from the brain. If, in contrast, the lesion is in a peripheral nerve, "flaccid paralysis" most frequently results, and the muscles are paralyzed in a relaxed state. This is because impulses cannot reach the muscles to cause them to contract.

Damage to the spinal cord that severs only a portion of the cord may result in paralysis, loss of sensation, or both, below the specific severed tracts. Though, in any given injury, damage is unlikely to create a precise **hemisection**—the severing of only the left or only the right side—of the spinal cord, knowing the effects of hemisection helps to determine the nature of an injury. In hemisection a specific pattern of impairment, the **Brown-Sequard syndrome**, results. All voluntary motor functions are lost below the site of the injury on the same side of the body as the injury. Touch and pressure sensations from the area below the injury are also lost on the same side as the injury because decussation of these tracts occurs at higher levels in the CNS; sensations of heat, cold, and pain are lost on the opposite side of the body because decussation of these tracts occurs at their lower ends. Knowledge of the pathways of spinal tracts and their decussations makes these effects predictable and helps neurologists to assess the nature of an injury.

Spinal shock follows severe trauma to the spinal cord.

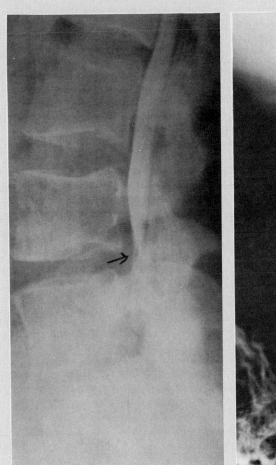
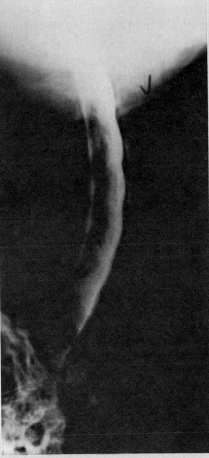

a   b

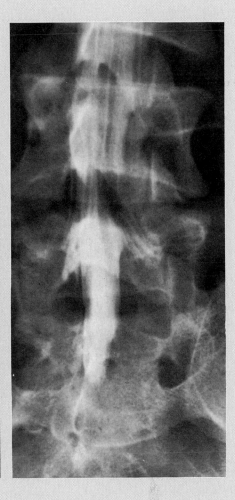

Figure 10.34 Cervical myelograms: (**a**) The single black arrow shows the location of an injury to the cord. (**b**) The two black arrows show the location of a displacement of cervical vertebrae that creates pressure on the spinal cord. (Courtesy of Alexandria Hospital, Alexandria, Virginia, Joyce R. Isbel, R.T.)

Figure 10.35 A myelogram of the lumbar region of the spine. (Courtesy of Alexandria Hospital, Alexandria, Virginia, Joyce R. Isbel, R.T.)

Any injury that leads to partial or complete severing of the cord is likely to cause spinal shock. At first, all cord reflexes in the area below the injury cease to function. The person loses bladder and bowel control, and arterial blood pressure drops precipitously in response to a change in body position, such as movement from a horizontal to a vertical position (postural hypotension). The cessation of reflex activities below the level of the injury is ascribed to the lack of signals that usually come from higher nerve centers to facilitate reflexes. Reflex arcs below the level of the injury are still intact and gradually, after a period ranging from several days to several months, resume function as they readjust to decreased input and become self-initiating.

The treatment of spinal cord injuries usually involves six to eight weeks in traction. Fractures of the vertebrae may be reduced by traction or may require surgical reduction. Electrical stimulation of muscles may be used in the absence of neural stimuli to maintain contractility, and isometric muscle retraining may be used to establish new neural pathways where damage is not too severe to prevent it. This retraining makes use of remaining undamaged neurons that had not previously been part of the regularly used pathways.

Until recently it was thought that the central nervous system had extremely limited ability to regenerate itself and repair damages. Experiments are now underway in animals to graft peripheral nerve tissue into the damaged region of the spinal cord. Such grafts provide sheaths through which some axons of the spinal cord seem to be able to reestablish connections. Without such sheaths the regeneration of spinal cord axons is prevented by the growth of glial cells, the scar tissue of the nervous system. Many problems remain to be solved before grafting can be used in humans, but the technique may eventually offer new hope for individuals sustaining spinal cord injuries.

Complications of spinal cord injury include urinary infections, decubitis ulcers (bed sores), and spinal deformity. Urinary infections can be controlled by antibiotics and by frequent drainage of the bladder, usually by catheterization (inserting a tube into the bladder) until urinary function is regained. Decubitis ulcers are prevented by adequate dietary protein and frequent movement of the injured person. However, the limitations on moving such individuals make it very difficult to prevent these ulcers. Children are especially susceptible to spinal deformity because their vertebral columns are still growing. Using frames in which the child can be held erect rather than wheelchairs helps to prevent deformity in the ambulatory phase of recovery.

Recovery of useful function (sensation, movement, or both) varies with the location and severity of the injury. When the cord is completely severed, the likelihood of useful recovery is small. Less than one in six patients regains any useful function. Nevertheless, victims of paraplegia whose injury is in the lower lumbar region can sometimes walk with good braces and crutches if they have strong trunk muscles. Given the severity of such injuries, it may seem surprising that patients regain any functions. Those who do appear to make use of autonomic pathways and branches of cranial nerves that have not been damaged. The prognosis for individuals with partially severed cords is better than for those with completely severed cords; almost half of the individuals with partial cervical lesions and four out of five with partial thoracolumbar lesions experience some useful recovery of function.

Rehabilitation of victims of spinal cord injury is an essential part of total care. Efforts are made to help the injured individuals make use of whatever functions they have to pursue a vocation, often in a sheltered workshop setting. Education of the person and his or her family is an important part of rehabilitation because their lifestyle may change markedly. Finally, special equipment to compensate for disabilities often makes the difference between independence or helplessness.

CHAPTER SUMMARY

(Chapter summary points and review questions are numbered to correspond to the numbered objectives in the text of each chapter.)

Organization and General Function

1. Describe the general organization of the nervous system.
    a. The central nervous system consists of the brain and spinal cord.
    b. The peripheral nervous system consists of all nerve fibers outside the CNS, including the sensory and motor fibers of the somatic system and the sympathetic and parasympathetic fibers of the autonomic system.
2. Explain briefly how the nervous system functions to maintain homeostasis.
    a. The nervous system detects changes in the external and internal environments, processes information, and regulates the responses of effectors (muscles and glands) to maintain homeostasis.
    b. The nervous system interacts with the endocrine system in accomplishing homeostasis.

Development

3. Describe the general development of the nervous system.
    a. The nervous system develops from ectoderm of the posterior surface of the embryo, first forming a neural tube and neural crests.
    b. The neural tube gives rise to the brain and spinal cord, the motor portions of the cranial and spinal nerves, the retina and optic nerves of each eye, and a portion of the pituitary gland.
    c. The cells of the neural crests give rise to the sensory neurons, the autonomic neurons, and the medulla of the adrenal gland.

Cells and Tissues

4. Distinguish between neurons and neuroglia, including Schwann cells; describe the structure, function, and location of neurons and of each type of neuroglia.
    a. Neurons are the signal-conducting cells of the nervous

system; neuroglia are the insulating and supporting cells.

b. Neurons:
   (1) have the structures shown in Figures 10.4 and 10.5
   (2) function by conducting impulses along their dendrites and axons
   (3) are located throughout the body in peripheral nerves as well as in the brain and spinal cord
c. Neuroglia:
   (1) constitute the connective tissue of the nervous system
   (2) include the myelin-producing Schwann cells of the PNS, the myelin-producing oligodendrocytes of the CNS, the supporting astrocytes of the CNS, the cavity-lining ependymal cells of the CNS, and the phagocytic microglia of the CNS

5. Describe the structure of nerves, tracts, ganglia, and nuclei.
   a. Nerves are bundles of nerve fibers, mostly axons, and their associated connective tissues; they are found in the PNS.
   b. Tracts are bundles of mostly myelinated fibers found in the CNS.
   c. Ganglia are aggregations of cell bodies associated with peripheral nerves.
   d. Nuclei are aggregations of cell bodies in the CNS.

Nerve Degeneration and Regeneration

6. Describe the process by which injured neurons degenerate and the process by which they may regenerate.
   a. Injured neurons in the PNS degenerate distal to an injury, as shown in Figure 10.9.
   b. Regeneration can occur if the cell body is intact and a channel to guide the growth of the axon remains.

Initiation and Conduction of Nerve Impulses

7. (a) Explain how the property of excitability contributes to the functioning of the nervous system; (b) describe the processes of initiation and conduction of an impulse along a neuron; (c) list and describe briefly the factors that affect the initiation and conduction of an impulse.
   a. The property of excitability—the ability of neurons to respond to a stimulus and to conduct an impulse—makes it possible for the nervous system to receive information and use it to regulate function.
   b. The processes of initiation and conduction of an impulse along a neuron occur as follows:
      (1) When a neuron is stimulated, the movement of ions across its membrane creates a change in the potential difference.
      (2) When a resting neuron is stimulated, a small number of sodium ions move into the cell, creating an action potential, which moves along the membrane as an impulse.
      (3) Following a wave of depolarization is a wave of repolarization, which prepares the neuron to receive another stimulus.

c. Factors that affect the generation and conduction of an impulse include strength of stimulus, summation, the all-or-none principle, refractoriness, saltatory conduction, myelination, and axon diameter.

Transmission of Impulses

8. Define synapse and neurotransmitter; distinguish between excitatory and inhibitory synapses.
   a. A synapse is a specialized area of communication between neurons.
   b. A neurotransmitter is the chemical that flows from the axon of the presynaptic neuron to receptor sites on the postsynaptic neuron.
   c. A synapse may be excitatory or inhibitory, depending on the nature of the interaction between the neurotransmitter and the postsynaptic receptor sites.

9. Describe the physiological properties of the transmission of a signal across a synapse, including the effect of multiple synapses on the same neuron.
   a. Signals are transmitted across a synapse as follows:
      (1) The impulse arrives at the distal end of the presynaptic axon and changes the permeability of the membrane to calcium ions.
      (2) Calcium ions diffuse into the neuron and cause synaptic vesicles to release a neurotransmitter into the synaptic cleft.
      (3) The neurotransmitter unites with the receptor sites on the postsynaptic neuron and causes a change in its membrane potential.
      (4) The transmitter is inactivated.
   b. Multiple synapses on the same neuron may:
      (1) create excitatory postsynaptic potentials (EPSPs) and facilitate transmission
      (2) create inhibitory postsynaptic potentials (IPSPs) and inhibit transmission
   c. In neuronal pools the combined effects of many synapses determine the net effect in the postsynaptic neuron.

Spinal Cord

10. Describe the structure of the spinal cord, including its major tracts.
    a. The spinal cord extends from the base of the brain to the second lumbar vertebra and gives rise to thirty-one pairs of spinal nerves.
    b. In cross section the spinal cord displays a butterfly-shaped area of gray matter, which contains large numbers of neuron cell bodies and synapses, and an outer area of white matter, which contains the myelinated spinal tracts.
    c. The properties of the spinal tracts are summarized in Table 10.2.

Meninges and Cerebrospinal Fluid

11. Describe the location, structure, and function of the meninges.
    a. The meninges are located in three layers around the central nervous system:
       (1) the outer dura mater, a tough protective covering
       (2) the middle arachnoid layer, a thin cobweblike structure
       (3) the inner pia mater, a delicate, highly vascularized membrane that follows the contours of the brain and spinal cord
    b. In addition to protecting the CNS, the meninges allow cerebrospinal fluid to move from the subarachnoid space to the dural sinuses.
12. Describe the location, composition, and function of cerebrospinal fluid.
    a. Cerebrospinal fluid, similar to plasma except for its high concentration of sodium ions, fills the ventricles of the brain, the central canal of the spinal cord, and the subarachnoid space.
    b. Cerebrospinal fluid acts as a shock absorber for the CNS and regulates the internal pressure within the cavities it fills.

Spinal Nerves

13. Describe the structure of spinal nerves, their distribution, and their arrangement into plexuses.
    a. Spinal nerves consist of sensory and motor fibers. They carry signals between the spinal cord and other parts of the body.
    b. The thirty-one pairs of spinal nerves are distributed as follows:
       (1) eight in the cervical region
       (2) twelve in the thoracic region
       (3) five in the lumbar region
       (4) five in the sacral region
       (5) one in the coccygeal region
    c. Plexuses, or networks of nerves, found in the cervical, brachial, lumbar, and sacral regions, distribute sensory signals to the CNS and distribute motor signals to coordinate the functions of the effectors supplied by the nerves of each plexus.

Reflexes

14. Describe the properties of a reflex arc.
    a. A simple reflex arc consists of a receptor, a sensory neuron, usually one or more interneurons, a motor neuron, and an effector.
    b. Through a reflex arc a stimulus can be received, and a stereotyped response made without conscious action.
15. Discuss briefly the withdrawal, crossed-extensor, and stretch reflexes, including the role of negative feedback in their function.

    a. The withdrawal reflex causes a part of the body to be withdrawn from the cause of an injury.
    b. The crossed-extensor reflex accompanies the withdrawal reflex and helps the body to maintain balance.
    c. Stretch reflexes regulate muscle contraction and help to maintain muscle tone.
    d. The role of negative feedback in reflexes is summarized in Figure 10.31.

Integrated Function of the Nervous System

16. Explain how the functions of the nervous system studied in this chapter contribute to homeostasis.
    a. The excitability of neurons and the signals carried by the nervous system help to regulate the body.
    b. In this chapter we have emphasized the reflex level of function and how it protects the body from injury and regulates muscle contraction and muscle tone.

Clinical Applications

17. Explain briefly the clinical significance of each of the following reflexes: Babinski, plantar, patellar, and Achilles reflexes.
    a. Reflexes may be clinically significant because they help the neurologist locate injuries to the nervous system.
    b. The following reflexes are frequently used to assess neurological function:
       (1) The Babinski and plantar reflexes assess function of the corticospinal tracts.
       (2) The patellar reflex assesses functioning of stretch receptors and facilitating impulses from higher centers.
       (3) The Achilles reflex detects damage to certain neurons or tracts in the lumbosacral region and abnormal thyroid function.
18. Discuss the nature of the malfunction in each of the following clinical conditions: (a) multiple sclerosis, (b) poliomyelitis, (c) neuritis, (d) neuralgia, (e) sciatica, and (f) meningitis.
    a. Multiple sclerosis involves a degeneration of myelin in the CNS.
    b. Poliomyelitis is a viral disease that causes destruction of the ventral horn (motor) neurons of the spinal cord.
    c. Neuritis is an inflammatory nerve lesion that may be caused by a variety of factors and that causes pain.
    d. Neuralgia is pain in an area innervated by the sensory portion of a peripheral nerve; the cause is difficult to determine, and sometimes the pain may be relieved only by severing the sensory nerve.
    e. Sciatica is a neuritis of the sciatic nerve, often caused by damage to an intervertebral disc in the lumbar area.
    f. Meningitis is an inflammation of the meninges, usually caused by an infection.

REVIEW

Important Terms

action potential (impulse)	neurotransmitter
afferent	nucleus
autonomic nervous system	paraplegia
axon	parasympathetic division
central nervous system	peripheral nervous system
conduction	plexus
contralateral	potential difference
decussation	quadriplegia
dendrite	receptor
depolarization	reflex
effector	refractory period
efferent	repolarization
EPSP	resting potential
facilitation	saltatory conduction
ganglion	Schwann cell
gray matter	signal
interneuron	soma
ipsilateral	somatic nervous system
IPSP	summation
meninges	sympathetic division
meningitis	synapse
myelin	tract
nerve	transmission
neuroglia	white matter
neuron	

Questions

1. What are the components of the CNS? The PNS?

2. How does the nervous system help to maintain homeostasis?

3. List the major steps in the development of the nervous system.

4. **a.** How do neuroglia differ from neurons?
   b. Describe the structure of a neuron and explain how its structure is suited to its function.
   c. What is the function of each type of neuroglia?

5. **a.** How do nerves differ from tracts?
   b. How do ganglia differ from nuclei?

6. List the steps in the processes of nerve degeneration and regeneration and the conditions under which they occur.

7. **a.** What is excitability?

b. What are the events in the initiation of a nerve impulse and the events that affect the ability of a neuron to conduct a second impulse?

c. Define: threshold, subthreshold, summation, all-or-none principle, absolute and relative refractory periods, and saltatory conduction.

8. What is a synapse? A neurotransmitter?

9. **a.** List in sequence the steps in the transmission of a signal across a synapse, including the inactivation of the transmitter.
   b. Describe the properties of neuronal pools.

10. **a.** Describe the gross anatomy of the spinal cord.
    b. What structures are seen in a cross–section of the spinal cord?

11. What is the structure of each of the meninges, and in what sequence are they arranged?

12. Where is cerebrospinal fluid found, and what is its function?

13. **a.** What is the relationship between spinal nerves and the spinal cord?
    b. Name the spinal nerves and larger peripheral nerves associated with each of the four major plexuses.

14. Explain what reflexes occur when you step on a tack.

15. Modify your explanation in (14) to illustrate a crossed-extensor reflex and a stretch reflex.

16. How do reflexes contribute to homeostasis?

17. What abnormality can be detected by assessing each of the following reflexes: Achilles? Babinski? patellar?

18. Describe briefly each of the following conditions: multiple sclerosis, poliomyelitis, neuritis, neuralgia, sciatica, and meningitis.

Problems

1. What effect might a long-term diet extremely low in sodium have (a) on the excitability of neurons, and (b) on the composition and amount of cerebrospinal fluid?

2. Use Table 10.2 to determine the most likely effects of the following injuries: (a) The gracile and cuneate tracts are damaged in the cervical area on the right side of the body. (b) The left lateral spinothalamic tract is damaged in the lumbar area. (c) The rubrospinal tract is damaged on both sides of the cord in the lumbar area. (d) The spinal cord is completely severed in the lumbar area.

REFERENCES AND READINGS

Arehart-Treichel, J. 1980. Spinal cord injuries. *Science News* 118:9 (July 7).

Arehart-Triechel, J. 1982. Probing the causes of MS. *Science News* 121:76 (January 30).

Bedbrock, G. M. 1979. Spinal injuries with tetraplegia and paraplegia. *Journal of Bone and Joint Surgery* 61–B:267 (August).

Guyton, A. C. 1981. *Textbook of medical physiology* (6th ed.). Philadelphia: W. B. Saunders.

Houk, J. C. 1979. Regulation of stiffness by skeletomotor reflexes. *Annual Review of Physiology* 41:99.

Iverson, L. L. 1979. The chemistry of the brain. *Scientific American* 241(3):134 (September).

Keynes, R. D. 1979. Ion channels in the nerve-cell membrane. *Scientific American* 240(3):126 (March).

Kostyuk, P. G., and Vasilenko, D. 1979. Spinal interneurons. *Annual Review of Physiology* 41:115.

Levi-Montalcini, R., and Calissano, P. 1979. The nerve-growth factor. *Scientific American* 240(6):68 (June).

Marx, J. L. 1980. Regeneration in the central nervous system. *Science* 209:378 (July 18).

Maugh, T. H. 1977. Multiple sclerosis: Genetic link, viruses suspected. *Science* 195:667 (February 18).

Maugh, T. H. 1977. Multiple sclerosis: Two or more viruses may be involved. *Science* 195:768 (February 25).

Maugh, T. H. 1977. The EAE model: A tentative connection to multiple sclerosis. *Science* 195:969 (March 11).

Morell, P., and Norton, W. T. 1980. Myelin. *Scientific American* 242(5):88 (May).

Prineas, J. W. 1979. Multiple sclerosis: Presence of lymphatic capillaries and lymphoid tissue in the brain and spinal cord. *Science* 203:1123 (March 16).

Schwartz, J. H. 1980. The transport of substances in nerve cells. *Scientific American* 242(4):152 (April).

Solomon, S. H. 1980. Brain peptides as neurotransmitters. *Science* 209:976 (August 29).

Stevens, C. F. 1979. The neuron. *Scientific American* 241(3):54 (September).

Victor, M., and Adams, R. D. 1981. *Principles of neurology* (2nd ed.). New York: McGraw-Hill.

11

NERVOUS SYSTEM: BRAIN AND CRANIAL NERVES

ORGANIZATION AND GENERAL FUNCTION

Objective 1. Describe the relationships of the brain and the cranial nerves to the rest of the nervous system and summarize the major functions of the brain and the cranial nerves.

As you read this sentence, many different activities are going on in your brain and cranial nerves. The largest part of your brain, the cerebrum, is concerned with thinking and memory and with receiving stimuli from all parts of the body, interpreting them, and initiating action. The next largest part, the cerebellum, is responsible for the coordination of muscular movements, and the remainder of the brain relays messages and controls activities of internal organs. These and other parts of the brain are shown in Figure 11.1.

Associated with the brain are twelve pairs of cranial nerves. These nerves carry sensory information from the sense organs located in the head to the brain; they carry motor impulses to the muscles of the head and some other parts of the body. The cranial nerves are part of the peripheral nervous system and are related to the brain as the spinal nerves are related to the spinal cord.

In this chapter we will consider the various activities of the brain and the cranial nerves in relation to the rest of the nervous system.

The functions of the brain have been a source of much puzzlement and confusion over the years. For centuries debate raged among learned people about whether the heart or the brain was the center of the intellect. Even when it became accepted that the brain was the organ in which conscious activities were controlled, it was thought by some that the cavities within the brain were filled with sensations and images. The tissues of the brain were relegated to the role of packing material. It was not until 1664 that Thomas Willis, a naturalist at Oxford University, stated the view that the cerebral cortex was the center of memory. At the end of the eighteenth century phrenology—the examination of external bumps on the skull—was used in an attempt to determine the function of different parts of the brain. Now known to be an unworkable scheme, phrenology nevertheless led to more scientific investigations. During the latter part of the nineteenth century several investigators used electrodes to stimulate the brain of experimental animals. (Some even used humans who happened to have a defect in the skull through which electrodes could be placed in their brains.) Through these studies many areas of the brain could be stimulated and their functions better understood.

The brain has been evolving in animals for millions of years, and the structure of the adult human brain contains structures that reflect such evolution. The stages in the embryonic development of the brain (already shown in Figure 10.2) parallel the three major evolutionary changes shown in Figure 11.2. The part of the brain that evolved first is termed the **reptilian brain**. The reptilian brain contains all the basic parts of the brain but includes very little of the cerebrum or cerebellum. The part that evolved next, the **limbic system**, seems to have capabilities for emotional experiences and possibly is able to determine the significance of perceived objects and events. For example, monkeys whose limbic system has been partially destroyed will eat hex nuts, bolts, and other nonfood items, presumably because their limbic system is no longer functioning to tell them what is food and what is not food. The limbic system is derived primarily from the forebrain of the embryo. The latest portion to evolve, the **neocortex**, or the neomammalian brain, makes up the largest part of the cerebrum in humans. Some portions of the neocortex are the last parts of the brain to complete development in the individual; these include the portion concerned with speech, and several areas, called association areas, involved with language, spatial abilities, memory, and planning. In humans some areas of the brain may not be fully developed until after ten years of age. Thus, it is understandable that children develop speech and other intellectual abilities over a period of time that correlates with the physiological development of their brains.

DEVELOPMENT

Objective 2. Summarize the embryonic development and the evolution of the brain.

Embryonic Development

Early in embryonic development the anterior end of the neural tube (shown in Figure 10.2, Chapter 10) enlarges and differentiates into three areas: the **forebrain** (prosencephalon), **midbrain** (mesencephalon), and **hindbrain** (rhombencephalon). Subsequently, the forebrain further differentiates into the telencephalon and the diencephalon, and the hindbrain further differentiates into the metencephalon and the myelencephalon. These embryonic divisions and the parts of the brain derived from them are listed in Table 11.1.

PARTS OF THE BRAINSTEM

Objective 3. Describe the location, structure, and function of (a) the medulla oblongata, (b) the pons, (c) the midbrain, (d) the thalamus, and (e) the hypothalamus.

The **brainstem**, continuous with the spinal cord and extending superiorly from it to the cerebrum, includes the medulla oblongata, pons, midbrain, thalamus, and hypothalamus (Figure 11.3)—essentially everything but the cerebellum and the telencephalon. A few other major structures are labeled in this figure; they will be discussed later.

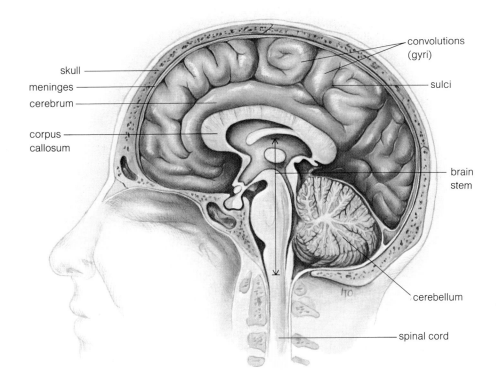

skull

meninges

cerebrum

corpus
callosum

convolutions
(gyri)

sulci

brain
stem

cerebellum

spinal cord

Figure 11.1 The general structure of the brain.

Throughout the brainstem are thousands of myelinated tracts and some aggregations of cell bodies called **nuclei**. The various areas of the brainstem operate below the level of consciousness, yet life is impossible without them.

Medulla Oblongata

In the **medulla oblongata** are numerous fibers (continuations of fibers to and from the spinal cord) and several important nuclei. Some of the nuclei of the medulla receive signals from fibers of the spinal tracts, integrate them with

other information, and then send the resulting signals on to the cerebellum or the thalamus. Other nuclei of the medulla—some of which are called centers—receive and integrate information from other parts of the brain and send out signals to control various functions. The **cardiac center** sends signals that regulate heart rate; the **vasomotor center** sends signals to the muscles of the blood vessels, causing the muscles to contract and the vessels to constrict; the **respiratory center** works in conjunction with centers in the pons to regulate the rate and depth of breathing. Still other centers in the medulla control functions such as coughing,

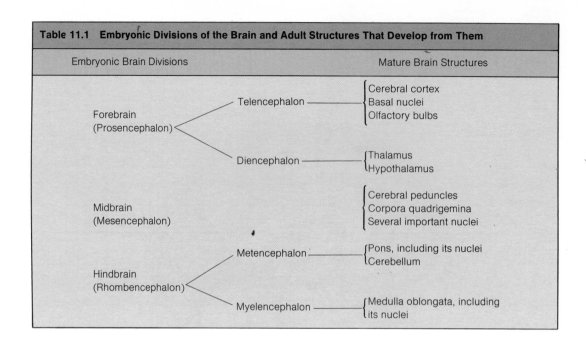

Table 11.1 Embryonic Divisions of the Brain and Adult Structures That Develop from Them		
Embryonic Brain Divisions		**Mature Brain Structures**
Forebrain (Prosencephalon)	Telencephalon	Cerebral cortex Basal nuclei Olfactory bulbs
	Diencephalon	Thalamus Hypothalamus
Midbrain (Mesencephalon)		Cerebral peduncles Corpora quadrigemina Several important nuclei
Hindbrain (Rhombencephalon)	Metencephalon	Pons, including its nuclei Cerebellum
	Myelencephalon	Medulla oblongata, including its nuclei

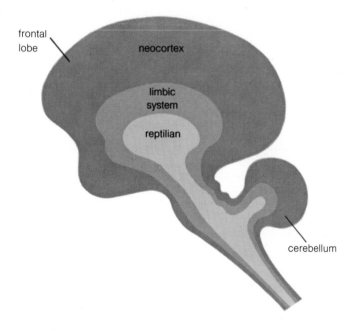

Figure 11.2 A schematic diagram of the three evolutionary parts of the brain.

sneezing, vomiting, swallowing, and hiccoughing. The nuclei of cranial nerves IX through XII are also found in the medulla. (Cranial nerves will be discussed later in this chapter.)

In the study of the spinal cord we noted that the gray matter occupies the central portion of the spinal cord, and the white matter occupies the peripheral portion. As the spinal tracts enter the medulla, they bend toward the midline so that the white matter intermingles with the gray matter throughout the brainstem. This arrangement blends into the segregated pattern present in the brain, where myelinated tracts occupy the central portion of the brain, and unmyelinated cell bodies and dendrites occupy the surface of the brain—just the opposite of the arrangement of the spinal cord.

Pons

In addition to the many fibers running through it from the medulla to the more superior parts of the brainstem, the **pons** also has fibers running horizontally. These fibers carry impulses between the two hemispheres of the cerebellum. Thus, the word *pons*, meaning bridge, is an appropriate name for this area of the brain. Many fibers that pass through the pons carry impulses between the cerebellum and the cerebrum. As will be explained later, these fibers are

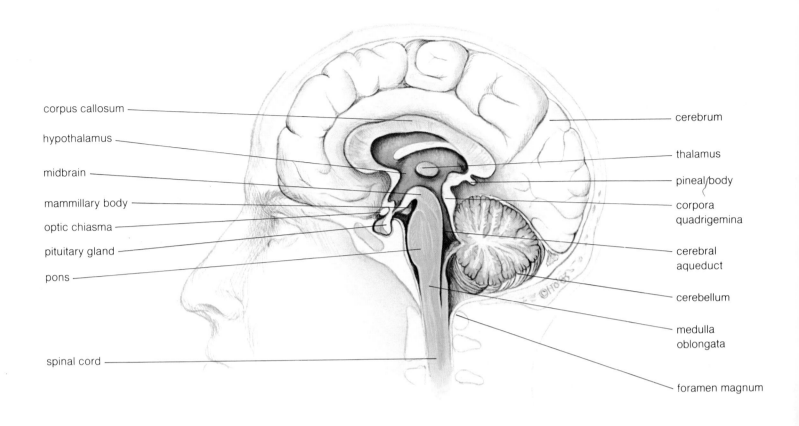

corpus callosum

hypothalamus

midbrain

mammillary body

optic chiasma

pituitary gland

pons

spinal cord

cerebrum

thalamus

pineal body

corpora quadrigemina

cerebral aqueduct

cerebellum

medulla oblongata

foramen magnum

Figure 11.3 A sagittal section through the brain, showing parts of the brainstem in color.

important in the coordination of voluntary movements. Nuclei of cranial nerves V through VIII are located in the pons, as are two of the respiratory centers.

Midbrain

The lower, or inferior, surface of the **midbrain** contains two bundles of fibers called the **cerebral peduncles**. They carry motor impulses from the cerebral cortex to the pons and spinal cord, and sensory impulses from the spinal cord to the thalamus. The upper, or superior, surface of the midbrain has two pairs of rounded protrusions collectively called the **corpora quadrigemina**. One pair, the **superior colliculi**, control reflexive movements of the head and eyeballs in response to visual and other stimuli. The other pair, the **inferior colliculi**, control reflexive movements of the head and trunk in response to auditory stimuli. The nuclei of cranial nerves III and IV that control movements of the eye are also located in the midbrain. Two other important nuclei are located in the midbrain: the **substantia nigra**, a dark area near the cerebral peduncles, and the **red nucleus**, located more posteriorly. Both of these nuclei are connected to the basal nuclei of the cerebrum and are concerned with motor functions.

Thalamus

The **thalamus**, which lies superior to the midbrain, contains many different nuclei, so it is composed primarily of gray matter. All sensory impulses except sensations of smell reach the cerebrum by way of the nuclei of the thalamus; the relay of such impulses is important in maintaining consciousness. Some nuclei of the thalamus also relay motor impulses from the cerebrum to the spinal cord. A few sensory impulses are processed in the thalamus without being relayed to the cerebral cortex—crude sensations of pain, temperature, and touch. Thus, the thalamus functions somewhat like a telephone switchboard by relaying impulses through its synapses, and occasionally acting as the "operator" by interpreting and responding to a message.

Hypothalamus

The **hypothalamus** lies below or inferior to the thalamus. It might be called the center for the maintenance of homeostasis because it regulates so many internal processes. It receives sensory impulses from the internal organs and uses this information to control the actions of the autonomic nervous system. As we shall see in Chapter 13, the autonomic nervous system regulates the activities of the visceral organs, blood supply to the muscles and skin, and even the size of the pupils of the eyes.

The hypothalamus also provides the anatomical connection between the nervous and endocrine systems, the two control systems of the body. This connection is through the hypophysis, or pituitary gland. The posterior part of the pituitary gland, which is derived from nervous tissue, is directly attached to the hypothalamus. The anterior pituitary gland lies next to and is physically (but not functionally) connected to the posterior pituitary. The hypothalamus is connected to the anterior pituitary by special blood vessels; it is connected to the posterior pituitary mainly by nerve fibers. These nervous and circulatory connections between the hypothalamus and the parts of the pituitary gland allow the hypothalamus to influence the pituitary gland. (The pituitary gland will be discussed with the endocrine system in Chapter 15.)

The hypothalamus is also influenced by the limbic system, the primitive part of the cerebrum. When the portion of the limbic system that is associated with emotions is stimulated, it sends signals to the hypothalamus. Such signals can cause a variety of responses because of the effects the hypothalamus can have on the autonomic nervous system and the pituitary gland. For example, you might consider fright an emotional response to a situation, but it has a physiological effect. When you are frightened, the

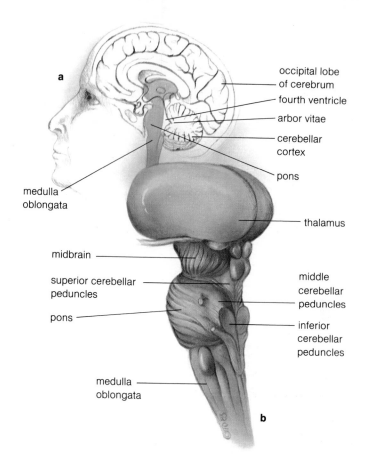

Figure 11.4 The cerebellum: (**a**) a sagittal section of the brain, showing the cerebellum, (**b**) the location of the cerebellar peduncles on the brainstem.

hypothalamus causes a portion of the autonomic system to respond to prepare the body to deal with the emergency. Blood pressure and heart rate increase, and the muscles receive more glucose and oxygen so they can contract forcefully over a long period of time with less susceptibility to fatigue. The hypothalamus also stimulates the pituitary gland to stimulate other glands in the body to respond to prolonged stress.

Other centers in the hypothalamus monitor body temperature and blood osmotic pressure and control effectors that maintain these functions at nearly constant levels by negative feedback. When body temperature rises or drops, the hypothalamus causes changes that bring the body temperature back to normal. Likewise, increasing blood osmotic pressure leads to the sensation of thirst, and fluids are consumed. Some of the water from the fluids enters the blood and reduces the osmotic pressure. Hunger and satiety centers are also present in the hypothalamus;

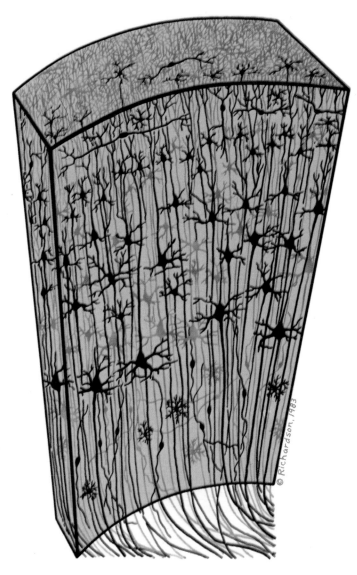

Figure 11.5 The cellular composition of the cerebellar cortex.

could not throw or catch a ball, write a word, or even walk in a straight line.

The second-largest part of the human brain, the **cerebellum** (Figure 11.4) is located inside the cranium under the occipital bones. It consists of two lateral hemispheres and a central worm-shaped part, the **vermis**. A cross-section of the hemispheres shows a branching treelike arrangement of gray and white matter called the **arbor vitae** (tree of life). The cerebellum is attached to the brainstem by three sets of fibers, the **superior, middle,** and **inferior cerebellar peduncles**. The superior peduncles connect the cerebellum with the midbrain, the middle peduncles connect it with the pons, and the inferior peduncles connect it with the medulla.

The cerebellum has an outer layer of gray matter called the **cerebellar cortex** (Figure 11.5). In the cortex are several kinds of neurons, of which the **Purkinje cells** are the most thoroughly studied. Each Purkinje cell may have as many as 100,000 synapses from other neurons on its dendrites. The axons of the Purkinje cells form many of the white myelinated tracts that run from the cerebellar cortex to the brainstem. These tracts also contain fibers that carry impulses to the cerebellar cortex. The net effect of the various cerebellar cells is to control and integrate muscular contractions.

The functions of the cerebellum are to coordinate movements and to help maintain posture and balance. All of its activities take place unconsciously. The cerebellum receives sensory impulses from the eyes and organs of balance as well as from sensory receptors in the muscles, tendons, and joints. It also receives collateral signals associated with motor signals for voluntary muscle action. Most of the output of the cerebellum is inhibitory. The actions of the cerebellum maintain muscle tone and integrate the contractions of the many separate muscles that are involved in complex movements. To accomplish this, the cerebellum adjusts the motor impulses in accordance with sensory information it is receiving. Thus, the cerebellum refines and coordinates voluntary movements.

these centers are discussed in Chapter 22. See Table 11.2 later in this chapter for a summary of the functions of the parts of the brainstem as well as other parts of the brain.

CEREBELLUM

Objective 4. Describe the location, structure, and function of the cerebellum.

You are never aware of the actions of your cerebellum, yet you depend on it for nearly every movement you make. If your cerebellum were not functioning properly, you

CEREBRUM

Objective 5. Describe the location, structure, and function of the cerebrum.

In everyday language the word brain is often used to mean the part of the cerebrum that carries out conscious thought processes. Except for some crude sensations that are interpreted in the thalamus, any object, event, or thought that has reached the level of awareness is processed in a part of the cerebrum; any intentional movement is initiated by the cerebrum. Other parts of the cerebrum carry out activities below the level of consciousness.

Structure and Function

The **cerebrum** is the largest and most complex of all the parts of the human brain. It consists of left and right hemispheres connected by a large bundle of myelinated fibers, the **corpus callosum** (see Figure 11.1), and other smaller fiber bundles. The outer several millimeters of the cerebrum consists of six layers of cell bodies in most areas. This layered arrangement of cell bodies, called the **cerebral cortex**, makes up the gray matter of the cerebrum. The interconnections among these cell bodies are far more complex than that in the cerebellum and are not well understood.

The surface of the cortex (Figure 11.6) is greatly folded. The upward folds, or **gyri** (singular, gyrus), alternate with the downward grooves, or **sulci** (singular, sulcus). The larger sulci, called **fissures**, divide each hemisphere into lobes. The **frontal, parietal, occipital,** and **temporal** lobes lie approximately beneath the skull bones of the same name. A very deep fissure, the **longitudinal fissure**, separates the two hemispheres.

A number of functional areas of the cortex have been identified (Figure 11.7), often by observing the effects of injuries to specific areas of the brain or by stimulating certain areas in the brains of animals. Some of our understanding of human brain function comes from stimulating selected areas of the human brain during brain surgery, as was initially done by the Canadian surgeon Penfield.

Each hemisphere is divided into an anterior and a posterior region by a **central fissure**. On either side of the central fissure are important functional areas. The **postcentral gyrus** in the parietal lobe, which lies immediately posterior

During brain surgery, the brain is sometimes stimulated to assure that vital parts of it are not disturbed during the surgical procedure. Such stimulation does not usually inflict pain because no pain receptors are present in the brain itself. Local anesthetics are used during the opening of the cranial cavity but the person remains awake during the brain stimulation. In this way the person can report what he or she experiences from stimulation of memory areas.

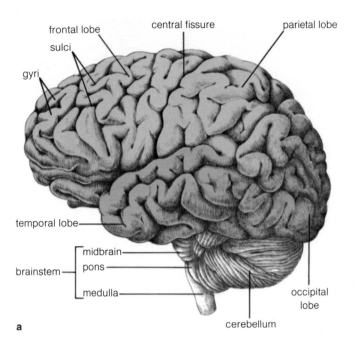

a

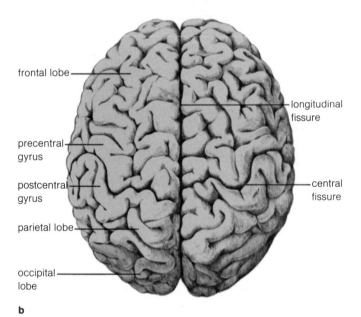

b

Figure 11.6   The external surface of the brain, showing the lobes of the cerebrum, gyri, sulci, and the relationships of the cerebrum to other parts of the brain: (**a**) lateral view, (**b**) superior view.

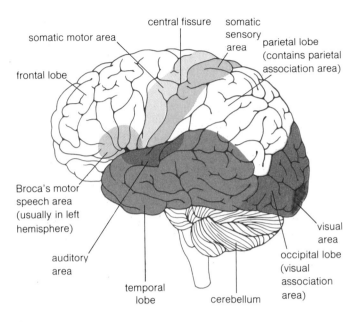

Figure 11.7 Some of the major functional areas of the cerebral cortex.

to the fissure, is devoted mainly to receiving sensory signals from the skin and from taste receptors; thus, it is called the **somatic sensory area**. The **precentral gyrus** in the frontal lobe, which lies immediately anterior to the fissure, is devoted mainly to initiating motor impulses that cause contraction of voluntary muscles; thus, it is called the **somatic motor area**. In addition, particular areas along each of these gyri are related to certain parts of the body, as shown in Figure 11.8. Labeled areas pertaining to special senses are discussed later in this chapter.

In the last chapter we considered how the tracts of the spinal cord carry signals to and from the brain (see Table 10.2). Now that we are familiar with structures in the brain, we can trace the main pathways of sensory and motor signals. Recall that all spinal tracts are paired, even though they may be shown on only one side of the figures that follow. Some pathways by which sensory signals are relayed to the brain are shown in Figure 11.9.

On the left side of the figure locate the gracile and cuneate fasciculi. These tracts carry signals from skin re-

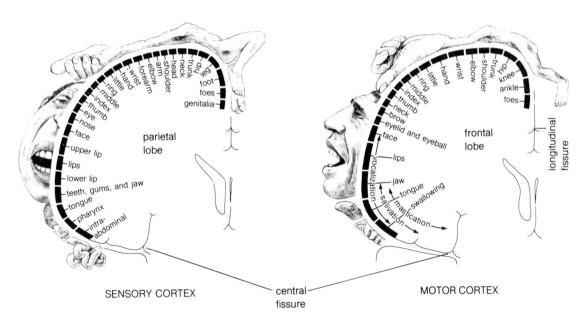

Figure 11.8 The location of sensory and motor areas of the cortex, with sketches of the parts of the body each portion serves. Each of the body parts in the figure is represented in proportion to the area of the cortex with which it is associated.

ceptors sensitive to fine touch and from muscle receptors that make it possible to sense body position. The cuneate fasciculus carries signals from the arms and trunk; the gracile fasciculus carries signals from the legs. In both cases branches of the sensory axon carry signals along the same side of the spinal cord to a nucleus in the medulla (the nucleus gracilis or the nucleus cuneatus), where they synapse with neurons whose axons decussate (cross over to the opposite side of the brainstem) and carry signals to the thalamus. From the synapses in the thalamus the signals are carried to the somatic sensory area of the cerebral cortex.

Also on the left side of Figure 11.9 find the spinocerebellar tracts. Signals from muscle spindles arriving in the posterior horn are relayed to spinocerebellar fibers and then travel along the same side of the spinal cord and brainstem to the cerebellar cortex. Information from these signals is used in the control of muscle tone and posture.

On the right side of Figure 11.9 find the lateral spinothalamic tract. Signals from pain and temperature receptors are sent to the posterior horn by way of peripheral sensory fibers. These fibers synapse with neurons of the lateral spinothalamic tracts; axons of these tracts decussate immediately and carry signals up the spinal cord and brainstem to the thalamus. Here they synapse with other neurons whose axons carry signals to the somatic sensory area of the cerebral cortex.

Also on the right side of Figure 11.9 find the anterior spinothalamic tract. Signals from crude touch and pressure receptors in the skin are carried by peripheral sensory fibers to the posterior horn, where they synapse with neurons of the anterior spinothalamic tract. These axons decussate and carry signals to the thalamus, where they synapse onto other neurons that carry signals to the somatic sensory area.

By way of these various sensory pathways information from sensory receptors is relayed to the cerebral cortex where touch, temperature, and pain signals are received, and information used to control muscle tone and posture is relayed to the cerebellum. All of this sensory information is processed in the cerebrum or cerebellum and used to determine what kind of motor signals will be sent out.

Some pathways by which motor signals are relayed from the brain to skeletal muscles are shown in Figure 11.10. On the left side of the figure find the lateral and anterior corticospinal tracts. Upper motor neurons of both of these tracts originate in the somatic motor area of the cerebral cortex and pass through the internal capsule (a bundle of nerve tracts in the white matter of the cerebrum), brainstem, and spinal cord, where they finally synapse onto lower motor neurons of the peripheral nervous system in the anterior horn of the spinal cord gray matter. Damage to an upper motor neuron can lead to spastic paralysis (paral-

ysis in the contracted state); damage to a lower motor neuron can lead to flaccid paralysis (paralysis in a relaxed state). Both of these tracts, which carry signals that stimulate voluntary muscle action, are often referred to as the **pyramidal tracts**. The lateral tract decussates in the **pyramid** of the medulla and is therefore often referred to as the pyramidal tract proper; the anterior tract decussates in the spinal cord near where its fibers form synapses with peripheral motor neurons. Sensory signals received in the brain that call for movement of skeletal muscles are relayed to one of these tracts (as well as to some other brain centers). About 85% of these corticospinal tracts are in the lateral bundles; the remainder are in the anterior bundles.

On the right side of Figure 11.10 find the rubrospinal tract, which originates in the red nucleus of the midbrain and passes through the remainder of the brainstem and spinal cord to the anterior horn, where it forms synapses with motor neurons of the peripheral nervous system. Signals carried by this tract help to control muscle tone and posture; such signals are typically initiated as a result of sensory information received by the cerebellum. Also on the right side of Figure 11.10 locate the reticulospinal tract, which originates in the reticular formation of the brainstem, decussates in the brainstem, and carries signals to the anterior horn, where the signals are relayed to peripheral motor neurons. These signals increase muscle tone and motor activity. Finally, locate the vestibulospinal tract on the right side of Figure 11.10. This tract originates in the vestibular nucleus of the medulla and carries signals without decussating to the anterior horn of the spinal cord, where its fibers synapse with peripheral motor neurons. Signals conveyed by this tract help to maintain equilibrium and balance. All of the tracts found on the right side of Figure 11.10 are referred to collectively as the **extrapyramidal tracts**. Many of the signals carried by these tracts are from centers concerned with coordination and balance, and they help to control and integrate the conscious signals carried by the pyramidal tracts.

To illustrate how sensory and motor signals are integrated, suppose you are sitting on an uncomfortable chair in a hot, stuffy classroom. Sensory signals arrive in the somatic sensory area of your brain by way of peripheral sensory neurons and various spinal tracts—allowing you to perceive sitting position via the gracile and cuneate fascicles, pressures from the uncomfortable chair via the anterior spinothalamic tracts, and the warmth of the room via the lateral spinothalamic tracts. Subconscious sensory signals via the spinocerebellar tracts provide the information to the cerebellum for maintaining your posture. As a result of all of these sensory signals, you decide to get up from your chair, walk to a window, and open it. To allow you to do these

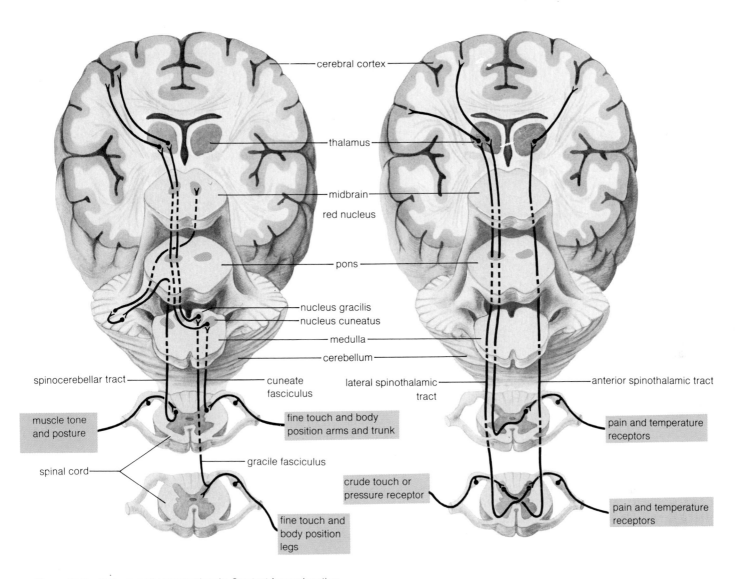

cerebral cortex

thalamus

midbrain
red nucleus

pons

nucleus gracilis
nucleus cuneatus

medulla
cerebellum

spinocerebellar tract

cuneate
fasciculus

lateral spinothalamic
tract

anterior spinothalamic tract

muscle tone
and posture

fine touch and body
position arms and trunk

pain and temperature
receptors

spinal cord

gracile fasciculus

crude touch or
pressure receptor

pain and temperature
receptors

fine touch and
body position
legs

Figure 11.9   Pathways of sensory signals. See text for explanation.

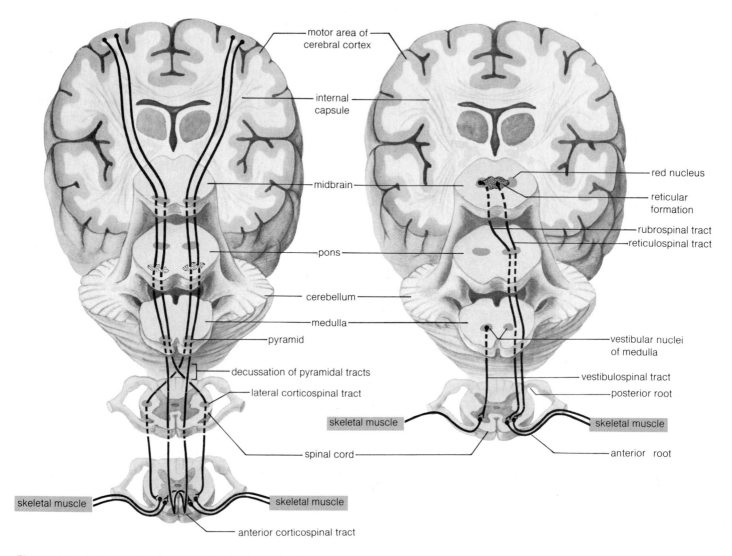

Figure 11.10 Pathways of motor signals. See text for explanation.

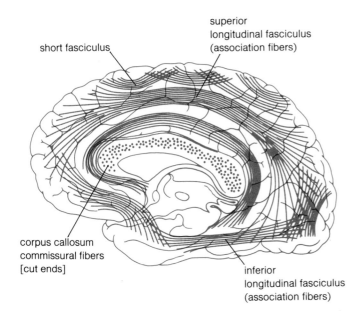

short fasciculus

superior
longitudinal fasciculus
(association fibers)

corpus callosum
commissural fibers
[cut ends]

inferior
longitudinal fasciculus
(association fibers)

Figure 11.11 Some pathways that connect the association areas of the cerebrum.

things, various motor signals are initiated in the somatic motor area of your brain and pass through the pyramidal tracts and peripheral motor neurons, causing contraction of the muscles required for you to walk and to open the window. Simultaneous signals from the cerebrum to the cerebellum initiate signals in the extrapyramidal tracts to maintain your balance and coordinate your movements. Thus, all of the spinal tracts described above are involved in sensing a situation and carrying out an appropriate action. Even so, this example is simplified; we have not considered important sensory input from your eyes and organs of balance and how these signals are integrated and used in coordinating movements.

In addition to the somatic sensory and motor areas other functional areas of the cerebrum include the **visual area** in the occipital lobe, the **auditory area** in the temporal lobe, and **Broca's motor speech area** in the frontal lobe (usually in the left hemisphere). (Refer back to Figure 11.7.) Sensory signals come from the retina of the eye via the thalamus to the visual area, where they are processed and then sent to the **visual association area**. The visual association area occupies most of the occipital lobe anterior to the visual area and is responsible for interpreting images received by the visual area. Sensory signals from the sound receptors in the inner ear are relayed via the thalamus to the auditory area and then to the **parietal association area**,

where they are interpreted. The auditory area, where spoken language is processed, is closely associated with Broca's motor speech area, where sentences are formulated and speech is initiated. However, the somatic motor area is also involved in the actual muscular movements required for speech. Thus, many interactions occur among the auditory area, Broca's area, and the somatic motor area as individuals receive spoken words and respond to them with other spoken words. People who have a defective Broca's area have seriously impaired speech; they can make noises and sometimes reply with a simple "yes" or "no," but they cannot formulate sentences.

Though briefly mentioned above, association areas deserve further comment. An **association area** is a portion of the cerebral cortex that neither receives direct sensory stimuli nor directly initiates motor impulses; instead, it appears to process and interpret sensory impulses. The association area in the frontal lobe seems to be concerned with such activities as planning for the future, solving problems, and determining appropriateness of behavior. The parietal association area interprets sizes, shapes, the quality of sensations, and other characteristics of objects touched. It also functions in the understanding of spoken words and the perception of one's body in relation to extrapersonal space. The temporal association area deals with remembering sensory experiences, especially things seen and heard, and interpreting new experiences in relation to what is remembered. Finally, the visual association area, as noted earlier, interprets visual images.

Tracts in the Cerebrum

Beneath the gray matter of the cortex is the white matter of the cerebrum, made up of three kinds of tracts, or bundles of fibers (Figure 11.11). **Association fibers** connect two functional areas of the cortex within the same hemisphere. Such fibers carry impulses between sensory and motor gyri and between sensory input areas and association areas, and between association areas. **Commissural fibers** connect the two hemispheres. The corpus callosum is the largest of the commissural tracts. **Projection fibers** carry impulses between the cerebral cortex and other parts of the central nervous system. An example of such tracts are the pyramidal tracts that carry signals from the somatic motor area through the spinal cord (see Figure 11.10).

Basal Nuclei

Deep inside the cerebrum are the **basal nuclei**, groups of cell bodies of neurons (Figure 11.12). Each nucleus is paired,

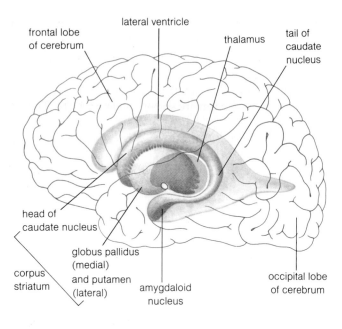

Figure 11.12 The location of the basal nuclei of the cerebrum.

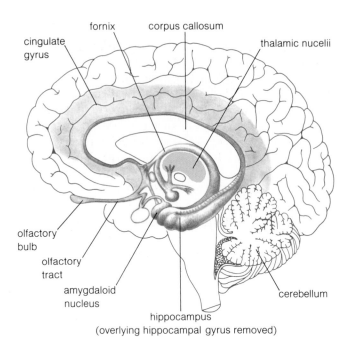

Figure 11.13 The major pathways of the limbic system.

and one member of each pair lies in each hemisphere. The largest nucleus is the **corpus striatum**. It includes the head of the **caudate nucleus**, the **globus pallidus**, and the **putamen**. The **amygdaloid nucleus** is attached to the tail of the caudate nucleus. These nuclei of the cerebrum are connected by fibers to each other and to other nuclei in the brainstem. The brainstem nuclei include the **subthalamic nuclei**, the substantia nigra, and the red nucleus of the midbrain.

The main function of the basal nuclei is to control muscle tone, often by inhibiting contractions. Their activities are coordinated with those of the cerebellum. The nuclei of the corpus striatum seem to work together to help control gross intentional movements, such as walking, that we normally perform automatically. These nuclei also appear to control muscle tone to allow specific fine muscle actions. For example, when you prepare to write something on a piece of paper, you position your arm in a certain way. Maintaining the appropriate tone in the muscles of the arm so you can use muscles of your hand to write is one of the functions of the basal nuclei. Destruction of the basal nuclei makes it impossible to maintain the arm in a position that allows the fine muscles of the hand to be used effectively. Damage to any of the nuclei of the basal ganglia can lead to the development of various kinds of tremors (involuntary movements).

Limbic System

The limbic system consists of some parts of the cerebrum and some parts of the brainstem (Figure 11.13). Two gyri of the cerebrum, the **cingulate gyrus** and the **hippocampal gyrus**, are part of the limbic system, as is the **hippocampus** (a nucleus). One of the basal nuclei, the amygdaloid nucleus, is also considered part of the limbic system. Some anatomists consider the anterior thalamic nuclei and the hypothalamus to be part of the limbic system, even though they are part of the brainstem. Note that the olfactory bulb and tract, which carry signals for sensing smell, are closely associated with the limbic system.

Other general functions of the limbic system include emotional aspects of behavior and some memory storage. In fact, emotions and memory seem to be closely associated. Learning experiments in monkeys show that, unless experience has either reward or punishment associated with it, the monkey is unlikely to remember it. It is thought that the hippocampus plays a role in determining what memories will be stored and that the emotional aspects of the experience affect what is remembered. Many different kinds of emotional experiences including rage, sexual arousal, aggressiveness, fear, and loss of fear have been associated with some part of the limbic system.

Many odors—the pleasant odor of a rose or the un-

Recent studies of the relationship of the limbic system to behavior have often made use of electrodes placed in selected areas of an animal brain. In some experiments the electrodes are placed so that the animal may stimulate its own brain by pressing a lever in its cage. In other experiments the animal is able to turn off stimulation or leave it on. By noting the effects of electrodes in specific areas, these studies have led to the location of pleasure or reward centers and punishment centers. Reward centers have been found in the hypothalamus, the amygdaloid nucleus, and some other areas of the basal nuclei and the thalamus. Some reward centers located in monkeys provide such satisfying stimuli that the animal will press a lever to receive stimulation up to 7000 times an hour. Punishment centers have been found in the thalamus and the hypothalamus. In some cases stimulation of a punishment or pain center inhibits a pleasure or reward center, thereby preventing the experiencing of pleasurable feelings.

A relatively new diagnostic technique called a CAT scan (computerized axial tomography) allows us to obtain radiographs (X rays) of selected sections through an organ. Some of the sections from such a scan of a human brain are shown in Figure 11.14. The technique might be used to detect a tumor or other abnormality. Here the frames from the scan are used to locate selected structures of the brain.

pleasant odor of spoiled food—elicit emotional feelings. One explanation of how odors are related to emotions is that the amygdaloid nucleus of the limbic system is connected to the olfactory bulb, a bundle of nerve fibers that carries signals from the smell receptors in the nasal epithelium to the cerebrum. Thus, signals from smell receptors may be relayed to the limbic system as well as to the cerebral cortex.

Reticular Formation

The **reticular formation** consists of columns of nuclei in the central core of the brainstem. Because it is concerned mostly with the control of wakefulness and sleep, it will be considered with those topics in the next chapter.

Summary of Brain Parts

The human brain is an exceedingly complex organ; the above discussion provides only a general overview of that organ. Table 11.2 summarizes the major parts of the brain and their functions.

CIRCULATION OF BLOOD AND CEREBROSPINAL FLUID

Objective 6. Describe the structure, location, and function of the ventricles of the brain and the blood vessels of the brain; explain how cerebrospinal fluid and blood circulate in the brain.

In the last chapter the arrangement of the meninges of the brain and spinal cord was described, and the location and function of the cerebrospinal fluid was discussed briefly. In this section we will consider the ventricles and blood vessels of the brain and relate their functions to the meninges and cerebrospinal fluid. Blood circulation in the brain is discussed here because of its intimate association with cerebrospinal fluid circulation.

Ventricles and Cerebrospinal Fluid

The **ventricles** consist of four hollow, fluid-filled spaces inside the brain (Figure 11.15). A **lateral ventricle** lies inside each hemisphere of the cerebrum. Each lateral ventricle is connected to the third ventricle by an **interventricular foramen**. The **third ventricle** consists of a narrow channel between the hemispheres through the area of the thalamus. It is connected by the **cerebral aqueduct (aqueduct of Sylvius)** in the midbrain portion of the brainstem to the fourth ventricle in the pons and medulla. The **fourth ventricle** is continuous with the central canal of the spinal cord. Three openings in the roof of the fourth ventricle, a pair of **lateral apertures** (foramina of Luschka) and a **median aperture** (foramen of Magendie) allow cerebrospinal fluid to move upward to the subarachnoid space that surrounds the brain and spinal cord.

The roof of each ventricle contains a network of capillaries called a **choroid plexus**. These capillaries receive blood from the small arteries of the pia mater. Cerebro-

Table 11.2   Major Parts of the Brain and Their Functions

Part	Function
Medulla oblongata	Receives and integrates signals from spinal cord and sends resulting signals to the cerebellum and thalamus
	Contains centers that regulate heart rate, blood pressure, repiratory rate, coughing, and some other involuntary movements
Pons	Relays impulses between the medulla and more superior part of the brain, between the hemispheres of the cerebellum, and between the cerebrum and cerebellum
	Contains centers that work with those in the medulla to regulate respiratory rate
Midbrain	Relays sensory impulses between spinal cord and thalamus and motor impulses between the cerebral cortex and the pons and spinal cord
	Controls reflexive movements of the head and eyeballs in response to visual stimuli and of the head and trunk in response to auditory stimuli
Thalamus	Contains many different nuclei through which it relays all sensory impulses (except sensations of smell) to the cerebral cortex
	Relays motor impulses from the cerebral cortex to the spinal cord
	Relays to the cerebral cortex impulses that maintain consciousness
	Processes some crude sensations
Hypothalamus	Receives sensory impulses from the internal organs by way of the thalamus and uses these impulses to control actions of the autonomic nervous system, thereby helping to maintain homeostasis
	Provides anatomical connection between the nervous and endocrine system by its relationship to the pituitary gland
	In combination with the limbic system participates in physiological response to emotional experiences
Cerebellum	Receives sensory information from the eyes; organs of balance; and receptors in muscles, tendons, and joints
	Uses sensory information to control and integrate complex voluntary muscular movements
Cerebrum	Contains areas that receive and process sensory information (somatic sensory area, visual area, auditory area) and that initiate motor impulses for voluntary movements (somatic motor area and speech area)
	Contains association areas where sensory information is interpreted, memories are stored, and complex processing occurs
	Contains tracts of association fibers, commissural fibers, and projection fibers
Limbic system	Contains basal nuclei, which control muscle tone
	Contains pleasure and punishment centers and so plays a role in emotional feelings
	Hippocampus plays a role in determining what memories will be stored
Reticular formation	Contains nuclei that are involved in wakefulness and sleep

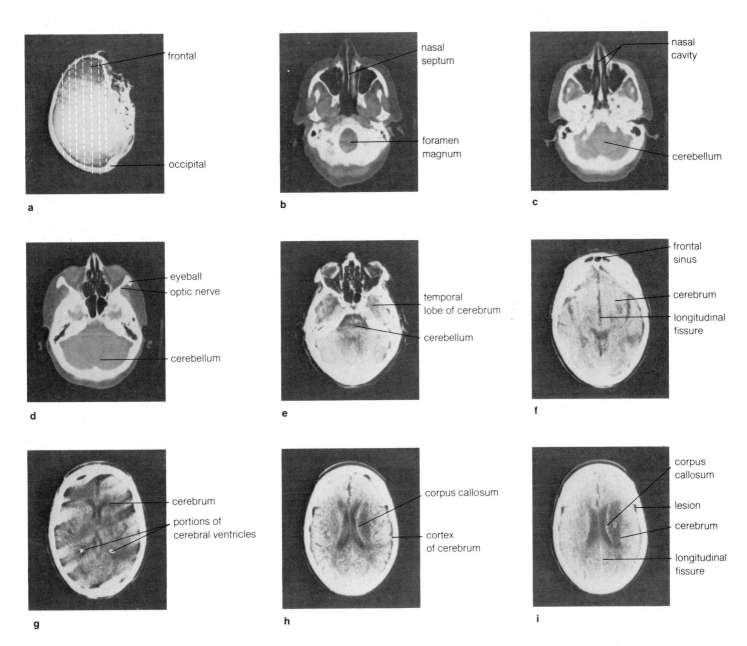

Figure 11.14 A CAT scan of the brain of an eighty-year-old woman: (**a**) a side view of the brain, with dotted lines showing the planes through the brain represented by individual frames from the scan, (**b**) a frame through the base of the brain (plane 1), (**c** through **h**) successive frames from the base of the brain toward the superior surface of the brain, (**i**) a frame from the scan showing a lesion in the left hemisphere of the cerebrum. (Courtesy of Alexandria Hospital, Alexandria, Virginia, Joyce R. Isbel, R.T.)

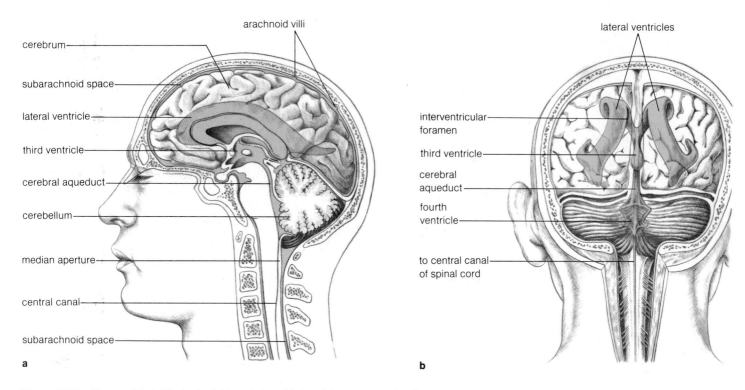

cerebrum

subarachnoid space

lateral ventricle

third ventricle

cerebral aqueduct

cerebellum

median aperture

central canal

subarachnoid space

arachnoid villi

a

lateral ventricles

interventricular foramen

third ventricle

cerebral aqueduct

fourth ventricle

to central canal of spinal cord

b

Figure 11.15 The ventricles of the brain: (**a**) lateral view, (**b**) dorsal view, presented as if the brain were transparent.

spinal fluid is secreted from each choroid plexus as follows. First, sodium ions are actively secreted into the ventricles. These ions, being positively charged, draw negatively charged ions, particularly chloride ions, into the ventricles. The presence of all these ions in the ventricular fluid increases its osmotic pressure within the ventricles and causes water to move by osmosis from the blood into the ventricles. The osmotic pressure of the cerebrospinal fluid remains about 160 mm Hg—about five times that of the blood.

Just as cerebrospinal fluid is constantly being formed, it is also constantly being reabsorbed into the blood. The openings in the roof of the fourth ventricle, the lateral and median aperatures, allow cerebrospinal fluid to reach the subarachnoid space. Arachnoid villi extend into this space, primarily over the dorsal surfaces of the hemispheres. Because of the high permeability of the arachnoid villi, cerebrospinal fluid freely passes through them into the dural sinuses.

Refer back to Figure 10.24 for a review of the location of the meninges and the spaces between them. Figure 11.16 summarizes the flow of cerebrospinal fluid.

Cerebrospinal fluid is found inside all the ventricles, in the central canal of the spinal cord, and in the subarachnoid

space around both the brain and spinal cord. The total volume of cerebrospinal fluid is about 150 milliliters. It is secreted at a rate of about 840 milliliters per day and reab-

Babies are sometimes born with a high cerebrospinal fluid pressure, often due to overproduction of fluid or an obstruction that prevents the outflow of fluid to the subarachnoid space. This condition is called **hydrocephalus**, which means water on the brain. In infants the bones of the skull have not completely developed and can easily be spread apart. If hydrocephalus is not treated, the fluid accumulates, and the skull becomes enlarged. The ventricles become even more enlarged than the skull so that the brain is flattened and pressed against the skull. The situation leads to brain damage if it is untreated. Hydrocephalus is now treated by placing a shunt in a ventricle of the brain to drain the cerebrospinal fluid into a vein to the heart or directly into the abdominal cavity (Figure 11.17).

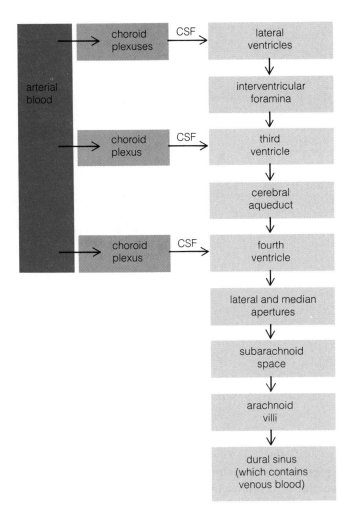

Figure 11.16 Flow of cerebrospinal fluid.

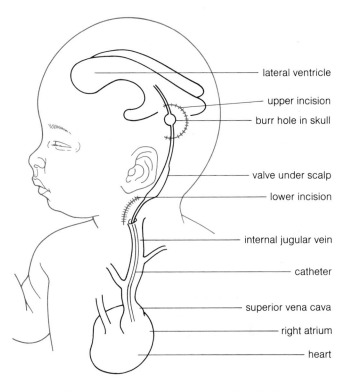

Figure 11.17 Hydrocephalus can be treated by placing a shunt between a cerebral ventricle and the heart or the abdominal cavity.

sorbed at the same rate, so the volume remains constant. Thus, the pressure within the ventricles and other cavities containing cerebrospinal fluid remains constant. However, conditions such as tumors, infections, and hemorrhages in the brain can disrupt the normal flow of cerebrospinal fluid, causing the pressure to change.

Cerebrospinal fluid acts as a shock absorber for the brain and spinal cord and may also contribute to nourishing brain tissue. When a person receives a blow to the head, the fluid absorbs the shock and minimizes the likelihood of damage to the nervous system. In a severe blow to the head fluid is pushed away from the side of the brain opposite the site of the blow, and the brain may hit the opposite cranial wall with sufficient force to cause tissue damage. As a result, the tissue damage occurs on the side of the brain opposite

the site of the blow. In such a concussion usually no permanent damage to brain tissue occurs. The injury may cause a massive electrical discharge within the brain tissue, but the mental confusion that results generally disappears after a few days.

Circulation of Blood in the Brain

A continuous supply of blood to the brain is essential for the cells to receive the glucose and oxygen they need and for wastes to be removed from them. Though most other tissues can metabolize fats as well as glucose, the brain normally requires glucose as its energy source. It has been estimated that the brain uses as much as 75% of the glucose consumed by the body.

The normal rate of blood flow through the brain is about 50 to 55 milliliters per 100 grams of brain tissue per minute. This amounts to about 15% of the total output of the heart when the body is at rest. Gray matter receives approximately six times as much blood as white matter. If the carbon dioxide concentration increases in the blood, it causes the acidity of the blood to increase, in turn causing the blood vessels of the brain tissue to dilate, and a larger volume of blood flows into the brain. Other substances, such as the metabolic product lactic acid, also increase the acidity of the blood and increase the blood flow to the brain. Though carbon dioxide concentration in the blood is the most sensitive regulator of blood supply to the brain, a decrease in oxygen concentration can also cause dilation of blood vessels. Severe brain damage occurs if the brain is deprived of its supply of oxygen and glucose for more than a few minutes.

Blood Vessels

The blood vessels that supply the brain include a pair of **internal carotid arteries**, which branch from the common carotid arteries in the neck, and a pair of **vertebral arteries**, which ascend to the brain on either side of the cervical vertebrae. As shown in Figure 11.18, the internal carotid arteries branch on each side of the brain to form left and right **anterior** and **middle cerebral arteries**. The paired vertebral arteries fuse into a single **basilar artery**, which in turn branches several times to form the paired **posterior cerebral arteries** and the arteries that supply the cerebellum and brainstem. The vertebral and carotid arteries join at the base of the brain via **communicating arteries** to form the **circle of Willis**, which permits blood to flow into any of the many vessels connected to it. In the event of a blockage of a blood vessel, blood can often flow in an alternate path, thus minimizing the damage to the brain because of the blockage. This problem will be discussed in more detail in Chapter 19.

Blood leaves the brain through many veins and the **dural sinuses**. The dural sinuses drain into the internal jugular veins (Figure 11.19).

The Blood–Brain Barrier

In most of the tissues of the body substances move freely between the capillaries (the smallest blood vessels) and the cells. However, in the tissues of the brain, except for parts of the hypothalamus, movement is limited by the structure of

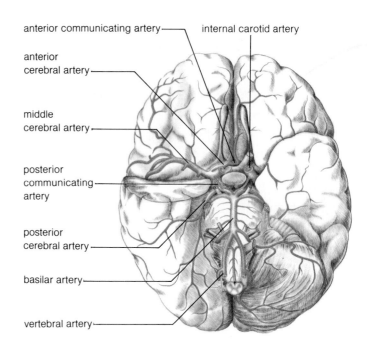

Figure 11.18 A ventral view of the brain, showing the distribution of arteries in the brain. The circle of Willis is formed by the anterior and posterior communicating arteries.

Arteriograms (Figure 11.20) can be made to determine the degree to which blood circulates through all the arteries of an organ. A dye that is opaque to X rays is injected into a major artery, and X-ray photographs of the artery and its branches are made as the dye circulates through them. An arteriogram of the brain might determine how adequately the cerebrum is supplied with blood. Failure of the dye to pass through all of the arteries of the cerebrum usually is due to blockage of one or more of these vessels. Blockage might be caused by deposits of fatty substances in the arterial wall (atherosclerosis, described in Chapter 19) or the presence of a blood clot.

the capillary walls and the surrounding connective tissue. These structures constitute the **blood–brain barrier** (Figure 11.21). The capillaries lack pores, or openings, that are found in the thin walls of other capillaries. Instead, the endothelial cells that make up the capillary wall are overlap-

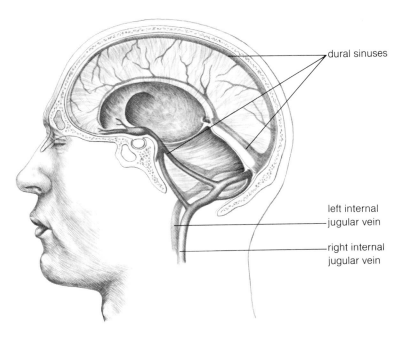

dural sinuses

left internal
jugular vein

right internal
jugular vein

Figure 11.19   A lateral view of the head, showing the location of the dural sinuses.

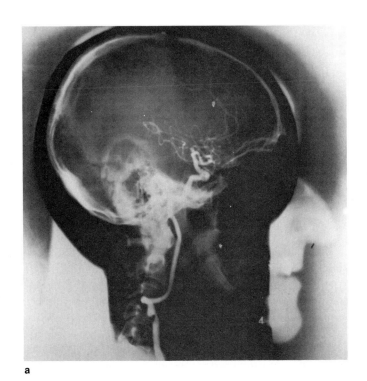

a

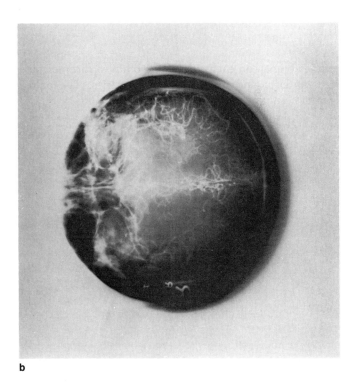

b

Figure 11.20   Arteriograms of the cerebrum: (**a**) a lateral view, showing dye in the internal carotid artery and in some of the arteries of the brain, (**b**) a frontal view of the cerebrum, showing dye in many of the arteries of the cerebrum. (Courtesy of Alexandria Hospital, Alexandria, Virginia, Joyce R. Isbel, R.T.)

ping, so that in some places the wall is two cells thick. Furthermore, the capillary is surrounded by a basement membrane, which in turn is partially surrounded by foot processes (cytoplasmic extensions) of an astrocyte, one of the glial cells of the brain. Substances leaving the capillaries of the brain, then, must pass through one or sometimes two cells in the capillary wall, the basement membrane, and often an astrocyte before reaching the fluids that surround the cells. This blood–brain barrier prevents many toxic substances that might be circulating in the blood from reaching the cells of the brain. It also makes it very difficult to deliver certain antibiotics and other types of medication to the cells of the brain.

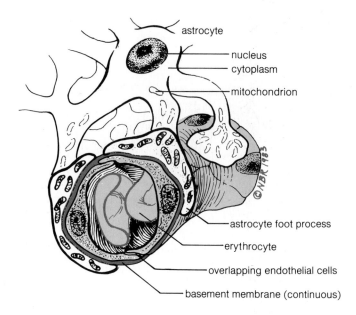

Figure 11.21 The structure of a capillary in the brain surrounded by an astrocytic foot process, showing how the blood–brain barrier is created.

Blood Flow and Cerebral Activity

Until recently studies of the functions of various parts of the cerebrum were based on experiments in which different points on the cortex were stimulated electrically and the behavioral effects observed. Now a new technique has been developed by Lassen and his colleagues in Denmark and Sweden. They inject a solution of the radioactive isotope xenon 133 into one of the main arteries of the brain, and use a radiation counter to monitor the arrival and departure of the radioactive substance as it circulates through the brain. Several hundred radiation detectors, each of which scans about 1 square centimeter of the cortex, are used. Computer techniques then create pictures of the variations in radioactivity in different parts of the brain (Figure 11.22). The colors in the pictures indicate the blood flow, and thus metabolic activity, of each area of the cortex. Dark gray indicates an average blood flow rate, light gray indicates flow rates as much as 20% below average, and color indicates flow rates up to 20% above average.

In resting subjects the brain is anything but at rest. The greatest metabolic activity is in the frontal area, where planning and problem solving appear to occur. This finding agrees with subjects' reports that they were thinking about problems or planning some kinds of future activities. Many of the studies of sensory perception and voluntary motor activity using this technique confirm findings from electrical stimulation studies. One surprising finding was that the left and right hemispheres were both active during speaking; earlier studies had shown that the functions of speech generally involved only one hemisphere, nearly always the left one. Furthermore, these investigators found that the act of reading aloud involves seven discrete centers in each hemisphere.

CRANIAL NERVES

Objective 7. List the twelve cranial nerves in order and describe the location and function of each.

The **cranial nerves** carry sensory and motor impulses to and from the brain. Each passes through a foramen in the skull as it runs between the organ it supplies and the brain. Unlike spinal nerves, cranial nerves lack dorsal and ventral roots. The twelve pairs of cranial nerves are identified by Roman numerals I through XII in order of their attachment from the front to the back of the brain. (Refer to Figure 11.23 as you read about each nerve.) The cranial nerves also have names that are associated with their functions. Some cranial nerves carry only sensory impulses. Several of the cranial nerves are called mixed nerves because they contain fibers of both types. The characteristics of the cranial nerves are summarized in Table 11.3.

The **olfactory nerves** (I) are sensory nerves. Their fibers run from the smell receptors in the nasal epithelium through the cribriform plate of the skull and enter the **olfactory bulbs**, which lie inferior to the frontal lobes of the cerebrum (Figure 11.23b). Here the fibers synapse with neurons of the olfactory tract. Fibers of the olfactory tract

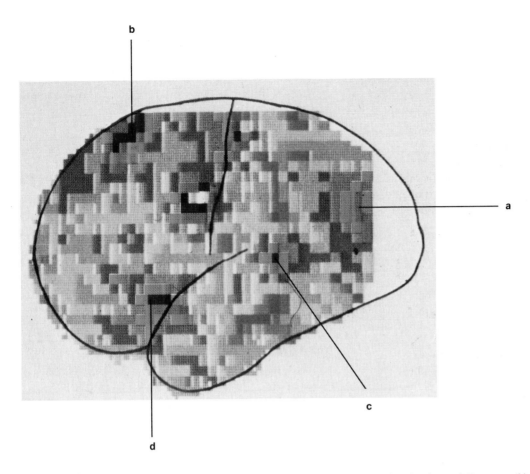

Figure 11.22 Reading silently activates four areas of the cerebral cortex: (**a**) the visual association area, (**b**) the supplementary motor area, (**c**) the frontal eye field, and (**d**) Broca's motor speech area. In this view of the left side of the cerebrum, through which blood containing radioactive xenon 133 is flowing, colored areas show above average blood flow, dark gray areas show average blood flow, and light gray areas show below average blood flow. (From N. A. Lassen, D. H. Invar, and E. Skinhøj, *Scientific American*, October 1978. Used by permission of N A. Lassen.)

carry impulses to the cerebral cortex and the limbic system. The pathway for smell is the only sensory pathway that does not pass through the thalamus.

The **optic nerves** (II) are also sensory nerves. They carry impulses related to sight from neurons in the retina of the eye to the optic chiasma, where the left and right optic nerves come together. Here the medial fibers of each nerve decussate and join the lateral fibers from the other nerve. The fibers pass through the optic chiasma without synapsing and form the optic tracts. These tracts end in a nucleus of the thalamus. Each fiber synapses with neurons of the

thalamic nucleus, and these neurons carry signals to the visual area of the cerebral cortex (Figure 11.23c). Some of the fibers from the optic nerves go to the superior colliculi of the midbrain, where they synapse with neurons that carry impulses to the cranial nerves III, IV, and VI, which are concerned with eye movements. In this way what is being seen contributes to the control of eye movements.

The **oculomotor nerves** (III) contain both sensory and motor fibers. The motor fibers extend from a nucleus in the midbrain to the muscle of the upper eyelid and four of the extrinsic eye muscles (Figure 11.23d). They control move-

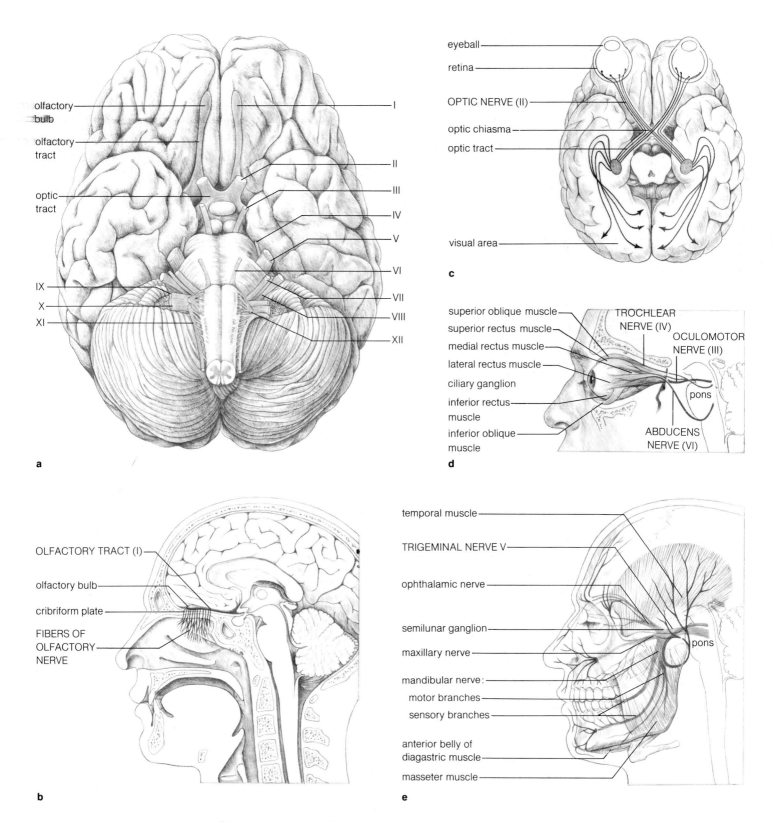

olfactory bulb

olfactory tract

optic tract

IX
X
XI

I

II
III
IV
V
VI

VII
VIII

XII

a

eyeball

retina

OPTIC NERVE (II)

optic chiasma

optic tract

visual area

c

superior oblique muscle

superior rectus muscle

medial rectus muscle

lateral rectus muscle

ciliary ganglion

inferior rectus muscle

inferior oblique muscle

TROCHLEAR NERVE (IV)

OCULOMOTOR NERVE (III)

pons

ABDUCENS NERVE (VI)

d

OLFACTORY TRACT (I)

olfactory bulb

cribriform plate

FIBERS OF OLFACTORY NERVE

b

temporal muscle

TRIGEMINAL NERVE V

ophthalamic nerve

semilunar ganglion

maxillary nerve

mandibular nerve :
motor branches
sensory branches

anterior belly of diagastric muscle

masseter muscle

pons

e

Figure 11.23 The cranial nerves: (**a**) a ventral view of the brain, showing the relationship of the cranial nerves to the brain, (**b**) I–olfactory nerve, (**c**) II–optic nerve, (**d**) III–oculomotor, IV–trochlear and VI–abducens nerves, (**e**) V–trige-

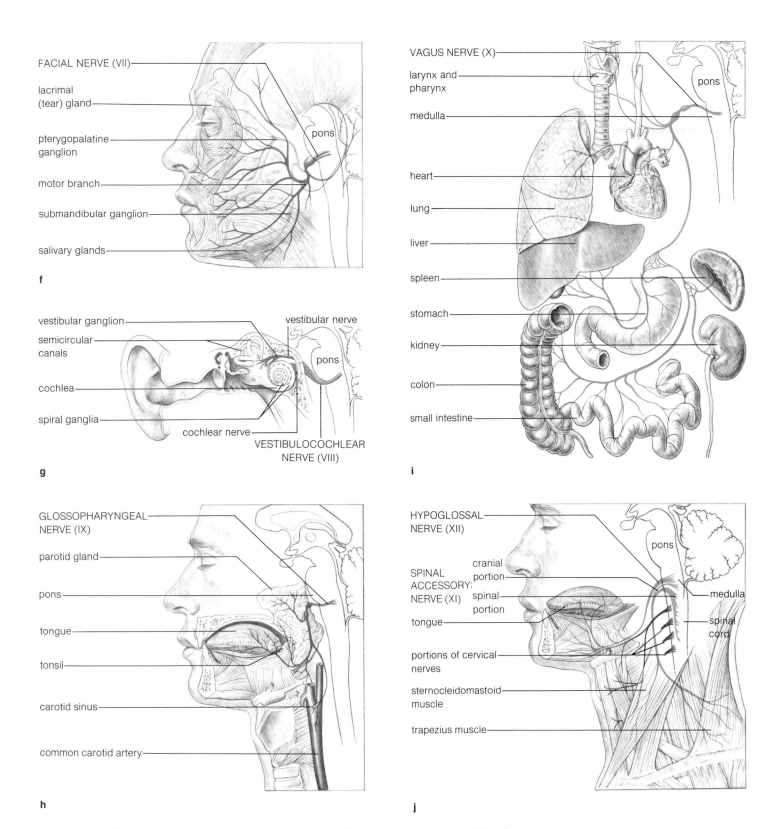

FACIAL NERVE (VII)

lacrimal (tear) gland

pterygopalatine ganglion

motor branch

submandibular ganglion

salivary glands

pons

f

vestibular ganglion

semicircular canals

cochlea

spiral ganglia

cochlear nerve

vestibular nerve

pons

VESTIBULOCOCHLEAR NERVE (VIII)

g

VAGUS NERVE (X)

larynx and pharynx

medulla

heart

lung

liver

spleen

stomach

kidney

colon

small intestine

pons

i

GLOSSOPHARYNGEAL NERVE (IX)

parotid gland

pons

tongue

tonsil

carotid sinus

common carotid artery

h

HYPOGLOSSAL NERVE (XII)

SPINAL ACCESSORY NERVE (XI)

cranial portion

spinal portion

tongue

portions of cervical nerves

sternocleidomastoid muscle

trapezius muscle

pons

medulla

spinal cord

j

minal nerve, (**f**) VII–facial nerve, (**g**) VIII–vestibulocochlear nerve, (**h**) IX–glossopharyngeal nerve, (**i**) X–vagus nerve, (**j**) XI–accessory and XII–hypoglossal nerves.

ments of the eyeball and eyelid. Some of the fibers of this nerve carry signals from the autonomic nervous system through the ciliary ganglion. They control the size of the pupil and the shape of the lens. (We will discuss both the autonomic nervous system and the structure of the eye in later chapters.) The sensory portions of the oculomotor nerves come from proprioceptors (detectors of position and movement) and detect length and tension in the various extrinsic eye muscles.

The **trochlear nerves** (IV), like the oculomotor, contain both sensory and motor fibers. They are the smallest of the cranial nerves. Motor fibers extend from a nucleus in the midbrain to the superior oblique muscle of each eye (Figure 11.23c). Sensory fibers convey signals from muscle proprioceptors.

The **trigeminal nerves** (V), the largest of the cranial nerves, are mixed nerves. The sensory portion of each nerve has three large branches, the **ophthalmic**, the **maxillary**, and the **mandibular nerves**. Each branch carries sensory impulses from the areas it serves, as shown in Figure 11.23e. The sensory branches come together to form the **semilunar**, or **gasserian**, **ganglion** and terminate on the ventrolateral surface of the pons. The motor portion of the trigeminal nerves begins as a separate root in the pons near the sensory portion. Motor fibers lie adjacent to sensory fibers of the mandibular nerve until they branch to the muscles of the mandible. These motor fibers control chewing movements.

The **abducens nerves** (VI) contain sensory and motor fibers. The motor fibers extend from a nucleus in the pons to the lateral rectus muscle of the eyeball. They work together with cranial nerves III and IV to control movements of the eyeball. Sensory fibers carry muscle length and tension information from the muscle to the pons (Figure 11.23d).

The **facial nerves** (VII) are mixed nerves (Figure 11.23f). Most of the sensory fibers come from the taste buds in the anterior two-thirds of the tongue and carry impulses to a nucleus in the pons. Taste sensations arriving in the pons are relayed to the thalamus and then to the gustatory area of the cerebral cortex. Some sensory fibers convey **muscle sense** impulses (those regarding muscle length and tension) from the face and scalp. Motor fibers run from a nucleus in the pons to the muscles of the face and scalp. They control movement of these muscles and thus facial expressions. Some motor fibers also stimulate the salivary glands to secrete saliva and the lacrimal gland to secrete tears. The fibers that go to glands are part of the autonomic nervous system.

The **vestibulocochlear nerves** (VIII) are primarily sensory; they have a few motor fibers whose function is unknown. Each has two branches, the cochlear, or auditory, branch and the vestibular branch. The **cochlear nerve** re-

ceives impulses from the sound receptors in the cochlea. The cell bodies of the cochlear nerve fibers are in the **spiral ganglion**, and their axons extend to a nucleus in the medulla, which in turn sends signals to the thalamus. The signals are relayed in the thalamus to the auditory areas of the cerebral cortex and to the cerebellum. The **vestibular nerve** originates in the semicircular canals and other structures of the inner ear that receive sensory information concerning balance. The cell bodies of the vestibular nerve are in the **vestibular ganglion**, and their axons extend to nuclei in the medulla and pons, from which signals are sent on to the thalamus. Some impulses are relayed to the cerebellum and some to the cerebral cortex. The distribution of this nerve is shown in Figure 11.23g.

The **glossopharyngeal nerves** (IX) are mixed nerves. Many of the sensory fibers originate in the taste buds of the posterior portion of the tongue and terminate in the thalamus (Figure 11.23h). Other sensory fibers carry muscle sense impulses from the muscles or signals from the carotid sinus, an organ in the wall of the carotid artery in the neck that is important in the regulation of blood pressure. The motor fibers extend from a nucleus in the medulla to the muscles of the pharynx and to the parotid salivary gland. They cause the muscles to contract and the gland to secrete saliva.

The **vagus nerves** (X) carry both sensory and motor fibers, primarily between the brain and the visceral organs (Figure 11.23i). The motor fibers begin in a nucleus of the medulla and terminate in muscles of the pharynx, the larynx, the respiratory and digestive tracts, and the heart. They stimulate all types of muscle: skeletal, smooth, and cardiac; their effects are important in the functioning of the autonomic nervous system discussed in Chapter 13. The sensory fibers carry impulses for pain and other sensations, including muscle sense from the same organs as are served by the motor fibers.

The **accessory nerves** (XI) carry motor and proprioceptive fibers (Figure 11.23j). Although this pair of nerves is classified with the cranial nerves, each originates partly in the medulla and partly from the cervical portion of the spinal cord. The medullary portion supplies the voluntary muscles of the soft palate, pharynx, and larynx that are used in swallowing. The spinal portion serves some of the muscles used to move the neck, shoulders, and rib cage. The sensory fibers carry muscle sense impulses back to the spinal cord and medulla.

The **hypoglossal nerves** (XII) also carry motor and proprioceptive fibers (Figure 11.23j). The motor fibers originate in a nucleus in the medulla and extend to the tongue. They control tongue movements involved in speech and in swallowing. Branches of the first three cervical nerves

Table 11.3 Characteristics of the Cranial Nerves

Nerve	Type	Pathways	Function
I Olfactory	Sensory	From nasal epithelium to olfactory bulb	Smell
II Optic	Sensory	From retina of eye to thalamus	Sight
III Oculomotor	Motor, proprioceptive*	From midbrain to four eye muscles; from ciliary body to midbrain	Movement of eyeball and eyelid; focusing; change in pupil size; muscle sense
IV Trochlear	Motor, proprioceptive	From midbrain to superior oblique muscle; from eye muscle to midbrain	Movement of eyeball; muscle sense
V Trigeminal	Mixed	From pons to muscles of mastication; from cornea, facial skin, lips, tongue, and teeth to pons	Chewing of food; sensations from organs of the face
VI Abducens	Motor, proprioceptive	From pons to lateral rectus muscle; from eye muscle to pons	Movement of eyeball; muscle sense
VII Facial	Mixed	From pons to facial muscles; from facial muscles and taste buds to pons	Facial expressions; secretion of saliva and tears; muscle sense; taste
VIII Vestibulo-cochlear or auditory	Sensory	Organs of hearing and balance to pons	Hearing, balance, and posture
IX Glossophar-yngeal	Mixed	From medulla to muscles of pharynx; pharyngeal muscles and taste buds to medulla	Swallowing, secretion of saliva; muscle sense; taste
X Vagus	Mixed	From medulla to viscera; from viscera to medulla	Visceral muscle movement; visceral sensations
XI Accessory or spinal accessory	Motor, proprioceptive	From medulla to throat and neck muscles; from muscles to medulla	Swallowing and head movements; muscle sense
XI Hypoglossal	Motor, proprioceptive	From medulla to muscles of tongue; tongue muscles to medulla	Speech and swallowing; muscle sense

*Proprioceptive = receiving sensations from muscles and joints denoting position and degree of contraction

join with the hypoglossal in serving parts of the tongue and some neck muscles. Sensory fibers carry muscle sense impulses back to the medulla.

NEUROTRANSMITTERS

Objective 8. List the major neurotransmitters of the central nervous system and cite examples of how each operates in the normal functioning of the nervous system.

In the last chapter we considered the transmission of signals across synapses and saw that a chemical substance is usually involved in such transmission. About thirty different chemical substances have been identified that might play a role in signal transmission in the central nervous system, most of them in the brain. You might ask why there are so many transmitters in the brain. We could begin to consider that question by noting the number of neurons and synapses in the human brain.

Brain Circuitry

Some scientists estimate that the brain contains 100 billion neurons. To get some idea of how enormous that number is, let us suppose that each cell has a length from dendrite to axon terminal of 1 millimeter. If 100 billion of such cells were placed end to end, they would reach around the earth's equator about ten times.

Scientists have also estimated that a typical neuron in the brain synapses with hundreds of other neurons. If the same transmitter were released at each of these synapses, and all of the postsynaptic receptor sites received that transmitter, there would be no way to distinguish one signal from another. This situation would be a little like many telephones having the same telephone number: Mass confusion would reign.

Such confusion is prevented in several ways. First, each transmitter acts only on a specific kind of receptor site on a postsynaptic neuron. Second, each neuron probably has several different kinds of receptors and responds to the transmitter at each receptor type in a different way. Third, the postsynaptic response at a single receptor is not strong enough to generate an impulse in the postsynaptic neuron; several similar receptors would need to receive signals to cause an effect on the neuron. Finally, the interaction of some transmitters with their receptors is excitatory, while the interaction of other transmitters with their receptors is inhibitory. Thus, the net effect on a cell is the sum of all of the excitatory and inhibitory signals it receives, as noted in our discussion of IPSPs and EPSPs in Chapter 10. This process, which involves a single neuron, represents the most basic level of **integration** within the nervous system. Thus, processing of information through the brain circuitry begins at the level of a single neuron, but complex circuits involve all of the above factors affecting each neuron in a given pathway.

Transmitters

Three transmitters—acetylcholine, norepinephrine, and gamma aminobutyric acid (GABA)—were discussed in Chapter 10. Here, we will consider the role of those transmitters in the central nervous system. We will also consider several other transmitters found only in the central nervous system.

In the central nervous system acetylcholine is the transmitter at some synapses in the spinal cord and at the synapses that activate the Purkinje cells of the cerebellum. Norepinephrine is thought to be the transmitter released by neurons in several different parts of the central nervous system, especially the limbic system. GABA is released by cerebellar Purkinje cells and participates in the coordination of motor activities.

Dopamine (DA) is an established transmitter of several kinds of neurons in the brain. It is released by many neurons in the substantia nigra of the midbrain, whose functions are concerned with motor control. Deficiencies of dopamine are thought to be the cause of Parkinson's disease, and excesses of it may be involved in mental disturbances such as schizophrenia. (Clinical conditions related to dopamine will be discussed in Chapter 12.)

Serotonin is released by several different groups of cells in the midbrain whose axons reach the hypothalamus, thalamus, and parts of the limbic system. It is also released at certain synapses in the spinal cord.

Glycine, a simple amino acid, is possibly released by some neurons in the spinal cord.

A variety of neuropeptides, short chains of amino acids found in the nervous system, have been identified over the past several years. They include thyrotropic-releasing hormone, luteinizing hormone–releasing hormone, somatostatin, vasopressin, and oxytocin—substances that will be considered in Chapter 15. Also included among the neuropeptides are endorphins and enkephalins. Endorphins and enkephalins are discussed in the essay at the end of this chapter.

How Transmitters Transmit

The study of the effects of neurotransmitters in the brain has led to an increased understanding of how postsynaptic neurons respond to stimulation by a transmitter. When a transmitter reaches an appropriate receptor on another neuron, it attaches to the receptor site. In most synapses that have been studied an excitatory transmitter–receptor interaction appears to activate a particular enzyme, which produces a "second messenger" inside the postsynaptic cell. For example, cyclic AMP has been suggested to be the second messenger in some cells.

Some chemical substances not normally present in the body can either mimic or block the action of a transmitter. If a substance forms a good fit with the receptor site, the cell may be unable to distinguish it from the normal transmitter, and it may mimic the action of the normal transmitter. If another chemical substance forms a fit with the receptor that is strong enough to maintain the attachment, it can antagonize the action of the normal transmitter—it does not fit well enough to have an effect on the cell, yet it ties up the receptor site so that the normal transmitter cannot reach it. Some hallucinogenic drugs have chemical structures similar to certain transmitters, suggesting that they attach to receptor sites but cause different effects than the normal transmitter. Some anesthetics may mimic inhibitory transmitter–receptor interactions, and the tranquilizer and muscle relaxant Valium seems to enhance the inhibitory effects of GABA.

This brief introduction to the complex topic of neurotransmitters in the central nervous system demonstrates the intricacy of patterns of signal transmission. It also provides background for the consideration of mental disturbances in Chapter 12. The study of neurotransmitters is one of the most active research fields in all of physiology; frequent new developments in this field should be anticipated.

CLINICAL TERMS

encephalitis (en"sef-al-i'tis)   inflammation of the brain, often caused by an infectious agent

tic douloureux (tik doo-loo-ro')   a spasmodic twitching of facial muscles accompanied by pain

vagotomy (va-got'o-me)   cutting of the vagus nerve

Essay: Endorphins and Enkephalins

Opium has been used for the relief of pain for many centuries. And for several centuries its addictive properties have been known. Over much of that time the search for nonaddictive opiates continued without success, but current research efforts are beginning to show promise. The finding of receptor sites with which opiates react in several areas of the brain has raised an interesting question: How can such sites exist when opiates are not natural body substances?

A separate line of research led to the discovery of beta-lipotropin, a hormone of the anterior pituitary gland that in some animals helps to mobilize fats from fat deposits for other cells to use for energy. Discoveries in recent years have shown that beta-lipotropin is a protein and that enzymes in the pituitary gland break it down into the hormone ACTH (see Chapter 15) and a variety of segments that have psychological and behavioral effects (Figure 11.24). These segments are the **endorphins** and **enkephalins**. It is now known that enkephalins can be synthesized independently of beta-lipotropin.

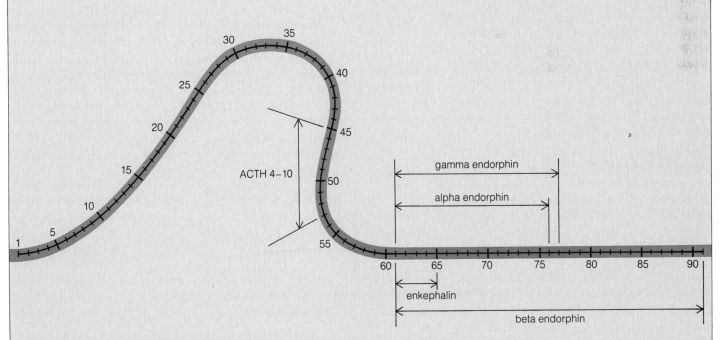

Figure 11.23   A diagram of a molecule of beta-lipotroptin, showing psychoactive fragments. Each of the ninety-one elements of this protein is a specific amino acid.

Table 11.4 Endorphins and Enkephalins

Name of Substance (amino acid fraction of beta-lipotropin)	Effects
ACTH 4-10 (47-53)	Improves memory and concentration in normal individuals; helps mentally retarded individuals comprehend situations; improves memory of senile individuals
Beta-endorphin (61-91)	Has powerful analgesic effect in mice and rats; in small sample of human trials countered depression and anxiety in mentally disturbed individuals, reduced hallucinations in some individuals suffering from schizophrenia; being studied for alleviation of pain in terminal cancer and for reducing withdrawal symptoms of opiates
Alpha-endorphin (61-76)	Has analgesic and tranquilizing effect in rats
Gamma-endorphin (61-77)	Produces violence, increased irritability, and increased sensitivity to pain in rats
Methionine-enkephalin (61-65) and leucine-enkephalin (61-64 + leucine)	Appear to be body's natural pain-relieving molecules; synthetic compounds similar to these have caused long-lasting pain relief in rats; natural enkephalins improve memory, induce pleasure, and in rats can initiate epilepsy

These two lines of research began to come together when it was discovered that the drug naloxone, which is used as an antidote to morphine, binds to the opiate receptor sites. One important question about the presence of opiate receptor sites was finally answered when it was found that enkephalins did, in fact, bind to the opiate receptor sites. In other words, natural constituents of the body that react with these sites have been identified.

It is now well established that enkephalins are transmitterlike substances of neuronal systems in the brain having to do with the perception of pain, as well as other brain functions. How they act is not fully understood, but their mechanism of action appears to be different from the inhibitory effects that generally cause hyperpolarization of postsynaptic neurons. One mechanism proposed is that enkephalins released at synapses bind to the presynaptic terminals of certain excitatory synapses, where they reduce the amount of transmitter released by an impulse in the presynaptic neuron. This type of inhibition, called **presynaptic inhibition**, may be involved in some of the pain-blocking actions that have been suggested for enkephalins.

CHAPTER SUMMARY

(Chapter summary points and review questions are numbered to correspond to the numbered objectives in the text of each chapter.)

Organization and General Function

1. Describe the relationships of the brain and the cranial nerves to the rest of the nervous system and summarize the major functions of the brain and the cranial nerves.
  a. The brain is part of the central nervous system, and the cranial nerves are part of the peripheral nervous system.
  b. The major functions of the brain include:
    (1) receiving sensory stimuli
    (2) thinking and memory storage, which occur in the cerebrum
    (3) coordination of muscular movements, which occurs primarily in the cerebellum
    (4) control of internal functions, which occurs primarily in the various parts of the brainstem

Development

2. Summarize the embryonic development and the evolution of the brain.
  a. The brain develops from the anterior end of the neural tube,

enlarging to form three areas: the forebrain, midbrain, and hindbrain.

b. The brain evolved in three major stages: the reptilian brain, the limbic system, and the neocortex.

Parts of the Brainstem

3. Describe the location, structure, and function of (a) the medulla oblongata, (b) the pons, (c) the midbrain, (d) the thalamus, and (e) the hypothalamus.

a. The brainstem consists of the medulla, pons, midbrain, thalamus, and hypothalamus; it is continuous with the spinal cord and forms the core of the brain.

b. The medulla oblongata, nearest the spinal cord, controls vital functions such as heart rate; blood pressure; respiration; and other functions such as coughing, sneezing, and swallowing.

c. The pons, located anterior to the medulla and adjacent to the cerebellum, transmits signals to and from the cerebrum and the cerebellum. The pons also helps to regulate respiration.

d. The midbrain relays signals to other parts of the brain and helps to control head and eye movements.

e. The thalamus acts as a relay center for transmitting signals to and from the cerebrum.

f. The hypothalamus acts as a center of homeostasis in that it regulates many internal processes and forms the connection between the nervous and endocrine systems.

Cerebellum

4. Describe the location, structure, and function of the cerebellum.

a. The cerebellum consists of two lateral hemispheres and a median vermis, all of which lie above the brainstem between the cerebrum and the medulla.

b. The functions of the cerebellum are to coordinate movements and to help maintain posture and balance.

Cerebrum

5. Describe the location, structure, and function of the cerebrum.

a. The cerebrum, the largest part of the human brain, consists of two hemispheres connected by the corpus callosum. It is located above the anterior brainstem in front of the cerebellum.

b. The outer cortex (gray matter) is only a few millimeters thick and consists of several layers of cell bodies, which are interconnected in complex ways. The inner white matter, which consists of myelinated tracts, makes up most of the volume of the cerebral hemispheres.

c. The cerebrum contains several lobes, each of which has one or more functional areas:

(1) The somatic sensory area in the parietal lobe receives signals from sensory receptors in the skin, muscles, and joints. These signals are relayed along spinal cord tracts.

(2) The somatic motor area in the frontal lobe sends signals to the effectors (mostly skeletal muscles). These signals are also relayed along spinal cord tracts.

(3) The visual area in the occipital lobe receives signals from the retina and sends them to the visual association area, also located in the occipital lobe.

(4) The auditory area in the temporal lobe receives signals from the sound receptors in the inner ear and relays them mainly to the parietal association area.

(5) Broca's motor speech area in the frontal lobe formulates sentences and initiates speech.

(6) Auditory areas, speech areas, and the somatic motor area act in a coordinated way to interpret speech and to formulate a spoken response.

(7) Association areas in other parts of the brain include the frontal association area, thought to be devoted to problem solving, and the temporal association area, thought to be concerned with memory and the interpretation of new experiences in relation to what is remembered. The visual association areas interpret visual signals, and the parietal association areas interpret auditory and touch signals and provide the sense of a body image.

d. The myelinated tracts of the cerebrum include:

(1) association fibers, which connect two functional areas in the same hemisphere

(2) commissural fibers, which connect the two hemispheres

(3) projection fibers, which carry signals between different parts of the central nervous system

e. The basal nuclei are a group of cell bodies of neurons imbedded deep in the cerebrum and the brainstem. The main function of the basal nuclei is to control muscle tone.

f. The limbic system consists of a network of fibers deep within the cerebrum that are concerned with emotional behavior and some aspects of memory. This system is also closely associated with the sense of smell.

g. The reticular system consists of a column of nuclei located in the central core of the brainstem but closely associated with the cerebrum. Its function is mainly to control sleep and wakefulness.

Circulation of Blood and Cerebrospinal Fluid

6. Describe the structure, location, and function of the ventricles of the brain and the blood vessels of the brain; explain how cerebrospinal fluid and blood circulate in the brain.

a. The brain contains four ventricles, one in each cerebral hemisphere, one in the midline of the thalamus, and one in the medulla and pons. All are filled with cerebrospinal fluid. All are connected with each other and with the central canal of the spinal cord and the subarachnoid space.

b. Cerebrospinal fluid is secreted by the choroid plexuses and reabsorbed through the subarachnoid villi into the dural sinuses. The circulation of cerebrospinal fluid is summarized in Figure 11.16.

c. Blood is supplied to the brain by the blood vessels shown in Figure 11.18. The blood–brain barrier controls the passage of substances from the blood into the tissues of the brain. The rate of blood flow through different portions of the brain is an indicator of cerebral activity.

Cranial Nerves

7. List the twelve cranial nerves in order and describe the location and function of each.
   a. The cranial nerves carry sensory and motor impulses to and from the brain. These nerves are listed in order, along with descriptions of their pathways and functions, in Table 11.3.

Neurotransmitters

8. List the major neurotransmitters of the central nervous system and cite examples of how each operates in the normal functioning of the nervous system.
   a. The brain contains a large number of different transmitters. The actions of the transmitters are determined by the nature of the interaction between the transmitter and the receptor site.
   b. The following transmitters have been described:
      (1) Acetylcholine appears to be released at some synapses in the spinal cord and by some neurons that activate the Purkinje cells of the cerebellum.
      (2) Dopamine is released by neurons in the substantia nigra whose functions are concerned with motor control.
      (3) Norepinephrine, serotonin, and GABA are also released by various neurons of the brain, and glycine appears to be released by some neurons in the spinal cord.

REVIEW

Important Terms

abducens nerve	Broca's motor speech area
accessory nerve	cardiac center
arbor vitae	cerebellar peduncles
association area	cerebellum
association fibers	cerebral aqueduct
auditory area	cerebral arteries
basal nuclei	cerebral peduncles
basilar artery	cerebrum
blood–brain barrier	circle of Willis
brainstem	commissural fibers

corpora quadrigemina	parietal lobe
corpus callosum	pons
cranial nerves	projection fibers
facial nerve	red nucleus
forebrain	respiratory center
frontal lobe	reticular formation
glossopharyngeal nerve	somatic motor area
gyrus	somatic sensory area
hindbrain	substantia nigra
hypoglossal nerve	sulcus
hypothalamus	temporal lobe
interventricular foramen	thalamus
lateral aperature	trigeminal nerve
limbic system	trochlear nerve
median aperature	vagus nerve
medulla oblongata	vasomotor center
midbrain	ventricles
occipital lobe	vermis
oculomotor nerve	vestibulocochlear nerve
olfactory nerve	visual area
optic nerve	

Questions

1. a. How are the brain and cranial nerves related to the rest of the nervous system?
   b. What are the major functions of the main parts of the brain?
   c. What is the major function of the cranial nerves?
2. a. Describe the embryonic development of the brain.
   b. What are the three levels of evolutionary development of the human brain?
3. a. Name the parts of the brainstem and tell where they are located.
   b. What are the major functions of each of the parts of the brainstem?
   c. Why is the hypothalamus appropriately called the center for the maintenance of homeostasis?
4. a. Where is the cerebellum, and what are its main parts?
   b. What is the general function of the cerebellum?
   c. Describe the arrangement of cells in the cerebellar cortex and the transmission of impulses through them.
5. a. Identify and give the function of the following parts of the cerebrum: (i) corpus callosum, (ii) cortex, (iii) somatic sensory area, (iv) somatic motor area, (v) visual area, (vi) auditory area, (vii) speech area, and (viii) the several association areas.
   b. Where are the basal nuclei, and what do they do?
   c. Where is the limbic system, and what does it do?

6. **a.** Trace the circulation of cerebrospinal fluid from the choroid plexus of the lateral ventricles to the dural sinuses.
   b. Trace the flow of blood from the internal carotid artery through the brain to the external jugular vein.
   c. What is the blood–brain barrier?
7. **a.** Name the twelve cranial nerves in order from the front to the back of the brain.
   b. What are the functions of each of the cranial nerves?
8. **a.** Name six neurotransmitters of the central nervous system.
   b. Explain briefly how transmitters might work.

Problems

1. Watch and listen to one minute of a television program. Say aloud and write down a one-sentence summary of what you learned from the program. List in sequence all of the neural pathways and parts of the brain that were involved in your receiving stimuli from the program and responding to them.

2. For at least five of the cranial nerves devise a simple, noninvasive test (one that does not require surgery or other disruption of body structures) to determine whether the nerve is functioning properly.

REFERENCES AND READINGS

Arehart-Treichel, J. 1978. The pituitary's powerful protein. *Science News* 114 (22):374 (November 25).

The Brain. 1979. A special issue of *Scientific American* 241 (3) (September).

Darien-Smith, I., Johnson, K., and Goodwin, A. 1979. Posterior parietal cortex: Relations of unit activity to sensorimotor function. *Annual Review of Physiology* 41:141.

Elde, R., and Hökfelt, T. 1979. Localization of hypophysiotropic peptides and other biologically active peptides within the brain. *Annual Review of Physiology* 41:587.

Guyton, A. C. 1981. *Textbook of medical physiology* (6th ed.). Philadelphia: W. B. Saunders.

Hawkins, R. A., and Biebuyck, J. F. 1979. Ketone bodies are selectively used by individual brain regions. *Science* 205:325 (July 20).

Holden, C. 1979. Paul MacLean and the triune brain. *Science* 204:1066 (June 8).

Imura, H., and Nakai, Y. 1981. "Endorphins" in pituitary and other tissues. *Annual Review of Physiology* 43:265.

Krulich, L. 1979. Central neurotransmitters and the secretion of prolactin, GH, LH, and TSH. *Annual Review of Physiology* 41:603.

Lassen, N. A., Ingvar, D. H., and Skinhøj, E. 1978. Brain function and blood flow. *Scientific American* 239(4):62 (October).

Llinás, R. R. 1975. The cortex of the cerebellum. *Scientific American* 232(1):56 (January).

Moss, R. L. 1979. Actions of hypothalamic-hypophysiotropic hormones on the brain. *Annual Review of Physiology* 41:617.

Nathanson, J. A., and Greengard, P. 1977. "Second messengers" in the brain. *Scientific American* 237(2):108 (August).

Siegel, G. J., Albers, R. W., Katzman, R., and Agranoff, B. W., eds. 1976. *Basic neurochemistry.* Boston: Little, Brown.

Snyder, S. H. 1977. Opiate receptors and internal opiates. *Scientific American* 236(3):44 (March).

Wilson, R. S. 1978. Synchronies in mental development: An epigenetic perspective. *Science* 202:939 (December 1).

12

NERVOUS SYSTEM: HIGHER ORDER FUNCTIONS

HIGHER ORDER FUNCTIONS

Objective 1. Identify higher order functions of the brain.

In Chapter 11 we considered the anatomy and basic functions of the brain. We also considered some aspects of language and some aspects of the processing of sensory and motor signals. Here we will consider **higher order functions**—functions that involve complex and highly integrated processing. These functions include sleep and wakefulness, learning, memory, emotions, and language. Although much remains to be learned about these functions, and much more is known than can be presented here, these topics will be given brief coverage.

SLEEP AND WAKEFULNESS

Objective 2. Describe how sleep and wakefulness are thought to be regulated, and explain the correlation of electroencephalograms with these processes.

Most of us take for granted our natural cyclic pattern of falling asleep and awakening. However, the internal regulation of sleep and wakefulness is a complex, poorly understood process. Certain structures in the brainstem (Figure 12.1) have been implicated in this process. The **reticular formation**, mentioned briefly in Chapter 11, consists of a diffuse column of nuclei in the central core of the brainstem. Among these nuclei are the **reticular activating system** (RAS), the **locus ceruleus**, the **pontine cells**, and the **raphe nuclei**. The role of these structures in sleep and wakefulness will be explained shortly. Because what we know about the activities of these nuclei is based in part on brain waves and electroencephalograms, we will consider those first.

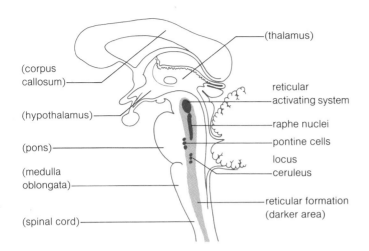

Figure 12.1 Some parts of the brainstem that have been implicated in the regulation of sleep and wakefulness. (Structures in parentheses are indicated as points of reference; they are not involved in the regulation of sleep and wakefulness.)

Brain Waves and Electroencephalograms

When electrodes are placed on various sites on an individual's scalp, electrical potential differences between brain sites can be observed and recorded on chart paper. The differences measured are the average of the **synaptic potentials** (EPSPs and IPSPs) between the various sites. Fluctuations in the potential differences, called **brain waves**, are measured in terms of frequency and amplitude. A record of brain waves over a period of time is called an **electroencephalogram** (EEG).

Table 12.1 presents the four different kinds of brain waves seen in normal EEGs. (Some of these waves and their

relationships to sleep are illustrated in Figure 12.3.) **Alpha waves** are rhythmic, synchronized waves that occur with a regular frequency of 8 to 13 cycles per second. These waves are characteristic of an individual who is awake but relaxed with eyes closed. **Beta waves** are also rhythmic, though irregular, waves; they occur at a frequency about twice that of alpha waves and at a lower amplitude. They are characteristic of an individual who is mentally alert. Beta waves are most frequently recorded from the frontal and parietal areas of the scalp. As these parts of the brain contain association areas that function during mental activities, beta waves and mental processes are correlated. **Theta waves** occur with a frequency of 4 to 7 cycles per second. They are most common in the temporal and parietal regions of the brains of children; they are rarely seen in normal, awake adults. Theta waves are seen in many brain disorders, but their presence does not necessarily indicate a disorder. **Delta waves**, occurring no faster than 3½ cycles per second and often as slowly as one every two or three seconds, are seen in infancy and in some kinds of brain disease. In adults delta waves are characteristic of normal deep sleep. Deep sleep is therefore slow-wave sleep.

Much of the information about the brain obtained through EEGs is purely descriptive. Using electroencephalograms to study the brain has been likened to standing outside a factory and trying to determine what is being made and how it is done from the noises that can be heard. We can correlate certain behaviors with certain EEG patterns without understanding the underlying mechanisms. Though EEGs do not tell us much about physiological processes, they have been used successfully to study sleep, to correlate with and to diagnose certain kinds of brain disease and to provide a definitive criterion for death. In patients receiving assistance from life-support systems to maintain respiration and circulation of blood, the complete absence of brain waves is accepted as evidence that death has occurred.

Table 12.1	Types of Brain Waves Seen in Electro-encephalograms	
Wave Type	Frequency (cycles/second)	Functional Status
Alpha	8–13	Awake but relaxed with eyes closed
Beta	14–25	Mentally alert
Theta	4–7	In children; rare in awake adults; in some brain disorders
Delta	⅓–3½	Deep sleep; infancy; serious brain disorders

Wakefulness

The awake state appears to be maintained by the reticular formation, and especially its anterior portion, the reticular activating system (RAS). Nuclei of the reticular formation are closely associated with many ascending and descending neural pathways between the parts of the brain and the spinal cord. The reticular formation receives signals from other parts of the brainstem and from the spinal cord, cerebellum, cerebral cortex, basal nuclei, and limbic system; it sends signals to the spinal cord, cerebellum, and cerebral cortex. When the RAS is stimulated by sensory signals, it relays signals to the cerebral cortex, and a state of arousal or wakefulness results. In turn, stimulation of the cerebral cortex causes the cortex to stimulate the RAS. This positive feedback in which the brain areas stimulate each other is an important factor in maintaining wakefulness (Figure 12.2).

Many different kinds of signals can be relayed to the cortex, and which signals actually reach the cortex can be influenced by the RAS. Though the exact mechanism by which the RAS influences the signals to be relayed to the cortex is not known, it is known that the RAS fails to relay weak signals and repetitive signals that form familiar patterns and does relay strong signals and novel signals. For example, a mother might sleep through a variety of noises but waken suddenly at the sound of a crying baby even though the cry might be less intense than other noises that failed to wake her. Thus, it is possible that emotional factors may affect the selection of signals the RAS relays.

Any unusual stimulus, such as the ringing of a telephone or doorbell, will usually rouse a sleeping person. One might be awakened by the phone but not by a siren, if sirens blaring in the night are a common occurrence. Even an individual who is awake and concentrating on some other task will probably be aware of a ringing bell. However, many fairly continuous stimuli will be ignored. Stimuli such as the hum of a motor or the presence of a light will not be relayed to the cortex. This screening out of stimuli is one form of **habituation**. Such habituation of sensory signals is controlled to a large degree by the RAS and is not related to fatigue of sensory receptor cells themselves.

Sleep

Sleep is a natural temporary absence of wakefulness from which the individual can be aroused. It is essential to good health in humans and other higher organisms, though its exact functions are not well understood. Research in sleep laboratories using electroencephalography and other techniques have identified five stages of sleep, characterized by patterns of eye movements and brain waves (Figure 12.3).

Four stages involve **non-rapid-eye-movement (non-REM) sleep**. In **stage 1** the individual experiences a drifting sensation, during which alpha waves are reduced in frequency and amplitude. If aroused from this drowsy state, most individuals will claim they were not really asleep. During this stage the activity of the RAS is somewhat reduced; its activity continues to decrease as deeper stages of sleep are achieved. In **stage 2** bursts of brain-wave activity with a frequency of about fifteen waves per second appear. These are called sleep spindles. In **stage 3** delta waves appear in the EEG, and heart rate, respiratory rate, blood

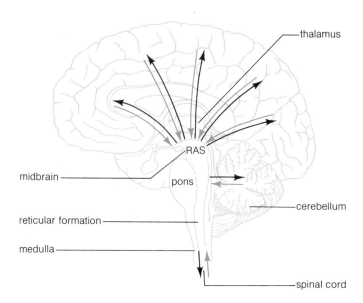

Figure 12.2 The reticular formation sends and receives signals from various parts of the brain. When stimulated, the reticular activating system sends impulses (shown in black) into the cortex. The cortex in turn sends impulses (shown in color) back to the RAS. This positive feedback mechanism is a major factor in maintaining wakefulness.

pressure, and body temperature decrease. In **stage 4** the sleeper is in deep, or oblivious, sleep, during which delta waves continue and physiological processes reach their lowest levels.

At intervals of 80 to 120 minutes the nature of sleep changes to what is called **paradoxical**, or **rapid-eye-movement (REM), sleep**. REM sleep is said to be paradoxical because the EEG takes on characteristics that resemble the beta waves of the awake, alert state. During this period of sleep the eyeballs move rapidly beneath the eyelids, and dreaming apparently occurs. Physiological processes increase to rates similar to the waking state but are often irregular. In these respects REM sleep is similar to wakefulness. Periods of REM sleep account for 90–120 minutes of a night's sleep; they usually last from 5 to 20 minutes, but they may last as long as 50 minutes toward the end of the sleep period. During a night's sleep four to six cycles of non-REM and REM sleep usually occur.

Perhaps you have suddenly awakened from a dream and for a moment were unable to move. This frightening experience illustrates the low resting tone of trunk and limb muscles during dreaming and the brief extension of this phenomenon into the waking state.

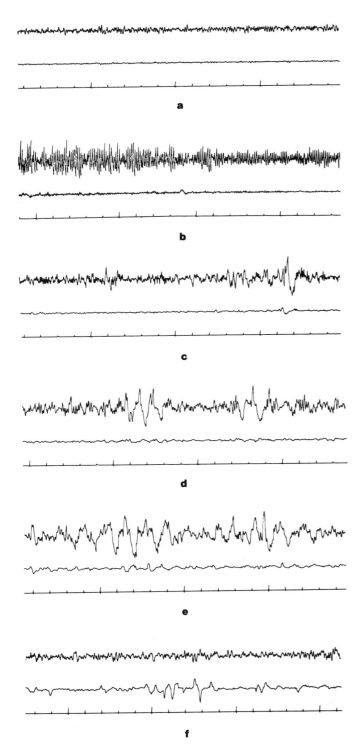

Figure 12.3 EEG records from a male college student. For each part of the record the top line is the EEG from one electrode on the scalp; the middle line is a record of eye movements; the bottom line is a time marker, indicating 1 second units: (**a**) relaxed awake, (**b**) stage 1 sleep, (**c**) stage 2 sleep, (**d**) stage 3 sleep, (**e**) stage 4 sleep, (**f**) REM or "paradoxical," sleep. (Records provided by T. E. LeVere.)

REM sleep differs from non-REM sleep in several ways. First, the sleeper is more difficult to arouse from REM than from non-REM sleep. Second, the muscle tone throughout the trunk and limbs is greatly depressed during REM sleep. Some studies report that involuntary twitches of skeletal muscles occur at irregular intervals, along with irregular eye movements; others indicate that the neurons controlling skeletal muscles become incapable of discharging, and only eye muscles remain capable of significant movement.

Studies of sleep deprivation illustrate another difference between REM and non-REM sleep. In sleep laboratories where individuals are carefully monitored, the encephalogram serves to distinguish the states of sleep. These individuals can be repeatedly awakened as they enter either REM sleep or non-REM sleep and thereby deprived of a particular sleep state for an entire night. The results of such studies show that individuals compensate for the type of sleep of which they were deprived during the next night or two of sleep and that a longer time is required to compensate for lost REM sleep than for lost non-REM sleep. The differences between REM and non-REM sleep are summarized in Table 12.2.

Theories of Sleep

Though most physiologists agree that sleep results from suppression of the RAS, how such suppression occurs is far from well understood. Furthermore, though many differences between REM and non-REM sleep can be observed, the mechanisms by which shifts from one state to another occur are likewise poorly understood. On the basis of what is now known, some of the attributes of the regulation of sleep and wakefulness seem to be as follows:

1. Neurons in the raphe nuclei, which release the transmitter serotonin, initiate both REM and non-REM sleep.

2. Neurons of the posterior one-third of the locus ceruleus, which release norepinephrine, suppress skeletal muscle tone during REM sleep, probably by acting in some way on the somatic motor cortex.

3. The pontine cells display spontaneous activity shortly before and during REM sleep and stimulate rapid eye movements. (These movements are not initiated by visual stimuli as they are during wakefulness; they seem to originate from some internal activity that occurs during sleep.)

4. Neurons in the middle one-third of the locus ceruleus appear to interact with the pontine cells: (a) During waking and non-REM sleep they inhibit the pontine cells

Table 12.2 A Comparison of REM and Non-REM Sleep

REM sleep	Non-REM sleep
EEG similar to wakeful, alert state	EEG shows damped alpha waves followed by delta waves
Muscle tone is inhibited, except in eye muscles	Muscle tone maintained
Dreaming occurs in this stage	No dreaming, though thoughts of recent events may be reported if sleeper is awakened from this phase
Respiration, heart rate, and blood pressure show irregular fluctuations	Respiration, heart rate, blood pressure, and body temperature show slight decreases
Sleeper is relatively difficult to arouse	Sleeper is relatively easy to arouse
Occurs in periods of 5–20 minutes but may last as long as 50 minutes	Occupies remainder of cycles of 80 to 120 minutes
Generally follows an initial period of non-REM sleep	Generally constitutes the first period of natural sleep
Accounts for 90–120 minutes of a typical adult's night's sleep (15–20%); accounts for half an infant's sleep	Accounts for the remainder of a typical adult's night's sleep (80–85%); accounts for half an infant's sleep
When sleeper is deprived of REM sleep, deficit is generally made up the next night; REM debt takes longer to be made up than non-REM debt	When sleeper is deprived of non-REM sleep, deficit is generally made up the next night; non-REM debt is made up more quickly than REM debt

and suppress the eye movements characteristic of REM sleep. (b) During REM sleep they cease to inhibit the pontine cells and thus allow spontaneous activity of the pontine cells to occur.

5. Several groups of neurons appear to be in some way involved in wakefulness and arousal. They include norepinephrine-secreting neurons in the anterior third of the locus ceruleus, dopamine-secreting neurons in the midbrain portion of the reticular activating system, and acetylcholine-secreting neurons of the cortex. (The last are probably involved in the positive feedback mechanism of wakefulness described earlier.)

6. Small polypeptides in cerebrospinal fluid, called "sleep factors," also may be involved in the initiation and regulation of sleep, but their functions remain obscure.

Though the above statements provide some understanding of sleep and wakefulness, much remains to be learned. For example, the details of what causes either set of raphe nuclei to begin to secrete serotonin are unknown, as are the interactions between the sets of nuclei that account for shifts in sleep phases. Further research is needed to determine how the various components of the sleep-wakefulness mechanisms are initiated and how they are integrated with each other.

Physiological Effects of Sleep

Sleep has effects on many structures in the body; by far the most significant are its effects on the nervous system. Sleep deprivation for a short period results in reduced attention span, impaired mental ability, and memory failure. Several days of sleep deprivation produces bizarre and psychotic behavior and causes the adrenal cortex to secrete hormones characteristic of stressful situations. In addition, a chemical similar to serotonin accumulates in the bloodstream; it is probably responsible for the hallucinations that sometimes occur after sleep deprivation. (The hallucinogen LSD is similar in structure to serotonin.) After prolonged sleep deprivation several days of longer than usual sleep periods are necessary to restore normal body functions. During these sleep periods the proportion of time spent in REM

Given the effects of sleep—or the lack of it—we have described, it is clear that we do need sleep. However, exactly why we need sleep is still unknown. The evolutionary theory of sleep proposes that, as our bodies evolved from ancestral animals, a mechanism was built in to force us to conserve energy when we would be relatively inefficient. Some evidence to support this theory comes from studies of animals that hibernate (enter a period of reduced metabolism and inactivity) during the winter months when food is scarce and the environment is hostile. Similarly, humans may sleep for part of each day to conserve energy and to allow the nervous system to recover its efficiency. By preventing us from attempting activities we are ill-prepared for, sleep may serve to keep us out of trouble at night.

sleep is greater than normal, indicating that REM sleep may be essential to restore the nervous system to normal functioning. Furthermore, some studies have shown that awakening sleepers at the point when they enter REM sleep worsens the effects of sleep deprivation. Sleep, especially REM sleep, seems to be involved in the resetting of homeostatic baselines in the central nervous system and in the consolidation of long-term memory.

LEARNING, MEMORY, EMOTIONS, AND LANGUAGE

Objective 3. Define the terms consciousness, learning, memory, and emotion; relate each to brain function.

Objective 4. Briefly describe the relationship between language and brain asymmetries.

Before learning, memory, and emotions can be considered, a definition of consciousness is needed. **Consciousness** is the state of being aware of objects, situations, or thoughts. When we are awake, we are conscious. When we are awake and alert, we can become aware of a new object, situation, or thought; we are in a position to learn something.

If we gain understanding or acquire a skill as a result of our experiences, we have learned. Thus, **learning** is the acquisition of a new skill or a new level of understanding as a result of experience. Learning may also be defined as a relatively permanent change in behavior recorded in the nervous system.

Memory is the ability to store and recall previous experiences. Learning and memory are therefore inseparable processes. It is by storing experiences in memory that we accumulate remembered experiences. Learning involves comparing new experiences with remembered experiences and gaining a new understanding; it makes use of the association areas in the brain as well as the memory storage areas. For example, at the beginning of this course you may have only vaguely understood the term homeostasis. The experience of studying this book has provided many examples of homeostasis. The accumulation of these experiences in memory should provide an expanded understanding of homeostasis. Each new example adds to that understanding.

Emotion is the affective, or feeling, aspect of experience. Almost every experience has an emotional component.

The purpose of the paragraphs that follow is to relate learning, memory, and emotion to what is known about the neurological processes that accompany these experiences. In this context it is important to realize that learning, memory, and emotion are abstract terms used to name observable behaviors and that it is not yet possible to relate these terms to specific cellular structures and functions. Thus, the best information available is limited to suggestions about parts of the brain that may be involved and about possible mechanisms that may or may not be confirmed by later research.

Memory Processes

Sensory receptors of various kinds receive stimuli and transmit signals to the brain, where they are interpreted. All of our conscious experience comes to our awareness by way of sensory signals, but some of these experiences are remembered longer than others. Determining what happens to sensory signals as they are stored in memory has been the subject of considerable research. Though much remains to be learned about the storage of experience in memory, many physiologists recognize three kinds of memory: sensory memory, short-term memory, and long-term memory.

Sensory memory is the retention of actual sensory images in the sensory areas of the brain for up to one second. For example, when you look out a window at a landscape and then close your eyes, the image of what you saw is sensory memory. It is thought that during this short period of time the brain scans the information in the sensory area and selects the portion that will be retained for further processing. The hippocampus seems to be involved in determining what is to be stored.

Short-term memory, or **primary memory**, is the memory of small fragments of information for a few seconds to a few minutes; unless transferred to long-term memory by practice, such information is soon forgotten. This type of information is limited to about seven bits of information, such as the seven digits of a telephone number or the words of a short sentence. Short-term memory allows one to remember a phone number long enough to dial it. Some physiologists believe that short-term memory is maintained by reverberating circuits within the neurons of the cerebral cortex. (These circuits were described in Chapter 10.)

Long-term memory is the memory of information for any period of time from minutes to years. Long-term memory is sometimes divided into two categories, secondary and tertiary memory. **Secondary memory** involves recent memory and includes things that are remembered from a few minutes to a few days. **Tertiary memory** often is so strongly established that it can be recalled very quickly throughout life. The things that you remember from the events of a day—things you might relate to your friends—are examples of secondary memory, whereas your name and address are examples of tertiary memory.

Theories about Long-Term Memory

Memories are stored in not one but several areas of the brain. Evidence for this statement comes from observations of individuals undergoing brain surgery who received only local anesthetic during the opening of the skull. When the surgeon stimulates different areas of the brain, the conscious individual may report different memories for each of several areas. Not only does memory involve different areas of the brain, but long-term memory may be accomplished by more than a single mechanism. It is almost certain that sensory and short-term memory involve different mechanisms than long-term memory.

One possible mechanism for some long-term memory storage may involve facilitated synaptic pathways, or **engrams**. Each time a signal travels a certain pathway, it may become easier for that pathway to be followed again. When a particular pattern of electrical activity that has occurred before is re-created, the person remembers the earlier event. If the theory of engrams is correct, it might explain the

A variety of memory defects have been observed in individuals who have sustained head injuries or other kinds of brain damage. For example, a person who sustained an injury in 1953 has, since that time, been unable to store new experiences in his memory. He fails to recognize doctors and other people who have worked with him. He can enjoy reading the same magazine article over and over because it is new to him each time. He must even be shown the way to the bathroom every time he needs to go. Another person has lost the ability to recognize faces—even those of close family members—yet he can recognize people by their voices or, given a photograph of a person, can draw a likeness of that person. The ability to remember voices indicates that all memory is not lost; the ability to draw a likeness from a photograph indicates there is no problem in seeing. Apparently, a particular area of the brain that matches visual images of the face with stored memories of faces doesn't work.

phenomenon of *déjà vu*—the sensation of having experienced a particular event before.

The possibility that long-term memory depends on continuous activity of neurons has been ruled out; the anesthesia, hypoxia (low oxygen supply), and other factors that reduce brain activity do not destroy long-term memories. Some physiologists have reported that RNA increases in certain neurons, suggesting that proteins are synthesized as memories are stored. They have speculated that the proteins may be used to increase the size or number of synapses of the neurons. Other physiologists contest these views and indicate that, although RNA and protein synthesis may occur with learning (and the storage of memories), these events have yet to be specifically related to memory storage.

Emotions

Emotions also play a part in learning and memory. As we noted in Chapter 11, the limbic system contains pleasure and reward centers, which some animals will learn to self-stimulate if electrodes are placed in their brains to make this possible. Several pathways of the reward system have been identified in the rat brain; of these pathways, fibers from the substantia nigra to the frontal cortex appear to be most associated with learning and memory. In experiments with rats stimulation of the substantia nigra or the cerebral cortex during training disrupts the animal's ability to remember the task one day later. However, if the animal is given the opportunity for self-stimulation of the reward system after learning, it engages in such stimulation and also remembers the task much better.

A possible location of pathways in humans analogous to those in rats is shown in Figure 12.4. The neurotransmitter in these pathways appears to be dopamine (DA). Experiments on the effects of various drugs on the dopamine synapses provide some tentative information on the function of the dopamine pathways. For example, as shown in Figure 12.5, reserpine impairs learning and memory by preventing the storage of dopamine in the secretory vesicles of the axons. Chlorpromazine causes similar impairment by blocking the receptor sites for dopamine. In contrast, amphetamines in small amounts facilitate learning and memory by stimulating the release of dopamine from synapses. Apomorphine, a chemical structurally similar to morphine, also facilitates learning and memory by stimulating dopamine receptors. Though the information available so far is insufficient to begin to design treatment programs for individuals with impaired learning and memory abilities, such programs may someday provide preventive or ameliorative therapy. Even without proven ap-

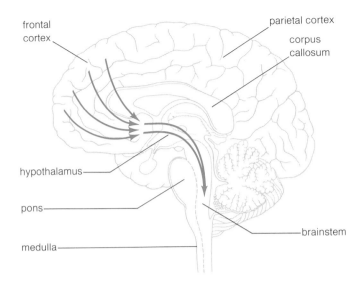

Figure 12.4 The possible pathways of the reward system of the human brain, based on studies of the rat brain.

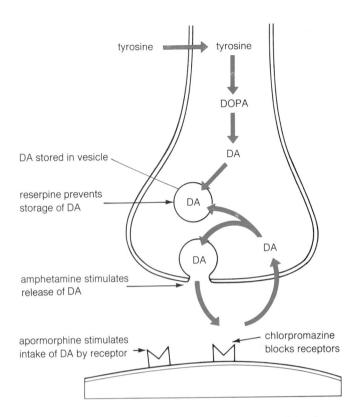

Figure 12.5 Effects of selected drugs on the transmission of signals at a dopamine-mediated (DA) synapse.

plications of this information, dopamine may be regarded as an extremely important factor in the brain's internal reward system that facilitates learning.

Another potent factor in the regulation of emotions is the group of opiatelike substances, the endorphins and enkephalins, introduced in Chapter 11. In contrast to the stimulating effect of dopamine, the opiatelike substances have a quieting effect. Dopamine and opiatelike substances seem to work together to create emotional good feeling. As was mentioned earlier, some of the endorphins and enkephalins also have been reported to stimulate learning and memory. Determining the exact relationships between dopamine and opiatelike substances and their effects constitute some of the many unsolved problems in neurophysiology.

Language and Brain Asymmetries

One of the first indications that the left and right hemispheres of the human brain were different was the observation by the French surgeon Paul Broca in 1861 that brain lesions causing speech disorders were generally located in the left hemisphere. Today, **brain assymetries**—hemispherical differences in structure and function—are well established. Understanding the capacities of different areas of the brain is useful in designing therapy for people with brain injuries.

Structural differences between the hemispheres include the somewhat larger left temporal lobe, variations in the pattern with which the spinal tracts decussate, or cross from one side to the other in the medulla, and differences in the brains of left- and right-handed individuals. For example, right-handed individuals are likely to have a left occipital lobe that is wider than the right lobe and a right frontal lobe that is wider than the left one. Differences in lobe size are much less frequent among left-handed individuals.

Functional differences parallel structural differences. One hemisphere is generally dominant over the other; that is, it controls many more human activities, especially those involving language. Language activities include formulating what is to be said or written, controlling speech or writing, and comprehending oral or written language. In over 90% of humans the left hemisphere is dominant; in the remainder either the right hemisphere is dominant or no dominance can be determined.

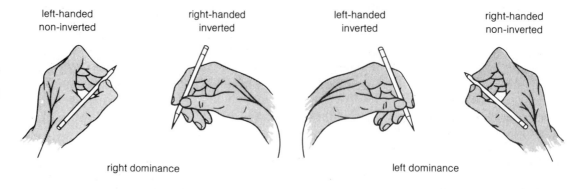

Figure 12.6 Writing position is correlated with cerebral dominance. (Redrawn with permission from J. Levy and M. Reid, *Science*, October 1976. Copyright 1976 by the American Association for the Advancement of Science.)

left-handed non-inverted   right-handed inverted   left-handed inverted   right-handed non-inverted

right dominance   left dominance

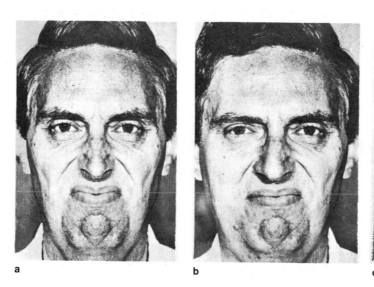

Figure 12.7 A face expressing disgust: (**a**) composite of left side of face, (**b**) original, (**c**) composite of the right side of same face. (Reproduced with permission from H. A. Sackeim, R. C. Gur, and M. C. Saucy, *Science*, October 1978. Copyright 1978 by the American Association for the Advancement of Science.)

a   b   c

Most studies of dominance have been based on observations of the effects of brain injuries, but EEG techniques are now being used. Studies using electrodes placed over the left and right sides of the head show that the activity is greater on the left side when an individual is using language or analyzing problems and greater on the right side when an individual is dealing with visual images or spatial problems or listening to music. These recent EEG studies, however, are able to detect activity on both sides of the brain during most activities. They tend to confirm the existence of dominance, but they also indicate that far more activity occurs in the right hemisphere during the use of language than had been supposed.

Hand preference is also associated with brain asymmetries. In most people right-handedness and left cerebral dominance occur together, but other combinations exist. The position of the hand during writing seems to help indicate dominance (Figure 12.6). According to measures of cerebral function, right-handed individuals who use the normal position and left-handed individuals who use the inverted position have dominant left hemispheres. Those who use the other two positions have dominant right hemispheres. Some individuals cannot be classified by writing position, and it is assumed that they probably do not have clearly defined dominance.

Even emotions seem to be related to hemispheric asymmetry. To determine this relationship, people expressing an emotion were photographed, and composite pictures consisting of the left side of the face and its mirror image or the right side of the face and its mirror image were made (Figure 12.7). The left side composites generally show stronger emotion than the right. Although innervation of facial muscles includes nerves from both sides of the brain serving each side of the face, there is some evidence that the right hemisphere exerts more control over emotional expression.

CLINICAL APPLICATIONS

Objective 5. For each of the following conditions describe the nature of the condition and how it is related to the nervous system: (a) parkinsonism, (b) manic-depressive psychosis, (c) schizophrenia, and (d) cerebral palsy.

Though great progress has been made in recent years in understanding the nature of many neurological disorders, much remains to be learned. In the short space devoted to such disorders below, it is possible to present only a few current ideas—ideas that may undergo revision as more is learned about the disorders.

Parkinsonism

Parkinson's disease, or **parkinsonism**, results from destruction of a significant portion of the substantia nigra, one of the basal nuclei of the brainstem. The symptoms include rigidity of a few or many muscles, resting tremors, and the loss of involuntary movements that normally occur as a part of intentional movements. For example, instead of the trunk and shoulder automatically adjusting to an appropriate position when one begins to write, the affected individual must deliberately assume the proper position. Persons with untreated parkinsonism walk with their heads bent forward and have a masklike facial expression; all their movements, whether walking or smiling, must be deliberately made (Figure 12.8).

The mechanism of the disease appears to be the loss of function of the inhibitory neurons in the substantia nigra, allowing oscillation between contraction and relaxation in the muscles. The neurotransmitter normally produced by the damaged neurons is dopamine, and thus a deficiency of dopamine is a characteristic of the disease. The substance L-dopa, structurally similar to dopamine, can be used to treat the disease. Unlike dopamine, L-dopa crosses the blood–brain barrier and reaches the substantia nigra, where it apparently compensates for the dopamine deficiency. This therapy is effective for only about three years after the onset of the disease.

Research is underway to identify other medications with more long-lasting effects. One line of research involves the grafting of dopamine-containing neurons from fetal rats into the experimentally destroyed substantia nigra of adult rats. Such grafts have been shown to reduce the detrimental effects of the destruction. If a similar technique could be developed for use in humans, it might prove a suitable way to treat parkinsonism. In addition, these experiments constitute the first successful grafting of brain tissue from one mammal to another, a significant accomplishment in itself.

Manic-Depressive Psychosis

Manic-depressive psychosis, or affective psychosis, is a severe mental disturbance in which great swings of mood occur, as the

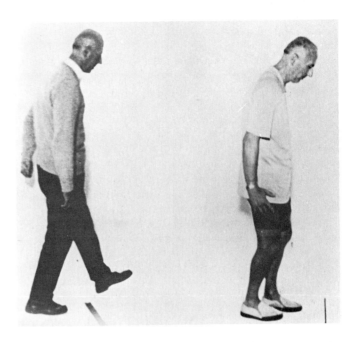

Figure 12.8 A person with Parkinson's disease before (left) and after (right) treatment with L-DOPA. (Reproduced with permission from J. W. Lance and J. G. McLeod, *A Physiological Approach to Clinical Neurology*, 2nd ed. (London: Butterworth, 1975), p. 168.)

name suggests, from manic (overactive) behavior to deep depression (dejection, absence of cheerfulness or hope). In many cases an individual experiences only depression without the manic phase. Furthermore, great variation exists in the degree to which either the manic or the depressive aspects of the disease are displayed by different people or by the same individual at different times.

Two theories of the cause of affective psychoses are related to neurotransmitters. Both are based on the idea that somehow there is an imbalance in the amount of neurotransmitter secreted by certain types of neurons in the brain. Susceptible neurons are generally located in the limbic system, the part of the brain most associated with emotion. The serotonin theory proposes that a deficiency of serotonin produces depression, and an excess of it produces mania. The norepinephrine theory proposes that a deficiency of norepinephrine produces depression, and an excess of it produces mania.

Both serotonin and norepinephrine are monoamines; that is, their molecular structure contains one amine group. (Dopamine is also a monoamine.) Cells that produce monoamine transmitters also contain an enzyme, monoamine oxidase (MAO), that can degrade each of the transmitters. Many of the efforts to treat affective disorders, particularly depression, are based on the use of drugs, such as hydrazine and its derivatives, that inhibit this enzyme. These drugs, called monoamine oxidase inhibitors, prevent the enzyme from acting, thereby allowing the concentration of the transmitter to build up.

Another group of medications, the tricyclic antidepressants, inhibit the reuptake of released norepinephrine back into the presynaptic knobs. They include imipramine (Tofranil) and amitryptyline (Elavil). Lithium, an inorganic ion related to sodium and potassium, has been used successfully to treat manic conditions and to stabilize the mood of patients who experience manic–depressive mood swings. Though its mode of action is not known, some evidence suggests that lithium may affect the movement of ions across cell membranes.

> Several types of seizures (abnormal discharges from brain neurons) occur in humans. Characteristic EEG patterns for a few such seizures are shown in Figure 12.9.

Schizophrenia

Schizophrenia is a complex set of disturbances in perception, thinking, and feeling; it may in fact be a set of several distinct but related diseases. Symptoms include detachment from reality, withdrawal, and disruption of communication with other people. Delusions and hallucinations are also common symptoms.

Several factors have been implicated in the pathology of schizophrenia. Schizophrenia tends to run in families, so a genetic predisposition toward the disease may exist. Viruslike agents have been found in the cerebrospinal fluid of some schizophrenic persons; it has been suggested that perhaps the viruslike agent is widely distributed and selectively affects individuals genetically predisposed to schizophrenia. Another factor that may cause schizophrenia in some instances is abnormalities in the structure of the brain, including enlarged ventricles, reversals in the normal asymmetries of the lobes of the brain, a thicker than normal corpus callosum, and an atrophied vermis. Enlargement of the ventricles is associated with aging but appears earlier in life in some schizophrenics. Reversal of symmetries (wider left frontal and right occipital lobes) is found in many schizophrenic people and in children suffering from language disorders.

It has also been reported that the brains of people with schizophrenia contain 50% more dopamine than normal brains; the excess is found almost exclusively in the limbic system. Therefore, one of the most common treatments for schizophrenia is the administration of antipsychotic drugs, such as chlorpromazine, that block the dopamine receptor sites. Though these drugs are effective in alleviating many of the symptoms of schizophrenia, they also appear to increase the number of dopamine receptor sites. A frequent side effect of long-term treatment with such drugs is the development of **tardive dyskinesia**, an assortment of involuntary movements such as facial twitches, rapid eye blinking, and tongue and lip movements. This pattern of disorders is similar to Parkinson's disease and may involve a deficiency of dopamine.

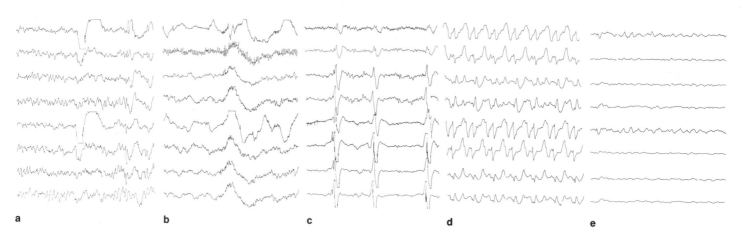

a   b   c   d   e

Figure 12.9 EEG patterns: (**a**) focal seizure (seizure caused by a lesion in a particular area of the brain) in four-year-old male who experienced birth trauma; (**b**) clinical seizure (seizure due to functional abnormality of the brain without the presence of a lesion) following hyperventilation in an eight-year-old child; (**c**) febrile encephalopathy (abnormal brain function caused by high fever) in a seventy-two-year-old person; (**d**) diffuse cerebral damage due to oxygen deprivation in a comatose seventy-nine-year-old person who had experienced cardiac arrest (heart stopped beating) and was resuscitated; (**e**) the EEG tracing of the oxygen-deprived person following the administration of the drug Valium, which suppressed the seizure activity and resulted in a nearly flat EEG. Such a tracing is typical of deep coma and indicates very little brain activity. (Courtesy of Dr. William Dolan, Arlington Hospital, Arlington, Virginia.)

Cerebral Palsy

Cerebral palsy includes a group of conditions in which abnormal functioning of the cerebrum causes muscular weakness, paralysis, and sometimes seizures. Although about one out of every 200 infants is affected to some degree with cerebral palsy, its causes are not well understood. A possible cause is lack of oxygen in the brain of the fetus prior to birth, during delivery, or shortly after birth. Several examples of the effects of cerebral palsy are shown in Figure 12.10, along with some therapies currently being used to help such children compensate for their disabilities.

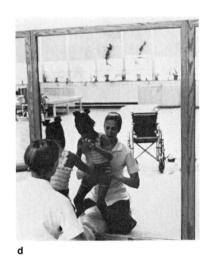
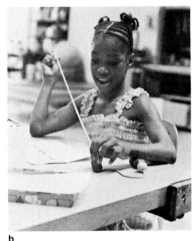
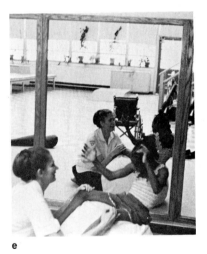
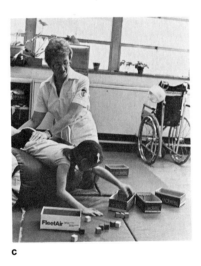
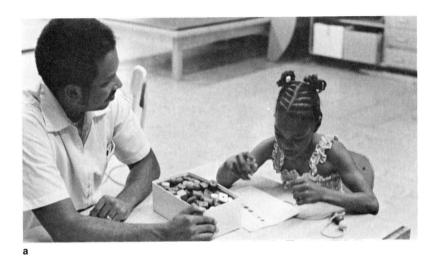

a

b

c

d

e

Figure 12.10 Physical therapy is useful in helping children affected by cerebral palsy to achieve more coordinated movements and to overcome to some degree the effects of their disabilities. (**a**) An occupational therapist helps an athetoid child who also has components of spasticity to string beads in sequence from left to right as a requisite for writing. The activity also stimulates motor planning, eye–hand coordination, and color discrimination. Athetosis results in involuntary movements of the extremities when purposeful activity is initiated. (**b**) The same child after successfully placing the proper bead on the string. (**c**) This child suffers from cerebral palsy resulting in ataxia and incoordination of all her muscles. To improve upper extremity function, the therapist is helping her to develop weight-bearing strength in her arms as she picks up blocks and puts them in shoe boxes. (**d**) The therapist is helping a child with athetoid spastic quadriplegia to develop hip and knee control. The activity involves moving from a sitting position on the bolster to a standing position and is done before a mirror to help the child to coordinate movements by seeing what she is doing. (**e**) Here, the therapist is helping the same child strengthen abdominal muscles by balancing on a large ball. (Photographs by author. Used with permission of the D.C. Public Schools, Department of Special Education, Sharpe Health School Administration, and the Department of Human Services of the District of Columbia.)

Clinical Terms

agraphia (ah-graf′e-ah)   inability to write because of a lesion in the brain

alexia (ah-lek′se-ah)   inability to read because of a lesion in the brain

amnesia (am-ne′se-ah)   loss of or lack of memory

aphasia (ah-fa′ze-ah)   inability to speak or write or inability to comprehend spoken or written language because of a lesion in the brain

coma (ko′mah)   a state of unconsciousness from which the individual cannot be roused

dyslexia (dis-leks′e-ah)   impaired ability to read because of a lesion in the brain, often involving reversal of letters in words

Essay: Learning Disabilities

Learning disabilities, minimal brain dysfunction, and hyperactivity are names for an ill-defined assortment of behaviors seen in children. The symptoms include overactive and impulsive behavior, short attention span, poor coordination, inability to delay gratification of wants, and poor academic performance in one or several areas. Statistically, boys are much more likely to be affected than girls. No single child is likely to display all of the symptoms, but it is estimated that between 6 and 10 million children in the United States suffer from some of them to the extent that their performance is impaired. Which of the labels is placed on a child suffering from these symptoms depends on which particular expert has examined the child.

Several conditions are excluded from the category of learning disabilities. Among the exclusions are mental retardation, strained family relationships, deprived environment, sensory impairments such as deafness or poor eyesight, and emotional problems. Children with learning disabilities often do display emotional disturbances, but these are thought to be the result of having to cope with the learning disability.

A typical learning-disabled child is a boy who resists getting ready for school in the morning, can't find his books, forgets his lunch, and may encounter a distraction on the way that keeps him from getting to school on time. When he gets there, he may be shunned by most of the other children because of his disorganized behavior and disheveled appearance. The teacher may be constantly telling him he could do better if he tried. He *is* trying, and he cannot understand why he cannot do as well as the other children. Eventually, frustration mounts, and emotional problems develop. Aggressive behavior may have been excessive since early childhood, but it is exacerbated by the frustrations of the school situation. Many behaviors of learning-disabled children would not be inappropriate in younger children, and any of the behaviors may appear occasionally in normal children. It is the persistence of the behaviors that distinguishes the learning-disabled child.

Causes

The present understanding of causes is as ill defined as the problem itself. Illnesses of the mother during pregnancy, birth injuries, and illnesses of the child may be causative factors. Heredity might play a part since three times as many boys as girls are affected. Moreover, a variety of minor physical abnormalities observable at birth seem to be predictive of future hyperactivity. These defects include more than one hair whorl, abnormalities in the shape or placement of one or both ears, a curved fifth finger, and variations in the spacing and length of the toes. A number of other ideas have been proposed, many of which are shrouded in controversy. They include diet, particularly the presence of food additives, and abnormalities in the way the body handles sugar.

Functional Deficits

At least two general types of functional deficits in the nervous system seem to exist, and they separate the class of learning disabilities into two categories. One, the attentional deficit, probably involves some structural or functional defect in the reticular activating system. Such a defect would account for short attention span and motor restlessness because of the inability of the RAS to exert normal controls.

The other deficit involves impaired ability to process information once it has been perceived. For example, disabled children may perceive a letter or geometric form as quickly as a normal child but have difficulty remembering what they have seen long enough to use the information. Keeping a word in mind long enough to say it, interpret its meaning, spell it, or write it down may be limited by some deficit in the interconnections within the brain. A sample of spelling and handwriting typical of many learning-disabled children is shown in Figure 12.11. One explanation for such a deficit is that both

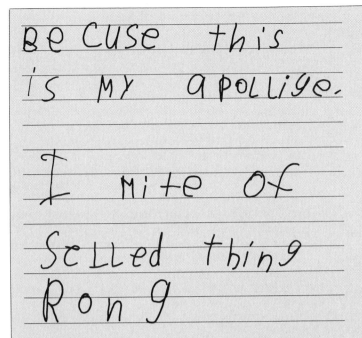

Be CUse this
is My apolliye.

I Mite oF

SeLLed thing
Rong

Figure 12.11 The ten-year-old boy who wrote this was unsure of his spelling ability.

hemispheres of the brain behave as right hemispheres, and thus the language symbols that are normally processed sequentially mainly in the left hemisphere are processed as spatially oriented material by both hemispheres.

Electroencephalograms of the brain activity of learning-disabled children often display minor variations from normal but lack sufficiently defined abnormalities for the diagnosis of severe pathology. Such findings have led to the term minimal brain dysfunction to describe the defects associated with learning disabilities. Whether the abnormal brain waves represent defective processing within the brain is unknown.

Treatment

One form of treatment involves the use of methylphenidate (Ritalin), an amphetaminelike drug, or amphetamines themselves. Such drugs appear to have a calming effect on most children, at least for the first few weeks of use, though their value has been questioned and their use is controversial. The effective dose for improving memory and school performance is about one-third the calming dose. At the maximum calming dose memory is impaired and heart rate and blood pressure increased. Long-term use may retard growth.

The calming effect of these stimulants has until recently been viewed as a paradox. When special arrangements were finally made to observe the effects of dextroamphetamine on normal boys, the drug was found to have a calming effect on them too. In fact, the drug sometimes has a calming effect on adults. Thus, stimulants are not specific treatments for hyperactivity.

Aside from the use of drugs other treatments that have been tried include diet, psychotherapy, and special educational programs. Diet seems to be effective in children who have some particular problem with certain foods, especially sugar, dyes, or other food additives. Psychotherapy may be effective in helping a youngster learn to cope with the frustrations that accompany a learning disability. Special educational programs often take advantage of modes of learning that are unimpaired and allow a child to proceed with a minimum of frustration. For example, the child who has difficulty with handwriting may be allowed to tape record lessons. Many children seem to outgrow their disabilities during adolescence. Others drop out of school, thus making their remaining disabilities less apparent. Until the nature of the defects within the brain are better understood, treatment will necessarily consist of attempting to cope with the symptoms instead of correcting the defect.

CHAPTER SUMMARY

(Chapter summary points and review questions are numbered to correspond to the numbered objectives in the text of each chapter.)

Higher Order Functions

1. Identify higher order functions of the brain.
   a. Higher order functions of the brain include sleep and wakefulness, learning, memory, emotions, and language functions.
   b. These functions are said to be higher order functions because they require complex and highly integrated brain function.

Sleep and Wakefulness

2. Describe how sleep and wakefulness are thought to be regulated, and explain the correlation of electroencephalograms with these processes.

a. Sleep and wakefulness are thought to be controlled by the reticular formation, which includes the following nuclei:
   (1) reticular activating system
   (2) locus ceruleus
   (3) pontine cells
   (4) raphe nuclei
b. Electroencephalograms, recordings of electrical potential differences between points on the scalp, show four distinct kinds of brain waves:
   (1) alpha waves, which are characteristic of an individual who is awake but relaxed with eyes closed
   (2) beta waves, which are characteristic of an individual who is mentally alert
   (3) theta waves, which are normal in children, and which in adults sometimes indicate a brain disorder
   (4) delta waves, which are characteristic of deep sleep, infancy, and some kinds of brain disease
c. Wakefulness seems to be maintained by the reticular activating system (RAS), which relays signals to the cerebrum and other parts of the brain. When the cerebral cortex is stimulated, it stimulates the RAS, and this positive feedback is an important factor in maintaining wakefulness.
d. Sleep, a natural temporary absence of wakefulness, is characterized by five stages:
   (1) Stage 1 consists of a period of drifting sensation, during which the RAS activity is somewhat reduced.
   (2) Stage 2 consists of a period during which sleep spindles appear in the electroencephalogram.
   (3) Stage 3 consists of a period during which delta waves appear and the rate of body functions decreases.
   (4) Stage 4 consists of a period of deep sleep, during which delta waves continue and body functions reach their lowest level.
   (5) Rapid-eye-movement (REM) sleep consists of a period of 5–20 minutes at intervals of 80–120 minutes, during which the EEG shows beta waves, the eyeballs move beneath the eyelids, dreaming occurs, and physiological processes increase in rate and become irregular.
e. Though the regulation of sleep and wakefulness is not fully understood, the following events appear to be involved:
   (1) Neurons in the raphe nuclei release serotonin and initiate both REM and non-REM sleep.
   (2) Neurons of the locus ceruleus and the pontine cells are also involved in sleep regulation.
   (3) Wakefulness and arousal seem to be controlled by norepinephrine-secreting neurons in the anterior third of the locus ceruleus, dopamine-secreting neurons in the RAS, and acetylcholine-secreting neurons of the cortex.
f. Physiological effects of sleep appear to involve a resetting of homeostatic baselines and the consolidation of long-term memory. Sleep deprivation reduces attention span, mental ability, and memory, and can lead to psychotic behavior.

Learning, Memory, Emotions, and Language

3. Define the terms consciousness, learning, memory, and emotion; relate each to brain function.
   a. Consciousness is the state of being aware of objects, situations, or thoughts.
   b. Learning is the acquisition of a new skill or a new level of understanding as a result of experience; it makes use of memories and association areas of the brain.
   c. Memory is the ability to recall previous experience.
      (1) Sensory memory lasts no more than one second and involves the brain scanning the information in the sensory area. The hippocampus appears to be involved in determining what is stored.
      (2) Short-term memory may involve reverberating circuits and lasts from a few seconds to a few minutes.
      (3) Long-term memory lasts from minutes to years and probably involves facilitated synaptic pathways, or engrams.
   d. Emotion is the feeling, or affective, aspect of experience and involves the limbic system.
4. Briefly describe the relationship between language and brain asymmetries.
   a. In over 90% of humans the left hemisphere is the dominant hemisphere in that it controls many higher functions.
   b. Language functions occur primarily in the left hemisphere of most individuals; hand preference is associated with hemispheric dominance.

Clinical Applications

5. For each of the following conditions describe the nature of the condition and how it is related to the nervous system: (a) parkinsonism, (b) manic-depressive psychosis, (c) schizophrenia, and (d) cerebral palsy.
   a. Parkinsonism is a disease in which muscle rigidity and resting tremors are caused by destruction of the substantia nigra and the resulting deficiency of dopamine. L-dopa is used to alleviate the symptoms as it can cross the blood–brain barrier and replace dopamine.
   b. Manic-depressive psychosis, or affective psychosis, involves disturbances in the mood of the patient. It is thought to be caused by imbalances in the neurotransmitters of the limbic system, most likely serotonin, norepinephrine, or both.
   c. Schizophrenia is a complex set of disturbances in thinking and feeling that may be due to excesses of dopamine in the limbic system, genetic predisposition, viruslike agents, or structural abnormalities in the brain. Drugs that block dopamine receptors are often used to treat schizophrenia; their long-term use often produces an assortment of involuntary movements called tardive dyskinesia.
   d. Cerebral palsy is a group of conditions in which abnormal functioning of the cerebrum causes muscular weakness, paralysis, and sometimes seizures. Its cause is unknown but may involve lack of oxygen near the time of birth.

REVIEW

Important Terms

alpha waves	long-term memory
beta waves	manic-depressive psychosis
brain asymmetries	memory
brain waves	non-REM sleep
cerebral palsy	parkinsonism
consciousness	pontine cells
delta waves	raphe nuclei
electroencephalogram	REM sleep
emotion	reticular activating system
engram	schizophrenia
higher order functions	sensory memory
learning	short-term memory
locus ceruleus	theta waves

Questions

1. What are the higher order functions of the brain?
2. a. What nuclei of the brain are involved in the regulation of sleep and wakefulness?
   b. What is an electroencephalogram?
   c. What are the main characteristics of the four kinds of brain waves?
   d. How is wakefulness thought to be maintained?
   e. What are the main characteristics of the five stages of sleep?
   f. What neurons are thought to be involved in the regulation of sleep and wakefulness, and what does each kind of neuron do?
   g. What are the physiological effects of sleep and of sleep deprivation?
3. a. Define learning, memory, and emotion.
   b. What part of the brain is involved in learning? In memory? In emotion?
   c. How do the types of memory differ from one another?
4. How are brain asymmetries associated with language?
5. a. What is the cause of parkinsonism, and how is it treated?
   b. What is manic-depressive psychosis, and what might cause it?
   c. What is schizophrenia, and what are some possible causes?
   d. What causes tardive dyskinesia?
   e. What is cerebral palsy?

Problems

1. Observe an animal or human child when it is asleep. Record eye movements seen through the eyelids and changes of position. Sometimes puppies make running movements with their legs during sleep. Note any such movements. Explain your observations on the basis of what you know about sleep.

2. For five minutes make a record of every thing you think about and every movement you make. After you finish your observations, add to your list all of the unconscious things that must have occurred (actions of proprioceptors, coordination in the cerebellum, and so on). Use your knowledge of the nervous system to explain what was happening inside your body as you engaged in the thoughts and actions.

REFERENCES AND READINGS

Adams, R. V. 1981. *Principles of neurology* (2nd ed.). New York: McGraw-Hill.

Anders, T. F., Carskadon, M. A., and Dement, W. C. 1980. Sleep and sleepiness in children and adolescents. *Pediatric Clinic of North America* 27(1):29 (February).

Buchbaum, M. S., Coursey, R. D., and Murphy, D. L. 1976. Biochemical high-risk paradigm: Behavioral and familial correlates of low platelet monoamine oxidase activity. *Science* 194:339 (October 15).

Burt, D. R., Creese, I., and Snyder, S. H. 1977. Antischizophrenic drugs: Chronic treatment elevates dopamine receptor binding in brain. *Science* 196:326 (April 15).

Cooper, J. R., Bloom, F. E., and Roth, R. H. 1978. *The biochemical basis of neuropharmacology* (3rd ed.). New York: Oxford University Press.

Davis, K. L., Mohs, R. C., Tinklenberg, J. R., Pfefferbaum, A., Hollister, L. E., and Kopell, B.S. 1978. Physostigmine: Improvement in long-term memory processes in normal humans. *Science* 201:272 (July 21).

Dole, V. P. 1980. Addictive behavior. *Scientific American* 243(6):138 (December).

Galaburda, A. M., LeMay, M., Kemper, T. L., and Geschwind, N. 1978. Right-left asymmetries in the brain. *Science* 199:852 (February 24).

Geschwind, N. 1979. Specializations of the human brain. *Scientific American* 241(3):180 (September).

Gillin, J. C., Mendelson, W. B., Sitaram, N., and Wyatt, R. J. 1978. The neuropharmacology of sleep and wakefulness. *Annual Review of Pharmacology and Toxicology* 18:563.

Greenburg, J. 1978. Cracking the cycles of depression and mania. *Science News* 114:367 (November 25).

Greenburg, J. 1978. Memory research: An era of good feeling. *Science News* 114:364 (November 25).

Greenburg, J. 1979. The schizophrenic brain: Rewriting the chapter. *Science News* 116:26 (July 14).

Hobson, J. A., Spagna, R.., and Malenka, R. 1978. Ethology of sleep studied with time-lapse photography: Postural immobility and sleep-cycle phase in humans. *Science* 201:1251 (September 29).

Kiester, E., Jr. 1980. Images of the night. *Science 80* 1(4):36 (May–June).

Kolata, G. B. 1978. Childhood hyperactivity: A new look at treatments and causes. *Science* 199:515 (February 3).

Kolata, G. B. 1979. Mental disorders: A new approach to treatment. *Science* 203:36 (January 5).

Levy, J., and Reid, M. 1976. Variations in writing posture and cerebral organization. *Science* 194:337 (October 15).

Loftus, E. F. 1979. The malleability of human memory. *American Scientist* 67:312 (May–June).

Marx, J. L. 1979. Parkinson's disease: Search for better therapies. *Science* 203:737 (February 23).

Miller, J. A. 1981. Brain-watch. *Science News* 119:76 (January 31).

Morrison, F. J., Giordani, B., and Nagy, J. 1977. Reading disability: An information-processing analysis. *Science* 196:77 (April 1).

Ramm, P. 1979. The locus coeruleus, catecholamines, and REM sleep: A critical review. *Behavioral and Neural Biology* 25:415 (April).

Rapaport, J. L., Buchsbaum, M. S., Zahn, T. P., Weingartner, H., Ludlow, C., and Mikkelsen, E. J. 1978. Dextroamphetamine: Cognitive and behavioral effects in normal prepubertal boys. *Science* 199:560 (February 3).

Routtenberg, A. 1978. The reward system of the brain. *Scientific American* 239(5):154 (November).

Sackeim, H. A., Gur, R. C., and Saucy, M. C. 1978. Emotions are expressed more intensely on the left side of the face. *Science* 202:433 (October 27).

Sprague, R. L., and Sleator, E. K. 1977. Methylphenidate in hyperkinetic children: Differences in dose effects on learning and social behavior. *Science* 198:1247 (December 23).

Tyrrell, D. A. J., Crow, T. J., Parry, R. P., Ferrier, I. N., Johnstone, E., Owens, D. G. C., and MacMillan, J. F. 1979. Possible virus in schizophrenia and some neurological disorders. *Lancet* 1(8121):839 (April 21).

Waldrop, M. F., Bell, R. Q., McLaughlin, B., and Halverson, C. F. 1978. Newborn minor physical anomalies predict short attention span, peer aggression, and impulsivity at age 3. *Science* 199:563 (February).

Wallace, P. 1975. Neurochemistry: Unraveling the mechanism of memory. *Science* 190:1076 (December 12).

Witelson, S. F. 1977. Developmental dyslexia: Two right hemispheres and none left. *Science* 195:309 (January 21).

13

AUTONOMIC NERVOUS SYSTEM

ORGANIZATION AND GENERAL FUNCTION

Objective 1. Describe the general organization of the autonomic nervous system and briefly explain its function.

When you are frightened, your heart races and you breathe rapidly. You can run faster and jump higher than at other times. When you are well fed, relaxed, and contented, your heart rate and breathing are slower. Unless you are highly motivated, you may find it difficult to get out of your easy chair to tackle a big job. These examples, of course, are extremes along a continuum of physiological activity that may occur in your body. Most of the time your body maintains itself somewhere between these extremes.

The **autonomic nervous system** (in association with the endocrine system) is primarily responsible for maintaining a nearly constant internal environment in your body, regardless of the changes that take place in the external environment. Though it is true that the autonomic nervous system makes it possible for you to respond to a frightening experience and to "unwind" after it is over, you spend only a small portion of your life in frightening circumstances. The ability of the autonomic nervous system to cope with extremes is important; its ability to continuously respond to small changes is even more important in controlling many of the functions of internal organs throughout life so that homeostasis is maintained.

The autonomic nervous system itself is a system of efferent motor nerves. However, afferent, sensory fibers from several different sources stimulate the autonomic nervous system. Impulses from sense organs are relayed to

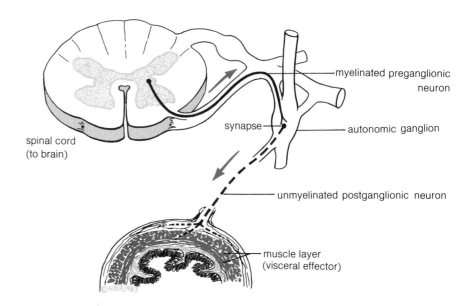

Figure 13.1   The arrangement of neurons in an autonomic pathway.

centers in the spinal cord, brainstem, and hypothalamus, where impulses are relayed again to autonomic neurons. In addition, the cerebral cortex itself can stimulate autonomic activity by exciting one of these centers. Sensory information from the internal organs travels along the vagus nerve and some afferent fibers of the spinal nerves to centers in the brain that initiate autonomic activity. These stimuli from the organs themselves constitute a kind of feedback in which information about the level of function of an organ is used to adjust its functional level.

All autonomic neural pathways are composed of two neurons: a preganglionic neuron and a postganglionic neuron. Impulses from the preganglionic neuron are transmitted by way of acetylcholine across a synapse in a **ganglion** to the postganglionic neuron (Figure 13.1). Preganglionic neurons are myelinated; postganglionic neurons are unmyelinated.

The properties of the autonomic nervous system are distinctly different from those of the somatic nervous system. The differences are summarized in Table 13.1.

The autonomic nervous system is divided into two parts: the **sympathetic division**, which originates in the thoracolumbar region of the spinal cord, and the **parasympathetic division**, which originates in the medulla, pons, and midbrain and the sacral region of the spinal cord. Thus,

Table 13.1 A Comparison of the Properties of the Somatic and Autonomic Nervous Systems	
Somatic	Autonomic
Innervates skeletal muscle.	Innervates smooth muscle, cardiac muscle, and glands.
Efferent axons synapse directly on effectors.	Efferent axons synapse in ganglia.
Innervation is always excitatory.	Innervation may be excitatory or inhibitory.
Transmitter is acetylcholine.	Transmitter is acetylcholine or norepinephrine.
Motor impulse leads to voluntary activity.	Motor impulse leads to involuntary activity.

these parts of the autonomic nervous system are sometimes referred to as the **thoracolumbar** and the **craniosacral** divisions, respectively. Fibers from each of the divisions of the autonomic nervous system supply nearly every one of the visceral organs (Figure 13.2). Branches of several pregan-

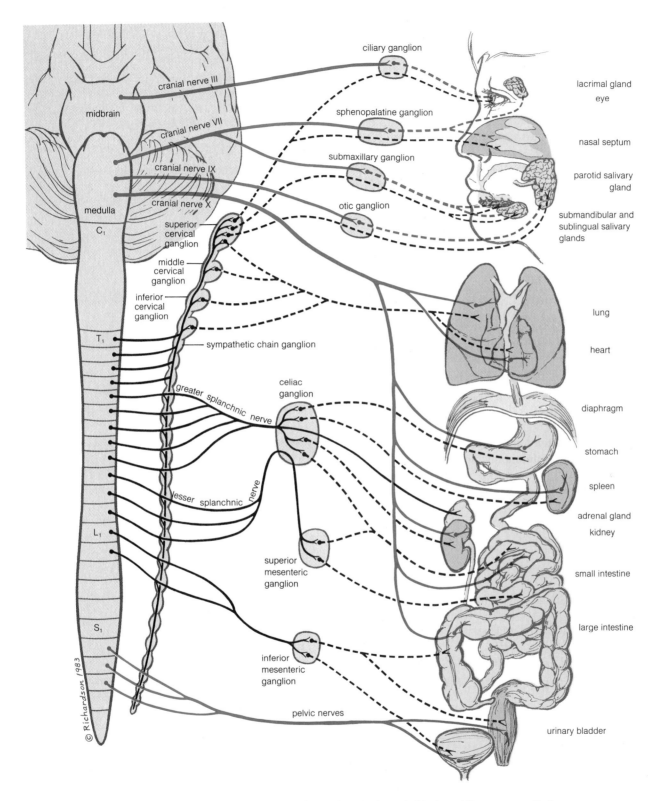

Figure 13.2 The autonomic nervous system. The sympathetic division is shown in black, and the parasympathetic division is shown in color. Preganglionic neurons are shown by solid lines and postganglionic by dotted lines.

glionic sympathetic fibers converge to form several important splanchnic nerves.

The general functions of the sympathetic division are to increase heart rate and respiratory rate, dilate bronchioles (small air passages in the lungs), stimulate sweating, increase the glucose level in the blood, and decrease the activities of the digestive tract. The general functions of the parasympathetic division are often the opposite of those of the sympathetic: to decrease heart rate and respiratory rate, increase digestive activities, and stimulate the storage of glucose in the liver.

The alternate stimulation of an organ by the sympathetic and parasympathetic divisions keeps the organ functioning within a narrow range of functional levels. This alternation contributes to the ability of the autonomic nervous system to maintain homeostasis. For example, your heart rate varies throughout the day, increasing as you engage in strenuous activity and decreasing as you relax. Yet the rate is kept within a range from about 70 to 110 beats per minute, going higher only when you engage in prolonged strenuous activity. Likewise, your body temperature, as we discussed in Chapter 5, is maintained within a narrow range around 37°C, rarely increasing or decreasing by more than a single degree.

DEVELOPMENT

Objective 2. Describe briefly the embryological development of the autonomic nervous system.

Before the end of the first month of embryonic development, groups of cells called the **neural crests** separate from the neural tube. (Refer back to Figure 10.2 in Chapter 10.) These cells migrate laterally and anteriorly from their original location to form two chains of ganglia, one on either side of the spinal cord. Some of these cells, the so-called chromaffin cells, migrate along a different path and form the medulla of the adrenal gland. Neural crest cells also give rise to several ganglia in the head region—the ciliary ganglion near the eye, for example. Subsequent growth of the spinal and cranial nerves establishes connections between the autonomic and other peripheral nerves.

NEUROTRANSMITTERS

Objective 3. Name the neurotransmitters of the autonomic nervous system and describe their interactions with their receptors.

Neurons of the autonomic nervous system synthesize and secrete neurotransmitters just as other neurons do. And like other transmitters, these must be inactivated to prevent continuous stimulation and to allow repolarization of the postsynaptic neurons. The different functions of the sympathetic and parasympathetic divisions of the autonomic nervous system are determined by the particular neurotransmitter released and how that transmitter interacts with the receptor it reaches (Figures 13.3 and 13.4).

Two neurotransmitters are found in the autonomic nervous system. Acetylcholine is released by all presynaptic neurons and by all parasympathetic postganglionic neurons (as well as by a few sympathetic postganglionic neurons). Neurons that release acetylcholine are said to be **cholinergic**. **Norepinephrine** (noradrenalin) is released by most sympathetic postganglionic neurons; such neurons are said to be **adrenergic**.

When acetycholine is released by cholinergic neurons, its effects are determined by the nature of the receptor with which it interacts. Two kinds of receptors exist: **nicotinic receptors** (so named because nicotine mimics the action of acetylcholine at such receptors) and **muscarine receptors** (so named because muscarine—a substance from toadstools—mimics the action of acetylcholine at these receptors). The actions of acetylcholine at such receptors are said to be nicotinic actions and muscarine actions, respectively.

Nicotinic receptors are found on both sympathetic and parasympathetic postganglionic neurons. The result of the interaction of acetylcholine with nicotinic receptors depends on the concentration of acetylcholine; small amounts stimulate and large amounts block transmission.

Muscarine receptors are found on organs innervated by postganglionic parasympathetic neurons—the heart, smooth muscle, and sweat glands. The result of the interaction of acetylcholine with muscarine receptors is muscle contraction or sweat secretion.

When norepinephrine is released by adrenergic neurons, its effects are similarly determined by the nature of the receptor with which it interacts. However, the action of norepinephrine is augmented by the release of both norepinephrine and **epinephrine** from the adrenal medulla (an organ associated with, but not part of, the sympathetic division). When the adrenal medulla is stimulated, it releases both of the hormones—epinephrine and norepinephrine—into the bloodstream, with epinephrine being released in quantities about four times as great as the quantity of norepinephrine. Compared with the rapid action of norepinephrine released by an axon directly into a tissue, epinephrine and norepinephrine released into the bloodstream are slower to act. However, their actions are more sustained because they circulate in the blood and stimulate the

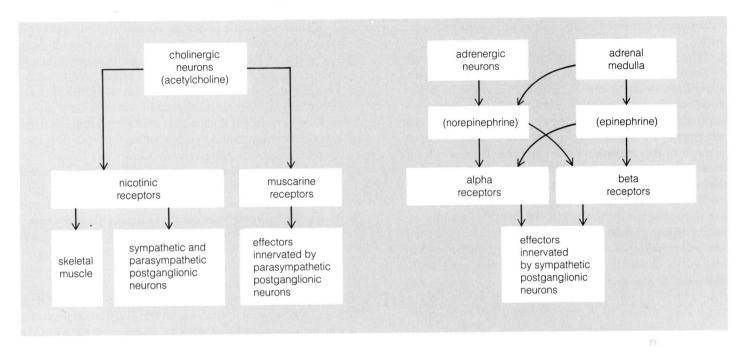

Figure 13.3 Summary of neurotransmitters and receptors involved in autonomic nervous system function.

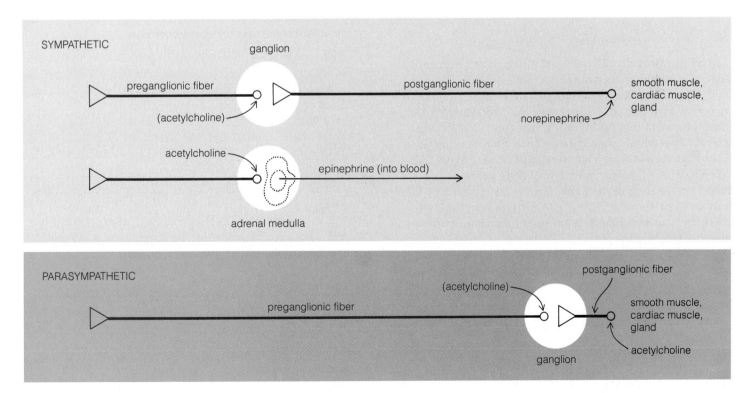

Figure 13.4 The fibers of the autonomic nervous system and their usual transmitters.

organs for several minutes before they are destroyed by the liver.

Organs that respond to epinephrine or norepinephrine (either via the blood or via sympathetic postganglionic neurons) have one or both of two kinds of receptors, **alpha receptors** and **beta receptors**. Epinephrine stimulates both alpha and beta receptors; norepinephrine stimulates alpha receptors to a greater extent than beta receptors. The effect of either of these transmitters on an organ depends on the quantity and sensitivity of each type of receptor found in the organ. The effects of stimulating alpha receptors include vasoconstriction, relaxation of intestinal smooth muscle, and dilation of the iris of the eye. The effects of stimulating beta receptors include vasodilation, acceleration of the heart rate and strengthening of its contraction, bronchodilation, relaxation of intestinal smooth muscle, and release of glucose and fatty acids into the blood.

SYMPATHETIC DIVISION

Objective 4. Describe the structure and functions of the sympathetic division.

Structure of the Sympathetic Division

The sympathetic division consists of the paired paravertebral **sympathetic chain ganglia**, the **preganglionic neurons**, and the **postganglionic neurons**. (Refer back to Figure 13.2.)

The cell bodies of the preganglionic neurons are in the lateral horns of the spinal cord. Their axons travel along a spinal nerve and through the myelinated **white communicating ramus** to one of the **sympathetic chain ganglia** (Figure 13.5). Here the axon takes one of three paths:

1. It may synapse directly with a postganglionic neuron in the chain ganglion.

2. It may extend through the chain ganglion to another ganglion, called a **prevertebral**, or **collateral**, **ganglion**. This ganglion lies nearer the visceral organ being served and is the site of the synapse between the preganglionic and postganglionic neurons.

3. It may extend upward or downward along the chain to another chain ganglion and either synapse directly or extend to a collateral ganglion.

Postganglionic neurons may have their cell bodies either in one of the chain ganglia or in one of the collateral ganglia. The axons of some of the postganglionic neurons, whose cell bodies are in the chain ganglia, extend along the unmyelinated **gray communicating ramus** and join one of the spinal nerves. Their axons terminate in the smooth muscle of blood vessels, sweat glands, or arrector pili muscles in the skin. Other postganglionic neurons extend from their synapse with a preganglionic neuron via splanchnic (visceral) nerves to blood vessels and smooth muscle within visceral organs.

The number of postganglionic fibers exceeds that of preganglionic fibers by about thirty to one. The stimulation of many postganglionic fibers by a single preganglionic fiber causes wide divergence of neural signals. For example, an impulse arriving in the celiac ganglion can be spread to several visceral organs (see Figure 13.2).

The distribution of nerves to the medulla of the adrenal gland is somewhat different from the distribution described above. The axons of preganglionic cells extend without a synapse from the spinal cord through the chain ganglia, along a splanchnic nerve, through the celiac ganglion, and directly to the adrenal medulla. The cells of the adrenal medulla are postganglionic cells, which release norepinephrine and epinephrine.

Functions of the Sympathetic Division

The sympathetic division works continuously and in conjunction with the parasympathetic division to maintain homeostasis. It makes small modifications in the functional level of different organs in accordance with the stimuli it receives from neural centers in the hypothalamus and other parts of the central nervous system, as described earlier. When the body is under stress, the entire sympathetic division is activated at once; the stimuli reaching the sympathetic division are stronger, and they stimulate the organs accordingly. Such stimuli have the following effects: The pupils dilate and the sweat glands become more active. The heart pumps faster and more forcefully. The air passages in the lungs (bronchi) and the blood vessels that serve the muscles dilate. The blood carries more nutrients, and its ability to clot is accelerated. The muscles of the digestive tract are relaxed, and the digestive secretions are greatly reduced even if there is food in the tract. Blood is diverted from the digestive tract and kidneys to the skeletal muscles, where it may be needed to supply oxygen and nutrients for strenuous activity. In extreme stress the kidneys produce a smaller volume of urine, thereby conserving fluid. Processes

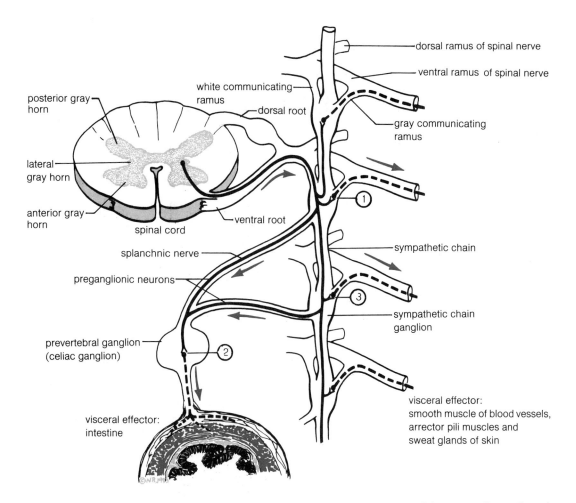

Figure 13.5 The arrangement of chain ganglia of the sympathetic nervous system and the nerve pathways through them. Synapses numbered 1, 2, and 3 are described in the text.

Labels in figure:
- dorsal ramus of spinal nerve
- ventral ramus of spinal nerve
- white communicating ramus
- dorsal root
- gray communicating ramus
- posterior gray horn
- lateral gray horn
- anterior gray horn
- spinal cord
- ventral root
- sympathetic chain
- splanchnic nerve
- preganglionic neurons
- sympathetic chain ganglion
- prevertebral ganglion (celiac ganglion)
- visceral effector: smooth muscle of blood vessels, arrector pili muscles and sweat glands of skin
- visceral effector: intestine

that provide energy for movement are accelerated. The effects of the sympathetic and the parasympathetic divisions are contrasted in Table 13.2.

PARASYMPATHETIC DIVISION

Objective 5. Describe the structure and functions of the parasympathetic division.

Structure of the Parasympathetic Division

The parasympathetic division consists of ganglia, preganglionic neurons, and postganglionic neurons. Although these are the same three components that are found in the sympathetic nervous system, they are arranged differently. (Refer back to Figure 13.2.) The cell bodies of the preganglionic neurons are located in the nuclei of certain cranial nerves or in the sacral portion of the spinal cord. Their axons extend to ganglia on or near the organs they serve, where they form synapses with the postganglionic neurons.

The postganglionic axons are usually short; they terminate only within the tissues of the organ they serve. Thus, parasympathetic innervation is more precise and less widespread than sympathetic innervation.

Functions of the Parasympathetic Division

Like the sympathetic division, the parasympathetic division acts continuously to maintain homeostasis. Generally, it works in opposition to the sympathetic division: A process that one division speeds up the other slows down and vice versa. When the parasympathetic division is strongly stimulated, the smooth muscles of the digestive tract become much more active, and the glands of the tract secrete copious quantities of digestive juices. The heart contracts more slowly, and the bronchi constrict. Some parasympathetic effects appear to be unrelated to the sympathetic effects. For example, the parasympathetic division stimulates the ciliary muscle of the eye and causes it to contract. This action reduces tension on the lens and allows it to focus on near objects. The sympathetic division has only a minor effect on the relaxation of the ciliary muscle.

Another function of the parasympathetic division is to cause dilation of the blood vessels in the clitoris and the penis and produce erection. This may be a reason that sexual performance is often impaired when individuals are under stress.

> The parasympathetic and not the sympathetic division stimulates the production of tears. Though tears may be associated with stress, they usually come after a stressful situation has been met, and the parasympathetic division has "taken over."

RELATIONSHIPS BETWEEN THE SYMPATHETIC AND PARASYMPATHETIC DIVISIONS

Objective 6. Explain how the sympathetic and parasympathetic divisions work together to maintain homeostasis.

Both the sympathetic and parasympathetic divisions are continually active. The basal rate of activity of each is called **sympathetic tone** or **parasympathetic tone**. For example, the actions of the sympathetic division maintain the diameter of the blood vessels at about half their widest diameter. A slight increase or decrease in the degree of sympathetic stimulation can change the diameters of the blood vessels of an organ. The actions of the parasympathetic division maintain functions such as the secretion of digestive juices and the tone of smooth muscle in the walls of the digestive tract. Contractions of these muscles (motility) move substances through the digestive tract. Small changes in the degree of parasympathetic stimulation regulates the flow of digestive juices and the motility of the digestive tract. These examples indicate that both systems are involved in maintaining homeostasis by responding to small changes on a continuous basis.

The two divisions are usually antagonistic. For example, the heart receives sympathetic stimulation that causes it to increase both its rate of beating and the strength of its contraction. At the same time, the heart receives parasympathetic stimulation that causes it to decrease its rate of beating. Thus the heart rate at any given time is the net effect of the two opposing forces.

Autonomic is actually a poor word to describe this system because it is far from autonomous, which means self-controlled. Both the sympathetic and the parasympathetic divisions are regulated by control centers in the brain, and several levels of control are imposed. Centers in the hypothalamus can stimulate either the sympathetic or the parasympathetic division and thereby can regulate a variety of physiological processes. Stimuli from higher centers in the limbic system can also stimulate the hypothalamus and in turn the autonomic nervous system. It is at this point in the "chain of command" that emotions can affect visceral functions. Finally, stimuli from the cerebral cortex have been found to exert influence on autonomic functions. Studies of individuals in meditative states have shown that their body processes respond in ways almost opposite to that of the sympathetic response. Thus, meditation appears to produce a generalized parasympathetic response, whereas fright or stress produce an integrated sympathetic response. These responses and other characteristics that distinguish the sympathetic and parasympathetic divisions are summarized in Table 13.3.

Table 13.2 Autonomic Effects on Various Organs

Organ	Effect of Sympathetic Stimulation	Effect of Parasympathetic Stimulation
Iris	Contract dilator muscle and dilate pupil	Contract constrictor muscle and constrict pupil
Ciliary muscle	None	Contract muscle and accommodate lens for near vision
Sweat glands	Stimulate secretion	None
Lacrimal glands	None	Secrete normal or excessive amount of tears
Salivary glands	Reduce amount of saliva	Increase amount of saliva
Respiratory system	Dilate passages	Constrict passages
Blood vessels of respiratory system	Dilate	Constrict
Heart	Increase heart rate and stroke volume	Decrease heart rate
Coronary vessels	Dilate	Constrict

Blood vessels of:
  Skeletal muscle
  Skin
  Digestive system
	
	Dilate
	Constrict
	Constrict
		
		None
		None
		Dilate

Adrenal medulla	Secrete epinephrine and norepinephrine	None
Liver	Increase breakdown of glycogen to glucose; decrease bile secretion	Increase storage of glycogen; increase bile secretion
Digestive glands (except salivary)	None	Increase secretion
Digestive tract	Decrease motility	Increase motility
Kidney	Constrict blood vesse's and decrease urine volume	None
Spleen	Contract and discharge stored blood	
Urinary bladder	Relax muscular wall	Contract muscular wall
Uterus	Inhibit contraction if nonpregnant, stimulate contraction if pregnant	Little effect
Sex organs	Constrict blood vessels of sperm passageways and cause ejaculation	Dilate blood vessels of clitoris and penis and cause erection
Arrector pili muscles	Contract and cause ''goose flesh''	None

Table 13.3   Comparison of Sympathetic and Parasympathetic Divisions

Sympathetic Division	Parasympathetic Division
Physiological Characteristics	*Physiological Characteristics*
Accelerated heart rate	Lowered heart rate
Increased blood pressure	Decreased blood pressure
Increased metabolic rate	Decreased metabolic rate
Increased oxygen consumption and respiratory rate	Decreased oxygen consumption and respiratory rate
Increase in intensity of beta waves in EEG	Increase of alpha waves in EEG
Increase in lactic acid in blood	Decrease in lactic acid in blood
Decrease in electrical resistance of skin	Increase in electrical resistance of skin
"Fight-or-flight" response	Meditation response*
Anatomical Characteristics	*Anatomical Characteristics*
Preganglionic neurons originate in thoracolumbar area	Preganglionic neurons originate in craniosacral areas
Contains chain ganglia and other visceral ganglia	Has ganglia very close to the organ supplied
Each preganglionic fiber forms synapses with many postganglionic fibers, so many organs are affected	Each preganglionic fiber forms synapses with only a few postganglionic fibers, and only one organ may be affected
Action is diffuse	Action limited to one or a few organs
Chemical Characteristics	*Chemical Characteristics*
Division is said to be adrenergic	Division is said to be cholinergic
Norepinephrine is the transmitter for most postganglionic fibers	Acetylcholine is the transmitter for postganglionic fibers
Adrenal medulla is stimulated to release epinephrine and norepinephrine	

*Some of the characteristics of the meditation response may be due to suppression of the sympathetic system rather than to action of the parasympathetic system. See Wallace and Benson (1972), cited at the end of this chapter.

CLINICAL APPLICATIONS

Objective 7. Distinguish between drugs that act on the sympathetic and the parasympathetic divisions and explain several conditions in which they might be used.

Six different categories of drugs can be distinguished on the basis of their site of action and their effects.

Sympathomimetic (adrenergic) drugs mimic the action of the sympathetic division. Norepinephrine and epinephrine act as sympathomimetic drugs by attaching to receptor sites, thus augmenting the action of the same naturally present chemicals. Other drugs, such as ephedrine, act in a similar way. When sympathomimetics bind to receptor sites, the body responds as though increased neural impulses were causing the release of neurotransmitters. Such drugs are sometimes used to treat individuals in shock, a state in which the blood pressure is severely depressed, because they elevate heart rate and blood pressure.

Other drugs, called **adrenergic blocking agents**, block the transmission of signals from postganglionic sympathetic axons to their receptor organs. Reserpine, a tranquilizer, blocks the synthesis and storage of norepinephrine. It is now rarely used because of its carcinogenic properties. Certain other drugs act by blocking the release of norepinephrine. When less neurotransmitter is released, fewer impulses are transmitted. Such a drug is sometimes used in treating hypertension.

Parasympathomimetic (cholinergic) drugs mimic the action of the parasympathetic division by attaching to receptor sites for acetylcholine. Pilocarpine is an example of such a drug. One of its actions is to increase the diameter of the canal of Schlemm, which drains aqueous humor from the eye, making it useful in the treatment of glaucoma (see Chapter 14). Anticholinesterases—drugs that inhibit cholinesterase, such as neostigmine and physostigmine—are indirectly parasympathomimetic. By slowing the action of cholinesterase, they effectively increase the duration of action of naturally occurring acetylcholine. Though such drugs can affect the parasympathetic nervous system, they are most often used in treating myasthenia gravis, a condition described in Chapter 8.

Atropine, a **cholinergic blocking agent**, is used to treat smooth muscle spasms and to dilate pupils during eye examinations. It blocks the action of the parasympathetic division, which normally maintains the pupil of the eye in a relatively constricted state. It also causes the ciliary muscle to relax and the lens of the eye to focus on distant objects. (More will be said about the eye in Chapter 14.) The advantages of atropine in eye examinations are to allow examination of the inside of the eye and to prevent the person from using the ciliary muscle during the testing of vision. In this way any lenses needed are prescribed for a relaxed, unstrained eye.

Certain drugs act at the synapses between the pre- and postganglionic fibers and affect the autonomic nervous system in ways that are not clearly sympathomimetic or parasympathomimetic.

Table 13.4 Some Drugs That Affect the Autonomic Nervous System		
Site of Drug Action	Drugs That Augment Activity	Drugs That Depress Activity
Synapses in ganglia—drugs have greater effect on sympathetic than on parasympathetic	Stimulate nicotinic receptors: nicotine Inhibit cholinesterase: physostigmine, neostigmine	Block transmission: tetramethylammonium ion
Endings of parasympathetic postganglionic neurons	Stimulate muscarine receptors: muscarine, pilocarpine Inhibit cholinesterase: physostigmine, neostigmine	Block transmission: atropine
Endings of sympathetic postganglionic neurons	Release norepinephrine: ephedrine, amphetamine	Interfere with norepinephrine storage: reserpine Prevent norepinephrine release: guanithidine (Ismelin) Compete with norepinephrine for receptor sites: methyldopa (Aldomet)
Alpha receptors	Stimulate receptors: phenylephrine (Neo-Synephrine)	Block receptors: phenoxybenzamine (Dibenzyline), phentolamine (Regitine)
Beta receptors	Stimulate receptors: isoproterenol (Isuprel)	Block receptors: propranolol (Inderal)

Nicotine stimulates ganglionic transmission of impulses and thus excites both sympathetic and parasympathetic fibers. Its effects include vasoconstriction of blood vessels in abdominal organs (a sympathetic effect) and increased intestinal motility (a parasympathetic effect). In contrast, a chemical substance called tetramethylammonium ion blocks the transmission of impulses from pre- to postsynaptic neurons in animals. Generally, drugs that act at the synapses in the ganglia affect the sympathetic nervous system to a greater extent than the parasympathetic system because of a greater resting sympathetic tone.

The actions of selected drugs affecting the autonomic system are summarized in Table 13.4.

Essay: Biofeedback

Until recently it was thought that the functions of the autonomic nervous system could not be consciously controlled. However, some autonomic functions have been brought under conscious control through operant conditioning, a kind of learning in which an individual (human or other animal) learns by trial and error, with responses followed by some kind of feedback. This feedback, usually a reward or a punishment, reinforces the learning. **Biofeedback** is feedback provided about an individual's own physiological processes. When presented immediately following efforts to control autonomic or other physiological functions, feedback can reinforce learning to perceive and control such functions.

Most people have little or no natural ability to perceive their own autonomic processes such as blood pressure or heart rate. Some even have difficulty perceiving tension in skeletal muscles. Experiments with biofeedback have been used successfully to improve perception of these processes and in many cases to help people learn to control them. Though much remains to be learned about biofeedback, some tentative ideas about its use are presented here.

What Responses Can Be Affected by Biofeedback?

Numerous experiments conducted with humans have shown that the following autonomic processes can be increased or decreased by the use of biofeedback: diameter of blood vessels, circulation of blood to the skin, sweating, heart rate and rhythm, blood pressure, salivation, and possibly gastrointestinal motility. Strong evidence exists to show that people can be taught to relax skeletal muscles by biofeedback. There is also some evidence that people can learn to increase or decrease alpha waves by receiving feedback from their EEGs. Because alpha waves increase in the wakeful, relaxed state, an increase in alpha waves presumably represents an increase in relaxation.

How Is Biofeedback Provided?

To provide biofeedback, some physiological process is monitored by an electronic device, and signals that indicate changes in the process are displayed for the individual. For example, an electrode is properly placed to sense the level of tension in a muscle. As the tension in the muscle changes, lights, sounds, or other signals indicate the changes. If lights are used, a red light might indicate high tension, a yellow light moderate tension, and a green light little tension. The individual watches the changes in the lights and attempts to perceive how the muscle feels when the green light is on and tries deliberately to keep the muscle in the state that makes the green light stay on. Alternatively, the pitch of a sound can be made to vary with the tension in the muscle, with higher pitches being related to higher tension and lower pitches to lower tension or relaxation.

Clicking sounds, in which the rate of the click is in proportion to the tension, can also be used.

Regardless of the physiological process monitored or the signal used, the purpose is to provide information or feedback about changes in the process. People use the information in two ways: (1) to learn how their bodies feel when the process increases or decreases, and (2) to learn to purposely cause the process to remain at the desired level.

Some Examples of the Use of Biofeedback

Headaches People who suffer from recurring tension or migraine headaches have been helped to reduce their pain by biofeedback. In tension headaches the muscles of the scalp, neck, and shoulders are contracted. Biofeedback helps the individual to recognize when the muscles are tense and to learn to relax the muscles.

The benefit of biofeedback in the treatment of migraine headaches was discovered quite accidentally when a woman susceptible to such headaches was participating in an experiment to learn to increase the temperature of her hands. During the experiment it was observed that increasing hand temperature alleviated the migraine headache, possibly by diverting blood from the head to the hands. Subsequently, it has been shown that about one-third of migraine sufferers are helped by this technique. Biofeedback directed toward controlling pulsation of scalp arteries has also proven effective in some cases. Here, the treatment is related to the cause in that much of the pain of migraine is attributed to pulsations of dilated arteries of the scalp and cranial cavity.

Hypertension The effect of biofeedback on hypertension (high blood pressure) has been studied in a limited number of people. The normal systolic blood pressure is about 120 mm Hg; the pressures in hypertensive individuals by definition exceed 140 mm Hg and frequently reach 180 mm Hg. Feedback from monitoring of both blood pressure and muscle tension have been effective in controlling hypertension. Such feedback has enabled some people to lower their blood pressure as much as 25 mm Hg. (See Chapter 19 for more information on hypertension.)

Other uses of biofeedback Feedback of heart rate has been used to treat heart arrhythmias (abnormal rates). Feedback of alpha brain waves (the waves produced in the awake but relaxed state) has been used to treat anxiety and to relieve pain. Monitoring other brain-wave patterns has helped susceptible individuals learn to recognize signs of impending seizures and ward them off. These and other applications of biofeedback have been tried in small numbers of people, with varying degrees of success. Further study is likely to lead to a better understanding of how people can be taught to recognize autonomic responses and control them.

CHAPTER SUMMARY

(Chapter summary points and review questions are numbered to correspond to the numbered objectives in the text of each chapter.)

Organization and General Function

1. Describe the general organization of the autonomic nervous system and briefly explain its function.
   a. The autonomic nervous system is divided into two parts:
      (1) the sympathetic division
      (2) the parasympathetic division
   b. The general function of the autonomic nervous system is to control the functions of the internal organs, thereby contributing to the maintenance of homeostasis.

Development

2. Describe briefly the embryological development of the autonomic nervous system.
   a. The autonomic nervous system develops from neural crest cells.
   b. During its development it establishes connections with internal organs and with other nerves.

Neurotransmitters

3. Name the neurotransmitters of the autonomic nervous system and describe their interactions with their receptors.
   a. Neurons of the autonomic nervous system synthesize and secrete neurotransmitters as other neurons do; transmitters also must be inactivated.
   b. Sympathetic and parasympathetic functions are determined by the transmitter released and by its interaction with receptors.
   c. Two neurotransmitters are released by the autonomic nervous system:
      (1) Acetylcholine is released by cholinergic neurons, which include (a) all preganglionic neurons, (b) all parasympathetic postganglionic neurons, and (c) a few sympathetic postganglionic neurons.
      (2) Norepinephrine is released by adrenergic neurons, which include most of the sympathetic postganglionic neurons.
   d. Receptors for acetylcholine include:
      (1) nicotinic receptors on postganglionic neurons of both the sympathetic and parasympathetic divisions, where the action of acetylcholine depends on its concentration
      (2) muscarine receptors on effectors innervated by parasympathetic neurons, where acetylcholine causes muscle to contract or glands to secrete

   e. Receptors for norepinephrine from postganglionic sympathetic neurons and for norepinephrine and epinephrine from the adrenal medulla include:
      (1) alpha receptors, which are stimulated more by norepinephrine than by epinephrine, resulting in vasoconstriction and relaxation of intestinal smooth muscle
      (2) beta receptors, which are stimulated mainly by epinephrine, resulting in vasodilation, increased heart rate and strength of contraction, bronchodilation, relaxation of intestinal smooth muscle, and release of glucose and fatty acids into the blood

Sympathetic Division

4. Describe the structure and functions of the sympathetic division.
   a. The sympathetic division consists of:
      (1) ganglia located in a paravertebral chain in the thoracolumbar region
      (2) preganglionic fibers that extend from the lateral horns of the thoracolumbar region of the spinal cord to the ganglia
      (3) postganglionic fibers that extend from the ganglion to the organ being served
   b. The sympathetic division:
      (1) interacts with the parasympathetic nervous system to regulate the functioning of internal organs
      (2) prepares the body to meet emergencies or stressful situations
      (3) is augmented by the action of the adrenal medulla

Parasympathetic Division

5. Describe the structure and functions of the parasympathetic division.
   a. The parasympathetic division consists of:
      (1) ganglia located in or near the organs they serve
      (2) preganglionic fibers that extend from the nuclei of cranial nerves or the sacral portion of the spinal cord to the ganglion
      (3) postganglionic fibers that extend from the ganglion to the organ being served
   b. The parasympathetic division:
      (1) works with the sympathetic division to regulate the functioning of internal organs
      (2) returns the body to normal functional levels after an emergency or stressful situation

Relationships between Sympathetic and Parasympathetic Divisions

6. Explain how the sympathetic and parasympathetic divisions work together to maintain homeostasis.
   a. Both systems act continuously, resulting in sympathetic tone and parasympathetic tone.
   b. Under normal circumstances these systems work together to make small changes in the functional levels of the internal organs.
   c. The actions of the sympathetic and the parasympathetic divisions are generally antagonistic—if one augments a function, the other usually diminishes it, and vice versa.
   d. During emergencies and stressful situations the sympathetic division prepares the body to meet the stress, and the parasympathetic division helps the body return to normal functional levels after the stressful situation is over.

Clinical Applications

7. Distinguish between drugs that act on the sympathetic and the parasympathetic divisions and explain several conditions in which they might be used.
   a. Drugs can act on the autonomic nervous system by stimulating or blocking transmission at postsynaptic fibers of the sympathetic or the parasympathetic division, or by stimulating or blocking transmission from preganglionic neurons to postganglionic neurons.
   b. Sympathomimetic (adrenergic) drugs can be used to treat patients in shock; adrenergic blocking agents are used as antihypertensive agents.
   c. Parasympathomimetic (cholinergic) drugs can be used in the treatment of glaucoma and myasthenia gravis; cholinergic blocking agents can be used to relax muscles within the eye.

Questions

1. a. What are the two parts of the autonomic nervous system?
   b. What is the main function of the autonomic nervous system?
2. From what embryonic cells is most of the autonomic nervous system derived?
3. a. What are the neurotransmitters of the autonomic nervous system, and from which neurons is each released?
   b. How do cholinergic and adrenergic neurons differ?
   c. Distinguish between nicotinic and muscarine receptors in location and function.
   d. Relate the adrenal medulla to the sympathetic division.
   e. Distinguish between alpha and beta receptors in sensitivity to epinephrine and norepinephrine and in function.
4. a. Describe the pathways of the fibers of the sympathetic division from lateral horns of the spinal cord to the effector organs.
   b. What are the specific effects of sympathetic stimulation that prepare the body for stressful situations?
5. a. How does the distribution of parasympathetic fibers differ from that of sympathetic fibers?
   b. What are the specific effects of parasympathetic stimulation that return the body to normal after a stressful situation?
6. What are six ways that drugs can act on the autonomic nervous system?

Problems

1. Suppose you are working in an emergency room and are called upon to give cardiopulmonary resuscitation for a period of time. Describe the role of your autonomic nervous system in helping you respond to the emergency.
2. After the emergency is over, you get a chance to relax a few minutes. Describe the role of the autonomic nervous system in your "recovery" from dealing with the emergency.

REVIEW

Important Terms

adrenergic	parasympathetic
biofeedback	parasympathomimetic
cholinergic	postganglionic
craniosacral	preganglionic
epinephrine	sympathetic
ganglion	sympathomimetic
norepinephrine	thoracolumbar

REFERENCES AND READINGS

Barsky, A. J. 1979. Patients who amplify bodily sensations. *Annals of Internal Medicine* 91:63 (July).

Bergersen, B. S. 1979. *Pharmacology in nursing.* St. Louis, Mo.: C. V. Mosby.

Ganong, W. F. 1981. *Review of medical physiology* (10th ed.). Los Altos, Calif.: Lange Medical Publications.

Guyton, A. C. 1981. *Textbook of medical physiology* (6th ed.). Philadelphia: W. B. Saunders.

Hardt, J. V., and Kamiya, J. 1978. Anxiety change through electroencephalographic alpha feedback seen only in high anxiety subjects. *Science* 201:79 (July 7).

Holden, C. 1980. Behavioral medicine: An emergent field. *Science* 209:479 (July 25).

Linford-Rees, W. 1979. A reappraisal of some psychosomatic concepts. *Psychotherapy and Psychosomatics* 31:9.

Miller, N. E. 1978. Biofeedback and visceral learning. *Annual Review of Psychology* 29:374.

Shapiro, D. 1979. Biofeedback and behavioral medicine: An overview. *Psychotherapy and Psychosomatics* 31:24.

Silverman, A. J. 1979. Field dependency, brain asymmetry, and psychophysiological differences. *Psychotherapy and Psychosomatics* 31:133.

Tarler-Benlolo, L. 1978. A role of relaxation in biofeedback training: A critical review of the literature. *Psychological Bulletin* 85(4):727.

Wallace, R. K., and Benson, H. 1972. The physiology of meditation. *Scientific American* 226(2):85 (February).

Wedding, D., and Tsushima, W. T. 1979. Clinical applications of biofeedback: A summary of research 1974–1978. *Hawaii Medical Journal* 38(1):9 (January).

14

SENSORY ORGANS

ORGANIZATION AND GENERAL FUNCTIONS

Objective 1. Describe the general properties of sensory receptors; distinguish among exteroceptors, proprioceptors, and visceroceptors, and among the types of stimuli they receive.

Your sense organs provide all the information you have about your external and internal environment—what is going on around you, the position of your body, how much your muscles are contracted, even where you have aches and pains. Humans and many other living things depend on sensory receptors to maintain homeostasis: To adapt to changes, you must first detect the changes, and this is what your sense organs do.

Sensory receptors detect changes. Sensory neurons associated with the sensory receptors carry signals to your central nervous system. Some of these signals go to your spinal cord or to parts of your brainstem, where they cause various motor responses. These processes, like the reflexes we considered in Chapter 10, go on without your being aware of them. However, some sensory signals go to your cerebral cortex, creating a conscious sensation. Sensations are then interpreted in light of what is remembered from other experiences. The interpretation of a conscious sensation is called **perception**.

As a result of perception you are able to interpret what you see, hear, smell, taste, or feel inside your body or on its surface. When you hear or read a new word, at first the word may have no meaning to you; however, you may be able to figure out what it means by the context in which it is used or by comparing it to words you already know. Analogously, when you have perceived something, you can consciously choose how you will respond to it, in part on the basis of your memory. You may use movement, speech, or perhaps only thought to respond. The sequence of sensory detection, perception, and action—carried out by sense organs, the cerebrum, and usually some muscles—allows you to detect and respond consciously to changes in your environment.

Properties of Receptors

All sensory receptors have certain properties in common. One, the property of **transduction**, is the *ability to convert a specific stimulus into an electrical signal*. A stimulus to which a receptor is sensitive causes the membrane of the receptor cell to depolarize. This depolarization of a receptor is called a **generator potential**. Though generator potentials in receptors and action potentials in neurons have some similarities, they also have some differences (see Table 14.1).

Another property of receptors is that they are *differentially sensitive to certain stimuli*. Each receptor is particularly sensitive to (has a low threshold for) one kind of stimulus and generally nonresponsive to (has a high threshold for) all other kinds of stimuli at normal intensities. For example, the receptor cells in the eye are sensitive to light, whereas the receptor cells in the taste buds are sensitive to certain chemicals. However, a strong blow to the head can stimulate light receptors and cause one to "see stars."

The generator potential produced by the stimulus may in turn trigger an action potential if it reaches threshold. The resulting *nerve impulse that is produced is the same for all receptors*. The quality of a sensation depends on which receptor is stimulated and where the nerve impulse is interpreted in the brain, and not on the nature of the nerve impulse itself. This property is called the **law of specific nerve energies**.

Given these three properties of receptors, you might wonder how differences in the intensity of stimuli are detected. For example, bright light can be distinguished from dim light, and a slightly sweet taste can be distinguished from a very sweet taste. A strong stimulus produces a greater number of nerve impulses per second (frequency of action potentials) than a weak stimulus. The number of impulses can be increased in two ways: (1) A strong stimulus may stimulate a large number of receptor cells, while a weak stimulus might excite only one or a few; or (2) a strong stimulus may cause a single receptor cell to send many impulses one after another, while a weak stimulus might cause only one or a few impulses to be conducted (Figure 14.1). This is because a strong stimulus produces a

Table 14.1	A Comparison of a Generator Potential and an Action Potential
Generator Potential	**Action Potential**
Can be additive; when a second stimulus arrives before a first stimulus is completed, the generator potential from the second stimulus is added to the depolarization caused by the first stimulus	Cannot be additive
Can produce a graded response; stronger or more frequent stimuli increase the amplitude of the generator potential	Does not produce a graded response; once the threshold for the action potential has been reached, an increase in the strength or frequency of stimuli has no effect on the size of the action potential
Has a highly variable duration, but exceeds 1 to 2 milliseconds; dependent on duration of stimulus	Has a nearly constant duration between 1 and 2 milliseconds; independent of stimulus
Has no refractory period (period required before next impulse can occur)	Has a refractory period of about 1 millisecond
Loses amplitude (diminishes in peak height) as it passes along the receptor cell and associated nerve fiber	Maintains constant amplitude as it passes along a nerve fiber

larger generator potential than a weak one; in turn, a larger generator potential produces a greater frequency of action potentials. This process results in the coding of information about the intensity of stimulation into the neural language of action potentials. Such coding is often referred to as **translation**.

Adaptation is yet a fourth property of receptor cells: *When a stimulus continues at a constant strength over a period of time, the rate at which a receptor generates nerve impulses decreases.* Though the exact mechanism for adaptation is unknown, it is known that receptors vary in their ability to adapt. Those that adapt slowly are called **slowly adapting receptors** and those that adapt rapidly are called **rapidly adapting receptors**. Slowly adapting receptors include pain receptors; receptors that detect changes in the amount of oxygen or carbon dioxide in the blood; and receptors in the muscles, tendons, and joints that provide feedback for the control of movement and sense of body position. Many slowly adapting receptors warn about potentially dangerous situations. Rapidly adapting receptors include those that detect pressure, touch, and smell.

Kinds of Receptors

Receptors can be classified according to where they are located or according to the kinds of stimuli they can receive.

By location, receptors fall into three categories. **Extero-ceptors** are usually located near the surface of the body, and they detect changes in the surroundings. Receptors for touch, heat, cold, light, and sound are examples of extero-ceptors. Bare nerve endings in the skin that detect pain are also exteroceptors. **Proprioceptors** are located in the muscles, tendons, and joints. They detect changes in the position of limbs and changes in muscle length and tension. **Visceroceptors** (enteroceptors) are located within organs of the body other than muscles, tendons, and joints. They detect pain, the degree of stretching of blood vessel walls, movements in the digestive tract, and similar sensations. Pain receptors (nociceptors) are found in nearly every tissue of the body. We usually are conscious of the activities of exteroceptors, but many of the impulses from propriocep-tors and visceroceptors are relayed to the cerebellum, brainstem, and other parts of the central nervous system besides the cerebral cortex.

Receptors can also be classified according to the type of stimuli they respond to. **Chemoreceptors** respond to changes in the concentration of chemicals. The receptors for taste and smell and the receptors that detect chemical changes in the blood are chemoreceptors. **Mechanorecep-tors** respond to mechanical changes such as changes in pressure or movement of fluids. The receptors for hearing, balance, touch, pressure, and the proprioceptors are all mechanoreceptors. **Thermoreceptors** respond to changes in temperature. They include the heat and cold receptors in the skin. **Photoreceptors** respond to light and are found only in the eye. **Nociceptors** (pain receptors) detect tissue damage. They usually consist of free nerve endings in the tissues, and the sensation of pain may be produced when they are stimulated. However, almost any stimulus can give rise to the sensation of pain if it is sufficiently intense.

All receptors detect stimuli and convert them into generator potentials. Each impulse travels along a basic sensory unit—receptor, nerve pathway, and interpreting unit. We become aware of nerve impulses from sense organs only when they arrive in the cerebral cortex. How they are processed there determines what kind of sensation we experience. Normally, signals from each kind of receptor

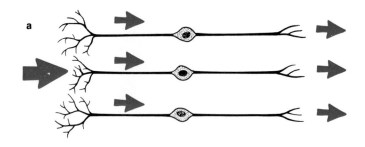

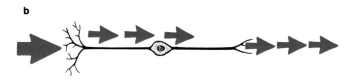

Figure 14.1 Mechanisms by which stimuli are increased in intensity: (**a**) Several neurons are stimulated simultaneously. (**b**) One neuron receives several stimuli in rapid succession.

are relayed to a specific area of the brain, where they are interpreted. For example, we interpret signals arriving in the visual area of the brain as sight, or signals sent to the tactile area as touch. If somehow the visual signals were routed to the tactile area, we would interpret them as touch even though our eyes would have been their origin. This illustrates that the impulses themselves are not specific for any particular sense.

In humans (and probably in many other animals, too) learning consists almost entirely of experience in the interpretation of sensory signals. Except for crude sensations, which may be interpreted in the thalamus, all conscious sensations are the result of interpretation of signals arriving in the cerebral cortex.

SKIN RECEPTORS

Objective 2. Distinguish among the types of sensory receptors in the skin on the basis of structure, function, and location.

Five different kinds of receptors have been identified in the skin (Figure 14.2). Some anatomists believe that

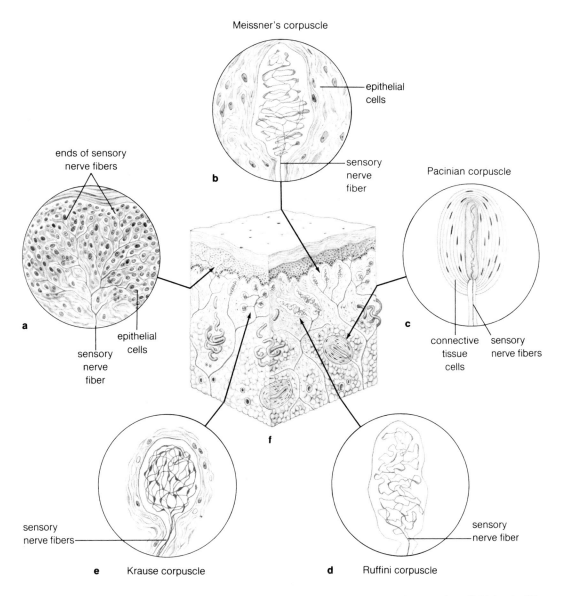

Figure 14.2 Sensory receptors found in the skin: (**a**) a free nerve ending, sensitive to pain or light touch, (**b**) a Meissner's corpuscle, also sensitive to touch, (**c**) a Pacinian corpuscle, sensitive to pressure, (**d**) a Ruffini corpuscle, sensitive to warmth, (**e**) a Krause corpuscle, sensitive to cold or extreme heat, (**f**) location of corpuscles.

additional kinds of receptors may be present in the skin, whereas others question whether all the ones that have been identified are actually functional. Lacking conclusive evidence to the contrary, we will discuss the five classical types of receptors.

Free sensory nerve endings (a) are distributed between cells of the epidermis. Most of these nerve endings are sensitive to pain, but some deep ones associated with hairs are sensitive to light touch. **Meissner's corpuscles** (b), located in the papillary layer of the dermis just below the epidermis, are also responsive to touch. A fairly strong stimulus is necessary to elicit a generator potential because the spherical corpuscle must be deformed to cause it to respond. **Pacinian corpuscles** (c) respond to strong pressure. These receptors are located deep within the reticular layer of the dermis. Because of their location and because of the heavy connective tissue sheath surrounding them, the Pacinian corpuscles require a much stronger stimulus than any other receptors. Pacinian corpuscles are also sensitive to vibrations.

Temperature sensations are detected by the **Ruffini corpuscles** (d) and the **Krause corpuscles** (e). Both are found in the dermis and in the subcutaneous tissues. A greater number of these receptors are found in the face and hands than in other skin areas. Wherever these receptors are found, the Krause corpuscles are far more numerous than the Ruffini corpuscles. The Ruffini corpuscles are stimulated by temperatures between 25°C and 45°C and are maximally stimulated at 37°C to 40°C. The Krause corpuscles are stimulated at temperatures from 15°C to 35°C and from 46°C to 50°C.

The perception of temperature involves not only the Krause and Ruffini corpuscles but the free nerve endings as well. The temperature perceived is a combination of the pattern of receptors stimulated and the strength of the stimuli. Figure 14.3 shows the rate of nerve impulse transmission from each kind of receptor at temperatures from 0°C to 60°C. Some important ideas expressed by the figure are as follows:

1. No sensation is felt when the skin temperature is below 0°C.

2. Up to about 12°C only pain can be felt.

3. Between 12°C and 25°C coldness is perceived from impulses generated by the Krause corpuscles.

4. Between 25°C and 35°C the temperature perceived is determined by the relative frequencies of impulses from Krause and Ruffini corpuscles.

5. Between 35°C and 45°C warmth is perceived from impulses generated by Ruffini corpuscles.

6. At about 46°C the sensation of paradoxical cold is felt. This is what you feel when you stick your foot into a bathtub full of hot water and perceive the sensation as cold.

7. Above 50°C only pain sensations are generated.

8. Above 60°C the skin receptors do not function.

Sensations from skin receptors reach the brain by several pathways. Sensations from facial skin travel along cranial nerves V and VII to the brain. Other nerve impulses from skin receptors enter the spinal cord by way of a posterior nerve root (Figure 14.4). Inside the spinal cord impulses travel along myelinated fibers of the dorsal column system (gracilis and cuneatus tracts) and the spinothalamic

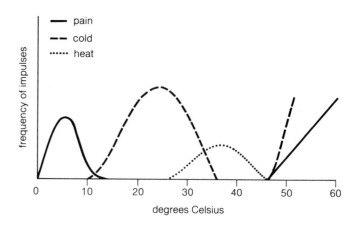

Figure 14.3 Signal conduction by various receptors occurs at temperatures from 0°C to 60°C.

tracts. Impulses that travel along the dorsal column system and ventral spinothalamic tract are relayed through the medulla, midbrain, and thalamus to the somatic sensory area of the cerebral cortex with great rapidity. Fine gradations in the intensity of stimuli can be distinguished, and the source of the sensations can be precisely localized. Sensations that are perceived through impulses traveling along these paths include fine touch sensations, vibrations, and pressure sensations. In contrast, impulses that travel the lateral spinothalamic tracts are relayed to the cerebral cortex with much less precise localization and at a relatively slow rate. Sensations that are perceived through impulses traveling along these tracts include crude touch, pressure, sensations of heat and cold, tickle, itch, and pain.

As the above description indicates, a complex assortment of sensations is derived from skin receptors. Though

It was once thought that the sensations of tickle and itch involved mild stimulation of the free nerve endings that normally transmit pain sensations. However, some small specialized fibers that carry tickle and itch sensations have been identified. Such sensations presumably help an organism to detect something crawling across the skin. Scratching relieves itching by removing the irritant or by stimulating free nerve endings or Pacinian corpuscles. When impulses from these receptors arrive in the brain, they apparently mask the impulses from the tickle and itch receptors.

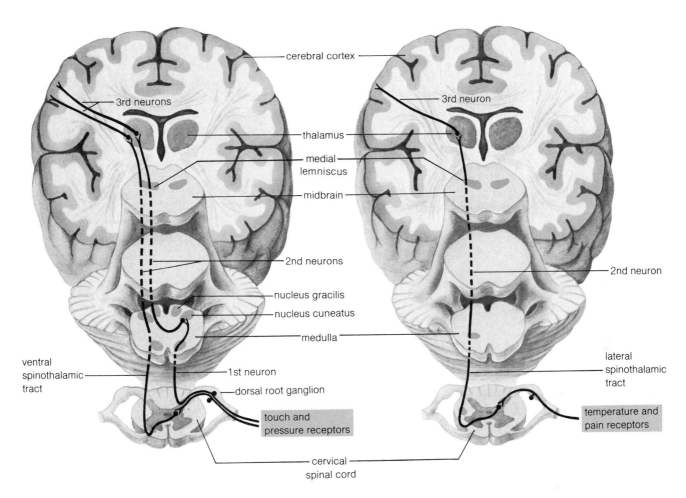

Figure 14.4 Pathways from skin receptors to the cerebrum: (**a**) Fine touch, vibrations, and pressure sensations travel rapidly along the dorsal column system (gracilis and cuneatus tracts) and the ventral spinothalamic tract to the thalamus and then to the somatic sensory area. (**b**) Crude touch, temperature, tickle, itch, and pain sensations travel more slowly along the lateral spinothalamic tract to the thalamus and then to various areas of the cortex.

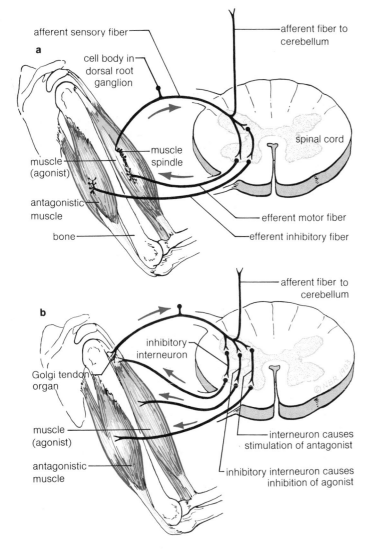

Figure 14.5 Pathways of impulses from proprioceptors: (**a**) muscle spindle, (**b**) Golgi tendon organ.

are responded to by the central nervous system.

Proprioceptors—found in muscles, tendons, and joints—have been described briefly in other chapters. **Muscle spindles**, located in skeletal muscles, and **Golgi tendon organs**, located in tendons, respond to stretching of muscles or tendons, respectively. In addition, **joint kinesthetic receptors** are found in the capsules of joints, where they detect the degree of bending of the joint.

Nerve impulses from proprioceptors follow several different pathways (Figure 14.5). The afferent neuron from the muscle spindle goes to the spinal cord, where it synapses directly with a motor neuron that goes to the same area of that muscle. This arrangement is the only known monosynaptic reflex pathway in the human body. Other axon branches of the same neuron synapse with interneurons. These interneurons synapse with motor neurons. They may inhibit motor neurons that control the contraction of antagonistic muscles or stimulate motor neurons of synergistic muscles. Still other branches of the axon travel up the spinal cord; it is through these pathways that sensory impulses are relayed to the cerebellum, where they provide information for the coordination of movement. The reflex pathway for the Golgi tendon organ always involves an interneuron; it differs from the muscle spindle pathway as shown in Figure 14.5b.

None of the afferent impulses from the proprioceptors reaches areas of the cerebral cortex that allow us to be conscious of them. What we are able to perceive about the position of joints and the tension in muscles comes from proprioceptors in the joints, from touch and pressure receptors in the skin, and from visual observations.

> One commonly used test for the function of proprioceptor pathways is to close your eyes and try to touch a fingertip to the end of your nose. Inability to do this denotes damage to a neural pathway normally involved in proprioception.

the perception of light, sound, taste, and smell are often thought of as the main sensory perceptions, the skin receptors are exceedingly important components of sensory perception because they can detect potentially dangerous environmental conditions.

PROPRIOCEPTORS

Objective 3. Review the structure, function, and location of proprioceptors and explain how stimuli from them

PAIN

Objective 4. Describe the qualities of pain, the locations of receptors, and the causes of pain; explain variations in reactions to pain and theories of analgesia.

Pain is normally a protective mechanism. Because pain receptors do not adapt to continuous stimulation, they provide persistent signals that some kind of tissue damage is occurring. In some cases pain persists in the absence of an identifiable cause, and an individual suffers from chronic pain that is difficult to relieve.

Pain can be classified qualitatively as **pricking, burning**, and **aching**. Pricking pain, felt when the skin is cut, pricked, or irritated, is transmitted to the somatic sensory area by small myelinated fibers. Burning pain, felt when the skin is burned, is transmitted to the reticular activating system by small, myelinated fibers or smaller, unmyelinated fibers. Burning pain is the most excruciating of all types of pain and, unlike pricking pain, often persists long after the injury. Aching pain is pain deep below the surface, and it may spread over a wide area. It is transmitted to the reticular activating system by small, unmyelinated, slowly conducting sensory fibers.

Most pain receptors are located in the skin, but some are found in the walls of arteries, in joint surfaces, in muscles, and in internal organs. The receptors in visceral organs are relatively sparsely distributed, but they can signal severe pain if a sufficiently large number of them are stimulated, as occurs in ulcers.

The direct cause of pain is thought to be the chemicals that are released from injured tissue. These chemicals, polypeptides called **kinins**, appear to stimulate the free nerve endings of the pain receptors as long as they are being released from the tissue. Another possible cause of pain is tissue **ischemia** (reduced bloodflow). It is possible that ischemia causes sufficient tissue damage to release various kinins.

Pain is not always felt where the tissue damage is occurring. Visceral pain in particular is often perceived as coming from another part of the body, a phenomenon called **referred pain** (Figure 14.6). It is thought that, in the mechanism of pain referral, branches of visceral pain fibers synapse in the spinal cord with some of the neurons receiving impulses from somatic pain fibers—that is, signals from somatic and visceral organs converge (Figure 14.7). When the visceral pain fibers are intensely stimulated, the brain may interpret the stimulus as if it came from the skin. This theory is supported by the observation that visceral referred pain is always felt in a somatic area innervated by the same spinal cord segment.

Headaches can result from a variety of causes, some of which involve referred pain. In fact, no headache is due to stimulation of pain receptors in the brain itself because the brain contains no pain receptors. As mentioned in Chapter 13, migraine headaches are thought to be caused by a spasm of some of the arteries that supply the brain as well as by arteries of the scalp. The pain results from pulsations

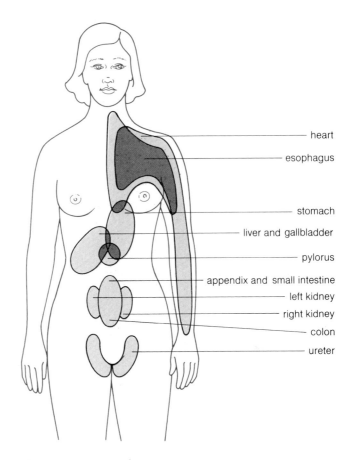

Figure 14.6 Areas on the surface of the body to which pain from internal organs may be referred.

in the dilated arteries that stimulate the pain receptors in the arterial walls. Tension headaches are caused by spasms of the muscles of the scalp and neck, but the pain may be referred so that some people feel it as an ache inside the head or as a tight band around the head. Infections of the sinuses and meninges and certain eye disorders can also cause headaches.

Studies of pain perception indicate that people show little variation in the sensitivity of their pain receptors. For example, when human subjects were exposed to gradually increasing skin temperature in a localized area, all first perceived pain at a temperature between 43.5°C and 47°C. Most perceived pain when their skin temperature reached 45°C, the temperature at which tissue destruction first begins to occur. Thus, we can conclude that variations in pain tolerance involve the reaction to pain and not the direct sensation of it.

Two related theories have been proposed to explain individual variations in reactions to pain. According to the **gating theory**, nonpain signals (such as those from mechanoreceptors in the skin that travel along large sensory fibers to the central nervous system) depress the transmission of pain signals from the same area of the body, or, in the case of referred pain, from other areas of the body. The degree of effectiveness of the nonpain signals to depress the pain signals contributes to the variations in reaction. According to the **endorphin theory**, pain stimuli cause the neural secretion of endorphins (discussed in Chapter 11), and the endorphins in turn minimize the individual's reaction to the pain stimuli. The ability of aspirin to relieve pain may come from stimulation of the production of endorphins. The chemical naloxone, which is known to block the action of endorphins, also blocks the action of aspirin as a pain reliever. Research is now in progress to develop synthetic enkephalins and endorphins for the relief of pain.

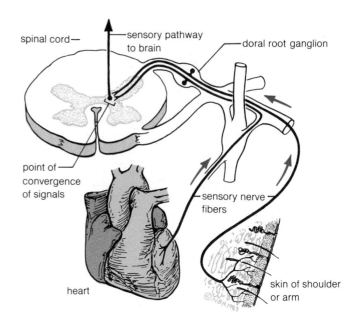

Figure 14.7 Possible mechanism for referred pain. Impulses originating in the heart travel the same pathway through the spinal nerve root as impulses originating in the skin of the shoulder and arm. They follow common nerve pathways to the cerebral cortex, where their source may be misinterpreted.

People differ widely in their ability to tolerate pain. These differences may be associated with the ability to ignore other types of sensations and with the need for sensory stimulation. Studies of responses to stimuli have made it possible to classify most people as reducers or augmenters. **Reducers** tend to minimize nearly all kinds of stimuli and have a relatively low need for stimulation. (All normal people require a certain level of stimulation to stay alert, as you might expect from your knowledge of the reticular activating system.) In contrast, **augmenters** tend to maximize stimuli and have a high need for sensory stimulation. As you might predict, reducers are able to endure more pain than augmenters.

CHEMICAL SENSES

Objective 5. Compare and contrast the senses of taste and smell in terms of structure, function, and location of receptors and interpretation of sensations in the brain.

The Sense of Taste

The receptors for the sense of taste are found in **taste buds**, mostly located on the tongue but also found on the soft palate and portions of the pharynx. Most of the taste buds are located within papillae that extend down into the epithelium of the tongue (Figure 14.8). Each taste bud opens onto the surface by way of a **taste pore**, through which chemicals reach the sensory receptors. Inside each taste bud are several receptors, called **taste (gustatory) cells**. Extending from each taste cell are several nerve endings, the **taste hairs**, sensitive to particular chemicals only when they are dissolved in the solutions that enter the taste pores. When the taste hairs are stimulated, they produce a generator potential in the taste cells, which synapse onto afferent nerve fibers. These fibers enter cranial nerves VII, IX, or X (depending on the part of the tongue or pharynx stimulated) and conduct impulses to the somatic sensory area of the cerebral cortex, where they are interpreted.

Only four distinct tastes can be distinguished; all other things we think we can taste are actually detected as smells. You might have noticed food tasting "flat" or having very little taste when your nose is congested from a cold or allergy. This shows how dependent on smell your appreciation of food really is.

The four basic tastes are sweet, sour, salty, and bitter. Though all of the taste buds are slightly sensitive to each of the four

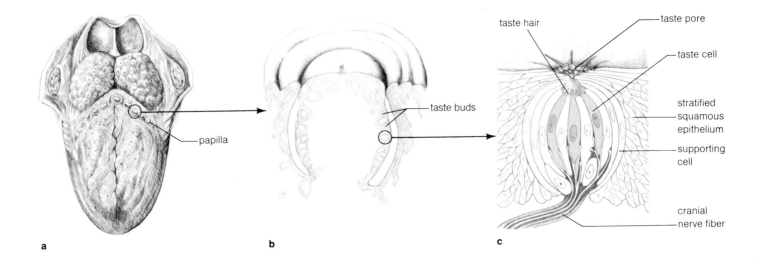

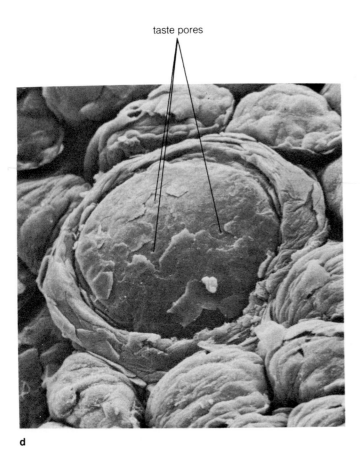

taste pores

Figure 14.8 Most taste receptors are located on the surface of the tongue (**a**) in taste buds (**b**). The structure of a taste bud is shown in (**c**). (**d**) A circumvallate papilla showing pores, × 488. (Photomicrograph reproduced with permission from *Tissues and organs: A text-atlas of scanning electron microscopy* by Richard G. Kessel and Randy H. Kardon. W. H. Freeman and Company. Copyright © 1979.)

basic tastes, those in certain areas of the tongue are particularly sensitive to one type of chemical (Figure 14.9). Taste buds on the tip of the tongue respond best to sweet substances such as sucrose and other sugars. Some chemicals, such as saccharine in low concentration, also stimulate these taste buds. The taste buds on the sides of the tongue are most sensitive to acids, which the brain interprets as being sour. Other taste buds on the tip and sides of the tongue are sensitive to salts, especially sodium chloride, or table salt. The taste buds at the back of the tongue are sensitive to bitter substances, such as quinine and saccharine in high concentration. Many substances that have a bitter taste are also poisonous or toxic, so the ability to taste them has a survival value.

The Sense of Smell

Compared to that of many other animals, the human sense of smell (olfactory sense) is quite limited; yet our ability to detect some chemicals through this sense exceeds that of most laboratory instruments. The receptors for the sense of smell are found in the **olfactory epithelium** of the lining of the nasal passages (Figure 14.10). These receptors are similar to those for taste in that they are thought to be stimulated by chemicals dissolved in water. The **olfactory cells** are specialized sensory neurons imbedded in the supporting cells of the epithelium. Extending from them into the nasal cavity are the **olfactory hairs**, or dendrites of the neurons. The axons extend through holes in the cribiform plate of the ethmoid bone and form synapses with neurons of the **olfactory bulb**. From the olfactory bulb impulses travel along the olfactory tract to the cerebrum, where they are inter-

Figure 14.9 Taste receptors in certain areas of the tongue are particularly sensitive to one of the four basic tastes: (**a**) sweet, which responds to sugars, (**b**) sour, which responds to acids, (**c**) salty, which responds to inorganic anions such as chloride, (**d**) bitter, which responds to certain inorganic cations.

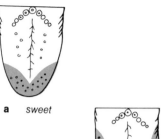
a *sweet*

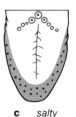
c *salty*

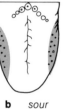
b *sour*

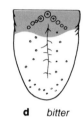
d *bitter*

preted in the medial aspect of the frontal lobe, in close association with the limbic system. The neural pathway for smell does *not* pass through the thalamus as all other sensory pathways do.

Though the manner in which olfactory receptors are stimulated is not well understood, one theory suggests that the shape of molecules and/or their electrical charge determines their smell. It is thought that receptor sites on the dendrites also have certain shapes or charges, and when a chemical fits onto a receptor, a generator potential is produced. This in turn can cause nerve impulses to be generated.

Attempts to classify odors have met with little success (probably because of the large number of odors and their subjective quality), but the following eight general groups have been identified: floral, musky, minty, camphoraceous (like the scent of camphor), pungent (like the scent of many spices), ethereal (like the scent of ether), fruity, and putrid (like the scent of decaying substances). Other categories may exist that have not yet been identified. Moreover, many sensations of smell may be combinations of several different types of odors, thus allowing humans to distinguish 2000 to 4000 different scents.

Studies of the human ability to identify odors have shown that three factors contribute to the ability to name an odorous substance. First, the more frequently individuals have encountered a substance, the more likely they are to identify it. Second, individuals can identify a substance for which they have known the name for a long time more easily than a substance for which they have only recently learned the name. Finally, aids in recalling the name of a new substance help people to identify its odor. Thus, it

appears that the interpretation of smells is partly a learned behavior.

Research in invertebrate animals has shown that chemical agents called pheromones affect the behavior of these animals. Male insects are attracted to females that emit a specific pheromone. Likewise, some infant vertebrate animals recognize their mothers by odor, and adult animals mark their territories or display their dominance by chemicals they emit through urine or sweat. Thus, the sense of smell could be important to group or to individual survival.

The ability to remember sights, sounds, and odors varies. Visual details of pictures are remembered with high accuracy over a short period of time but are forgotten after several months. In contrast, smells are not remembered quite as well as visual details over a short time but are still remembered even a year later. The name may not be remembered, but the odor is perceived as familiar and is often associated with an emotion. These findings suggest that, as the impulses from the smell receptors pass through the limbic system, the center of the brain most concerned with emotions, an association between an odor and an emotion may be created.

The senses of taste and smell are compared in Table 14.2.

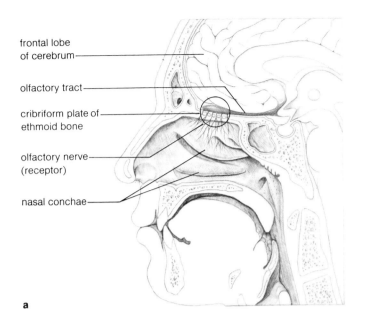

frontal lobe
of cerebrum

olfactory tract

cribriform plate of
ethmoid bone

olfactory nerve
(receptor)

nasal conchae

a

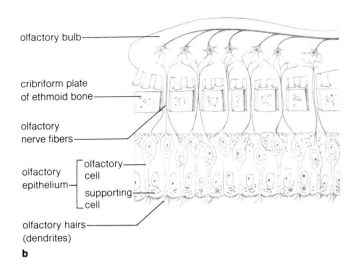

olfactory bulb

cribriform plate
of ethmoid bone

olfactory
nerve fibers

olfactory
epithelium — olfactory
cell

supporting
cell

olfactory hairs
(dendrites)

b

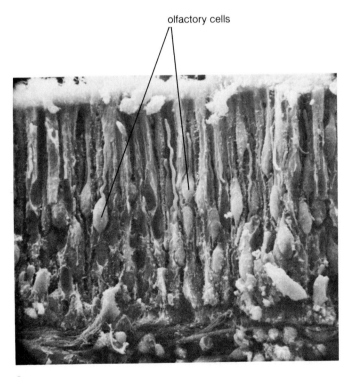

olfactory cells

c

Figure 14.10 The olfactory receptors are located in the nasal cavity (**a**). An enlargement of a portion of the olfactory area (**b**) shows the arrangement of cells and nerve fibers. (**c**) Olfactory epithelium showing olfactory cells, $\times$ 676. (Photomicrograph reproduced with permission from *Tissues and organs: A text-atlas of scanning electron microscopy* by Richard G. Kessel and Randy H. Kardon. W. H. Freeman and Company. Copyright © 1979.)

Table 14.2 Comparison of the Senses of Taste and Smell		
Characteristic	Taste	Smell
Receptor sensitivity	A few specific chemicals	Many different chemicals
Adaptation	Rapid	Rapid
Reduction with aging	Small because taste cells are continually replaced	Significant because olfactory cells that die are not replaced
Signals from receptors	Travel via cranial nerves VII, IX, and X to thalamus and then to cerebrum	Travel via cranial nerve I to limbic system before going to cerebrum

Subliminal odors are odors that are detected by receptors but are not consciously perceived. Researchers think that subliminal odors might be involved in human reproductive function. For example, some studies indicate that the menstrual cycles of women who live or work together in close association become synchronized after some time. It has been suggested that subliminally detected chemical variations in sweat and vaginal secretions might be the cause.

VISION

Objective 6. Describe the external and internal structures of the eye and their locations and functions.

Objective 7. Distinguish between black-and-white and color vision in terms of structure, function, and location of receptors.

Objective 8. Describe how signals are transmitted from the eye to the brain and how they are interpreted in the brain.

Objective 9. Trace the path of light waves through the eye and explain how they are focused on distant and near objects naturally and with the aid of corrective lenses.

Objective 10. Explain how the structure and function of the eye are altered in cataract and in glaucoma; briefly describe how these conditions are treated.

The eye is the organ of sight. You can demonstrate how important vision is by blindfolding yourself for even as short a time as half an hour and attempting to perform your usual activities. Many of us tend to take our sight for granted; yet to live without vision requires a great amount of adaptation and courage.

External Structure of the Eye

Though the light-sensitive cells are located deep inside the eye, many other external and internal structures aid in focusing light, moving the eyeball, and protecting the eye. The external structures of the eye are shown in Figure 14.11.

The eyes lie in pear-shaped orbits formed from bones of the skull. Each eye is protected by an upper and a lower **eyelid**, each of which has **eyelashes** along its unattached surface. Beneath the skin of each eyelid is the orbicularis oculi muscle, which closes the eye when it contracts. The upper eyelid also contains the levator palpebrae superioris muscle, which is responsible for lifting the upper lid. The inner surface of each eyelid and parts of the eyeball are covered with mucous membrane, the **conjunctiva**, which helps to protect and keep the eyeball moist. It is this membrane that becomes inflamed in conjunctivitis, or "pink eye."

The eye muscles Each eye has six **extrinsic eye muscles**. These muscles originate from the bones of the orbit and insert by tendons to the tough outer covering of the eyeball. Their function is to move the eyeball. The four rectus muscles move the eyeball in the direction indicated by their names. The **superior rectus** rotates the eyeball superiorly, the **inferior rectus** rotates it inferiorly, the **medial rectus** rotates it medially, and the **lateral rectus** rotates it laterally. The oblique muscles are attached to the eyeball by way of a pulley arrangement so that they move the eyeball in two directions simultaneously. The **superior oblique** rotates the eyeball downward and away from the midline. The **inferior oblique** rotates it upward and away from the midline. Although each eye muscle has a specific action, most eye movements involve the use of more than one muscle. Eye movements are also coordinated: Both eyes normally move together. The coordinated movement of the eyes is accomplished by the contraction of certain muscle pairs in the two eyes at the same time their antagonists are relaxed. To move the eyes to the left, the lateral rectus of the left eye and the medial rectus of the right eye contract, while their antagonists relax. **Strabismus**, also referred to as squint and cross-eye, is a condition in which these muscles fail to cause the eyes to move in proper coordination.

The lacrimal apparatus The **lacrimal apparatus** (Figure 14.11b) of each eye consists of a **lacrimal gland** and its numerous ducts, the **superior** and **inferior canaliculi**, a **lacrimal sac**, and a **nasolacrimal duct**. The lacrimal gland is located in the orbit on the superior, lateral surface of the eyeball. It continuously secretes tears medially and downward on to the surface of the eyeball, where the tears serve to keep the surface moist. Excessive secretion is stimulated by nerve fibers from the parasympathetic nervous system. Tears are collected by the canaliculi and emptied into the medial lacrimal sac, from which they drain by way of the nasolacrimal duct into the nasal cavity. In addition to their lubricating function, tears also have an antibacterial function. They contain **lysozyme**, an enzyme that helps to destroy bacteria that get into the eyes. Glandular cells in the conjunctiva also secrete a mucous substance that is a component of tears.

Internal Structure of the Eye

The eye is a hollow, spherical structure about 2.5 centimeters in diameter. Its wall is composed of three layers—the outer fibrous tunic, the middle vascular tunic or uvea, and the internal tunic. Its layers and internal structures are shown in Figure 14.12.

The outer tunic The outer tunic is divided into the **sclera**, which covers most of the eyeball, and the **cornea**, a transparent portion that forms the anterior one-sixth of the eyeball. The sclera, or white of the eye, contains many collagen fibers and forms a tough, protective outer covering. The cornea admits and helps to focus light waves as they enter the eye. It contains no blood vessels and thus must obtain oxygen from the air or by diffusion from adjacent fluids and tissues. The cornea was one of the first organs to be successfully transplanted because its lack of blood vessels prevents it from reacting antigenically and being rejected. (See Chapter 20 for a discussion of antigenic reaction.)

The vascular layer The vascular layer (uvea) consists of the **choroid coat**, the **ciliary body**, and the **iris**. The choroid coat lies adjacent to the sclera and contains numerous blood vessels that supply nutrients and oxygen to the other tissues. It also contains pigmented cells that absorb light and prevent it from being reflected within the eyeball.

The ciliary body extends toward the inside of the eye from the choroid coat. It is composed of the **ciliary muscles** and the **ciliary processes**. Attached to the ciliary body are the **suspensory ligaments**, which are in turn attached to the

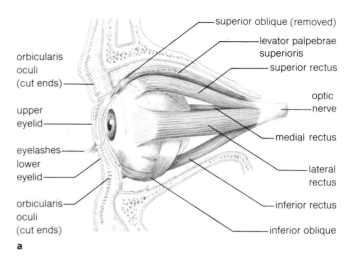

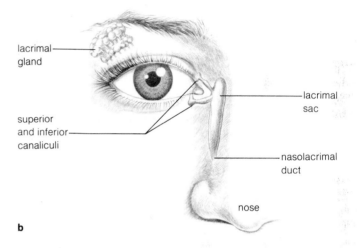

Figure 14.11 The external structure of the eyeball: (**a**) lateral view of the eyelids and extrinsic muscles of the eye, (**b**) the lacrimal apparatus of the right eye.

capsule that surrounds the lens of the eye. The capsule and ligaments, together with the ciliary body, hold the lens in place.

The lens The **lens** is a transparent, biconvex, elastic structure that bends light waves as they pass through its surfaces. It is composed of epithelial cells that have large amounts of clear cytoplasm in the form of fibers. Its capsule is composed of layers of intercellular protein. The lens can change shape from moment to moment and, by doing so, focus light waves onto the retina from objects at different distances from the eye. Because it grows throughout life, the lens can

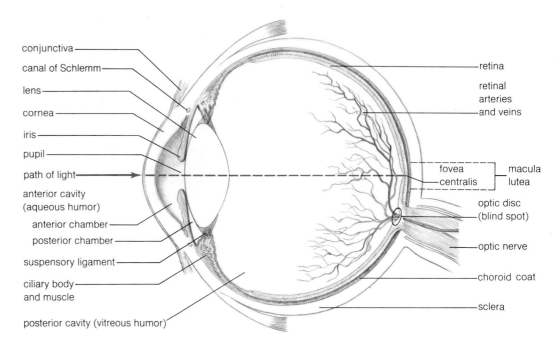

conjunctiva
canal of Schlemm
lens
cornea
iris
pupil
path of light
anterior cavity
(aqueous humor)
anterior chamber
posterior chamber
suspensory ligament
ciliary body
and muscle
posterior cavity (vitreous humor)

retina
retinal
arteries
and veins
fovea
centralis
macula
lutea
optic disc
(blind spot)
optic nerve
choroid coat
sclera

Figure 14.12 A mid-sagittal section through the eyeball showing the layers of its wall and its internal structure.

also change shape from year to year, thereby accounting for changes in vision.

How the lens changes shape is explained by the action of the ciliary muscles (Figure 14.13c). These smooth muscles are arranged partly in a circular pattern around the ciliary processes and partly in a bundle extending from the sclera to the middle of the suspensory ligament. When the muscles contract, they pull the choroid coat forward and relax the tension on the suspensory ligament. This in turn loosens the tension on the lens capsule and allows the elastic lens itself to assume a more spherical shape. When the ciliary muscles relax, tension in the suspensory ligament tightens the lens capsule around the lens and causes it to assume a more flattened shape. Note that the changes in the shape of the lens are passive, dependent only on the elasticity inherent in the structure of the lens. The ability of the lens to become more spherical and focus light from near objects on the retina is called **accommodation**. This process is discussed in the next section of this chapter.

The iris The **iris**, a part of the middle layer of the eye, is a disc-shaped structure that extends from the ciliary body across the eyeball in front of the lens (refer back to Fig-

Changes in pupil size are generally related to changes in the amount of light entering the eyes, but changes in emotional state and attitude can also affect pupil size. For example, when hungry people are shown food, their pupils dilate significantly, but when people who have recently eaten are shown food, their pupils dilate only slightly or even constrict. In another experiment two photographs of the same woman were prepared with the pupils enlarged in one photograph and reduced in the other. Participants in the experiment were asked to select the photograph in which the woman appeared more sympathetic or happier. They usually chose the photograph with the enlarged pupils. When asked in which photograph the woman appeared more angry or sad, they usually chose the photograph with the constricted pupils. These results seem to confirm what ladies of nobility knew many years ago when they used the drug belladonna to dilate their pupils. Belladonna, which means beautiful lady, got its name from this particular use, though the drug has medical uses as well.

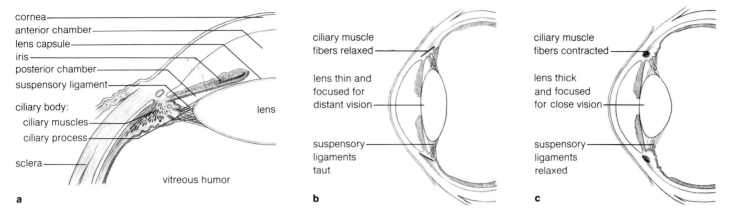

Figure 14.13 The components of the vascular layer: (a) The lens is attached to the ciliary body by the lens capsule and the suspensory ligament. (b) The ciliary muscles decrease the tension on the suspensory ligament when they contract and increase the tension when they relax.

ure 14.12). The iris forms the colored part of the eye; it has an opening in the center called the **pupil**. It contains two sets of smooth muscle fibers, a circular set near the pupil and a more peripheral, radial set (Figure 14.14). The iris controls the amount of light entering the eye by the radial muscles contracting in dim light and the circular muscles contracting in bright light. Both of these sets of muscles are under the control of the autonomic nervous system. Sympathetic stimulation causes the radial muscle to contract and the pupil to dilate, or get larger. Parasympathetic stimulation causes the circular muscle to contract and the pupil to constrict.

The anterior cavity As shown in Figure 14.12, the lens, suspensory ligament, and ciliary body divide the eye into an **anterior cavity** and a **posterior cavity**. The anterior cavity is further divided into an **anterior chamber** and a **posterior chamber**, which are separated by the iris and interconnected through the pupil. The epithelium of the ciliary process continuously secretes a watery fluid, the **aqueous humor**, which helps to maintain the shape of the front part of the eye and provides nutrients to the lens and cornea. Once secreted, this fluid travels from the posterior chamber through the pupil into the anterior chamber. From there it drains through the **canal of Schlemm** into a vein (Figure 14.15).

The internal tunic (retina) The internal tunic of the eyeball, the **retina**, contains the light-sensitive cells. It extends from the ciliary body around the back of the eyeball. As shown in Figure 14.12, the area of the retina that is stimulated most

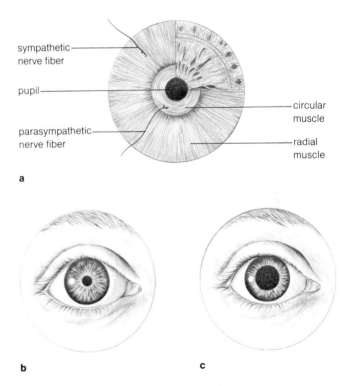

Figure 14.14 (a) The iris contains radial muscle fibers that are innervated by sympathetic nerves and circular muscle fibers that are innervated by parasympathetic nerves. (b) The circular muscles contract in bright light and constrict the pupil. (c) The radial muscles contract in dim light and dilate the pupil.

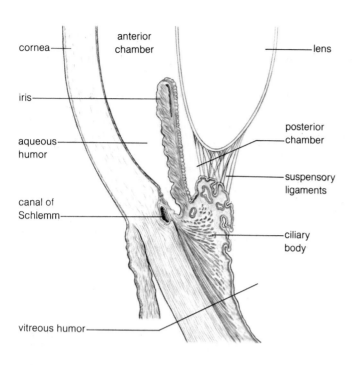

Figure 14.15 The aqueous humor secreted by the ciliary body travels from the posterior chamber through the pupil to the anterior chamber, where it drains into the canal of Schlemm.

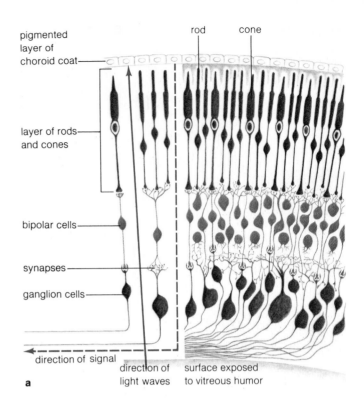

Figure 14.16 (**a**) Light waves pass through the eye and through the transparent neurons of the retina to the back of the eye, where they stimulate the rods and cones. Electrical signals are then conducted back through the retina by way of the bipolar cells to ganglion cells, whose axons are the fibers of the optic nerve. (**b**) Cross section of the retina, × 593. (Photomicrograph reproduced with permission from *Tissues and organs: A text-atlas of scanning electron microscopy* by Richard G. Kessel and Randy H. Kardon. W. H. Freeman and Company. Copyright © 1979.)

directly by light rays is a slight depression called the **fovea centralis**. This is the area of sharpest vision because of the high density of cone receptor cells and the absence of other retinal cells. The fovea lies in the center of a yellow area called the **macula lutea**. At the back of the eyeball, just medial to the fovea, is the **optic disc**, or **blind spot**. Here the nerve fibers from the light-sensitive cells leave the eyeball to form the optic nerve. An artery and a vein also pass through the optic disc. This area is called the blind spot because it is devoid of receptor cells.

The retina contains two types of receptor cells, the **rods** and the **cones**, and several types of neurons, including the **bipolar cells** and the **ganglion cells** (Figure 14.16). Light passes through the eye and through the transparent neurons of the retina to stimulate the rods and cones. When stimulated by light, the rods and cones develop a generator po-

tential that is hyperpolarizing, unlike the depolarizing generator potentials described earlier. This generator potential regulates the release of chemical neurotransmitters from the receptor terminals onto bipolar cells, causing their membrane potentials to change. Bipolar cells in turn release transmitter onto ganglion cells. The ganglion cells become depolarized, and action potentials are generated. The ganglion cells are the first cells in the sequence to generate action potentials, and their action potentials are conducted along their axons to the brain. The **optic nerve** consists of a bundle of all of the axons of ganglion cells. The retina also contains other types of neurons that provide for the lateral transfer of signals from one portion of the retina to other portions. Some of these cells may make inhibitory synapses onto bipolar or ganglion cells. Thus, light stimulation of one area of the retina may inhibit impulse generation by gan-

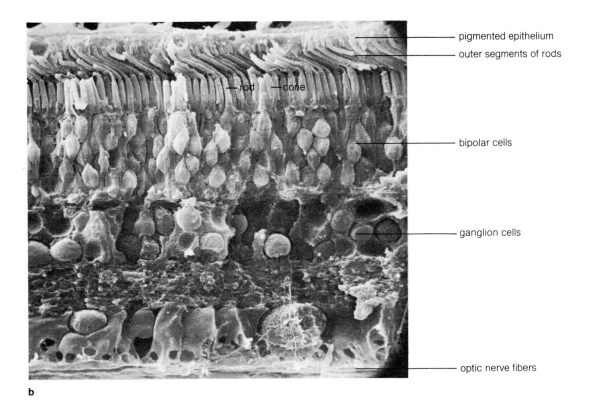

— pigmented epithelium
— outer segments of rods

— rod — cone

— bipolar cells

— ganglion cells

— optic nerve fibers

b

glion cells in another part of the retina. This kind of interaction may play a role in detecting contrast between different parts of the visual image.

The posterior cavity   The space inside the retina and behind the lens is filled with a jellylike substance called the **vitreous humor**. This humor fills the entire posterior cavity. It helps to maintain the shape of the eyeball and also contributes to intraocular pressure (pressure inside the eyeball). Unlike the aqueous humor, the vitreous humor cannot be replaced in any significant quantity. Therefore, in puncture wounds of the eye it is important to prevent the escape of vitreous humor.

The internal structures of the eye are summarized in Table 14.3.

Receptors

Each human eye contains about 125 million rods and about 5.5 million cones (Figure 14.17). The cones are most con-

centrated in the fovea centralis and become less dense from the fovea outward. The rods are absent from the fovea and macula but are present in the remainder of the retina. Both rods and cones contain light-sensitive pigment molecules that change shape when they absorb light waves. This change in shape initiates a series of chemical reactions resulting in the production of a substance that changes the permeability of the receptor cell membrane and thus produces a generator potential.

Rods   Rods are much more sensitive to light than cones, so they can be stimulated by dim light. They detect the intensity of light but do not detect colors. What we see as shades of gray are a function of the light intensity detected by the rods.

Rods contain a light-sensitive pigment, **rhodopsin**, which is synthesized from vitamin A. (Dietary deficiencies of this vitamin can lead to night blindness and impaired vision in dim light.) In the presence of light rhodopsin undergoes a chemical transformation, as described in the paragraph above, which leads to the production of a gener-

Table 14.3 Internal Structures of the Eye

Structure	Anterior Portion	Function	Posterior Portion	Function
Fibrous tunic	Cornea	Admit and refract light	Sclera	Protect
Vascular tunic	Ciliary body	Accommodation	Choroid coat	Provide blood supply and absorb light
	Iris	Regulate light entry		
Internal tunic	None		Retina	Receive stimuli and transmit impulses
Cavities	Anterior cavity	Aqueous humor helps maintain shape of eye, lens and cornea, and refracts light	Posterior cavity	Vitreous humor helps maintain shape of eye and refracts light
Lens	Separates anterior and posterior portions, focuses light			

When a person's eyes must remain dark-adapted, as when driving a car or piloting an airplane at night, red lights to which the rods are insensitive are used to illuminate instrument panels. When a person with dark-adapted eyes steps into a brightly lighted area, as from a darkened theater to a lobby, a sudden barrage of action potentials is sent through the optic nerve, causing discomfort.

ator potential. The resulting signal is transmitted by synapses from the rod cells through the bipolar cells to the ganglion cells, where action potentials are generated and sent by the optic nerve to the brain.

After transformation rhodopsin can be resynthesized by a process that requires ATP (Figure 14.18). In dim light the resynthesis of rhodopsin is able to keep pace with its utilization, and the eye is said to be **dark-adapted**. However, in bright light rhodopsin is used up rapidly. The sensitivity to light is greatly decreased, and the eye is said to be **light-adapted**.

Cones   Whereas the rods do not function well in bright light, the cones operate in moderate to bright light and are able to detect all the colors in the visible light spectrum.

There appear to be three different kinds of cones, each of which contains a different light-sensitive pigment. Cones that contain erythrolabe are most sensitive to red light, those that contain chlorolabe are most sensitive to green light, and those that contain cyanolabe are most sensitive to blue light. Combinations of these three colors of light produce all the colors humans can see. The nature of the chemical reactions that occur when the cone pigments are exposed to light are not as well understood as those involving rhodopsin, but it is supposed that a similar set of reactions occurs in these pigments and that vitamin A is required. The perception of any single color or pattern of colors is thought to be due to the type and number of cones that are stimulated and the way the impulses are interpreted in the brain.

Apart from the focusing power of the cornea and lens, the cones determine the eye's resolving power. The ability to discriminate two points that are very close together depends on there being at least one unstimulated cone between the cones that are stimulated by light from two points. Otherwise, we see the two points as a single point. Two points one meter away from the viewer must be separated by about 1 millimeter to be distinguishable.

Transmission of Visual Impulses to the Brain

Once rods and cones have been stimulated and impulses have been generated in ganglion cells, those impulses travel

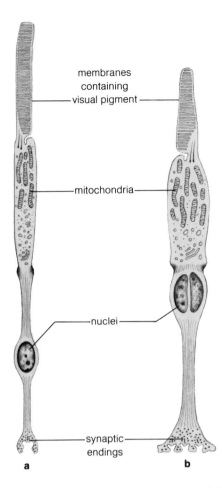

Figure 14.17 The receptor cells of the retina: (**a**) rod cell, (**b**) cone cell.

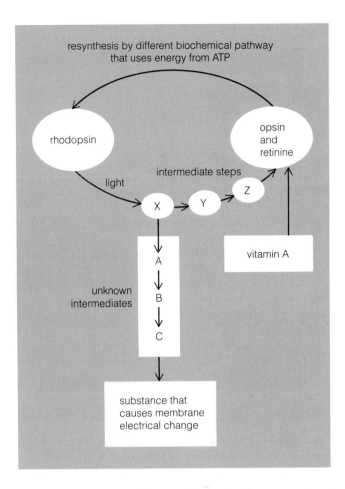

Figure 14.18 The effect of light on rhodopsin. The regeneration of rhodopsin proceeds counterclockwise.

Color blindness is thought to result from the absence or partial deficiency of one of the pigments normally found in the cones or from an abnormality in the chemical structure of a pigment. Though there are several kinds of color blindness, the most common type, which affects the perception of reds and greens, is due to an abnormal, recessive gene on the X-chromosome. (See Chapter 27 for more information on the genetics of color blindness.) Males are most frequently affected by color blindness because they carry a single X-chromosome. In fact, 70% of males are at least partially color blind. Females, who have two X-chromosomes, may have one chromosome with a gene for normal color vision and thus be unaffected by the presence of an abnormal gene on the other chromosome. In rare instances females inherit two abnormal genes and are color blind.

out the fibers of the optic nerve. At the base of the brain just anterior to the pituitary gland, the fibers from the medial half of each retina cross to the contralateral side of the brain. The area in which this crossing takes place is called the **optic chiasma**. The resulting left and right **optic tracts** pass to the ipsilateral thalamic nucleus, where the fibers of the tracts synapse with neurons that pass to the ipsilateral sides of the **primary visual cortex**, or visual area. The optic tracts contain fibers from the lateral retina of the same side and the medial retina of the opposite side (Figure 14.19). In the primary visual cortex information from the light-sensitive receptors is processed. Signals are then relayed to the visual association area, where they are interpreted.

In humans and some other animals both eyes can be focused on the same visual field, producing **binocular vision** (Figure 14.20). When impulses from both eyes arrive in the visual cortex, they can be compared. Because the angle with which each eye views an object is slightly different, the information from each eye is slightly different. These slight

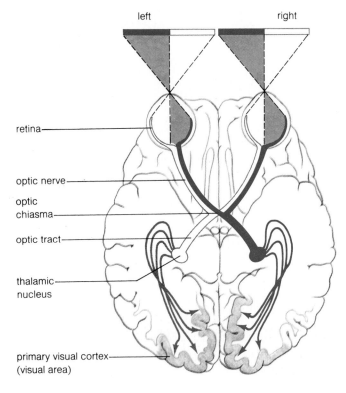

retina

optic nerve

optic
chiasma

optic tract

thalamic
nucleus

primary visual cortex
(visual area)

Figure 14.19 The pathway of neurons from the retina to the primary visual cortex.

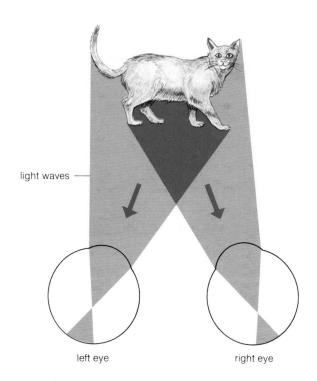

light waves

left eye

right eye

Figure 14.20 Binocular vision provides the visual cortex with slightly different images from each eye.

differences are used by cells in the visual cortex to perceive distance, depth, and the height and width of objects. Individuals who have lost the sight of one eye have difficulty judging distances and depth because their visual cortex lacks the information to make the comparisons.

Individuals with strabismus, or cross-eye, often are unable to focus both eyes on the same field of vision. If such a condition goes untreated, the brain eventually ignores the input from one eye; what is perceived is limited to information relayed from the eye whose muscular movements are better controlled. Effective vision is eventually lost in the repressed eye. Thus, it is important to diagnose and treat strabismus early.

Visual Perceptions

As noted at the beginning of this chapter, sensory receptors detect objects and events in the environment, and the cerebrum perceives these objects and events. In visual perception, and to some extent in other perceptions, the brain adds

information from memory and makes an interpretation that goes beyond the sensory information. As shown in Figure 14.21, the brain perceives transparency where none actually exists or a figure that is merely implied by the arrangement of other objects. When we perceive an optical illusion, we do so because there are at least two plausible and logical interpretations of the visual image in the brain. In Figure 14.22 the young girl's chin is the old woman's nose. We can perceive one or the other but not both at the same time because our brain can make only one interpretation at a given time.

Path of Light through the Eye and How It Is Focused

You are able to see things because light is reflected from them or because they are emitting light rays. When light rays pass from one medium to another, they are bent, or refracted (Figure 14.23). This is because of variations in the speed of light as it moves through different materials.

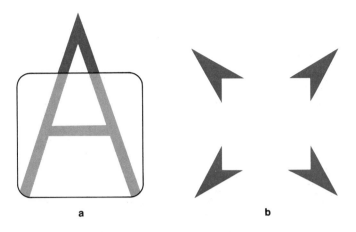

a   b

Figure 14.21 You probably see the letter "A" partially covered by a transparent screen in (**a**) and a clear square with arrows at the corners in (**b**). Actually, the letter "A" is printed in two shades, and your brain perceives transparency. The arrows in (**b**) are simply arranged in such a way that your brain perceives the contours of a square where no square actually exists.

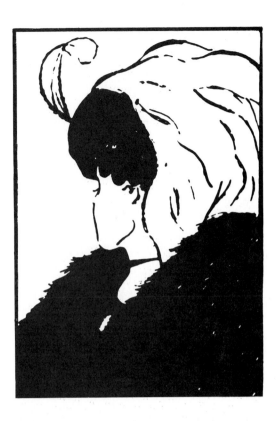

Figure 14.22 An optical illusion showing "my wife and my mother-in-law," as depicted by W. E. Hill in 1915.

Light rays from a point source such as a very tiny light bulb diverge as they pass from the source. The divergent rays are refracted at four different points as they travel from the air outside the eye to the retina: (1) the interface between the air and the cornea, (2) the interface between the cornea and the aqueous humor, (3) the interface between the aqueous humor and the lens, and (4) the interface between the lens and the vitreous humor. Though we normally think of the lens as the main structure for focusing light as it passes through the eye, its power to refract light is far less than that of the cornea. Most of the bending of light rays occurs as the rays pass from the air to the tissue of the cornea. Thus, the cornea acts as the "crude focusing" structure and the lens as the "fine focusing" structure.

Light reflected from an object (indicated as an arrow labeled X–Y–Z in Figure 14.23) enters the eye and is similarly bent by the cornea and the lens. It is focused on the retina as an upside down, left–right reversed image. Receptor cells receive the stimuli and transmit them to the brain, where the image is interpreted as right-side-up and correctly oriented left to right.

Light waves from distant objects (farther than 6 meters from the eye) travel in nearly parallel paths. They require very little bending by the lens after they have passed through the cornea to be focused on the retina (Figure 14.24). Light waves from close objects (nearer than 6 meters from the eye) are more divergent and require greater bending by the lens to be brought into focus on the retina.

When the eyes are focused on a near object, the ciliary muscles contract and allow the lens to become thicker. When the lens is rounded, it bends the light waves to a greater degree and causes them to focus on the retina. The ciliary muscles can contract in degrees and regulate the shape of the lens so as to bring near objects into focus regardless of their precise distance from the eye. During this process of **accommodation** two other events occur that help to create a sharp image of a near object. The pupils constrict and the eyes converge, as both medial rectus muscles contract slightly so that both eyes are directed toward the near object.

Most animals do not have the power to accommodate to seeing close objects sharply. A special modification of the

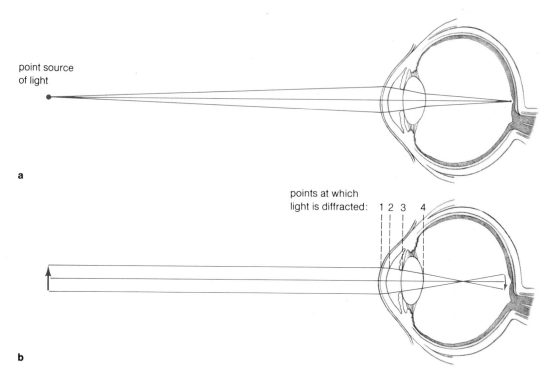

a

b

Figure 14.23 The pathway of light through the eye: (**a**) from a point source of light, (**b**) from an object that reflects light from its surface.

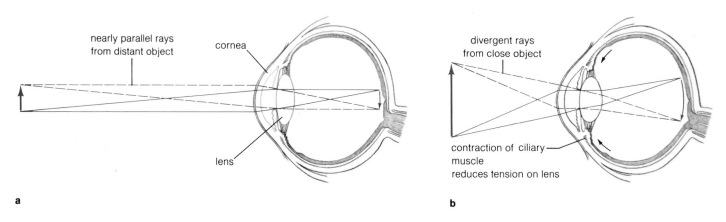

a

b

Figure 14.24 The lens of the human eye can accommodate to light waves from (**a**) distant objects or (**b**) close objects.

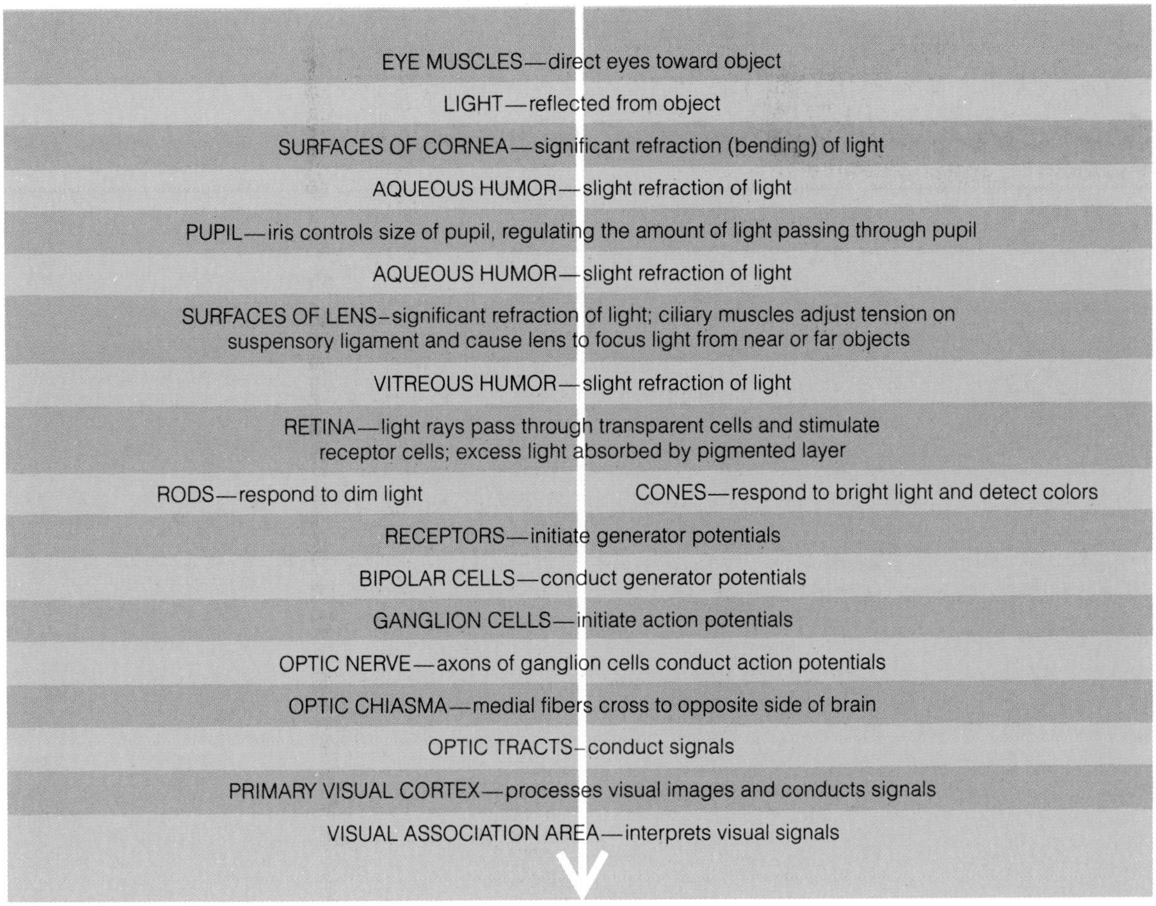

EYE MUSCLES—direct eyes toward object

LIGHT—reflected from object

SURFACES OF CORNEA—significant refraction (bending) of light

AQUEOUS HUMOR—slight refraction of light

PUPIL—iris controls size of pupil, regulating the amount of light passing through pupil

AQUEOUS HUMOR—slight refraction of light

SURFACES OF LENS—significant refraction of light; ciliary muscles adjust tension on
suspensory ligament and cause lens to focus light from near or far objects

VITREOUS HUMOR—slight refraction of light

RETINA—light rays pass through transparent cells and stimulate
receptor cells; excess light absorbed by pigmented layer

RODS—respond to dim light   CONES—respond to bright light and detect colors

RECEPTORS—initiate generator potentials

BIPOLAR CELLS—conduct generator potentials

GANGLION CELLS—initiate action potentials

OPTIC NERVE—axons of ganglion cells conduct action potentials

OPTIC CHIASMA—medial fibers cross to opposite side of brain

OPTIC TRACTS—conduct signals

PRIMARY VISUAL CORTEX—processes visual images and conducts signals

VISUAL ASSOCIATION AREA—interprets visual signals

Figure 14.25 A summary of the events of vision.

ciliary muscles allows humans to do this, but doing so places a strain on those muscles. Thus, when you are using your eyes to focus on close objects for long periods of time, it is a good idea to look away and focus on distant objects periodically to allow the ciliary muscles to relax.

The events of normal vision are summarized in Figure 14.25.

Defects in Vision

As we have noted, the elasticity of the lens allows it to change shape. However, with aging the lens becomes less elastic and thus less able to accommodate to focusing on close objects. This condition, **presbyopia** (literally "elder vision"), can be corrected by the use of lenses that bend light rays sufficiently to compensate for the loss of elasticity of the lens.

Other structural irregularities that require the use of corrective lenses are nearsightedness, or **myopia**; farsightedness, or **hypermetropia**; and **astigmatism** (Figure 14.26).

These terms are in contrast to **emmetropia**, or normal refraction of the eye.

A person with myopia can see close objects relatively well but has difficulty focusing on distant objects. In myopic individuals the eyeballs are longer than normal, causing the light rays to focus in front of the retina, especially if they enter the eyes as parallel rays from distant objects. Images can be made to focus on the retina by placing a concave lens in front of the natural lens. A concave lens causes the light rays to diverge before they enter the eye. Then, as they pass through the cornea and lens, they are bent so they converge on the retina and not in front of it.

Hypermetropia is just the opposite of myopia. The person can see distant objects but has difficulty focusing on close objects. The eyeballs are shorter than normal, and the focal point of the light rays lies behind the retina. In this case a convex lens is used to increase the convergence and cause the image to fall on the retina.

Astigmatism causes fuzzy images to be projected on the retina. Due to irregularities in the surface of the cornea

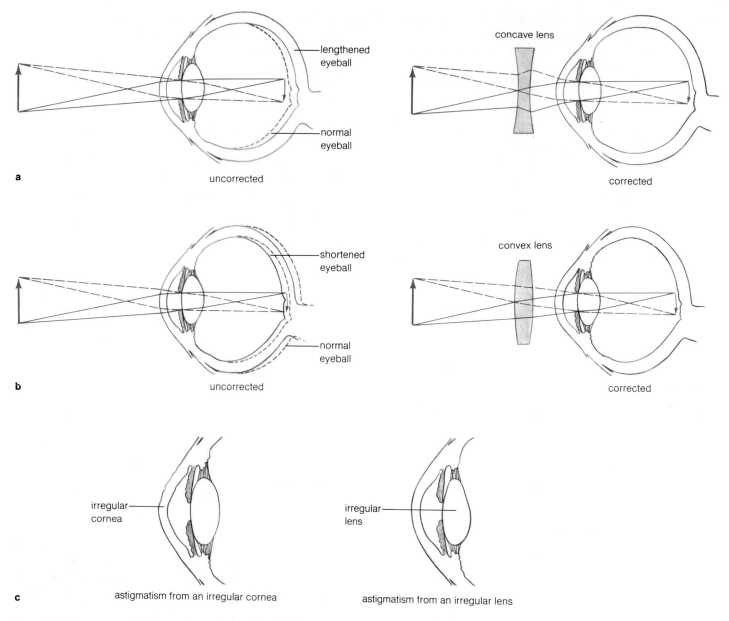

Figure 14.26 How corrective lenses change the bending of light waves in (**a**) myopia, (**b**) hypermetropia, (**c**) astigmatism.

or the lens or both, not all rays from a particular object are focused on the retina. Corrective lenses may compensate for the uneven curvature of these surfaces and cause the image to be projected evenly on the retina. Refer back to Table 14.3 for a summary of the functions of the parts of the eye.

Applications

Two common clinical conditions that involve parts of the eye are cataract and glaucoma. Both can cause blindness.

In **cataract** the cells of the lens lose their transparency and become cloudy or opaque to light. In the normal lens the light waves that strike it pass through with very little scattering. However, because of changes in the lens proteins in the formation of a cataract, light waves tend to scatter when they strike an altered area of the lens. Cataracts are most common in the elderly, though they can occur at any age, even appearing as a congenital condition. Two types of cataract can be distinguished by the location of the opaque area. In a nuclear cataract the central portion of the lens becomes opaque; in a cortical cataract the outer portion is altered. In some patients both areas are altered, or one type may progress to the other.

The treatment of cataract involves the surgical removal of the affected lens. Contact lenses have been used to replace the lens, and focal distances adjusted by the use of external glass lenses in eyeglass frames. The surgical implantation of a plastic replacement lens inside the eyeball (a recently developed technique) offers promise for even better vision following cataract surgery.

Like cataract, **glaucoma** is a condition that is more common in older people. Untreated, it invariably leads to blindness. Worldwide, it is the major cause of blindness. In glaucoma the pressure in the anterior cavity of the eye increases to an abnormal level, exerting pressure on the posterior cavity and greatly reducing the blood supply to the retina. Lack of nutrients because of the reduced blood supply ultimately damages the nerve cells of the retina. Simple methods exist for measuring the pressure inside the eyeball. When excessive pressure is detected, several treatments may be used to reduce the pressure, including the use of drugs to increase the rate of drainage of aqueous humor or the removal of a portion of the iris to improve the flow of the fluid. If the pressure is due to blockage of the canal of Schlemm, a new canal can be created surgically (refer back to Figure 14.15).

> The incidence of cataract is higher in diabetic individuals than in nondiabetic individuals of the same age. It is thought that abnormalities in glucose metabolism cause the osmotic pressure to increase in the lens tissue, thus hastening the cataract formation process.

HEARING

Objective 11. Describe the external and internal structures of the ear that relate to hearing and give their locations and functions.

Objective 12. Trace the path of sound waves through the ear and explain how they are transmitted and converted to nerve impulses.

Objective 13. Distinguish between conduction deafness and nerve deafness in terms of altered structure and function and method of treatment.

Objective 14. Describe the qualities of sound and how they are detected in the receptor cells and interpreted in the brain.

Senses that operate at a distance—like hearing, sight, and smell—are important for survival. For example, if you were in a burning building and could rely only on your temperature receptors, by the time you could feel the heat of the fire, it might be too late to escape. You might smell smoke, but you certainly would hear ringing alarms and sirens. Thus, your sense of hearing can be important to your survival—but it is also important in helping you to sense less extreme conditions. Because of your sense of hearing you can enjoy music, hear what others say to you, detect sounds that mean a meal is nearly ready to be served, or experience the pleasure of a crackling fire in the fireplace on a cold winter's evening.

The Structure of the Ear

The ear, as the organ of hearing, is divided into three portions, the **outer ear**, the **middle ear**, and the **inner ear** (Figure 14.27). The inner ear also contains structures that provide for a sense of equilibrium or balance. (Those structures will be considered in the next section of this chapter.)

The outer ear The outer ear consists of an outer flaplike structure, the **pinna**, or auricle (commonly called just "the ear"); the ear canal, or **external auditory meatus**; and a thin cone-shaped structure, the eardrum, or **tympanic membrane**. The pinna consists of thick elastic cartilage covered with skin. The external auditory meatus, part of which can be seen from outside the body, is a tube formed from the temporal bones of the skull, cartilage, and a thin layer of skin. The skin contains numerous touch and pain receptors and near the surface opening has hairs and **ceruminous glands**. These modified sebaceous glands secrete **cerumen**, or earwax. Both the hairs and the wax help to prevent foreign objects from entering the ear canal. At the inner end of the ear canal is the tympanic membrane, which marks the separation of the outer and the middle ear. It can be seen from the surface only with a special tool, called an otoscope. When sound waves passing through the ear canal reach this membrane, they set it into vibration.

In many animals the pinna can be moved to collect sound waves coming from different directions and direct them into the external auditory meatus. Its efficiency in humans is limited, though some individuals become adept at "wiggling their ears."

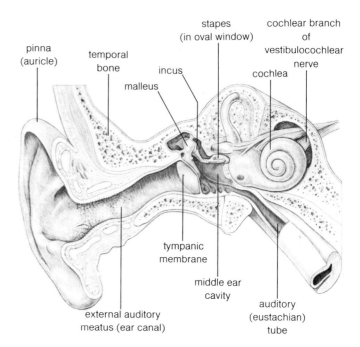

Figure 14.27 The structure of the ear.

The middle ear The middle ear is a small cavity in the temporal bone lined with epithelium and filled with air. Of its five openings three are associated with the conduction of vibrations, and two communicate with other organs. The openings concerned with conducting vibrations are covered with membranes: the **tympanic membrane** and the membranes of the **oval window** and the **round window**. Between the tympanic membrane and the oval window are the **ear ossicles**, or bones of the middle ear (Figure 14.28): the **malleus** (hammer), **incus** (anvil), and **stapes** (stirrup). Vibrations from the tympanic membrane are transmitted to the malleus, the handle of which is attached to the membrane, then to the incus, and finally to the stapes. The incus is attached by ligaments to both the malleus and the stapes. The footplate of the stapes fits into the oval window and transmits vibrations to the membrane covering that window. A third membrane-covered opening, the round window, allows for equalization of pressure in the fluid-filled inner ear when the oval window is set in vibration.

Two other openings in the middle ear are the **auditory (eustachian) tube**, which opens into the pharynx, and the **tympanic antrum**, which opens into the mastoid cells of the temporal bone. The auditory tube allows for the equalization of pressure in the middle ear cavity with atmospheric pressure.

Microorganisms can enter the middle ear cavity through the auditory tube and frequently can cause infections. Likewise, microorganisms can move on into the mastoid cells by way of the tympanic antrum.

The inner ear The inner ear consists of a **bony labyrinth**, a series of passageways within the petrous portion of the temporal bone, and a **membranous labyrinth** that lies within the bony one (Figure 14.29). The space between the membranous and bony labyrinths is filled with a fluid called **perilymph**, and the membranous labyrinth is filled with a similar fluid called **endolymph**. The labyrinths are organized into three parts: the cochlea, the vestibule, and the semicircular canals. Of these only the cochlea is concerned with hearing; the other parts are concerned with balance.

The **cochlea** is shaped like a snail shell—a spiral with

2¾ turns, as shown in Figure 14.29. A cross-section of the cochlea (Figure 14.30) shows that it contains a bony supporting structure, the **modiolus**, and three passageways, the **scala vestibuli**, the **scala tympani**, and the **scala media**, or **cochlear duct** (a). The diagram of the "unwound" cochlea (b) shows that the scala vestibuli and the scala tympani are joined at the apex by a small opening, the **helicotrema**. Both of these passageways are filled with perilymph. The cochlear duct lies between the scalae and is filled with perilymph. The partition between the scala tympani and the cochlear duct is called the **basilar membrane**; that between the scala vestibuli and the cochlear duct is called the **vestibular membrane**.

Within the cochlear duct is the **organ of Corti**, where the receptor cells of hearing are located (c). This long organ extends the full length of the cochlear duct and is therefore sometimes called the spiral organ. It consists of **supporting cells** and **hair cells** that rest on the basilar membrane and a **tectorial membrane** that rests on the hairlike projections of the hair cells. These hairlike projections receive vibrations and cause the hair cells (receptor cells) to produce generator potentials. The hair cells make synaptic connections onto the cochlear branches of the vestibulocochlear nerve. The structure of the labyrinths is summarized in Table 14.4.

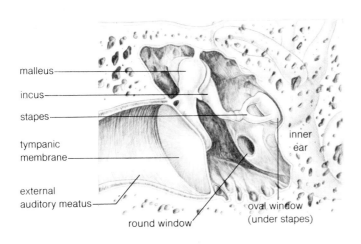

malleus

incus

stapes

tympanic
membrane

external
auditory meatus

inner
ear

round window

oval window
(under stapes)

Figure 14.28 The bones of the middle ear. Not shown in the figure are the ligaments that hold the bones to each other and to the membranes.

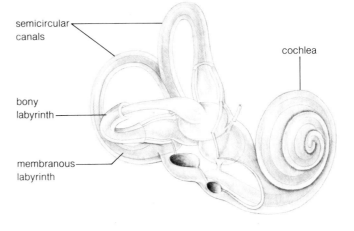

semicircular
canals

cochlea

bony
labyrinth

membranous
labyrinth

Figure 14.29 The inner ear consists of a bony labyrinth within which is the membranous labyrinth.

Path of Sound Waves and Nerve Impulses

Sound is transmitted through the atmosphere by the movement of air molecules. A disturbance in the air—called a sound wave—causes adjacent air molecules to move; consequently, sound can travel for miles as long as the moving molecules can cause other molecules to move. After sound waves strike the pinna, they enter the external auditory meatus, where they strike the tympanic membrane and cause it to vibrate. The vibrations of the tympanic membrane are transferred to the bones of the middle ear, which begin to vibrate. The bones act as a lever system and amplify, or increase the intensity of, the vibrations by about 3 decibels (units of sound intensity). The tympanic membrane has a much larger surface than the membrane of the oval window, to which the bones transmit vibrations. The transmission of vibrations from a larger to a smaller surface amplifies them by about 23 decibels—a greater degree than the lever action of the bones themselves. Therefore, the sound waves are transmitted to the perilymph in a much amplified state. Here, they move as pressure waves through the fluid of the scala vestibuli to the apex of the cochlea and back through the scala tympani to the round window. Intense pressure waves in the perilymph can cause the membrane of the round window to bulge out into the cavity of the middle ear. Pressure waves in the perilymph are transmitted to the cochlear duct, where they deflect the basilar membrane into the scala tympani. Movement of the basilar membrane causes the hairlike projections of the hair cells to move in relation to the tectorial membrane. In some way movement of the hair cell projections produces a generator potential in the hair cell. This signal regulates the release of chemical transmitter substances from the hair cells onto afferent endings of the cochlear nerve. Here, action potentials are produced and conducted along a branch of the cochlear nerve (which joins the vestibular nerve to become the vestibulocochlear nerve). Signals are then transmitted via several nuclei, including the thalamus, to the auditory area of the brain, where they are interpreted as sound. The pathway for sound vibrations is summarized in Figure 14.31.

Deafness

Deafness may be partial or complete and may be caused by damage to the conduction system or to the nerve fibers or receptor cells. **Conduction deafness** can be due to such a simple cause as accumulation of wax in the ear. Removal of wax is a simple procedure, although it is best performed by

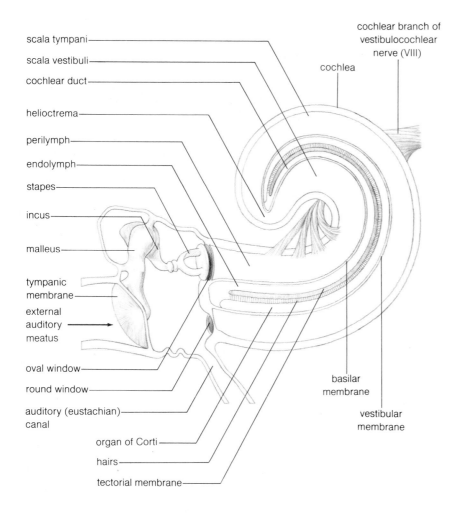

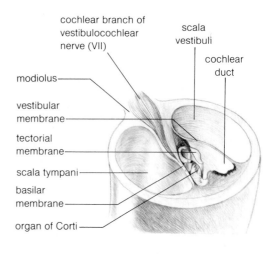

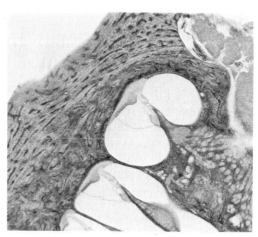

a

b

a health professional; otherwise, the tympanic membrane may be damaged. Conduction deafness may also come from a more complex cause such as otosclerosis, in which the bones of the middle ear become fused together and fail to transmit vibrations. Otosclerosis can be treated surgically by chipping away bone that holds the ossicles together and sometimes by replacing the stirrup with a metal or plastic prosthesis that is made free to vibrate against the oval window.

Another cause of conduction deafness is damage to or destruction of the tympanic membrane. In many cases a ruptured tympanic membrane will grow back across the opening and repair itself to some degree. However, extensive damage may leave enough scar tissue that hearing is permanently impaired.

Some hearing aids amplify sound so that hearing occurs even with limited conduction. It is possible to use a hearing aid to conduct sound through the bones of the skull instead of through the normal channel. When we hear the sound of our own voices, we are hearing partly by the conduction of vibrations through the bones of our skull as well as through the air. This is why our own voices sound different to us than to others.

Nerve deafness results from damage to receptors or nerve fibers. It can be caused by excessive exposure to loud noises, tumors, or other kinds of brain damage. Some loss of function in the cochlear nerve accompanies aging. Though no effective treatment is available for most kinds of nerve deafness, electronic devices someday may be feasible.

Qualities of Sound

Sound has three qualities that are significant in our study of hearing: pitch, intensity, and timbre.

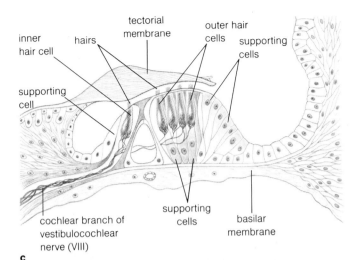

inner hair cell | supporting cell | hairs | tectorial membrane | outer hair cells | supporting cells | supporting cells | basilar membrane | cochlear branch of vestibulocochlear nerve (VIII)

c

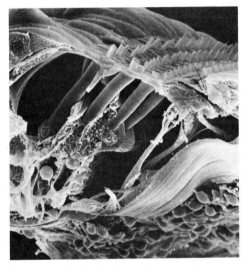

d

Table 14.4 Summary of the Structure of Labyrinths

Bony Labyrinth	Membranous Labyrinth
Vestibule—section of bony labyrinth nearest middle ear. Oval and round windows, semicircular canals, and cochlea open into vestibule.	Utricle—part of the membranous labyrinth contained in the vestibule. Contains endolymph; the macula, an organ of balance; and branches of the vestibular nerve. Saccule—another part of the membranous labyrinth contained in the vestibule. Contains endolymph and macula.
Cochlea—bony spiral tube that contains the receptor cells for hearing.	Cochlear duct—membranous structure within the cochlea. Contains endolymph, organ of Corti, and branches of the vestibular nerve.
Bony semicircular canals—three half-circle structures that contain the receptor cells for balance.	Membranous semicircular canals—contained within the bony semicircular canals. Contain endolymph; cristae, the organs of balance; and branches of the vestibular nerve.

Figure 14.30 The structure of the cochlea: (**a**) unwound, and in longitudinal section, (**b**) cross section diagram and photomicrograph × 25, (**c**) the organ of Corti, (**d**) scanning electron microscope photograph of organ of Corti. (**b**: photograph by author; **d**: photograph courtesy of Dr. Goran Bredberg.)

Pitch is determined by the frequency of vibrations, higher frequencies producing higher pitched sounds. The normal human ear is sensitive to frequencies from about 20 to 20,000 hertz (vibration cycles per second), depending on loudness. The range of pitches on a piano is from about 30 to 4,000 hertz, only a portion of the total range of hearing.

Intensity, or loudness, is measured in decibels, an arbitrary scale on which an increase of ten units represents a tenfold increase in loudness, so that a 20 decibel increase represents a 100-fold increase in intensity. For example, the ticking of a watch makes a sound of about 20 decibels, and conversation between two people sitting close together makes a sound of about 70 decibels. Thus, conversation is 100,000 times as loud as the ticking watch. Sounds above 100 decibels, such as those made by a pneumatic hammer, electronically amplified music, and airplanes during takeoff, can cause permanent damage to the cochlea. The **attenua-**

tion reflex helps to protect against inner ear damage during loud noises. In this reflex small muscles of the middle ear pull the stapes outward and the malleus inward to make the ossicles rigid. This can reduce sounds by 30 to 40 decibels. However, it fails to protect against very sudden loud noises as the reflex takes several hundred milliseconds to occur.

Timbre is a quality of sound that comes from additional vibrations of higher frequencies (called harmonics) superimposed on a basic tone. For example, when the same note or pitch is sounded on several different musical instruments, each instrument produces its own quality of sound. You can easily tell the difference among the sounds of a piano, a trumpet, a violin, and a saxophone, even when each instrument is playing the same tone. These differences are due to the different set of vibrations, or pattern of harmonics, that each instrument produces; such differences create the timbre of a sound.

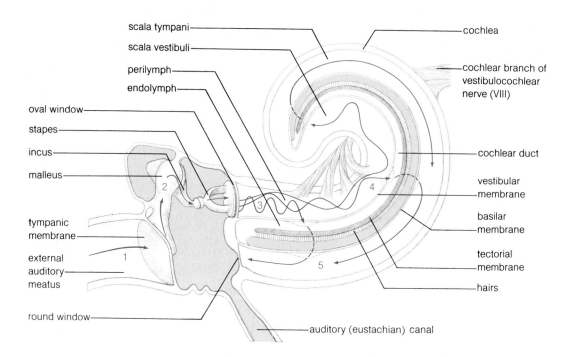

scala tympani

scala vestibuli

perilymph

endolymph

oval window

stapes

incus

malleus

tympanic membrane

external auditory meatus

round window

cochlea

cochlear branch of vestibulocochlear nerve (VIII)

cochlear duct

vestibular membrane

basilar membrane

tectorial membrane

hairs

auditory (eustachian) canal

Figure 14.31 The transmission of sound vibrations through the ear: (**1**) Sound vibrations in air pass through the external auditory meatus and set the tympanic membrane vibrating. (**2**) Vibrations are transferred to the bones of the middle ear and amplified as they reach the oval window. (**3**) Vibrations of the oval window set the fluid of the scala vestibuli in vibration. (**4**) Vibrations of this fluid cause certain portions of the basilar membrane to bulge into the cochlear duct. The movement of the basilar membrane stimulates the hair cells of the organ of Corti and causes impulses to be conducted along the cochlear nerve. (**5**) Vibrations of the fluid of the scala vestibuli are transferred to the scala tympani and dissipated as the round window bulges out toward the middle ear.

How Qualities of Sound Are Detected

Pitch is detected by the organ of Corti, which consists of over 20,000 strands of cells that run perpendicular to the length of the organ. Because of differences in the thickness of these strands, it is believed that portions of the organ of Corti vibrate selectively according to the pitch of the sound being transmitted to them. The portion of the basilar membrane nearest the base of the cochlea vibrates best in response to high-pitched sounds, while the portion at the apex vibrates best in response to low-pitched sounds (Figure 14.32). Thus, different populations of hair cells, and different nerve fibers, are stimulated by different sound frequencies. Signals from particular regions of the organ of Corti arrive in particular locations in the brain.

Intensity is also detected in the organ of Corti. Louder sounds cause greater movement of the basilar membrane, which in turn causes an increase in the frequency of im-

pulses transmitted from the receptor to the cochlear nerve fibers and from there to the auditory area of the brain.

Timbre is detected in the same way as pitch. However, several areas of the organ of Corti are stimulated simulta-

Frequent exposure to loud sounds can cause damage to the sensitive organ of Corti. Operators of pneumatic hammers, workers subjected to loud noises in factories and airports, and even rock musicians often wear earplugs or other devices to protect their ears. Rock concert goers, disco dancers, and other people who regularly expose themselves to loud sounds—no matter how pleasurable they think these experiences are—should also protect their ears.

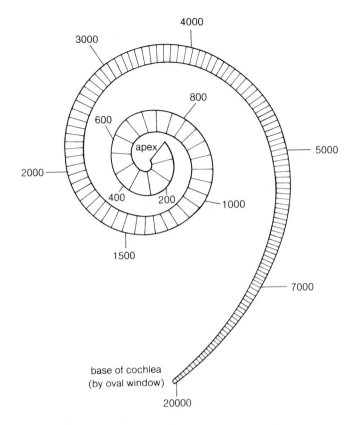

Figure 14.32 The location of hair cells in the organ of Corti, showing the pitch to which each area is most sensitive. Numbers are in hertz (cycles per second).

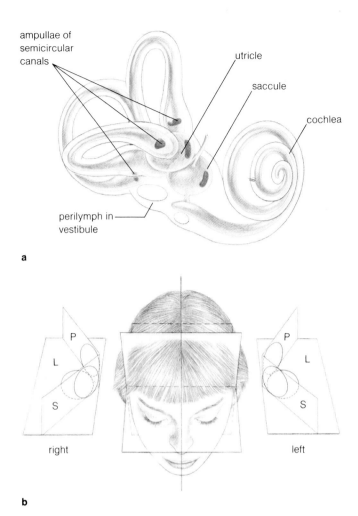

Figure 14.33 (**a**) The organs of static equilibrium are the utricle and possibly the saccule, located in the vestibule of the inner ear. The organs of dynamic equilibrium are the semicircular canals. (**b**) A diagram of the orientation of the semicircular canals.

neously, and then the patterns of impulses in different fibers are transmitted to the brain.

Think for a moment of the great variety of pitches, intensities, and timbres produced by a symphony orchestra. The fact that you can distinguish which instruments are playing, recognize several pitches simultaneously, and detect variations in intensity provides some idea of the complexity of the information that can be processed by the organ of Corti and associated areas of the brain.

BALANCE

Objective 15. Distinguish between static and dynamic balance, or equilibrium, in terms of the structures involved and their locations and functions.

Objective 16. Describe how sensations from the organs of balance are transmitted to and interpreted in the brain.

Objective 17. Discuss the causes of and treatments for (a) motion sickness and (b) Meniere's disease.

The Organs of Balance

The organs of balance, located in the inner ear, consist of the **saccule**, the **utricle**, and the three **semicircular canals** (Figure 14.33). Located in the vestibule, the saccule and utricle are concerned with static equilibrium. They provide information about position when the head is stationary. The

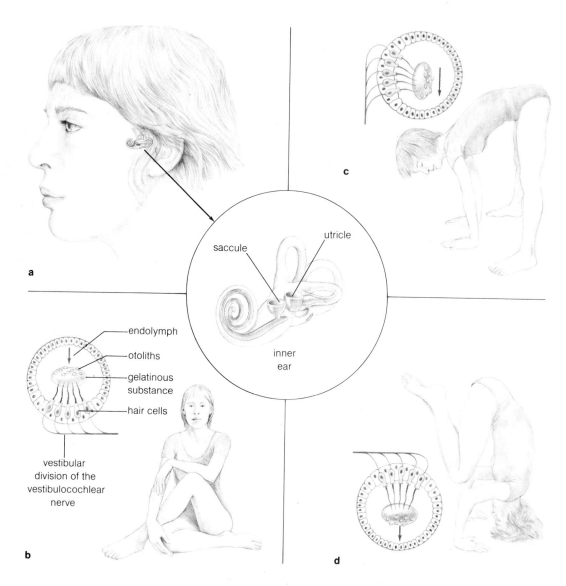

Figure 14.34 Static equilibrium is provided by the utricle and possibly also the saccule (**a**). In the walls of these structures is a macula (**b**), consisting of hair cells with projections into the gelatinous mass that contains otoliths. The projections of the hair cells are deflected when the head is in a horizontal position (**c**) and "weighted down" when the head is upside down (**d**).

semicircular canals, in contrast, provide information about changes in position.

Static equilibrium   Inside the utricle is a structure called the **macula** (Figure 14.34). The macula contains hair cells, the hairs of which are imbedded in a gelatinous substance. Also within the gelatinous substance are particles of calcium carbonate called **otoliths** (literally, ear stones). The otoliths cause the gelatinous substance to be heavier than the en-

dolymph that fills the remainder of the cavity within the macula. A similar structure in the saccule may operate in the same way as the one in the utricle, but its function in humans is open to question.

The hair cells of the macula are responsive to the force of gravity. When the head is in an upright position, gravity causes the gelatinous mass containing the otoliths to press upon the hair cells. When the position of the head is changed, the gelatinous mass shifts position, and the hair-

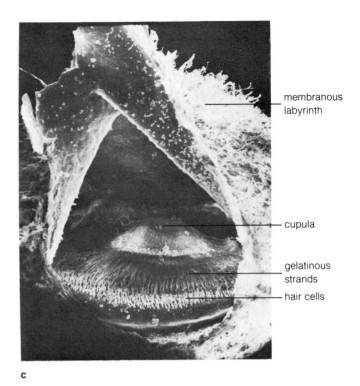

superior semicircular canal

semicircular duct within canal

posterior semicircular canal

ampulla and receptor

lateral semicircular canal

a

membranous labyrinth

cupula

gelatinous strands

hair cells

c

cupula

hairlike projections

hair cells of crista

nerve fibers

b

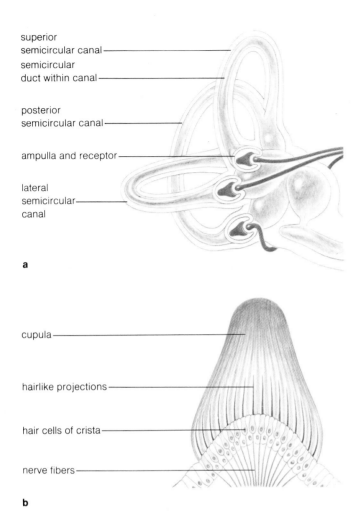

Figure 14.35 The organs of dynamic equilibrium are the semicircular canals (**a**). Each canal contains an ampulla (**b**), which contains hair cells (the cristae) with projections into a gelatinous mass, the cupula, (**c**) an open ampulla showing the cupula, gelatinous strands, and hair cells, × 113. (Photomicrograph reproduced with permission from *Tissues and organs: A text-atlas of scanning electron microscopy* by Richard G. Kessel and Randy H. Kardon. W. H. Freeman Company. Copyright © 1979.)

like projections of the hair cells are bent. Bending of the projections produces a generator potential in the hair cells, which make chemical synapses onto afferent nerve fibers. Action potentials are generated in the nerve fibers and transmitted via the **vestibular branch** of the vestibulocochlear nerve to motor areas of the medulla and cerebellum. Impulses generated by the motor areas coordinate body movements with the position of the head. These impulses, called **positional reflexes**, maintain the body in an upright

position. Some impulses also go to the cerebrum, where they create awareness of position.

The macula also can respond in a limited way to movement. If the position of the head is changed abruptly, the gelatinous mass moves more slowly than the whole head. The hairlike projections are bent, and an impulse is generated.

Dynamic equilibrium   Each of the three semicircular canals lies in a plane roughly perpendicular to the other two, somewhat like the arrangement of the floor and the two adjacent side walls in the corner of a room. Consequently, the endolymph in the duct of at least one of the canals is affected by any kind of movement. Each canal contains a structure called an **ampulla**, located in an enlarged area of the semicircular duct, at one end of the canal. Inside an ampulla are many hair cells with their hairlike projections imbedded in a gelatinous mass. The group of hair cells is called a **crista**, and the gelatinous mass is called the **cupula** (Figure 14.35).

The hair cells of each crista respond to rotary or angular movements of the endolymph; those hair cells in canals in the plane of movement receive maximal stimulation. Because the canals on the two sides of the head are symmetrical, turning the head displaces fluid toward the ampulla on one side and away from it on the other side. Nodding the head stimulates hair cells in the anterior canals and deflects fluid away from the ampullae in the posterior canals. When the head is first set in motion, a slight lag occurs before the endolymph begins to move. You can demonstrate this kind of lag by quickly picking up a full glass of water with a sweeping motion. Some of the water will lag behind and spill out of the glass. The lag in the movement of the endolymph causes the cupula to move in the opposite direction of the head movement. The movement of the cupula bends the projections on the hair cells, producing a generator potential in the hair cells. These cells synapse onto nerve fibers and cause impulses to be relayed to the brain, particularly the cerebellum. Here, motor impulses are generated that maintain balance and coordination during starting, stopping, or turning movements. These movements are called **acceleratory reflexes**. Impulses to the cerebrum create awareness of motion.

The receptors in the semicircular canals not only detect specific movements as described above, they also detect changes in movement. After the initial lag in the flow of endolymph when movement begins, the endolymph begins to flow at the same rate the head is moving, and the cupula is no longer displaced. As long as the rate of movement is constant, the number of impulses generated by the cristae remains at a minimum. For example, when a vehicle you are riding in first begins to move, you experience a strong sensation of movement. However, after the vehicle has been moving at a constant speed for a period of time, you are only slightly aware of the movement. When there is a change in the rate or direction of movement, the cristae are again stimulated, and they generate many sensory impulses. You quickly become aware that there has been a change in the movement.

Applications

Two disturbances in the function of the organs of balance are motion sickness and Meniere's disease.

Motion sickness Motion sickness is a temporary disturbance in the functioning of the semicircular canals and does not involve any structural damage or defect. It results from repetitive changes in the rate and direction of movement and from conflicting vestibular and visual signals—for example, the constantly shifting head position experienced while riding in a boat combined with the sight of a relatively stationary horizon. The exact nature of the disturbance is not well understood, but holding the head in a fixed position and fixing the eyes on a single point seem to alleviate symptoms for some people. When turning rapidly, dancers keep their eyes on one object by turning their heads rapidly and quickly refocusing on the same object. This minimizes changes in the visual field and helps them to avoid becoming dizzy. Drugs such as Dramamine, Bonamine, and Marezine can be used to prevent and relieve symptoms of motion sickness.

Meniere's disease Meniere's disease is caused by irritation or damage to the inner ear, leading to the accumulation of an excess of endolymph. If the semicircular canals are affected, dizziness and loss of equilibrium result. If the cochlea is affected, ringing (tinnitus) and other noises in the ears or deafness can result. Conditions that can lead to Meniere's disease include infection, trauma, allergy, and cardiovascular diseases. No permanent cure exists for this disease, but drugs can be used to control the dizziness.

CLINICAL TERMS

ametropia (ah-met-ro′pe-ah) any imperfection in the refraction of light in the eye

blepharitis (blef-ar-i′tis) inflammation of the eyelids

diplopia (dip-lo′pe-ah) seeing double images of single objects

hemianopia (hem″e-an-o′pe-ah) blindness in half the field of vision of one or both eyes

iritis (i-ri′tis) inflammation of the iris

keratitis (ker-at-i′tis) inflammation of the cornea

labyrinthitis (lab″ir-in-thi′tis) inflammation of the labyrinth of the inner ear

mastoiditis (mas-toid-i′tis) inflammation of the antrum and cells of the mastoid process of the temporal bone

nystagmus (nis-tag′mus) an involuntary rapid movement of the eyeball in any direction

otitis media (o-ti'tis me'de-ah)   inflammation of the middle ear

ptosis (to'sis)   drooping of the upper eyelids from nerve or muscle damage

retinitis pigmentosa (ret-in-i'tis pig-men-to'sah) a disorder caused by the inability of choroid cells to remove debris from sensory cells; eventually results in blindness

retinoblastoma (ret''in-o-blas-to'mah)   a tumor derived from retinal cells

tinnitus (tin-i'tis)   ringing in the ears

trachoma (trak-o'mah) an infectious inflammation of the conjunctiva

vertigo (ver'ti-go)   a sensation in which the surroundings appear to revolve around the individual, or the feeling that the individual is revolving in space; not synonymous with dizziness

Essay: Acupuncture

Acupuncture has been in use in China for 4000 years. It is one of two branches of Chinese traditional medicine, the other being herbal medicine. Acupuncturists treat disease and pain by inserting special needles at loci—traditionally located points on the body; the technique itself reportedly does not cause pain. Acupuncture techniques have been known in the Western world since the sixteenth century and have been practiced in France and a few other countries off and on since then, but it is only since the recent improvement of relations with China that acupuncture has come into the limelight in the United States. As a result, several interesting and important questions have been raised concerning acupuncture. Is it a kind of hypnosis? What are acupuncture loci, and can they be objectively observed? Can acupuncture reduce pain and, if so, how? What are the possible clinical applications of acupuncture?

Is Acupuncture Related to Hypnosis?

Because it is difficult to separate the effects of hypnosis and other psychic phenomena from the effects of acupuncture in humans, a tentative answer to this question comes from research on animals. Over 400 abdominal and other surgical operations have been performed on horses and other large animals at the Peking Municipal Veterinary Hospital using acupuncture anesthesia with a reported rate of 95% of those subjected to acupuncture becoming successfully anesthetized. Success rates are lower in humans, but experience in China shows that acupuncture anesthesia was effective in about 80% of more than 1000 cases. Many of these operations have been witnessed by Western observers who confirm the Chinese reports. It would appear from these figures that acupuncture anesthesia is more effective in animals, which are presumably unaffected by hypnosis, than in humans. Because a higher percentage of animals than humans were anesthetized by acupuncture, one might even conclude that psychic factors in humans tend to interfere with acupuncture anesthesia.

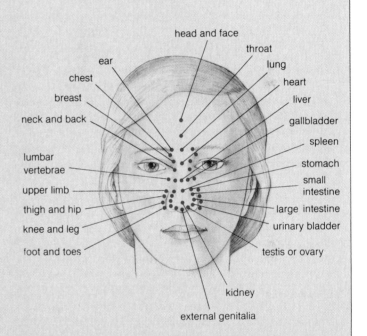

Figure 14.36 The distribution of nose acupuncture points and organs they affect, according to *Acupuncture Anesthesia*, 1975, Department of Health, Education and Welfare Publication No. (NIH) 75–784.

Loci and Meridians

According to tradition, there are certain acupuncture points, or loci, distributed over the surface of the body (365 in number) at which stimulation can be effectively applied to reduce pain or to restore health in corresponding areas. The nose loci are shown in Figure 14.36. Also according to tradition, a set of lines called meridians connect the various loci.

Some of the first evidence for a physical basis for loci and meridians was discovered in the 1950s by a Japanese medical student, Nakatani. After developing a simple technique for measuring electrical resistance on the skin, he located 370 points on the human body surface that have a lower resistance (or a higher electrical conductance) than the surrounding areas. Nakatani went on to locate the most highly conductive points and establish lines connecting them. To his amazement, his map of conductive points and lines corresponded remarkably well with the loci and meridians of acupuncture.

Nakatani also observed that the conductive points were especially conductive when the body was in an unhealthy state. One explanation for this is based on two observations: (1) Most electrical conductance in the body occurs through the pores of the skin, and, (2) when an organ is diseased, stimulation of the sympathetic division of the nervous system causes dilation of the pores in areas where nerve pathways from visceral organs and skin overlap. (This is a phenomenon similar to referred pain.) Nakatani continued his experimentation by injecting various drugs that affect the autonomic nervous system and measuring their effects on skin resistance. He found that resistance was reduced by drugs that stimulated the sympathetic nervous system or that suppressed the parasympathetic system. Conversely, resistance was increased by drugs with opposite actions. Thus, the physical existence of acupuncture loci and meridians appears to have been confirmed and a relationship between electrical resistance and the autonomic nervous system demonstrated.

Other researchers have determined that the number of nerve endings in loci is greater than in surrounding areas, and that many of these points lie over nerve plexuses, or points at which the superficial nerves from each side of the body meet.

Acupuncture and Pain

If acupuncture can produce surgical anesthesia, it is clearly able to reduce pain. How it does so has been the subject of many studies since the mid-1960s. All experimental data collected so far support the idea that the effects of acupuncture are mediated in some way through the nervous system. Placement of electrodes in certain areas of the thalamus of various animals has shown that pain signals are received there and that acupuncture can inhibit the pain discharge waves. Pain signals are also received in the hypothalamus, and these too can be damped by acupuncture. The latter finding further indicates a possible relationship between acupuncture and the autonomic nervous system, which is controlled largely by the hypothalamus.

Studies of pain stimuli and acupuncture stimuli singly and in combination have shed some light on the theory of pain gating. As has been explained earlier, impulses or signals from sensory receptors can vary in frequency. When two signals converge, the signal at the lower frequency will be suppressed. The greater the difference in frequencies, the more complete the suppression of the lower frequency signal. Consequently, the higher the frequency of a pain signal, the more difficult it is to suppress. The fact that predictable effects of the meeting of two signals have been observed supports the gating theory of pain suppression and suggests that a "gate" may be the meeting point of two signals. The observation of several points where signals converge suggests that multiple gates probably exist. It follows that, when acupuncture signals have a higher frequency than pain signals arriving at the same gate, they will suppress the pain signals.

Studies of the concentration of neurotransmitters and hormones during acupuncture suggest that acetylcholine, norepinephrine, epinephrine, and some pituitary hormones may be responsible for the sustained effects of acupuncture stimulation. These chemicals may cause the release of endorphins, which in turn might reduce the effect of pain signals.

Other Effects of Acupuncture—Possible Clinical Uses

In addition to surgical anesthesia and pain relief, acupuncture has other effects. Some studies have shown significant increases in the number of white blood cells several hours after acupuncture, although other studies have shown similar effects after stimulation of points other than the acupuncture points. Case histories in China and animal studies elsewhere have demonstrated that acupuncture can reduce blood pressure. The mechanism by which the pressure is reduced may be by inhibition of the sympathetic nervous system. Recent reports from China indicate that acupuncture is now being used to treat schizophrenia, and that about three-fourths of the patients have shown improvement. Some American physicians are also studying its use in schizophrenia. One possible explanation for the reported effect of acupuncture on schizophrenia is that it reduces the level of input to the reticular activating system and therefore lowers cortical activity.

Acupuncture could be a useful alternative or concurrent form of therapy in many conditions. Unlike drugs used to control pain or treat symptoms, acupuncture apparently has no harmful side effects. In cases where drug sensitivity is present, acupuncture could be a valuable anesthetic or therapeutic agent. Should further research confirm the effects of acupuncture and offer an acceptable explanation of its mechanism of action, it may become more accepted by Western health professionals as a safe anesthetic and a valid form of treatment.

CHAPTER SUMMARY

(Chapter summary points and review questions are numbered to correspond to the numbered objectives in the text of each chapter.)

Organization and General Functions

1. Describe the general properties of sensory receptors; distinguish among exteroceptors, proprioceptors, and visceroceptors, and among the types of stimuli they receive.
- **a.** The general properties of sensory receptors include:
  - **(1)** the ability to convert a specific stimulus into a generator potential
  - **(2)** differential sensitivity to specific kinds of stimuli
  - **(3)** the generation of the same kind of nerve impulses regardless of the nature of the receptor
  - **(4)** varying abilities to adapt to continuous stimuli
- **b.** Receptors may be classified by location as:
  - **(1)** exteroceptors, which detect changes in the external environment
  - **(2)** proprioceptors, which detect changes in muscles, tendons, and joints
  - **(3)** visceroreceptors, which detect changes in internal organs
- **c.** Receptors may be classified according to the type of stimuli to which they respond as:
  - **(1)** chemoreceptors, which respond to chemicals
  - **(2)** mechanoreceptors, which respond to mechanical stimuli
  - **(3)** thermoreceptors, which respond to temperature changes
  - **(4)** photoreceptors, which respond to light
  - **(5)** nociceptors, which respond to tissue damage
- **d.** Regardless of the nature of stimuli and how they are received, all perceptions are the result of the interpretation of patterns of nerve impulses in the cerebral cortex.

Skin Receptors

2. Distinguish among the types of sensory receptors in the skin on the basis of structure, function, and location.
- **a.** Several types of skin receptors exist.
  - **(1)** Free sensory nerve endings in the epidermis are sensitive to pain.
  - **(2)** Meissner's corpuscles in the dermis are responsive to touch.
  - **(3)** Pacinian corpuscles in the dermis are responsive to pressure.
  - **(4)** Krause corpuscles in the dermis and subcutaneous tissues are responsive to cold and extremely warm temperatures.
  - **(5)** Ruffini corpuscles in the dermis and subcutaneous tissues are responsive to moderately warm temperatures.

- **b.** Each receptor, when stimulated, sends signals through specific tracts of the spinal cord to specific sensory areas of the cerebral cortex, where the signals are interpreted.

Proprioceptors

3. Review the structure, function, and location of proprioceptors and explain how stimuli from them are responded to by the central nervous system.
- **a.** Signals from neuromuscular spindles go to the spinal cord, where they directly stimulate a motor neuron, and also stimulate interneurons, which lead to stimulation or inhibition of other motor neurons.
- **b.** Signals from receptors in tendons and joints eventually reach the cerebral cortex, where they help us to perceive position of our limbs.

Pain

4. Describe the qualities of pain, the locations of receptors, and the causes of pain; explain variations in reactions to pain and theories of analgesia.
- **a.** Pain, normally a protective mechanism, can be described as pricking, burning, or aching.
- **b.** Pain receptors are located mostly in the skin but are also found in arteries, joints, and internal organs.
- **c.** Pain is thought to be caused by the release of chemicals from injured tissues, but it is not always felt at the site of the injury because it can be referred.
- **d.** Variations in the response to pain appear to be due to a person's interpretation of it and not to variations in the sensitivity of the receptors.
- **e.** Reactions to pain have been explained by two theories:
  - **(1)** the gating theory
  - **(2)** the endorphin theory

Chemical Senses

5. Compare and contrast the senses of taste and smell in terms of structure, function, and location of receptors, and interpretation of sensations in the brain.
- **a.** Taste receptors:
  - **(1)** are hair cells found in the taste buds
  - **(2)** can detect salt, sweet, sour, or bitter tastes
  - **(3)** require that substances tasted be dissolved in water
  - **(4)** relay signals to cranial nerves and thence to the cerebral cortex

b. Smell receptors:
  (1) are hair cells found in the nasal epithelium
  (2) can detect many different odors, which have been classified into seven categories
  (3) require that substances smelled be dissolved in water
  (4) relay signals via the olfactory nerves to the limbic system and the cerebral cortex

Vision

6. Describe the external and internal structures of the eye and their locations and functions.
  a. The external structures of the eye include:
    (1) eyelids and eyelashes, which are protective structures
    (2) extrinsic eye muscles, which rotate the eyeball and assist in directing the eyes toward specific visual fields
    (3) the lacrimal apparatus, which produces tears, keeps the eyeball moist, and helps to remove foreign matter from the surface of the eyeball
  b. The internal structures of the eye are arranged in three layers:
    (1) The outer tunic consists of the protective sclera and the transparent cornea, which admits and helps to focus light.
    (2) The middle tunic consists of the vascular choroid coat; the ciliary body, which helps to regulate tension on the lens and produces aqueous humor; and the iris, which regulates the amount of light entering the eye.
    (3) The internal tunic consists of the retina, the layer in which the light-sensitive rods and cones are found.
  c. The inside of the eye is divided by the lens, suspensory ligament, and ciliary body into two cavities:
    (1) The anterior cavity, which contains aqueous humor, is separated by the iris into the anterior chamber and the posterior chamber
    (2) The posterior cavity, which contains vitreous humor, helps to maintain the shape of the eyeball
  d. The lens is a transparent structure that can change shape according to the tension placed on it by the ciliary body and the suspensory ligament; it helps to focus light on the retina.
7. Distinguish between black-and-white and color vision in terms of structure, function, and location of receptors.
  a. Black-and-white vision is accomplished by the rods.
    (1) Rods are located in greater numbers in the periphery of the retina.
    (2) Rods are responsive to dim light.
  b. Color vision is accomplished by the cones.
    (1) Cones are located predominantly in the macula lutea and fovea centralis.
    (2) Cones are sensitive to bright light and can detect color.
    (3) Color blindness is due to the genetically determined absence or abnormality of certain pigments in the cones.
  c. Both rods and cones contain light-sensitive pigments that change shape when exposed to light; the change in shape causes chemical reactions that lead to the production of a generator potential.
8. Describe how signals are transmitted from the eye to the brain and how they are interpreted in the brain.
  a. Fibers of the optic nerve travel from the retina to the optic chiasma, where the fibers from the medial retina of each eye cross and go to the opposite side of the brain.
  b. The optic tracts lead to nuclei in the thalamus, from which signals are sent to the primary visual cortex for further processing.
  c. Signals are then relayed to the visual association area, where final interpretation is made.
9. Trace the path of light waves through the eye and explain how they are focused on distant and near objects naturally and with the aid of corrective lenses.
  a. Light is focused as it passes through the surfaces of the cornea and the lens; the lens changes shape to accommodate to distant and near objects.
  b. In an emmetropic eye light is focused sharply on the retina.
  c. In presbyopia the lens has lost some of its power of accommodation; corrective lenses compensate so that both near and distant objects can be seen clearly.
  d. In hypermetropia the eyeball is shorter than normal; corrective lenses cause light rays to converge on the retina instead of behind it.
  e. In myopia the eyeball is longer than normal; corrective lenses cause light rays to diverge and focus on the retina instead of in front of it.
  f. In astigmatism the surfaces of the lens or cornea (or both) are irregular; corrective lenses compensate for the irregularities.
10. Explain how the structure and function of the eye are altered in cataract and in glaucoma; briefly describe how these conditions are treated.
  a. In cataract the lens loses its transparency. Cataract is treated by surgically removing the lens and compensating by the use of external lenses.
  b. In glaucoma pressure inside the eyeball increases, usually because the canal of Schlemm is blocked. Glaucoma is treated by drugs that decrease the amount of fluid in the eye or by surgery that creates a means for fluid to drain from the eye.

Hearing

11. Describe the external and internal structures of the ear that relate to hearing and give their locations and functions.
  a. The ear, or organ of hearing, is divided into the outer, middle, and inner ear.
  b. The outer ear consists of:
    (1) the pinna, which collects sound waves
    (2) the external auditory meatus, a canal through which sound waves pass

(3) the tympanic membrane, a membrane that separates the outer and middle ear and transmits vibrations from the outer to the middle ear

c. The middle ear:
(1) contains the ear ossicles—the malleus, incus, and stapes, which transmit vibrations to the oval window
(2) has openings to the pharynx and inner ear (at the oval and round windows)

d. The inner ear consists of:
(1) a bony labyrinth, the cochlea
(2) a membranous labyrinth filled with endolymph inside the bony one
(3) a space between the labyrinths filled with perilymph

e. The cochlea consists of:
(1) a bony modiolus
(2) the scala vestibuli
(3) the scala tympani
(4) the cochlear duct, which contains the basilar membrane, tectorial membrane, and the organ of Corti, where the receptor cells are located

12. Trace the path of sound waves through the ear and explain how they are transmitted and converted to nerve impulses.
a. Sound waves travel through air in the outer ear, are transmitted across the tympanic membrane to the middle ear ossicles, then across the membrane of the oval window to the fluids of the inner ear.
b. Pressure waves in the fluid of the scala vestibuli cause movement of the basilar membrane, which in turn causes the hair cells of the organ of Corti to move in relation to the tectorial membrane.
c. Movement of the hair cells in relation to the tectorial membrane initiates a nerve impulse in the cochlear portion of the vestibulocochlear nerve.
d. The impulse travels to the auditory portion of the cerebrum, where it is interpreted.

13. Distinguish between conduction deafness and nerve deafness in terms of altered structure and function and method of treatment.
a. Conduction deafness is caused by a defect or obstruction in the outer or middle ear that prevents sound waves from reaching the inner ear. It can be treated by removing the obstruction or by correcting the defect, usually by freeing the ear ossicles to vibrate or by providing a hearing aid that bypasses the obstruction.
b. Nerve deafness results from damage to the organ of Corti or to the nerve fibers. It cannot at present be treated effectively.

14. Describe the qualities of sound and how they are detected in the receptor cells and interpreted in the brain.
a. The qualities of sound are:
(1) pitch, the frequency of sound vibrations, which are detected by specific areas of the organ of Corti
(2) intensity, the loudness in decibels of a sound, which is detected by the organ of Corti according to the frequency of impulses generated
(3) timbre, the pattern of impulses detected by the organ of Corti

b. Sounds are relayed to the brain and interpreted as follows:
(1) Sounds of different pitches are relayed to different sites in the brain.
(2) Loudness is interpreted by the number and frequency of impulses arriving in the brain.
(3) Timbre is interpreted by the pattern of impulses sent from the organ of Corti.

Balance

15. Distinguish between static and dynamic balance, or equilibrium, in terms of the structures involved and their locations and functions.
a. Static equilibrium is detected by hair cells in the macula of the utricle, and possibly the saccule. These cells respond to the force of gravity.
b. Dynamic equilibrium, the response to changes in position of the head, is detected by hair cells in the cristae of the semicircular canals.

16. Describe how sensations from the organs of balance are transmitted to and interpreted in the brain.
a. Impulses from the organs of balance are relayed to the cerebellum, where they stimulate responses that maintain balance and coordination.
b. Impulses from the organs of balance also are relayed to the cerebrum, where they provide information about position and movement of the head.

17. Discuss the causes of and treatments for (a) motion sickness and (b) Meniere's disease.
a. Motion sickness is a temporary disturbance of the interaction between the semicircular canals and visual signals. It can be prevented or alleviated by certain drugs.
b. Meniere's disease is caused by damage to the inner ear and results in dizziness and/or deafness. No permanent cure is available, but drugs can alleviate symptoms.

REVIEW

Important Terms

accommodation
adaptation
anterior cavity
anterior chamber
aqueous humor
astigmatism
binocular vision
canal of Schlemm
cataract
cerumen
chemoreceptor
choroid coat
ciliary body
cochlea
cochlear duct
conduction deafness
cones
conjunctiva
cornea
dynamic equilibrium
ear ossicles
emmetropia
exteroceptor
free sensory nerve endings
generator potential
glaucoma
hypermetropia
iris
ischemia
kinin
Krause corpuscles
lacrimal apparatus
law of specific nerve
energies
lens

mechanoreceptor
Meissner's corpuscles
myopia
nerve deafness
nociceptor
olfactory cells
optic chiasma
organ of Corti
oval window
Pacinian corpuscles
perception
photoreceptor
posterior cavity
posterior chamber
presbyopia
proprioceptor
referred pain
retina
rhodopsin
rods
round window
Ruffini corpuscles
saccule
sclera
semicircular canals
static equilibrium
strabismus
taste cells
thermoreceptor
transduction
translation
tympanic membrane
utricle
visceroceptor
vitreous humor

Questions

1. **a.** What are the properties of a receptor?
    b. How are stimuli classified by the location of a receptor?
    c. How are they classified by the nature of a stimulus?

2. How are sensations from the skin detected and interpreted in the brain?

3. How are sensations from proprioceptors detected and interpreted in the brain?

4. **a.** What are the qualities of pain?
    b. Where are pain receptors located, and how is referred pain produced?
    c. How can individual differences in reaction to pain be explained?

5. **a.** Compare the structure and location of the receptors for taste and smell.
    b. Why does food taste flat when you have a cold?
    c. Which kinds of chemicals are detected by taste cells and which by olfactory cells?
    d. How are impulses from taste cells transmitted to the brain?
    e. How are impulses from olfactory cells transmitted to the brain, and how might there be emotional reactions to smells?

6. **a.** What are the structures that protect the eye?
    b. How do the extrinsic muscles work to move the eyes together?
    c. Name the layers of the eyeball and the structures found in each layer.
    d. What is the function of each of the structures listed in (c)?
    e. Where is the lens located, and what does it do?
    f. Name the cavities of the eyeball, their fluids, and their functions.

7. **a.** Describe the function of the rods.
    b. Describe the function of the cones.

8. **a.** How are sensations transmitted to the brain, and how are they interpreted?
    b. What is the difference between the reception and perception of signals?

9. **a.** Trace the path of light through the eye and explain how an image from a distant object and from a near object is focused on the retina.
    b. What deviation from normal is present in the following conditions, and how is it corrected with lenses? (1) presbyopia, (2) myopia, (3) hypermetropia, and (4) astigmatism.

10. **a.** What is a cataract, and how is it treated?
    b. What is glaucoma, and how is it treated?

11. **a.** Describe the structure of the external ear and tell how it contributes to hearing.
    b. What structures are located in the middle ear, and what do they do?
    c. What structures other than those in (b) are in communication with the middle ear?
    d. What is the structure of the inner ear?

e. What are the parts of the organ of Corti, and where are they located?

12. a. What three media are involved in the transmission of sound waves?

b. How does the effect of a sound wave get from the air outside the pinna to the auditory cortex?

13. a. What is the difference between conduction deafness and nerve deafness?

b. Why should you avoid exposure to sounds over 100 decibels?

14. a. What are the three qualities of sound?

b. Describe what happens in your ears and your auditory cortex when you listen to a symphony orchestra.

15. a. What is the difference between static and dynamic balance?

b. What are otoliths?

c. How is the detection of the force of gravity different from the detection of motion?

16. What is the role of the cerebellum and of the cerebrum in responding to sensory impulses from the organs of balance?

17. Discuss motion sickness and Meniere's disease.

Problems

1. Suppose you have a mild headache but go ahead with your studying. As you get interested in your work, you forget all about your headache. Explain in physiological terms how this might happen.

2. Compare the location of eyeglasses and contact lenses to the focusing structures of the eye and explain why vision can be better corrected in some cases with contact lenses.

3. Some people claim to be tone deaf and say they cannot sing a melody. Using what you know about hearing, perception, and speech, list some kinds of malfunctions that might produce tone deafness.

REFERENCES AND READINGS

Anonymous. 1979. Electric pain control: It's endorphin. *Science News* 115:38 (January 20).

Anonymous. 1979. Sticking it to schizophrenia. *Science News* 115:167 (March 17).

Bahill, A. T., and Stark, L. 1979. The trajectories of saccadic eye movements. *Scientific American* 240(1):108 (January).

Bizzi, E. 1974. The coordination of eye-hand movements. *Scientific American* 231(4):100 (October).

Buchsbaum, M. S. 1978. The sensoristat in the brain. *Psychology Today* 11(12):96 (May).

Cain, W. S. 1979. To know with the nose: Keys to odor identification. *Science* 203:467 (February 2).

Deutsch, D. 1975. Musical illusions. *Scientific American* 233(4):92 (October).

Favreau, O. E., and Corballis, M. C. 1976. Negative aftereffects in visual perception. *Scientific American* 235(6):42 (December).

Geographic Health Studies Program, John E. Fogarty International Center for Advanced Study in the Health Sciences. 1975. *Acupuncture anesthesia*. Washington, D.C.: U.S. Department of Health, Education and Welfare (DHEW Publication No. (NIH) 75-784).

Glickstein, M., and Gibson, A. R. 1976. Visual cells in the pons of the brain. *Scientific American* 235(5):90 (November).

Greenburg, J. 1979. Psyching out pain. *Science News* 115:332 (May 19).

Hess, E. H. 1975. The role of pupil size in communication. *Scientific American* 233(5):110 (November).

Hopson, J. L. 1979. Scent and human behavior: Olfaction or fiction? *Science News* 115:282 (April 28).

Johansson, G. 1975. Visual motion perception. *Scientific American* 232(6):76 (June).

Kanizsa, G. 1976. Subjective contours. *Scientific American* 234(4):48 (April).

Land, E. H. 1977. The retinex theory of color vision. *Scientific American* 237(6):108 (December).

Marx, J. L. 1977. Analgesia: How the body inhibits pain perception. *Science* 195:471 (February 4).

Metelli, F. 1974. The perception of transparency. *Scientific American* 230(4):91 (April).

Miller, J. A. 1978. Vision's brain. *Science News* 114:372 (November 25).

Pert, C. B., and Pert, A. 1976. (D-ala^2)-met-enkephalinamide: A potent, long-lasting synthetic pentapeptide analgesic. *Science* 194:330 (October 17).

Regan, D., Beverley, K., and Cynader, M. 1979. The visual perception of motion in depth. *Scientific American* 241(1):136 (July).

Rushton, W. A. H. 1975. Visual pigments and color blindness. *Scientific American* 232(3):64 (March).

Sekuler, R., and Levinson, E. 1977. The perception of moving targets. *Scientific American* 236(1):60 (January).

Trotter, R. A. 1979. Acupuncture for analgesia and . . . *Science News* 116:296 (October 27).

van Heyningen, R. 1975. What happens to the human lens in cataract. *Scientific American* 233(6):70 (December).

Wei, L. Y. 1979. Scientific advances in acupuncture. *American Journal of Chinese Medicine* 7(1):53.

15

ENDOCRINE SYSTEM

ORGANIZATION AND GENERAL FUNCTION

Objective 1. Describe the location of each of the endocrine glands and their general function as a system.

Objective 2. Explain the mechanisms of action of hormones, including the role of prostaglandins and cyclic nucleotides.

Objective 3. Explain how hormone actions are regulated.

The **endocrine system**, like the nervous system, is involved in communication, control, and integration of body functions. However, the endocrine system acts more slowly than the nervous system. The various endocrine glands synthesize and release chemicals called **hormones** into the bloodstream, and these chemicals can travel great distances to exert their regulatory effects on the cells of the body. Nerve cells also release chemicals, but these chemicals, called neurotransmitters, usually travel only short distances at synapses. The functions of both the endocrine and the nervous systems are closely related, and they work together to maintain homeostasis.

The endocrine system consists of a number of ductless glands located in various parts of the body. These glands are called endocrine glands because they release their secretions directly into blood vessels that run through the glands. (The prefix *endo* means within.) These glands are not to be confused with the exocrine glands, such as the sweat and oil glands of the skin, which release their secretions externally through ducts (see Figure 15.1).

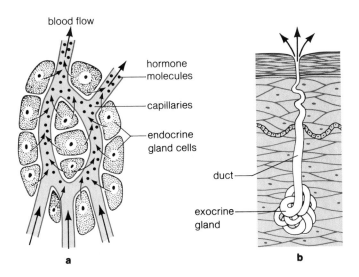

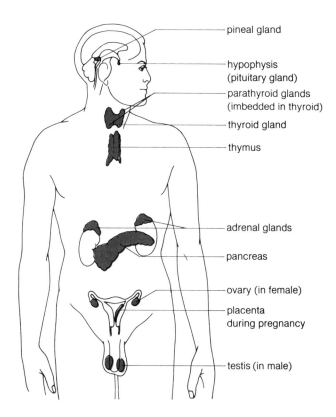

Figure 15.1 (**a**) An endocrine gland releases chemical substances called hormones into the capillaries that run through the gland. (**b**) An exocrine gland releases its secretions through a duct.

Figure 15.2 The glands of the endocrine system are located in various parts of the body.

The glands of the endocrine system (Figure 15.2) include the hypophysis (pituitary), thyroid, parathyroids, adrenals, pancreas, and gonads (or sex glands). The placenta, thymus, kidneys, digestive tract, and pineal gland also function partly as endocrine structures.

The chemical regulation provided by the endocrine system is closely integrated with the regulation by nerve impulses provided by the nervous system. The functions of the endocrine and nervous systems are compared in Table 15.1.

Mechanisms of Action of Hormones

Hormones cause their effects by changing the rate of certain cellular processes. For example, the pancreatic hormone insulin causes most cells (except those in the brain and certain other organs) to increase the rate at which they take glucose from the blood. Thyroid hormones increase the metabolic rate of cells. Hormones are secreted spontaneously, but certain stimuli can increase or decrease the rate

of secretion. Once in the bloodstream, a hormone can reach almost any cell in the body. However, each hormone affects only certain kinds of cells, which make up that hormone's **target organ**. Some hormones have more than one target organ.

How hormones produce their physiological effects is the subject of much current research. Many chemicals besides the hormones themselves have been implicated in hormone action. Furthermore, it is clear that hormones do not all act in the same way. Although many unanswered questions remain, it is possible to describe in a general way the mechanism of action of two major groups of hormones, the steroids and the polypeptide hormones. (Refer to Figures 15.10 and 15.21 for the general structure of these hormones.)

Steroids are relatively small molecules that are synthesized from the chemical precursor cholesterol. They are lipid soluble and easily pass through cell membranes. In nontarget organs steroids pass through the membrane in both directions with equal ease. In target organs steroids dif-

Table 15.1	A Comparison of the Functions of the Endocrine and Nervous Systems	
Characteristic	Endocrine	Nervous
Nature of message	Chemical hormone acting over long distance	Nerve impulse and chemical transmission at synapses
Mode of transmission	Bloodstream	Conduction on neurons and transmission across synapses
Effects	Changes the rate of metabolic activities of affected cells	Changes membrane potential of affected cells; carries sensory and motor signals; is involved in consciousness, learning, memory, emotion, and control of movements
Time for effects to occur	Relatively long	Relatively short
Duration of effects	Relatively prolonged	Relatively brief, except memory storage

On the basis of our understanding of steroid action, new interpretations of some endocrine abnormalities are possible. Instead of being due to excesses or deficiencies of the hormones themselves, some abnormalities may be due to variations in the quantity of receptor molecules available. For example, testicular feminization (a condition in which male secondary sex characteristics fail to develop) may be due to an absence, deficiency, or defect in the receptor protein for the male sex hormone. Similarly, hormone-dependent tumors, such as certain kinds of breast tumors, have estrogen receptor proteins. If these receptors could be rendered nonfunctional by an antihormone (an inactive substance similar to the hormone) binding to the receptors, the hormone might be unable to stimulate the tumor, and it would cease to grow. Finally, the possibility exists that new kinds of contraceptives could be developed that prevent conception by interfering with the receptor proteins for hormones essential to the reproductive process.

fuse into cells but do not leave them. Inside the cells they attach to receptor molecules in the cytoplasm. The presence of these receptor molecules determines which hormone can act on the cell: The cells of the target organ for a particular steroid have specific receptor molecules that combine with the steroid hormone.

When a steroid hormone has entered a cell and formed a complex with a receptor molecule, the complex moves to the nucleus of the cell. The presence of the complex somehow causes receptor molecules to be retained in the nucleus, where they bind directly to the chromosomes. In particular, the receptor molecules bind to the nonhistone proteins of the chromosomes. These proteins appear to have two subunits, one of which binds directly to the DNA and somehow activates a gene. The activated gene synthesizes RNA, and the eventual result is the production of a particular protein inside the cell. This mechanism is summarized in Figure 15.3.

The **polypeptide hormones**, which include insulin and most of the hormones of the pituitary gland, exert their effects by mechanisms quite different from those of ste-

roids. These relatively large molecules exert their effects by binding to receptor sites on the surface of the cells of their target organs. Chemical events are initiated by the presence of the hormone–receptor complex on the cell membrane. Within minutes of the binding of the hormone to the receptor, alterations in the rate at which materials move across membranes may occur due to changes in permeability. Over the next few hours the hormone may cause the activation of enzymes in the cell by first activating cyclic nucleotides or protein kinases.

Role of Cyclic Nucleotides and Protein Kinases

Recent research has shown that many of the physiological effects of hormones (and neurotransmitters) are mediated through the phosphorylation of proteins. Enzymes called protein kinases phosphorylate (add a phosphate group to) the proteins, using energy from ATP. These enzymes, which are of course proteins, are activated by phosphorylation to carry out specific reactions within the cell. The reactions that occur produce the physiological effects of the hormones or neurotransmitters. For example, hormones that cause the breakdown of stored lipids do so by activating an enzyme called hormone-sensitive lipase. Hormones that cause glucose to be released do so by activating an

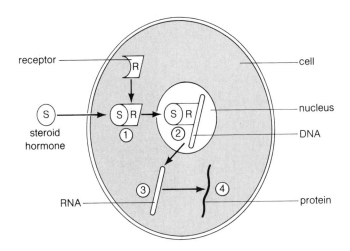

Figure 15.3 The possible action of steroid hormones probably involves (**1**) the formation of a hormone–receptor complex inside the cell, (**2**) the movement of the complex to the nucleus, where it activates a gene, (**3**) the production of RNA, and (**4**) the production of a protein.

enzyme that degrades glycogen. Similarly, some neurotransmitters cause degradation of glycogen. The fact that the effects of both hormones and neurotransmitters are mediated through similar mechanisms provides an interesting example of the close relationship between the two control systems of the body.

How the chemicals (hormones and neurotransmitters) exert their effects to cause the phosphorylation of proteins is still the subject of much current research. Three possible mechanisms are shown in Figure 15.4. Insulin and steroid hormones appear to activate a protein kinase enzyme. Peptide hormones and neurotransmitters such as serotonin, dopamine, epinephrine, and norepinephrine generally activate the enzyme adenylate cyclase. Once activated, this enzyme breaks down ATP and releases cyclic AMP. (Cyclic AMP, a second messenger molecule, was discussed in Chapter 3.) Cyclic AMP activates some protein kinases. Some other neurotransmitters activate the enzyme guanylate cyclase, which catalyzes the conversion of GTP (guanosine triphosphate) to cyclic GMP. Cyclic GMP, another second messenger molecule, activates other protein kinases.

Many observations concerning hormones and their actions can be explained by noting that the different mechanisms for phosphorylation of proteins are sometimes synergistic and sometimes antagonistic. They constitute a complex set of on–off switches that regulate cell function. Furthermore, specific proteins are activated by each hormone or neurotransmitter. When a particular chemical reaches its specific receptor, the complex produced activates the proper enzymes for the formation of a cyclic nucleotide (cyclic AMP or cyclic GMP). It is assumed that these cyclic nucleotides are compartmentalized within cells so that they cause the phosphorylation of the correct proteins. Many cells are the target organs of more than one hormone. Without the chemical specificity a single hormone might conceivably have many effects within a cell. With the specificity it is assured that when one peptide hormone leads to the production of cyclic AMP, the end result is the physiological effect of that hormone and no other.

As we have seen, hormones combine with receptors either on the surface of the cell or inside the cell. It is thought that one way cells react to high concentration of a hormone is to reduce the number of usable receptor molecules. How the receptors become inactive is not fully understood, but it is likely that some surface receptors sink below the surface and that many kinds of surface and internal receptors change their molecular configuration.

Some hormones affect not only the number of their own receptors but also the number of receptors for other hormones. For example, studies of the effect of excess thyroid hormones in rats have shown that the number of receptors for epinephrine in heart cells increases in proportion to the degree of excess of thyroid hormones. This same phenomenon also appears to occur in humans because hyperthyroid patients tend to have higher than normal heart rates. The increased heart rate might be explained by an increased sensitivity of the heart cells to epinephrine.

Prostaglandins

Prostaglandins (Figure 15.5) are a group of closely related substances derived from a twenty-carbon unsaturated fatty acid called arachidonic acid. Prostaglandins behave somewhat like hormones. Because they were first found in semen (which is produced partly by the prostate gland), they were named prostaglandins. However, they have been isolated from most mammalian tissues, and it is likely that they can be synthesized in the membrane of nearly every cell.

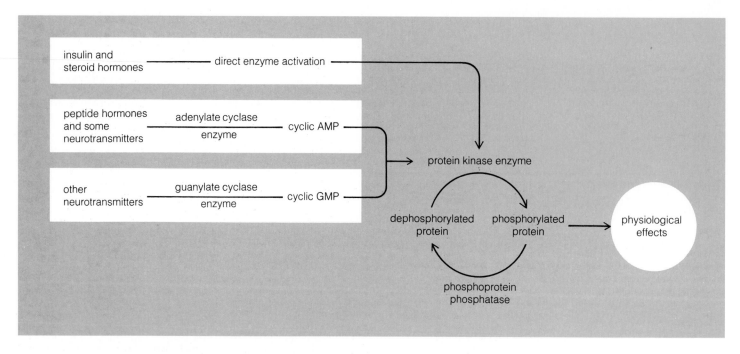

Figure 15.4 A diagram of the possible role of cyclic phosphates and phosphorylated proteins in mediating the effects of hormones and neurotransmitters. The protein kinase enzymes are the key enzymes in the creation of phosphorylated proteins, which are thought to be directly involved in producing the specific physiological effects of each hormone. They can be activated directly or by the production of cyclic AMP or cyclic GMP.

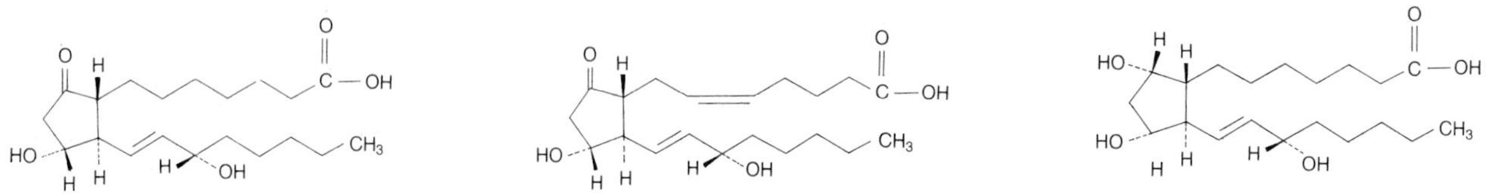

PGE₁

PGE₂

one kind of PGF

Figure 15.5 The chemical structure of some prostaglandins.

When prostaglandin E (PGE) is present in the membrane, the rate of production of cAMP increases. A similar relationship between prostaglandin F (PGF) and cGMP has been reported.

PGE and PGF are antagonistic to each other in controlling cellular functions. For example, when the concentration of PGF and therefore cGMP increases, blood vessels become constricted. When the concentration of PGE and therefore cAMP increase, blood vessels become dilated. In addition, PGE dilates bronchial passages, and PGF constricts them. Thus, the balance between these two types of prostaglandins is important in maintaining homeostasis in many different physiological processes.

Other functions of PGEs are to increase the permeability of blood vessel walls, inhibit the aggregation of blood platelets in blood clotting, act as a sedative, and increase body temperature. It is now thought that the fever-reducing effect of aspirin may be due to its inhibition of PGE synthesis. Both PGEs and PGFs have been shown to contract uterine smooth muscle. In fact, the pregnant uterus is more sensitive to prostaglandins than to oxytocin (a hormone that is involved in labor) during the first two trimesters of pregnancy. Both PGEs and PGFs have been tried as agents to induce abortion. Serious complications often accompany their use during the first trimester, but they seem to be safe and effective during the second trimester and for the induction of labor.

Though the prostaglandins behave like hormones, and in fact have been called "tissue hormones," they do not meet the requirements for true endocrine products for two reasons. First, they are not produced by discrete glands. Second, they are metabolized so rapidly after they are released that they can affect only cells near the site of their production and cannot travel in the blood for any significant distance. The properties that make them dissimilar to hormones make them similar to neurotransmitters. Yet they cannot be classified as neurotransmitters because they are produced by many cells that are not nerve cells, and they do not act across synapses. Prostaglandins appear to be a unique class of regulators, and much remains to be learned about them.

Table 15.2	Embryonic Origin of the Endocrine Glands and the Chemical Nature of Their Secretions	
Gland	Embryonic Origin	Chemical Nature of Secretion
Adenohypophysis	Ectoderm	Proteins or polypeptides
Neurohypophysis	Ectoderm	Polypeptides
Adrenal medulla	Ectoderm	Amines derived from one amino acid
Thyroid	Endoderm	Modified amino acids
Parathyroids	Endoderm	Polypeptides
Pancreas	Endoderm	Proteins or polypeptides
Adrenal cortex	Mesoderm	Steroids
Gonads	Mesoderm	Steroids

DEVELOPMENT

Objective 4. Identify the embryonic germ layer from which each endocrine gland is derived and relate its embryological origin to the chemical nature of its secretions.

Some endocrine glands are derived from each of the embryonic germ layers (see Table 15.2). The formation of the pituitary gland (hypophysis) involves ectoderm from both the floor of the brain and the epithelial roof of the mouth (Figure 15.6). The neural ectoderm becomes the neurohypophysis; the part from the mouth (Rathke's pouch) becomes the adenohypophysis and the intermediate lobe of the pituitary. The intermediate lobe of the pituitary gland releases melanocyte-stimulating hormones. Though these hormones cause the dispersion of pigment granules in cells called melanocytes in fish, amphibians, and reptiles, their function (if any) is unclear in humans. Therefore, the poorly developed intermediate lobe of the human pituitary will receive no further consideration.

The thyroid, parathyroids, and pancreas are derived from pouches in the endodermal lining of the digestive tract and thus originate from endoderm. The adrenal medulla, which originates with the autonomic nervous system from the neural crests, is formed from ectoderm. The adrenal cortex and gonads are formed from mesoderm.

The chemical nature of the secretions of endocrine glands is related to their embryonic origin. With the exception of the thyroid gland, which secretes modified amino acid hormones, all of the glands of endodermal origin secrete hormones that consist of proteins or polypeptides. Glands of ectodermal origin secrete hormones that are proteins, polypeptides, or modified amino acids. Glands of mesodermal origin secrete steroids.

PITUITARY GLAND

Objective 5. Describe the location and structure of the pituitary gland and the source, function, and regulation of each of its hormones.

Objective 6. Summarize the relationship between the pituitary and the brain.

Objective 7. Explain the nature of the malfunction in common pituitary disorders.

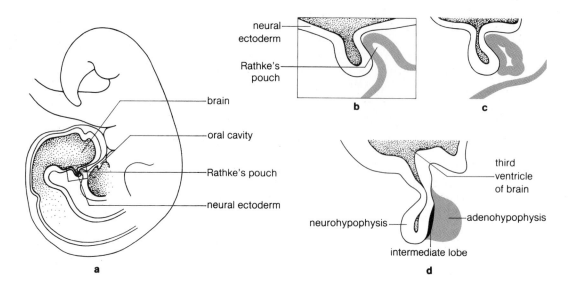

Figure 15.6 The pituitary gland is formed from Rathke's pouch, an ectodermal structure in the roof of the mouth, and neural ectoderm (**a**) and (**b**). Rathke's pouch separates from the mouth and comes to lie adjacent to the neural portion of the pituitary (**c**). The adenohypophysis and the intermediate lobe are derived from Rathke's pouch, and the neurohypophysis is derived from neural ectoderm (**d**).

Location and Structure

The **pituitary gland**, or **hypophysis**, (Figure 15.7) is an organ about 1.2 to 1.5 centimeters in diameter and weighing only about half a gram. Located just inferior to the hypothalamus, the pituitary is protected by the sella turcica of the sphenoid bone. The pituitary gland, as noted in the discussion of development, is really two glands, the **adenohypophysis** and the **neurohypophysis**. Both are closely associated with the hypothalamus, the part of the brain that regulates endocrine function and integrates it with neural function. The neurohypophysis is directly connected to the hypothalamus by the hypothalamic–hypophyseal tract, a nerve tract in the infundibulum, or stalk of the neurohypophysis. The adenohypophysis is closely associated with the hypothalamus by way of the hypothalamic-hypophyseal portal system, veins that carry blood from capillaries in the hypothalamus to capillaries in the adenohypophysis.

The hormones released from the neurohypophysis are manufactured not there, but rather in certain hypothalamic neurons. The hormones move down the axons that make up the nerve tracts and are stored in the terminals of the axons in the neurohypophysis until they are released into the blood. Therefore, the neurohypophysis is a storage area for hormones produced by the hypothalamus. The hypothalamus thus is capable both of conducting impulses and of secreting hormones.

Hormones of the Adenohypophysis

Six distinct hormones of significance in humans are synthesized in the adenohypophysis and secreted from it. A seventh hormone may also be produced there (see Figure 15.8).

Growth hormone Growth hormone (GH), a protein also called somatotropin or somatotropic hormone, stimulates the release of somatomedins, which stimulate the growth of body cells until adult size has been reached and maintain adult size thereafter.

Growth hormone increases the rate at which cells take up amino acids and use them to synthesize proteins. It also stimulates the release of fat from fat cells and the breakdown of glycogen to glucose in the liver. These functions

Growth hormone has been synthesized recently in the laboratory using recombinant DNA. In this technique the gene containing information for the synthesis of the hormone is combined with the DNA of living bacterial cells. The bacterial cells thereby produce growth hormone along with other metabolic products.

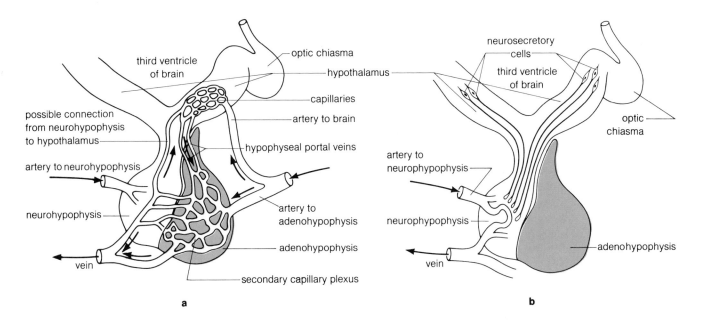

Figure 15.7 The pituitary gland really consists of two glands, the adenohypophysis and the neurohypophysis. It also has (**a**) circulatory and (**b**) neural connections with the hypothalamus. The circulatory connection constitutes the pituitary portal system.

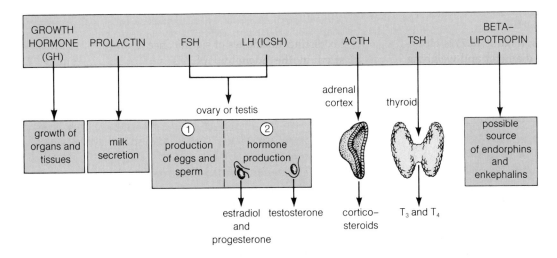

Figure 15.8 The hormones of the adenohypophysis and their effects.

are important in the maintenance of the normal concentration of blood glucose between meals and in response to stress.

Prolactin **Prolactin**, or lactogenic hormone, is also a protein. It stimulates milk secretion in mammary glands that have already been prepared for milk production by other hormones, including estradiol, progesterone, corticosteroids, and insulin. Milk production will be discussed in more detail in Chapter 29.

Follicle-stimulating hormone **Follicle-stimulating hormone** (FSH) stimulates the development of an ovum, or egg, in females each month. It also stimulates cells of the ovaries to produce estrogens. In males this hormone aids in the maturation of sperm. The hormone is a glycoprotein (contains carbohydrate as well as protein).

Luteinizing hormone **Luteinizing hormone** (LH), or **interstitial-cell-stimulating hormone** (ICSH) as it is called in the male, is also involved in regulating the reproductive system. In females it works with estrogens to cause the release of ova from the ovaries and to prepare the uterus for implantation should an ovum be fertilized. This glycoprotein hormone also stimulates the secretion of progesterone by the ovary and the development of the mammary glands in preparation for milk secretion. In males ICSH stimulates the development of the interstitial cells of the testes and causes them to produce testosterone. Both FSH and LH are discussed in more detail in Chapter 28.

Adrenocorticotropic hormone **Adrenocorticotropic hormone** (ACTH) acts on the cortex of the adrenal gland and regulates the production and secretion of several of its hormones, especially the corticosteroids. Corticosteroids in turn stimulate the release of fats and glucose and help the body to resist stress. (The mechanisms of these actions will be discussed in Chapters 23 and 26.) ACTH is a polypeptide containing thirty-nine amino acids in a single chain.

Thyroid-stimulating hormone **Thyroid-stimulating hormone** (TSH), a protein also called thyrotropin, stimulates the thyroid gland to synthesize and secrete its hormones.

Beta-lipotropin Although it has not been proven to have a specific effect in humans, **beta-lipotropin** has been isolated from the pituitary glands of various animals. As mentioned in Chapter 11, the endorphins and enkephalins are specific portions of the beta-lipotropin molecule. It may be that the adenohypophysis is a source of these substances. Some evidence also exists that the synthesis of these substances occurs in the brain itself, so the exact relationship between the adenohypophysis and the brain regarding beta-lipotropin and its components is not yet understood.

Regulation of Hormones of the Adenohypophysis

For each of the established hormones of the adenohypophysis, regulating hormones have been isolated from the hypothalamus, and the chemical structure of some of these hormones has been determined. The actions of the regulating hormones are summarized in Table 15.3. Most of them seem to be small polypeptides produced in neurosecretory cells of the hypothalamus and released into the blood

Table 15.3 Regulating Hormones from the Hypothalamus		
Hormone	Abbreviation	Function
Thyroid-stimulating hormone-releasing hormone	TRH	Stimulate release of TSH
Adrenocorticotropic hormone-releasing hormone	CRH	Stimulate release of ACTH
Follicle-stimulating-hormone-releasing hormone*	FSH-RH	Stimulate release of FSH
Luteinizing-hormone-releasing hormone*	LH-RH	Stimulate release of LH
Growth-hormone-releasing hormone	GH-RH	Stimulate release of GH
Growth-hormone-inhibiting hormone (somatostatin)	GH-IH	Inhibit release of GH
Prolactin-releasing hormone	PRH	Stimulate release of prolactin
Prolactin-inhibiting hormone	PIH	Inhibit release of prolactin

*These two factors—FSH-RH and LH-RH—are now believed to be the same substance, a small peptide molecule that stimulates the release of FSH under some circumstances and LH under other circumstances.

vessels of the hypothalamic–hypophyseal portal system through which they travel to the secretory cells of the adenohypophysis.

What regulates the **releasing** and **inhibiting** hormones is another important issue in understanding the regulation of the function of the adenohypophysis. Both neural impulses and hormonal influences can affect the neurosecretory cells of the hypothalamus. Thus, stress and anxiety can stimulate the hypothalamic cells by increasing neural signals. Hormones circulating through the blood of the hypothalamus can also stimulate the hypothalamic cells. Their effects usually provide negative feedback.

Negative feedback, an important kind of regulatory mechanism discussed in Chapter 1, is an inhibition of a response by the product of that response (Figure 15.9). In some instances the secretions of the hypothalamus are suppressed by negative feedback, but in most instances the secretions of the pituitary gland are affected directly. For example, as shown in Figure 15.9, when the concentration of thyroid hormones in the blood reaches a certain level, they

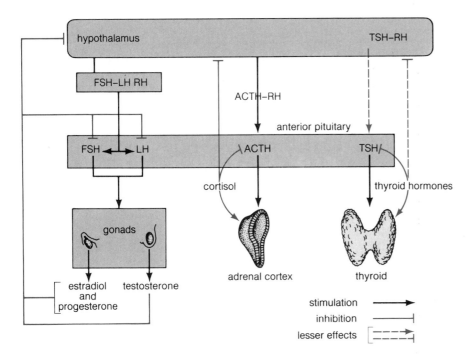

Figure 15.9 Examples of negative feedback in the regulation of the function of the anterior pituitary gland and glands it affects. Feedback into the hypothalamus is most important in the regulation of sex hormones, moderately important in the regulation of the adrenal cortex hormones, and only slightly important in the regulation of the thyroid hormones.

inhibit further secretion of TSH from the pituitary. The decrease in TSH reduces the amount of stimulation received by the thyroid gland and thereby reduces the amount of thyroid hormones released. Thus, the products of the response (thyroid hormones), through their action on the pituitary, inhibit their own further production.

Other examples of negative feedback on the pituitary include inhibition of the release of ACTH by the presence of hormones from the adrenal cortex, inhibition of the release of FSH by the presence of estrogens, and inhibition of the release of LH (ICSH) by the presence of progesterone (testosterone). In fact, all gonadal hormones can inhibit both FSH and LH.

Hormones of the Neurohypophysis

Two hormones are stored in the neurohypophysis—oxytocin and antidiuretic hormone, or vasopressin, both of which are small polypeptides (Figure 15.10). These hormones (or neurosecretions) are released in much the same way as the regulating hormones. After being synthesized in the cell bodies of neurons of the hypothalamus, they travel to the ends of the axons. When released from the axons into the blood, they act directly as hormones. No releasing hormone is involved.

Oxytocin **Oxytocin** stimulates contraction of smooth muscle of the uterus and the contractile cells near the ducts of mammary glands. Suckling and distention of the cervix and vagina stimulate the release of oxytocin. In females it is released in large quantities during sexual intercourse, labor, and lactation. Oxytocin is important in the initiation of labor and in the maintenance of productive uterine contractions during labor. In fact, it is sometimes used to induce or to speed up labor. No function for oxytocin has been identified in males.

Antidiuretic hormone **Antidiuretic hormone** (ADH), also called **vasopressin**, has two functions, one of which is sug-

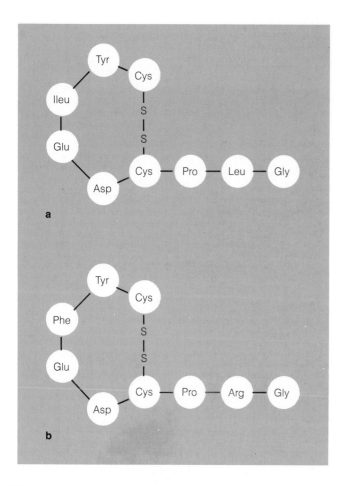

Figure 15.10 The amino acid composition of polypeptide hormones (**a**) oxytocin and (**b**) antidiuretic hormone.

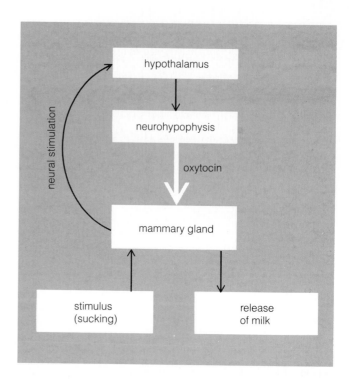

Figure 15.11 A neural-hormonal feedback loop. The sucking of an infant stimulates receptors in the nipple of the mammary gland. Impulses travel to the hypothalamus, where they stimulate the release of oxytocin from the neurohypophysis. Oxytocin travels in the blood to the mammary gland and stimulates the release of milk.

gested by each of its names. It prevents excess loss of water in urine—the antidiuretic effect. It also causes a modest degree of constriction of blood vessels—the vasopressor effect. The mechanisms of these actions are as follows: When the blood becomes concentrated and exerts an increased osmotic pressure, osmoreceptors in the hypothalamus detect this change and stimulate the release of ADH; ADH increases the amount of water returned to the blood by the kidneys. When the blood pressure drops, pressure receptors similarly cause increased release of ADH, and blood vessels constrict.

Regulation of Hormones of the Neurohypophysis

At the beginning of labor oxytocin release is stimulated by nerve impulses from the distended cervix. Before the onset

of labor oxytocin is released, but progesterone renders the uterus unresponsive to it. When, at the end of pregnancy, the progesterone concentration drops, oxytocin is able to exert its effect. During breast feeding the infant's sucking of the nipple causes nerve impulses to be sent to the hypothalamus. These impulses cause oxytocin to be released, and the oxytocin in turn causes milk to be ejected from the mammary gland. The release of milk by the sucking of an infant is an example of a direct neural-hormonal positive feedback loop (Figure 15.11).

The regulation of ADH is accomplished by cells in the hypothalamus, which detect changes in the osmotic pressure of the blood. When these cells detect that the osmotic pressure of the blood is high, they stimulate the release of ADH, thereby causing water to be added to the blood. Pain and stress also can create neural stimuli that cause the release of ADH (see Chapter 25).

Table 15.4 Some Pituitary Disorders

Disorder	Possible Cause	Hormone	Excess or Deficiency	Effects
Pituitary dwarfism	Destruction or congenital deficiency of GH-producing cells	Growth hormone	Deficiency	Small but well-proportioned body; sexual immaturity
Giantism	Pituitary tumor before adult size is reached	Growth hormone	Excess	Large, well-proportioned body
Acromegaly	Pituitary tumor after adult size is reached	Growth hormone	Excess	Disproportionate increase in size of bones of face, hands, and feet
Diabetes insipidus	Damage to the hypothalamus	ADH	Deficiency	Excessive excretion of dilute urine
High blood level of ADH	Excessive stimulation of ADH-secreting neurons or pituitary tumor	ADH	Excess	Excessively dilute blood and low plasma sodium

Pituitary Disorders

Abnormalities in body size often involve excesses or deficiencies in the amount of growth hormone produced. Abnormalities in the amount of ADH produced also lead to certain kinds of disorders in the composition of the blood. Selected pituitary disorders are summarized in Table 15.4. One condition, acromegaly, is illustrated in Figure 15.12.

THYROID GLAND

Objective 8. Describe the location and structure of the thyroid gland and the source, function, and regulation of its hormones.

Objective 9. Explain the nature of the malfunction in common thyroid disorders.

Structure and Location

The **thyroid gland** (Figure 15.13) is located inferior to the thyroid cartilage. The left and right lobes of the gland surround the larynx; the isthmus, which connects the lobes, lies in the anterior midline of the body. The gland is well supplied with blood vessels, which branch from the common carotid arteries and return blood to the internal jugular veins.

The microscopic anatomy of the thyroid gland (Figure 15.14) shows thyroid follicles composed of cuboidal epithelium and filled with a substance called **colloid**. Colloid consists of a protein called thyroglobulin, to which the

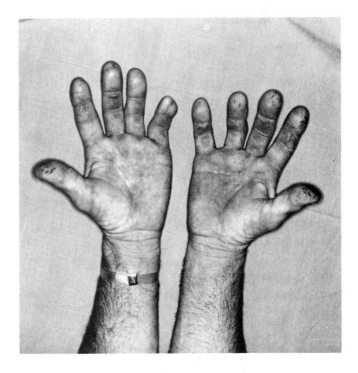

Figure 15.12 The hands of an individual suffering from acromegaly. Notice the unusually thick fingers. (Armed Forces Institute of Pathology negative number 72–14615.)

hormone molecules are attached. The thyroid gland can store enough hormone in the colloid to supply the body for about two months. Some of the cells around the follicles, the parafollicular c-cells, produce calcitonin, a hormone that will be discussed later.

Thyroid Hormones

The thyroid hormones are synthesized from iodine and the amino acid tyrosine. Small amounts of dietary iodine are essential for synthesis to occur. Both **thyroxine** (tetraiodothyronine, or T_4) and **triiodothyronine** (T_3) have hormone activity (Figure 15.15); however, T_3 is the more active of the two. T_4 traveling in the blood is probably converted to T_3 in the target cells. Both hormones are unusual in that they are modified amino acids that are bound to proteins for transport in the blood.

Both T_3 and T_4 regulate metabolism. They increase the rate of oxygen consumption and thus the rate at which carbohydrates are used and proteins are broken down. They also increase the rate at which fats are used. All of these processes increase the rate at which heat is given off, and thus they raise the body temperature. Both hormones also work with growth hormone to help regulate growth, especially of nervous tissue.

Production of T_3 and T_4 is regulated in several ways. Though the hypothalamus plays a role in regulating thyroid

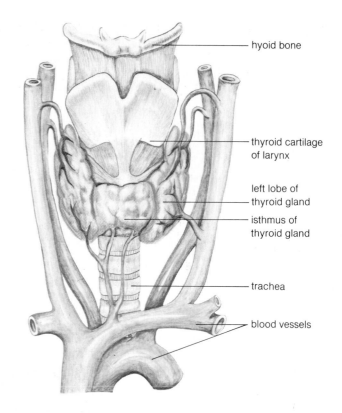

Figure 15.13 The thyroid gland consists of two lobes and an isthmus across the trachea.

Figure 15.14 The microscopic anatomy of the thyroid gland, × 183. (Armed Forces Institute of Pathology negative number 56–5264–738450.)

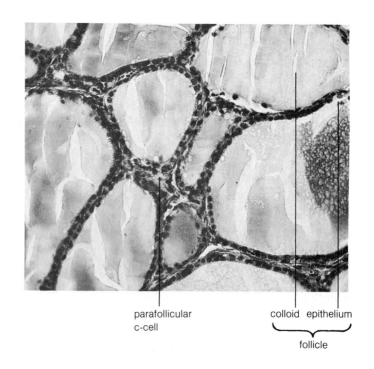

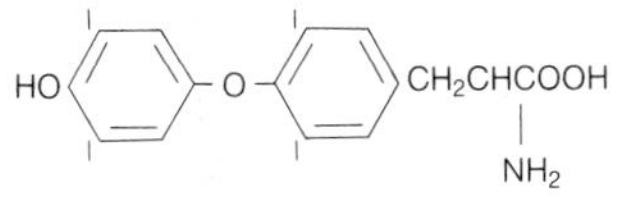

Figure 15.15 The structure of the hormones (**a**) thyroxine (T_4), and (**b**) triiodothyronine (T_3).

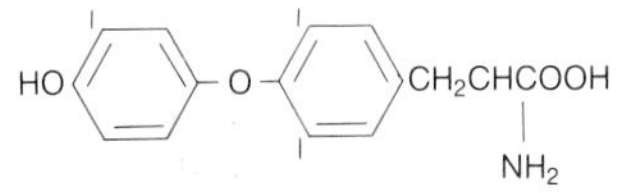

function, the primary regulatory mechanism involves cells in the adenohypophysis that detect the concentrations of T_3 and T_4 in the blood. When they are too low, TSH is released from the adenohypophysis. TSH travels to the thyroid gland and stimulates synthesis and release of T_3 and T_4. When the concentrations of these hormones become elevated, they have a negative feedback effect on the adenohypophysis, and the chain of events leading to release of the hormones is inhibited. (Refer back to Figure 15.9.) Several other factors can influence thyroid activity. For example, pregnancy increases the production of thyroid hormones.

People who live in cold climates have a higher level of thyroid activity than those who live in warm climates. Thus, the body responds to changes in the external environment and regulates thyroid activity (and other functions) to maintain body temperature.

Calcitonin

Calcitonin is secreted from c-cells of the thyroid gland when the calcium concentration in the blood is high, and it stimulates the uptake of calcium by the bones. Because calcitonin works with parathyroid hormone in the regulation of blood calcium it will be discussed along with the discussion of the parathyroids.

Thyroid Disorders

Disorders of the thyroid gland are not uncommon. They may be due to an excess of thyroid hormones (hyperthyroidism) or to a deficiency of them (hypothyroidism). Several tests of thyroid function are available, the most reliable of which is the measurement of the concentrations of T_3 and

T_4 in the blood. The rate at which the thyroid gland manufactures its hormones can be measured by giving a person a dose of radioactive iodine and measuring the radioactivity of the thyroid gland over the next twenty-four hours.

Hypothyroidism can be present at birth or can develop later in life. Hypothyroidism in an infant is called **cretinism;** if not treated, it leads to mental retardation, impaired growth, low body temperature, and abnormal bone formation. The symptoms do not usually appear at birth because the infant has received a supply of thyroid hormones from the mother's blood during development. However, it is necessary to detect the symptoms in the first month of life and begin treatment with thyroid hormones if the infant is to develop normally. Hypothyroidism that develops after growth and development is complete is called **myxedema**. This disorder is characterized by accumulation of fluids in the tissues (edema), a low level of T_3 and T_4 in the blood, sluggishness, mental slowness, and weight gain. The condition can be effectively treated with thyroid hormones.

Simple, or **endemic**, **goiter** is a form of hypothyroidism in which the gland becomes enlarged. It occurs in particular geographic areas in which human diets are deficient in iodine, but it can be prevented by the use of iodized salt. The mechanism for the enlargement of the gland when iodine is lacking is as follows: First, the gland fails to produce sufficient quantities of the hormones because it lacks iodine; second, the pituitary releases excess quantities of TSH because the low blood concentration of thyroid hormones fails to inhibit it; and finally, the gland enlarges under the stimulation of TSH. It is as if the gland were increasing in size so as to produce more of its hormones.

Several different forms of **hyperthyroidism** exist; two will be discussed here. **Graves' disease** (Figure 15.16a) is characterized by weight loss, slightly elevated body temperature, excitability, exophthalmia (protrusion of eyeballs because of fluid accumulation behind them), and diffuse goiter. In this disease a substance called long-acting thyroid stimulator (LATS) is produced, probably through an autoimmune reaction (see Chapter 20). LATS causes many follicles within the gland to release excess T_3 and T_4; this widespread effect on the gland constitutes the diffuse goiter. **Toxic goiter** (Figure 15.16b) differs from Graves' disease in that, though LATS is not produced, isolated areas (nodules) within the gland release excess T_3 and T_4 in spite of any regulatory mechanism that would normally prevent them from releasing the hormones. Hyperthyroidism can be treated by the use of drugs that antagonize the formation of thyroid hormones, by surgical removal of part of the gland, or by administration of a sufficient quantity of radioactive iodine to destroy some of the gland cells.

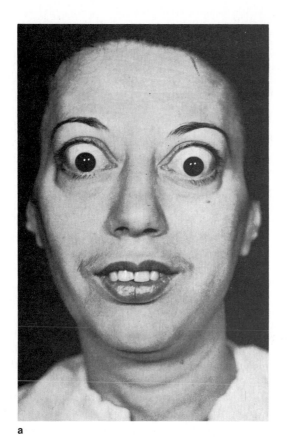

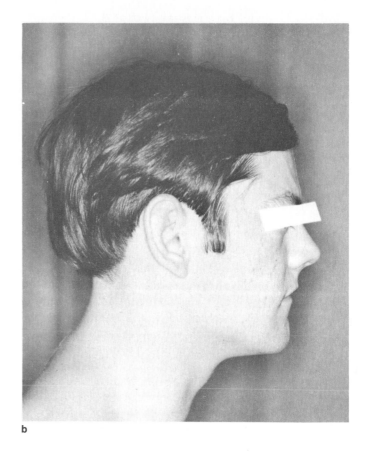

a

b

Figure 15.16 Hyperthyroid conditions: (**a**) An individual suffering from Graves' disease. (Reproduced with permission from Robbins, S. L., and Cotran, R. S., 1979. *Pathological Basis of Disease*. Philadelphia: W. B. Saunders.) (**b**) An individual with a goiter caused by hyperthyroidism. (Armed Forces Institute of Pathology negative number 72–14994.)

PARATHYROID GLANDS

Objective 10. Describe the location and structure of the parathyroid glands and the source, function, and regulation of their hormone.

Objective 11. Explain the nature of the malfunction in parathyroid disorders.

Location and Structure

The **parathyroid** glands (Figure 15.17) consist of at least four separate glands located on the posterior surface of the lobes of the thyroid gland. Each of these groups of cells is encapsulated with connective tissue and measures approximately 6 × 3 × 1 millimeters. Internally, the glands consist of densely packed cords of epithelial cells well supplied with

blood vessels. The epithelial cells synthesize and secrete parathyroid hormone.

Parathormone

Parathormone, or parathyroid hormone (PTH), is the hormone produced by the parathyroid glands. It is a large polypeptide hormone that helps to regulate the metabolism of calcium and certain other minerals. It does not seem to be regulated by the pituitary gland.

With respect to calcium metabolism parathormone and calcitonin have antagonistic effects. It is their combined actions, along with vitamin D action, that maintain homeostasis with respect to calcium. As shown in Figure 15.18, when the calcium level in the blood drops, the parathyroid releases parathormone. Parathormone increases the rate of

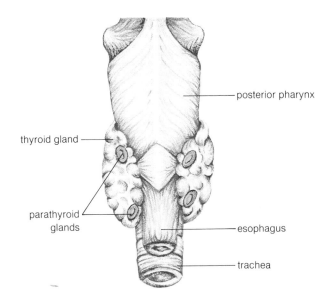

thyroid gland —

parathyroid
glands

— posterior pharynx

— esophagus

— trachea

Figure 15.17 The parathyroid glands lie on the posterior surface of the thyroid gland.

calcium absorption from the intestine, decreases the rate of calcium excretion from the kidneys, and causes calcium to be taken from the bones and returned to the blood. All of these effects increase the amount of calcium in the blood. When the calcium level in the blood reaches a high level, the calcium has two effects. It provides negative feedback to the parathyroid glands and causes a decrease in the secretion of parathormone. At the same time, it stimulates the thyroid gland to secrete calcitonin. Calcitonin causes calcium to be absorbed in smaller amounts, excreted in larger amounts, and moved from the blood to the bones, thus reducing the amount of calcium in the blood. The combined effects of these two hormones normally maintain the blood calcium level within a narrow range.

Parathormone also decreases the phosphate level in the blood by stimulating the kidneys to eliminate phosphate in the urine. In addition, it increases the absorption of both phosphates and magnesium from the intestinal tract, and it stimulates the osteoclasts (bone-destroying cells) to break down bone and release both calcium and phosphates. Osteoclasts are especially quick to respond to small quantities of parathormone and destroy bone. Because the action of parathormone in causing the excretion of phosphates is greater than its action in bringing it into the blood, the net

effect of the hormone is to increase calcium and decrease phosphate in the blood.

The actions of parathormone and vitamin D are intimately associated. Parathormone enhances calcium absorption from the intestine indirectly by its action on vitamin D, stimulating the kidneys to convert one form of vitamin D (D_3) to another form (1,25-dihydroxycholecalciferol). The latter form acts to increase the absorption of calcium from the intestine.

Curiously, vitamin D seems to be able to cause calcification in some circumstances and bone destruction in others. Which action it has depends on the amount of calcium available and a variety of other factors. When individuals are given large doses of vitamin D, large amounts of bone are destroyed. Doses of parathormone also stimulate bone destruction, but in the absence of vitamin D the parathormone causes far less bone destruction. Though the exact mechanisms of action of parathormone and vitamin D are not known, it is clear that they interact to regulate bone resorption. The action of vitamin D in promoting the calcification of bone seems to be that it increases the concentration of calcium in extracellular fluids.

Parathyroid Disorders

Hypoparathyroidism, due to a deficiency of parathormone, may be caused by injury to the glands or their surgical removal, sometimes in conjunction with thyroid surgery. The primary effect of hypoparathyroidism is the lowering of the blood calcium level. This lowering of calcium lowers the threshold and causes neurons to depolarize more easily and the number of nerve impulses to increase. Muscle twitches and spasms result, producing the clinical picture of **tetany**. If the muscles of respiration are affected, death by suffocation can result.

Hyperparathyroidism, due to an excess of parathormone, is usually caused by a tumor of the parathyroids. Since one of the effects of parathormone is the breakdown of bone, when an excess of the hormone is present, bones become soft and some of the bone substance is replaced by fibrous connective tissue. An excess of parathormone also causes calcium to be deposited in the kidneys. Analyses of the content of kidney stones sometimes suggests the presence of a parathyroid tumor.

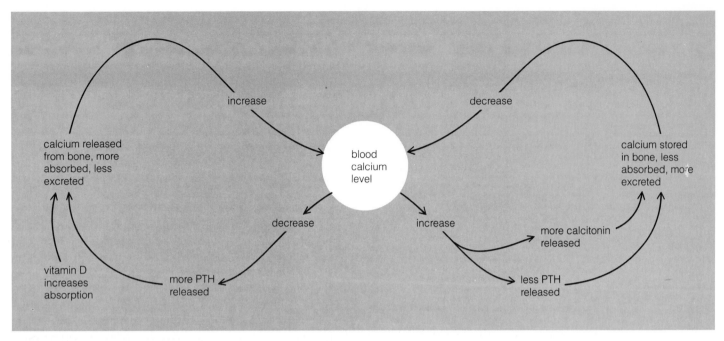

Figure 15.18 Blood calcium concentration is regulated by the effects of parathormone (PTH), calcitonin, and vitamin D.

ADRENAL GLANDS

Objective 12. Describe the location and structure of the adrenal glands and the source, function, and regulation of their hormones.

Objective 13. Explain the nature of the malfunction in adrenal disorders.

Location and Structure

The adrenal glands are paired structures located superior to the kidneys (Figure 15.19). Each gland, which measures about 5 × 3 × 1 centimeters, consists of an inner medulla and an outer cortex. As noted in the discussion of development, these parts of the adrenal gland are derived from two different embryonic sources. In fact, they are really two separate glands that happen to be in close physical association.

The **adrenal medulla** (Figure 15.20a) consists of chromaffin cells derived from the neural crest and directly responsive to stimulation by preganglionic sympathetic fibers of the autonomic nervous system. These cells are surrounded by venous sinuses into which the hormones are released. The hormones travel quickly through the blood to target organs.

The **adrenal cortex** (Figure 15.20b) consists of three distinct layers of cells surrounded by a fibrous capsule, all of which are derived from mesoderm. From the capsule inward, the layers are the **zona glomerulosa**, the **zona fasciculata**, and the **zona reticularis**. Each layer has distinct cell types that secrete particular hormones. Cells in the glomerulosa produce hormones called mineralocorticoids; cells in both the fasciculata and the reticularis produce glucocorticoids or sex hormones.

Hormones of the Adrenal Medulla

The hormones of the adrenal medulla are **epinephrine** (adrenalin) and **norepinephrine** (noradrenalin). Epinephrine and norepinephrine are the preferred terms in the United States. Epinephrine, which makes up about four-fifths of the medulla's secretions, is made in the gland by the addition of a methyl group to norephinephrine. The functions and regulation of these hormones has been discussed in Chapter 13. Although the action of the hormones is of greater duration than neural stimulation, it is limited to no more than three minutes after their release into the blood—the length of time it takes for the hormones to be inactivated by enzymes in the liver and other tissues.

No known endocrine disorders exist that can be traced directly to a deficiency of hormones from the medulla, but

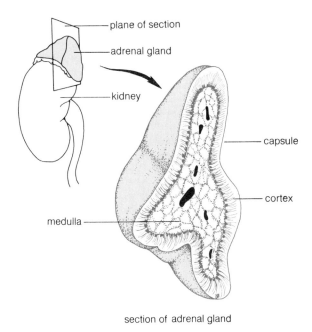

plane of section

adrenal gland

kidney

capsule

cortex

medulla

section of adrenal gland

Figure 15.19 Each adrenal gland is located superior to the kidney and is composed of a cortex and a medulla.

medullary tumors sometimes cause excess secretion. The symptoms are the same as those for excessive sympathetic activity, and treatment usually involves removing the tumor.

Hormones of the Adrenal Cortex

Mineralocorticoids **Mineralocorticoids**, as the name implies, are responsible for the regulation of mineral metabolism. The mineralocorticoid of major importance in humans is **aldosterone** (Figure 15.21a). Like all of the hormones of the adrenal cortex, aldosterone is a steroid. Its primary function is to regulate the sodium content of the body. As shown in Figure 15.22, aldosterone is secreted when the sodium level is low. It acts on the kidneys to cause more sodium to be returned to the blood and more potassium to be excreted. As the sodium concentration in the blood increases, water follows it by osmosis, so the blood volume also increases. Consequently, the effect of aldosterone is to increase both sodium and water in the blood. Other mechanisms involved in fluid regulation will be explained in Chapter 25.

Glucocorticoids As their name suggests, **glucocorticoids** affect carbohydrate metabolism; however, they also affect

the metabolism of proteins and fats. The glucocorticoid with the greatest activity is cortisol (Figure 15.21b). **Cortisol** stimulates the liver to synthesize carbohydrates from non-carbohydrates such as amino acids and glycerol. Thus, it helps to regulate the concentration of glucose in the blood, protecting against low blood sugar between meals. Cortisol also stimulates the degradation of proteins within cells and causes the concentration of amino acids in the blood to increase. A third effect of cortisol is to stimulate the breakdown of fats in adipose tissue and release fatty acids into the blood. The increase in fatty acids causes many cells to use relatively less glucose. Though the mechanism by which it acts is not well understood, cortisol also counteracts some of the effects of inflammation. When tissue is inflamed, the permeability of the capillaries increases, and fluids accumulate in the spaces between the cells. Lysosomes also may release enzymes from injured cells. Cortisol seems to counteract these changes, perhaps by reducing the permeability of capillaries and making the lysosomal membranes more stable. Cortisol is also concerned in the body's response to stress, but this topic will be discussed in Chapter 26.

Androgens Sex hormones that resemble testosterone (Figure 15.21c) or estradiol are released from the inner two layers of the adrenal cortex. Larger quantities of male than female hormones are produced. These male hormones, called **androgens**, are important in the development of a male fetus. Though the genetic sex is determined by the chromosomes in a fertilized egg, a male fetus will develop normal male characteristics only if the fetal gonads and adrenal glands produce sufficient quantities of androgens.

Regulation of Hormones of the Adrenal Cortex

The production of aldosterone from the glomerulosa appears to be controlled by the concentration of potassium in the blood, by renin from the kidney, and by a peptide in the blood called angiotensin. The details of the regulation of aldosterone will be discussed in Chapter 25.

The other two layers of the adrenal cortex are controlled by ACTH, as described earlier in this chapter (see Table 15.3). Mainly cortisol, but other glucocorticoids as well as the sex hormones, exert negative feedback on the anterior pituitary and the hypothalamus to regulate the activity of these parts of the adrenal cortex.

Disorders of the Adrenal Cortex

Deficiencies of either aldosterone or cortisol are known, and sometimes both occur together. **Addison's disease** (Fig-

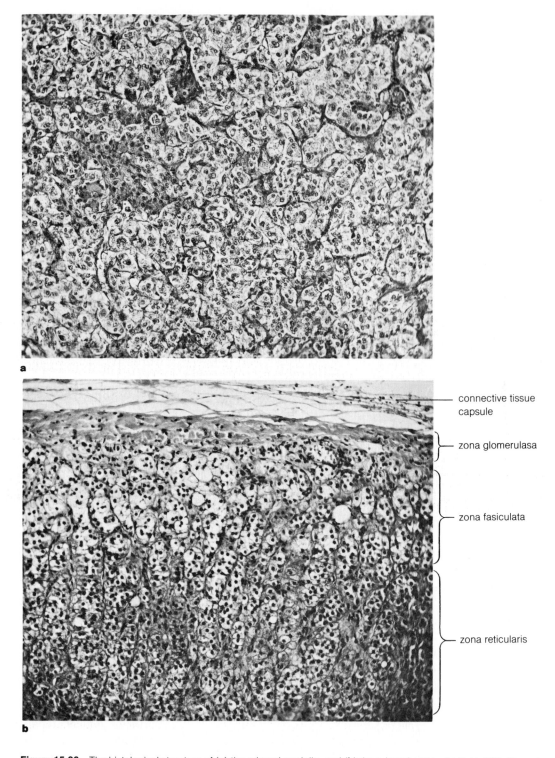

Figure 15.20 The histological structure of (**a**) the adrenal medulla, and (**b**) the adrenal cortex, both × 125. (Armed Forces Institute of Pathology negative numbers 525470-53-7472 (**a**) and 525470-53-7473 (**b**).

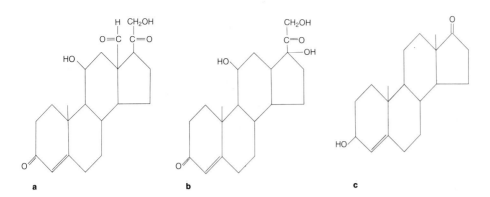

Figure 15.21 Some steroid hormones of the adrenal cortex: (**a**) aldosterone, (**b**) cortisol, (**c**) an androgen.

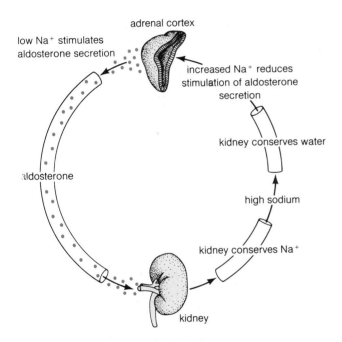

Figure 15.22 Aldosterone regulates the sodium and water in body fluids.

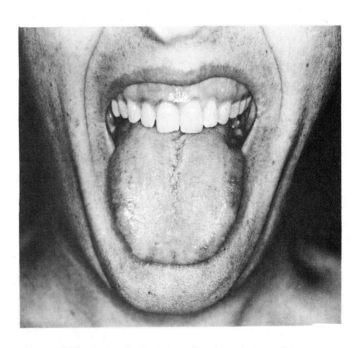

Figure 15.23 Spots of pigment on the skin, gums, and tongue are characteristic of an individual suffering from Addison's disease. (Armed Forces Institute of Pathology negative number 70–13320.)

ure 15.23) results from a loss of function of all three zones of the adrenal cortex. The lack of glucocorticoids leads to anemia, muscular weakness, and fatigue. Sometimes the concentration of potassium in the blood is above normal and the concentration of sodium below normal, so mineralocorticoids as well as glucocorticoids are affected. In the absence of the negative feedback of cortisol, the pituitary secretes excess amounts of ACTH. Because ACTH also

stimulates melanocytes to produce pigment, a bronzing of the skin independent of sun exposure is often a symptom of Addison's disease.

Excesses of all the types of adrenocortical hormones are known; most have been found to be caused by a tumor of the cortex that may affect more than one layer of cells. **Hyperaldosteronism** leads to excess sodium in the blood and depletion of potassium from the blood. As fluid accumulates in the tissues, hypertension, or high blood pressure, develops. **Cushing's syndrome** (Figure 15.24) is due to an excess of cortisol and leads to such symptoms as obesity, particularly in the trunk, and a moon-shaped face. Diabetes often occurs with this disease. The **adrenogenital syndrome** is marked by an excess of androgens. It varies in its effects, depending on the age and sex of the affected individual. For example, prepubertal females may have abnormalities of the genitals, especially partially formed male structures. Adult females will develop masculine characteristics— deeper voice, a beard, and enlargement of the clitoris (a structure homologous to the penis). Prepubertal males may undergo precocious sexual development, with enlargement of the penis and other sexual characteristics early in childhood. Adult males may have undiagnosed adrenal tumors because their bodies are already masculine and the masculinizing effects of the tumor go unnoticed.

PANCREAS

Objective 14. Describe the location and structure of the pancreas and the source, function, and regulation of its hormones.

Objective 15. Explain the nature of the malfunction in pancreatic disorders.

Location and Structure

The **pancreas** (Figure 15.25) lies inferior to the stomach in a bend of the duodenum, as shown in Figure 15.2. It is both an exocrine and an endocrine gland. A large pancreatic duct runs through the gland, carrying enzymes and other exocrine digestive secretions from the pancreatic acinar cells to the small intestine. The tissue of the pancreas has, in addition to the acinar cells, groups of cells called **islets of Langerhans**, which produce endocrine secretions (Figure 15.26). Four kinds of cells have been identified in the islets: (1) A-cells, which produce glucagon; (2) B-cells, which produce insulin; (3) D-cells, which produce somatostatin, a growth-hormone-inhibiting hormone and (4) F-cells, which produce pancreatic polypeptide (PP). About three-fourths of the cells of the islets are B-cells.

Hormones of the Pancreas

Glucagon **Glucagon** is a polypeptide that stimulates the release of glucose and elevates the blood sugar level. It acts

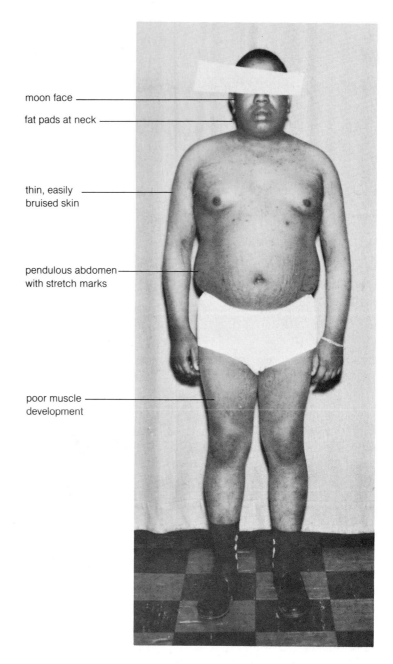

moon face ——

fat pads at neck ——

thin, easily bruised skin ——

pendulous abdomen —— with stretch marks

poor muscle development ——

Figure 15.24 Typical symptoms of Cushing's syndrome. (Armed Forces Institute of Pathology negative number 63–9617.)

by stimulating the liver to convert stored glycogen into glucose. Glucagon is controlled by feedback in accordance with the level of glucose in the blood: When the blood sugar rises, the secretion of glucagon is suppressed; when it drops, the secretion of glucagon is stimulated.

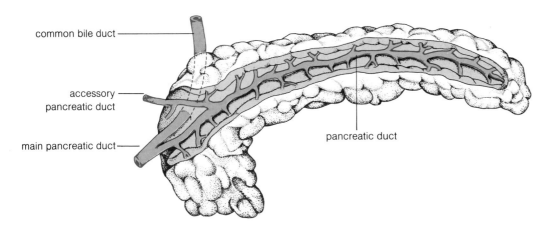

common bile duct

accessory pancreatic duct

main pancreatic duct

pancreatic duct

Figure 15.25   Gross anatomy of the pancreas.

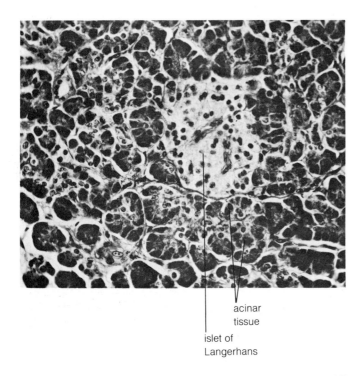

acinar tissue

islet of Langerhans

Figure 15.26   Microscopic anatomy of the pancreas, × 206. (Armed Forces Institute of Pathology negative number 71–9195.)

Insulin   **Insulin** is a polypeptide whose action is antagonistic to that of glucagon. Insulin decreases the level of glucose in the blood. It acts by increasing the rate at which glucose is transported out of the blood and into cells and by stimulating muscle cells to take up sugar from the blood and convert it to glycogen. Like glucagon, insulin is primarily regulated by feedback from the blood glucose concentration. When the blood sugar level drops, the secretion of insulin is suppressed; when the blood sugar level increases, the secretion of insulin is stimulated.

Complexity of blood sugar regulation The interaction of insulin and glucagon in regulating blood glucose is shown in Figure 15.27. However, these hormones are only two of many that are involved in regulating blood glucose level. For example, growth hormone, epinephrine, and cortisol all increase the blood glucose level and thereby stimulate the production of insulin. Somatostatin inhibits the secretion of both insulin and glucagon. These are but a few examples of the components of the complex process by which blood glucose is regulated. The process is discussed in more detail, along with carbohydrate metabolism, in Chapter 23.

Other hormones of the pancreas Both somatostatin and pancreatic polypeptide are relatively newly discovered hormones of the pancreas, and both are still being studied. Biochemically, both are polypeptides. It now appears that pancreatic polypeptide inhibits the release of digestive secretions of the pancreas. **Somatostatin**, the same substance as growth-hormone-inhibiting hormone from the hypothalamus, is produced not only by the pancreas and hypothalamus but also by some cells of the digestive tract. One of the actions of somatostatin seems to be to suppress the release of other hormones from the pancreas. It also appears to suppress the release of hormones from the digestive tract. These hormones, which include substances such as gastrin, will be discussed briefly later in this chapter and in more detail in Chapter 22. A third effect of somatostatin is to reduce the rate at which triglycerides are absorbed from the intestine after a fatty meal.

Disorders of the Pancreas

By far the most common endocrine disorder of the pancreas is **diabetes mellitus**, now recognized to exist in two forms: insulin-dependent and non-insulin-dependent. The insulin-dependent form is caused by a failure of the B-cells to produce adequate amounts of insulin; the non-insulin-dependent form appears to involve failure of insulin to facilitate the movement of glucose into cells. In both disorders the blood glucose concentration is elevated above the normal range of 80 to 100 milligrams per 100 milliliters of blood to 300 or more milligrams per 100 milliliters of blood. Some of the glucose is excreted in the urine, and water follows the glucose, causing excessive urination and dehydration of body tissues. Because fat instead of glucose is metabolized, acidic products of fat metabolism accumulate in the blood. Insulin-dependent diabetes is the more severe form of the disease: It appears earlier in life than the other form and requires insulin for treatment. Non-insulin-dependent diabetes appears relatively late in life and can

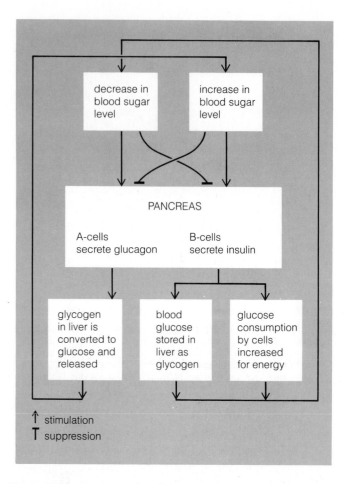

Figure 15.27 Glucagon and insulin help to regulate the blood glucose concentration, and the blood glucose concentration in turn feeds back to regulate the secretion of glucagon and insulin.

often be controlled by limiting carbohydrate in the diet or by the use of oral hypoglycemics (drugs that apparently stimulate the action of insulin.) A tendency toward non-insulin-dependent diabetes appears to be inherited as an autosomal recessive characteristic (see Chapter 27). Diabetes mellitus is discussed in more detail in Chapter 24.

Hypoglycemia occurs when the blood glucose level falls below normal. Theoretically, it may be caused by an excess of insulin, a deficiency of glucagon, or a failure of the secretion of the two hormones to completely regulate the blood sugar. Some individuals have been found to have few or no A-cells and thus are deficient in glucagon, whereas others produce excess quantities of insulin usually because of a tumor of the B-cells. The presence of excess insulin is more correctly referred to as hyperinsulinism. By far the greatest number of individuals who are bothered by mild symptoms of hypoglycemia probably have a slight irregularity in the way insulin, glucagon, or perhaps other hormones function to regulate the blood glucose concentration.

> The symptoms of hypoglycemia include weakness, tremors, a cold sweat, headache, and dizziness. They can be as mild as what everyone experiences after not eating for several hours or severe enough to cause bizarre behavior and even coma. The most common treatment for mild to moderate hypoglycemia is a high-protein, low-sugar diet consumed in numerous small meals each day. Hypoglycemia is sometimes a sign of an early stage of diabetes mellitus, as the pancreas becomes erratic in its insulin production.

GONADS

Objective 16. For each of the gonads name the hormones they secrete and give the major function of each hormone.

The gonads are the sex glands, the ovaries and the testes. They produce ova and sperm and also secrete hormones. In the female the **ovaries** are located in the pelvic cavity in close proximity to the oviducts and the uterus. The hormones produced by the ovaries include estradiol, progesterone, and relaxin. **Estradiol** stimulates the development of female secondary sex characteristics during puberty and maintains them through the reproductive years of adult life. It also stimulates maturation of ova (in the ovaries) and development of the uterine lining and the mammary glands. **Progesterone** stimulates further development of the uterine lining and mammary glands. It is also required for the formation of the placenta and for the maintenance of pregnancy. Both estradiol and progesterone are required for ovulation. **Relaxin**, secreted only during the later stages of pregnancy, helps soften ligaments, especially those that hold the pubic symphysis together. It may also affect other ligaments; if it affects a woman's foot ligaments, she may experience an increase in shoe size following a pregnancy.

In the male the **testes**, located in the scrotum, secrete the hormone **testosterone**, which is necessary for the development of male secondary sex characteristics and for their maintenance throughout reproductive life. It is also an extremely potent growth hormone.

The details of how these hormones act and how they are regulated will be discussed in Chapter 28.

OTHER ENDOCRINE STRUCTURES

Objective 17. Describe the location, structure, and endocrine activity of each of the following: (a) placenta, (b) thymus, and (c) pineal gland.

Objective 18. Give examples of hormones from the digestive tract and other sources.

Placenta

During pregnancy the placenta provides for the exchange of nutrients and wastes between the mother and the developing fetus. It also has some endocrine functions. Five hormones have been isolated from it: estradiol, progesterone, **human chorionic gonadotropin** (HCG), **chorionic growth-hormone-prolactin**, and a hormone with a **thyroid-stimulating** activity. Estradiol and progesterone have the same roles as in the nonpregnant state, and progesterone also helps to maintain pregnancy. HCG stimulates the ovary to continue its production of these hormones; it is also the hormone on which most pregnancy tests are based. The other hormones listed above have effects similar to their counterparts in the pituitary gland. The placenta will be discussed in more detail in Chapters 28 and 29.

Thymus

The **thymus** gland is located beneath the sternum and between the lungs. Although it will be discussed in more detail in Chapter 20, it is mentioned here because it does appear to have an endocrine function. Its hormone, **thymosin**, stimulates the development of certain kinds of white blood cells involved in producing immunity.

Pineal Gland

The **pineal gland** is located between the cerebral hemispheres, where it protrudes from the roof of the third ventricle. It consists of **pineal cells** and supporting glial cells. Though the function of the gland is still the subject of current research, it is known to secrete one hormone, **melatonin**. Melatonin concentration in the blood appears to follow a diurnal (day–night) cycle as it rises in the evening and through the night and drops to a low around noon.

Serotonin, a neurotransmitter found in other locations in the brain, is also found in the pineal gland.

Research evidence is accumulating to support the idea that the pineal gland may be involved in regulating cyclic phenomena in the body. This topic is considered in the essay on biorhythms later in this chapter.

Hormones from Other Sources

Traditionally, the term hormone was used to describe chemical secretions from discrete endocrine glands, but over the years chemicals from other sources have been found to have regulatory effects. **Renin**, a hormone (actually an enzyme) produced by certain cells of the kidney, helps to regulate blood pressure, as described in Chapter 25. Another substance from the kidney, renal erythropoietic factor, activates the blood protein **erythropoietin**, which stimulates the production of erythrocytes, as described in Chapter 16. Certain cells of the lining of the digestive tract produce hormones such as **gastrin**, **secretin**, and **cholecystokinin**, as described in Chapter 22. Prostaglandins, described earlier in this chapter, might also be called hormones because they do have regulatory effects. They are produced by many kinds of cells. Finally, carbon dioxide, produced by all cells as a by-product of metabolism, travels in the blood to sensors in the medulla and hypothalamus and helps to regulate respiration. It is not truly a hormone, but it can have a hormonelike action.

The functions of the endocrine system are summarized in Table 15.5.

Table 15.5 Summary of Endocrine Functions

Gland	Hormones	Target Organs	Major Effects	Negative Feedback	Disorders
Adenohypophysis	Growth hormone (somatotropin)	Cells	Growth, maintenance of adult size, protein synthesis, release of fats and glucose		Dwarfism, giantism, acromegaly.
	Prolactin	Mammary glands	Milk secretions		
	Follicle-stimulating hormone	Ovary	Maturation of ovum and production of estrogen in female	Estrogen	
		Testes	Maturation of sperm in male		
	Luteinizing hormone (interstitial-cell-stimulating hormone)	Ovary	Release of ova	Progesterone	
		Uterus	Prepare for implantation		
		Mammary glands	Prepare for milk secretion		
			Development of interstitial cells and production of testosterone	Testosterone	
	Adrenocorticotropic hormone	Adrenal cortex	Release of hormones from adrenal cortex	Cortisol	
	Thyroid-stimulating hormone	Thyroid gland	Synthesis and release of thyroid hormones	Thyroid hormones	
Neurohypophysis	Oxytocin	Smooth muscle of uterus and mammary ducts	Initiate labor, release milk		
	Antidiuretic hormone (vasopressin)	Kidney tubules	Conserve water	Blood osmotic pressure	Diabetes insipidus, dilute blood and low blood sodium
		Smooth muscle of blood vessels	Raise blood pressure slightly	Blood pressure	
Thyroid	Thyroxine and tri-iodothyronine	Cells	Increase O_2 consumption and rate of use of nutrients, increase body temperature	Thyroid hormones suppress TSH	Cretinism, myxedema, goiter, Graves' disease
	Calcitonin	Blood calcium	Uptake of calcium into bones	Low blood calcium	

Gland	Hormones	Target Organs	Major Effects	Negative Feedback	Disorders
Parathyroids	Parathormone	Intestine Kidneys Blood calcium	Increase absorption of calcium Decrease excretion of calcium Remove calcium from bones	High blood calcium	Hyperparathyroidism, hypoparathyroidism
Adrenal medulla	Epinephrine and norepinephrine	Organs affected by sympathetic stimulation	Same as sympathetic stimulation but of longer duration		Tumors of adrenal medulla
Adrenal cortex	Aldosterone	Kidneys, blood sodium and potassium	Increase sodium reabsorption, increase potassium secretion, increase blood volume	Low blood potassium, renin, angiotensin II	Hyperaldosteronism
	Cortisol	Cells, especially liver	Synthesis of carbohydrate from other substances, breakdown of protein and fat, antiinflammatory effect	High cortisol suppresses ACTH	Addison's disease Cushing's syndrome Adrenogenital syndrome
	Androgens	Male fetus	Masculinization		
Pancreas	Glucagon	Blood glucose	Increase blood glucose	High blood glucose	Diabetes mellitus
	Insulin	Cells, especially liver, fat, and muscle; blood glucose	Entry of glucose into cells, decrease blood glucose	Low blood glucose	Hypoglycemia
	Somatostatin (growth hormone inhibiting hormone)	Pancreas	Suppress release of pancreatic and digestive hormones		
	Pancreatic polypeptide	Pancreas	Inhibit release of pancreatic digestive enzymes		
Ovaries	Estradiol	Ova, uterus, female secondary sex characteristics	Maturation of ova; development of uterine lining, mammary glands, and secondary sex characteristics	High estradiol suppresses FSH-LH-RH and FSH	
	Progesterone	Uterine lining and mammary glands	Formation of placenta, maintenance of pregnancy	High progesterone suppresses FSH-LH-RH and LH	
	Relaxin	Pubic symphysis	Softening of ligaments		
Testes	Testosterone	Cells, secondary sex characteristics	Growth, development of secondary sex characteristics	High testosterone suppresses FSH-LH-RH and ICSH	
Placenta	Human chorionic gonadotropin	Ovary	Stimulate hormone production		
	Chorionic growth hormone-prolactin	Cells	Similar to pituitary counterparts		
Thymus	Thymosin	Blood cells	Involved in immunity		
Pineal gland	Melatonin	Cyclic phenomena?	Regulate cyclic phenomena?		
Kidney	Renin	Blood pressure	See Chapter 25		
	Renal erythropoietic factor	Erythrocytes	See Chapter 16		
Digestive tract	Gastrin	} See Chapter 22			
	Secretin				
	Cholecystokinin				

CLINICAL TERMS

Hashimoto's thyroiditis   an inflammation of the thyroid gland, probably caused by an autoimmune reaction

hirsutism (her'sūt-izm)   abnormal hairiness

neuroblastoma (nu''ro-blas-to'mah)   a malignant tumor consisting of neural tissue, often involving sympathetic nervous system tissue in the adrenal medulla

pheochromocytoma (fe-o-kro''mo-si-to'mah)   a tumor of the adrenal medulla or chromaffin tissue elsewhere in the body that secretes excessive amounts of epinephrine

pituitary cachexia (kak-eks'e-ah)   a general ill health, weakness, and wasting caused by pituitary failure; Simmonds' disease

Waterhouse-Friderichsen syndrome   a sudden severe disease caused by a meningococcus; causes fever, coma, and hemorrhage, especially in the adrenal glands

---

Essay: Biorhythms

That many of the activities of living things are influenced by the time of day and the season of the year is well known. Even some physiological processes such as sleep and wakefulness clearly have a normal daily cycle. Less obvious is the fact that many other physiological processes are time-related and cyclic. All of these cycles are called **biorhythms**.

As data has accumulated to demonstrate cyclic processes in living things, research has been directed toward determining how the processes are regulated. Although many questions remain, it now seems that interactions between an organism and several subtle environmental factors are likely to be involved in regulation. The environmental factors include light, temperature, the moon and tides, and the earth's electromagnetic field. Of these light has been the most thoroughly investigated and two different kinds of light-related cycles observed. One of these cycles is called a **circadian rhythm**, or daily cycle. (*Circa* means around and *dia* refers to day.) The other—the **seasonal cycle**—appears to be determined by changes in the length of daylight through the seasons.

The term **biological clock** has been used to denote the regulatory mechanism for biorhythms. To qualify as a biological clock, a regulator must have two qualities: (1) It must be able to relay time-related information so that it influences physiological processes, and (2) it must have a mechanism to allow resetting. Given the present amount of information on cyclic processes, it is unlikely that any single organ constitutes *the* biological clock. Rather, several organs are probably involved, with one perhaps having a kind of "pacemaker" role in coordinating the activities of the others.

Biorhythms Based on Birthdate

The popular interest in biorhythms based on one's birthdate and the presumed existence of several cycles at various intervals throughout life requires some comment. It has been claimed that certain "critical days" occur in which a person is accident prone or subject to other disasters and that at other critical days the person is capable of above-average performance. Some quasi-scientific studies have attempted to demonstrate these cycles and critical days. However, these studies generally lack adequate controls, and they certainly have no basis in any known physiological processes. Furthermore, there are no known factors that could possibly account for the stipulated length of the cycles, and no known factors that could possibly reset them. It also seems rather unlikely that the cycles, based only on the passage of a certain number of days, could predict in any meaningful way the complex processes involved in an individual human being's mental, physical, or emotional state.

Below, we'll consider biorhythms and mechanisms that have been more carefully studied and confirmed.

Effects of Light on the Human Body

Animal studies indicate that light is likely to be a factor in regulating biorhythms in humans. Three kinds of effects of light on humans have been studied: photochemical, neural, and neuroendocrine.

In our study of the skin in Chapter 5, we considered the role of the skin in synthesizing vitamin D in the presence of sunlight. In addition to the fact that ultraviolet rays from the sun can cause sunburn, certain photochemical reactions can cause skin rashes in sensitized individuals.

Neural and neuroendocrine effects of light have also been observed. For example, the cortisol level in the blood of humans shows rhythmic variation over a twenty-four-hour period. It is generally highest in the morning shortly after waking and lowest in the evening. When people change schedules so that they are awake at night and sleeping during the day, the cortisol rhythm shifts to the new rhythm, but it takes from five to ten days to do so. Blind people do not seem to have a reliable rhythmic variation in cortisol level: Though there are peaks and valleys in the blood cortisol concentrations, they are not attuned to a twenty-four-hour cycle. Thus, it appears that light received by the eyes somehow resets the cortisol cycle. The normal daily peaks for cortisol and other constituents of human blood and urine are shown in Figure 15.28. It is not known whether these cycles are produced by light or simply reset or entrained by light.

Role of the Pineal Gland

In many animals, and probably in humans, too, the pineal gland appears to work with the hypothalamus to regulate biorhythms. Two of the chemicals that have been isolated from the gland, melatonin and serotonin, seem to be involved in the regulatory process. The activity of an enzyme, **N-acetyltransferase**, may be the controlling factor. Serotonin is acted on by the enzyme and converted to an intermediate compound. This compound is readily converted to melatonin by another enzyme, but the activity of N-acetyltransferase seems to be the key enzyme controlling the conversion.

Melatonin has been shown to influence both circadian rhythms and seasonal rhythms. The size of the sex glands of several animals varies in relation to the length of daylight at different seasons of the year, and this process appears to be mediated by melatonin. Melatonin also seems to affect daily periods of locomotor activity, daily variations in body temperature, and periods of sleep and wakefulness. Unfortunately, data on pineal gland function in humans is extremely limited. However, the above examples have demonstrated that melatonin could be the means by which time-related data is transmitted so as to influence physiological processes.

Now let us look at the resetting mechanism. As mentioned earlier, the activity of N-acetyltransferase seems to be the controlling factor. In animal studies its activity has been shown to rise as light intensity decreases and to reach a peak during darkness. As the enzyme activity peaks, the supply of melatonin in the pineal gland also reaches a high level, and the serotonin supply is depleted. As light intensity increases, the activity of the enzyme decreases; concurrently, melatonin concentration drops, and serotonin is replenished. Thus, light and darkness turn the enzyme off and on and continuously reset the process each day.

Melatonin has also been shown to have a twenty-four-hour rhythm in humans, as measured by excretion in the urine. This reaches a peak during the night and is at its lowest level in the afternoon. Studies of women who have been blind since the first year of life suggest that melatonin may have an effect on

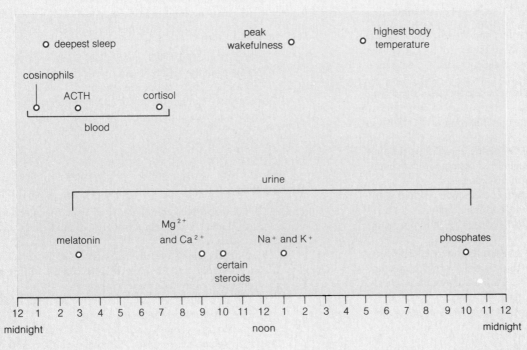

Figure 15.28 The peak times of secretion of various chemicals and other physiological parameters. These data represent averages for a large group of individuals; particular individuals may show peaks at slightly different times.

the maturation of the ovaries, as this group reached sexual maturity earlier than normal females. Other observers noted many years ago that young boys who had pineal tumors that interfered with the function of the pineal reached puberty earlier than normal.

Performance Cycles

Human performance has been shown to be somewhat dependent on biorhythms. Studies comparing rhythms in normal light-and-dark cycles and rhythms under constant conditions have been made. Rhythms under constant conditions of either light or darkness are called **free-running rhythms** because they are not reset by changes in light and darkness. These rhythms have been shown to retain a circadian period but tend to be slightly longer than twenty-four hours. Studies of **jet lag**, the effects of travel across several time zones, show that the resetting of circadian cycles requires about four days after a westbound flight over nine time zones and about six days after an eastbound flight over the same number of time zones. These measures are based on the time needed to reestablish normal cycles of body temperature, performance, and excretion of sodium and other products in the urine. Since the westbound flight increases the perceived daylength, the inclination for free-running cycles to exceed twenty-four hours may account for this difference. The body seems to be able to compensate for westward flights more easily than eastward flights because it generally has a free-running cycle of more than twenty-four hours. Regardless of the level of understanding of the exact mechanisms for adjustments to changes in day–night cycles, factors that change these cycles clearly have physiological effects.

Conclusion

Biorhythms seem to lead to efficient function by regulating activity to coincide with environmental conditions. By influencing activities so that the body responds appropriately to the environment, these cycles indirectly help to maintain homeostasis. We might say that biorhythms cause the body to "make hay while the sun shines."

CHAPTER SUMMARY

(Chapter summary points and review questions are numbered to correspond to the numbered objectives in the text of each chapter.)

Organization and General Function

1. Describe the location of each of the endocrine glands and their general function as a system.
   a. The locations of the specific endocrine glands are shown in Figure 15.2.
   b. The general function of the endocrine glands is to produce chemicals called hormones, which contribute to the chemical regulation of physiological processes.
2. Explain the mechanisms of action of hormones, including the role of prostaglandins and cyclic nucleotides.
   a. Several mechanisms are involved in the actions of hormones:
      (1) Steroids generally enter target cells and form complexes with receptors, after which they attach to a chromosome in the nucleus of the cell and influence protein synthesis.
      (2) Polypeptide hormones have short-term effects on the transport of substances across the cell membrane; these effects are mediated by a hormone-receptor complex at the cell membrane.
      (3) Polypeptide hormones have long-term effects on the enzyme activities inside cells; these effects are apparently mediated by the hormone-receptor complex activating membrane-bound enzymes that produce "second messengers."
   b. Prostaglandins and cyclic nucleotides usually serve as intermediates in the action of a hormone.
3. Explain how hormone actions are regulated.
   a. Factors that regulate the actions of hormones include the receptors, prostaglandins, and cyclic nucleotides.
   b. Phosphorylation of proteins may be involved in hormone regulation.

Development

4. Identify the embryonic germ layer from which each endocrine gland is derived and relate its embryological origin to the chemical nature of its secretions.
   a. The pituitary gland and the adrenal medulla are derived from ectoderm, and their secretions consist of proteins, polypeptides, or modified amino acids.
   b. The gonads and adrenal cortex are derived from mesoderm, and their secretions are steroids.
   c. Other major endocrine glands are derived from endoderm, and their secretions are proteins, polypeptides, or modified amino acids.

Pituitary Gland

5. Describe the location and structure of the pituitary gland and the source, function, and regulation of each of its hormones.
   a. The pituitary gland rests in the sella turcica at the base of the brain. It is composed of two major parts, the adenohypophysis and the neurohypophysis.
   b. The hormones of the adenohypophysis and their functions are:
      (1) growth hormone, which stimulates growth and maintains body size
      (2) prolactin, which stimulates lactation in the developed mammary gland
      (3) follicle-stimulating hormone, which stimulates estrogen production and the maturation of ova in females and the development of sperm in males
      (4) luteinizing hormone, which stimulates progesterone secretion and the release of ova in females or (under the name of interstitial-cell-stimulating hormone) stimulates testosterone production and the development of the interstitial cells that produce the hormone in the male
      (5) adrenocorticotropic hormone, which stimulates the adrenal cortex
      (6) thyroid-stimulating hormone, which stimulates the thyroid gland
   c. These hormones of the adenohypophysis are regulated by hormones released by the hypothalamus and by negative feedback from hormones of the glands each hormone stimulates.
   d. The hormones of the neurohypophysis are produced in the hypothalamus and stored in the neurohypophysis.
   e. The hormones of the neurohypophysis and their functions are:
      (1) Oxytocin, which stimulates uterine muscle to contract, especially during labor, and which stimulates cells near the ducts of the mammary glands to contract during lactation
      (2) Antidiuretic hormone, or vasopressin, which acts to cause sodium and water to be returned to the blood from the kidney filtrate and which has a small effect on increasing the blood pressure.
   f. Hormones of the neurohypophysis are regulated mainly by neural impulses acting on the hypothalamus.
6. Summarize the relationship between the pituitary and the brain.
   a. Neural stimuli can affect the hypothalamus and cause the release of regulating hormones that affect the adenohypophysis and the release of hormones from the hypothalamus to the neurohypophysis.
   b. The integration of neural and endocrine regulatory mechanisms is accomplished mainly through the relationships between the hypothalamus and the pituitary gland.
7. Explain the nature of the malfunction in common pituitary disorders.
   a. Certain pituitary disorders are summarized in Table 15.4.

Thyroid Gland

8. Describe the location and structure of the thyroid gland and the source, function, and regulation of its hormones.
   a. The thyroid gland is located below the larynx and surrounds the trachea.
   b. The hormones thyroxine and triiodothyronine regulate the metabolic rate in all cells.
   c. Thyroxine and triiodothyronine are regulated mainly by the release of TSH from the adenohypophysis, which they regulate by negative feedback.
   d. The hormone calcitonin helps to regulate the calcium concentration in the blood.
9. Explain the nature of the malfunction in common thyroid disorders.
   a. Hypothyroidism, called cretinism in the young and myxedema in older individuals, is caused by a deficiency of thyroid hormones.
   b. Hyperthyroidism (Graves' disease and toxic goiter) is caused by an excess of thyroid hormones.
   c. Simple goiter is caused by a lack of iodine in the diet.

Parathyroid Glands

10. Describe the location and structure of the parathyroid glands and the source, function, and regulation of their hormone.
    a. The parathyroid glands are imbedded in the posterior part of the thyroid gland.
    b. Their hormone, parathormone, regulates the concentration of calcium and certain other minerals in the blood.
    c. Parathormone is regulated by negative feedback from the increased concentration of calcium in the blood.
11. Explain the nature of the malfunction in parathyroid disorders.
    a. Hypoparathyroidism, a deficiency of parathormone, leads to reduced calcium concentration in the blood and to tetany.
    b. Hyperparathyroidism, an excess of parathormone, leads to an increase in the concentration of calcium in the blood.

Adrenal Glands

12. Describe the location and structure of the adrenal glands and the source, function, and regulation of their hormones.
    a. The paired adrenal glands are located one above each kidney. Each consists of two separate glands, the medulla and the cortex. The cortex is further divided into an outer layer, which produces aldosterone, and middle and inner layers, which both produce glucocorticoids and sex hormones.
    b. The medulla secretes epinephrine and norepinephrine, whose functions were discussed in Chapter 13.
    c. The cortex secretes:
       (1) aldosterone, which helps to regulate the metabolism of sodium and potassium

(2) glucocorticoids, which help to regulate carbohydrate metabolism and contribute to the body's resistance to stress

(3) sex hormones, which contribute to the development of maleness

d. Hormones of the adrenal cortex are regulated as follows:

(1) Aldosterone is regulated by angiotensin, potassium, and renin.

(2) Other adrenocortical hormones are regulated primarily by ACTH.

13. Explain the nature of the malfunction in adrenal disorders.

a. Addison's disease results from a deficiency of cortisol.

b. Hyperaldosteronism results from an excess of aldosterone.

c. Cushing's syndrome results from an excess of cortisol.

d. Adrenogenital syndrome results from an excess of sex hormones from the adrenal cortex.

Pancreas

14. Describe the location and structure of the pancreas and the source, function, and regulation of its hormones.

a. The pancreas is located below the stomach in a bend of the duodenum.

b. In addition to cells that produce digestive secretions, the pancreas contains islets of Langerhans, which in turn contain four kinds of cells:

(1) A-cells, which produce glucagon

(2) B-cells, which produce insulin

(3) D-cells, which produce somatostatin

(4) F-cells, which produce pancreatic polypeptide

c. The functions of the hormones of the pancreas are as follows:

(1) Glucagon raises the blood glucose concentration.

(2) Insulin lowers the blood glucose concentration and stimulates the uptake of glucose by cells.

(3) Somatostatin appears to suppress the release of other hormones produced by the pancreas.

(4) Pancreatic polypeptide inhibits the release of digestive secretions from the pancreas.

d. Insulin and glucagon are regulated in part by the concentration of glucose in the blood which influences the secretory cells by negative feedback. Many other hormones are involved in the regulation of blood sugar.

15. Explain the nature of the malfunction in pancreatic disorders.

a. Diabetes mellitus is due to deficiency or inactivity of insulin.

b. Hypoglycemia may be caused by an excess of insulin, a deficiency of glucagon, or a failure of these hormones to completely regulate the blood sugar.

Gonads

16. For each of the gonads, name the hormones they secrete and give the major function of each hormone.

a. The ovaries or female gonads secrete:

(1) estradiol, which stimulates the development and maintenance of female secondary sex characteristics and the development of ova, the uterine lining, and the mammary glands

(2) progesterone, which further stimulates development of the uterine lining and mammary glands and maintains pregnancy

(3) relaxin, which softens the ligaments of the pubic symphysis in pregnancy

b. The testes or male gonads secrete testosterone, which stimulates the development and maintenance of male secondary sex characteristics and stimulates growth.

c. These hormones and their regulation are discussed in more detail in Chapter 28.

Other Endocrine Structures

17. Describe the location, structure, and endocrine activity of the following: (a) placenta, (b) thymus, and (c) pineal gland.

a. Hormones of the placenta help to maintain pregnancy.

b. The thymic hormone, thymosin, is involved in the development of cells that produce immunity.

c. The hormones produced by the pineal gland appear to be involved in biorhythms.

18. Give examples of hormones from the digestive tract and other sources.

a. Hormones from the digestive tract include gastrin, secretin, and cholecystokinin.

b. Hormones from the kidney include renin and renal erythropoietic factor.

c. Prostaglandins and carbon dioxide might be included in the category of hormones because they have regulatory functions.

REVIEW

Important Terms

adenohypophysis	beta-lipotropin
adrenal cortex	calcitonin
adrenal medulla	circadian
adrenocorticotropic hormone	cortisol
	endocrine
aldosterone	epinephrine
androgen	follicle-stimulating hormone
antidiuretic hormone (vasopressin)	
	glucagon

glucocorticoid

growth hormone

hormone

human chorionic gonadotropin

hypophysis

insulin

luteinizing hormone

melatonin

mineralocorticoid

negative feedback

neurohypophysis

norepinephrine

oxytocin

pancreas

parathormone

parathyroid

pineal gland

placenta

prolactin

prostaglandin

somatostatin

target organ

thymus

thyroid gland

thyroxine

triiodothyronine

Questions

1. **a.** Name the major endocrine glands and tell where each is located.
   b. What is the general function of the endocrine system?

2. **a.** What is the most likely mechanism of action of a steroid hormone?
   b. What is the most likely mechanism of action of a polypeptide hormone?
   c. What are the roles of cyclic phosphates and protein kinases in hormone action?
   d. What is the role of prostaglandins in hormone action?

3. What factors may be involved in the regulation of hormone action?

4. **a.** Which glands are derived from each of the germ layers?
   b. How are the chemical structures of hormones related to the germ layer of the gland that produces them?

5. **a.** Where is the pituitary located?
   b. How are the two parts of the pituitary related?
   c. Name the hormones of the adenohypophysis and give the function of each.
   d. How are the hormones of the adenohypophysis regulated?
   e. What are the hormones of the neurohypophysis?
   f. Why would you not expect the hormones of the neurohypophysis to be regulated by releasing hormones?
   g. What is negative feedback?

6. Discuss the relationships between the pituitary and the brain.

7. **a.** How would you distinguish between acromegaly and giantism?
   b. If a patient had a low blood level of ADH, what disease would you suspect?

8. **a.** Where is the thyroid gland located?
   b. What is the colloid found in the thyroid gland?
   c. What is the function of thyroxine, and how is it regulated?
   d. What is the function of calcitonin, and how is it regulated?

9. **a.** If you had a chance to observe the behavior of a patient with a goiter, how would you go about determining the cause of the goiter?
   b. Contrast the symptoms, causes, and treatments for hypothyroidism and hyperthryoidism.

10. **a.** Where are the parathyroid glands?
    b. What is the function of parathormone?
    c. How do parathormone and calcitonin contribute to the regulation of the calcium concentration in the blood?

11. **a.** What might happen to a person if hypoparathyroidism were untreated? Why?
    b. What happens to the bones, blood, and kidneys in hyperparathyroidism?

12. **a.** Where are the adrenal glands located?
    b. Explain how an adrenal gland can be said to be two glands in one.
    c. What is the function of epinephrine, and how is it regulated?
    d. What are the three layers of the adrenal cortex, and what hormones are produced by each?
    e. How are the hormones in (d) regulated?

13. What diagnosis would you make on the basis of the following laboratory reports on patients?
    a. Low blood concentration of aldosterone or cortisol
    b. High blood concentration of aldosterone
    c. High blood concentration of cortisol
    d. High blood concentration of adrenal sex hormones

14. **a.** Where is the pancreas located, and what are its functions?
    b. What are the islets of Langerhans, and what kinds of cells do they contain?
    c. What is the source and function of glucagon?
    d. What is the source and function of insulin?
    e. What is the role of blood sugar concentration in regulating these hormones?

15. **a.** What is diabetes mellitus, and how is it different from diabetes insipidus?
    b. What is hypoglycemia?

16. Name the hormones produced by each of the gonads.

17. What is the endocrine function of each of the following?
    a. Placenta
    b. Thymus
    c. Pineal gland

18. Name some other hormones and tell where they are produced and what they do.

Problems

1. Suppose an overweight person comes to you complaining of fatigue. You suspect an endocrine disorder. Which disorders would you look for? What additional information would you want about the person? (If possible, indicate which laboratory tests you would order.)

2. If the person complained of fatigue but was not overweight, what disease(s) would you suspect might be present?

3. How would any of the following symptoms help you to narrow down the possible causes of a disease: (a) bronze-colored skin, (b) extreme thirst, (c) complaints of being cold, (d) poor healing of wounds?

REFERENCES AND READINGS

Anonymous. 1979. Labs vie for human growth hormone. *Science News* 116:22 (July 14).

Aschoff, J. 1978. Features of circadian rhythms relevant for the design of shift schedules. *Ergonomics* 21(10):739.

Binkley, S. 1979. A timekeeping enzyme in the pineal gland. *Scientific American* 240(4):66 (April).

Binkley, S. A., Riebman, J. B., and Reilly, K. B. 1978. The pineal gland: A biological clock in vitro. *Science* 202:1198 (December 15).

Blank, M. S., Panerai, A. E., and Freisen, H. G. 1979. Opioid peptides modulate luteinizing hormone secretion during sexual maturation. *Science* 203:1129 (March 16).

Brown, F. A., Jr. 1972. The "clocks" timing biological ryhthms. *American Scientist* 60:756 (November–December).

Brownstein, M. J., Russell, J. T., and Gainer, H. 1980. Synthesis, transport, and release of posterior pituitary hormones. *Science* 207:373 (January 25).

Deguchi, T. 1979. Circadian rhythms of serotonin N-acetyltransferase activity in organ culture of chicken pineal gland. *Science* 203:1245 (March 23).

Fink, G. 1979. Feedback actions of target hormones on hypothalamus and pituitary, with special reference to gonadal steroids. *Annual Review of Physiology* 41:571.

Greiner, A. C., and Chan, S. C. 1978. Melatonin content of the human pineal gland. *Science* 199:83 (January 6).

Guillemin, R. 1978. Peptides in the brain: The new endocrinology of the neuron. *Science* 202:390 (October 27).

Hedlund, L., Lischko, M. M., Rollag, M. D., and Niswender, G. D. 1977. Melatonin: Daily cycle in plasma and cerebrospinal fluid of calves. *Science* 195:686 (February 18).

Katzenellenbogen, B. S. 1980. Dynamics of steroid hormone receptor action. *Annual Review of Physiology* 42:17.

Klein, R., and Armitage, R. 1979. Rhythms in human performance: 1½-hour oscillations in cognitive style. *Science* 204:1326 (June 22).

Kolata, G. B. 1977. Hormone receptors: How are they regulated? *Science* 196:747 (May 13).

Kolata, G. B. 1978. Polypeptide hormones: What are they doing in cells? *Science* 201:895 (September 8).

Krieger, D. T., and Liotta, A. S. 1979. Pituitary hormones in the brain: Where, how, and why? *Science* 205:366 (July 27).

Labrie, F., Borgeat, P., Drouin, J., Beaulieu, M., Lagacé, L., Ferland, L., and Raymond, V. 1979. Mechanism of action of hypothalamic hormones in the adenohypophysis. *Annual Review of Physiology* 41:555.

Langs, D. A., Erman, M., and DeTitta, G. T. 1977. Conformations of prostaglandin $F_{2\alpha}$ and recognition of prostaglandins by their receptors. *Science* 197:1003 (September 2).

Marx, J. L. 1975. Learning and behavior (I): Effects of pituitary hormones. *Science* 190:367 (October 24).

Marx, J. L. 1975. Learning and behavior (II): The hypothalamic peptides. *Science* 190:544 (November 7).

McCarthy, J. A. 1978. Prostaglandins: An overview. *Advances in Pediatrics* 25:121.

McEwen, B. S. 1976. Interactions between hormones and nerve tissue. *Scientific American* 235(1):48 (July).

McEwen, B. S. 1980. Binding and metabolism of sex steroids by the hypothalamic-pituitary unit: Physiological implications. *Annual Review of Physiology* 42:97.

Meites, J. 1977. The 1977 Nobel Prize in physiology or medicine. *Science* 198:594 (November 11).

O'Malley, B. W., and Schrader, W. T. 1976. The receptors of steroid hormones. *Scientific American* 234(2):32 (February).

Oppenheimer, J. H. 1979. Thyroid hormone action at the cellular level. *Science* 203:971 (March 9).

Pacold, S. T., Kirsteins, L., Hojvat, S., and Lawrence, A. M. 1978. Biologically active pituitary hormones in the rat brain amygdaloid nucleus. *Science* 199:804 (February 17).

Quabbe, H. J. 1977. Endocrine concomitants of the sleep–wake rhythm in man. *Environmental Endocrinology*, Proceedings of an International Symposium, Montpellier, France, July 11–15, p. 124.

Romijn, H. J. 1978. The pineal, a tranquilizing organ? *Life Sciences* 23(23):2257.

Schally, A. V. 1978. Aspects of hypothalamic regulation of the pituitary gland. *Science* 202:18 (October 6).

Schally, A. V., Kastin, A. J., and Arimura, A. 1977. Hypothalamic hormones: The link between brain and body. *American Scientist* 65:712 (November–December).

Schusdziarra, V., Zyznar, E., Rouiller, D., Boden, G., Brown, J. C., Arimura, A., and Unger, R. H. 1980. Splanchnic somatostatin: A hormonal regulator of nutrient homeostasis. *Science* 207:530 (February 1).

Silva, J. E., and Larsen, P. R. 1977. Pituitary nuclear 3,5,3'-triiodothyronine and thyrotropin secretion: An explanation for the effect of thyroxine. *Science* 198:617 (November 11).

Sterling, K., Milch, P. O., Brenner, M. A., and Lazarus, J. H. 1977. Thyroid hormone action: The mitochondrial pathway. *Science* 197:966 (September 2).

Turner, C. D., and Bagnara, J. T. 1976. *General endocrinology.* New York: Holt, Rinehart and Winston.

Wurtman, R. J. 1975. The effects of light on the human body. *Scientific American* 233(1):69 (July).

UNIT FOUR

HOMEOSTATIC SYSTEMS

The internal systems of the body carry out many processes that help to maintain homeostasis, and their activities are controlled by the nervous and endocrine systems described in Unit Three. How these internal systems function and are regulated to maintain homeostasis is a theme that runs through all the chapters in Unit Four.

We will begin our study with the transport system, which includes the blood (Chapter 16), heart (Chapter 17), and blood vessels (Chapters 18 and 19). We will see how nutrients, gases, wastes, and other substances move throughout the body and how control mechanisms maintain their concentrations within a narrow range. Our study of the lymphatic system (Chapter 20) will show how that system assists with transport and also plays a role in the development of immunity. When we study the respiratory system (Chapter 21), we will see how gases are exchanged with the external environment and with the cells of the body to maintain oxygen and carbon dioxide homeostasis.

Our study of digestion (Chapter 22), metabolism (Chapter 23), and nutrition (Chapter 24) will show us what happens to nutrients as they are prepared for transport, how they are used by cells, and what nutrients are needed to maintain a healthy body. When we consider the urinary system (Chapter 25), we will see how the kidneys rid the body of metabolic wastes and help to regulate the composition of the blood.

Finally, Chapter 26 will show us how fluids, electrolytes, and pH are regulated and will summarize the nature of homeostatic mechanisms and the effects of stress on them.

16

CARDIOVASCULAR SYSTEM: BLOOD

ORGANIZATION AND GENERAL FUNCTIONS

Objective 1. (a) Describe the organization of the circulatory system and the role of blood in it; (b) name the main components of blood and list the major functions of blood.

The heart pumps blood through the circulatory system, an extensive closed system of blood vessels that carry blood to and from nearly every cell in the body. The components of the circulatory system are blood, the heart, and the blood vessels. Blood will be considered in this chapter, the heart and the blood vessels in the next three chapters.

Blood is the fluid that is transported through the blood vessels of the circulatory system as the heart contracts. Blood consists of formed elements (cells or cell fragments) suspended in a liquid called **plasma**. The formed elements are the **erythrocytes**, or red blood cells; the **leukocytes**, or white blood cells; and the **platelets**, a particular kind of cell fragment (Figure 16.1). The various types of leukocytes will be discussed later. As mentioned in Chapter 4, blood is classified as a connective tissue because it is composed of cells in a (fluid) matrix.

Erythrocytes are by far the most prominent of the formed elements seen in a microscopic view of a drop of blood. Normally, they make up 40% of the blood volume in females and 45% of the blood volume in males. The volume of erythrocytes in the blood is an important measure of the oxygen-carrying capacity of blood. Determining this volume, called the **hematocrit**, is a routine part of the laboratory study of blood.

The human body contains about five liters of blood, the amount varying according to body size and the amount of fat stored in the body. Blood usually comprises about 8% of the total body weight; thus, an average-sized adult male would have slightly more than five liters of blood in his body and an average-sized adult female slightly less than five liters. When a person donates a pint of blood, about 10% of the total blood volume is removed. Through a variety of homeostatic mechanisms we shall consider later, the body replaces the lost plasma in two or three days and the lost blood cells in three or four weeks.

The functions of blood include transport, protection, and regulation. Blood carries nutrients, including vitamins and minerals, oxygen, carbon dioxide, waste products, and hormones. It protects against the invasion of microorganisms and damage from toxic substances. Through its clotting mechanism blood helps to prevent its own loss. The regulation of blood composition by the nervous system helps to regulate the water content of the cells, the pH of body fluids, body temperature, and the concentration of many other substances in the body. The functions of blood—which are essential to human survival—are summarized in Table 16.1.

DEVELOPMENT

Objective 2. Describe the development of the formed elements of blood.

The formed elements of the blood—erythrocytes, leukocytes, and platelets—are constantly lost through a variety of processes. These elements are replaced as they are destroyed so that a relatively constant number of each is maintained.

Hemopoiesis, or **hematopoiesis**, is the general process by which all blood cells and platelets are formed. In the embryo blood cells first develop in the yolk sac. In the fetus, as the embryo is called after the second month of development, blood cells form in a variety of tissues, including the bone marrow, liver, spleen, thymus gland, and lymph nodes. In the adult blood cells develop primarily in the bone marrow, where all the formed elements can be produced.

The formed elements of the blood are derived from an undifferentiated cell type, the **stem cell**. Stem cells differentiate into five types of cells whose names end in "blast," denoting that the cells are in the process of further differentiation. Lymphoblasts give rise to both large and small **lymphocytes**; monoblasts give rise to **monocytes**. Myeloblasts differentiate along three separate lines, giving rise to **basophils**, **neutrophils**, and **eosinophils**. Together, these last three cell types are classified as **polymorphonuclear (PMN) cells** because of the great variation in the shapes of

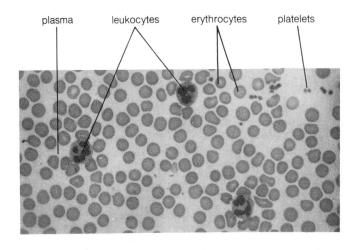

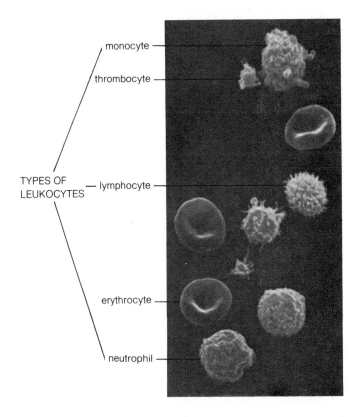

Figure 16.1 (**a**) Blood consists of plasma (the liquid portion); and erythrocytes, leukocytes, and platelets (the formed elements). (**b**) Three-dimensional shapes of cells can be seen in a scanning electron micrograph. (Photomicrographs reproduced with permission from William A. Jensen (**a**) and from *Tissues and organs: A text-atlas of scanning electron microscopy* by Richard G. Kessel and Randy H. Kardon. W. H. Freeman and Company. Copyright © 1979 (**b**).)

Table 16.1 The Functions of Blood

Functions	Examples
Transport of:	
Nutrients	Glucose, amino acids, vitamins, and minerals are carried to nearly all cells.
Oxygen	Oxygen is transported from the lungs to all cells of the body by the erythrocytes.
Carbon dioxide	Carbon dioxide is transported from cells to lungs.
Waste products	Urea, uric acid, and other waste products are carried from cells to the liver, lungs, and kidneys.
Hormones	Hormones are carried from an endocrine gland to target organs.
Protection against:	
Invasion of microorganisms	Leukocytes engulf and destroy some microorganisms. Antibodies react with specific antigens, such as those on microorganisms.
Damage from toxic substances	Some toxic substances are carried to the liver, where they are rendered nontoxic, and then to the kidneys, where they are excreted. Some toxic substances are inactivated by antitoxins.
Blood loss	The clotting mechanism seals off blood vessels. Substances released from platelets initiate clotting after tissue injury.
Regulation of:	
Water content of cells	Centers in the hypothalamus detect changes in the osmotic pressure and cause the blood to gain or lose water, thereby maintaining water equilibrium between blood and cells.
pH of body fluids	Certain neural centers detect carbon dioxide concentration and regulate the pH of body fluids indirectly. (An excess of carbon dioxide causes acid to accumulate.)
Body temperature	Temperature sensors in the hypothalamus detect changes in body temperature and act to increase or decrease blood flow to skin.

their nuclei (see Figure 16.2). They are distinguished by their staining properties when treated with laboratory dyes, or stains. Basophils accept a basic stain (pH greater than 7), eosinophils accept eosin (an acid stain), and neutrophils do not stain well with either kind of stain.

In addition to producing leukocytes, stem cells in the bone marrow also give rise to erythrocytes. In the differentiation process first a nucleated cell is produced; after gradually decreasing in size and losing its nucleus, the cell becomes a **reticulocyte**, the immediate precursor of an erythrocyte. Significant numbers of reticulocytes in circulating blood indicate that erythrocytes are being destroyed prematurely, and immature cells are being released into

circulation before they have completed differentiation. Such a condition might follow severe blood loss. Completely differentiated erythrocytes are biconcave disc-shaped cells lacking nuclei; they carry oxygen (and some carbon dioxide).

Normally, the rate of production of new erythrocytes equals the rate at which old erythrocytes are dying—2.5 million per second! Even at this rate only about 1/120 of the body's erythrocytes die each day. When production of erythrocytes is not keeping pace with their destruction, they decrease in number, and the oxygen-carrying capacity of the blood decreases. Certain cells in the kidneys detect the lack of oxygen and release a substance called **renal**

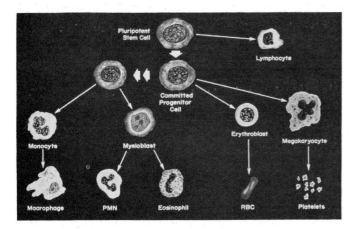

Figure 16.2 The differentiation of the formed elements of blood from stem cells. The polymorphonuclear (PMN) cell further differentiates to form neutrophils and basophils, as well as eosinophils. (Courtesy of Robert Chilcote, M. D., University of Chicago.)

Table 16.2	Normal Numbers of Formed Elements in Human Blood	
Element		Normal Numbers per Microliter*
Erythrocytes		
Adult male		4.6 to 6.2 million
Adult female		4.2 to 5.4 million
Infant		5.0 to 5.1 million
Leukocytes		*5000 to 9000*
Neutrophils	50–70%	
Eosinophils	1–4%	
Basophils	0.1%	
Monocytes	2–8%	
Lymphocytes	20–40%	
Platelets		*250,000 to 300,000*

*1 microliter = 1/1,000,000 liter

erythropoietic factor (REF). REF activates a plasma globulin, **erythropoietin**, which travels in the blood to the bone marrow, where it stimulates the development and release of new erythrocytes. Iron, vitamins such as folic acid and vitamin B_{12}, and intrinsic factor from the stomach are also essential for the production of erythrocytes.

Finally, stem cells form **megakaryocytes**, which fragment and give rise to platelets. Platelets are important in the clotting of blood.

BLOOD AS A TISSUE

Objective 3. List the components of blood, their characteristics, and the amounts of each component normally present.

Of the total blood volume approximately 45% is formed elements, and the remaining 55% is plasma. Due to the presence of cells, blood is in fact thicker than water—about five times as thick. It contains the numbers of formed elements listed in Table 16.2.

Plasma

Plasma is the fluid that remains when the formed elements are removed from blood. Plasma is more than 90% water and contains electrolytes (inorganic ions), proteins, gases, nutrients, waste products, hormones, and clotting factors

(Table 16.3). In contrast to plasma, **serum** is the fluid that remains after both the formed elements and the clotting factors have been removed from blood.

Of the substances in plasma, electrolytes, gases, some nutrients, and waste products are dissolved in the water of the plasma (a passive process), while other substances are attached to carrier proteins of the plasma (an active process). For example, cholesterol, which is relatively insoluble in water, is attached to proteins to form lipoproteins. Two kinds of lipoproteins carry cholesterol: the low-density lipoproteins (LDLs) and the high-density lipoproteins (HDLs).

Various types of plasma proteins protect and regulate the body in three important ways. First, antibodies confer immunity against infectious diseases and help to destroy foreign substances. Second, several factors, including fibrinogen and prothrombin, cause blood to clot should a leak develop in a vessel. Finally, large proteins, especially albumin, contribute to the osmolarity of the blood: They are important in "pulling" fluid back into the blood after it has filtered out of the small blood vessels (capillaries) that pass adjacent to the cells.

Table 16.3 Constituents of Plasma	
Constituent	Amount/Concentration*
pH	7.35 to 7.45
Water	90% of plasma
Electrolytes (inorganic)	<1% of plasma
Na^+	142 mEq/l (142 mmol/l)
K^+	4 mEq/l (4 mmol/l)
Ca^{2+}	5 mEq/l (2.5 mmol/l)
Mg^{2+}	3 mEq/l (1.5 mmol/l)
Cl^-	107 mEq/l (107 mmol/l)
HCO_3^-	27 mEq/l (27 mmol/l)
Phosphate (mostly HPO_4^{2-})	4 mEq/l (2 mmol/l)
SO_4^{2-}	1 mEq/l (0.5 mmol/l)
Gases	about 1% of plasma
CO_2	60 ml/100 ml plasma
O_2	0.2 ml/100 ml
N_2	0.9 ml/100 ml
Nutrients	about 3% of plasma
Glucose and other carbohydrates	100 mg/100 ml
Amino acids	40 mg/100 ml
Lipids	500 mg/100 ml
Cholesterol	150–250 mg/100 ml
Vitamins	traces
Trace elements	traces
Waste products	about 1% of plasma
Urea	<20 mg/100 ml
Creatinine	<1 mg/100 ml
Uric acid	5 mg/100 ml
Bilirubin	0.2–1.2 mg/100 ml
Proteins	6% of plasma (2.5 mmol/l)
Albumins	4.5 g/100 ml
Globulins	2.5 g/100 ml
Fibrinogen	0.3 g/100 ml
Hormones	traces

*Concentrations for some substances are expressed in both millimoles (mmol) and milliequivalents (mEq). One millimole is one-thousandth of a gram molecular weight of a substance. For substances that have a valence of 1, mEq and mmol are equal; for substances that have a valence of 2, 2 mEq equal 1 mmol.

Lipoproteins of different densities can be separated by ultracentrifugation. Because 80% of cholesterol is carried in LDLs, the HDLs have received little attention until recently. However, it now appears that individuals with relatively high levels of HDLs (and therefore lower levels of LDLs) may be at less risk of heart disease and atherosclerosis (deposits of lipids in blood vessel walls). Further research is needed to understand how transport of lipids is related to their potential for damaging the circulatory system, but what is known demonstrates the importance of understanding how much and in what form substances are carried in the plasma.

Erythrocytes

Erythrocytes (Figure 16.3) are about 7½ μm in diameter and 2 μm thick. Circulating erythrocytes not only lack nuclei; they also lack mitochondria, microtubules, and the machinery for synthesizing protein. Moreover, these cells have a very large surface area for their volume, allowing for easy gas exchange and for deformability as they pass through narrow capillaries. Because they lack a nucleus, erythrocytes are unable to reproduce themselves and have a short life span of about 120 days. During that time they travel a total distance of about 300 miles through the blood vessels, passing through capillaries whose diameter is smaller than the diameter of the erythrocyte. The flexible, deformable membrane allows the cells to assume a rod shape as they pass through narrow capillaries and to return to a disc shape in larger vessels.

A protein called **spectrin** forms a layer on the inner surface of the erythrocyte membrane and provides the cell durability that other cells attain from their microtubules. When erythrocytes are deficient in spectrin, as has been observed in some anemias, the cells become spherical and have difficulty passing through small capillaries, especially within the spleen. Such cells become trapped and are destroyed.

The principal component of the erythrocyte cytoplasm is **hemoglobin**, a pigment that is bright red when oxygenated. This pigment gives erythrocytes their red color and their name, red cells. Hemoglobin (Figure 16.4) consists of a large protein molecule, called a **globin**, into which four molecules of **heme** are imbedded. Each heme group contains an iron atom that can form an attachment to an oxygen molecule. Because each heme group can carry one O_2 molecule, each molecule of hemoglobin can carry four O_2 molecules. The presence of red cells containing hemoglobin increases the oxygen-carrying capacity of blood to about seventy times the amount of oxygen that could be carried dissolved in the plasma without red cells. Hemoglobin also transports carbon dioxide. Because the carbon dioxide binds to the globin portion of the molecule, hemoglobin can carry oxygen and carbon dioxide simultaneously. Ordinarily, red cells traveling from the lungs to other tissues carry mostly oxygen. In the tissues the red cells exchange oxygen for carbon dioxide and carry mostly carbon dioxide back to the lungs. When not oxygenated, the erythrocytes have a darker, bluish-red color.

Carbon monoxide (CO) is a particularly deadly gas for it can bind to hemoglobin more tightly than can oxygen (O_2). Because carbon monoxide is colorless and odorless, people can be overcome by it before they know what is happening. The signs of carbon monoxide poisoning are extremely flushed or red appearance of the skin (because CO-bound hemoglobin is bright red); euphoria or exaggerated delight that may border on hysteria; followed by sleepiness, coma, and death. If the victim is discovered before death has occurred, blood transfusions may be given to put erythrocytes capable of carrying oxygen into the blood. As CO binds more tightly than O_2, simply administering oxygen may not help.

Faulty gas heaters can produce toxic levels of carbon monoxide indoors. Carbon monoxide concentration in outdoor air is one of the measures of air pollution.

Phagocytic cells of the liver, spleen, and bone marrow digest dead erythrocytes. These phagocytes separate hemoglobin into heme and globin, further digesting the globin

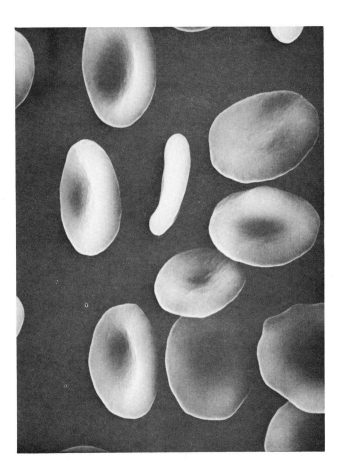

Figure 16.3   A scanning electron micrograph of erythrocytes. (Courtesy of Amanda Tuley and Robert Chilcote, M.D., University of Chicago, Comprehensive Study of Sickle Cell Disease Center.)

to amino acids, which can be used to synthesize other proteins. Iron is separated from the heme and returned to the plasma, where it attaches to a protein called **transferrin**. Transferrin carries the iron to the bone marrow, where it is reused in making new erythrocytes, or to the liver, where it is combined with a protein and stored as **ferritin**. The remainder of the heme is processed mainly in the liver, first to the bile pigment **biliverdin**, then to another bile pigment, **bilirubin**, which is secreted in bile. Bile enters the digestive tract, and some is excreted, ridding the body of the products of heme breakdown (Figure 16.5). Thus, some components of hemoglobin are conserved for future use; the breakdown of erythrocytes is less wasteful than it might at first have seemed. Individuals with anemia resulting from rapid red cell destruction do not need iron, and those receiving frequent blood transfusions to offset erythrocyte destruction

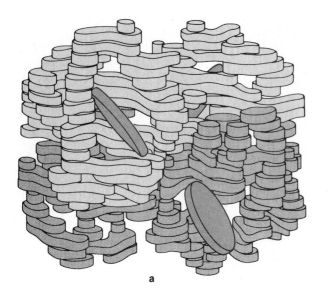

a   b

Figure 16.4 (**a**) The three-dimensional structure of a hemoglobin molecule as deduced from X-ray diffraction studies. The protein portion consists of four chains of amino acids, two alpha chains shown in light gray and two beta chains shown in dark gray. Three of the four heme groups are shown as colored discs. (**b**) The molecular structure of heme. Note the iron atom in the center of the molecule.

may acquire harmful excesses of iron. Iron supplements are needed only when bleeding is the cause of anemia, as in injuries or excessive blood loss during menstruation.

Leukocytes

Leukocytes are the largest of the formed elements in blood. Neutrophils, eosinophils, basophils, monocytes, and lymphocytes are all derived from stem cells (see Figure 16.2). The percentages of each type of leukocyte in normal blood are given in Table 16.2.

Neutrophils, the most numerous of all leukocytes, guard the skin and mucous membranes of the body. They increase in number during an infection but live only a few days after they are released into the bloodstream and generally function within the tissues. Injured cells release a substance that stimulates neutrophils circulating in capillaries near the site of an injury to leave the capillary and enter the tissue. By a process called **diapedesis** neutrophils deform and elongate and squeeze through pores between the cells of a capillary wall. Once at the site of an injury, neutrophils phagocytize and kill microorganisms and, in turn, die themselves. Macrophages, phagocytic cells de-

rived from monocytes, clean up the debris from dead and injured cells.

Eosinophils may act as phagocytes, but they probably have other functions, including detoxification of foreign proteins, the turning-off of inflammatory reactions, and the breakdown of antigen–antibody complexes after immune reactions have occurred.

Basophils, though not phagocytic, do play a role in the body's defense mechanisms. They release histamine into injured tissue and thereby initiate the inflammatory process (see Chapter 4). Basophils closely resemble connective tissue mast cells, which also release histamine.

Monocytes function like neutrophils; they are active phagocytes and are especially likely to digest larger debris. Lymphocytes circulate in the blood, but most are found in lymphoid tissues. They function in the development of immunity. Lymphocytes and monocytes are emptied into the blood along with lymph that has collected in the lymph vessels. (Lymph, lymph vessels, and immunity will be described in Chapter 20.) From the blood these cells move by diapedesis to the tissues and are returned to the lymph vessels. Because of this recycling it is difficult to estimate the longevity of lymphocytes and monocytes. However, lymphocytes labeled with radioactive tracers have been found

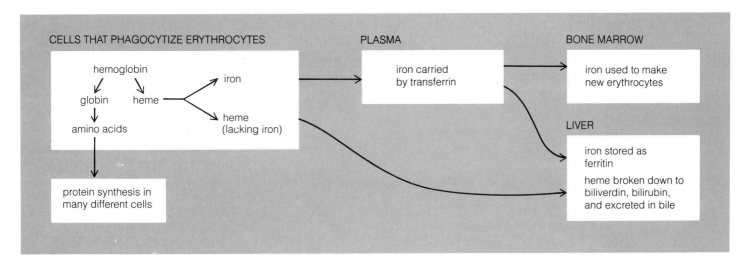

Figure 16.5 Several components of hemoglobin from the breakdown of erythrocytes are reused by the body.

CELLS THAT PHAGOCYTIZE ERYTHROCYTES

hemoglobin
→ globin   heme
globin → amino acids
heme → iron
heme → heme (lacking iron)
amino acids → protein synthesis in many different cells

PLASMA

iron carried by transferrin

BONE MARROW

iron used to make new erythrocytes

LIVER

iron stored as ferritin

heme broken down to biliverdin, bilirubin, and excreted in bile

in the blood 100 to 300 days after labeling, and some researchers believe they may circulate for years.

Platelets

Platelets, also called **thrombocytes**, are cell fragments only 2 to 4 μm in diameter. They initiate the sequence of reactions that causes blood clotting. When an injury occurs or a roughened area exists within a blood vessel, platelets adhere to the exposed collagen molecules in the area. Their role in hemostasis, the arrest of bleeding, will be discussed later in this chapter. Being cell fragments, platelets are short-lived and are completely replaced about every five to ten days.

DISORDERS OF ERYTHROCYTES AND LEUKOCYTES

Objective 4. Describe the causes and effects of each of the following types of disorders: (a) anemias, (b) polycythemia, (c) leukemias, and (d) infectious mononucleosis.

Anemias

Anemia is a decrease in the number of erythrocytes or a lack of hemoglobin. Several different kinds of anemia exist, but only a few of the more common types will be considered here. All anemias produce some of the same symptoms. Because the oxygen-carrying capacity of the blood is diminished, the affected individual tires easily during exercise and may complain of lack of energy.

Nutritional anemia If the diet lacks sufficient quantities of iron or the iron in the diet is not properly absorbed from the intestine, the bone marrow will be unable to produce erythrocytes that contain adequate amounts of hemoglobin. A variety of vitamin deficiencies also cause anemia (see Chapter 24).

Hemorrhagic anemia When a person suffers excessive loss of blood, the resulting anemia is called hemorrhagic anemia. It can be caused by severe injury, bleeding ulcers, or excessive menstrual flow. Sudden excessive blood loss can be fatal, and prolonged loss of small amounts of blood can produce chronic anemia. Blood transfusions can be used to treat acute hemorrhagic anemia, but correcting the cause is a better treatment for chronic conditions.

Hemolytic anemia   In hemolytic anemia the cell membranes of many erythrocytes rupture and pour their contents into the plasma. Erythroblastosis fetalis, and transfusion reactions discussed later in this chapter, cause this type of anemia, as do certain parasites (malaria) and toxins (streptococcal infections).

Aplastic anemia   X rays and other forms of radiation and some drugs can damage bone marrow and suppress hemopoiesis. Aplastic anemia occurs when red blood cell production fails. (The term *aplastic* is derived from the roots *a*, meaning not, and *plasia*, meaning to form.) In leukemia excessive production of white cells in bone marrow suppress normal red cell production. The treatment of leukemia suppresses white cell division, removing the cause of red cell suppression. Such treatment is difficult because it requires sufficient chemotherapy or radiation therapy to suppress the malignant cells without suppressing normal cell production. Bone marrow transplants from compatible siblings to aplastic recipients are sometimes used today.

Pernicious anemia   In some individuals the glands of the stomach lining fail to produce a substance called intrinsic factor, which is required for the absorption of vitamin B_{12} from the intestinal tract. The resulting deficiency of the vitamin is called pernicious anemia. Vitamin B_{12} is essential for the formation of erythrocytes, and without it the erythrocytes are abnormally large and irregular in shape. Their membranes are especially fragile, and they have a shorter than normal lifespan. Individuals with pernicious anemia

may receive vitamin B_{12} injections at regular intervals throughout life, thus bypassing the absorptive difficulty.

Sickle cell anemia   In sickle cell anemia a mutant gene directs the synthesis of abnormal hemoglobin molecules. Though the abnormal hemoglobin molecule differs from normal hemoglobin by only a single amino acid, it affects the function of erythrocytes significantly. After such hemoglobin molecules unload oxygen in the tissues, the molecules tend to stick to one another, forming fibrils within the erythrocytes. These fibrils deform the red cells into a sickle shape, hence the name of the disease (Figure 16.6). The abnormally shaped cells aggregate in the blood vessels and block circulation. Pain in bones and joints, probably due to occluded vessels, is a common complaint of individuals with sickle cell anemia. Treatment includes transfusions to replace the damaged cells and medications to alleviate pain.

Individuals who have sickle cell anemia have inherited an abnormal gene from each of their parents. As genes occur in pairs, some individuals have one sickle cell gene and one gene for normal hemoglobin; they are said to have sickle cell trait. Though they do not have anemia, they can transmit the defective gene to their offspring. (See Chapter 27 for a discussion of mechanisms of inheritance.)

Polycythemia

In contrast to anemia, **polycythemia** is a condition in which abnormally large numbers of erythrocytes are produced. As much as 65% of the volume of the blood may be composed of cells, and the proportion of plasma is correspondingly

---

Hemolytic anemia can be caused by an autoimmune reaction in which the individual's body forms antibodies against its own red blood cells. In hemolytic anemia erythropoietin is produced in larger than normal quantities, increasing red cell production to compensate for premature destruction and releasing immature red cells into the blood stream. Jaundice, a yellowing of the skin due to the accumulation of bilirubin, may be seen in severe cases. Treatment is directed toward removing the causative agent if possible. Transfusions are used only in severe cases where compensation has failed or destruction has accelerated.

The sickle cell gene is most common in populations whose ancestors came from subtropical Africa, from the Mediterranean area, or from parts of Asia—areas where the parasitic disease malaria was once common. The presence of one sickle cell gene greatly increases one's resistance to malaria because erythrocytes containing parasites sickle and are removed by the spleen. In an area where the population was exposed to malaria, many who did not have the gene died of malaria. The surviving population therefore includes a large proportion of individuals who carry one sickle cell gene.

reduced. The blood is viscous and flows slowly through the blood vessels. In spite of the fact that there are many erythrocytes, the tissues fail to receive enough oxygen because of the slow movement of the blood. A malignancy of the red cells is one cause of polycythemia. High volumes of red cells can also be caused by prolonged, strenuous activity at high altitudes, but this condition is not thought to be pathological.

Leukemias

Leukemia is a cancerous disease of the white blood cell–forming tissues. In its acute form it can lead to death in a matter of months, but in its chronic form it can allow survival for years.

Two major types of leukemia have been identified, lymphoid and myeloid. In **lymphoid** leukemia the lymphocytes of the lymph nodes or other lymphatic tissues produce large numbers of abnormal cells called lymphoblasts. In **myeloid** leukemia the bone marrow produces large numbers of immature neutrophils and other leukocytes. The bone marrow activity is diverted to producing leukemic cells rather than other cells, leading to anemia, decreased platelets and bleeding, and a tendency to develop bacterial infections because of the reduced numbers of normal neutrophils. Regardless of the type, leukemia is characterized by abnormal leukocytes, many of which are not fully mature cells.

Infectious Mononucleosis

Infectious mononucleosis, sometimes called the kissing disease because it is transmitted through close contact, most frequently affects children and young adults. It is caused by Epstein-Barr virus, which infects lymphocytes and nasal and pharyngeal cells.

Symptoms of infectious mononucleosis include a severe sore throat, enlarged lymph nodes, fever, and tiredness. The disease is mentioned here because it causes a significant increase in the number of leukocytes in circulation and an increase in the percentage of lymphocytes. A diagnostic test is based on the fact that an antibody in the blood of individuals with infectious mononucleosis clumps, or agglutinates, sheep red blood cells. Treatment involves alleviating the symptoms and watching for complications. Complications are rare, but they may include rupture of the spleen, neurological disorders, hepatitis, and autoimmune reactions affecting red cells or platelets. Recovery usually takes several weeks and is generally complete.

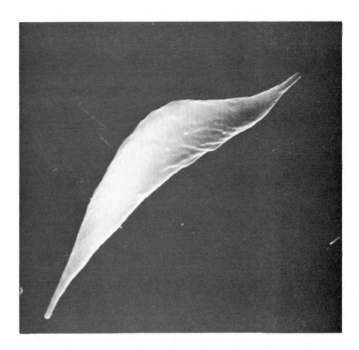

Figure 16.6   A scanning electron micrograph of a sickled erythrocyte. (Courtesy of Amanda Tuley and Robert Chilcote, M.D., University of Chicago, Comprehensive Study of Sickle Cell Disease Center.)

Before the 1960s acute lymphoid leukemia, the most common form of childhood leukemia, was almost invariably fatal. Since that time several chemotherapeutic drugs used in combination have been found effective in producing remissions of the disease. During the remissions the patients are symptom free. In most cases complete remissions for several years are now obtained. Researchers at St. Jude Children's Research Hospital in Memphis, Tennessee, followed the fates of over 600 children treated between 1962 and 1975. Of these patients 44% were completely free of the disease for two and one-half years, at which time they stopped therapy. Among these disease-free patients 80% have not had a relapse in four years following the cessation of therapy, and none of the patients that remained healthy for four years had a later relapse. Similar results have been obtained by investigators of the Children's Cancer Study Group at major university hospitals across the United States. They find that, in groups of children between the ages of two and ten with a white cell count under 10,000, given proper therapy, more than 80% are free of the disease five years later.

BLOOD TYPES AND TRANSFUSIONS

Objective 5. Describe the nature of ABO and Rh blood types; explain their roles in transfusions and in ascertaining parentage.

Like all cell membranes, the membranes of erythrocytes contain glycoproteins, some of which behave as antigens. An **antigen** is a substance, usually a protein, that can stimulate the production of another specific kind of protein, called an **antibody**, that will react specifically with the antigen. Once produced, antibodies circulate in the blood as part of the gamma globulins, a group of plasma proteins. Because they are involved in immunity, antigens and antibodies will be discussed in more detail in Chapter 20.

Here we are interested in antigens that are present on the membranes of erythrocytes, and in antibodies in the plasma that are capable of reacting with those antigens. The antigens found on erythrocytes determine a person's blood type. In normal human blood antibodies that react with the antigens are not present; the inadvertent mixing of bloods that contain a matching antigen and antibody causes what is known as a transfusion reaction. Because such a reaction agglutinates human erythrocytes, the antigens are sometimes called **agglutinogens** and the antibodies **agglutinins**.

The ABO Blood Types

The **ABO blood types** are based on the presence of two antigens or agglutinogens, designated A and B. If a person's erythrocytes have antigen A, the person has type A blood; if they have antigen B, the person has type B blood. If both antigens A and B are present, the blood is type AB; if neither is present, the blood is type O.

Which antigens are present on the erythrocytes is determined by information in the individual's genes. The actual combination of genes a person has for a given trait is called the **genotype** for that trait. Each person has two genes that determine the ABO genotype from among the three kinds of genes that may be present. These three genes are called A, B, and O. Genes A and B provide information for the synthesis of antigens A and B, respectively; gene O lacks the information needed to make any antigen. Thus, the possible genotypes are AA, AO, BB, BO, AB, and OO. Genotypes AA and AO produce type A blood, genotypes BB and BO produce type B blood, genotype AB produces type AB blood, and genotype OO produces type O blood. The blood type is called the **phenotype**—the observable characteristic produced by the genotype. Note that the A phenotype can be produced by two genotypes: AA and AO. The same is true for the B phenotype. (See Chapter 27 for more information on inheritance of genetically determined characteristics.)

Antibodies, or agglutinins, for both A and B antigens exist. We will call these antibodies a and b, respectively. Note that gene O produces no antigen, so there is no corresponding antibody o. As we shall see in Chapter 20, the particular antibodies present in plasma are allowed to develop during embryonic life so that an individual normally has no matching antigens and antibodies. For example, the plasma of a person with type A blood contains antibody b, and the plasma of a person with type B blood contains antibody a. Type AB blood contains neither antibody, and type O blood contains both a and b antibodies. Thus, an individual's plasma contains all the types of a and b antibodies it can without causing agglutination. Information about genes, antigens, and antibodies is summarized in Table 16.4 and Figure 16.7.

The ABO blood types are not equally distributed among the races of humans. Large numbers of Oriental people have type B blood, and many native Americans have type O blood. The percentages of blood types among whites and blacks in the United States are presented in Table 16.4.

If blood is mixed in such a way as to bring together matching antigens and antibodies, the red blood cells will agglutinate. Though some **agglutination** can take place in all the combinations listed under agglutination in Table 16.4, the more serious transfusion reactions occur when the antigens of donor cells match antibodies of the recipient's plasma. The larger volume of recipient blood compared to the volume of donor blood provides a great number of antibodies that are able to agglutinate donor cells. Reactions may occur when the antigens of the recipient's cells match the antibodies in the donor blood, but these are generally less serious. In this case there are large numbers of recipient cells, and the plasma of the donor blood is diluted as it is transfused; the likelihood of small numbers of donor antibodies agglutinating large numbers of the recipient's cells is minimal.

The most serious consequence of a transfusion reaction is **renal** (kidney) **failure**, which may involve at least three factors: (1) As red blood cells are destroyed, they release a substance that causes constriction of blood vessels, especially those in the kidney. (2) Small blood vessels may become blocked. (3) Large quantities of hemoglobin and red cell membranes damage renal tissue.

The possible problems entailed in antigen–antibody matching in transfusions have led to the concepts of universal donors and universal recipients. Individuals with type O blood have been called "universal donors" because their blood contains neither A nor B antigens. Conversely, people with type AB blood have been called "universal

Table 16.4 Characteristics of ABO Blood Types

Blood Type	Genes	Agglutinogens on Cells	Agglutinins in Plasma	Agglutination		Distribution	
				Plasma Causes Agglutination of Blood Types:	Cells Agglutinated by Plasma of Blood Types:	Whites % population	Blacks % population
A	AA, AO	A	b	B, AB	B, O	41	27
B	BB, BO	B	a	A, AB	A, O	10	20
AB	AB	AB	none	none	A, B, O	4	7
O	OO	none	a, b	A, B, AB	none	45	46

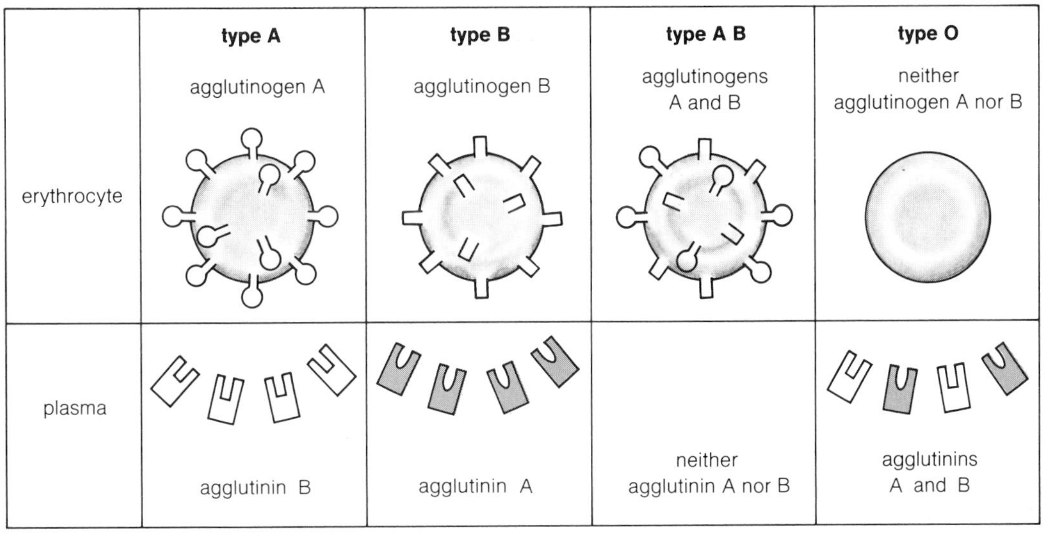

Figure 16.7 Agglutinogens (antigens) and agglutinins (antibodies) for each of the blood types in the ABO system. Note that antigens are on the erythrocytes, and antibodies are in the plasma.

recipients" because their blood contains neither a nor b antibodies. However, application of the concepts of universal donor and universal recipient is not a sufficient precaution in transfusions because there are many other types of antigens and antibodies in human blood. In addition to the Rh blood types to be discussed in the next section, human blood contains other antigens such as M, N, Kell, Duffy, Lewis, and Lutheran. The presence of each antigen is genetically determined and, though transfusion reactions are rare, they cannot be ignored.

Today, bloods are carefully cross-matched before each transfusion is given. Cross-matching involves mixing a sample of the recipient's cells with donor plasma and mixing a sample of the donor cells with the recipient's plasma. If no agglutination occurs in either mixture, the transfusion can safely proceed.

The Rh Blood Types

Rh blood type is another important consideration in the matching of blood for transfusion. Named for the Rhesus monkey, where it was first identified, the Rh factor, like A, B, and other factors, consists of antigens on the membranes of the erythrocytes. A person who has an Rh antigen on the red blood cells is said to be Rh-positive, and one who does not is said to be Rh-negative. Unlike the ABO group, where nonmatching antibodies are normally present (b in type A blood, for example), Rh antibodies are not normally present in human blood. They are produced only by Rh-negative individuals in response to the presence of Rh antigen. Should an Rh-negative person accidentally receive a transfusion that contains Rh antigens, the person's body will begin to make Rh antibodies. Furthermore, if an Rh-negative mother gives birth to an Rh-positive infant, the condition **erythroblastosis fetalis** may occur in subsequent pregnancies involving an Rh-positive fetus. As shown in Figure 16.8, the antigens and antibodies behave as follows:

1. During a first pregnancy red cells bearing antigens from an Rh-positive fetus might enter the Rh-negative mother's blood system when the placenta separates from the uterine wall at the time of delivery and cause the mother's body to produce Rh antibodies.

2. During a second or subsequent pregnancy anti-Rh antibodies from the mother's blood cross the placenta, where they react with and damage the red blood cells of the Rh-positive fetus.

An Rh-negative woman can have an Rh-positive child only if the father contributes an Rh-positive gene to the child. About 12% of U.S. marriages are between an Rh-negative woman and an Rh-positive man. Overall, the chances of such couples having an Rh-positive child are about 3 in 5. A father who carries two Rh-positive genes will always contribute such a gene to his offspring, and all offspring will be Rh-positive; a father who carries one Rh-positive gene and one Rh-negative gene has a 50% chance of transmitting an Rh-positive gene to each child.

Erythroblastosis fetalis was once a life-threatening condition, and the fetus often required a complete blood transfusion at birth to provide it with red blood cells not bearing the Rh antigen and to remove plasma containing the Rh antibody. Today, an Rh-negative mother is given a gamma globulin containing Rh antibodies that inactivates fetal Rh antigens that may have entered her body. This treatment must be given within 72 hours after delivery, abortion, or miscarriage of each Rh-positive fetus from an Rh-negative mother so that the mother's antibody-producing system will not be stimulated by fetal red cells to begin producing antibodies against the Rh antigen. When the treatment is used, Rh-negative mothers can expect to give birth to normal Rh-positive infants in the future. If the treatment is not used, each subsequent pregnancy involving an Rh-positive fetus will probably result in a fetus more seriously affected than the one before. The increasing damage to the fetus occurs as the mother's body produces larger numbers of antibodies with each subsequent exposure to the Rh antigen.

Use of Blood Types in Ascertaining Parentage

The blood type of a child is determined by the genes inherited from its parents. Information about which antigens are present in the mother's and the child's blood helps to determine which antigens the father could have. For example, if a child has type AB blood and the mother has type A blood, the father must have either type B or AB blood. Tests involving only ABO blood types may prove a man *not* to be the father of a child, but they cannot necessarily prove that he *is* the father. Tests involving antigens from infant and maternal tissues other than blood now provide more precise information about the antigens the father must have; these tests increase the likelihood of determining parentage.

HEMOSTASIS AND ITS DISORDERS

Objective 6. Describe the process of hemostasis and distinguish between the extrinsic and intrinsic mechanisms of blood clotting.

Objective 7. Explain how the following are related to hemostasis: (a) anticoagulants, (b) hemophilia, and (c) thrombi and emboli.

Hemostasis

Hemostasis is the arrest of bleeding. Any animal with a circulatory system must have a mechanism to stop bleeding when a blood vessel is severed. Furthermore, this mechanism must not interfere with the normal circulation of blood; that is, it must not arrest the flow except when there is an injury.

Three processes are involved in hemostasis following injury to a small blood vessel: (1) blood vessel spasm, (2) formation of a platelet plug, and (3) coagulation of the blood around the injury.

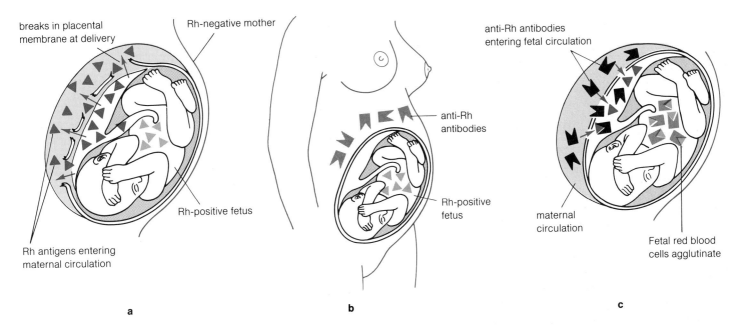

Figure 16.8 Erythroblastosis fetalis. (**a**) Red cells bearing antigens from an Rh-positive fetus cross the placenta, usually during delivery, and enter the mother's bloodstream. (**b**) Unless treated with Rh antibodies to react with the antigens, the mother's body produces antibodies that will damage the red blood cells of a future fetus. (**c**) If a subsequent pregnancy occurs in an untreated mother, antibodies will enter the fetal circulation during development and destroy many of the fetus's red blood cells.

Blood vessel spasm   When a small vessel (an arteriole or a venule) is injured, the smooth muscle in its walls contracts. The contraction apparently is stimulated directly by the injury and possibly also by nerve impulses from the pain receptors in the injured tissue. The contraction may be sufficient to close the severed ends of the blood vessel and press the linings of the vessel together. A stickiness of the lining cells (endothelium) helps to hold them together. The duration of the contraction may exceed half an hour; it lasts longer in larger vessels than it does in smaller ones.

Formation of a platelet plug   Platelets normally move freely through the lumen (internal channel) of blood vessels. However, if there is a roughened endothelial surface and underlying collagen is exposed, platelets adhere to the collagen. The adhering platelets are somehow stimulated to release several kinds of chemicals, one of which is adenosine diphosphate (ADP). ADP increases the stickiness of the platelets so that circulating platelets adhere to those already attached to the collagen. In this example of positive feedback (stickiness produces more stickiness) the clump of platelets rapidly increases in size. The platelets also release epinephrine and serotonin, both of which stimulate further constriction of the blood vessels.

The processes of blood vessel spasm and platelet plug formation are summarized in Figure 16.9.

Coagulation of blood   Although bleeding from small injuries may be stopped by the above processes, blood coagulation usually occurs as a part of hemostasis. Two mechanisms for the initiation of blood coagulation exist, the extrinsic mechanism that is triggered by injury and the intrinsic mechanism that is triggered by abnormalities in the linings of blood vessels. Regardless of the mechanism of initiation, the two pathways converge, and the final steps of the coagulation process are the same (Figure 16.10): The end product is a blood clot. Coagulation factors are listed in Table 16.5.

The **extrinsic mechanism** of blood coagulation is activated by tissue damage. In addition to causing blood vessel spasm and platelet plug formation, the damaged tissue releases a lipoprotein, **thromboplastin**. With the help of calcium ions and other coagulation factors, thromboplastin activates factor X.

The **intrinsic mechanism** of blood coagulation is activated by the presence of small ruptures or roughened areas along the internal surfaces of blood vessels. Platelets adhere to these areas and release platelet coagulation factors into the plasma. Both platelet factors and plasma factors participate in a cascade of reactions, which activate factor X.

Once factor X is activated, the pathways converge. A protein, **prothrombin**, is normally present in the blood. Prothrombin is activated by coagulation factors and becomes **thrombin**. Another inactive protein, **fibrinogen**, is also normally present in the plasma.

Thrombin and certain coagulation factors cause fibrinogen to be activated and become **fibrin**, the substance of the clot. It is a fibrous protein that forms a loose meshwork over the injured area. Blood cells become trapped in the meshwork, reinforce the platelet plug, and close off the opening.

After a half-hour or more, the clot retracts and becomes smaller and more dense. This retraction is thought to be due to the action of platelets trapped in the clot. As the fibrin filaments gather around the platelet aggregation, the platelets send out cytoplasmic processes that attach to the fibrin and pull the fibers closer together. When a clot forms in a test tube, fluid is squeezed from the clot. This fluid, plasma minus the substances involved in clot formation, is called serum.

Blood clots are temporary structures that seal off a damaged area until healing can take place. As healing occurs, the clots themselves are dissolved by an enzyme called **plasmin**. Inactive plasmin circulates in the plasma along with other inactive factors until there is an injury. At the time of the formation of thromboplastin, coagulation factor XII activates plasmin, small amounts of which become trapped in the clot. Plasmin is a slow-acting proteolytic enzyme that gradually dissolves away the clot as tissue repair is taking place.

The coagulation factors   As shown in Table 16.5, each of the substances involved in the coagulation mechanisms has a factor number. It should be noted that factor IV consists of calcium ions. Though this factor is involved in some way in many of the steps in the clotting process, it is generally available in sufficient quantities in blood that deficiency is not a problem. It should also be noted that factors II, VII, IX, and X require vitamin K for their synthesis. Therefore, vitamin K is essential to the normal clotting of blood. It is often given before surgery to individuals who might have deficient intake or absorption of this vitamin.

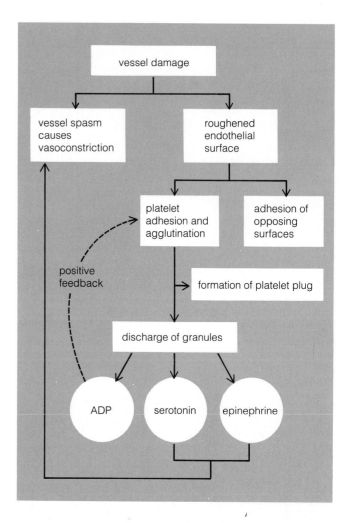

Figure 16.9   Summary of the events involved in hemostasis prior to blood coagulation.

Anticoagulants   **Anticoagulants** are substances that reduce the ability of blood to clot by interfering with any of the reactions in the clotting mechanisms. Anticoagulants are used to reduce clotting in individuals who are susceptible to clot formation. In addition, they are used in the laboratory to prevent blood samples from clotting before certain tests can be run on them. Heparin, a substance produced by the body, interferes with the activation of several clotting factors. It can be injected into the body or used in the laboratory. Another substance, dicumarol, competes with vitamin K and interferes with the synthesis of factors V and VII in the liver. It takes up to two days to act, but it has a longer lasting effect than heparin and can be taken orally. Most laboratory anticoagulants bind to calcium ions in the blood and thus interfere with the clotting reactions. They include sodium citrate and ammonium oxalate.

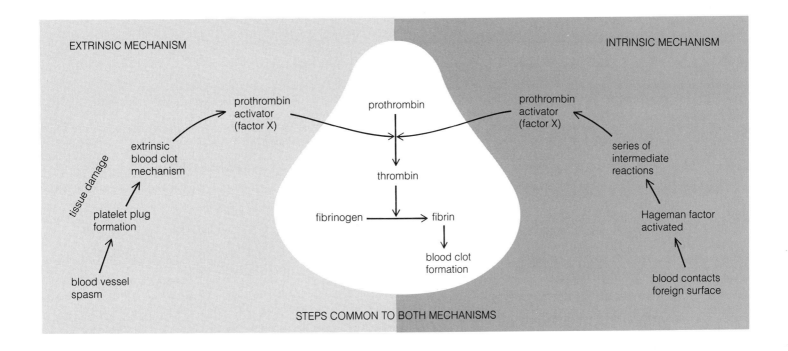

EXTRINSIC MECHANISM

INTRINSIC MECHANISM

prothrombin
activator
(factor X)

prothrombin

prothrombin
activator
(factor X)

extrinsic
blood clot
mechanism

thrombin

series of
intermediate
reactions

tissue damage

fibrinogen → fibrin

platelet plug
formation

Hageman factor
activated

blood clot
formation

blood vessel
spasm

blood contacts
foreign surface

STEPS COMMON TO BOTH MECHANISMS

a

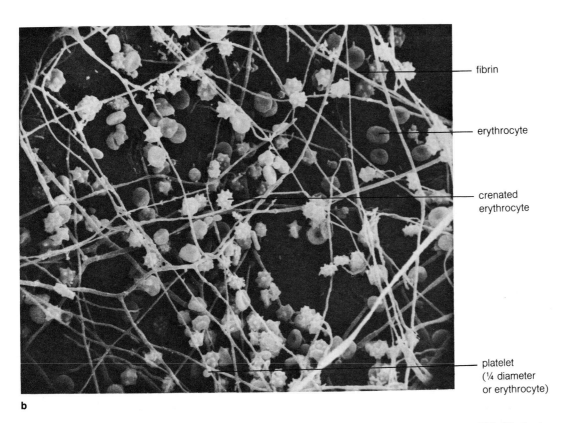

fibrin

erythrocyte

crenated
erythrocyte

platelet
(¼ diameter
or erythrocyte)

b

Figure 16.10 (**a**) Mechanism of blood coagulation, (**b**) a thrombus, or clot, within a blood vessel, × 598. (Photomicrograph reproduced with permission from *Tissues and organs: A text-atlas of scanning electron microscopy* by Richard G. Kessel and Randy H. Kardon. W. H. Freeman and Company. Copyright © 1979.)

Table 16.5 Blood Coagulation Factors

Number	Factor Name	Nature and Origin	Function
I	Fibrinogen	Protein synthesized in liver	Precursor of fibrin, the substance of the clot
II	Prothrombin	Protein synthesized in liver; synthesis requires vitamin K	Precursor of thrombin, which converts fibrinogen to fibrin
III	Thromboplastin	Lipoprotein formed from tissues or platelet disintegration	Catalyzes thrombin formation
IV*	Calcium ions	Inorganic ion present in plasma	Necessary for reactions in all stages of process
V	Proaccelerin or labile factor	Protein synthesized in liver	Required for extrinsic and intrinsic mechanisms
VI	(Number no longer used; substance now thought to be the same as V)		
VII	SPCA (serum prothrombin conversion accelerator)	Substance synthesized in liver; synthesis requires vitamin K	Necessary for extrinsic mechanism
VIII	Antihemophilic factor	Globulin synthesized in liver and other tissues; absence is inherited disorder, hemophilia A	Necessary for intrinsic mechanism
IX	PTC (plasma thrombo-plastin component), or Christmas factor	Protein synthesized in liver; absence is inherited disorder, hemophilia B; synthesis requires vitamin K	Necessary for intrinsic mechanism
X	Stuart-Power factor	Substance synthesized in liver; synthesis requires vitamin K	Necessary for extrinsic and intrinsic mechanisms
XI	PTA (plasma thrombo-plastin antecedent)	Protein synthesized in liver	Necessary for intrinsic mechanism
XII	Hageman factor	Source unknown; proteolytic enzyme	Necessary for intrinsic mechanism and to activate plasmin
XIII	FSF (fibrin stabiliz-ing factor)	Source unknown	Renders fibrin insoluble
Pf_1	Platelet accelerator	Platelets; same as factor V	Accelerates action of platelets
Pf_2	Thrombin accelerator	Platelets; phospholipid	Accelerates thrombin formation
Pf_3	Platelet thrombo-plastic factor	Platelets; phospholipid	Necessary for intrinsic mechanism
Pf_4	Platelet factor 4	Platelets	Binds heparin, a natural anticoagulant, during clotting

*IV no longer used; referred to simply as Ca^{2+}

Disorders of Hemostasis

Hemophilia   **Hemophilia** is a group of related inherited diseases. In each type a genetic defect prevents the synthesis of one of the coagulation factors. The most common, hemophilia A, is due to the absence of factor VIII. Next most common, Christmas disease, or hemophilia B, is due to the absence of factor IX. Both of these conditions are inherited as sex-linked, recessive characteristics and affect males almost exclusively. The missing factors are all essential for the intrinsic mechanism of clotting. Symptoms of hemophilia generally include ease of internal bleeding from even mild injuries, especially in joints where vessels are continually subject to twisting and distortion.

Thrombi and emboli   A **thrombus** is a clot that has formed within an intact blood vessel. An **embolus** is a thrombus that has broken away from the site of formation and is traveling within the blood vessels. Several theories have been proposed to explain the formation of clots in intact blood vessels. Roughened areas in the lining of blood vessels seem to be the most likely initiators of the clotting process. Platelets adhere to these areas just as they do to injured areas. Once a small group of platelets has adhered to an area, the conditions are set for the clot to enlarge. Two other causes include sluggish blood flow, particularly in the leg veins because of defective valves or lack of activity, and inflammations in any vessels due to infections or toxic substances.

Once a clot has formed, it is potentially dangerous. If it remains attached (a thrombus), it can occlude a vessel and reduce blood supply to surrounding tissues. If it breaks loose (an embolus), it can travel to a smaller but essential vessel and occlude it.

CLINICAL TERMS

citrated whole blood   blood to which citrate has been added to prevent coagulation by binding to calcium

disseminated intravascular coagulation   a disorder in which extensive clotting in some parts of the body and hemorrhage in other parts of the body occur simultaneously

embolism (em'bol-izm)   the blocking of a blood vessel by a clot that has been traveling in the blood, as from a vessel in the leg to one in the lungs

eosinophilia (e″o-sin-o-fil'e-ah)   the presence of excessive numbers of eosinophils, often associated with allergies or worm infestations

hemolysis (hem-ol'is-is)   the rupture of erythrocytes, releasing hemoglobin

macrocytosis (mak″ro-si-to'sis)   the presence of abnormally large erythrocytes

microcytosis (mik″ro-si-to'sis)   the presence of abnormally small erythrocytes

neutrophilia (nu-tro-fil'e-ah)   the presence of excessive numbers of neutrophils, often associated with an infection

purpura (pur'pu-rah)   the presence of purplish patches on the skin and mucous membranes as a result of ruptured subcutaneous blood vessels

septicemia (sep-tis-e'me-ah)   the presence of pathogenic bacteria in the blood

thrombosis (throm-bo'sis)   the formation of a clot (thrombus) that remains in a blood vessel or heart chamber where it was formed

Essay: The Role of Blood in Diagnosis and Therapy

Blood plays an exceedingly important role in the diagnosis of human disease as it is easily obtained and circulates to all tissues, thereby reflecting their physiological state. Chemical tests and counts of the various kinds of blood cells provide information about abnormalities in nearly every system of the body. Furthermore, blood tests can be performed on a small sample of blood with a minimum of discomfort and inconvenience to the individual involved.

From years of accumulated observations, the normal range of concentrations is known for an enormous number of substances found in the blood. Some of the substances most frequently studied are described in Table 16.6.

Counts of the numbers of red blood cells and white blood cells in a given volume of blood are also used for diagnostic purposes. Excesses of white blood cells often indicate a bacterial infection. A differential count, in which the percentages of each type of leukocyte are determined, can be used in the diagnosis of leukemia, mononucleosis, various bacterial and viral infections, worm infestations, and other diseases. Counts of both red and white cells are used to diagnose leukemia, and the morphology of the red cells themselves may suggest sickle cell or other kinds of anemia. The hematocrit, or packed cell volume, is also related to the number of red blood cells. Because most of the cells in blood are red blood cells, the volume of cells in a centrifuged sample of blood provides a reasonably accurate measure of the number of red cells when the cells are of normal size. Platelet counts can also be done; a reduced platelet count may indicate an aplastic bone marrow or overly rapid destruction by antibodies.

Finally, serological (serology = study of serum) tests are available to determine the presence of many different kinds of antibodies. Some of these tests are helpful, for example, in diagnosing autoimmune diseases.

Though blood is useful for these and other diagnostic purposes, its value in therapy should not be overlooked. Nearly all medications reach the cells they affect by traveling through the bloodstream. One of the reasons some medications are given round the clock is that to be effective their concentration must be maintained at a nearly constant high level in the bloodstream. For this reason extensive research is underway to develop implantable drug-delivery systems. Some of these involve the surgical implantation of a drug pellet, the placement of a reservoir that can be refilled with a hypodermic syringe, or a pump filled with a fluorocarbon propellant that maintains a constant pressure and thus a constant supply of the drug.

In some circumstances natural components of the blood can be used therapeutically. For example, heparin is used to prevent or limit the ability of the blood to clot.

Blood itself in such forms as red cells, plasma, or platelets has therapeutic uses. Transfusion to compensate for blood loss following injuries or surgery is the most common of these uses. Individuals with platelet deficiencies sometimes can be treated with platelet transfusions, leaving the remaining fractions of the same blood for use in treating others. Certain fractions can be used to replace clotting factors missing in individuals with hemophilia. Blood plasma alone can be used to increase the blood volume following hemorrhage with little risk of a transfusion reaction if blood typing facilities are not available or the correct type of blood cannot be found.

Recent advances in the development of synthetic blood have made possible its use as a substitute for real blood, at least experimentally. Synthetic blood consists of an emulsion of

Table 16.6 Blood Components and Their Use in Diagnosis and Management of Disease	
Blood Component	Used in Diagnosis and Management of:
Glucose	Diabetes mellitus, hypoglycemia
Cholesterol, lipids and lipoproteins	Heart and blood vessel diseases
Proteins	Kidney disease, malnutrition, impaired amino acid absorption
Enzymes	Tissue damage, which allows enzymes to leak into blood
Uric acid	Gout, kidney disease
Bilirubin	Excessive breakdown of erythrocytes, liver disease, blockage of bile ducts
Blood urea nitrogen (BUN)	Kidney failure
Electrolytes (Na^+, K^+, Cl^-, etc.)	Kidney function, metabolic function
Blood gases (CO_2 and O_2)	Kidney and lung function
pH	Acidosis, alkalosis
Hormones	Endocrine disorders

perfluorocarbons—hydrocarbons in which some of the hydrogen atoms have been replaced by fluorine atoms. These perfluorocarbons are able to carry large quantities of oxygen to the cells of the body until additional blood becomes available. Tests with healthy volunteers have so far shown no harmful side effects from the use of synthetic blood. Synthetic blood may provide an answer to the problem of treating individuals whose religious or other beliefs prevent them from receiving blood or those for whom the appropriate type of blood is not available.

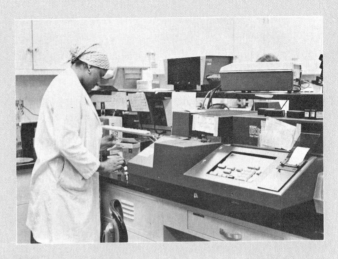

Figure 16.12 The equipment shown here is used to measure blood urea nitrogen, uric acid, calcium, and glucose. The technician is preparing to place a sample in the machine. (Photograph by author; arrangements courtesy of Children's Hospital National Medical Center, Washington, D.C.)

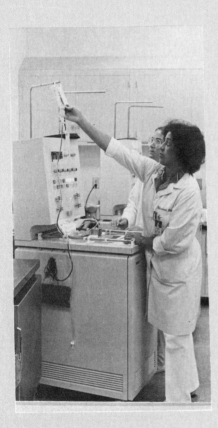

Figure 16.11 A student looks on as a technician operates a blood washing machine. Blood is often washed in this manner prior to transfusion to remove fragments of dead white and red blood cells. Students receive valuable experience by assisting technicians in a laboratory. (Photograph by author; arrangements courtesy of Childrens Hospital National Medical Center, Washington, D.C.)

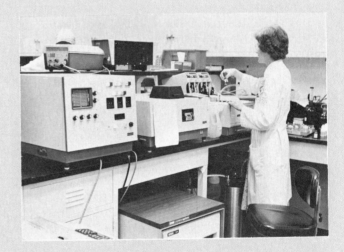

Figure 16.13 The technician in this photograph is analyzing the enzymes found in a blood sample. Elevated enzymes are indicative of tissue damage; the particular enzyme that is elevated may indicate which tissue is damaged. For example, if liver cells are being destroyed by some disease process, specific enzymes from liver cells are found in the blood. (Phogograph by author; arrangements courtesy of Childrens Hospital National Medical Center, Washington, D.C.)

CHAPTER SUMMARY

(Chapter summary points and review questions are numbered to correspond to the numbered objectives in the text of each chapter.)

Organization and General Functions

1. (a) Describe the organization of the circulatory system and the role of blood in it; (b) name the main components of blood and list the major functions of blood.
   a. The circulatory system consists of:
      (1) the heart that pumps blood through the circulatory system
      (2) a closed system of blood vessels that carry blood to and from nearly every cell in the body
      (3) blood, the fluid inside the blood vessels
   b. The main components of blood include:
      (1) formed elements—erythrocytes, leukocytes, and platelets
      (2) plasma, the liquid portion of blood, which contains many important substances
   c. The functions of blood include:
      (1) transport of nutrients, gases, waste products, and hormones
      (2) protection against invasion of microorganisms and damage from toxic substances
      (3) clotting, which prevents blood loss
      (4) participation in the regulation of the water content of cells, the pH of body fluids, and body temperature

Development

2. Describe the development of the formed elements of blood.
   a. Hemopoiesis, or hematopoiesis, is the formation of blood cells.
   b. Erythrocytes, leukocytes, and platelets are formed from stem cells in the bone marrow of an adult, as shown in Figure 16.2.
   c. In the fetus blood cells also form in the liver, spleen, thymus gland, and lymph nodes.

Blood as a Tissue

3. List the components of blood, their characteristics, and the amounts of each component normally present.
   a. In normal blood approximately 55% is plasma, and the remainder consists of cells and platelets.
   b. The liquid plasma is the carrier of many substances including gases, electrolytes, nutrients, hormones, and wastes. Some substances, especially cholesterol, are carried on proteins in the plasma.

   c. Other proteins in the plasma are involved in maintaining osmotic pressure, in immunity, and in the blood-clotting mechanism.
   d. Erythrocytes:
      (1) contain hemoglobin, the carrier molecule for oxygen and some carbon dioxide
      (2) live about 120 days in circulation and are replaced at a rate of about 2.5 million cells per second
   e. As erythrocytes die, their hemoglobin is degraded, the iron and amino acids reused, and the heme converted to bilirubin and subsequently excreted.
   f. Among the leukocytes neutrophils and monocytes are active phagocytic cells, while lymphocytes are primarily concerned with the development of immunity.
   g. Platelets are important in the clotting mechanism.
   h. The normal amounts of components of blood are summarized in Tables 16.2 and 16.3.

Disorders of Erythrocytes and Leukocytes

4. Describe the causes and effects of each of the following types of disorders: (a) anemias, (b) polycythemia, (c) leukemias, and (d) infectious mononucleosis.
   a. Anemia is a deficiency in the number of erythrocytes or a lack of hemoglobin; it can have a variety of causes. Its main effects are derived from the deficient oxygen-carrying capacity of the blood.
   b. Polycythemia, an excess of erythrocytes, may be caused by malignancy or the normal compensation for prolonged strenuous activity at high altitude.
   c. Leukemias are cancerous diseases in which excessive quantities of abnormal leukocytes are produced and replace the normal elements of bone marrow; their effects are due to poor function of leukoctyes and lack of other blood elements.
   d. Infectious mononucleosis, caused by a transmissible virus, is a disease of the young; its effects are produced by infecting lymphocytes and nasal and pharyngeal cells.

Blood Types and Transfusions

5. Describe the nature of ABO and Rh blood types; explain their roles in transfusions and in ascertaining parentage.
   a. Erythrocytes have proteins on their surfaces that act as antigens, and plasma contains antibodies.
   b. Blood types are identified by the antigens on the red cell surfaces.
   c. Transfusion reactions result from mixing matching antigens and antibodies and the subsequent agglutination of red blood cells.

d. Rh-negative mothers sometimes produce antibodies that damage the red cells of a developing Rh-positive fetus, causing erythroblastosis fetalis.

e. Parentage can sometimes be established by determining the blood types of mother, child, and possible fathers.

Hemostasis and Its Disorders

6. Describe the process of hemostasis and distinguish between the extrinsic and intrinsic mechanisms of blood clotting.

   a. Hemostasis, the arrest of bleeding, involves:

   (1) blood vessel spasm

   (2) formation of a platelet plug

   (3) coagulation of blood

   b. Coagulation can be initiated by extrinsic or intrinsic factors:

   (1) Extrinsic factors are released when tissue is injured.

   (2) Intrinsic factors are released when roughened areas or leaks develop within blood vessels.

   c. Coagulation results in the formation of a clot of fibrin. Many different chemical substances are involved in the process.

7. Explain how the following are related to hemostasis: (a) anticoagulants, (b) hemophilia, and (c) thrombi and emboli.

   a. Anticoagulants are substances that interfere with the clotting mechanism.

   b. Hemophilia is a group of inherited diseases in which one of the coagulation factors is missing.

   c. Thrombi and emboli are abnormal clots in intact blood vessels.

REVIEW

Important Terms

agglutination	hemophilia
anemia	hemopoiesis
antibody	hemostasis
anticoagulant	leukemia
antigen	leukocyte
basophil	lymphocyte
diapedesis	lymphoid
embolus	megakaryocyte
eosinophil	monocyte
erythrocyte	myeloid
erythropoietin	neutrophil
fibrin	plasma
fibrinogen	platelet
hemoglobin	polycythemia

prothrombin	thromboplastin
serum	thrombus
thrombin	

Questions

1. a. Of what does blood consist?

   b. What are the major functions of blood?

   c. What would happen to the body if an excessive amount of blood were lost?

2. a. What is hemopoiesis?

   b. What embryonic and adult tissue types can give rise to formed elements in the blood?

3. a. What substances are found in plasma?

   b. What are the functions of plasma?

   c. Describe the distinguishing characteristics of each of the formed elements in the blood.

   d. Define diapedesis, phagocytosis, and mast cell.

   e. What use might be made of knowing the normal values for each of the constituents of human blood?

   f. What happens to erythrocytes after they have circulated for about four months?

4. a. What is anemia?

   b. What are some factors that can produce anemia?

   c. How is it that cells are oxygen deficient in polycythemia?

   d. What is leukemia, and how can individuals with the disease have lowered resistance to infection?

5. a. Describe the antigens and antibodies found in the following blood types: A-Rh positive, B-Rh negative, AB-Rh positive, and O-Rh negative.

   b. Explain what happens in a transfusion reaction.

   c. How can erythroblastosis fetalis be prevented?

6. a. What is hemostasis, and what are the three processes involved in it?

   b. What is the difference between the intrinsic and the extrinsic blood-clotting mechanisms?

7. a. What is the difference between an internal and an external anticoagulant?

   b. What is hemophilia?

   c. Why are thrombi and emboli dangerous?

Problems

1. In first aid to an injured person pressure is often applied to a bleeding wound. Use your knowledge of physiology to explain how pressure stops bleeding.

2. Suppose you are working as a laboratory technician. How would you go about determining whether a certain person can receive a transfusion of a particular sample of blood? How would you distinguish anemia from leukemia? How would you distinguish a bacterial infection from infectious mononucleosis?

REFERENCES AND READINGS

Anonymous. 1979. Childhood leukemia: A 40 percent cure. *Science News* 115:133 (March 3).

Anonymous. 1979. Framework protein for blood cell flux. *Science News* 116:86 (August 4).

Anonymous. 1980. Predicting leukemia relapses. *Science News* 117:9 (January 5).

Arehart-Treichel, J. 1980. Artificial blood. *Science News* 117:237 (April 12).

Blackshear, P. J. 1979. Implantable drug-delivery systems. *Scientific American* 241(6):66 (December).

Guyton, A. C. 1981. *Textbook of medical physiology* (6th ed.). Philadelphia: W. B. Saunders.

Jaques, L. B. 1979. Heparin: An old drug with a new paradigm. *Science* 206:528 (November 2).

Marx, J. L. 1979. The HDL: The good cholesterol carrier. *Science* 205:677 (August 17).

Maugh, T. H. 1979. Blood substitute passes its first test. *Science* 206:205 (October 12).

Perutz, M. F. 1978. Hemoglobin structure and respiratory transport. *Scientific American* 239(6):92 (December).

Tilkian, S. M., Conover, M. B., and Tilkian, A. G. 1979. *Clinical implications of laboratory tests*. St. Louis, Mo.: C. V. Mosby.

Till, J. E. 1981. Cellular diversity in the blood forming system. *American Scientist* 69:522 (September–October).

Zucker, M. B. 1980. The functioning of blood platelets. *Scientific American* 242 (6): 86 (June).

17

CARDIOVASCULAR SYSTEM: THE HEART

ORGANIZATION AND GENERAL FUNCTION

Objective 1. Describe the general plan of the heart, its location, and its general function in the circulatory system.

Make a clenched fist. Slowly count to 70, opening and closing your fist with each count. Your heart is about the size of your clenched fist, and it contracts and relaxes about 70 times per minute throughout your life. Though the muscles of your hand would ache after a few minutes of contracting 70 times per minute, your heart is able to contract continually at that rate without fatigue. These contractions over a lifetime do enough work to lift a 10 ton weight to a height of 10 miles.

The heart is an important component of the circulatory system. It pumps the blood through the blood vessels (to be discussed in Chapters 18 and 19). It is a cone-shaped, hollow, muscular organ, measuring about 12 centimeters from base to apex, 9 centimeters in width at its widest point, and 6 centimeters in thickness. Inside, the heart consists of four chambers separated by valves and septa.

Skeletal landmarks that can be palpated (felt) through the skin help to define the location of the heart (Figure 17.1). The bulk of the heart lies beneath the sternum between the second and sixth ribs; the apex, or point, of the heart extends to the left of the sternum.

Internally, the heart is located in the thorax between the lungs in a cavity called the **mediastinum** (Figure 17.2). Within this cavity the heart itself is enclosed in a tough, loose-fitting membrane, the **pericardial sac**.

The heart is connected to the major blood vessels of the body, and these vessels are in turn connected to smaller vessels. Together, the heart and blood vessels form a closed

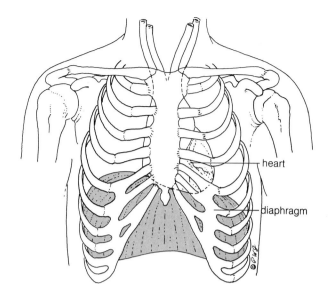

Figure 17.1 The location of the heart in relation to the ribs and sternum.

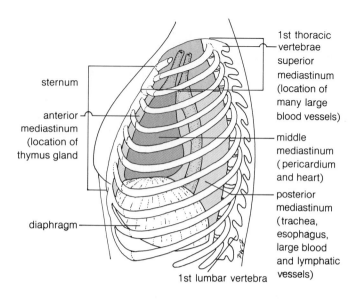

Figure 17.2 The location of the heart within the mediastinum, as seen in side view. The lungs have been removed in this figure.

system of tubes that carry blood to all parts of the body. The heart consists of two side-by-side pumps that force blood through the blood vessels. In this chapter we will consider the structure and function of the heart. Some aspects of the regulation of the circulation of blood through the heart will be considered in Chapter 19.

DEVELOPMENT

Objective 2. Describe the embryonic development of the heart.

Between the third and fifth weeks of development the heart consists of a simple, pulsating tube that receives blood from veins and pumps it out into arteries (Figure 17.3a). During the fifth week of development the heart grows rapidly and becomes S-shaped. It also twists around so that the venous end, which receives blood from the venae cavae, comes to lie behind and slightly superior to the arterial end. Septa (separating walls of tissue) grow inside the tube, dividing it into two tubes. Each tube develops into a "pump," one destined to supply the respiratory portion of the lungs through the pulmonary artery, the other to supply the remainder of the body through the aorta. The single tube is divided into the aorta and the pulmonary artery at about the

time that the arterial end of the heart is divided into two ventricles. At the same time the venous end is divided into two atria (plural of atrium). The atria are distinct by the end of the seventh week of development, but an opening, the **foramen ovale**, persists between them until birth. Likewise, a connection, the **ductus arteriosus**, persists between the aorta and the pulmonary artery. These openings permit blood to circulate through the body of the fetus, with about 15% of the blood passing through the lungs. During development the placenta (and not the lungs) functions as a respiratory organ for the fetus. The heart is the first major organ to become functional during embryonic development.

TISSUES

Objective 3. (a) Describe the tissue layers of the heart and the pericardium; (b) describe the properties of cardiac muscle.

The heart wall consists of three layers—the **endocardium**, the **myocardium**, and the **epicardium**, or visceral pericardium. The heart is surrounded by the **pericardial sac**, or **parietal pericardium**, which consists of two layers, the serous pericardium and the fibrous pericardium (Figure 17.4).

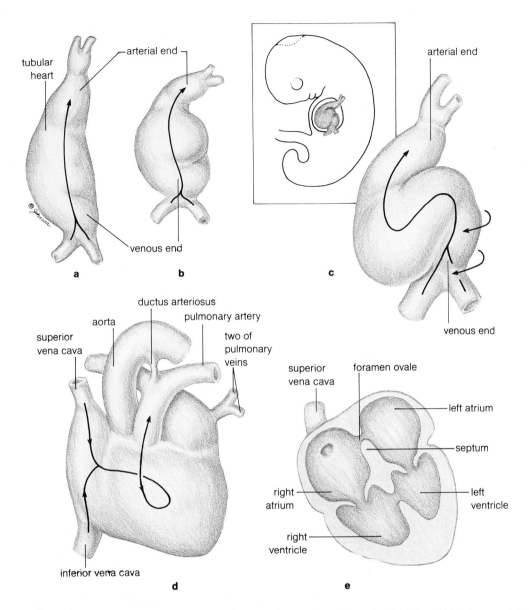

Figure 17.3 The development of the heart: (**a**) tubular heart at about five weeks, (**b**), (**c**), and (**d**) subsequent stages in the development of the heart over the next several weeks, (**e**) a section through the heart showing the development of the septum that divides the heart into four chambers.

The endocardium, a glistening membrane that lines the cavities and forms the valves of the heart, consists of a single layer of endothelial cells on the surface and several underlying layers of elastic connective tissue and smooth muscle cells. The endocardium is thicker in the atria than in the ventricles and is continuous with the linings of the blood vessels.

Beneath the endocardium in some parts of the heart is the specialized tissue, derived from muscle tissue, that is responsible for initiating and conducting impulses to cause the heart muscle to contract. It will be discussed in more detail later.

The myocardium, the muscular part of the heart, makes up about three-fourths of the heart's bulk. It is

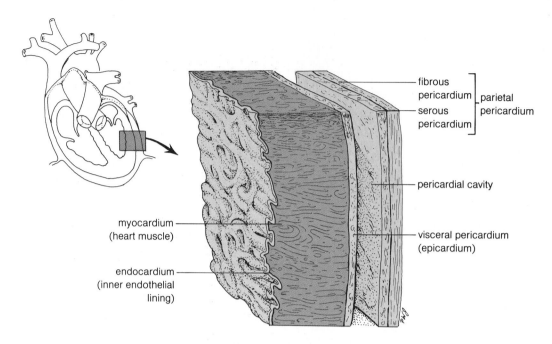

Figure 17.4 The tissue layers of the heart and pericardium.

composed of cardiac muscle. **Cardiac muscle** is similar to skeletal muscle in that it has striations, but it has several distinctive characteristics. Cardiac muscle contains myofilaments composed of actin and myosin like those in skeletal muscle and has a sarcoplasmic reticulum and T-tubules, which are found at the Z-lines, one per sarcomere. In contrast to long, multinucleated fibers of skeletal muscle, the fibers of cardiac muscle are branched and consist of a series of cells connected to each other by **intercalated discs**. (Refer back to Figure 4.19, Chapter 4.) The electrical resistance across intercalated discs is much less (1/400) than that across the external membranes of cardiac muscle fibers; ions flow freely across the intercalated discs, and action potentials easily move from one cardiac cell to the next. Because of the ease with which action potentials move across intercalated discs, cardiac muscle behaves as a syncytium (a multinucleate cellular mass that acts as a functional unit).

The myocardium is divided into two functional syncytia, the atrial syncytium and the ventricular syncytium, separated by the fibrous endocardial tissue of the heart valves. Each syncytium contracts separately, but the separate contractions are coordinated by the specialized conductive tissue of the myocardium.

The epicardium, or visceral pericardium, is a serous membrane that covers the muscular part of the heart. It is continuous with the serous portion of the parietal pericardium. Both of these serous membranes secrete a watery fluid into the space between them, the pericardial cavity. This serous secretion, the **pericardial fluid**, lubricates the surfaces of the membranes and reduces friction when the heart contracts and relaxes.

The pericardial sac, or parietal pericardium, includes not only the serous layer but also a fibrous layer, which gives it strength. The fibrous layer protects the heart.

Sometimes the pericardial membranes become inflamed so that they stick together and form adhesions. This condition is called **pericarditis**. The pericardial cavity can also become engorged with fluid or blood, producing a condition called **cardiac tamponade**. This excess fluid interferes with the filling of the chambers of the heart between contractions and greatly reduces the heart's efficiency.

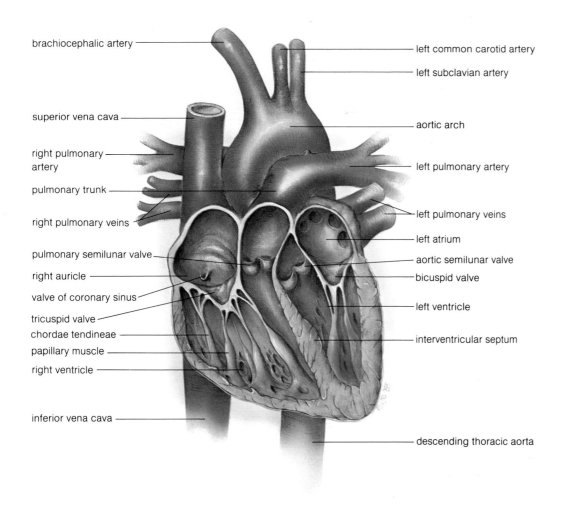

brachiocephalic artery

left common carotid artery

left subclavian artery

superior vena cava

aortic arch

right pulmonary artery

left pulmonary artery

pulmonary trunk

right pulmonary veins

left pulmonary veins

left atrium

pulmonary semilunar valve

aortic semilunar valve

right auricle

bicuspid valve

valve of coronary sinus

left ventricle

tricuspid valve

chordae tendineae

interventricular septum

papillary muscle

right ventricle

inferior vena cava

descending thoracic aorta

Figure 17.5   The internal anatomy of the heart in cross section, viewed anteriorly.

ANATOMY OF THE HEART

Objective 4. Describe the general anatomical plan of the heart and trace the flow of blood through the heart chambers.

Objective 5. Describe the circulation of blood through the heart wall itself.

The heart is a small but complex organ. To understand its function we will need to consider both its internal and its external structure.

Internal Anatomy of the Heart

The heart (Figure 17.5) is divided into left and right halves, each half operating as a separate pump. The right half re-
ceives blood from the systemic circulation (all of the organs except the lungs) and pumps blood to the lungs. The left half receives blood from the pulmonary circulation (lungs) and pumps it into the systemic circulation.

Each half of the heart has two chambers, an **atrium** and a **ventricle**. In addition each atrium has a flaplike appendage called an **auricle**. The left and right atria are separated by the **interatrial septum**; the left and right ventricles are separated by the **interventricular septum**. Other structures labeled in Figure 17.5 will be discussed later in this chapter or in Chapter 18.

Though both ventricles contract at the same time, the left one contracts with greater force than the right one. The wall of the left ventricle contains more muscle and is noticeably thicker than the wall of the right ventricle. Blood is ejected into the systemic circulation by way of the aorta at a pressure about five times as great as the pressure under which it is pumped into the pulmonary circulation. This great pressure in the aorta provides sufficient force to propel the blood through the entire systemic circulation. In spite of the pressure difference the volume of blood passing through each side of the heart is the same.

Several other features of the heart are of importance. A depression in the interatrial septum, the **fossa ovalis**, marks the location of the embryonic foramen ovale. Internally, the muscle mass of the atria is separated from the muscle mass of the ventricles by connective tissue rings that surround the valves (Figure 17.6). These rings separate the electrical activity of the atria and the ventricles. Externally, the atria and ventricles are separated by the **coronary sulcus**. Several heart blood vessels located in or near the sulcus are labeled in Figure 17.6.

Four valves control the flow of blood through the heart (see Figures 17.5 and 17.6). The valve between the right atrium and the right ventricle, the **tricuspid valve**, has three flaps, or **cusps**. Other names for this valve are the right atrioventricular valve or the right **A-V valve**. When it is open, blood can flow from the right atrium to the right ventricle. When the valve is closed, blood cannot flow into the ventricle, nor can it be pushed back into the atrium when the ventricle contracts. Thin fibrous strands, the **chordae tendineae**, connect the cusps of the valve to columns of muscle, the **papillary muscles**, which are attached to the inner wall of the ventricle. This system of cords and muscles prevents the cusps of the valves from being pushed back into the atrium and turned inside out when the ventricle contracts. In a normal heart the cords and muscles passively allow the pressure of the blood to cause the valve to completely close off the atrioventricular opening during ventricular contraction. A similar valve is located between the left atrium and left ventricle. It is called the **bicuspid valve** (because it has two cusps), mitral valve, left atrioventricular, or **left A-V valve**. It too has cords and papillary muscles that prevent backflow of blood into the left atrium just as the tricuspid does on the right side.

Two other valves, the **semilunar valves**, determine the direction of flow of blood from the ventricles to the arteries. Each of these valves has three half-moon-shaped cusps, hence the name semilunar. The **pulmonary semilunar valve**, located between the right ventricle and the pulmonary artery, prevents the backflow of blood from the artery into the ventricle after a contraction of the heart. Likewise, the **aortic semilunar valve** lies between the left ventricle and the aorta. The semilunar valves have no system of muscles and cords; instead, the cusps have depressions that fill with

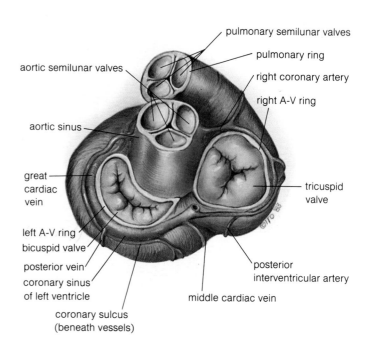

Figure 17.6 The valves of the heart and their supporting fibrous rings, as seen in a cutaway superior view after the removal of the atria.

Abnormal sounds called **heart murmurs** are heard when the valves fail to close properly, or when excessive turbulence is created in the blood inside a chamber. For example, in aortic stenosis, a condition in which the aortic valve is abnormally small, pressure builds up inside the left ventricle—sometimes as much as three or four times the normal pressure. As a result of this high pressure great turbulence is created within the ventricle at the root of the aorta as blood passes the aortic valve. This turbulence causes intense vibration in the wall of the aorta—loud enough to be heard without the use of a stethoscope in severe cases. In some other heart murmurs the cusps of the valves fail to close completely, and blood is allowed to flow back into the chamber from which it came, causing a blowing or swishing noise.

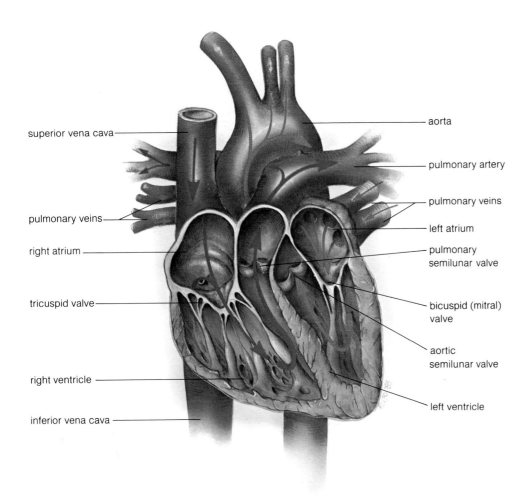

superior vena cava

pulmonary veins

right atrium

tricuspid valve

right ventricle

inferior vena cava

aorta

pulmonary artery

pulmonary veins

left atrium

pulmonary semilunar valve

bicuspid (mitral) valve

aortic semilunar valve

left ventricle

Figure 17.7   The pathway of blood through the heart.

blood and cause the cusps to close the blood vessel. Regardless of the structure or location, valves permit blood to flow through the heart in one direction only.

Turbulence in blood as the valves of the heart close makes sound, often described as a "lubb-dupp," that is audible with a stethoscope. The "lubb" is associated with the closing of the A-V valves and the "dupp" with the closing of the semilunar valves. The coordination of the opening and closing of the valves will be discussed with the cardiac cycle later in this chapter.

Flow of Blood through the Heart

As shown in Figure 17.7, blood from the superior and inferior venae cavae enters the right atrium. It passes through the tricuspid valve to the right ventricle and is pumped out

of the heart through the pulmonary semilunar valve into the pulmonary artery. Blood in the pulmonary artery circulates through the lungs, where it is oxygenated (the hemoglobin is saturated with oxygen), and returns to the heart through the pulmonary veins. This time it enters the left atrium and passes through the bicuspid valve to the left ventricle. From here it is pumped out of the ventricle through the aortic semilunar valve into the aorta. From the aorta blood passes through the systemic circulation and returns to the heart by way of the venae cavae.

Even though the heart consists of two separate pumps, these pumps work together. Both atria contract at the same time, forcing blood into their respective ventricles. Then the ventricles contract simultaneously, forcing blood into the arteries. The alternate opening and closing of valves when the atria contract and when the ventricles contract is shown in Figure 17.8.

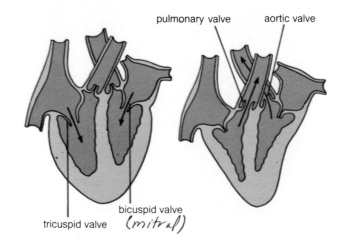

pulmonary valve   aortic valve

tricuspid valve   bicuspid valve
(mitral)

Figure 17.8 (**a**) The tricuspid and bicuspid valves open when the atria contract. (**b**) The tricuspid and bicuspid valves close, and the semilunar valves open, when the ventricles contract.

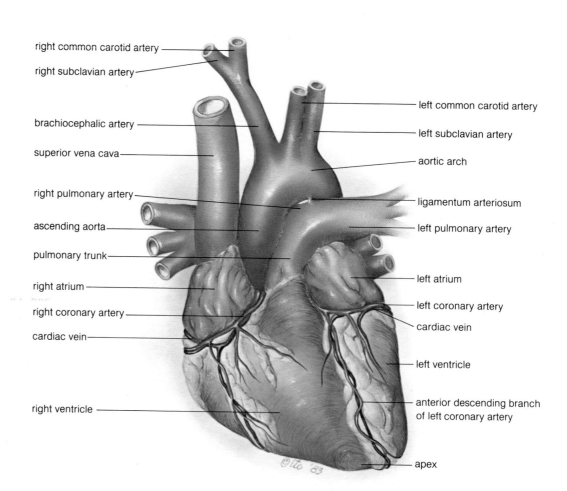

right common carotid artery

right subclavian artery

brachiocephalic artery

superior vena cava

right pulmonary artery

ascending aorta

pulmonary trunk

right atrium

right coronary artery

cardiac vein

right ventricle

left common carotid artery

left subclavian artery

aortic arch

ligamentum arteriosum

left pulmonary artery

left atrium

left coronary artery

cardiac vein

left ventricle

anterior descending branch of left coronary artery

apex

Figure 17.9 An anterior, external view of the heart.

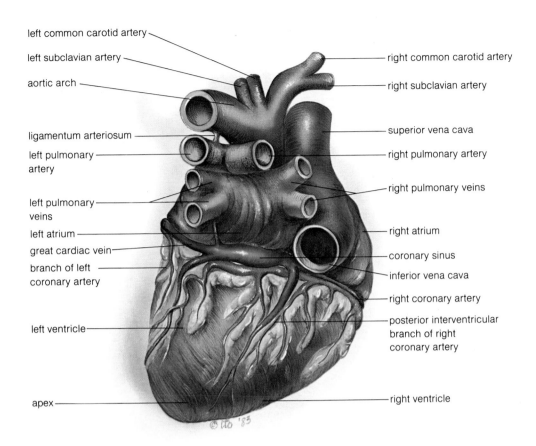

left common carotid artery

left subclavian artery

aortic arch

ligamentum arteriosum

left pulmonary artery

left pulmonary veins

left atrium

great cardiac vein

branch of left coronary artery

left ventricle

apex

right common carotid artery

right subclavian artery

superior vena cava

right pulmonary artery

right pulmonary veins

right atrium

coronary sinus

inferior vena cava

right coronary artery

posterior interventricular branch of right coronary artery

right ventricle

Figure 17.10   A posterior, external view of the heart.

External Anatomy of the Heart

In an anterior view (Figure 17.9) the outer walls of portions of each of the four chambers can be seen. The site at which the **right coronary artery** branches from the aorta is also visible. The **left coronary artery** also branches from the aorta very near the heart and passes beneath the pulmonary artery; it can be seen passing between the left and right ventricles and between the left atrium and ventricle to the posterior side of the heart. Also visible in this figure is the **ligamentum arteriosum**, a band of fibrous tissue between the aortic arch and the pulmonary artery. This structure is what remains of the ductus arteriosus of embryonic life.

In a posterior view of the heart (Figure 17.10) branches of both coronary arteries can be seen. The **great cardiac vein** collects blood from smaller veins and carries it to the coronary sinus. The great vessels that carry blood to and from the heart are also shown in these figures.

Circulation of Blood through Heart Muscle

Like any other cells of the body, the cells of the heart muscle itself must have a supply of nutrients and oxygen and a means of getting rid of wastes. Although the chambers of the heart are filled with blood, only the endocardium is nourished by that blood. The left and right coronary arteries and their branches supply blood to the heart muscle. As shown in Figure 17.9, these arteries branch from the base of the ascending aorta as it leaves the heart. They traverse the anterior surface of the heart in the grooves shown in the figure and pass to the posterior surface, where their branches **anastomose**, or join together. The anastomoses make it possible for blood from one artery to enter the capillary network normally served by the other, an important factor in maintaining a blood supply to the cells of the heart when a vessel becomes blocked. Numerous branches from the main arteries carry blood to the capillary

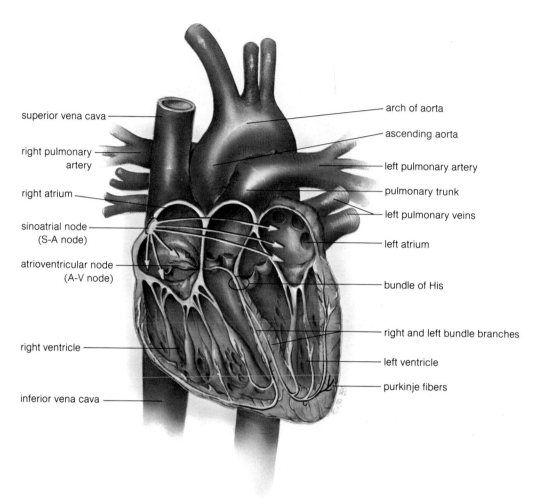

superior vena cava

right pulmonary artery

right atrium

sinoatrial node (S-A node)

atrioventricular node (A-V node)

right ventricle

inferior vena cava

arch of aorta

ascending aorta

left pulmonary artery

pulmonary trunk

left pulmonary veins

left atrium

bundle of His

right and left bundle branches

left ventricle

purkinje fibers

Figure 17.11 The conduction system of the heart: (**a**) Impulses are initiated by the S-A node and pass through the muscle cells of the atria, causing the atria to contract. (**b**) Some of these impulses reach the A-V node and stimulate it to send impulses along the bundle of His and the Purkinje fibers. (**c**) Impulses pass from the Purkinje fibers through the muscle cells, causing a wave of contraction to pass over the ventricles.

networks among the muscle cells.

After passing through the capillaries, blood enters the cardiac veins, which are located adjacent to the branches of the arteries. Many of the veins unite to form a large vessel, the **coronary sinus**, located on the posterior surface of the heart. This sinus carries blood from the heart wall and empties it directly into the right atrium. Other veins, especially those from the wall of the right ventricle, return blood directly to the right ventricle. About 30% of the blood that reaches the myocardium passes into short vessels called

sinusoids within the myocardium. From these sinusoids blood passes directly into the cavities of the ventricles. It is important to note that all the blood that passes through the heart tissue itself is returned to the chambers of the heart rather than to the venae cavae.

Blood flows in vessels of the heart muscle only when the heart is relaxed; contraction compresses the vessels and prevents the flow. So the heart muscle is continuously nourished and supplied with oxygen even though the blood flows through the tissues only five-eighths of the time.

PHYSIOLOGY OF THE HEART

Objective 6. Explain the initiation and regulation of the heartbeat.

Objective 7. Describe the normal cardiac cycle, including the way it appears in an electrocardiogram.

Objective 8. Define cardiac output in terms of heart rate and stroke volume and discuss the factors that regulate cardiac output.

Initiation and Regulation of the Heartbeat

Normally, the parts of the heart beat in an orderly sequence: First the atria contract, then the ventricles contract. This orderly sequence is maintained by a **conduction system**, consisting of heart muscle cells that are specialized to initiate and conduct action potentials. Other heart muscle cells—the contractile cells—are normally stimulated to contract in the proper sequence by action potentials delivered to them by cells of the conduction system. However, cardiac muscle cells have an inherent ability to contract in the absence of stimulation.

The conduction system   The **conduction system** of the heart (Figure 17.11) consists of the sinoatrial node, or S-A node; the atrioventricular node, or A-V node; the atrioventricular bundle, or bundle of His, and the Purkinje fibers.

The **S-A node** is located in the wall of the right atrium near where the superior vena cava enters it. This area in the embryo is called the **sinus venosus**, hence the name sinoatrial. The cells of the S-A node have an inherent ability to depolarize spontaneously and rhythmically. These cells have a resting potential of −55 to −60 millivolts instead of the −80 to −90 millivolts found in most other heart cells. S-A node cells have a low potential because their membranes naturally allow large numbers of sodium ions to leak into the cells. This resting potential is unstable and gradually undergoes depolarization caused by a slow decrease in membrane permeability to potassium. This slow depolarization is called the pacemaker potential, or diastolic depolarization. It causes the membrane potential to reach a threshold level for an action potential.

Once this threshold of −45 to −50 millivolts is reached, an action potential is generated. When this occurs, sodium ions rush into the cells, and total depolarization of the membranes occurs rapidly. The membranes remain depolarized for about 0.1 second, after which the permeability of the membranes to potassium increases and their permeability to sodium decreases. Return to the resting potential occurs as potassium ions move out of the cells. When the

resting potential is regenerated, the membranes' permeability to potassium again decreases, causing a gradual membrane depolarization. Another cycle in the automatic rhythmicity of the S-A node cells is initiated. The process is repeated continuously throughout life, establishing the resting heart rate at about seventy-two beats per minute. When the heart rate is above or below this rate, the S-A node is being influenced by neural or chemical factors. However, its ability to continuously depolarize and repolarize is inherent in the properties of the membranes of the cells of the S-A node.

The action potential generated by the depolarizing cells of the S-A node spreads through the muscle cells of the atria. As noted earlier, this cell-to-cell conduction is facilitated by the intercalated discs. The action potential causes the atria to contract in a wave that passes from the area of the S-A node *toward* the ventricles, but not *to* them, because of the connective tissue rings between the atria and ventricles. (Refer back to Figure 17.6.) Blood is thus pushed from the atria into the ventricles on each side of the heart at the same time. Because the action potentials from the S-A node are generated at a greater frequency than in any other part of the heart's conducting system, the S-A node determines the frequency of the heart beat and is thus known as the **pacemaker**. As the pacemaker, the S-A node sets the rate of contraction of the entire heart and synchronizes the action of the atria and ventricles.

The **A-V node**, located on the right side of the interatrial septum just superior to the ventricles, receives impulses from the S-A node. These impulses cause the A-V node to depolarize. After a short delay due to its own slow conductivity, the A-V node relays impulses to the specialized cells of the **bundle of His** in the interventricular septum. These cells carry the action potential across the nonconductive connective tissue of the septum. The bundle of His divides into left and right **bundle branches** and ultimately into **Purkinje fibers**. Impulses from the many branches of the Purkinje fibers stimulate the muscle cells of

Isolated cardiac muscle cells in laboratory cultures contract rhythmically without external stimulation. As such cells grow in culture, they form sheets, and the membranes of adjacent cells come in contact with one another. Then the whole sheet of cells begins to contract rhythmically, with waves of contraction passing over the sheet. The contractility of the cells becomes synchronized without external regulation.

the ventricles to depolarize and contract. The ventricles contract in a sudden wave that begins at the apex of the heart and travels through the ventricles, forcing blood out of the heart.

Each portion of the conduction system has its own inherent rate of depolarization. If no pacesetting stimuli are received from the S-A node, the A-V node generates impulses at a rate of forty to sixty times per minute. And in the absence of other stimuli the Purkinje fibers generate impulses at a rate of fifteen to forty times per minute. Even the muscle cells themselves can sometimes spontaneously generate impulses. Groups of muscle cells that generate such impulses are called **ectopic foci**. (Ectopic means located in a site other than the normal one.) Ectopic foci are responsible for some kinds of abnormal heart rates, or arryhthmias (discussed later in this chapter). Ectopic foci can initiate heart rates of 200 to 300 beats per minute and override impulses being generated by the S-A node.

Refractory period of the heart All muscle cells have a **refractory period**, a period during an action potential when a second stimulus will not normally generate a second action potential. The refractory period is divided into the **absolute refractory period**, during which no stimulus can affect the muscle, and a later **relative refractory period**, during which only a suprathreshold (unusually strong) stimulus can stimulate the muscle. In skeletal muscle the absolute refractory period is short (1 to 2 milliseconds), but in cardiac muscle the absolute refractory period is extremely long (about 300 milliseconds). The long refractory period prevents cardiac muscle from being stimulated repeatedly without undergoing relaxation between contractions. This allows time for the heart chambers and the blood vessels of the heart wall to refill between contractions; it also allows the heart muscle to relax between contractions. The properties of cardiac muscle, including its refractory properties, are compared with those of skeletal muscle in Table 17.1.

The Electrocardiogram

An **electrocardiogram** (ECG or EKG) is a record of the electrical activity associated with the contraction of cardiac muscle (Figure 17.12). Such records are useful in assessing the manner in which impulses from the conduction system pass through the heart and in detecting electrical abnormalities. During the time when action potentials are spreading over the atria, some parts of the atria are already depolarized, and other parts are yet to be depolarized. The surfaces of depolarized cells have a negative charge relative to the surfaces of cells yet to be depolarized. This creates a battery

Table 17.1	A Comparison of Cardiac and Skeletal Muscle Fibers	
Characteristic	Cardiac Fibers	Skeletal Fibers
Nature of control	Involuntary	Voluntary
Arrangement of fibers	Branched	Unbranched
Microscopic appearance	Striated	Striated
Intercalated discs	Present	Absent
Arrangement of T-tubules	1 per sarcomere, located at Z-line	2 per sarcomere, located at A-I junctions (see Chapter 8)
Duration of action potential	150 to 300 msec	1 to 5 msec
Contraction time	150 to 300 msec	40 msec
Absolute refractory period	150 to 300 msec	1 to 2 msec

ffect—a negative and a positive "pole." The voltage of this "battery" is sufficient to be conducted to the surface of the body and detected as the **P wave** of the ECG. Subsequently, when the action potentials are spreading over the ventricles, another electrical potential gradient, or "battery," is established, and detected as the **QRS complex** of the ECG. Its voltage is greater than the P wave because the ventricles have a much larger muscle mass than the atria. The placement of electrodes for the three most commonly used ECG leads is shown in Figure 17.12. Wires from the leads are connected to a machine called an **electrocardiograph**, and a tracing—the electrocardiogram—is produced.

A normal electrocardiogram (Figure 17.12b–d) consists of a P wave, a QRS complex, and a T wave, spaced as shown. The letters are arbitrarily selected and do not stand for any particular words. Such a tracing is produced each time the heart contracts and relaxes—about once every 0.8 second. The P wave occurs following the initiation of a stimulus in the S-A node and represents the depolarization of the atria. The QRS complex follows the excitation of the A-V node and represents the depolarization of the ventricles. The **T wave** represents the repolarization of the ventricles. Repolarization of the atria occurs during the QRS complex and is obscured by the stronger electrical signals from depolarization of the ventricles. The **P-Q interval** (sometimes re-

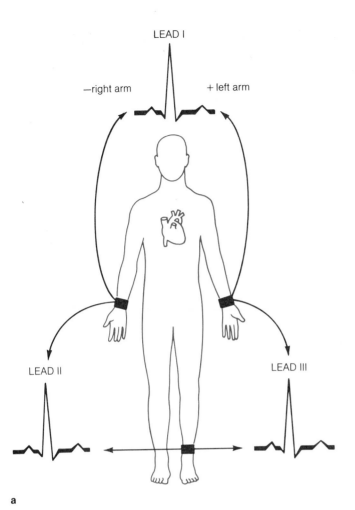

LEAD I

−right arm   + left arm

LEAD II   LEAD III

a

ferred to as the **P-R interval**) represents the time between the initiation of atrial contraction and the initiation of ventricular contraction. We can use this understanding of an electrocardiogram to help us follow the events in the cardiac cycle.

Cardiac Cycle

The **cardiac cycle** consists of one heartbeat, or one cycle of contraction and relaxation of the cardiac muscle. It has a pumping phase and a filling phase. Pumping occurs during contraction; filling occurs during relaxation. Though some texts use systole and diastole to refer to the atria as well as the ventricles, we will use **systole** to refer to ventricular contraction, and **diastole** to refer to ventricular relaxation. At a typical resting heart rate of seventy-two beats per minute, each cycle takes about 0.80 second. The details of the cardiac cycle are shown in Figure 17.13. Though both sides of the heart go through the cycle at the same time, only pressures and volumes for the left side of the heart are given in the diagram. Refer to the figure as you read the following description of the cardiac cycle.

Though the heart beats continuously—that is, goes from one cardiac cycle to the next—a single cycle can be divided into five phases for study.

Phase 1: Atrial contraction   At the time an impulse is initiated in the S-A node, the heart is relaxed and the atria are filled with blood. The atrioventricular valves (tricuspid and bicus-

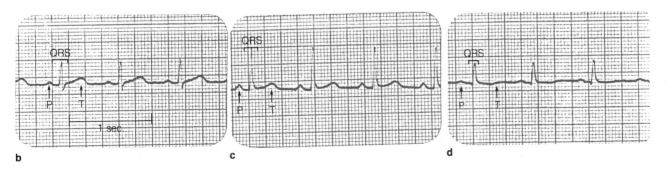

b   c   d

Figure 17.12 An electrocardiogram is a record of the electrical discharges associated with the contraction of the cardiac muscle. (**a**) Several different patterns of electrode placement can be used to obtain an electrocardiogram, and each produces a different shaped tracing. The placement of the positive and negative electrodes for three commonly used leads is shown here. (**b**) Normal EKG using lead I, (**c**) normal EKG using lead II, (**d**) normal EKG using lead III. The background "graph paper" is marked so that the distance across five heavy blocks (twenty-five light blocks) equals 1 second. (EKGs courtesy of Arlington Hospital, Arlington, Virginia.)

pid) are open, and the ventricles are about three-fourths full of blood. The impulse from the S-A node causes depolarization of the atria (seen as a P wave) and **atrial contraction**. During the 0.10 second of the contraction the atrial pressure increases, and a small amount of blood is pushed into the ventricles. Atrial contraction is not essential to life because it accounts for only about one-fourth of the blood flow to the ventricles, the remainder flowing passively.

Phase 2: Isovolumetric ventricular contraction   Toward the end of the first 0.10 second of the cycle, the impulse from the S-A node has passed through the A-V node, and the ventricles begin to depolarize. This depolarization is seen as the QRS complex on the electrocardiogram. Systole begins. The first 0.05 second of systole is called **isovolumetric ventricular contraction** because the volume of blood in the ventricle does not change. This phase occupies the time between the closing of the atrioventricular valves and the opening of the semilunar valves. Because the A-V valves bulge into the atria, atrial pressure increases slightly. Turbulence in ventricular blood at the time the A-V valves close causes the first heart sound detected through a stethoscope—the "lubb" of "lubb-dupp."

Phase 3: Ventricular ejection   When the pressure in the ventricles exceeds the pressure in the pulmonary arteries and the aorta, the semilunar valves open, and blood is ejected from the ventricles. This phase, **ventricular ejection**, lasts about 0.25 second from the time the semilunar valves open until they close. The ventricular pressure rises during the first part of this phase, and the ventricular volume declines rapidly as the blood is ejected from the ventricle. Arterial pressure rises correspondingly but remains elevated somewhat longer. Toward the end of systole the volume of the ventricles has dropped to its lowest level, and the pressure in the ventricles and the arteries declines. During ventricular ejection 70 to 90 milliliters of blood are ejected from each ventricle. This phase ends when the arterial pressure exceeds the ventricular pressure and the semilunar valves close.

Phase 4: Isovolumetric ventricular relaxation   For about 0.05 second between the closing of the semilunar valves and the opening of the A-V valves, the ventricles begin to relax; the ventricular blood volume remains constant and at its lowest level (about 50 milliliters). This is called **isovolumetric ventricular relaxation**. The closing of the aortic semilunar valve causes a brief rise in aortic pressure (the dicrotic notch), followed by a rebound positive pressure wave. The second heart sound may be heard through a stethoscope at this time—the "dupp" of "lubb-dupp."

Phase 5: Ventricular filling   When the A-V valves open, the ventricles fill with blood. This phase, **ventricular filling**, lasts about 0.35 second, as blood flows passively from the atria to the ventricles. Filling is rapid during the first 0.1 second and slower during the remainder of this phase. Toward the end of this phase a new impulse is initiated in the S-A node, and the beginning of a new P wave marks the start of another cardiac cycle.

Cardiac Output

Cardiac output is the amount of blood pumped from each ventricle per minute. *The volume of blood moving from the left ventricle to the aorta is the same as the volume of blood moving from the right ventricle to the pulmonary artery.* Thus, cardiac output refers to the volume pumped from either ventricle. It is the product of the number of heartbeats per minute and the volume of blood pumped by one ventricle during a contraction. Cardiac output equals heart rate times stroke volume. For example, at a normal heart rate of 72 beats per minute and an average volume of 70 milliliters per beat, the cardiac output is 5040 milliliters per minute—about 5 liters per minute, or the equivalent of the total body blood volume.

Though the above values are typical for a normal resting adult, several factors can alter them. During strenuous exercise the heart rate may easily reach 150 beats per minute, and the stroke volume can reach 120 milliliters, increasing the cardiac output to 18 liters per minute. In trained athletes the cardiac output can go as high as 35 liters per minute—seven time the total blood volume!

Cardiac output is controlled by a combination of factors, some of which affect the heart rate and some of which affect the stroke volume (see Figure 17.14).

Control of heart rate   The **heart rate** is determined by the frequency of firing of the S-A node. This pacemaker has its own intrinsic firing rate, but its rate is subject to modification by both neural and hormonal factors.

The neural factors involve both sympathetic and parasympathetic fibers of the autonomic nervous system. The sympathetic fibers that innervate the heart arise from chain ganglia in the thoracic area and carry impulses to the S-A and A-V nodes. Parasympathetic fibers are located in the vagus nerve; they also innervate both nodes. Sensory (afferent) impulses are carried from several organs to the **cardiovascular center** in the medulla. Because this center regulates both heart action and dilation and constriction of blood vessels, it will be discussed in Chapter 19.

The hormone epinephrine, released from the adrenal medulla, stimulates the heart to beat faster and more force-

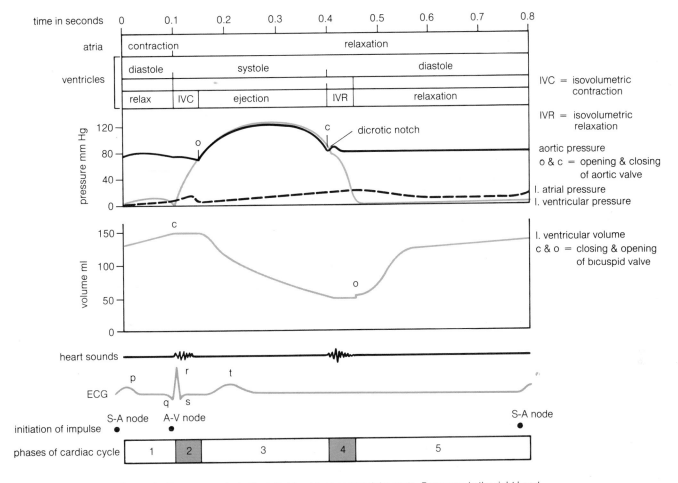

Figure 17.13 The cardiac cycle. Pressures refer to the left side of the heart and the aorta. Pressures in the right heart and pulmonary artery are lower than the ones shown here. (See text for explanation of figure.)

fully. It is released when the body is under stress and during strenuous exercise.

Heart rate is also affected by changes in body temperature, electrolytes in the blood plasma, and hormones other than epinephrine. However, these effects are relatively small compared to the effects of epinephrine in the blood and the effects of the autonomic nervous system.

Control of stroke volume The **stroke volume** is the difference between the volume of blood in the ventricle before systole (the end-diastolic volume) and the volume of blood in the ventricle after systole (the end-systolic volume). Any factor that increases the amount of blood in the ventricle before systole generally causes an increase in the stroke volume. Experiments with animals have shown that, when the end-diastolic volume is caused to increase, the walls of the

ventricles are stretched and the force of the contractions also increase. The increase in strength of contractions as a result of stretching the walls of the ventricles is known as **Starling's law of the heart**. An increase in the amount of blood being returned to the heart (venous return) will cause an increase in the amount of blood in the ventricles. And according to Starling's law of the heart, this factor contributes to increasing stroke volume. Conversely, a decrease in venous return will cause a decrease in stroke volume.

Sympathetic stimulation and epinephrine from the adrenal gland also increase stroke volume. In addition to reaching the S-A node and increasing heart rate, sympathetic nerve fibers reach the individual cells of the myocardium, where they increase the strength of contraction of the muscle fibers. Norepinephrine from the sympathetic nerve endings or epinephrine from the blood plasma have the

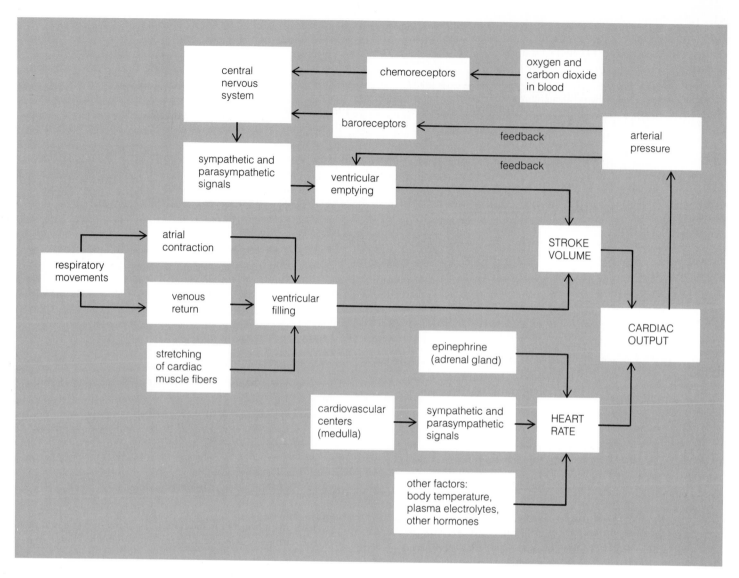

Figure 17.14 Factors involved in regulating cardiac output.

same effect—that of stimulating muscle fibers to contract more vigorously. Movements of the lungs during respiration also affect the return of venous blood to the heart and thus affect atrial and ventricular contraction.

Feedback Many of the factors that determine cardiac output are in turn influenced by the cardiac output. The arterial pressure resulting from the cardiac output is detected by baroreceptors (described in Chapter 19). The baroreceptors relay signals by way of the central nervous system to the heart, where they affect ventricular rate and contraction. In addition, chemoreceptors (described in Chapter 21) detect

changes in blood carbon dioxide and oxygen concentrations. These chemoreceptors relay signals by way of the central nervous system to the heart, where they too affect ventricular emptying.

Cardiac output as a component of circulation Cardiac output is an integral part of the total functioning of the circulatory system. Cardiac output is affected by blood pressure in various vessels and changes in the osmotic pressure and carbon dioxide content of the blood. How these and other factors are integrated into the overall functioning of the circulatory system will be considered in Chapter 19.

CLINICAL APPLICATIONS

Objective 9. Define and discuss briefly the causes, effects, and treatment of (a) myocardial infarction, (b) heart failure, (c) arrhythmias, and (d) congenital heart defects.

Myocardial Infarction

Myocardial infarction is the medical term for what is commonly called a heart attack. When a branch of one of the coronary arteries becomes occluded (blocked), the flow of blood to the tissues served by that branch is stopped. The myocardial cells receive no blood or so little blood that they cease to function, and the tissue is said to be **infarcted**. An infarction may be caused by the deposition of fatty substances in the lumen of the blood vessel to the extent that blood flow is blocked. Often a blood clot forms on the roughened surface of the vessel wall over the fatty deposits.

A less serious but similar condition, **ischemic heart disease**, occurs when one or more vessels are not completely blocked, but the blood flow is reduced. **Ischemia** is a condition of reduced blood flow. The painful condition called **angina pectoris** results from ischemia in myocardial tissue. It often occurs when an individual has engaged in some form of activity that places greater demand on the myocardium than its limited blood supply will accommodate. Nitroglycerine tablets alleviate the pain of angina by dilating the blood vessels of the heart and other organs. Such dilation increases blood flow through the coronary arteries. At the same time it reduces arterial pressure and hence reduces the demands placed on the heart.

Myocardial infarction results from a sudden and more extensive blocking of blood flow than occurs in angina. Once the infarction has occurred, blood seeps into the area from anastomosing blood vessels. The blood vessels dilate, and blood accumulates in them. Flow is sluggish, and the blood contains little or no oxygen. If only a small area is infarcted, a collateral blood supply may become established before the cells die; in this case the heart muscle will not be permanently damaged. If the area of infarcted tissue is extensive, it becomes divided into a central portion of dead fibers, a surrounding zone of nonfunctional cells, and an outer zone of ischemic cells (Figure 17.15). During the healing process fibrous tissue replaces the dead cells, including some of the cells in the nonfunctional area that died during the healing process. Cells in the ischemic area recover their function as collateral blood vessels grow into the area and reestablish blood flow. Many of the cells in the nonfunctional area will become functional again if they receive a blood supply before they die.

The degree of tissue damage resulting from a myocardial infarction can be assessed by measuring the amount of the enzyme serum glutamic-oxaloacetic transaminase (SGOT) in the blood. This enzyme is present in fairly high concentrations in heart muscle cells. When heart cells die, they release the enzyme into the blood. The concentration of SGOT becomes elevated about 8 hours after an infarction and continues to rise until 24 to 36 hours after the attack. If no further tissue damage occurs, the SGOT level begins to drop. However, if another infarction occurs, the SGOT level will become elevated again. Tissue damage can be monitored by following the blood concentration of SGOT in the first few days following an infarction. Several other enzymes released into the blood also can be monitored to assess damage and repair of cardiac muscle.

The victim of a myocardial infarction suffers severe, heavy chest pain and is usually placed on complete bed rest and given oxygen. The extra oxygen allows the limited amount of blood passing through the heart muscle to deliver more oxygen to the heart cells. As the patient recovers from the attack, it is important to minimize the stress placed on the heart. Thus, the patient's mobility is greatly curtailed while the infarcted tissue heals.

The incidence of myocardial infarction is higher in men than in women and is rarely seen in women before menopause. It has been suggested that estrogens may have a protective effect on the heart, although at this time the nature of their effect is not understood.

Several possible treatments for myocardial infarction are in experimental stages. The enzyme hyaluronidase, which digests the cementing substances between cells, has been tested experimentally in animals. It appears to reduce the size of the infarcted area below what would have been expected from the degree of tissue injury inflicted on the animal. However, its mode of action is not yet known.

Since the discovery that ischemic tissue accumulates liposomes, membrane-bound particles filled with lipids, it has been suggested that such particles could be prepared in the laboratory and laden with drugs or metabolites. These liposomes could then serve as carriers of selected substances to the injured tissue. It has also been discovered that prostacyclin, a naturally occurring and potent prostaglandin, has beneficial effects on infarcted tissue. These effects include reducing systemic blood pressure without changing heart rate, lowering the resistance of blood vessels to the flow of blood through them, inhibiting platelet aggregation that might cause clots to form in blood vessels, and reducing the release of enzymes from lysosomes of injured cells. All these effects contribute to minimizing the tissue damage following a myocardial infarction.

Heart Failure

Heart failure occurs when the cardiac output is insufficient to provide an adequate blood supply to the tissues. Unless failure is total, some blood continues to be pumped. It may be acute (sudden in onset and severe) or chronic. Acute heart failure often follows a myocardial infarction because the damaged muscle pumps blood less efficiently. As the infarction heals and the heart

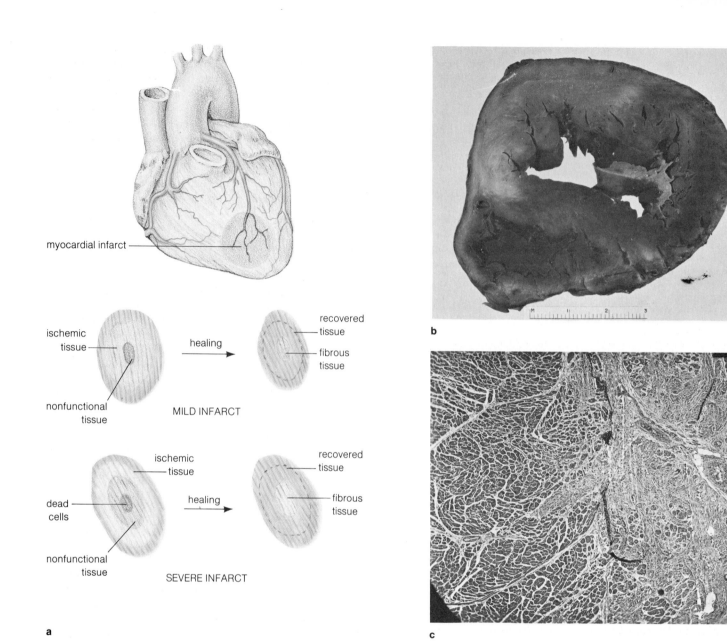

a

myocardial infarct

ischemic tissue

nonfunctional tissue

healing

recovered tissue

fibrous tissue

MILD INFARCT

dead cells

ischemic tissue

nonfunctional tissue

healing

recovered tissue

fibrous tissue

SEVERE INFARCT

b

c

Figure 17.15 (**a**) The process of tissue damage and healing following a myocardial infarction. (**b**) A cross-section of the heart following the death of the individual three days after a myocardial infarction. Notice the white areas in the wall of the heart where blood supply was impaired. (Armed Forces Institute of Pathology negative number 60–6123.) (**c**) A photomicrograph of a healed myocardial infarction, × 33. Notice the fibrous tissue on the left side of the figure where the infarction has healed. (Armed Forces Institute of Pathology negative number 61–3009.)

becomes able to pump enough blood to adequately supply the patient's tissues, the heart failure is reversed. In chronic heart failure there is a gradual deterioration of the cardiac output. It may be due to hypertension, coronary artery disease, diseases or defects in the valves, or congenital lesions.

The symptoms of heart failure differ depending on whether the failure is in the left or right side of the heart or in both. In left-sided heart failure blood backs up in the left atrium and into the pulmonary vessels, causing accumulation of fluids in lung tissue and labored breathing. In right-sided heart failure blood backs up in the systemic veins and causes fluids to accumulate in the body tissues. Any kind of heart failure decreases the cardiac output, lowers renal blood flow, and thereby reduces the efficiency of the kidneys in removing excess fluids and wastes from the blood. Thus, for several reasons fluids accumulate in the tissues of the body causing edema and congestion in the tissues. This phenomenon gave rise to the name **congestive heart failure**.

When the cause of heart failure is a defective valve, the condition can be corrected by repairing the valve surgically. When the cause is some more generalized condition, treatment with drugs can alleviate the symptoms. Diuretics and digitalis may be used independently or together. Diuretics increase kidney excretion and thereby help to remove fluids from edematous areas and reduce the excessive load on the heart. Digitalis increases the strength of the contractions of the heart and increases cardiac output. It is also useful for treating arrhythmias that may accompany heart failure.

Arrhythmias

An **arrhythmia** is any disturbance in the rate of the heartbeat. Arrhythmias frequently follow myocardial infarction or heart failure, and they are often produced by ectopic foci. They also occur when there is a defect in the conduction system of the heart. Figure 17.16 shows electrocardiograms of a normal heart rhythm (a) and a variety of arrhythmias (b through g).

Sinus arrhythmias indicate an alteration in the rate at which signals are initiated by the S-A node. This rate may be irregular (b), slower than normal—bradycardia (c), or faster than normal—tachycardia (d). **Bradycardia** is an abnormally slow heart rate, usually below 60 beats per minute. It can be caused by heart block (discussed below), by abnormally low body temperature, or by excessive parasympathetic stimulation. Athletes often have slower than normal heart rates because their hearts have unusually high stroke volumes. Bradycardia from this cause is of no medical concern because the tissues are being adequately nourished. **Tachycardia** is an abnormally rapid heart beat, usually in excess of 100 beats per minute. It can be caused by abnormally high body temperature (fever), by excessive sympathetic stimulation, or by ectopic foci. Ectopic foci also cause premature ventricular contractions—contractions that are initiated in the ventricles independently of impulses from the S-A node (e).

Heart block arrhythmias are due to a defect in the conduction system such that the impulses do not follow the normal conduction pathway. If some of the impulses from the S-A node fail to reach the A-V node, the atria contract more often than the ventricles. Should the atrial contraction rate also be greatly increased, atrial flutter results (f). If the impulses in the conduction pathway fail to be transmitted in one or both of the bundles of His, contraction of the affected ventricle(s) is disrupted. For example, in left bundle branch block, the contraction of the left ventricle is abnormal. If the atrial contraction rate simultaneously increases, sinus tachycardia also occurs (g).

Flutter and Fibrillation

Flutter is a condition in which a chamber of the heart is beating regularly but rapidly at a rate of 250 to 300 beats per minute. Because the chamber does not have time to fill between beats, flutter is an extremely inefficient heart beat, and cardiac output is greatly reduced. Unless the heart rate can be returned to normal by the use of medications, it may lead to **fibrillation**, a condition in which the heart muscle is contracting very rapidly but in an uncoordinated fashion. Various regions of the heart beat at their own independent rhythms. Ventricular fibrillation is immediately life threatening unless it can be stopped by **defibrillation**. A machine called a defibrillator is used to do this. It passes a strong electrical current through the body and momentarily stops the heart. After the defibrillating shock, the heart sometimes spontaneously reestablishes a normal sinus rhythm, the rhythm regulated by the S-A node.

The drug digitalis is frequently used to treat arrhythmias. In addition to strengthening the contractions of the heart, it also causes the beats to become more regular. One of the drawbacks of digitalis is that it is highly toxic. A small amount may correct and prevent arrhythmias, but a slightly larger amount may actually induce arrhythmias.

For patients with persistent arryhthmias an artificial pacemaker can be used to correct the condition. This device consists of a stimulator implanted under the skin from which electrodes extend to the heart. The stimulator is operated by a battery that must be replaced about once every five years (or once every ten years for the new atomic-powered battery).

Congenital Heart Defects

Congenital heart defects—anatomical abnormalities in the heart seen in newborn infants—often result in seriously impaired heart function. Many of these defects are thought to be caused by infections of the mother such as rubella (German measles) or medications used by the mother during pregnancy, especially at the time the heart of the embryo is developing. Although heart defects may pose an immediate threat to the survival of the infant, other defects often accompany them. An agent that can cause

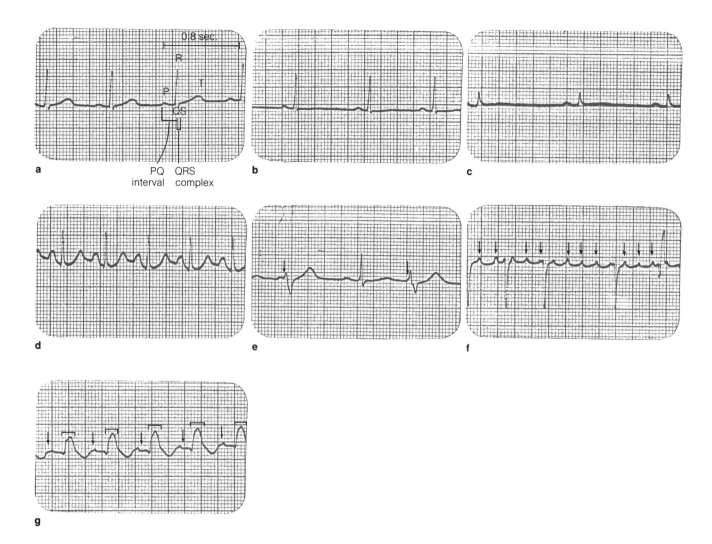

Figure 17.16 Electrocardiograms: (**a**) normal with P, QRS, and T waves indicated; (**b**) sinus arrhythmia in which distance between P waves varies, as might occur with metabolic or electrolyte abnormalities (see Chapter 26); (**c**) sinus bradycardia with flattening of the T wave; (**d**) sinus tachycardia with sharply defined P and T waves; (**e**) premature ventricular contractions with normal wave in between caused by ectopic foci in the ventricle initiating impulses independently of the S-A node; (**f**) atrial flutter with partial heart block, in which several P waves may occur between each QRS complex—the multiple P waves give the EKG a saw-toothed appearance (atrial flutter), and the absence of QRS complexes associated with each P wave indicates that not all the P waves are being transmitted to the A-V node (QRS complexes are inverted because of a different placement of leads); (**g**) sinus tachycardia with left bundle branch block—excessively rapid P waves with distorted QRS complexes because impulses are not transmitted through fibers of the bundle of His to the left ventricle. (Courtesy of Arlington Hospital, Arlington, Virginia.)

a heart defect may also cause defective development of other organs.

Three major groups of congential heart defects can be defined in terms of their effects on heart function: (1) stenosis, or narrowing, of a channel of blood flow in the heart or a closely associated vessel; (2) a left-to-right shunt, which allows blood to bypass the systemic circulation; and (3) a right-to-left-shunt, which allows blood to bypass the pulmonary circulation.

Coarctation of the aorta (Figure 17.17a), a constriction (stenosis) of the aorta, causes the left ventricle to work excessively hard to force blood into the aorta. The effects are essentially the same as those described for aortic stenosis, a condition which can also be due to abnormal development.

Left-to-right shunting can be caused by a patent ductus arteriosus (Figure 17.17b), an atrial septal defect (c), or a ventricular septal defect (d). A **patent ductus arteriosus** consists of a connection between the pulmonary artery and the aorta. This connection is normally present in fetal life, where it allows blood to go from the pulmonary artery to the aorta without circulating through the uninflated lungs. Resistance to flow in the fetal lungs causes high pressure in the pulmonary artery that forces blood through the ductus arteriosus into the aorta. At birth when the lungs expand, the pressure is higher in the aorta than in the pulmonary artery and blood flow is reversed in the ductus arteriosus. Normally, the ductus arteriosus becomes occluded within a few hours to a few days after birth, probably because the high oxygen content of blood in the aorta constricts muscle in the wall of the ductus. If the ductus fails to close blood is recycled through the pulmonary circulation and after several years the entire heart becomes greatly enlarged. This enlargement is due to the increased pumping activity required to maintain adequate systemic blood flow while at the same time pumping two to three times the normal amount of blood through the pulmonary circulation. Surgical ligation (tying off) of the ductus arteriosus corrects this condition.

An **atrial septal defect** is often caused by failure of the foramen ovale to close. Like the ductus arteriosus, the foramen ovale provides a way for blood to bypass the pulmonary circulation during fetal life. At birth a valve normally occludes the foramen ovale and prevents movement of blood between the atria. The slightly higher pressure in the left than the right atrium normally keeps the valve closed until the opening is permanently sealed by the growth of fibrous tissue. If the foramen ovale fails to close or if a more extensive defect exists in the interatrial septum, significant left-to-right shunting may occur. If not surgically repaired by open-heart surgery, enlargement of the heart is followed by death from right ventricle failure and accumulation of fluids in the lungs.

A **ventricular septal defect**, an opening in the intraventricular septum allows blood to flow from the left to the right ventricle when the ventricles contract, increasing the pressure in the right ventricle to near that in the left ventricle. Like an atrial septal defect, a ventricular septal defect can be repaired by open-heart surgery. If it is not repaired, the walls of the right ventricle become as thick as those in the left ventricle and much of the pumping action of the heart is devoted to pumping blood through the defect and recycling it through the pulmonary circulation.

The **tetralogy of Fallot** (Figure 17.17e)—a condition in which four different defects of the heart occur simultaneously—creates right-to-left shunting. The defects are: (1) the aorta originates from the right ventricle or both ventricles, (2) the pulmonary artery is stenosed, (3) an intraventricular septal defect allows blood to flow from the left to the right ventricle and to the aorta or directly into the aorta when it is located over the septal defect, and (4) the right ventricle becomes greatly enlarged. The main physiological effect of these defects is that as much as three-fourths of the blood may be pumped from the right ventricle into the aorta without passing through the pulmonary circulation and being oxygenated. The infant affected by the tetralogy of Fallot is cyanotic, sometimes called a "blue baby." In recent years surgical procedures have been developed to correct the multiple defects, greatly increasing the life expectancy of the individual.

Clinical Terms

antiarrhythmic (an-tĭ-a-rith'mik) drug   a substance that helps to restore a normal rhythm or to prevent arrhythmias

asystole (ah-sis'to-le)   inability of the heart to perform a complete contraction

cardiomegaly (kar''de-o-meg'al-e)   enlargement, or hypertrophy, of the heart

congestive heart failure   inability of the heart to pump an adequate amount of blood because of accumulation of fluids around the heart or in the lungs

cor pulmonale (kor pul''mo-nă'le)   failure of the right side of the heart because of obstructed blood flow in the lungs

palpitation (pal-pi-ta'shun)   a sudden increase in the heart rate that is felt by the individual

Figure 17.17 Some common congenital defects of the heart: (**a**) coarctation (narrowing) of the aorta; (**b**) patent ductus arteriosus; (**c**) atrial septal defect; (**d**) ventricular septal defect; (**e**) tetralogy of Fallot.

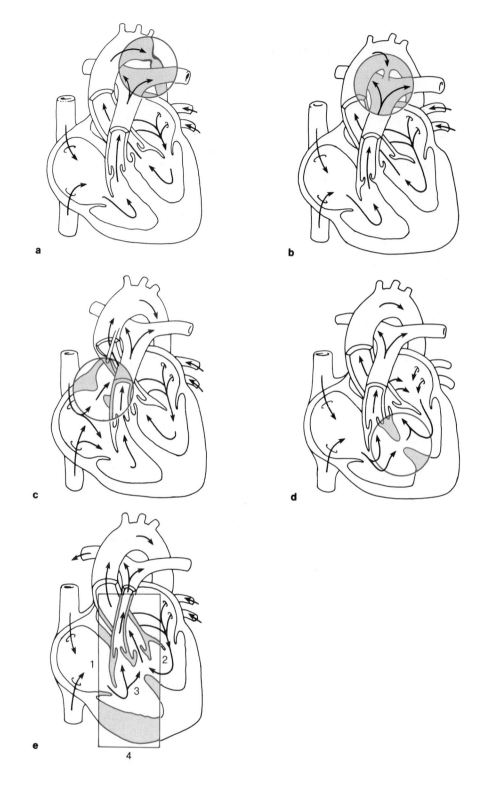

Essay: The Framingham Study—Factors That Contribute to Heart Disease

The Framingham study, which began in 1948 in Framingham, Massachusetts, was one of the nation's first long-term epidemiological studies exploring the effects of personal habits and environment on heart disease. Epidemiology concerns the incidence, distribution, and control of disease. At the beginning of the study, 5127 men and women aged thirty to sixty-two were enrolled. Every two years for the next twelve years each of these individuals was examined for the development of coronary heart disease.

It was reasoned that, because habits and environmental factors can be changed, knowledge of their role in coronary heart disease would be helpful in preventing the disease. The factors considered in the study included level of physical activity, body weight, cigarette smoking, blood pressure, blood cholesterol level, vital capacity, pulse rate, and alcohol consumption. Much of the data collected was based on subjects' reports on their own habits during and prior to the study. Relying on the memory of the subjects allowed for some error in the study, and other variables such as degree of physical activity were not precisely quantifiable. Nevertheless, even with these shortcomings the study has led to some important findings.

Of the factors studied excessive cigarette smoking, obesity, and sedentary living showed the highest correlation with the development of coronary heart disease. Over the period of the study the mortality rate due to coronary heart disease among sendentary men was twice as great as that among more active men. However, activity level showed little relationship to the development of angina pectoris or coronary insufficiency.

Men whose body weight exceeded their optimum weight by 20% or more were twice as likely to develop angina pectoris as those whose weight was within 10% of normal. Sudden death from heart disease among the obese (more than 20% overweight) was nearly five times as frequent as among those whose body weights were less than 20% above normal. On the other hand, recent analyses of Framingham data show greatest longevity among the somewhat (10%–20%) overweight group.

Heart attacks of any kind were about twice as frequent among heavy cigarette smokers as among nonsmokers. Curiously, cigar and pipe smokers and ex-smokers had a lower incidence of heart attacks than nonsmokers. The mortality rate from coronary heart disease increased in direct proportion to the number of cigarettes smoked per day, but the number of years the subjects had smoked did not seem to be related to coronary mortality.

Measures of systolic blood pressure, serum cholesterol, and vital capacity (the amount of air a subject can move in and out of the lungs) were made. When smokers were compared with nonsmokers, the smokers showed an excess risk of heart attack at any level of blood pressure, serum cholesterol, and vital capacity. High cholesterol (over 250 mg%) and high systolic blood pressure (over 160 mm Hg) seem to make their own independent contributions to increasing the risk of heart attack. Considering the three abnormalities—cigarette smoking, high cholesterol, and high systolic blood pressure—the more of these abnormalities a person has, the higher the risk of heart attack.

Among the factors found not to influence an individual's risk of developing coronary heart disease were use of alcohol, number of hours of sleep, marital status, and family size.

In 1965 another study was begun with 1319 of the participants in the original Framingham study. Among these participants were 352 housewives, 387 working women, and 580 men. Each participant completed a 300 item questionnaire that assessed employment and occupational status, personality type, stress the individual was experiencing, reactions to anger, sociocultural mobility, and family responsibilities. All participants were aged forty-five to sixty-four and free from coronary heart disease at the beginning of the study. Working women were defined as those who had worked outside the home for more than half their adult lives. The categorization of women as housewives or working women provided an opportunity to study the effects of employment on women.

The incidence of coronary heart disease was not significantly different among housewives and working women. When the women in clerical occupations (secretaries, bank clerks, and sales personnel) were compared to other women (employed and unemployed), the clerical workers were seen to have a much higher risk of developing coronary heart disease. The women in clerical positions who had children and were married to men doing blue-collar work showed the greatest risk. Among the items on the questionnaire those relating to suppressed hostility, having a nonsupportive boss, and lack of job mobility were the best predictors of heart disease. In contrast to these findings it was found that single working women had the lowest risk of heart disease of any group in the sample. Thus, among women employment per se is not related to increased risk of coronary heart disease. Rather, it appears that the kind of employment and the stresses from the combination of employment, marriage, and children are factors that contribute to heart disease among women.

The Framingham Study has been successful in identifying some effects of personal habits and environment on heart disease. Its contribution to reducing the incidence of such disease depends on individuals making use of its findings.

CHAPTER SUMMARY

(Chapter summary points and review questions are numbered to correspond to the numbered objectives in the text of each chapter.)

Organization and General Function

1. Describe the general plan of the heart, its location, and its general function in the circulatory system.
   a. The heart is a hollow muscular organ located in the mediastinum.
   b. Its function is to pump blood to all parts of the body.

Development

2. Describe the embryonic development of the heart.
   a. The heart develops first as a straight tube and then as a curved tube, and then becomes partitioned to form a four-chambered structure.
   b. The foramen ovale and the ductus arteriosus allow blood to pass through the heart with only 15% entering the fetal pulmonary circulation.

Tissues

3. (a) Describe the tissue layers of the heart and the pericardium; (b) describe the properties of cardiac muscle.
   a. The layers of the heart wall include the endocardium, the myocardium, and the epicardium.
   b. The heart is surrounded by the pericardial sac, which has a fibrous layer and a serous layer continuous with the epicardium.
   c. The pericardial cavity, filled with pericardial fluid, lies between the heart and the pericardial sac.
   d. Cardiac muscle has several distinctive characteristics:
      (1) Its fibers undergo extensive branching.
      (2) Its cells are connected by intercalated discs through which action potentials easily move.
      (3) Other characteristics are summarized in Table 17.1.

Anatomy of the Heart

4. Describe the general anatomical plan of the heart and trace the flow of blood through the heart chambers.
   a. The heart consists of a left and a right pump, each of which has an atrium and a ventricle.
   b. The left and right sides of the heart are separated by the interatrial and interventricular septa.
   c. Valves separate the atria from the ventricles and the ventricles from the arteries leaving the heart:

(1) The tricuspid valve separates the right atrium and ventricle.
(2) The bicuspid (mitral) valve separates the left atrium and ventricle.
(3) These valves have cusps, chordae tendineae, and papillary muscles.
(4) Semilunar valves, which have cusps but no chordae tendineae or papillary muscles, separate the right ventricle from the pulmonary artery and the left ventricle from the aorta.
   d. Blood enters the heart from the venae cavae and passes through the following structures:
      (1) right atrium
      (2) tricuspid valve
      (3) right ventricle
      (4) semilunar valve to the pulmonary artery and lung tissue
      (5) from lung tissue and pulmonary veins to the left atrium
      (6) bicuspid (mitral) valve
      (7) left ventricle
      (8) semilunar valve to the aorta

5. Describe the circulation of blood through the heart wall itself.
   a. Blood reaches the myocardium by way of the left and right coronary arteries, their branches, and the capillaries of the myocardium.
   b. Capillaries of the myocardium are drained by sinusoids or veins:
      (1) Sinusoids return blood directly to the ventricles.
      (2) Veins return blood to the right atrium by way of the great coronary vein and coronary sinus.

Physiology of the Heart

6. Explain the initiation and regulation of the heartbeat.
   a. The heartbeat is initiated by the sinoatrial (S-A) node, which sends impulses to:
      (1) the atrioventricular (A-V) node
      (2) the bundle of His
      (3) the Purkinje fibers
   b. The heart rate is regulated by the S-A node (pacemaker), which coordinates the impulses to the ventricles.
   c. The refractory period of cardiac muscle is much longer than that of skeletal muscle.

7. Describe the normal cardiac cycle, including the way it appears in an electrocardiogram.
   a. The cardiac cycle (summarized in Figure 17.14) consists of five phases:
      (1) atrial contraction
      (2) isovolumetric ventricular contraction
      (3) ventricular ejection

(4) isovolumetric ventricular relaxation

(5) ventricular filling

b. The electrocardiogram, a record of electrical discharges associated with the contractions of the cardiac cycle, consists of:

(1) a P wave, seen as the action potential passes over the atria, stimulating contraction

(2) a QRS complex, seen as the ventricles are stimulated to contract

(3) a T-wave, which represents the repolarization of the ventricles (Repolarization of the atria is obscured by the QRS complex.)

8. Define cardiac output in terms of heart rate and stroke volume and discuss the factors that regulate cardiac output.

a. Cardiac output, the amount of blood pumped from each ventricle per minute, is the product of heart rate times stroke volume.

b. The cardiac output of a normal resting adult is about 5 liters per minute, but the cardiac output during exercise, especially in trained athletes, is much higher.

c. Factors that affect cardiac output are summarized in Figure 17.15.

Clinical Applications

9. Define and discuss briefly the causes, effects, and treatment of (a) myocardial infarction, (b) heart failure, (c) arrhythmias, and (d) congenital heart defects.

a. Myocardial infarction, usually caused by blockage of coronary arteries, is an ischemic area of cardiac muscle in which some muscle cells die. Treatment is aimed at supplying oxygen to the damaged cells and reducing the amount of work done by the heart during the healing process.

b. Heart failure, caused by hypertension, coronary artery disease, defective valves, or congenital lesions, is a condition in which the cardiac output is insufficient to provide an adequate blood supply to the tissues. Diuretics are used to remove excess fluids from the tissues, and digitalis is used to strengthen the heartbeat and prevent arrhythmias. Surgery may be used to repair defective valves or bypass diseased coronary arteries.

c. Arrhythmias are disturbances in the heart rate; they often follow a myocardial infarction but can be caused by ectopic foci. Digitalis and sometimes the implantation of an artificial pacemaker are used to treat arrythmias.

d. Congenital heart defects are abnormalities in the structure of the heart due to defective development. Infections such as rubella and medications used by the pregnant mother may cause defects. Treatment usually involves surgery to repair the defects in the heart.

REVIEW

Important Terms

arrhythmia	heart failure
atrial contraction	heart rate
atrium	infarction
auricle	ischemia
A-V node	isovolumetric ventricular contraction
A-V valve	
bradycardia	isovolumetric ventricular relaxation
cardiac cycle	
cardiac output	myocardium
congenital heart defects	pacemaker
coronary arteries	pericardium
coronary sinus	S-A node
diastole	semilunar valves
ectopic foci	stroke volume
electrocardiogram	systole
endocardium	tachycardia
epicardium	ventricle
fibrillation	ventricular ejection
flutter	ventricular filling

Questions

1. a. What is the shape and size of the heart?
   b. Where is the heart located?
   c. What is the major function of the heart?

2. a. How does the heart develop from a single tube to a four-chambered structure?
   b. What are the foramen ovale and the ductus arteriosus?

3. a. What are the three layers of the heart wall?
   b. Where is the pericardial cavity, and how does it fill with fluid?
   c. What is the location and function of the pericardial sac?

4. a. Describe the location and structure of the chambers and valves of the heart.
   b. Trace the flow of blood through the chambers of the heart.

5. Trace the flow of blood through the myocardium.

6. a. List the parts of the conduction system of the heart in sequence from where the impulse is initiated.
   b. What is a pacemaker?
   c. What are ectopic foci, and how do they affect the conduction of impulses through the heart?
   d. How is the refractory period of cardiac muscle different from that of skeletal muscle?

7. **a.** What is an electrocardiogram?
   b. Describe the phases of the cardiac cycle in terms of what is happening to the muscle itself, the valves, and the pressures within the chambers and arteries.
   c. Relate the cardiac cycle to the electrocardiogram and to the heart sounds.

8. **a.** What is cardiac output?
   b. How is the heart rate regulated?
   c. How is stroke volume regulated?

9. **a.** What is a myocardial infarction, and how does the heart recover from such damage?
   b. What is heart failure, and how is it treated?
   c. Distinguish among the various kinds of arrhythmias.
   d. Discuss the nature of common congenital heart defects.

Problems

1. Apply the concepts of this chapter to explain why arrhythmias might follow a myocardial infarction.

2. Suppose you are treating a person who has difficulty breathing, a low urinary output, and tissue edema (fluid collection). Why would you or would you not order an ECG? An SGOT? What would you expect to learn from either of these diagnostic tests?

3. Another person has had an ECG taken. The tracing shows no correlation between the P waves and the QRS complexes. What condition might cause such results? What might be done to treat the person immediately? If the condition persists, what long-term treatment might be used?

4. What would happen if the volume of blood moving from the heart to the aorta were not the same as that moving from the heart to the pulmonary artery?

REFERENCES AND READINGS

Alpert, N. R., Hamrell, B. B., and Mulieri, L. A. 1979. Heart muscle mechanics. *Annual Review of Physiology* 41:521.

Caride, V. J., and Zaret, B. L. 1977. Liposome accumulation in regions of experimental myocardial infarction. *Science* 198:735 (November 18).

Cranefield, P. F., and Wit, A. L. 1979. Cardiac arrythmias. *Annual Review of Physiology* 41:459.

Guyton, A. C. 1981. *Textbook of medical physiology* (6th ed.). Philadelphia: W. B. Saunders.

Haynes, S., and Feinleib, M. 1980. Women, work, and coronary heart disease: Perspectives from the Framingham heart study. *American Journal of Public Health* 70(2):133 (February).

Jarvik, R. K. 1981. The total artificial heart. *Scientific American* 244(2):74 (January).

Kannel, W. B. 1966. *Habits and coronary heart disease: The Framingham heart study.* Bethesda, Md.: National Heart Institute.

Lefer, A. M., Ogletree, M. L., Smith, J. B., Silver, M. J., Nicolaou, K. C., Barnette, W. E., and Gasic, G. P. 1978. Prostacyclin: A potentially valuable agent for preserving myocardial tissue in acute myocardial ischemia. *Science* 200:52 (April 7).

Levy, M. N., Martin, P. J., and Stuesse, S. L. 1981. Neural regulation of the heart beat. *Annual Review of Physiology* 43:443.

Maclean, D., Fishbein, M. C., Maroko, P. R., and Braunwald, E. 1976. Hyaluranidase-induced reductions in myocardial infarct size. *Science* 194:199 (October 8).

Marx, J. L. 1980. Coronary artery spasms and heart disease. *Science* 208:1127 (June 6).

Pollack, G. H. 1977. Cardiac pacemaking: An obligatory role of catecholamines. *Science* 196:731 (May 13).

Somberg, J. C., and Smith, T. W. 1979. Localization of the neurally mediated arrhythmogenic properties of digitalis. *Science* 204:321 (April 20).

Sperelakis, N. 1979. Propagation mechanisms in heart. *Annual Review of Physiology* 41:441.

Stumpf, W. E., Sar, M., and Aumuller, A. 1977. The heart: A target organ for estradiol. *Science* 196:319 (April 15).

Vary, T. C., Reibel, D. K., and Neely, J. R. 1981. Control of energy metabolism of heart muscle. *Annual Review of Physiology* 43:419.

Zelis, R., Flaim, S. F., Liedtke, A. J., and Nellis, S. H. 1981. Cardiocirculatory dynamics in the normal and failing heart. *Annual Review of Physiology* 43:455.

18

CARDIOVASCULAR SYSTEM: BLOOD VESSELS

ORGANIZATION AND GENERAL FUNCTION

Objective 1. Describe the general plan of the circulatory system and list its major functions.

After blood is pumped out of the heart, it circulates throughout the entire body in a closed system of blood vessels and subsequently returns to the heart. These vessels form a complex set of pathways through which blood flows near every cell in the body. The passage of blood through the vessels is regulated in ways that provide an increased blood supply to metabolically active tissues when they need it without depriving any other tissues. Thus, all cells receive nutrients and get rid of wastes according to their needs. In addition to transporting blood, the blood vessels help to regulate the blood pressure and to control the relative amount of blood going to the various tissues.

The general plan of the circulatory system (Figure 18.1) consists of the heart, arteries that carry blood away from the heart, capillaries that allow exchange of substances between blood and the cells, and veins that carry blood back to the heart. Two major circuits exist in the circulatory system: (1) The pulmonary circuit, which carries blood from the right ventricle to the capillaries of the lungs and back to the left atrium, and (2) the systemic circuit, which carries blood from the left ventricle to the capillaries of all other parts of the body and back to the right atrium. In most cases blood passes through only one set of capillaries from the time it leaves the heart until it returns. However, blood leaving the intestinal organs is transported through the hepatic portal system from capillaries of the intestinal organs to another set of capillaries in the liver. After passing through the second set of capillaries, blood is returned to the right atrium.

DEVELOPMENT

Objective 2. Describe briefly the development of the blood vessels.

Blood vessels are derived from the embryonic tissue mesoderm. They originate as cords of cells during the third week of embryonic development. A lumen forms within each cord of cells so that a tube is created, and each tube becomes a blood vessel. Each vessel is lined with endothelium, a layer of squamous epithelium of mesodermal origin. Supporting tissues and smooth muscle come to surround some of the tubes later in development. Eventually, the tubes extend throughout all the tissues of the embryo as thousands of branches are formed by budding. Although there is a typical arrangement of the major blood vessels in the human body, many variations are seen in the distribution of the smaller vessels. These variations are due to the somewhat random pattern of budding that occurs as the embryo develops.

Extensive early development of blood vessels in the human embryo is essential to survival because the human ovum contains very little stored food material. Consequently, the embryo quickly establishes a circulatory system that is in close contact with the maternal blood of the placenta. Throughout the remainder of the developmental period, it receives nutrients and gets rid of wastes by the passage of materials between the fetal and maternal blood across membranes in the placenta. By the end of the third week of embryonic development, the blood vessels of the human embryo have arrived at the stage shown in Figure 18.2. Even though human embryos have almost no yolk, they develop a yolk sac with many blood vessels like vertebrate embryos that have a large yolk containing stored nutrients.

TISSUES OF BLOOD VESSELS

Objective 3. Describe the structure of each type of blood vessel and explain how structure is related to function.

Three major types of blood vessels, differing in both structure and function, are found in the body: arteries, capillaries, and veins. The general structure of each is shown in Figure 18.3.

Arteries and Arterioles

Arteries consist of three coats of tissue (tunicae) that surround the lumen in concentric circles. The walls of the arteries are thicker than the walls of any other vessels, and their thickness helps them to withstand the high pressures exerted on them by the blood they carry from the heart. The inner coat of an artery, the **tunica interna**, or **intima**, consists of a single layer of epithelial cells called the **endothelium**; a thin layer of areolar connective tissue; and a thin layer of elastic connective tissue. The middle and thickest coat of an artery, the **tunica media**, consists of elastic connective tissue and smooth muscle. The outer coat of an artery, the **tunica externa**, or **adventitia**, consists of white fibrous connective tissue with a few elastic fibers and smooth muscle cells. Large arteries are themselves supplied with blood vessels that nourish their thick walls. These vessels are called the **vasa vasorum**, or vessels of a vessel.

The structure of an artery is closely related to its function. The largest arteries receive blood from the heart under high pressure. These arteries are especially well supplied with elastic fibers, particularly in the tunica media, so that the walls of the arteries stretch to accommodate the sudden arrival of a large amount of blood ejected into them from the heart. Because of their **elasticity** such arteries spring back to their former diameter, forcing the blood to move on down the artery. Over and over, with each heartbeat, elastic arteries stretch and spring back.

In arteries farther away from the heart much of the elastic layer is replaced by smooth muscle. The wall of a muscular artery can contract and cause the lumen to become smaller. Such contraction leads to **vasoconstriction**; conversely, relaxation leads to **vasodilation**. By changing the degree of vasoconstriction or vasodilation, the muscular arteries regulate the size of their lumens, thereby determining the distribution of blood in various vessels and maintaining nearly constant blood pressure as the blood gets farther from the heart. The dimensions of arteries and other blood vessels are summarized in Figure 18.4.

Arteries branch and rebranch many times as they traverse the tissues. Most tissues receive blood from more than one arterial branch, and sometimes branches rejoin as they pass through the tissues. The rejoining of branches is called an **anastomosis**. By providing alternate pathways for blood to reach any given tissues, anastomoses help to assure that a tissue will receive blood even when one of the vessels that supplies it is blocked. Such alternate pathways are referred to as **collateral circulation**.

Arterioles are vessels smaller than arteries that also carry blood away from the heart. A gradual transition in the thickness of vessel walls occurs, so it is difficult to determine exactly where an artery becomes an arteriole. Arterioles carry blood to the smallest of all vessels, the capillaries. In many tissues the junctions of arterioles with capillaries are marked by the presence of **precapillary sphincters**, short

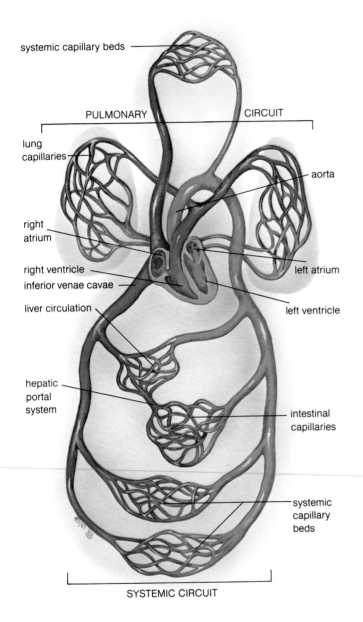

Figure 18.1 The general plan of the circulatory system.

systemic capillary beds

PULMONARY CIRCUIT

lung capillaries

aorta

right atrium

right ventricle

inferior venae cavae

left atrium

liver circulation

left ventricle

hepatic portal system

intestinal capillaries

systemic capillary beds

SYSTEMIC CIRCUIT

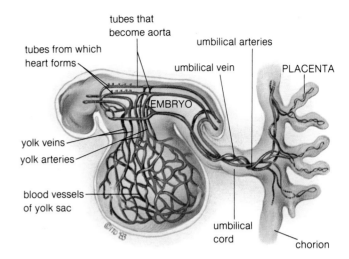

Figure 18.2 The structure of the circulatory system of the human embryo at about three weeks.

tubes that become aorta

tubes from which heart forms

umbilical arteries

umbilical vein

PLACENTA

EMBRYO

yolk veins

yolk arteries

blood vessels of yolk sac

umbilical cord

chorion

Capillaries

Capillaries are thin-walled vessels with an inside diameter of 4 to 12 microns (μ). Their average diameter of 8 μ is just large enough to allow red blood cells to pass through single file. The walls of the capillaries consist of a single layer of endothelial cells continuous with the endothelial lining of the arterioles and venules. Each arteriole branches into many capillaries so that a **capillary network** (Figure 18.5) is formed. This network is so extensive that nearly every cell in the body has a capillary passing very near it.

The thin wall of the capillary is well suited to its function—the exchange of materials between the blood and the cells. Because of its thinness many substances pass from the blood through the capillary wall and into the extracellular fluids that surround the cells. Likewise, many substances from the extracellular fluids pass through the capillary walls and enter the blood. The cells that make up the wall of a capillary are loosely joined so that some substances may easily pass between the cells. Even white blood cells can force their way between the endothelial cells. However, as we shall see later, red blood cells and large protein molecules normally do not leave the capillaries.

Specialized kinds of capillaries are found in certain parts of the body. For example, the capillaries through which large quantities of substances are filtered out of the blood in the kidney are **fenestrated**—perforated with thousands of small holes (*fenestra* = window). These holes facilitate filtration. The capillaries of the brain are covered by a

segments of the blood vessel in which the smooth muscle layer is particularly thick. This muscle allows the vessel to expand or contract and control the entry of blood into the capillaries it serves. When the muscle is completely contracted, blood is prevented from entering the associated capillaries. The precapillary sphincters are extremely important in regulating the relative amounts of blood entering many tissues of the body at any given time.

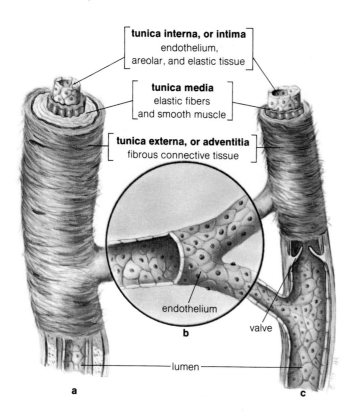

tunica interna, or intima
endothelium, areolar, and elastic tissue

tunica media
elastic fibers and smooth muscle

tunica externa, or adventitia
fibrous connective tissue

endothelium

valve

lumen

a

b

c

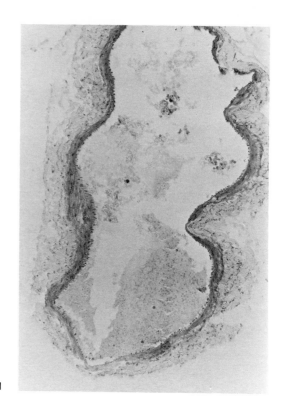

d

Figure 18.3 The general structure of (**a**) an artery, (**b**) a capillary, (**c**) a vein; the capillary is shown larger than is proportional to the size of the artery and vein. (**d**) A cross section of an artery, × 100, (**e**) a cross section of a vein, × 100. (Photographs by author.)

basement membrane and glial cells, as noted in Chapter 11. In some tissues, especially the liver, capillaries are enlarged to form **sinusoids**. Sinusoids have a much larger diameter than capillaries, though their walls are about the same thickness. Sinusoids are lined with phagocytic cells, which remove foreign material from the blood as it passes through the sinusoids. Circulation is slow through sinusoids because of their large total cross-sectional area (see Chapter 19) so there is ample time for phagocytosis to occur.

Veins and Venules

Like arteries, **veins** consist of three coats of tissue (see Figure 18.3). However, they have lesser amounts of elastic tissue and smooth muscle than the arteries but more fibrous connective tissue than arteries. Veins are not subject to receiving blood under high pressure. In fact, the pressure in veins is only barely sufficient to cause the blood to return to the heart.

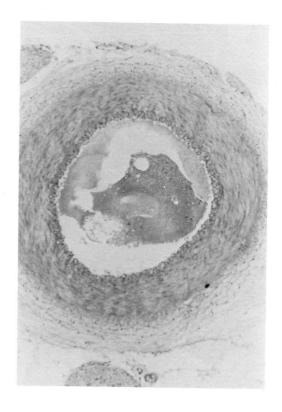

e

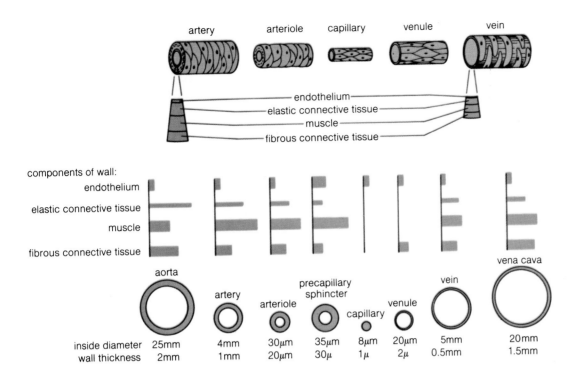

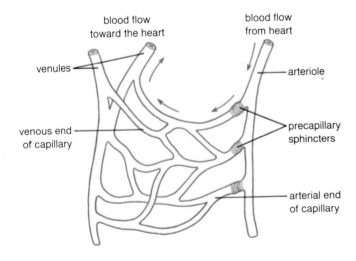

Figure 18.4   A summary of the sizes and structures of the wall of various blood vessels.

Figure 18.5   A capillary network, showing the relationship of arterioles, precapillary sphincters, capillaries, and venules.

Two factors assist in the movement of blood through the veins—valves and muscular contractions. **Valves** (Figure 18.6), specialized structures in the walls of veins, allow blood to flow toward the heart but prevent the backflow of blood away from the heart. Various movements help to push blood foward in the veins. Some breathing movements create negative intrathoracic pressure and thus help to move blood through the thorax. Walking movements, especially

Standing motionless for long periods of time deprives the veins of the assistance of muscular movements to push blood along. Thus, people who must be on their feet should walk around to help keep blood circulating in the legs. They might also stand first on one foot and then on the other, or periodically flex their knees.

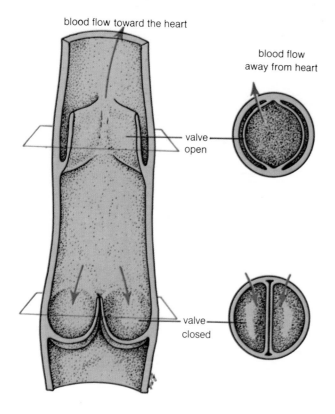

blood flow toward the heart

blood flow away from heart

valve open

valve closed

Figure 18.6 The location and structure of the valves of a vein.

the contractions of the calf muscles, apply pressure to the veins and help to push blood through them. Blood that is pushed upward by muscle contractions is prevented from falling back by the valves.

Like arteries, veins vary in diameter. Tiny **venules** collect blood from the capillaries and carry it to larger venules and eventually to the veins. Veins also sometimes have very large lumens; in this case they are called **sinuses**. They are similar to the sinusoids of the capillaries in two ways. In addition to having large lumens, sinuses consist mostly of endothelium without the protective outer coats. Venous sinuses are found in several locations—the liver, spleen, brain, and heart. The **dural sinuses** lie beneath the dura mater, where they drain blood from the brain, and the **coronary sinus** lies on the posterior surface of the heart.

The sizes and structure of the walls of veins and venules are summarized in Figure 18.4.

The walls of veins can be stretched by prolonged periods of standing or by the stresses of pregnancy. When such stretching occurs, the valves no longer close the lumen of the vein, and backflow occurs. The backflow causes additional stretching, and eventually the walls are greatly weakened and the veins distended. Such distended veins are called **varicose veins**. When veins in the anal canal are similarly distended, they are called **hemorrhoids**.

ANATOMY OF BLOOD VESSELS

Objective 4. Locate and identify the major blood vessels of the human body.

Objective 5. List the special characteristics of the circulation of blood through (a) the brain, (b) the lungs, (c) the intestinal organs and liver, (d) the spleen, (e) the kidneys, (f) the muscles, (g) the skin, and (h) the fetus.

Arteries of the Systemic Circulation

The aorta and the major arteries of the systemic circulation are shown in Figure 18.7. More detailed diagrams of the distribution of some arteries are shown in Figures 18.8 through 18.13. Table 18.1 provides an overview of the major arteries and the regions of the body to which they carry blood. Tables 18.2 through 18.7 provide more detail about the arteries and the regions of the body they supply.

Veins of the Systemic Circulation

The superior and inferior venae cavae and the veins that drain into them make up the venous portion of the systemic circulation. In general, the veins follow the same pathways as the arteries. Figures 18.14 through 18.19 and Tables 18.8 through 18.13 provide information on the venous circulation.

Vessels of the Pulmonary Circulation

As you learned in the chapter on the heart, blood from the right ventricle goes to the lungs and is returned to the left atrium. This pathway is called the **pulmonary circulation** (Figure 18.20). Blood going through the pulmonary circula-

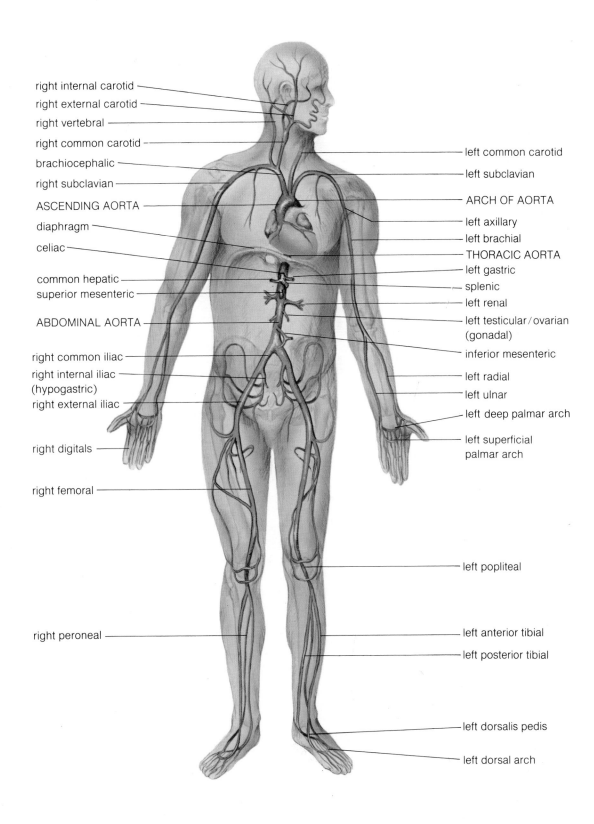

right internal carotid

right external carotid

right vertebral

right common carotid

brachiocephalic

right subclavian

ASCENDING AORTA

diaphragm

celiac

common hepatic

superior mesenteric

ABDOMINAL AORTA

right common iliac

right internal iliac
(hypogastric)

right external iliac

right digitals

right femoral

right peroneal

left common carotid

left subclavian

ARCH OF AORTA

left axillary

left brachial

THORACIC AORTA

left gastric

splenic

left renal

left testicular / ovarian
(gonadal)

inferior mesenteric

left radial

left ulnar

left deep palmar arch

left superficial
palmar arch

left popliteal

left anterior tibial

left posterior tibial

left dorsalis pedis

left dorsal arch

Figure 18.7 An anterior view of the aorta and major arteries.

Table 18.1 The Branches of the Aorta	
Artery	Region of Body Served
Ascending Aorta	
Coronary (right and left)	Heart muscle
Arch of the Aorta	
Brachiocephalic (right)	
Right common carotid	Right side of head and neck
Right subclavian	Right shoulder and arm
Left common carotid	Left side of head and neck
Left subclavian	Left shoulder and arm
Thoracic Aorta	
Intercostals	Intercostal and chest muscles
Superior phrenics	Diaphragm
Bronchials	Nonrespiratory portion of bronchi and lungs
Esophageals	Esophagus
Abdominal Aorta	
Inferior phrenics	Diaphragm
Celiac	Liver, stomach, spleen, and pancreas
Superior mesenteric	Small intestine, ascending and transverse colon
Suprarenals	Adrenal (suprarenal) glands
Renals	Kidneys
Gonadals (ovarian or testicular/spermatic)	Ovaries or testes
Inferior mesenteric	Transverse, descending, and sigmoid colon; rectum
Common iliacs	
Internal iliacs	Urinary bladder, muscles of buttocks, uterus or prostate gland
External iliacs	Hip and leg

tion, passes through the capillaries of the respiratory membranes of the lungs. Here the blood exchanges gases with the air in the lungs, losing carbon dioxide and gaining oxygen. Blood enters the **pulmonary trunk** from the right ventricle. The pulmonary trunk divides into the **right** and **left pulmonary arteries**, which carry blood to the right and left lungs. These arteries branch into the lobar branches and then into many smaller arteries and arterioles, finally reaching capillary size. After passing through the capillaries, the blood enters small venules, veins, and finally the **pulmonary veins**. Two pulmonary veins drain blood from each lung; all four carry blood to the left atrium. The arteries carry unoxygenated blood, and the veins carry oxygenated blood. Only in the pulmonary circulation is this the case; in all other parts of the body (except in fetal circulation), arteries carry oxygenated blood and veins carry unoxygenated blood.

Special Characteristics of Circulation through Various Regions of the Body

Brain Three anatomical properties of the brain and skull contribute to the special characteristics of circulation of blood to and from the brain. First, the arteries at the base of the brain are arranged in a circle, the **circle of Willis**, described in Chapter 11. This circle of blood vessels provides alternate pathways for blood to enter the brain. If one vessel is blocked because of an embolus or obstruction, the blood can often use an alternate pathway to reach all the parts of the brain. Second, the passage of materials from the blood vessels to the cells of the brain is controlled by the **blood-brain barrier**, also described in Chapter 11. This barrier prevents many substances from entering the tissue of the brain, though these substances can enter other tissues. Third, the **skull** provides a chamber around the brain and its blood vessels. Because the skull is noncompressible, the veins inside the brain are not subject to compression from rapid changes in external pressure as are veins in many other parts of the body.

About 15% of the total blood volume is in the brain at all times, regardless of whether the person is engaging in exercise, mental activity, or sleep. The gray matter receives about six times as much blood as the white matter. However, different areas within the brain may receive more blood than others, depending on the mental activities that are taking place. For example, when light is shined in the eyes, the relative amount of blood going to the occipital region of the brain increases. In children the blood flow to the brain is higher than it is in adults—over 100 milliliters/minute per 100 grams of brain tissue compared with

50 to 55 milliliters/minute per 100 grams of brain tissue in adults.

Brain tissue is especially sensitive to reductions in the concentrations of glucose and oxygen and to increases in the concentration of carbon dioxide. Glucose is the primary energy source for brain cells, and these cells cannot readily shift to fat as a source of energy if they are deprived of glucose. Oxygen is essential for the metabolism of glucose; brain cells deprived of oxygen for more than three to five minutes sustain permanent damage. Though glucose and oxygen are exceedingly important for normal brain function, it is the concentration of carbon dioxide that plays a major role in the regulation of blood flow to the brain. If the carbon dioxide concentration increases (as always occurs when oxygen is being used rapidly), the excess carbon dioxide causes dilation of the arteries and increases the flow of blood to the brain.

Table 18.2	Arteries of the Head, Neck, and Brain
Artery	Region of Body Served
Common carotid	
External carotid	Thyroid gland; salivary glands; tongue; neck, throat, scalp, and facial muscles; jaws and teeth.
Internal carotid	Anterior and middle cerebral arteries supply the cerebrum; other branches supply pituitary, eyeball and eye muscles, lacrimal gland and nasal cavity.
Vertebral	Spinal cord and vertebrae of the neck. Left and right vertebrals join to form the basilar artery, which supplies the occipital lobe of the cerebrum and the cerebellum.

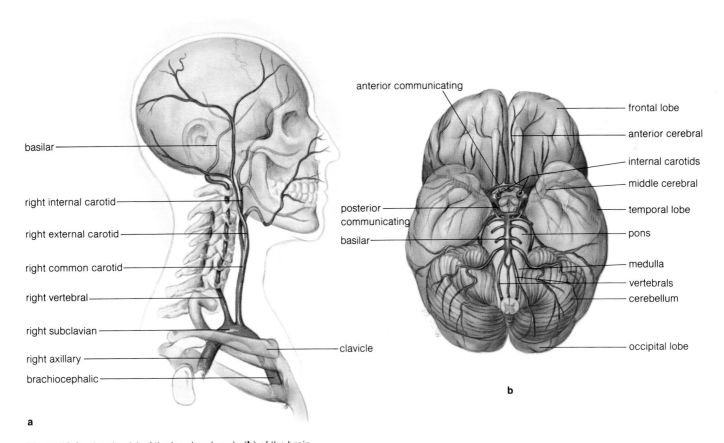

Figure 18.8 Arteries (**a**) of the head and neck, (**b**) of the brain.

Table 18.3	Arteries of the Shoulder and Arm
Artery	Region of Body Served
Subclavian	
Dorsoscapular	Muscles and skin of shoulder and upper back
Internal thoracic (mammary)	Muscles and skin of chest and upper abdomen; breast, membranes of the thoracic cavity, pericardium
Axillary	Continuation of subclavian beyond first rib; muscles of the chest and shoulder, head of humerus and shoulder joint
Brachial	Continuation of axillary beyond shoulder joint; branches supply humerus, muscles and skin of upper arm; frequently used for blood pressure measurements; branches into radial and ulnar distal to the elbow
Radial	Branches supply elbow and muscles of forearm on the thumb side; bones and joints of the wrist
Ulnar	Branches supply elbow and muscles of forearm on ulnar side; bones and joints of the wrist
Palmar arches	Anastomoses of branches of radial and ulnar arteries; branches from the palmar arches supply the digits; create extensive collateral blood supply to hand

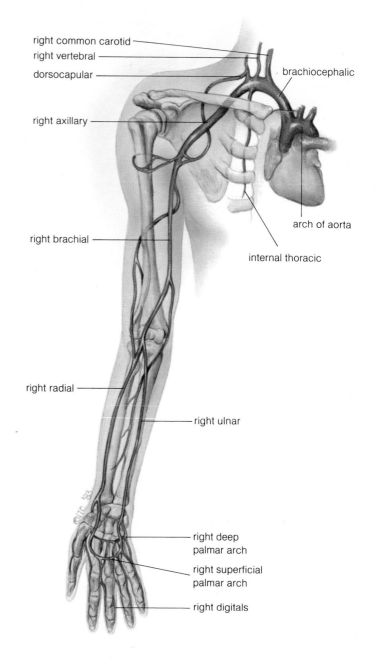

Figure 18.9 Arteries of the shoulder and arm.

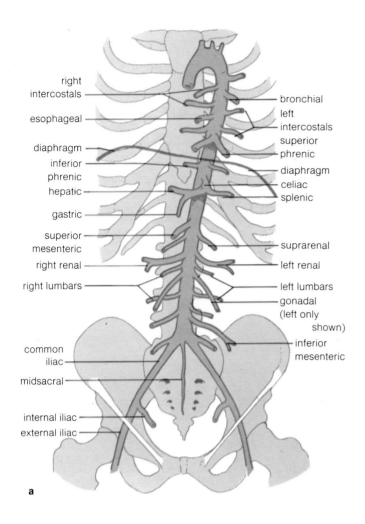

right
intercostals
esophageal
diaphragm
inferior
phrenic
hepatic
gastric
superior
mesenteric
right renal
right lumbars

common
iliac

midsacral

internal iliac
external iliac

bronchial
left
intercostals
superior
phrenic
diaphragm
celiac
splenic

suprarenal
left renal
left lumbars
gonadal
(left only
shown)
inferior
mesenteric

a

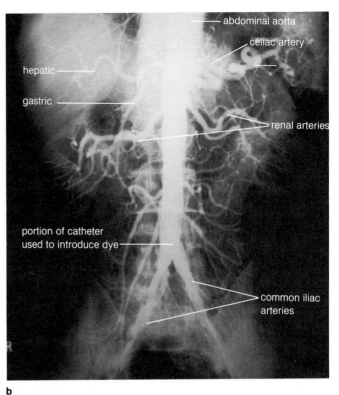

abdominal aorta
celiac artery
hepatic
gastric
renal arteries
portion of catheter
used to introduce dye
common iliac
arteries

b

Figure 18.10 The major arteries branching from the descending aorta: (**a**) a diagram of the positions of the arteries, (**b**) an arteriogram showing some of the major branches of the abdominal aorta. An arteriogram is made by injecting a dye that is opaque to X rays into an artery and X ray photographing the artery and its branches as the dye passes through them. (Arteriogram courtesy of Alexandria Hospital, Alexandria, Virginia, Joyce R. Isbel, R.T.)

Table 18.4 Arteries of the Descending Aorta	
Artery	Region of Body served
Bronchial	Airways, nonrespiratory portion of lungs
Intercostals	Spinal cord, skin and muscles of the back and chest, including intercostal muscles, breasts
Esophageal	Esophagus
Superior phrenic	Diaphragm
Inferior phrenic	Diaphragm
Celiac (see Table 18.5)	
Superior mesenteric (see Table 18.6)	
Suprarenal	Adrenal gland
Renal	Kidneys and ureters; a pair of very large arteries responsible for transporting large quantities of blood through kidneys for waste removal and electrolyte balance
Gonadal (ovarian or testicular, sometimes called spermatic)	Gonads
Inferior mesenteric (see Table 18.6)	
Lumbar	Muscles and skin of lumbar region; lumbar vertebrae
Common iliac (see Table 18.7)	
Midsacral	Sacral vertebrae and rectum

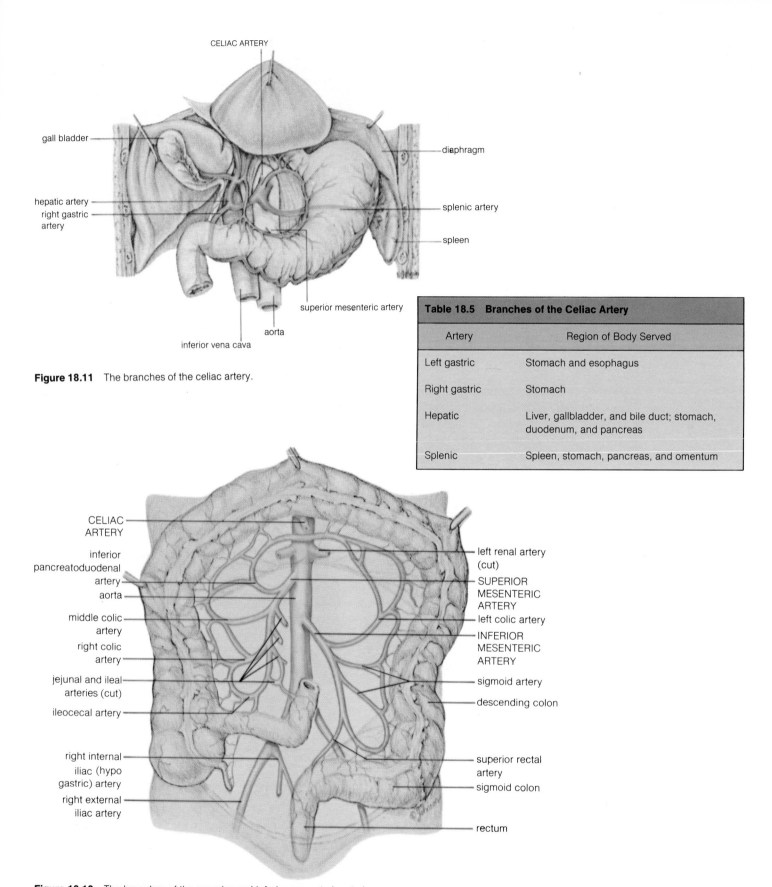

CELIAC ARTERY

gall bladder

hepatic artery
right gastric
artery

diaphragm

splenic artery

spleen

superior mesenteric artery

inferior vena cava

aorta

Figure 18.11   The branches of the celiac artery.

Table 18.5	Branches of the Celiac Artery
Artery	Region of Body Served
Left gastric	Stomach and esophagus
Right gastric	Stomach
Hepatic	Liver, gallbladder, and bile duct; stomach, duodenum, and pancreas
Splenic	Spleen, stomach, pancreas, and omentum

CELIAC ARTERY

inferior pancreatoduodenal artery

aorta

middle colic artery

right colic artery

jejunal and ileal arteries (cut)

ileocecal artery

right internal iliac (hypo gastric) artery

right external iliac artery

left renal artery (cut)

SUPERIOR MESENTERIC ARTERY

left colic artery

INFERIOR MESENTERIC ARTERY

sigmoid artery

descending colon

superior rectal artery

sigmoid colon

rectum

Figure 18.12   The branches of the superior and inferior mesenteric arteries.

Table 18.6 Branches of the Superior and Inferior Mesenteric Arteries

Artery	Region of Body Served
Superior mesenteric	
Intestinal	Many branches to the walls of the small intestine
Inferior pancreatoduodenal	Pancreas and duodenum
Ileocecal	Ileum and cecum
Right colic	Ascending colon
Middle colic	Transverse colon
Inferior Mesenteric	
Left colic	Descending colon
Sigmoid	Descending and sigmoid colon
Superior rectal	Rectum

Table 18.7 The Arteries of the Pelvic Area and Leg

Artery	Region of Body Served
Common iliac	Forms left and right branch from abdominal aorta near the sacrum
Internal iliac (hypogastric)	Pelvic organs, skin and muscles of pelvic area
External iliac	Becomes the femoral artery as it passes to the area of the thigh
Femoral	Muscles of the upper thigh; forms many anastomoses with external iliac and with arteries of the lower leg
Popliteal	Continuation of femoral artery as it passes into the popliteal fossa behind the knee; branches to form the anterior and posterior tibial arteries
Anterior tibial	Skin and muscles of anterior leg and dorsum (upper surface) of foot
Posterior tibial	Skin and muscles of posterior leg, ankle joint, heel, and sole of foot
Dorsalis pedis, dorsal arch, and plantar arch	Anastomosing vessels that serve the midportion of the foot and give rise to branches that serve the toes

Lungs   The lungs receive blood from two sources—the pulmonary arteries and the bronchial arteries. As we have seen, the pulmonary arteries carry blood to the respiratory membranes, where it is oxygenated, and the pulmonary veins return oxygenated blood to the heart. The bronchial arteries, one going to the left lung and two to the right lung, carry blood to the bronchi and other parts of the lungs that conduct air to and from the respiratory membranes. Blood from the bronchial arteries nourishes the nonrespiratory tissues of the respiratory system. (We will consider the circulation of blood through the lungs in more detail in Chapter 21.)

Intestinal organs and liver   Blood enters the intestinal organs by way of the celiac, superior mesenteric, and inferior mesenteric arteries (refer back to Figures 18.11 and 18.12). Oxygenated blood from the celiac artery goes directly to the liver by way of the hepatic artery. The remainder of the blood from these arteries goes first to the capillaries of an organ of the digestive tract or the spleen, where it supplies oxygen and nutrients to the tissues. Blood leaving the capillaries of the digestive tract enters one of several veins that empty into the hepatic portal vein (refer to Figure 18.18). The **hepatic portal vein**, like any other **portal vein**, carries blood from one set of capillaries to another—in this case from the digestive tract to the liver. The hepatic portal vein is the largest blood vessel in the body that does not attach directly to the heart.

Much of the blood carried by the hepatic portal vein comes from the capillaries of the small intestine, where nutrients are absorbed. Thus, the blood is heavily laden with glucose, amino acids, and other nutrients. These nutrients are carried to the liver, where some are stored and others are processed before they are delivered to the tissues.

The liver receives an extremely large portion of the cardiac output—nearly 30%. It also serves as a blood reservoir, retaining up to 500 milliliters of blood in its sinuses. In times of stress stimulation by the sympathetic nervous sys-

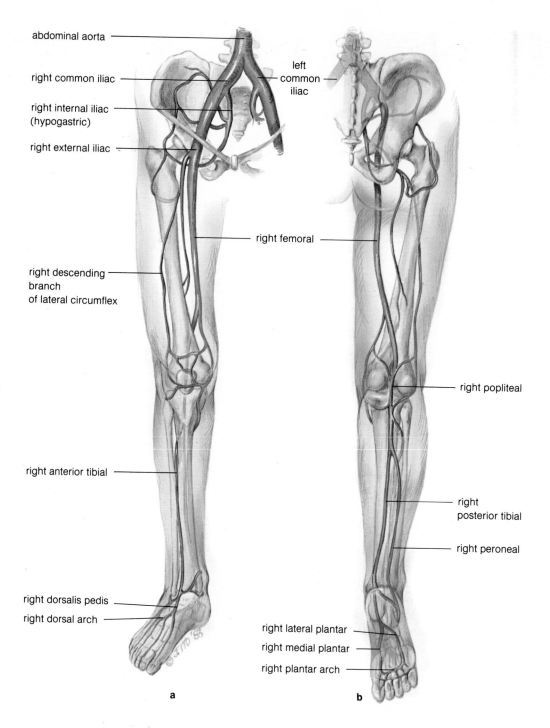

abdominal aorta

right common iliac

right internal iliac
(hypogastric)

right external iliac

left common iliac

right femoral

right descending
branch
of lateral circumflex

right popliteal

right anterior tibial

right posterior tibial

right peroneal

right dorsalis pedis

right dorsal arch

right lateral plantar

right medial plantar

right plantar arch

a

b

Figure 18.13 The arteries of the pelvic area and leg: (**a**) diagram of anterior view, (**b**) diagram of posterior view, (**c**) arteriogram of pelvic area after injection of dye, (**d**) arteriogram of thigh, showing dye in arteries adjacent to and within the femur, (**e**) arteriogram of the knees, (**f**) arteriogram of the legs and ankles. Figures (**c**) through (**f**) were taken in sequence as the injected dye passed from the pelvic area to the ankles. (Arteriograms courtesy of Alexandria Hospital, Alexandria, Virginia, Joyce R. Isbel, R.T.)

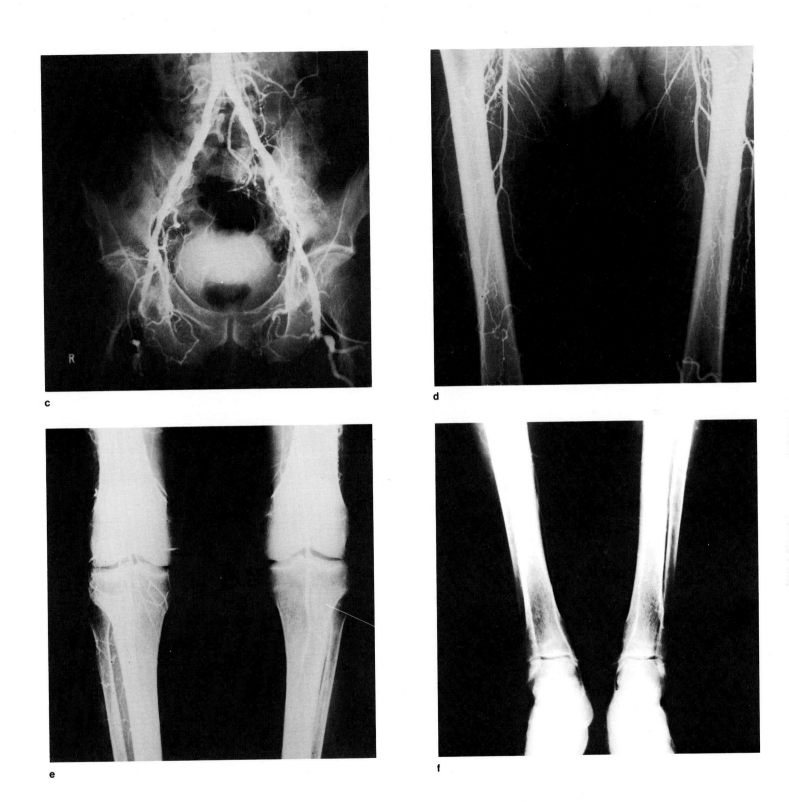

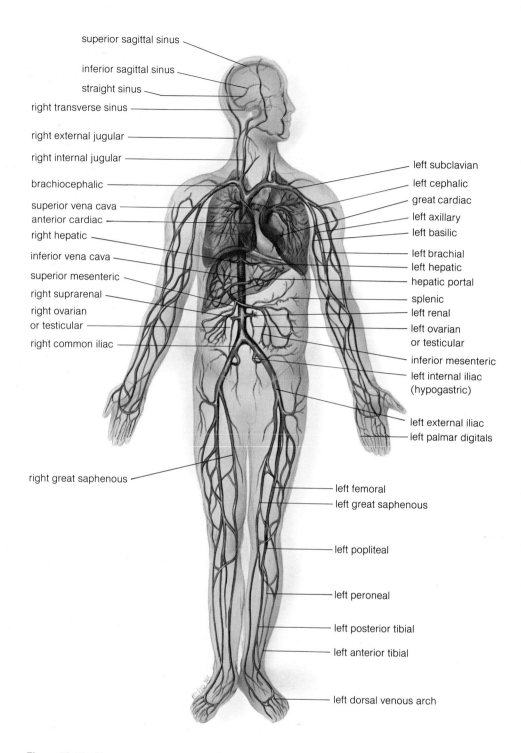

superior sagittal sinus

inferior sagittal sinus

straight sinus

right transverse sinus

right external jugular

right internal jugular

brachiocephalic

superior vena cava

anterior cardiac

right hepatic

inferior vena cava

superior mesenteric

right suprarenal

right ovarian or testicular

right common iliac

right great saphenous

left subclavian

left cephalic

great cardiac

left axillary

left basilic

left brachial

left hepatic

hepatic portal

splenic

left renal

left ovarian or testicular

inferior mesenteric

left internal iliac (hypogastric)

left external iliac

left palmar digitals

left femoral

left great saphenous

left popliteal

left peroneal

left posterior tibial

left anterior tibial

left dorsal venous arch

Figure 18.14 The major veins of the human body in anterior view.

Table 18.8	Veins Draining into the Superior and Inferior Venae Cavae	
Vein	**Region of Body Served**
Superior Vena Cava	
Azygos	Thorax
Brachiocephalic (innominate)	Head, neck, and arms
Internal jugular	Inside of skull and brain
External jugular	Skin and muscles of scalp and face
Subclavian	Shoulder and arm
Inferior Vena Cava	
Hepatic	Liver
Suprarenal	Adrenal gland
Renal	Kidneys
Gonadal (ovarian or testicular/spermatic)	Gonads
Common iliac	Pelvic area and legs

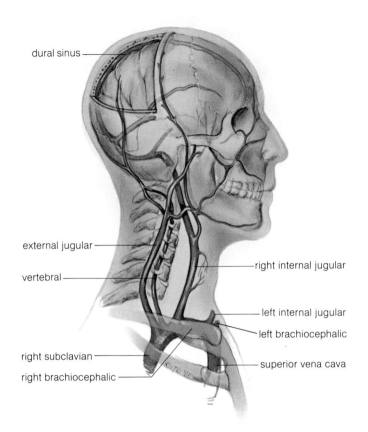

Figure 18.15 Veins of the head, neck, and brain.

tem can cause the liver to release as much as 300 milliliters of blood into the circulation. The details of circulation within the liver are considered in Chapter 22.

Spleen Circulation of the blood through the spleen, as noted above, involves the celiac artery and the hepatic portal vein. However, the spleen itself has some special circulatory characteristics. The spleen is made up of lymphatic tissue and contains many large sinusoids with phagocytic cells along the walls. These cells destroy worn out red blood cells as they pass through the sinusoids. Because of the many sinusoids the spleen also contains a large volume of blood. As blood oozes through the sinusoids, many blood cells become trapped in the sinusoids. When the body is under stress, stimulation by the sympathetic nervous system can cause blood vessels in the spleen to constrict, ejecting up to 250 milliliters of blood into the systemic circulation. Because this blood contains large numbers of red blood cells, its release into the circulation can increase the volume of red cells in circulation by 3 to 4%.

Table 18.9	Veins Draining the Head, Neck, and Brain
Vein	**Region of Body Served**
Brachiocephalic (left and right)	Receives blood from all other veins of head, neck, and brain
Internal jugular	Receives blood from dural sinuses inside cranial cavity
External jugular	Receives blood from salivary (parotid) glands, skin and muscles of the face, scalp, and neck
Vertebral	Receives blood from the cerebellum

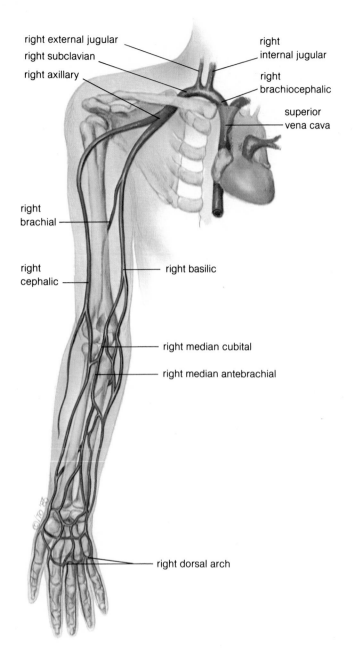

right external jugular
right subclavian
right axillary
right internal jugular
right brachiocephalic
superior vena cava
right brachial
right basilic
right cephalic
right median cubital
right median antebrachial
right dorsal arch

Figure 18.16 Veins of the shoulder and arm.

Table 18.10	Veins Draining the Shoulder and Arm
Vein	Region of Body Served
Subclavian	Drains into the brachiocephalic; receives the cephalic and axillary veins
Cephalic	Drains the radial side of upper arm and forearm
Axillary	Drains the brachial and basilic veins
Brachial	Drains the skin and muscles of the posterior upper arm
Basilic	Drains the medial side of the lower arm; receives the median cubital and median antebrachial
Dorsal arch	Anastomoses of larger veins in the hand; also drains the digits

Kidneys   The kidneys receive large quantities of blood by way of the renal arteries. As we shall see in Chapters 25 and 26, the kidneys remove wastes from the blood and also adjust the concentration of various constituents of the blood. Under resting conditions about 22% of the left ventricular cardiac output goes through the kidneys.

Muscles   The amount of blood flowing through the muscles is highly variable, depending on the amount of muscular contraction that is taking place. Each 100 grams of tissue receives 4 to 7 milliliters of blood per minute during rest and 50 to 75 milliliters during exercise. Muscle fibers in the walls of the arterioles themselves can be stimulated to contract or relax and thus regulate the amount of blood that is delivered to the muscles. When an individual is engaging in strenuous muscular activity, these arterioles dilate and allow a large quantity of blood to enter the capillaries of the muscles. When an individual is at rest, these arterioles constrict and reduce the amount of blood circulating through the muscles. Dilation of arterioles during exercise is caused primarily by changes in skeletal muscle metabolism. Changes in sympathetic nervous system activity and blood oxygen concentration may also regulate blood flow in these vessels during exercise.

Skin   As in the muscles, arterioles in the skin can also constrict or dilate. The constriction and dilation of skin arterioles is important in the regulation of body temperature. When the body temperature rises, the blood vessels

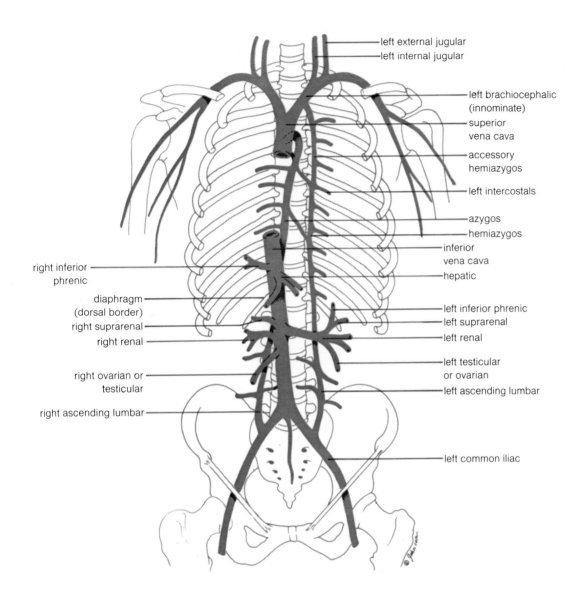

left external jugular
left internal jugular
left brachiocephalic (innominate)
superior vena cava
accessory hemiazygos
left intercostals
azygos
hemiazygos
inferior vena cava
hepatic
left inferior phrenic
left suprarenal
left renal
left testicular or ovarian
left ascending lumbar
left common iliac

right inferior phrenic
diaphragm (dorsal border)
right suprarenal
right renal
right ovarian or testicular
right ascending lumbar

Figure 18.17 Veins of the thorax and abdomen.

Table 18.11   Veins Draining the Thorax and Abdomen

Vein	Region of Body Served
Superior Vena Cava	
Azygos	Drains into superior vena cava; serves as a collateral vessel for draining thoracic and abdominal skin and muscles
Brachiocephalic	
Hemiazygos	Drains into brachiocephalic; also serves as a collateral vessel for draining thoracic and abdominal skin and muscles
Ascending lumbar	Drains into hemiazygos; drains blood from lumbar skin and muscles
Inferior Vena Cava	
Right inferior phrenic	Diaphragm
Hepatic	Drains liver, which receives all blood from organs of the digestive tract (see Table 18.12)
Right suprarenal	Adrenal gland
Right renal	Kidney
Right ovarian or testicular	Gonad
Left renal	Receives branches from left inferior phrenic, left suprarenal, and left ovarian or testicular, in addition to draining kidney
Common iliac	Receives blood from pelvic area and leg; also receives left ascending lumbar, which forms a collateral pathway for the return of blood to the venae cavae

Table 18.12   Veins of the Hepatic Portal System

Vein	Region of Body Served
Hepatic portal vein	Receives blood from organs of the digestive system; transports blood to the liver, where it is circulated through hepatic sinusoids and carried to the hepatic veins
Splenic	Drains blood from the spleen and stomach to the hepatic portal vein
Superior mesenteric	Drains blood from the small intestine and part of the large intestine to the hepatic portal vein
Inferior mesenteric	Drains blood from part of the large intestine to the splenic vein

Table 18.13   Veins of the Pelvis and Leg

Vein	Region of Body Served
Common iliac	Drains into inferior vena cava
Internal iliac (hypogastric)	Drains pelvic organs and skin and muscles of the pelvic area
External iliac	Drains all of the veins of the leg into the common iliac
Deep femoral	Drains the deep muscles and bones of the leg; becomes the popliteal behind the knee; drains the peroneal vein, the anterior tibial, and the posterior tibial
Great saphenous	Drains the medial superficial skin and muscles of the leg
Dorsalis pedis, dorsal arch, and plantar arch	Establish collateral circulation through the foot and drain the digits

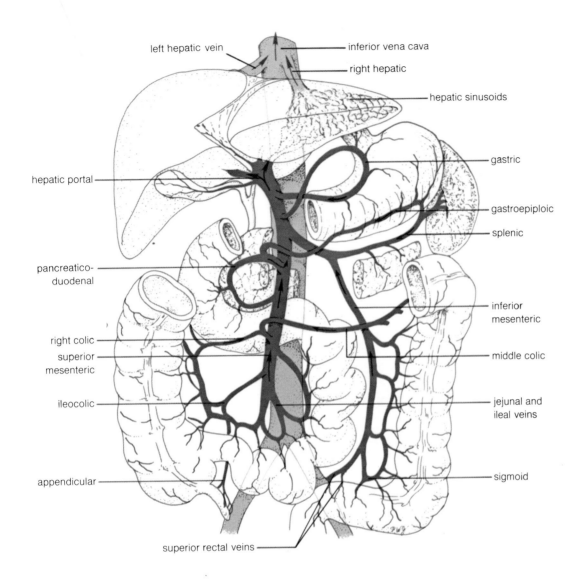

left hepatic vein

inferior vena cava

right hepatic

hepatic sinusoids

gastric

hepatic portal

gastroepiploic

splenic

pancreatico-
duodenal

inferior
mesenteric

right colic

middle colic

superior
mesenteric

ileocolic

jejunal and
ileal veins

appendicular

sigmoid

superior rectal veins

Figure 18.18   Veins of the hepatic portal system. Arrows show the direction of the flow of blood.

dilate and allow more blood (as much as 2500 milliliters/minute) to pass through capillaries near the surface of the skin. Heat is then lost through the skin. When the body temperature falls, the blood vessels constrict and limit the amount of blood passing through the capillaries, and heat is conserved. Blood vessels of the skin and muscles often either constrict or dilate simultaneously because exercise is a main cause of an increase in temperature and inactivity is a main cause of a decrease in temperature. Blushing, initiated by the sympathetic nervous system, results from dilation of blood vessels in the skin of the face.

Fetus   The circulation of blood through a developing fetus deviates from the circulation after birth in four ways (Figure 18.21). Fetal blood is delivered to the placenta through a pair of **umbilical arteries** and returned to the fetus through a single **umbilical vein**. The umbilical vein joins the hepatic portal vein near the liver. Most of the blood from the placenta and the fetal digestive organs passes through the **ductus venosus** to the inferior vena cava, bypassing the liver. Of the blood entering the right atrium, some goes to the right ventricle and some through the **foramen ovale** to the left atrium. Only the blood going to the right ventricle

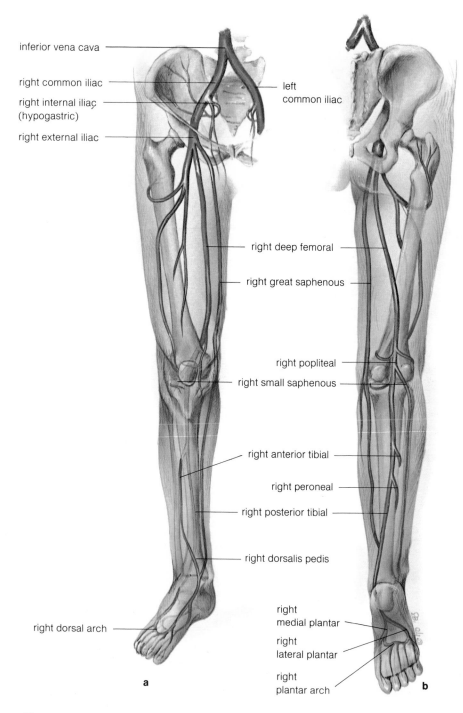

inferior vena cava

right common iliac

right internal iliac
(hypogastric)

right external iliac

left
common iliac

right deep femoral

right great saphenous

right popliteal

right small saphenous

right anterior tibial

right peroneal

right posterior tibial

right dorsalis pedis

right
medial plantar

right
lateral plantar

right
plantar arch

right dorsal arch

a

b

Figure 18.19 Veins of the pelvic area and leg: (**a**) diagram of anterior view, (**b**) diagram of posterior view, (**c**) X ray of venous flow through the right common iliac vein and its branches. Note the constriction in the right external iliac. (X ray courtesy of Alexandria Hospital, Alexandria, Virginia, Joyce R. Isbel, R.T.)

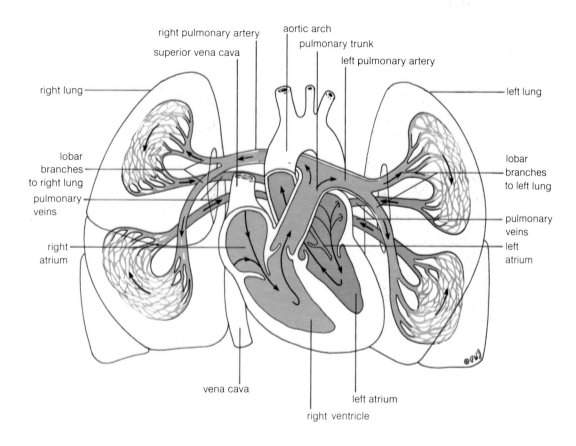

right pulmonary artery

aortic arch

superior vena cava

pulmonary trunk

left pulmonary artery

right lung

left lung

lobar
branches
to right lung

lobar
branches
to left lung

pulmonary
veins

pulmonary
veins

right
atrium

left
atrium

vena cava

left atrium

right ventricle

Figure 18.20 The pulmonary circulation. Arteries carrying unoxygenated blood are shown in gray. Veins carrying oxygenated blood are shown in color.

passes through the pulmonary artery; much of the blood in the pulmonary artery passes through the **ductus arteriosus** to the aorta, bypassing the pulmonary circulation. The umbilical vessels, ductus venosus, foramen ovale, and ductus arteriosus function only in the fetus, where they provide for the circulation of blood through the placenta and for limiting the circulation of blood through the fetal liver and lungs (Figure 18.21b).

Many functions carried out after birth by the infant's liver are carried out before birth by the mother's liver. Nutrients are processed and made ready for absorption across the placenta, and toxic substances that might enter the mother's body are often detoxified, thereby minimizing the effect of such substances on the fetus. The fetal liver is too immature to perform these functions; in fact, it has

difficulty metabolizing the breakdown products of its own worn-out red blood cells. Consequently, many newborn infants, especially premature ones, show signs of jaundice.

Though the fetal liver is limited in function, it does require nutrients and oxygen. In addition to supplying nutrients, the maternal blood passing through the placenta supplies the fetus with oxygen and removes carbon dioxide and some other wastes from the fetal blood. Thus, the placenta serves as a respiratory organ for the fetus and to some extent as a kidney, too.

Modifications in the circulation of blood through the fetal heart are related to the fact that the fetal lungs do not function as respiratory organs. About two-thirds of the blood entering the right atrium passes through the foramen ovale and bypasses the pulmonary circulation. Some of the

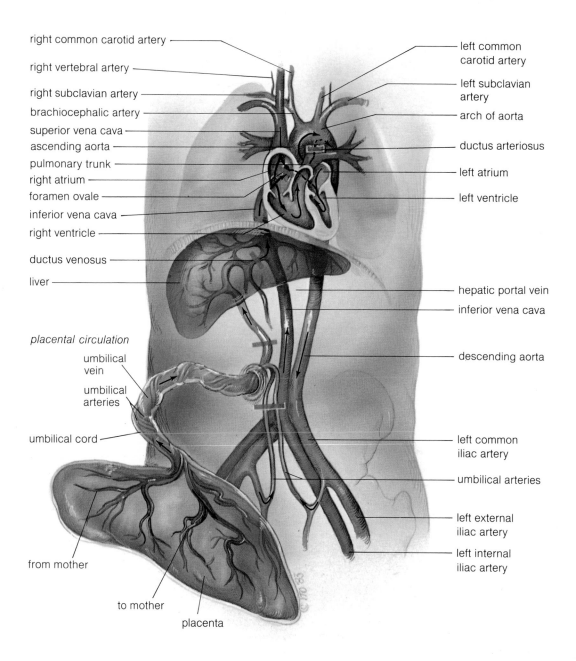

right common carotid artery

right vertebral artery

right subclavian artery

brachiocephalic artery

superior vena cava

ascending aorta

pulmonary trunk

right atrium

foramen ovale

inferior vena cava

right ventricle

ductus venosus

liver

placental circulation

umbilical vein

umbilical arteries

umbilical cord

from mother

to mother

placenta

left common carotid artery

left subclavian artery

arch of aorta

ductus arteriosus

left atrium

left ventricle

hepatic portal vein

inferior vena cava

descending aorta

left common iliac artery

umbilical arteries

left external iliac artery

left internal iliac artery

Figure 18.21 (**a**) The circulation of blood through a fetus. The bars across blood vessels indicate sites through which blood no longer flows after birth. (**b**) Diagram of pathways of blood within a fetus.

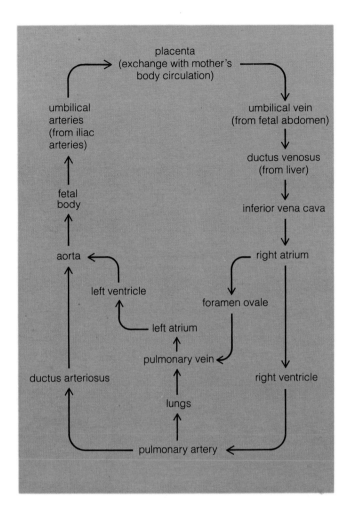

blood that leaves the heart by way of the pulmonary artery enters the aorta by way of the ductus arteriosus. Only enough blood passes through the pulmonary circulation to nourish the developing lung tissue.

The remainder of the fetal circulation is the same as postnatal circulation, except that blood entering the internal iliac arteries passes through extensions of these arteries, the umbilical arteries, and blood returning from the placenta arrives via the umbilical vein.

Shortly after birth several events take place that alter the fetal circulation and establish the neonatal circulation. The tying of the umbilical cord blocks the flow of blood through all of the umbilical vessels; these vessels atrophy and become fibrous ligaments. Within one to three hours after birth the muscular wall of the ductus venosus contracts, blocking the passage of blood through it. With the expansion of the lungs as breathing begins, the blood vessels within the lungs dilate. Increased blood flow to the lungs alters the pressures in the chambers of the heart. The pressure in the left atrium becomes greater than the pressure in the right atrium. A flap of tissue on the left side of the interatrial septum closes over the foramen ovale, and the higher pressure in the left atrium holds the flap in place. Over a period of a few months the flap adheres to the septum, and the closure becomes permanent. For a few hours to a few days after birth the ductus arteriosus remains open, but the higher pressure in the aorta causes the flow through the ductus arteriosus to go from the aorta to the pulmonary artery. Eventually, the ductus arteriosus atrophies, and all fetal connections between the pulmonary and systemic circulations are closed off.

CLINICAL TERMS

aneurysm (an'u-rizm)   a saclike dilation of a blood vessel

claudication (klaw-dik-a'shun)   limping or lameness often associated with blood vessel disease in a leg

cyanosis (si-an-o'sis)   bluishness of the skin, usually due to insufficient oxygenation of the blood

hematoma (hem-at-o'mah)   a solid mass of clotted blood in a tissue caused by leakage of blood vessels

shunt   to turn aside or divert; passage between the sides of the heart or between two blood vessels, as in an arteriovenous shunt

CHAPTER SUMMARY

(Chapter summary points and review questions are numbered to correspond to the numbered objectives in the text of each chapter.)

Organization and General Function

1. Describe the general plan of the circulatory system and list its major functions.
   a. The circulatory system consists of the heart, blood, and blood vessels.
   b. The blood vessels are arranged in two main circuits:
      (1) the pulmonary circuit
      (2) the systemic circuit
   c. The main function of the circulatory system is to transport substances to and from all the cells of the body.

Development

2. Describe briefly the development of the blood vessels.
   a. Blood vessels begin development as cords of cells that hollow out to form tubes.
   b. The tubes become distributed to all tissues by budding.

Tissues of Blood Vessels

3. Describe the structure of each type of blood vessel and explain how structure is related to function.
   a. The three main types of blood vessels are:
      (1) arteries, which carry blood away from the heart
      (2) veins, which carry blood toward the heart
      (3) capillaries, which pass near cells and exchange substances
   b. Arteries consist of:
      (1) a tunica interna (intima), which includes a single layer of cells called the endothelium, a thin layer of connective tissue, and a thin internal elastic membrane
      (2) a tunica media, which includes elastic connective tissue and smooth muscle
      (3) a tunica externa (adventitia), which consists of fibrous connective tissue
      (4) Large arteries are supplied with smaller blood vessels, vasa vasorum
   c. Arterioles are small blood vessels that branch from arteries and carry blood to capillaries. At their junction with capillaries they have precapillary sphincters, short segments with a thick layer of smooth muscle.
   d. Capillaries:
      (1) are about 8 μ in diameter
      (2) consist of endothelium, which allows exchange of substances with the tissues

      (3) may be fenestrated or enlarged to form sinusoids
   e. Veins:
      (1) have the same three layers as arteries, but contain more connective tissue and less elastic tissue and smooth muscle
      (2) may be enlarged to form sinuses
      (3) contain valves, which prevent backflow of blood
      (4) are assisted in maintaining blood flow by skeletal muscle contractions
   f. Venules are small blood vessels that connect capillaries and veins.

Anatomy of Blood Vessels

4. Locate and identify the major blood vessels of the human body.
   a. Major blood vessels of the systemic circulation include:
      (1) the aorta and its branches (listed in Table 18.1)
      (2) the superior and inferior venae cavae and their branches (listed in Table 18.8)
   b. Vessels of the pulmonary circulation include:
      (1) the pulmonary artery and its branches
      (2) the pulmonary veins and their branches
   c. The hepatic portal vein carries blood from the digestive organs and spleen to the liver (see Table 18.12).
   d. Other vessels are named in Tables 18.2 through 18.7, 18.9 through 18.11, and 18.13.

5. List the special characteristics of the circulation of blood through (a) the brain, (b) the lungs, (c) the intestinal organs and liver, (d) the spleen, (e) the kidneys, (f) the muscles, (g) the skin, and (h) the fetus.
   a. In the brain:
      (1) arteries at the base of the brain form the circle of Willis, which provides alternate pathways for blood to enter the brain
      (2) the blood–brain barrier prevents many substances in the blood from entering the brain tissue
      (3) the skull, being noncompressible, prevents veins of the brain from being compressed by atmospheric pressure
      (4) about 15% of the blood volume is in the brain at all times
      (5) brain tissue is especially sensitive to changes in glucose and oxygen supply
   b. In the lungs:
      (1) respiratory membranes receive blood from the pulmonary circulation
      (2) nonrespiratory portions of the lungs are nourished by the bronchial arteries
   c. In the intestinal organs and liver:
      (1) the digestive organs and spleen receive oxygenated blood from branches of the aorta and are drained by branches of the hepatic portal vein

(2) blood in the hepatic portal vein carries many nutrients from the digestive organs to the liver

d. In the spleen:

    (1) large sinusoids store blood that can be released into circulation when the body is under stress

    (2) phagocytic cells in the linings of the sinusoids destroy worn out erythrocytes

e. In the kidney:

    (1) wastes are filtered from the blood

    (2) the concentrations of various substances in the blood are adjusted

f. In the muscles:

    (1) blood flow varies greatly—increasing during exercise and decreasing during rest

    (2) dilation of blood vessels during exercise is caused primarily by changes in muscle metabolism

g. In the skin:

    (1) blood vessels dilate when the body temperature is elevated and constrict when the body temperature is lowered

    (2) skin blood vessels are therefore important in temperature regulation

h. In the fetus:

    (1) the umbilical vein carries blood from the placenta to the fetus, and the umbilical arteries carry blood from the fetus to the placenta

    (2) the foramen ovale and the ductus arteriosus allow blood to bypass the pulmonary circulation

    (3) at birth umbilical circulation ceases, and the pathways that bypass the lungs close so that blood is oxygenated in the lungs

REVIEW

Important Terms

adventitia	tunica externa
anastomosis	tunica interna
arteriole	tunica media
artery	valve
capillary	vasa vasorum
collateral circulation	vasoconstriction
endothelium	vasodilation
fenestrated	vein
portal vein	venule
precapillary sphincter	See tables for names of major
sinus	blood vessels.
sinusoid	

Questions

1. a. What is the difference between the systemic and the pulmonary circulation?

  b. What are the main functions of the circulatory system?

2. a. How do blood vessels supply every cell in the body?

  b. Why does a human embryo require a blood supply early in development?

3. a. How do the walls of arteries and veins differ, and how do they resemble each other?

  b. What is the function of vasa vasorum, and what does it have in common with a coronary artery?

  c. How do the properties of elasticity and contractility account for the behavior of arteries, arterioles, and veins?

  d. Define anastomosis, collateral circulation, and precapillary sphincter.

  e. How is the structure of a capillary related to its function?

  f. What is the function of the valves in the veins, and why are valves not necessary in arteries?

  g. How do sinuses and sinusoids differ, and how are they alike?

4. a. Trace the flow of blood from the celiac artery to the external jugular vein.

  b. Trace the flow of blood from the internal carotid artery to the renal vein.

  c. Trace the flow of blood from the subclavian artery to the great saphenous vein.

5. a. What special characteristics are found in the circulation of blood through the brain, the lungs, the intestinal organs, and the spleen?

  b. Under what conditions would the volume of blood in the muscles and in the skin change?

  c. Trace the flow of blood from the placenta through a developing fetus and back to the placenta.

Problems

1. Describe in as much detail as possible what happens in the various blood vessels in your body when you engage in strenuous exercise.

2. Combine what you have learned in this chapter and others to explain all the changes that occur in the circulatory system of an infant at the time of birth and the few days following birth.

REFERENCES AND READINGS

Gray, H. 1973. *Anatomy of the human body* (29th American ed.). C. M. Goss, ed. Philadelphia: Lea and Febiger.

Sparks, H. V., and Belloni, F. L. 1978. Local vascular regulation. *Annual Review of Physiology* 40: 67.

19

CARDIOVASCULAR SYSTEM: CIRCULATION

PRINCIPLES OF CIRCULATION

Objective 1. State the principles of pressure, flow, and resistance in fluids as they apply to the circulation of blood.

The principles of pressure, flow, and resistance that apply to the flow of a fluid through a tube also apply to the flow of blood through a blood vessel.

Flow is the volume of fluid moving through a tube in a given period of time. **Pressure** is force per unit area—the force tending to push fluid through a tube. **Resistance** is the force that tends to oppose the flow. Fluid flows from one point to another along a tube because of a pressure decrease. Flow is directly proportional to the change in pressure; that is, the greater the driving pressure, the greater the flow. On the other hand, as resistance increases, flow decreases; flow is therefore said to be inversely proportional to resistance. These ideas are summarized in the following equation:

$$\text{flow (milliliters/minute)} = \frac{\text{change in pressure}}{\text{resistance}}$$

Resistance Resistance to movement is mainly the result of friction within the moving liquid and between the moving liquid and the stationary tube. Resistance to the flow of blood is determined by the cross-sectional area, the length of the blood vessel, and the viscosity of the blood.

The greatest single factor affecting the resistance in a vessel is cross-sectional size. This size is expressed in terms of the vessel's internal radius, which is half its internal diameter. Resistance is inversely proportional to the fourth power of the radius (Figure 19.1).

$$\text{resistance} = \frac{1}{\text{radius}^4}$$

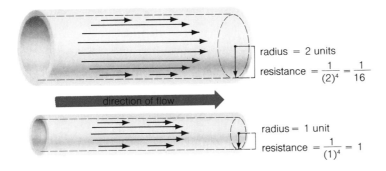

Figure 19.1 The effect of the internal radius of a vessel on resistance when pressure and other factors are held constant.

radius = 1 unit
P_{in} ——— P_{out}
length = x

radius = 1 unit
P_{in} ——— P_{out}
length = 2x

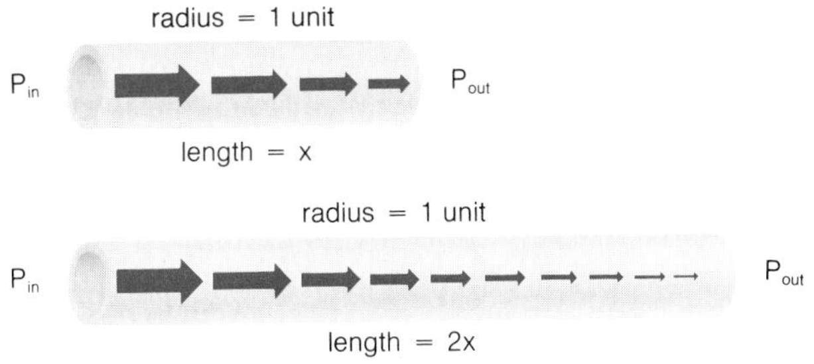

Figure 19.2 The effect of the length of a vessel on resistance. When P_{in} (pressure of blood entering the vessel) is the same for both vessels, P_{out} (pressure of blood leaving vessel) is less in the longer vessel. When the difference between P_{in} and P_{out} is the same for both vessels, the flow in the shorter (× length) vessel is twice as great as the flow in the longer (2 × length) vessel.

For example, the resistance offered by a vessel with a radius of 1 unit is $1/(1)^4$ or 1; the resistance offered a vessel with a radius of 2 units is $1/(2)^4$ or 1/16. Thus, the vessel with the radius of 2 units has a resistance of only 1/16 that of the vessel with the radius of 1 unit. Consequently, large vessels in the body give much less resistance to flow than small vessels, provided pressure and other factors are held constant.

Resistance is also affected by the length of a vessel. Other factors being equal, the resistance of a vessel is directly proportional to its length (Figure 19.2). The resistance encountered by blood flowing through a vessel of length 2X is twice that encountered by a vessel of length X because the fluid molecules encounter twice as much friction-creating vessel surface. Assuming that both vessels have the same radius and the same input pressure (P_{in}), the output pressure (P_{out}) at the end of the longer vessel will be less than the pressure at the end of the shorter vessel. However, if pressure is maintained so that the change in pressure from P_{in} to P_{out} is the same for both vessels, the flow through the shorter vessel will be twice that through the longer vessel because the shorter vessel has only half the resistance.

Viscosity **Viscosity** has a small effect on the flow of blood. Viscosity, a fluid's own internal resistance to flow, is a measure of the degree of difficulty the molecules of the

fluid have in sliding over one another. At the same pressure difference between the input and the output ends of a vessel, a viscous fluid (like molasses) flows much more slowly than a less viscous fluid (like water). Because of the presence of blood cells and large molecules, blood is about five times more viscous than water, but much less viscous than molasses. Normally, the viscosity of blood remains nearly constant, but diseases that increase or decrease the number of cells or other constituents in blood can alter its viscosity. Conditions such as polycythemia and sometimes leukemia greatly increase the blood's viscosity.

Pressure As we have seen, flow is proportional to the pressure difference between one point in a vessel and another point farther along the vessel. Pressure is generated by the contractions of the ventricles pushing blood into the blood vessels. In general, the pressure in vessels decreases from the high pressure in the aorta to the low pressure in the venae cavae (Figure 19.3). Blood pressure will be discussed further in the next section.

Cross-sectional area Cross-sectional area, an important factor in understanding the circulation of blood, is equivalent to the size of the lumen of a tube. Notice that in Figure 19.4 the cross-sectional area of the large vessel is about 114 square millimeters—much larger than any of its branches. However, the total cross-sectional area of the eight branches shown is about twice as great as that of the large vessel. This diagram represents the situation we might find in the body as a large artery branches into eight smaller arteries. But the branching in the body does not stop with the smaller arteries. Additional branching occurs to form arterioles and then capillaries. The estimated total cross-sectional area of each type of blood vessel is shown in Table 19.1. The cross-sectional area increases about 1000 times from the aorta to the capillaries.

Velocity **Velocity** is the distance traveled in a given time, or the speed of the moving fluid. It is proportional to flow divided by the total cross-sectional area of the vessels:

$$\text{Velocity} = \frac{\text{flow}}{\text{total cross-sectional area}}$$

As shown in Figure 19.3, the velocity of blood varies from relatively high in the arteries to very low in the capillaries, with an intermediate velocity in the veins. Velocity decreases as the total cross-sectional area increases. This is analogous to the flow of water in a river. At a point in the river where the channel is narrow, velocity is rapid; as the channel widens, the velocity decreases. Should the channel narrow again, the velocity would increase. Likewise, in blood vessels velocity is rapid in the aorta and larger arteries, slow in capillaries, and faster in veins—but never as fast as in arteries.

Flow As noted earlier, flow is the volume of fluid moving through a tube in a given period of time. Over the whole circulatory system total flow is constant. The amount of blood leaving the ventricles is the same as the amount of blood entering the atria. In one minute the same number of milliliters of blood flows through arteries, capillaries, and veins. As blood passes from arteries to arterioles, the number of milliliters of blood passing through a single arteriole is less than the number of milliliters of blood passing through a single artery, but because of the greater number of arterioles flow is constant.

Figure 19.3 and Table 19.2 summarize the relationships of the various factors involved in circulation.

CIRCULATION IN ARTERIES AND ARTERIOLES

Objective 2. Define blood pressure, pulse, pulse pressure, and mean arterial pressure.

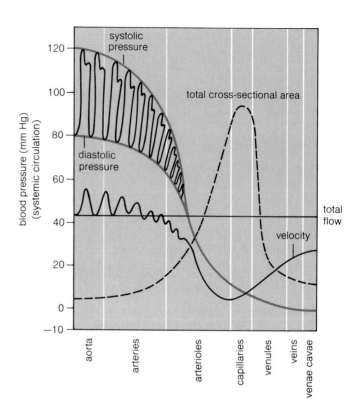

Figure 19.3 The interrelationships among pressure, cross-sectional area, velocity, and flow through blood vessels. The scale at the left applies to pressure only; other variables are not expressed quantitatively, and only relative changes are indicated.

Table 19.1 Cross-sectional Area of Different Classes of Blood Vessels	
Class of Vessel	Total cross-sectional Area (mm²)
Aorta	250
Small arteries	2000
Arterioles	4000
Capillaries	250,000
Venules	25,000
Small veins	8000
Venae cavae	800

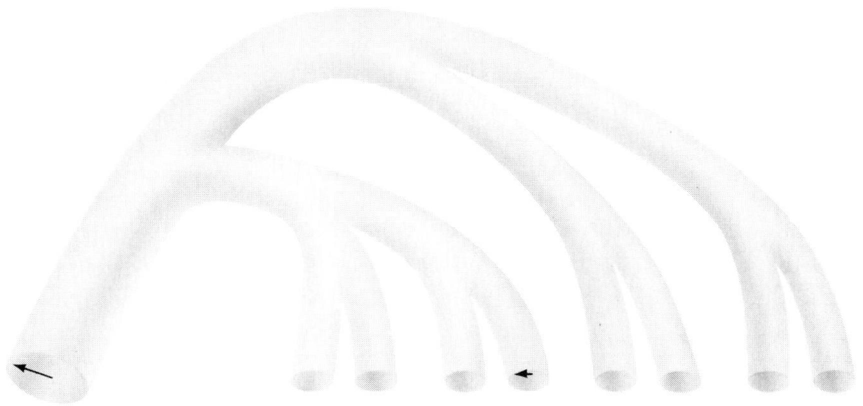

radius (r) = 6mm
r^2 = 36mm^2
cross-sectional area =
πr^2 = 3.14 × 36mm^2 = 114mm^2

r = 3mm
r^2 = 9mm^2
total cross-sectional area =
3.14 × 9mm^2 × 8 tubes = 226mm^2

Figure 19.4 Cross-sectional area of blood vessels increases as the vessels branch.

Table 19.2 Summary of the Principles of Circulation

	Definitions	Concepts
Flow	volume of fluid moving through a tube in a given period of time	Total flow is constant; an equal volume of blood is flowing through all types of vessels at all times.
		In any particular vessel flow is directly proportional to pressure and inversely proportional to resistance.
Pressure	force per unit area tending to push a fluid through a tube	Because of the rhythmic contractions of the heart, pressure is high and pulsating in the arteries and arterioles, lower in the capillaries, and lowest in the venules and veins.
Resistance	force tending to oppose the flow of a fluid through a tube	Resistance is affected by the radius and length of vessels. Resistance is inversely proportional to the fourth power of the radius of the vessel; thus, large vessels have much less resistance than small ones. Other factors being equal, resistance is proportional to the length of the vessel. When two vessels have the same input pressure, the output pressure is lower in the longer vessel.
Viscosity	a fluid's own internal resistance to flow	Viscosity impedes flow, other factors being equal.
		Total cross-sectional area is lowest in arteries, highest in capillaries, and intermediate in veins.
Velocity	distance traveled in a given time; the speed of a moving fluid	Velocity is high and pulsating in arteries, is low in arterioles nearest capillaries and in capillaries, and gradually increases in venules and veins.
		Constant total flow is maintained throughout the circulatory system, though there are many variations in pressure, resistance, velocity, and cross-sectional area.

Objective 3. Explain how circulation is regulated in arteries and arterioles.

Blood Pressure

It was noted earlier that the pressure varies in different types of blood vessels. When we speak of blood pressure, we are usually referring to arterial pressure—or more precisely to two arterial pressures, the systolic pressure and the diastolic pressure. These pressures reflect changes in pressure as the heart goes through the cardiac cycle. The **systolic pressure** is the maximum pressure developed in the arteries during the systolic phase of the cardiac cycle; the **diastolic pressure** is the minimum pressure in the arteries that occurs at the end of the diastolic phase of the cardiac cycle (see Chapter 17). Because the left ventricle contracts with greater force than the right ventricle, the pressures in the aorta are greater than the pressures in the pulmonary trunk.

Blood pressures are measured as the height of a column of mercury that the pressure will support, expressed in millimeters of mercury (mm Hg). Normal adult male systemic pressures are a systolic pressure in the range of 120 mm Hg and a diastolic pressure in the range of 80 mm Hg. Corresponding normal adult female pressures are in the range of 110 to 70, respectively. Pulmonary pressures are about one-fifth the systemic pressures. Though blood pres-

To measure human systemic blood pressure a **sphygmomanometer** and a **stethoscope** are needed. The cuff of the sphygmomanometer is placed around the upper arm over the brachial artery and inflated to a pressure greater than the systolic pressure. This completely blocks the flow of blood through the artery. Air is then slowly released from the cuff, and the pressure on the artery is reduced. As the cuff pressure reaches the systolic pressure, blood starts to spurt through the compressed artery under the cuff. The turbulence of the blood creates a sound that can be heard with a stethoscope. The pressure registered on the sphygmomanometer at the time the first sound is heard is the systolic blood pressure. As more and more air is released from the cuff, the sounds continue until they become muffled and difficult to hear. The pressure shown on the sphygmomanometer at the point at which the sounds become greatly muffled is the diastolic pressure. When the pressure in the cuff is lower than the diastolic pressure, no sounds are heard because the smooth flow of blood through an artery makes no sound. The events in the brachial artery related to the measurement of blood pressure are summarized in Figure 19.5.

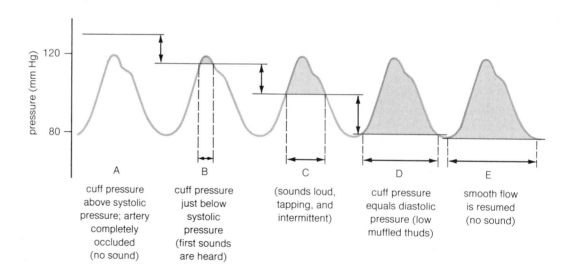

A	B	C	D	E
cuff pressure above systolic pressure; artery completely occluded (no sound)	cuff pressure just below systolic pressure (first sounds are heard)	(sounds loud, tapping, and intermittent)	cuff pressure equals diastolic pressure (low muffled thuds)	smooth flow is resumed (no sound)

Figure 19.5 The events that take place in the brachial artery and how they relate to sounds heard during the measurement of blood pressure. Systolic pressure, normally 110 to 120mm Hg, is recorded at B and diastolic pressure, normally 70 to 80mm Hg, at D.

sure is usually measured in an artery, venous pressure can be measured. It is much lower (0–5 mm Hg) and does not reflect the systolic and diastolic fluctuations seen in arteries.

Pulse and Pulse Pressure

Pulse is a detectable movement that results from the expansion and recoil of an artery due to the pressure differences within the vessel. The pulse rate is exactly the same as the heart rate because an artery pulses every time the heart beats. Pulse is usually taken on the radial artery in the wrist, but it can be taken on any artery that flows near enough to the surface of the body to be palpated (felt). Often a pulse can be felt in the common carotid artery. **Pulse pressure** is the difference between the systolic and diastolic pressures; at a systolic pressure of 110 mm Hg and a diastolic pressure of 70 mm Hg, the pulse pressure is 40 mm Hg. The pulse that can be felt in an artery comes from the difference between these two pressures.

Mean Arterial Pressure

Because the arterial pressure is continuously changing throughout the cardiac cycle, it is sometimes useful to have an average value for the arterial pressure. **Mean arterial pressure**—the average pressure driving blood through the systemic circulation—is such a value. The mean arterial pressure is estimated by adding one-third of the pulse pressure to the diastolic pressure. For example, for an individual at rest with a blood pressure of 122/80, the mean arterial pressure is 80 + 14 = 94.

Physiologically, the mean arterial pressure (MAP) is the product of the cardiac output (CO) times the peripheral resistance (PR): MAP = CO × PR. As explained in Chapter 17, cardiac output is the amount of blood being pumped from the heart (stroke volume × heart rate). **Peripheral resistance** is the force impeding the flow of blood in the peripheral vessels. It is the overall effect of all of the factors that contribute to resistance. The mean arterial pressure can be altered by any factor that alters the cardiac output or the peripheral resistance—heart rate, stroke volume, dilation or constriction of peripheral vessels, and many other factors. Keeping in mind the factors that affect mean arterial pressure will help you understand the discussion of the regulation of circulation.

Regulation of Circulation in Arteries

The walls of arteries are constructed to withstand variations in pressure. When the heart pumps a large quantity of blood into an artery, the elastic walls stretch to accommodate the increased volume of blood it now contains. The force of this stretched artery wall then drives the blood on toward the capillaries. Farther from the heart muscle in the arterial walls help to maintain constant blood pressure by dilating or constricting as needed.

Regulation of Circulation in Arterioles

Compared to arteries, arterioles have a much greater ability to change the size of their lumens. Therefore, they are major determinants of peripheral resistance and can act to direct the distribution of blood to various organs. These vessels are wrapped with smooth muscle fibers, and they can constrict or dilate markedly (Figure 19.6). Whenever metabolic activity in a tissue increases, as often happens in cardiac and skeletal muscles, the arterioles respond by dilating and allowing much more blood to enter those tissues. Figure 19.7 shows the variation in blood flow to different tissues during rest and during exercise.

The factors that control dilation and constriction of arterioles include chemical changes in the blood within the arteriole and in the tissues, and nervous and endocrine factors. Although the details of exactly how chemical changes cause immediate dilation or constriction of an arteriole are not known, it is clear that oxygen, carbon dioxide, pH, and certain ions are involved. Oxygen deficit, an excess of carbon dioxide, or lowered pH cause dilation. When sympathetic nerve fibers in the walls of arterioles are stimulated, the arterioles constrict; when they are inhibited, the arterioles dilate. Therefore, sympathetic fibers control both **vasoconstriction** and **vasodilation**. Vasopressin causes constriction of arterioles. Epinephrine causes vasodilation of arterioles leading to some capillary beds and vasoconstriction of others. Though significant, the effects of epinephrine are modest in comparison to the effects of the sympathetic nervous system and the direct responses to the chemical composition of the environment of the vessel wall.

CIRCULATION IN CAPILLARIES

Objective 4. Explain how the exchange of materials between capillaries and tissues takes place.

The exchange of materials between the capillaries and the tissues is an important function of the circulatory system; the rest of the system merely gets the blood to and from the capillaries. Although only about 5% of the total blood volume is in the capillaries at any given time, it is that portion of the blood that is carrying out the exchange

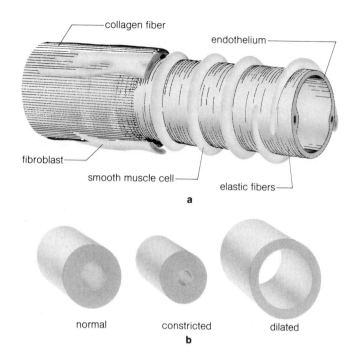

Figure 19.6 The structure of the wall of an arteriole (a) is related to (b) its ability to become constricted or dilated.

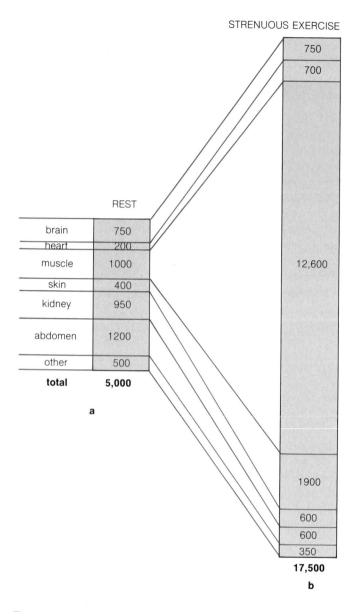

Figure 19.7 The variations in blood volume delivered to different tissues during (a) rest and (b) exercise, expressed in milliliters/minute.

function of the circulatory system. Most capillaries are only about 1 millimeter long, but taken together, they have an extremely large total cross-sectional area. They are arranged so that they come within 20 to 30 μ of all the cells of the body. Thus, materials can readily move from capillary to cell and from cell to capillary. The walls of the capillaries further facilitate movement because their squamous epithelial cells are arranged in a single layer, and the cells have tiny pores between them.

Flow of Blood through Capillaries

The entry of blood into capillaries is controlled by the **precapillary sphincters**. By opening and closing, these sphincters work with the smooth muscle of the arterioles to control the flow of blood through the capillaries. Because of their very small diameter the capillaries have high resistance. This resistance causes the blood to move slowly through them but does not impede overall circulation because there is such a large number of capillaries. The relationship between total cross-sectional area and velocity is shown in Figure 19.8: Blood in an arteriole moves three

volume units in one second, while blood in the capillaries moves only one volume unit in one second. The cross-sectional area of the arteriole is two times that of each capillary, but there are six capillaries. Thus, in one second six of the volume units shown in the figure move through the arteriole, and six of the volume units move through the capillaries. In other words, flow is constant, even though cross-sectional area and velocity differ.

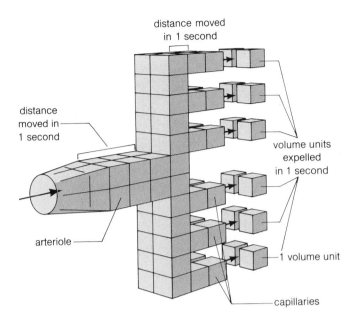

distance moved
in 1 second

distance
moved in
1 second

volume units
expelled
in 1 second

arteriole

1 volume unit

capillaries

Figure 19.8 Relationships between cross-sectional area and velocity of flow in arterioles and capillaries.

Movement of Materials out of and into Capillaries

Before the cells of the body can receive nutrients carried by the blood or return wastes to it, the blood must come in close proximity to the cells. However, substances moving between capillaries and cells must pass through the interstitial fluids surrounding all cells. Pressures in the capillaries and the interstitial fluids determine the movement of fluids between the capillaries and the tissue fluids.

We have already discussed in Chapter 3 the factors that affect the movement of materials across cell membranes—between interstitial fluids and cells. Movement between capillaries and the interstitial fluids occurs primarily by pressure gradients, gases being moved by diffusion. The exact pressures in a capillary vary with the location of the capillary (skin, muscle, or other location) and with physiological conditions (blood pressure, composition of blood, or other factors). Pressures reported in Figure 19.9 represent a hypothetical capillary provided for illustrative purposes.

Blood moving in a capillary exerts two kinds of pressures: hydrostatic pressure and oncotic pressure. Blood **hy-**

drostatic pressure is the blood pressure—the pressure that remains from the constant pumping of the heart. By the time blood reaches the arterial end of the capillary, the hydrostatic pressure is about 35 mm Hg. This pressure, sometimes called filtration pressure, tends to push substances out of the capillary. By the time blood reaches the venous end of the capillary, the hydrostatic pressure has dropped to about 16 mm Hg, mostly because of the resistance to flow encountered as the blood passes through the narrow capillary. In contrast, the blood **oncotic pressure**, the osmotic pressure created by colloids in the blood, tends to draw substances into the blood. Because most of the substances that exert oncotic pressure remain in the blood at all times, the blood oncotic pressure remains relatively constant at about 25 mm Hg.

Interstitial fluids also exert hydrostatic and oncotic pressures, but their effects on the movement of materials into and out of the capillaries are small compared to the effects of pressures in the blood.

As shown in Table 19.3, the force that changes most as blood passes through the capillary is the blood hydrostatic pressure. At the arterial end of the capillary it creates a **net outward pressure** of about 10 mm Hg, which pushes fluids out of the capillary. At the venous end of the capillary the blood hydrostatic pressure has dropped so that there is a **net inward pressure** of about 9 mm Hg, which draws fluids into the capillary.

As a result of pressure differences only about 90% of the fluid forced out of the capillary at the arterial end is returned at the venous end. As we shall see in Chapter 20, lymphatic vessels interspersed through the interstitial spaces collect the excess fluid and return it to the blood.

Though pressure differences at the arterial and venous ends of capillaries are important in the movement of water and some dissolved substances, *diffusion* (see Chapter 3) is also important in the movement of substances between the capillaries and the interstital fluids, *and* between the interstitial fluids and the cells. In diffusion substances move along a concentration gradient from higher to lower concentration. Oxygen diffuses out of the capillaries, through the interstitial fluid, and into the cells; as oxygen leaves the blood, hemoglobin releases some of its bound oxygen. Carbon dioxide diffuses out of the cells, through the interstitial fluid, and into the capillaries. Glucose diffuses out of the capillaries and into the interstitial fluid, where it is transported by carrier molecules into the cells. Fat-soluble substances diffuse through the capillary walls by dissolving in the lipids of the cell membranes, and ions and water-soluble substances pass through pores between the endothelial cells of the capillaries.

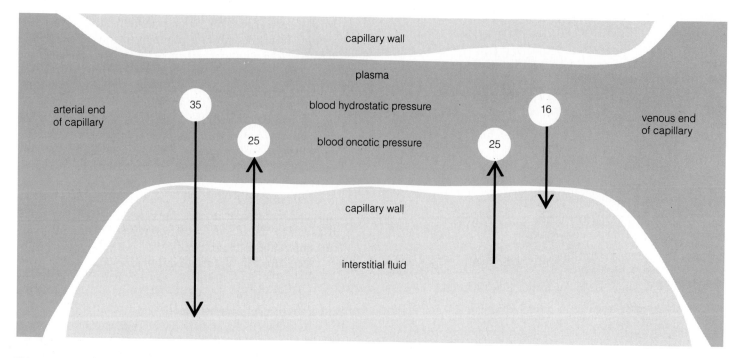

Figure 19.9 Pressures in mm Hg that affect movement of fluids out of and into capillaries. Arrows indicate direction of movement, and their lengths indicate the pressure.

Table 19.3 Forces Moving Fluids into and out of Capillaries (expressed as pressures in mm Hg)	
Forces at the Arterial End of a Capillary	Forces at the Venous End of a Capillary
Blood hydrostatic pressure moving fluids out ------- 35	Blood hydrostatic pressure moving fluids out --------- 16
Blood oncotic pressure moving fluids in --------- 25	Blood oncotic pressure moving fluids in ---------- 25
Net outward pressure --- 10	Net inward pressure ------- 9

CIRCULATION IN VENULES AND VEINS

Objective 5. Explain how circulation is regulated in the venules and veins.

In the small venules that receive blood from the capil-

laries, the hydrostatic pressure remaining from the pumping of the heart is only about 10 mm Hg. In comparison to the mean arterial pressure of more than 90 mm Hg, this is a small pressure that must carry the blood back to the heart. By the time the blood reaches the right atrium, the pressure is near zero. Thus, a small but important pressure gradient exists along the venules and veins as blood moves toward the right atrium.

About 60% of the total blood volume is in the veins at any time, and valves in the veins and muscle contractions help to move this large volume of blood toward the heart. When the smooth muscle in the walls of the veins contracts, it raises the pressure in the veins. The contraction of skeletal muscles adjacent to the veins also pushes blood toward the heart as valves prevent backflow. Finally, movements of the diaphragm during breathing apply pressure to the inferior vena cava. As the diaphragm contracts, pressure increases in the abdomen and decreases in the thorax, pushing blood from the abdominal vena cava to the thoracic vena cava and on to the right atrium.

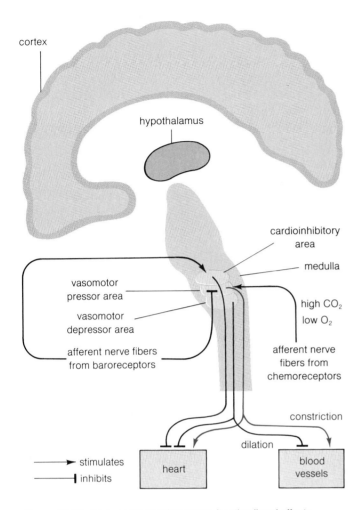

cortex

hypothalamus

cardioinhibitory area

medulla

vasomotor pressor area

vasomotor depressor area

high CO₂ low O₂

afferent nerve fibers from baroreceptors

afferent nerve fibers from chemoreceptors

constriction

dilation

stimulates

inhibits

heart

blood vessels

Figure 19.10 The cardiovascular center, its stimuli and effects.

INTEGRATED FUNCTION OF THE CIRCULATORY SYSTEM

Objective 6. Explain the role of the following in the integrated function of the circulatory system: (a) control centers in the brain, (b) baroreceptors, (c) chemoreceptors, and (d) local factors.

Objective 7. Explain how circulatory function is altered by (a) exercise and (b) a change in posture.

Control Centers in the Brain

The **cardiovascular center** in the medulla consists of a fairly large diffuse area of interconnected neurons that receive signals from other parts of the central nervous system and from baroreceptors and chemoreceptors (discussed below). These neurons send efferent signals through sympathetic or parasympathetic fibers to the heart and blood vessels, regulating heart function and blood pressure in accordance with physiological demands. For the purpose of understanding its various effects, the cardiovascular center can be divided into three areas: (1) the cardioinhibitory area, (2) the vasomotor pressor area, and (3) the vasomotor depressor area (Figure 19.10). (These areas are not anatomically distinct.)

The **cardioinhibitory area** is stimulated by signals from baroreceptors in response to an increase in blood pressure. The cardioinhibitory area then sends signals to the heart that cause the heart rate to decrease. Though no specific cardioacceleratory area exists, excitement and other stimuli directly stimulate the sympathetic fibers that lead to the heart, causing the heart rate to increase.

The **vasomotor pressor area** and the **vasomotor depressor area** act reciprocally to maintain **vasomotor tone**, the degree of constriction of vessels. When stimulation of the pressor area increases or stimulation of the depressor area decreases, there is an increase in the constriction of the arterioles and a rise in blood pressure. Veins may also constrict, increasing the amount of blood returned to the heart. In contrast, when stimulation of the pressor area decreases (and stimulation of the depressor area increases), arterioles become less constricted and blood pressure decreases.

The relative degree of stimulation of the pressor and depressor areas is determined by several factors. Stimuli from the baroreceptors when blood pressure is high act on the vasomotor centers to cause dilation of blood vessels. They also decrease cardiac output until the blood pressure returns to normal. Stimuli from chemoreceptors when the carbon dioxide concentration in the blood is high or the oxygen concentration low act on the vasomotor centers to cause constriction of the blood vessels and increased cardiac output. Stimuli from the hypothalamus cause dilation of skin blood vessels when body temperature is high and constriction of skin blood vessels when body temperature is low. Emotional stimuli also affect blood vessels in the skin, causing vasodilation (blushing) or vasoconstriction (paleness).

Baroreceptors

Baroreceptors, or **pressoreceptors**, are sensitive to stretch, usually caused by slight increases in blood pressure (Figure 19.11). One set of baroreceptors is located in the caro-

tid sinus, an area of the common carotid artery near where it branches into the external and internal carotids. Another set of baroreceptors is located in the walls of the aortic arch. These baroreceptors send out impulses continuously. If the blood pressure drops, the rate at which signals are generated also drops; if the blood pressure rises, the rate at which signals are generated increases. The signals are transmitted to the cardiovascular center in the medulla, where they affect both vasomotor tone and heart rate. When pressure is high, the frequency of impulses is also high, and the inhibition of vasoconstriction and the slowing of the heart rate is at its maximum. When pressure is low, the frequency of impulses is also low, vasoconstriction is no longer inhibited, and the heart rate is no longer slowed.

The baroreceptors adapt to altered pressure in only a few days. Consequently, these receptors are of little value in controlling blood pressure in individuals with hypertension (high blood pressure) because they respond to the elevated pressure as if it were the "normal" pressure.

> Massage of the carotid sinus is sometimes used as a means of slowing the heart rate during an attack of tachycardia. Untrained individuals should not attempt to massage the carotid sinus because improperly performed massage can lead to *complete* cardiac arrest (cessation of heart contractions).

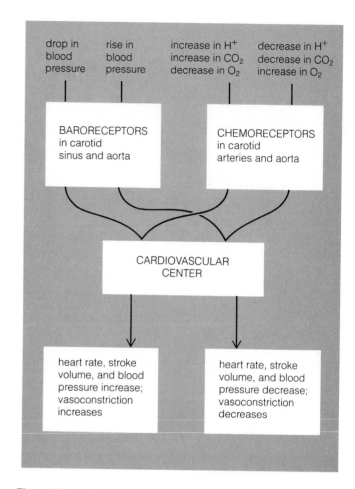

Figure 19.11 Role of baroreceptors and chemoreceptors in regulating heart function and blood pressure.

Chemoreceptors

In addition to the baroreceptors the carotid arteries and aorta contain an additional set of specialized receptors, the **chemoreceptors** (Figure 19.11) which are responsive to the concentrations of oxygen, carbon dioxide, and hydrogen ions. Although these structures are important primarily in the regulation of breathing, they can affect blood pressure. A decrease in oxygen or an increase in carbon dioxide or acid causes an increase in the blood pressure and heart rate. These chemoreceptors are discussed in more detail in Chapter 21.

Local Control of Circulation

Though regulation of circulation is accomplished primarily by the cardiovascular center, baroreceptors, and chemoreceptors, local factors within specific tissues also are involved. Blood vessels in skeletal muscles receive few sympathetic nerve fibers and thus are minimally affected by signals from the cardiovascular center. Metabolism in active muscles causes increased temperature; increased oxygen use; and increased accumulation of carbon dioxide, lactic acid, and other metabolites. These metabolic products cause vasodilation and decrease peripheral resistance in blood vessels supplying the muscles. Thus, the blood supply to active muscles increases independently of any signals from the cardiovascular system. Likewise, epinephrine from the adrenal glands (in addition to that released by the sympathetic nerve fibers) decreases peripheral resistance in blood vessels of muscle and increases it in blood vessels of the skin. Furthermore, a group of chemicals known as **kinins**, formed in certain glands when they are actively secreting, cause vasodilation in the glands and increase the blood flow through active glands. As we shall see in Chapter 25,

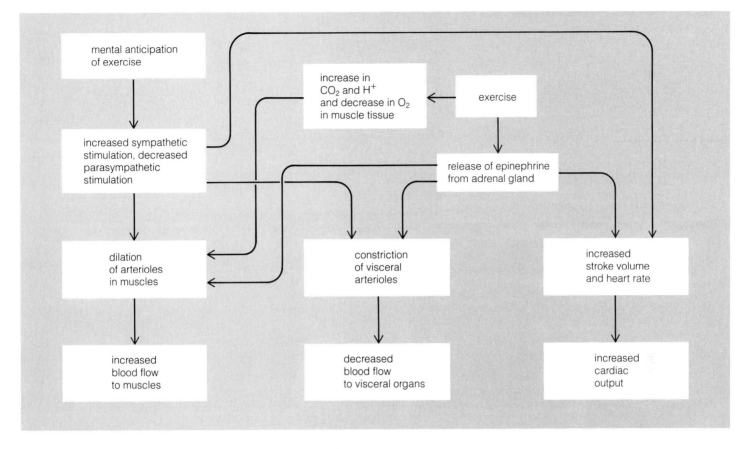

Figure 19.12 A flow chart of the regulatory events in the cardiovascular system in response to exercise.

the kidney responds to changes in blood pressure and controls the activation of angiotensin, a powerful vasoconstrictor. Finally, chemical substances taken into the body can affect peripheral resistance; for example, nicotine acts as a vasoconstrictor, and alcohol acts as a vasodilator.

Effect of Exercise on Circulatory Function

The volume of blood delivered to the muscles greatly increases during exercise. Even the mental anticipation of exercise causes an increase in sympathetic stimulation and a decrease in parasympathetic stimulation. When exercise begins, epinephrine is released from the adrenal glands, increasing cardiac output and decreasing peripheral resistance in the blood vessels of skeletal muscle. Because blood

flows along the path of least resistance, the volume of blood going to the muscles increases. This increased blood flow is the result of both the increased blood volume in the dilated vessels of the muscles and the increased cardiac output. Figure 19.12 summarizes these processes. In individuals who engage in regular exercise the cardiovascular system adapts to the increased demands of the muscles: As noted in Chapter 8, the resting heart rate decreases, and the maximum cardiac output during exercise increases.

Effects of Gravity and Posture on Circulatory Function

Gravity affects the pressure in both arteries and veins. Compared to the pressure at the level of the heart, the

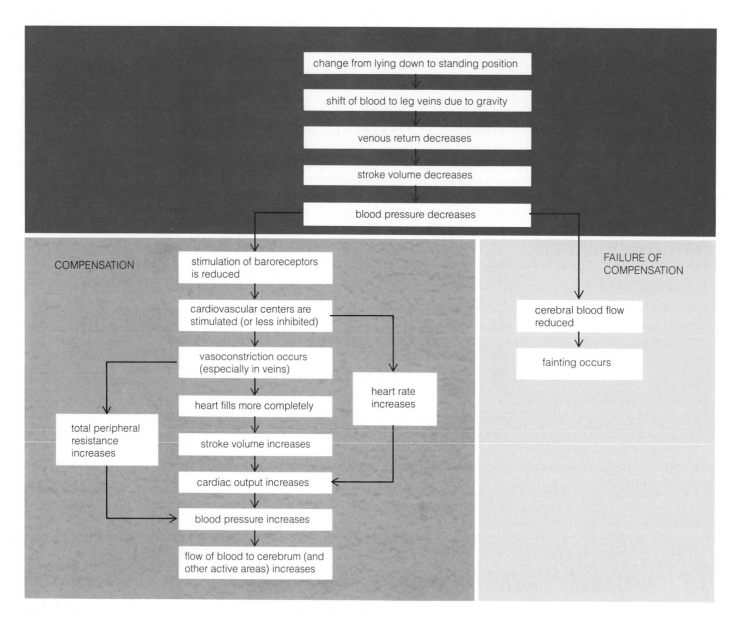

Figure 19.13 Effects of moving from a lying to a standing position, and how these effects are compensated by the cardiovascular system.

pressure in any vessel above the heart is lower, and the pressure in any vessel below the heart is higher. For example, in a human 160 centimeters tall standing in an upright position, when the mean arterial pressure at heart level is 100 mm Hg, the mean arterial pressure in a large artery in the head is 62 mm Hg, and the mean arterial pressure in a large artery in the foot is 180 mm Hg. Similar but smaller pressure differences occur in veins. In contrast, in a human lying down most of the blood vessels are nearly level with the heart, and gravity has little effect on pressures.

When a person changes from a lying to a standing position, the force of gravity causes blood to collect in the veins below the heart. This causes a decrease in the venous return and a concurrent decrease in stroke volume. When the stroke volume decreases, the blood pressure also drops.

The compensatory mechanisms that overcome the drop in blood pressure begin with the decrease in the rate at which baroreceptors send inhibitory impulses to the cardiovascular center. With the removal of this inhibition the heart rate accelerates. In addition, the veins constrict and cause an increase in venous return. Together, these effects increase the heart rate and stroke volume and therefore the cardiac output. The decrease in baroreceptor inhibition also results in vasoconstriction and an increase in total peripheral resistance. When the cardiac output and the total peripheral resistance increase, the mean arterial pressure will increase toward normal. If these compensatory mechanisms fail to respond quickly enough, the blood flow to the brain decreases suddenly, and fainting occurs. Such a condition is called **postural hypotension**. These mechanisms are summarized in Figure 19.13.

CLINICAL APPLICATIONS

Objective 8. Explain how circulatory function is altered by (a) atherosclerosis, (b) hypertension, (c) emotional stress, (d) hemorrhage, and (e) cerebrovascular accident.

Objective 9. Describe the general circulatory effects of (a) myocardial infarction and (b) congestive heart failure.

Atherosclerosis

Atherosclerosis is a condition in which some of the arteries are hardened and their lumens narrowed by the deposition of **atheromatous plaque** (Figure 19.14). Though much research has been done to determine how this plaque is formed, the mechanism is still poorly understood. It is clear that the plaque consists of smooth muscle cells and fat-laden cells, which accumulate in excess beneath the degenerating endothelial layer. The plaque also contains connective tissue, fibrinogen, and crystals of cholesterol. It can completely occlude an artery, but it is more likely to partly occlude and roughen the artery so that clotting is initiated. The blood clot may then occlude the artery completely.

One theory of the formation of plaque suggests that cholesterol or thrombi (blood clots) are converted into plaque mostly as a result of their irritation of arterial walls. However, this theory is not supported by electron microscope studies of plaque formation because little or no lipid is found in the early stages of plaque formation. Moreover, smooth muscle fibers are found in areas of the artery wall where healing is taking place.

A relatively new theory hypothesizes that a mutated cell initiates plaque formation. If this theory is correct, then the search for causes of atherosclerosis should be among mutagens—those factors that can cause mutations, such as chemicals, viruses, and ionizing radiations. Some of these mutagens are carried on blood lipoproteins, so the role of lipoproteins in transporting mutagens may explain why high blood lipid concentrations are correlated with atherosclerosis.

Much research has focused on the relationship between cholesterol in the blood and atherosclerosis. Some animal studies have shown that increasing cholesterol in the diet is often correlated with the development of plaque. Other studies have shown a correlation between reduced blood cholesterol and regression of plaque. However, by no means have all studies supported these findings. The role of cholesterol and other lipids in atherosclerosis remains unclear. It is considered in somewhat more detail in the essay at the end of this chapter.

Hypertension

Hypertension, or high blood pressure, is defined as a resting arterial pressure exceeding 140/95 over a prolonged period of time. Figure 19.15 shows the range of pressures that have been observed in different age groups. Elevation of the diastolic pressure above 95 mm Hg rather than elevation of systolic pressure above 140 mm Hg seems more important in the development of cardiovascular disorders, though elevation of either pressure can

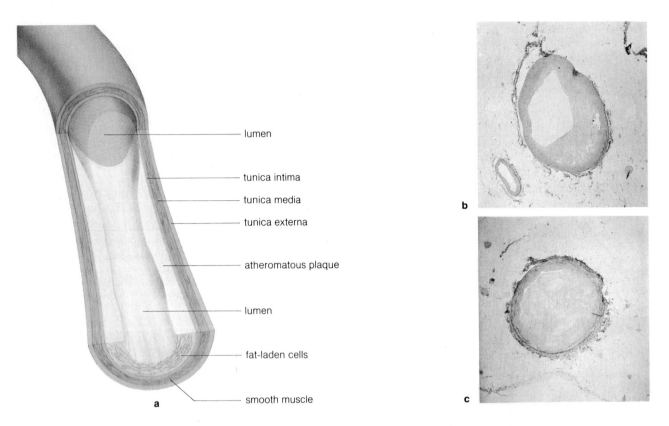

Figure 19.14 Atheromatous plaque: (**a**) a drawing of a portion of an artery showing the location of the plaque in relation to the normal layers of the artery, (**b**) a photomicrograph of an artery partially occluded with plaque, × 13.8 (Armed Forces Institute of Pathology negative number 58–4604), (**c**) a photomicrograph of an artery almost completely occluded with plaque, × 12 (Armed Forces Institute of Pathology negative number 61–5786.)

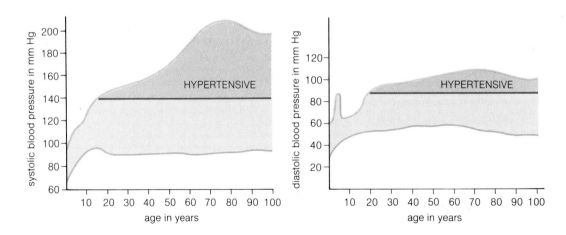

Figure 19.15 Range of normal and hypertensive pressures for different ages in the population.

lead to health problems. Disorders that can result from untreated hypertension include heart failure, kidney damage, and cerebrovascular accident (occlusion or rupture of a cerebral artery, sometimes called a stroke).

Hypertension is classified as **essential**, or **primary, hypertension** when the exact cause is unknown, and as **secondary hypertension** when the cause is known—in other words, the hypertension is secondary to another factor. About 90% of all cases of hypertension are essential hypertension. The remaining 10% are due to excess secretion of epinephrine by the adrenal medulla, aldosterone by the adrenal cortex, or renin by the kidney (the last is called **renal hypertension**). These mechanisms will be discussed in Chapter 25.

Essential hypertension cannot be cured, but it can be treated. The problems of treating hypertension involve identifying the individuals who need treatment and encouraging them to continue treatment once it is initiated. Because the initial symptoms of hypertension are gradual in onset, many people develop dangerously high blood pressures before they discover they have the disorder. Treatment generally involves the use of drugs that block the action of the sympathetic nervous system and thereby dilate the arterioles or that cause the excretion of excessive tissue fluids. Dietary sodium is sometimes restricted. The control of hypertension involves continuous treatment for life. Many individuals tend to terminate their medications when they begin to feel better. However, because the medications do not cure hypertension, they must be taken regularly to keep the disorder under control and to keep symptoms from recurring.

Emotional Stress

Emotional stress usually affects the higher brain centers and may stimulate sympathetic nerve impulses. These impulses cause constriction of arterioles and increase arterial blood pressure. Thus, emotional stress contributes to hypertension. Such impulses also cause constriction of veins, increased venous pressure, and increased venous return, thereby increasing heart rate, stroke volume, and thus cardiac output. These effects were described in Chapter 13 as the fight-or-flight effects of sympathetic stimulation.

Depending on the response of the higher brain centers, a sudden emotional stimulus can cause effects opposite to those described above. The activity of the sympathetic nervous system is suddenly suppressed, and the blood vessels lose their tone. The arterial pressure decreases, the veins fail to constrict, and venous return is reduced. Heart rate and stroke volume decrease, and therefore so does cardiac output. Insufficient cardiac output is called **shock**. If the person is standing, the flow of blood to the brain is decreased, and fainting occurs. Since fainting places the person in a lying-down position, the act of fainting initiates the compensatory mechanisms of increasing blood flow to the brain. Attempting to keep the person upright works against the compensatory mechanism.

Hemorrhage

Hemorrhage, or excessive loss of blood, may cause **hypovolemic shock**—shock due to decreased blood volume. A person in shock has ashen pale, cool skin, and a rapid, weak pulse. The loss of blood decreases both the arterial and venous pressures. The effect of lowered venous pressure is to reduce cardiac filling and thereby to reduce cardiac output and arterial pressure. The lowering of arterial pressure reduces the firing rate of the baroreceptors, an event that initiates the action of the compensatory mechanisms.

When the decrease in the firing rate of baroreceptors is detected in the cardiovascular center, signals are sent by sympathetic nerve fibers to the heart, veins, and arterioles. At the same time, parasympathetic signals decrease. The heart rate, stroke volume, and therefore cardiac output increase. Constriction of arterioles occurs, which, together with the increase in cardiac output, tends to increase arterial pressure toward normal. If these corrective mechanisms are insufficient to compensate for the blood loss, the person will require a transfusion.

The effects of hemorrhage and the body's compensatory mechanisms are summarized in Figure 19.16.

Cerebrovascular Accident

A **cerebrovascular accident** (CVA), sometimes referred to as a stroke, is the sudden interruption of blood flow to a portion of the brain because of an occlusion or rupture of a cerebral blood vessel. Occlusion may result from atherosclerosis or an embolism. When blood flow is interrupted, brain cells succumb to the deficiency of oxygen and glucose in a matter of minutes. Paralysis, loss of speech, and other impairments accompany a CVA. The location of the CVA and the extent of damage determine the seriousness of the effects.

Recovery of function is limited by the degree of collateral circulation that is established and whatever reestablishment of function the neurons of the brain can accomplish. New techniques of microsurgery have offered ways to prevent impending strokes. Arteriograms can be used to locate arteries that are partly occluded. If the affected artery is in the neck or outside the cranium, it can be opened and the occluding plaque removed. If the artery is within the cranial cavity, the blood supply to the brain can be increased by attaching one of the scalp arteries to the occluded artery at a point beyond the occlusion. These techniques require very tiny instruments and a surgical microscope; only in the last few years has such equipment been available.

The selection of individuals for microsurgery is based on their previous history of mild brain ischemia. It now seems clear that most stroke victims have one or more such attacks before they have a permanently damaging stroke. If the surgery can be performed after the warning signs appear, the person can often be spared the disabling effects of a stroke.

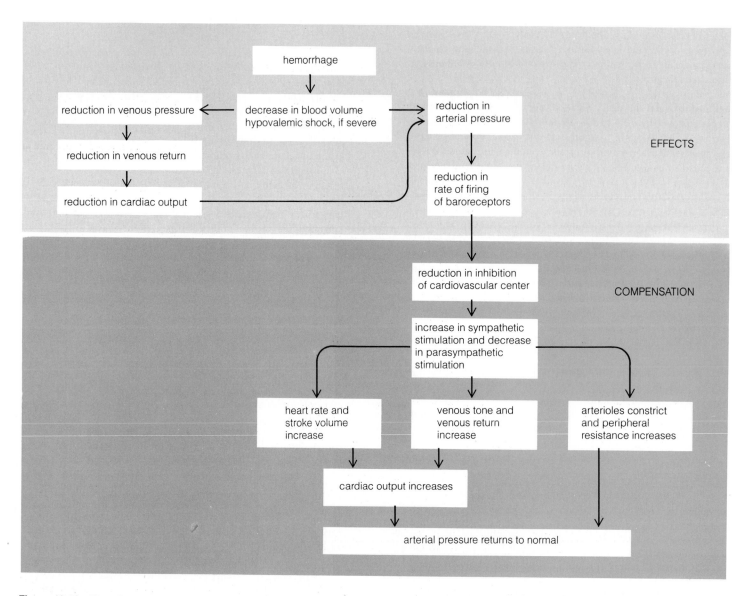

Figure 19.16 The effects of hemorrhage and hypovolemic shock and the compensatory mechanisms related to these conditions.

Circulatory Effects of Myocardial Infarction

We have already considered the effects of a myocardial infarction on the heart muscle and the circulation of blood through it. In addition, a myocardial infarction produces general circulatory effects. Because the pumping action of the heart is impaired, the cardiac output decreases, and serious hypotension (low blood pressure) results. One effect of myocardial infarction seems to be the inhibition of the sympathetic and the stimulation of the parasympathetic nervous systems. Such a response is inappropriate to compensate for hypotension; in fact, it exacerbates the already lowered blood pressure and cardiac output rather than enhancing it. However, it reduces the workload on the heart and may spare the muscle tissue further damage. If the heart is seriously damaged, it may be increasingly overworked in spite of the reduced load, and complete heart failure may eventually result.

Circulatory Effects of Congestive Heart Failure

Heart failure, as noted in Chapter 17, is the inability of the heart to pump a supply of blood sufficient to meet the body's demands. As the heart's ability to contract weakens, blood is still being delivered to it, and it becomes engorged with blood. Engorgement of the left ventricle leads to engorgement of the left atrium, and blood backs up in the pulmonary circulation. Excess fluid leaves the blood and accumulates in the tissues of the lungs, increasing the distance gases must diffuse. This fluid accumulation constitutes the congestion of congestive heart failure. Exchange of oxygen and carbon dioxide is impaired. Not only is cardiac output decreased, but the oxygen content of the blood is also decreased. Blood pressure decreases, and the flow of blood to the kidneys is impaired. The kidneys fail to remove wastes efficiently or to adjust the concentration of sodium and other substances in the blood. Accumulation of sodium further exacerbates the edema in pulmonary and other tissues. Increased volume of tissue fluids interferes with the movement of substances from the capillaries to the cells. All in all, the normal function of the circulating blood in delivering substances to cells is seriously impaired.

Clinical Terms

antihypertensive (an″-te-hi-per-ten′siv) **drug**   a substance that helps to reduce blood pressure

endarterectomy (end″-ar-ter-ek′to-me)   the removal of the inner wall of an artery to reduce occlusion of the vessel

phlebothrombosis (fleb″o-throm-bo′sis)   inflammation of a vein caused by a thrombus; thrombus is easily detached to become an embolus

phlebotomy (fleb-ot′o-me)   the opening of a vein for the removal of blood

thrombectomy (throm-bek′to-me)   the removal of a venous thrombus

thrombophlebitis (throm″bo-fleb-i′tis)   inflammation of a vein that results in the formation of a thrombus

vasodilator (vas-o-di′la-tor) **drug**   a substance that increases the diameter of blood vessels

Essay: Risk Factors in Heart and Blood Vessel Diseases

Cardiovascular diseases—diseases of the heart and blood vessels—are the leading cause of death among Americans. In this country each year nearly 1 million people die of these diseases, more than twice as many as die from cancer. Another 27 million are afflicted in some way by cardiovascular disease. Because of the serious threat to life and the physical impairments caused by these diseases, much research has gone into identifying risk factors that contribute to their development. It is the purpose of this essay to describe these factors and evaluate their contributions to the development of cardiovascular disease.

As we have already seen, hypertension and atherosclerosis, which are themselves cardiovascular diseases, are often precursors of more serious disorders such as cerebrovascular accidents, myocardial infarctions, and heart failure. One of the most effective steps that can be taken to reduce the risk of more serious cardiovascular disease is to bring hypertension under control. Other steps that may reduce risks include controlling the dietary intake of cholesterol and sodium and avoiding behaviors that are correlated with the development of cardiovascular disease.

Risk factors can be divided into those over which an individual has no control (age, sex, and heredity) and those over which an individual might exercise some control (weight, exercise, tobacco smoking, and diet). We will consider what is currently known about the contribution of these factors to the development of cardiovascular diseases.

Age and sex   Under age 55 men are known to be more prone to myocardial infarction than women, but over that age women are equally prone to the disorder. It has been suggested that female hormones secreted prior to menopause may in some way protect women from myocardial infarction.

It is also known that the number of degenerated smooth muscle cells in arterial walls increases with age as a supposedly natural part of the aging process. Thickening of arterial walls has been shown to occur over time in animals even when the animals were maintained experimentally on a low-fat, cholesterol-free diet.

Heredity   Epidemiologists and cardiologists have noted that the incidence of heart and blood vessel diseases is higher in some families than in others. Though some familial similarities might be due to similar lifestyles, it is thought that genetic factors are involved. As we shall see in the discussion of cholesterol and fats, hereditary factors are certainly involved in the body's metabolism of these substances and thus are at least indirectly related to cardiovascular disorders.

Weight Excessive body weight seems to contribute to the development of cardiovascular disease. However, follow-up studies on the longevity of participants in the Framingham Study (cited in Chapter 17) have shown that moderately (10 to 20%) overweight individuals in the study have had a lower mortality rate than either the thinnest or the most obese individuals. The number of capillaries the heart must pump blood through is far larger in overweight individuals than in individuals of normal weight; over a period of years these extra miles of capillaries add up to a significant amount of constant strain on the heart. Another important aspect of obesity is that the obese person's diet is likely to contain fairly large amounts of fat. As we shall see, excessive fat appears to contribute to cardiovascular disease.

Tobacco smoking Tobacco smoking, especially cigarette smoking, has been correlated with both cancer and cardiovascular disease. Though there has been a decrease in the number of cigarettes smoked by the American population and a shift to low-tar, low-nicotine cigarettes, the contribution of cigarettes to the risk of heart disease is still high. It is thought that the carbon monoxide in the smoke of even milder cigarettes may contribute to the risk of heart disease, though it may not contribute to the risk of cancer.

Exercise Experts are not entirely in agreement about the benefits of exercise in reducing the risk of cardiovascular disease. In trained athletes the stroke volume of the heart is significantly increased, and the heart rate at rest is correspondingly reduced. The effect of training such as jogging in nonathletes is to increase the strength of contraction and the stroke volume. More research is needed to determine how important exercise is in lowering the risk of cardiovascular disease.

Diet Cholesterol and fats have been implicated in cardiovascular disease for some time; recently excessive intake of methionine (in proteins) and vitamin B_6 deficiency also have been implicated.

Determinants of blood cholesterol concentrations include: (1) how much is in the food we eat, (2) how much is manufactured in the body, (3) how much is excreted in the feces, and (4) how much the cells of the body use. Of these four determinants the amount manufactured in the body accounts for 75%. Therefore, reducing cholesterol intake can have only limited effect on blood cholesterol concentration, especially since limiting intake stimulates synthesis in the body. Some individuals are genetically programmed to produce more cholesterol than others, and this may be one of the hereditary factors in heart and blood vessel disease. Limiting fats also may have only a modest effect on blood cholesterol because the body can use carbohydrates as well as fats to make cholesterol. Recent studies have focused on determining how cholesterol is carried in the blood. The cholesterol carried in low-density lipoproteins (LDLs) includes the part that is made in the body and carried to the cells. The cholesterol carried in high-density lipoproteins (HDLs) seems destined to be transported to the intestine and removed from the body in the feces. Therefore, the amount of LDL in the blood is a much better predictor of risk of cardiovascular disease than total blood cholesterol or total blood lipids.

Methionine, an amino acid in protein, is an essential component of the diet because our bodies cannot synthesize it, and it is needed to make body proteins. However, when it is ingested in excess, it is metabolized to another amino acid, homocysteine. In the presence of an adequate amount of vitamin B_6, homocysteine is converted to a nontoxic substance, cystathionine, and excreted. However, without enough vitamin B_6 homocysteine accumulates in the blood and theoretically may be involved in the formation of atherosclerotic deposits in the blood vessels. Should this theory be confirmed, atherosclerosis might be controlled by limiting the amount of methionine in the diet to that needed for protein synthesis or by providing enough vitamin B_6 to assure that homocysteine does not accumulate in the blood.

Blood pressure Hypertension is seen in nearly all victims of cardiovascular disease. It is not known whether hypertension initiates atherosclerosis, but it does seem to accelerate the process. Substances that are related to both hypertension and atherosclerosis (renin, angiotensin, sodium, and epinephrine) may contribute to the development of both disorders. One encouraging finding has to do with the regression of atherosclerotic lesions. It seems that lowering blood pressure and blood lipid concentration results in regression of the lesions. This fact is important in encouraging individuals with atherosclerosis to follow dietary recommendations and to continue medication for hypertension.

Conclusion From this brief review it is clear that, while we cannot change our age, sex, or heredity, we can reduce the risk of cardiovascular disease by choosing a lifestyle that minimizes the risks from controllable factors—weight, smoking, diet, exercise, and blood pressure.

CHAPTER SUMMARY

(Chapter summary points and review questions are numbered to correspond to the numbered objectives in the text of each chapter.)

Principles of Circulation

1. State the principles of pressure, flow, and resistance in fluids as they apply to the circulation of blood.
   a. The principles of circulation are summarized in Table 19.2.

Circulation in Arteries and Arterioles

2. Define blood pressure, pulse, pulse pressure, and mean arterial pressure.
   a. Blood pressure is the pressure with which the heart pushes blood through the vessels. In arteries:
      (1) systolic pressure is the highest pressure developed during the ejection of blood from the ventricles
      (2) diastolic pressure is the lowest pressure reached during ventricular relaxation
   b. Pulse is a detectable movement that results from the expansion and recoil of an artery due to pressure changes produced by the beating heart.
   c. Pulse pressure is the difference between systolic and diastolic pressures.
   d. Mean arterial pressure is the average pressure driving blood through the arteries.
3. Explain how circulation is regulated in arteries and arterioles.
   a. Circulation from the pulsatile action of the heart is made continuous by the elasticity of the walls of the large arteries.
      (1) They are distended when the ventricles force blood into them.
      (2) They recoil during diastole and force blood toward the capillaries.
   b. Circulation through the arterioles is regulated by smooth muscle in their walls and by precapillary sphincters.
      (1) Smooth muscle contracts and causes vasoconstriction.
      (2) Smooth muscle relaxes and causes vasodilation.
      (3) Precapillary sphincters control the entry of blood into specific capillaries.

Circulation in Capillaries

4. Explain how the exchange of materials between capillaries and tissues takes place.
   a. The capillaries perform the main function of the circulatory system—the exchange of materials between the blood and the cells and the exchange of gases in the lungs.
   b. Blood hydrostatic pressure, blood oncotic pressure, and diffusion determine how exchange will occur:

(1) Blood hydrostatic pressure causes movement of materials from the capillaries.
(2) Blood oncotic pressure causes water and dissolved materials to be drawn into the capillaries.
(3) Diffusion is the main force that causes movement through capillary walls of small soluble molecules.

Circulation in Venules and Veins

5. Explain how circulation is regulated in the venules and veins.
   a. Very little pressure from the heart's pumping action remains in the blood flowing through the veins.
   b. Flow in venules and veins is assisted by:
      (1) contraction of smooth muscle in the walls of the vessels
      (2) valves that prevent the backflow of blood
      (3) contraction of skeletal muscles adjacent to the veins
      (4) breathing movements

Integrated Function of the Circulatory System

6. Explain the role of the following in the integrated function of the circulatory system: (a) control centers in the brain, (b) baroreceptors, (c) chemoreceptors, and (d) local factors.
   a. Control centers in the brain consist of a diffuse network of neurons called the cardiovascular center, which includes:
      (1) a cardioinhibitory area that decreases cardiac function
      (2) a vasomotor pressor area and a vasomotor depressor area that act reciprocally to maintain vasomotor tone and to dilate or constrict arterioles according to signals from chemoreceptors and baroreceptors
   b. Baroreceptors respond to small changes in blood pressure and relay signals to the cardiovascular center.
      (1) When pressure increases, they send larger numbers of signals, which reduce cardiac output and cause vasodilation.
      (2) When pressure decreases, they send fewer signals, which allow cardiac output to increase and vasoconstriction to occur.
   c. Chemoreceptors respond to changes in the carbon dioxide and oxygen concentrations in the blood; though they are important primarily in the regulation of breathing, they do regulate circulation by:
      (1) increasing heart function and vasodilation when carbon dioxide is elevated or oxygen lowered
      (2) decreasing heart function and vasodilation when carbon dioxide is lowered or oxygen elevated
   d. Local factors such as increased carbon dioxide, decreased oxygen, or increased body temperature, especially in active muscles, cause local vasodilation, as do epinephrine and kinins when they are released.

7. Explain how circulatory function is altered by (a) exercise and (b) a change in posture.

    a. During exercise sympathetic stimulation, epinephrine, and other local factors increase the blood flow to the muscles and decrease that going to the visceral organs; increased sympathetic activity also increases cardiac output.

    b. When a person changes position from lying to standing, the force of gravity reduces venous return and blood pressure drops. When baroreceptors respond, they cause an increase in cardiac output and blood pressure.

Clinical Applications

8. Explain how circulatory function is altered by (a) atherosclerosis, (b) hypertension, (c) emotional stress, (d) hemorrhage, and (e) cerebrovascular accident.

    a. Atherosclerosis—hardening and occlusion of arteries—reduces the blood supply to affected tissues.

    b. Hypertension, a condition in which the resting systemic arterial pressure persistently exceeds 140/95, places an excessive workload on the heart and can lead to various circulatory disorders.

    c. Emotional stress may cause either excessive sympathetic stimulation or sudden excessive parasympathetic stimulation.

    d. Hemorrhage, a sudden loss of blood, results in lower cardiac output, lower blood pressure and, if severe enough, hypovolemic shock.

    e. A cerebrovascular accident, or stroke, is a sudden interruption of blood flow in an artery in the brain because of atherosclerosis, an embolus, or a rupture in the artery.

9. Describe the general circulatory effects of (a) myocardial infarction and (b) congestive heart failure.

    a. Both myocardial infarction and congestive heart failure affect the heart and the vascular system.

    b. In a myocardial infarction blood supply to a portion of the myocardium is blocked, and the affected tissue becomes ischemic and some cells die. Performance of the heart is reduced, so cardiac output is reduced.

    c. In congestive heart failure fluids accumulate in pulmonary and other tissues. Exchange of substances in the lungs and other tissues is decreased, and kidney function is impaired.

REVIEW

Important Terms

baroreceptors	cardiovascular center
cardioinhibitory area	carotid sinus
cerebrovascular accident	pressure
chemoreceptors	pulse
diastolic pressure	pulse pressure
flow	resistance
hemorrhage	shock
hydrostatic pressure	sphygmomanometer
hypertension	systolic pressure
hypovolemic shock	vasoconstriction
mean arterial pressure	vasodilation
oncotic pressure	vasomotor depressor area
peripheral resistance	vasomotor pressor area
postural hypotension	vasomotor tone
precapillary sphincter	

Questions

1. a. How is the flow of blood affected by pressure and by resistance?

    b. Assuming constant pressure, how is the resistance in a vessel 2 millimeters in diameter different from resistance in one 8 millimeters in diameter?

    c. Assuming constant pressure, how does the resistance over a length of 20 centimeters of a vessel differ from the resistance over 10 centimeters of a vessel?

    d. Use pressure, blood vessel cross-sectional area, and velocity to explain how flow remains constant over the entire circulatory system.

2. a. How does the systolic blood pressure differ from the diastolic pressure?

    b. Why do pulmonary pressures differ from systemic pressures?

    c. Describe what happens in the brachial artery when blood pressure is being measured.

    d. What is pulse pressure?

    e. If the systolic pressure is 125 mm Hg and the diastolic pressure is 77 mm Hg, what is the mean arterial pressure?

3. a. How is circulation through arteries regulated?

    b. How do the arterioles undergo vasoconstriction and vasodilation?

4. a. What characteristics of the structure of capillaries allow them to carry out their function?

    b. Use blood hydrostatic pressure and blood oncotic pressure to explain the movement of materials out of and into capillaries.

    c. Apply what you know about capillary exchange to explain what would happen when the tissue contains excess fluid; when the blood hydrostatic pressure is either elevated or lowered.

5. Explain how the structure of veins is related to their function.

6. **a.** What is vasomotor tone, and how is it maintained?
   b. What is the effect of the cardioinhibitory area?
   c. How do baroreceptors regulate heart rate?

7. **a.** Describe the effects of exercise on the circulatory system.
   b. What is postural hypotension, and how does the body normally prevent it?

8. **a.** Apply what you know about atherosclerosis and hypertension to explain how each might aggravate the other.
   b. How can emotional stress lead to either hypertension or shock?
   c. Explain how the body compensates for hemorrhage.
   d. How is a cerebrovascular accident like a myocardial infarction, and how is it different?

9. **a.** Suppose you are working with a person who has suffered a myocardial infarction. List all the effects this condition might have on the circulatory system and explain how you would detect these effects.
   b. Suppose you are working with a person who is suffering from congestive heart failure. Again, describe the effects and how you would observe them.

Problems

1. If the heart is pumping 5 liters of blood per minute, what is the total flow through each type of blood vessel?

2. Now that you have studied the effect of exercise on the circulatory system, refer back to and evaluate the exercise program in Chapter 9. How could participating in such a program be beneficial to the circulatory system? Under what circumstances could it be harmful?

REFERENCES AND READINGS

Arehart-Treichel, J. 1979. Microsurgery. *Science News* 115:237 (April 7).

Benditt, E. P. 1977. The origin of atherosclerosis. *Scientific American* 236(2):74 (February).

Brody, M. J., Haywood, J. R., and Trow, K. B. 1980. Neural mechanisms in hypertension. *Annual Review of Physiology* 42:441.

Coleridge, H. M., and Coleridge, J. C. G. 1980. Cardiovascular afferents involved in regulation of peripheral vessels. *Annual Review of Physiology* 42:413.

Donald, D. E., and Shepherd, J. T. 1980. Autonomic regulation of the peripheral circulation. *Annual Review of Physiology* 42:419.

Duling, B. R., and Klitzman, B. 1980. Local control of microvascular function: Role in tissue oxygen supply. *Annual Review of Physiology* 42:373.

Faden, A. J., and Holaday, J. W. 1979. Opiate antagonists: A role in the treatment of hypovolemic shock. *Science* 205:317 (July 20).

Fein, J. M. 1978. Microvascular surgery for stroke. *Scientific American* 238(4):59 (April).

Folkman, J. 1976. The vascularization of tumors. *Scientific American* 234 (5):59 (May).

Gore, R. W., and McDonagh, P. F. 1980. Fluid exchange across single capillaries. *Annual Review of Physiology* 42:337.

Granger, D. N., and Kvietys, P. R. 1981. The splanchnic circulation: Intrinsic regulation. *Annual Review of Physiology* 43:409.

Gruberg, E. R., and Raymond, S. A. 1979. Beyond cholesterol: A new theory of atherosclerosis. *Atlantic Monthly* 243:59 (May).

Heymann, M. A., Iwamoto, H. S., and Rudolph, A. M. 1981. Factors affecting changes in the neonatal systemic circulation. *Annual Review of Physiology* 43:371.

Hilton, S. M., and Spyer, K. M. 1980. Central nervous regulation of vascular resistance. *Annual Review of Physiology* 42:399.

Iwatsuki, K., Cardinale, G. C., Spector, S., and Udenfriend, S. 1977. Hypertension: Increase of collagen biosysthesis in arteries but not in veins. *Science* 198:403 (October 28).

Johansson, B. 1981. Vascular smooth muscle reactivity. *Annual Review of Physiology* 43:359.

Kolata, G. B. 1979. Is labile hypertension a myth? *Science* 204:489 (May 4).

Kolata, G. B., and Marx, J. L. 1976. Epidemiology of heart disease: Searches for causes. *Science* 194:509 (October 29).

Kontos, H. A. 1981. Regulation of cerebral circulation. *Annual Review of Physiology* 43:397.

Kummerow, F. A. 1979. Nutrition imbalance and angiotoxins as dietary risk factors in coronary heart disease. *American Journal of Clinical Nutrition* 32(1):58.

Lewis, L. A., and Naito, H. K. 1978. Relation of hypertension, lipids, and lipoproteins to atherosclerosis. *Clinical Chemistry* 24(12):2081 (December).

Markovitz, D. C., and Fernstrom, J. D. 1977. Diet and uptake of aldomet by the brain: Competition with natural neutral amino acids. *Science* 197:1014 (September 2).

Marx, J. L. 1976. Atherosclerosis: The cholesterol connection. *Science* 194:711 (November 12).

Marx, J. L. 1976. Hypertension: A complex disease with complex causes. *Science* 194:821 (November 19).

Needleman, P., Kulkarni, P. S., and Raz, A. 1977. Coronary tone modulation: Formation and actions of prostaglandins, endoperoxidases, and thromboxanes. *Science* 195:409 (January 28).

Olsson, R. A. 1981. Local factors regulating cardiac and skeletal muscle blood flow. *Annual Review of Physiology* 43:385.

Rudolph, A. M. 1979. Fetal and neonatal pulmonary circulation. *Annual Review of Physiology* 41:383.

Voors, A. W., Berenson, G. S., Dalferes, E. R., Webber, L. S., and Shuler, S. E. 1979. Racial differences in blood pressure control. *Science* 204:1091 (June 8).

20

LYMPHATICS AND IMMUNITY

ORGANIZATION AND GENERAL FUNCTIONS

Objective 1. Describe the organization and general functions of the lymphatic system.

The lymphatic system is closely related to the circulatory system. Though the lymphatic system has no heart, it does have a system of blind-ended tubes, the lymphatic vessels, a fluid called lymph, and a variety of lymphatic tissues. The lymphatic vessels make up a conducting system that carries fluid from the extracellular spaces to the blood circulatory system. When extracellular fluid enters a lymphatic vessel, it is called lymph. Lymph contains many of the same components found in blood plasma. The lymphatic tissues include the lymph nodes, thymus gland, tonsils, and spleen. The appendix and the Peyer's patches of the intestine also contain lymphatic tissue. Though all lymphatic tissues together weigh less than 2 kilograms, they contain 2 trillion cells.

Lymphatic tissues consist mainly of a network of reticular fibers in which many lymphocytes are found. Of these tissues the lymph nodes, scattered throughout the body, are most numerous. They are connected to lymphatic vessels, and lymph flowing through the vessels also flows through the lymph nodes. As lymph passes through the lymph nodes, microorganisms and other foreign substances are removed from the fluid. The spleen and tonsils may be thought of as large lymph nodes.

One of the major functions of the lymphatic system is to collect extracellular fluid and return it to the blood. Extracellular fluid contains proteins and fluid that are lost from and not reabsorbed into the blood capillaries. Because of the large pores in the lymph capillaries, the small number of

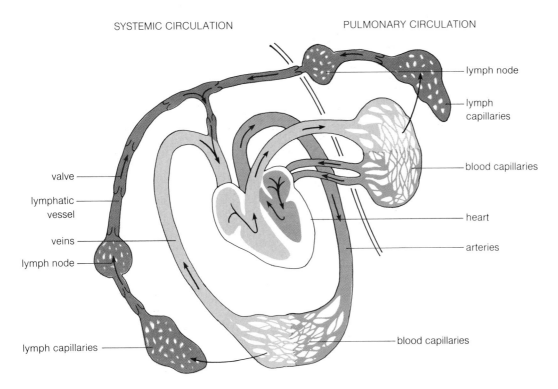

SYSTEMIC CIRCULATION   PULMONARY CIRCULATION

lymph node

lymph capillaries

blood capillaries

valve

lymphatic vessel

veins

heart

lymph node

arteries

lymph capillaries

blood capillaries

Figure 20.1 A schematic diagram showing the relationship of the lymphatic system to the blood circulatory system.

protein molecules that left the blood easily enter these capillaries and are carried back to the blood through the lymphatic vessels. The relationship between the lymphatic and the circulatory systems is shown in Figure 20.1.

Another major function of the lymphatic system is to defend the body against the invasion of microorganisms. It does this in two ways: Some of its cells phagocytize the microorganisms, and other cells produce antibodies. Antibodies react with antigens on the surface of the microorganisms and inactivate them, kill them, or increase their chance of being phagocytized.

FLUID AND TISSUES

Objective 2. Describe the nature of lymph.
Objective 3. Describe the tissues of the lymphatic vessels, lymph nodes, thymus, tonsils, and spleen.

Lymph

Lymph is a tissue fluid (extracellular fluid) that has entered a lymphatic vessel. Lymph contains all the constituents of blood except erythrocytes and platelets. The amount of protein in lymph is less than in plasma because filtration pressure pushes only small numbers of protein molecules out of the blood capillaries. On the other hand, the number of lymphocytes is much higher in lymph than in blood because many lymphocytes are formed in lymphatic tissues from stem cells that migrated to those tissues from the bone marrow.

Lymphatic Tissues

Lymphatic vessels The lymphatic vessels begin as saclike, blind-ended tubes called **lymph capillaries** (Figure 20.2). These capillaries are about 50 μm in diameter (larger than

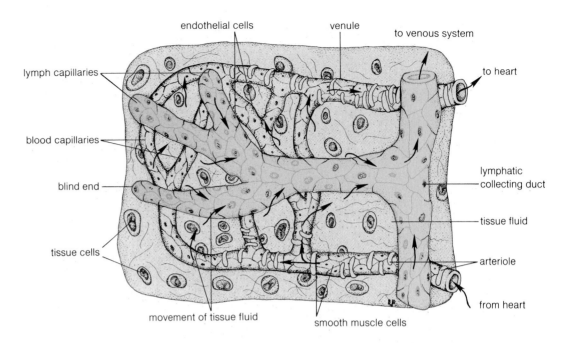

Figure 20.2 The location and structure of lymph capillaries, collecting ducts, and lymphatics.

blood capillaries) and have walls made of a single layer of endothelial cells, just as blood capillaries have. The lymph capillaries are distributed throughout the body so that they pass very near almost all the cells of the body.

Lymph capillaries drain into larger vessels called **collecting ducts**, which in turn drain into the largest vessels, called **lymphatics**. The lymphatics are similar to veins except that their walls are thinner and contain more valves than veins. Some collecting ducts and all lymphatics contain smooth muscle.

Lymph nodes   **Lymph nodes**, situated along the lymphatics, are bean-shaped organs that vary in size from 1 to 25 millimeters in diameter. They have **afferent lymphatic vessels** carrying lymph to them and **efferent lymphatic vessels** carrying lymph from them (Figure 20.3). Each lymph node is covered by a fibrous connective tissue **capsule** and is filled with a network of reticular connective tissue. Within the lymph node lymph flows through large, thin-walled vessels called **lymph sinuses**. Cells in the germinal centers give rise to lymphocytes, some of which will become the antibody-producing cells. The walls of the lymph sinuses are lined with phagocytic cells.

Spleen   The **spleen**, the largest of the lymphatic tissue masses, is located in the upper left quadrant of the abdom-

inal cavity. Internally, it is divided into lobules. Like a lymph node, it is covered with a fibrous connective tissue capsule and has an inner reticular network (Figure 20.4). The reticular network consists of **red pulp** and **white pulp**. Blood from the splenic artery enters venous sinusoids of the red pulp. As blood circulates through the red pulp, dead erythrocytes are phagocytyzed. The white pulp consists of

Lymph nodes are subject to several pathological processes. Though they play an important role in fighting infection, the lymph nodes themselves may become infected. When this occurs, the lymph node may contain a pus-filled abscess surrounded by inflamed tissue. A similar condition can result from an allergic reaction. Lymph nodes may also be affected directly or indirectly by malignancy. Hodgkin's disease and leukemia affect the lymph nodes directly. In other forms of cancer malignant cells may break away from a primary tumor and enter the lymph. They are especially likely to lodge and multiply in lymph nodes. Thus, many of the lymph nodes of the body become secondary sites of malignant growth.

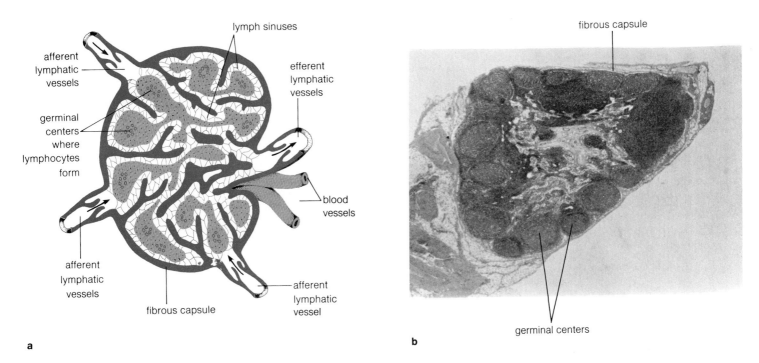

Figure 20.3 The structure of a lymph node, shown in cross-section: (**a**) diagram, (**b**) photomicrograph, × 19. (Photograph by author.)

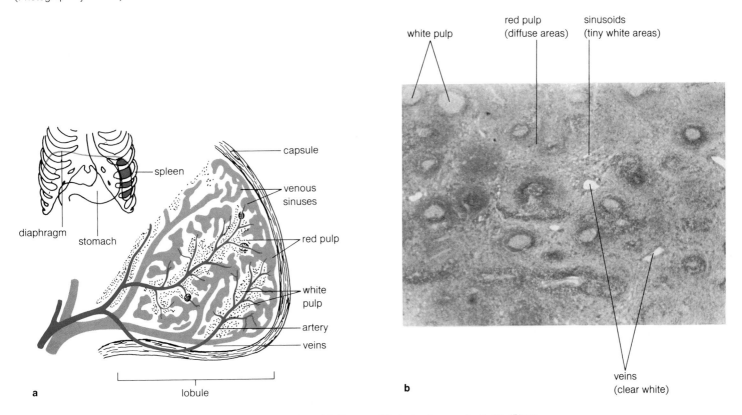

Figure 20.4 The structure of the spleen, shown in cross-section: (**a**) diagram, (**b**) photomicrograph, × 18. (Photograph by author.)

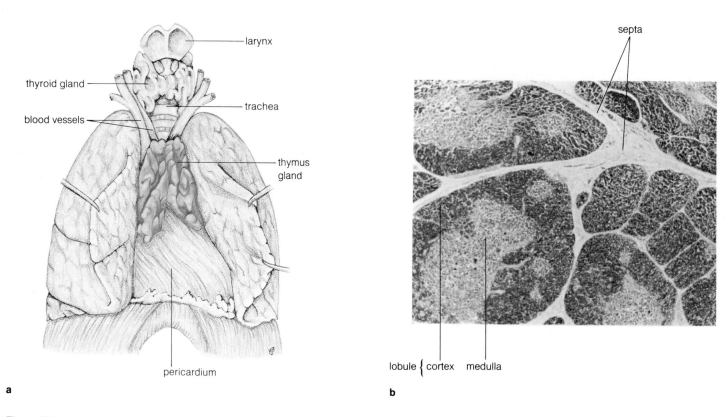

a

b

Figure 20.5 (**a**) The location of the thymus gland, (**b**) thymus from human fetus, × 18. (Photograph by author.)

lymphatic tissues arranged around blood vessels. Lymphocytes called B-lymphocytes are produced by the spleen and other lymphatic tissues.

Thymus The thymus gland (Figure 20.5), a two-lobed structure located in the mediastinum, is covered by a thin fibrous capsule and divided internally into many lobules. Each lobule consists of epithelial cells and lymphocytes. The thymus is generally large in infancy and childhood but begins to regress during adolescence. Large numbers of a special kind of lymphocyte, the T-lymphocyte, are produced in the thymus. It is thought that the thymus also produces a hormone, **thymosin**, which stimulates the development of the T-cells. Several other hormones have recently been isolated from the thymus gland; their actions are under investigation.

Tonsils **Tonsils** are masses of lymphatic tissue imbedded in the mucous membranes of the respiratory tract. (Their locations are described more precisely in Chapter 21.) The tonsils function much like any other lymph node to phago-

cytize foreign substances from the lymph. Sometimes, however, they become overloaded with microorganisms flowing through them and themselves become inflamed and enlarged. When the tonsils enlarge so that they make breathing difficult or when they become chronically infected, they may be removed by a tonsillectomy. Tonsillectomies are performed less frequently today than in the past because the tonsils are now known to be important in the body's defense against infection.

ANATOMY OF THE LYMPHATIC SYSTEM

Objective 4. Locate and identify the vessels and nodes of the lymphatic system.

The small lymph vessels that drain the lymph capillaries carry lymph to larger vessels (Figure 20.6). The **thoracic duct** begins as an enlarged area in a lymph vessel called the **cysterna chyli**, into which lymph from the intestinal and iliac lymph nodes drains. The thoracic duct receives other

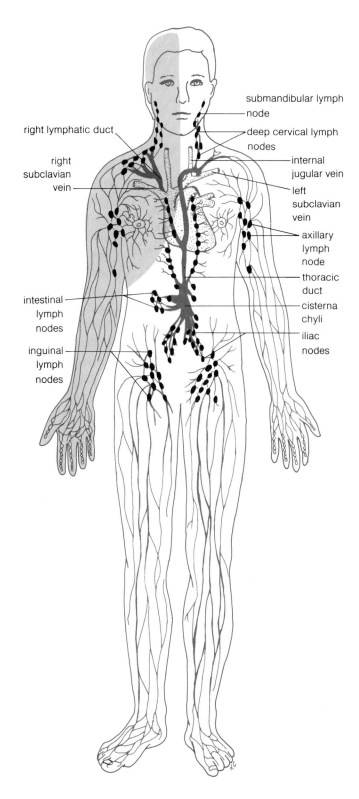

Figure 20.6 The location of the major lymphatic vessels and lymph nodes. The shaded area in the figure shows the portion of the body drained by the right lymphatic duct.

small branches as it carries lymph toward the left subclavian vein. It drains lymph from all parts of the body except the right arm and shoulder, part of the right thorax, and the right side of the head and neck. Lymph from these parts of the right side of the body is drained by the **right lymphatic duct** into the right subclavian vein.

Groups of lymph nodes are interposed along the lymphatics and are particularly concentrated in several areas. The **deep cervical lymph nodes** are located along the internal jugular veins. The **submandibular lymph nodes** are located along the lower border of the mandible. Both of these groups of lymph nodes become enlarged and painful to the touch when the body is fighting an infection. This is because the nodes themselves become inflamed as they defend the body against an infectious organism. The **axillary lymph nodes** are located in the armpit and chest area. Because they drain the tissue of the mammary glands they can be responsible for the spread of malignant cells from the breast. The **inguinal lymph nodes** are located in the groin area and drain the legs and the genital area. In addition, many small individual lymph nodes are scattered throughout the body.

PHYSIOLOGY OF THE LYMPHATIC SYSTEM

Objective 5. Explain the functions of the lymphatic system and describe how lymph moves through the system.

The lymphatic system has no pump like the heart in the circulatory system. Movement of lymph through the lymphatic vessels is produced by the contraction of the myoepithelial lining of the lymph vessels and by the contraction of adjacent skeletal muscles. The contractions of skeletal muscles, including those of the respiratory system, apply pressure to the lymph capillaries and smaller lymphatic vessels. Lymph is pushed toward the main lymphatic ducts. Valves in the lymphatics (shown in Figure 20.1) prevent the backflow of lymph in much the same way that valves in the veins prevent backflow of blood.

Proteins enter the interstitial fluid in the liver and intestine and, to a lesser extent, in all tissues. The lymphatic system returns these proteins to the blood at the subclavian veins. In twenty-four hours one-fourth to one-half of the total amount of plasma protein is returned to the blood. More fluid leaves the blood capillaries than is returned to them, and the lymphatic system also returns this fluid to the blood. Over twenty-four hours two to four liters of interstitial fluid are returned to the blood.

If the lymphatics fail to return lymph to the blood, fluid accumulates in the tissues, and **edema** is produced. Edema may be caused by obstructions in the lymphatic system, excessive capillary pressure, too little protein in the blood, or injuries that cause fluids to accumulate in the tissues.

IMMUNITY

Objective 6. Distinguish among nonspecific defense mechanisms (nonspecific immunity) and the types of specific immunity.

Objective 7. Explain the function of nonspecific defense mechanisms, including tissue response to injury.

Objective 8. Describe the formation and function of antibodies in humoral immunity.

Objective 9. Describe the formation and function of cell-mediated immunity.

Objective 10. Distinguish among the various kinds of active and passive immunity.

Specific versus Nonspecific Immunity

The word immune comes from the Latin *immunis*, which means free from burden. In general usage we say that people are immune to a disease when their bodies are able to resist reinfection after they have once had the disease or have been vaccinated against it. For example, if you have had chickenpox or have received polio vaccine, you are immune to those diseases. However, the same physiological mechanisms that confer immunity can sometimes produce unpleasant or even harmful effects. Allergies and autoimmune diseases are examples of such effects.

Though the above examples are what most people understand when they think of **immunity**, the body's overall immune mechanisms perform a variety of tasks to defend the body against infection and to help maintain homeostasis.

The actions of the immune system can be divided into two general types: nonspecific defense mechanisms (nonspecific immunity) and specific immunity. **Nonspecific defense mechanisms** come into play in response to any kind of tissue injury or to the presence of any foreign substance. **Specific immunity** develops in response to exposure to an **antigen**, a specific foreign substance such as a protein on the surface of a microorganism. Specific immunity can be further divided into humoral immunity and cell-mediated immunity. **Humoral immunity** is conferred by **antibodies**, complex proteins that circulate in the plasma and react with specific antigens. (The fluids of the body are sometimes called humors; thus, immunity that results from

factors in the blood is called humoral immunity.) **Cell-mediated immunity** is conferred by lymphocytes that have been sensitized to particular antigens.

Nonspecific Defense Mechanisms

As we saw in Chapter 5, the body is protected from invasion by microorganisms first by the skin. Glands in the skin secrete substances that are toxic to many bacteria. In addition, the mucous membranes of the digestive, respiratory, and urinary tracts secrete mucus, which traps microorganisms and creates a barrier to the entry of chemical substances. Furthermore, some of these membranes are ciliated, and the cilia sweep foreign substances out of the tracts. Should any microorganisms or foreign substances penetrate the barrier created by the skin and mucous membranes, an inflammatory response occurs and phagocytic cells move toward the invaders and attempt to engulf them. The pH of the tissue fluids and lysozymes released from damaged cells also may help to destroy invading microorganisms. All these defenses are nonspecific. That is, they operate in the same way regardless of which organism or foreign substance has invaded the body.

Inflammatory response Though the inflammatory response was discussed in some detail in Chapter 4, we will review it briefly here. The nonspecific barriers are reasonably efficient in guarding the body against invaders, but a few microorganisms are continuously penetrating the barriers. Small-scale inflammatory responses are occurring all the time, and we are usually unaware of these numerous minor invasions. However, whenever there is tissue injury from any one of many possible causes, an observable inflammatory response is initiated. The steps in this response are as follows:

1. Tissue injury and entry of microorganisms

2. Vasodilation in the blood vessels near the site of the injury

3. Increase in permeability of blood vessel walls, allowing proteins, fluids, and white blood cells to enter injured tissue

4. Phagocytosis of microorganisms and tissue debris

5. Tissue repair.

Let us look at this process in more detail.

When tissue is injured, histamine, prostaglandins, and other chemicals called kinins are released. They cause the dilation of blood vessels in the area of the injury and increase the permeability of the capillaries. What we observe as a swollen, reddened area around an injury is created by increased blood flow to the area and the accumulation of fluid in the tissue. The pain and heat associated with inflammation are the result of these two phenomena. The blood-clotting mechanism also operates where blood vessels have been broken.

After about half an hour neutrophils begin to pass through the capillary walls into the tissues. It is thought that they are attracted to the injured area by the same substances that cause the vascular changes. Later, macrophages (monocytes that have matured) also enter the tissue, but how they are attracted is not clearly understood. Once these phagocytic white blood cells have entered the injured tissue, they begin to engulf and digest microorganisms, dirt, and other foreign matter in the wound, and the debris left by dying cells. Finally, fibroblasts become active and secrete collagen fibers that form scar tissue. The epithelium of the skin grows over the injured area. This process is summarized in Figure 20.7.

Specific Immune Response

Three characteristics distinguish the specific immune response from the nonspecific responses: (1) specificity, (2) heterogeneity, and (3) memory. **Specificity** refers to the fact that the immune system can distinguish one antigen from another. **Heterogeneity** refers to the many different kinds of specific antibodies and other cell products that are produced by the immune system even in response to the same antigen. **Memory** is the property of the immune system that allows it to respond rapidly and defend the body against an antigen to which it has previously reacted.

The cells that make the specific immune response possible are lymphocytes. These lymphocytes arise in the red bone marrow as precursors of two cell types: B-cells and T-cells. Precursor B-cells are transformed into **B-cells** in the fetal liver and possibly in the fetal spleen. Precursor T-cells migrate to the thymus gland, where, probably under the influence of the thymic hormone thymosin, they differentiate into at least three different kinds of **T-cells**—the T-effectors, the helper T-cells, and the suppressor T-cells. Both B-cells and T-cells subsequently migrate to the lymph nodes and bone marrow. B-cells, assisted by the helper T-cells and the suppressor T-cells, produce humoral immunity. Humoral immunity is mediated through antibodies produced by the B-cells circulating in the blood and is most effective in defending the body against the bacterial infections and the extracellular phase of viral infections (before the viruses invade cells). The T-effectors produce cell-

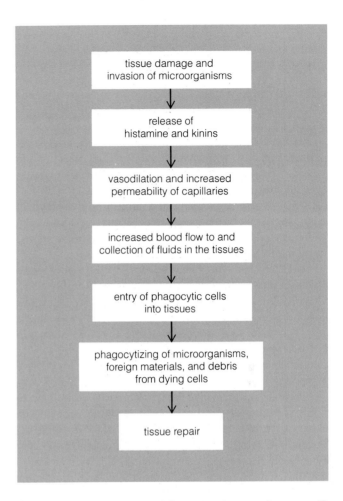

Figure 20.7 A summary of the inflammatory response in nonspecific defense mechanisms.

mediated immunity. Cell-mediated immunity occurs at the cellular level and is most effective in defending the body against fungi, intracellular viral infections, parasites, foreign tissue (from organ transplants, for example), and cancer.

Humoral immunity Humoral immunity depends on the ability of B-cells to recognize specific antigens, usually proteins or other substances not normally present in the body. A great many different kinds of B-cells exist in the body, and current evidence suggests that they arise from stem cells (precursors of blood cells).

The mechanism by which B-cells recognize antigens and react to them is as follows: Each B-cell has receptor sites for a specific antigen on its surface. When an antigen attaches to the receptor site of a B-cell, the B-cell is stimulated to divide. The daughter cells become **plasma cells**. Plasma cells then begin to manufacture proteins called antibodies, which can combine with the specific antigen that stimulated their production because each antibody has a specific shape complementary to the antigen. Each plasma cell releases into the blood thousands of antibody molecules per minute for the few days that it stays alive and active. As some plasma cells die, others are produced so that, once the body is exposed to a particular antigen, antibodies are produced against that antigen as long as the antigen is present in the body. Antibodies, also called **immunoglobulins**, are an important component of the plasma proteins called the gamma-globulins. However, immunoglobulins also are found in locations outside the blood.

Each antibody molecule consists of four polypeptide chains (Figure 20.8), two long or **heavy chains** and two short or **light chains**. Much of the length of each chain of immunoglobulins consists of the same sequence of amino acids, but each chain also has a variable segment. The properties of the variable segments determine which specific antigen can bind to the antibody. On the basis of the structural characteristics of the chains, immunoglobulins (Igs) can be classified into five groups. IgG, the main immunoglobulin in the blood, is responsible for reacting with many foreign antigens that may enter the blood. IgA, found in tears and intestinal secretions, helps to prevent foreign antigens from entering the body. IgE is involved in a variety of allergic reactions. The functions of the remaining two groups, IgM and IgD, are not yet well understood.

Antibodies may have several effects, and they are assisted by other proteins such as complement and opsonins. Complement is a set of plasma proteins (enzymes) that participate in inflammatory reactions. Opsonins are proteins that coat microorganisms, making them susceptible to phagocytosis. Some antibodies neutralize toxins produced by infectious agents; some, with the help of complement, cause lysis of the membranes of invading cells; some, with the aid of opsonins, foster phagocytosis. In one way or another antibodies cause destruction of the substance containing the antigen.

Many B-cells appear to be regulated by the helper T-cells and the suppressor T-cells. Helper T-cells seem to stimulate the B-cells to produce antibodies against some antigens, but some B-cells are T-cell independent and require no help from the T-cells. Suppressor T-cells may have several modes of operation. They may directly prevent B-cells from acting, or they may prevent the helper T-cells from stimulating the B-cells. Finally, they may suppress the T-effectors that are involved in cell-mediated immunity (to be described below).

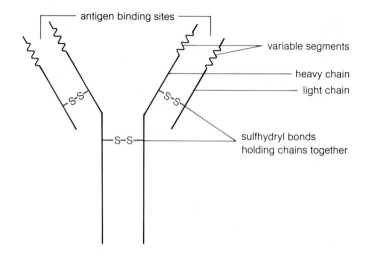

Figure 20.8 The general structure of an immunoglobulin.

As a part of the initial or **primary response** to an antigen, some of the B-cells become memory cells, capable of later recognizing the specific antigen to which they have been sensitized. These memory cells remain in the lymph nodes after an infection has abated. Any time a microorganism with its specific antigen invades the body again later, the memory cells produce a clone of B-cells. (A **clone** is a colony of identical cells produced from a single cell.) These B-cells produce antibodies, as already described. However, in second and subsequent infections antibodies are present in the circulation sooner and in greater numbers than during the initial infection. This is called a **secondary response**.

Cell-mediated immunity   In contrast to humoral immunity, cell-mediated immunity is produced by the T-effector cells. When such a T-cell is exposed to a particular antigen, it is stimulated to produce many more T-cells like itself that are sensitive to the particular antigen. This constitutes a clone of T-cells. Such sensitized T-cells attach to the cell that contains the antigen. Though many details about the action of T-cells remain to be discovered, one mechanism is that T-effectors produce substances called lymphokines, which destroy the cell to which the T-cells are attached. T-cells that become attached to cells containing the antigen are destroyed along with the invading cell, but other T-cells of the same clone remain in the body ready to proliferate whenever the antigen they recognize is present. Thus, T-cells "remember" an antigen to which they have been exposed just as B-cells do. In addition to producing lymphokines, T-cells also stimulate the inflammatory response.

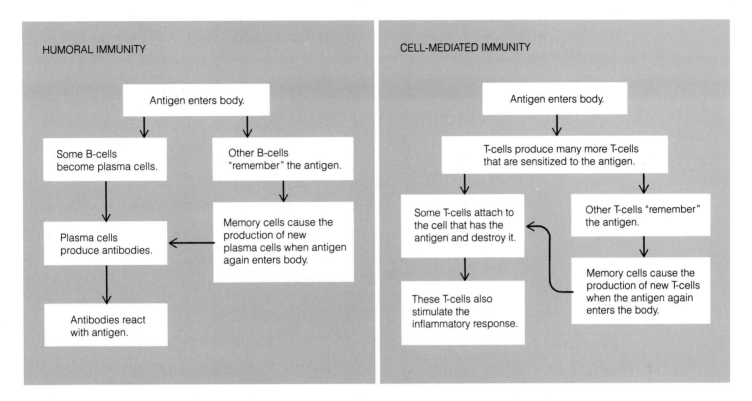

HUMORAL IMMUNITY

Antigen enters body.

Some B-cells become plasma cells.

Other B-cells "remember" the antigen.

Plasma cells produce antibodies.

Memory cells cause the production of new plasma cells when antigen again enters body.

Antibodies react with antigen.

CELL-MEDIATED IMMUNITY

Antigen enters body.

T-cells produce many more T-cells that are sensitized to the antigen.

Some T-cells attach to the cell that has the antigen and destroy it.

Other T-cells "remember" the antigen.

These T-cells also stimulate the inflammatory response.

Memory cells cause the production of new T-cells when the antigen again enters the body.

Figure 20.9 A summary of humoral and cell-mediated immunity, the two kinds of specific immunity.

The processes of humoral and cell-mediated immunity are summarized in Figure 20.9.

Kinds of Active and Passive Immunity

Immunity is **active** when the body has been stimulated to form specific antibodies against a particular antigen. Such immunity destroys microorganisms that carry the antigen. Active immunity may be acquired by having a disease or by receiving a vaccine. Vaccines may contain dead organisms or attenuated (weakened) organisms, but the organism must be able to stimulate the lymphocytes to produce specific antibodies; toxoid vaccines contain weakened toxins capable of stimulating lymphocytes. (Table 20.1 gives examples of the different kinds of vaccines.) To acquire active immunity, the body must be stimulated to produce its own antibodies and memory cells.

Immunity is **passive** when ready-made antibodies from another person or animal are introduced. The immunity acquired in this passive way is only temporary, because the recipient's B-cells have not been stimulated to

Table 20.1 Active Component of Vaccines

Component	Type of Organism	Examples of Diseases
Killed organisms	Bacterium	Whooping cough, typhoid fever
	Virus	Poliomyelitis (Salk vaccine)
Attenuated (weakened) organisms	Virus	Measles, smallpox, poliomyelitis (Sabin vaccine), yellow fever
Weakened toxins	Toxin-producing bacterium	Tetanus, botulism, diphtheria

Table 20.2 Immunization Program for Young Children*

Disease	Recommended Schedule of Immunization	Method Used	Duration of Protection after Completion of Recommended Schedule
Diphtheria	2, 4, 6, and 18 months and 4–6 and 14–16 years (DPT inoculation)	Toxoid (a toxin rendered nontoxic that retains immunological effect	About 10 years
Pertussis (whooping cough)**	Same as diphtheria (DPT inoculation)	Killed organism	About 10 years
Tetanus (lockjaw)	Same as diphtheria (DPT inoculation)	Toxoid	About 10 years
Polio	2, 4, 6, and 18 months and 4–6 years	Killed or attenuated organism	About 10 years
Rubella (German measles)	15 months	Attenuated organism	Probably for life
Rubeola (red measles)	15 months (can be given with rubella)	Attenuated organism	Probably for life
Mumps	15 months (with rubella)	Attenuated organism	Probably for life

*Until recently smallpox immunization was recommended for all young children, but many epidemiologists now believe that the disease has been nearly eradicated and immunization is no longer needed. However, immunization may be a means of maintaining eradication of the disease.
**Pertussis vaccine is usually not given after five years of age.

produce active immunity. The antibodies (immunoglobulins) in an individual's blood plasma are found in the gamma-globulin fraction, a component of plasma containing protein molecules of a particular size and nature. The gamma-globulin fraction from many blood samples can be pooled and injected into a person in need of temporary immunity. Because the pooled gamma-globulin has many different kinds of antibodies in it, it offers the patient temporary protection against a variety of diseases. It is given after exposure to a serious disease such as hepatitis or measles and generally prevents or lessens the severity of the disease. Fetuses acquire passive immunity from the mother's antibodies that cross the placenta.

Another kind of passive immunity is acquired by breastfed babies. Breast milk contains antibodies made by the mother's body. These antibodies react with microorganisms in the infant's intestinal tract and may also have other immunological effects. Breast milk seems to be particularly effective in preventing newborn diarrhea caused by some strains of the bacterium, *Escherichia coli*. This organism is a normal inhabitant of the adult intestinal tract, though it may cause disease in adults if it invades other tissues.

Childhood immunization is an important part of preventive health care. Table 20.2 summarizes the immunization program that is currently recommended for young children.

Objective 11. Discuss the relationship of immune reactions to (a) transplant rejection, (b) defense against cancer, (c) allergy, and (d) autoimmune disease.

Transplant Rejection

Early animal experiments in tissue transplanting often involved skin grafts. The grafts at first appeared healthy, but in a few days to weeks they became inflamed and dropped off the recipient's body. First thought to be the result of infection, this reaction is now known to be immunological and is called a host versus graft reaction. Antigens in the donor tissue elicit the production of T-effector cells (more so than B-cells), and the T-effector cells attack and destroy the donor cells.

It is now known that the cells of any individual have a set of antigens that are unique to that individual. These are called **histocompatibility antigens** (*histo* = tissue). Only identical twins have exactly the same histocompatibility antigens. These antigens are located on the surfaces of all nucleated cells, including those of any organ or tissue to be transplanted. If the antigens of the donor tissue are foreign to the body of the recipient, as they likely would be in a randomly chosen pair of people, T-cells will be produced and destroy the donor tissue.

To minimize this reaction, laboratory techniques have been developed for tissue matching before transplanting an organ. Prospective transplant recipients have their tissues typed by a procedure somewhat like blood typing, although lymphocytes rather than erythrocytes are used. There are hundreds of possible combinations of tissue antigens—far more than the number of blood types. When a donor organ becomes available, the potential recipient whose tissue most closely matches that of the donor organ is chosen to receive it. Thus, the possibility of the organ being rejected is reduced.

Drugs that suppress the immune system are also used to reduce the recipient's response to the donor organ. However, these drugs suppress both T-cells and B-cells, and the individual's immunity to infections is decreased as well. Consequently, transplant recipients sometimes succumb to secondary infections, even though the transplant may have been successful. Methods are currently being developed to provide antibodies to the recipient's T-cells called antilymphocytic serum, thereby selectively suppressing the production of T-cells without suppressing the recipient's antibody production.

Defense against Cancer

Cancer cells, which may have been caused to mutate by chemical carcinogens or viruses, may have antigens that are different from normal cells of the body. One of the functions of T-cells appears to be to recognize and destroy these abnormal cells. According to the

An abnormal condition related to transplant rejection sometimes occurs in pregnant females. Though proteins do not normally pass across the placenta, in a few cases they do. Mother and baby have some common proteins, but each also has proteins that the other does not have. If fetal proteins that are foreign to the mother enter her blood through the placenta, her body will make antibodies to these proteins. If these antibodies then cross the placenta and reach the fetus, fetal tissues can be damaged. It is thought that this process may account for some otherwise unexplained stillbirths and spontaneous abortions.

Because the structure of the normal placenta allows some proteins to cross the membranes, it is possible that antigens from the mother will enter the fetus. However, an immune reaction does not occur in this case because the immune system of the fetus is immature and incapable of producing significant numbers of antibodies.

immune surveillance theory, this seek-and-destroy mechanism is a natural one that prevents mutated cells from developing into cancers. If this theory is correct, in a lifetime each of us has within our body many different potentially malignant cells. A cancer develops when the T-cells fail to identify and destroy the mutated cell.

This theory is being used by some researchers to develop vaccines they believe will cause the immune system to destroy those cancer cells that the natural mechanism has failed to detect. One of the drawbacks to the development of such vaccines is that malignant cells produce substances that inhibit the production of T-cells. Further research is needed to determine whether this particular immunological therapy for cancer will be a useful technique. Other research is underway to develop a specific interferon that can be used to treat cancer. Interferon, a protein that fights viral infection, will be discussed in the essay at the end of this chapter.

Allergy

An allergy is a sensitivity to an antigen that normally does not produce an immunological response. Thus, allergy is sometimes called **hypersensitivity**—the person is more sensitive than usual to certain substances. Some allergies are thought to be inherited, although an allergic individual may have an allergy not expressed by either parent. What may be inherited is the tendency to be allergic; those who have inherited the tendency are likely to develop allergies under certain physiological and environmental conditions. Unfortunately, little is known about what conditions trigger the development of allergies.

An antigen that causes an allergic reaction is called an **allergen**. When the tissues of an individual first come in contact with the allergen, the allergen stimulates the production of special types of antibodies, the IgE immunoglobulins. These antibodies attach to cells called **mast cells**, which contain histamine. When the person subsequently comes in contact with the allergen, the antibody-coated mast cells attach to the allergen and release histamine. Histamine causes vasodilation, contraction of smooth muscle (especially in the respiratory passages), and increased permeability of capillaries. Eosinophils also usually increase in number in the blood and tissue fluids.

These reactions produce the symptoms of allergy: runny nose, collection of fluid in tissues, constriction of bronchioles of the lungs in asthma, itching, and other symptoms. Because of the increase in the numbers of eosinophils, nasal secretions can be used to determine whether the runny nose is due to an allergy. If it is, large numbers of eosinophils will be found in the secretions.

Sometimes an allergic reaction can lead to an immediately life-threatening condition, **anaphylactic shock**. In this condition the mast cells release histamine and other substances. Sudden and extensive vasodilation causes pooling of blood in the peripheral vessels, a precipitous drop in blood pressure, and a greatly decreased cardiac output. Unless immediate treatment (usually with epinephrine) is provided, death may occur.

Autoimmune Disease

Autoimmune disease is a condition in which a person becomes hypersensitive to antigens on cells of his or her own body. This abnormal condition raises the question of how the body determines what cells belong to it and what cells are foreign to it. One theory is that during embryological development some of the B-cells attach to each of the antigens that are normally present in the embryo. Somehow these cells are then made inactive; by the time an infant is born, any cells capable of reacting with any of the infant's own antigens have been destroyed or inactivated. This is called the clonal deletion theory.

In autoimmune disease the ability to recognize "self" has been lost for certain antigens on body cells. As a result of some disease processes body cells elicit a response from the immune system, and the body begins to destroy some of its own cells. Diseases thought to involve autoimmune reactions include rheumatic fever, rheumatoid arthritis, and myasthenia gravis. In rheumatic fever tissues of the heart and joints are affected. In rheumatoid arthritis the joints are the primary site of damage. And in myasthenia gravis the patient develops an immune reaction to the acetylcholine receptors in skeletal muscles. Some types of diabetes in which the beta cells of the pancreas are destroyed may also be caused by an autoimmune reaction. At present, treatment of autoimmune diseases is limited to attempting to alleviate symptoms. No means of preventing the immune reactions exists.

Clinical Terms

agammaglobulinemia (a-gam-ma-glob″-u-lin-e′me-a) the inability to produce antibodies because of a sex-linked recessive trait

anaphylaxis (an-af-il-aks′is) a severe allergic reaction upon second exposure to a substance to which an individual has been sensitized

diGeorge syndrome a defect in the ability to produce T-cells, leading to a deficiency in cell-mediated immunity

elephantiasis (el″ef-an-ti′as-is) an inflammation and blockage of lymph ducts due to a worm infestation

lymphadenectomy (lim″fad-en-ek′to-me) the surgical removal of lymph glands

lymphedema (lim-fe-de′mah) collection of fluid in soft tissues because of an excess of lymph

lymphoma (lim-fo′mah) any tumor consisting of lymphatic tissue

splenectomy (sple-nek′to-me) surgical removal of the spleen

splenomegaly (sple-no-meg′al-e) enlargement of the spleen

stem cell immunodeficiency a severe deficiency in immunity due to the absence of cells that give rise to lymphocytes

Essay: Interferon

As early as the 1930s it had been observed that infection with one virus prevented for a time any infection by another virus. Then in the 1950s a substance was discovered that protected cells against viral infections. This substance, named **interferon**, is released by cells that have been infected with a virus; it travels to other cells and causes them to resist viral infection by the same or a different virus. Interferon appears to attach to the cell surface and stimulate cells to produce a second substance that actually inhibits reproduction of the virus. Viruses usually alter the cell's nuclear apparatus, causing it to make viruses; such interference is prevented by the substance released by interferon.

Some of the properties of interferon were determined shortly after its discovery. Interferon is a protein of fairly low molecular weight. It reacts with cells, not viruses. Furthermore, it makes cells resistant to many different kinds of viruses. Experiments with interferon from different organisms indicated that each species produces its own kind of interferon. For example, interferon from chick cells had no effect on cells from other organisms. Efforts to purify interferon led to the discovery that a single species might have several different types of interferon. For example, interferon produced by human fibroblasts (cells that make connective tissue) is different from interferon produced by human white blood cells.

Other properties of interferon have been more difficult to determine. Purification has been especially difficult, primarily because interferon tends to stick to other proteins. Because a very small amount of interferon is effective, tests for its activity are positive even when it is contaminated with another protein. Recent advances in purification techniques have made it possible to prepare relatively pure interferon. Nevertheless, it is extremely expensive to prepare even small quantities.

Other studies have focused on determining how interferon acts. It appears that, once interferon is released from a cell, it binds to cell-surface receptors on neighboring cells. Interferon, then, does not actually enter cells. It appears to act in somewhat the same way as some hormones, working from the surface of the cell to cause the production of an antiviral protein inside the cell. This mechanism is consistent with the observation that a very small amount of interferon can induce resistance to viruses. One molecule attached to a receptor site could cause the cell to produce many molecules of the antiviral protein.

If antiviral protein is produced by the above mechanism, the next question is, how does that protein cause cells to resist viral infection? Because it has been observed that viruses do enter cells that are producing antiviral protein, it seems likely that the protein interferes with the viruses's ability to synthesize either nucleic acid or protein that it needs to replicate itself once inside the cell. Studies have shown that some viruses are prevented from making nucleic acid, and others are prevented from making protein.

Since small amounts of interferon have become available, it has been used in a variety of therapeutic situations, but only a few individuals have been treated because of the scarcity and high cost of interferon. Interferon seems not to be of any great benefit to people suffering from colds or influenza, its only effect being to delay the onset of symptoms. Other applications offer greater promise. For example, individuals who have a chronic form of hepatitis are susceptible to relapses and can spread the disease to others. Interferon appears to be effective in preventing both the relapses and the spread of the disease.

Interferon shows greatest promise in the treatment of cancer. Tests on a form of bone cancer have shown that, after the bulk of the cancerous tissue is destroyed by radiation or removed by surgery, interferon seems to reduce the incidence of metastasis. The mechanism by which it acts is unknown, but it is possible either that interferon suppresses the cancer cells because they contain some unidentified virus or that interferon in some way interferes with the growth of cancer cells.

Interferon has been produced in the laboratory from cultures of human fibroblasts or white blood cells. Some researchers are working on synthesizing the protein. Late in 1979 Charles Weissman and his colleagues at the University of Zurich developed a recombinant DNA technique by which they could cause bacteria to produce a human interferon. They isolated genes from human cells, selecting those genes most likely to produce interferon. They inserted the genes into bacterial DNA. Finally, they put the modified DNA into bacterial cells and cultured the cells. Each bacterium produced a separate colony, and the cells in some of the colonies contained the interferon gene.

The problem then became one of determining which colonies were capable of producing interferon. By a complex sequence of steps the investigators finally obtained a product from some colonies that they thought contained interferon. This product was introduced into cultures of human cells, and the cultures were later infected with viruses. If the cells were resistant, the researchers concluded that interferon had been added.

Now that the steps in this process have been worked out, it is possible to employ bacteria to make interferon for therapeutic use in humans. As this essay is being written, the main problem is to learn to increase the yield of interferon. By the time you read it, much progress will likely have been made both in increasing yields from bacterial production of interferon and in biochemical synthesis of it.

CHAPTER SUMMARY

(Chapter summary points and review questions are numbered to correspond to the numbered objectives in the text of each chapter.)

Organization and General Functions

1. Describe the organization and general functions of the lymphatic system.
   a. The lymphatic system consists of lymph, lymphatic vessels, and masses of lymphatic tissue.
   b. The functions of the lymphatic system are to return proteins and tissue fluids to the blood and to produce immunity.

Fluid and Tissues

2. Describe the nature of lymph.
   a. Lymph is extracellular fluid that has entered a lymph vessel; it is similar in composition to blood plasma.
3. Describe the tissues of the lymphatic vessels, lymph nodes, thymus, tonsils, and spleen.
   a. Lymphatic vessels include:
      (1) saclike, blind-ended, thin-walled lymph capillaries, which are larger and more permeable than blood capillaries
      (2) collecting ducts, which collect lymph from the capillaries and whose walls may contain smooth muscle
      (3) lymphatics, which collect lymph from the collecting ducts and whose walls contain smooth muscle and valves
   b. Lymph nodes consist of reticular connective tissue and lymph sinuses that receive lymph from afferent lymphatic vessels and drain into efferent lymphatic vessels.
   c. The spleen contains red pulp and white pulp.
      (1) Worn-out erythrocytes are phagocytized as blood circulates through the red pulp.
      (2) White pulp surrounds the blood vessels.
      (3) B-lymphocytes are made in the spleen and other lymph tissues.
   d. The thymus, located in the mediastinum,
      (1) is composed of epithelial cells and lymphocytes
      (2) produces T-lymphocytes from precursor cells
      (3) produces the hormone thymosin, which probably activates T-cells
   e. The tonsils, masses of lymphatic tissue imbedded in the mucous membranes of the respiratory tract, phagocytize foreign substances in the lymph.

Anatomy of the Lymphatic System

4. Locate and identify the vessels and nodes of the lymphatic system.

   a. All smaller lymph vessels drain into one of two ducts.
      (1) The thoracic duct begins as the cysterna chyli, which drains lymph from the abdominal area and legs and subsequently receives vessels that drain the left arm, thorax, neck, and head.
      (2) The right thoracic duct drains the right arm, thorax, neck, and head.
   b. Lymph nodes are interposed along the lymphatics throughout the body but are especially concentrated in the cervical, submandibular, axillary, and inguinal regions.

Physiology of the Lymphatic System

5. Explain the functions of the lymphatic system and describe how lymph moves through the system.
   a. Lymph moves through the lymphatic system by:
      (1) contraction of the myoepithelium of the lymph vessels
      (2) contraction of adjacent skeletal muscles
      (3) prevention of backflow by valves in the lymph vessels
   b. The functions of the lymphatic system include:
      (1) the return of proteins and fluid from the interstitial spaces to the blood
      (2) phagocytizing foreign substances that enter the blood
      (3) contributing to immunity

Immunity

6. Distinguish among nonspecific defense mechanisms (nonspecific immunity) and the types of specific immunity.
   a. Nonspecific defense mechanisms include:
      (1) phagocytosis
      (2) the inflammatory response to injury or the invasion of microorganisms
   b. Specific immunity includes
      (1) the production of humoral antibodies
      (2) cell-mediated immunity
7. Explain the function of nonspecific defense mechanisms, including tissue response to injury.
   a. The response to tissue injury includes:
      (1) the release of histamine and kinins, which cause vasodilation and increased permeability of capillaries
      (2) the migration of white blood cells to the injured area
      (3) the collection of tissue fluids in the injured area
      (4) the phagocytizing of microorganisms, foreign substances, and debris from dying cells
      (5) tissue repair
   b. Other factors involved in nonspecific defense mechanisms include:
      (1) skin secretions
      (2) mucus and cilia of mucous membranes

8. Describe the formation and function of antibodies in humoral immunity.
   a. Precursor cells from bone marrow produce B-cells.
   b. Each clone of B-cells produces a specific antibody by the following steps:
      (1) An antigen reacts with the receptor sites on a sensitive B-cell.
      (2) The B-cell divides, and the daughter cells become plasma cells.
      (3) Plasma cells release thousands of antibodies specific for the antigen that induced their production.
   c. Some B-cells are retained as memory cells, which are capable of producing more antibodies when challenged by the same antigen.
9. Describe the formation and function of cell-mediated immunity.
   a. Precursor cells from bone marrow are activated in the thymus gland to form three kinds of T-cells:
      (1) T-effectors
      (2) helper T-cells
      (3) suppressor T-cells
   b. Helper T-cells and suppressor T-cells help to regulate the activity of B-cells.
   c. T-effectors act as follows:
      (1) When activated by an antigen, a T-effector divides and forms a clone.
      (2) Cells of the clone attach to the cell that contains the antigen and produce chemicals called lymphokines, which destroy the antigen-containing cell and the T-cell.
      (3) T-cells also stimulate the inflammatory response.
   d. Some T-effectors sensitized by a specific antigen remain and serve as memory cells.
10. Distinguish among the various kinds of active and passive immunity.
    a. Active immunity is produced by an individual's B-cells in response to:
       (1) having a disease
       (2) receiving a vaccine
    b. Passive immunity is produced by temporarily receiving antibodies from another individual through:
       (1) injections of gamma-globulin
       (2) placental transfer
       (3) breast milk

Clinical Applications

11. Discuss the relationship of immune reactions to (a) transplant rejection, (b) defense against cancer, (c) allergy, and (d) autoimmune disease.
    a. Transplant rejection is due to the recipient's body producing T-cells against surface antigens on the cells of the donor tissue.
    b. Tests for histocompatibility and drugs to suppress immunological reactions minimize the probability of tissue rejection.

   c. According to the immune surveillance theory, the body defends itself against cancer by producing T-cells that destroy cells with abnormal surface antigens.
   d. Allergy is a hypersensitivity to certain antigens called allergens.
   e. Symptoms of allergy are due to histamine released from mast cells when the antibodies on their surfaces react with the allergen.
   f. Autoimmune disease occurs when an individual becomes allergic to some of his or her own tissues.

REVIEW

Important Terms

allergen	light chain
autoimmune disease	lymph
B-cells	lymph node
cell-mediated immunity	lymphatic tissue
clone	lymphatic vessel
heavy chain	plasma cells
histocompatibility antigen	red pulp
humoral immunity	spleen
immune surveillance theory	T-cells
immunity	thymus
immunoglobulin	tonsils
interferon	white pulp

Questions

1. a. What are the components of the lymphatic system?
   b. What are the functions of the lymphatic system?

2. How does lymph resemble blood plasma, and how is it different from blood plasma?

3. a. Compare lymphatic vessels to blood vessels.
   b. List the main characteristics of each kind of lymphatic tissue.

4. a. Trace the flow of lymph from each of the following locations back to the circulatory system: (1) legs, (2) intestine, (3) right arm, (4) left side of head.
   b. Where are concentrations of lymph nodes found?

5. a. How does lymph move through the vessels?
   b. What is the function of the lymph nodes?
   c. What is edema, and how might it be caused?

6. What is the difference between specific and nonspecific immunity?

7. Describe the steps in the inflammatory response.

8. a. Describe how humoral antibodies are formed.
   b. How are new antibodies formed when the same antigen appears again?

9. a. Describe how T-cells are formed and how they function.
   b. How are new T-cells formed when the same antigen appears again?
   c. Why is T-cell immunity called cell-mediated immunity?

10. a. What is the difference between active and passive immunity?
    b. How is active immunity acquired?
    c. How is passive immunity acquired?

11. a. Explain how transplanted organs can be rejected and describe some ways to minimize the chance of rejection.
    b. What are histocompatibility antigens?
    c. How does the body defend itself against cancer?
    d. What is an allergy, and how are its symptoms related to immunology?
    e. What is an autoimmune disease?
    f. What is one theory of how the immune system is prevented from destroying cells that are normally present in the body?

Problems

1. Use what you know about the lymphatic system to explain why tonsils often become inflamed when a person's body is fighting an infection.

2. Suppose that you are working in a family health clinic. Devise a method to assure that all infants and young children in the neighborhood receive the appropriate immunizations.

REFERENCES AND READINGS

Anonymous. 1980. Interferon: Gene-splicing triumph. *Science News* 117:52 (January 26).

Arehart-Treichel, J. 1980. The human sweetbread. *Science News* 117:52 (January 26).

Bellanti, J. A. 1979. *Immunology: Basic processes.* Philadelphia: W.B. Saunders.

Burke, D. C. 1977. The status of interferon. *Scientific American* 236(4):42 (April).

Capra, J. D., and Edmunson, A. B. 1977. The antibody combining site. *Scientific American* 236(1):50 (January).

Carter, S. K. 1976. Immunotherapy of cancer in man. *American Scientist* 64:418 (July–August).

Cunningham, B. A. 1977. The structure and function of histocompatibility antigens. *Scientific American* 237(4):96 (October).

Eisen, H. N. 1980. *Immunology.* New York: Harper & Row.

Henderson, D. A. 1976. The eradication of smallpox. *Scientific American* 235(4):25 (October).

Hood, L. E., Weissman, I. L., and Wood, W. B. 1978. *Immunology.* Menlo Park, Calif.: Benjamin/Cummings.

Hopson, J. L. 1980. Battle at the isle of self. *Science 80* 1(3):77 (March–April).

Marx, J. L. 1978. Antibodies (I): New information about gene structure. *Science* 202:298 (October 20).

Milstein, C. 1980. Monoclonal antibodies. *Scientific American* 243:66 (October).

Pittard, W. B., III. 1979. Breast milk immunology. *American Journal of Diseases in Children* 133:83 (January).

Raff, M. C. 1976. Cell-surface immunology. *Scientific American* 234(5):30 (May).

Rose, N. R. 1981. Autoimmune diseases. *Scientific American* 244(2):80 (February).

Talmage, D. W. 1979. Recognition and memory in the cells of the immune system. *American Scientist* 67:173 (March–April).

U.S. Department of Health, Education and Welfare. 1977. *Parents' Guide to Childhood Immunization.* Washington: DHEW Publication No. (OS) 77–50058.

Yelton, D. E., and Scharff, M. D. 1980. Monoclonal antibodies. *American Scientist* 68:510 (September–October).

21

RESPIRATORY SYSTEM

ORGANIZATION AND GENERAL FUNCTIONS

Objective 1. Describe the overall plan of the respiratory system and explain its general functions.

You would live no more than a few minutes without oxygen and only a little longer if your cells had no way to rid themselves of toxic carbon dioxide. All the cells of the body require a continuous supply of oxygen to metabolize food and obtain energy; during metabolism carbon dioxide is produced and must be efficiently removed from the cells.

The main function of the respiratory system is to move oxygen from the atmosphere to the blood and to remove carbon dioxide from the blood to the atmosphere. This involves two processes—breathing and external respiration. **Breathing**, or **ventilation**, is the mechanical process by which air is moved into and out of the lungs. **External respiration** is the process by which gases are exchanged between the blood and the air.

Though the respiratory system is involved only in breathing and external respiration, the total process of **respiration** includes two other processes—internal respiration and cellular respiration. **Internal respiration** is the process by which gases are exchanged between the blood and the cells. Because internal respiration involves the same principles of **gas exchange** as external respiration, it will be considered in this chapter. **Cellular respiration**, the process by which cells use oxygen for metabolism and produce carbon dioxide as a waste product, will be discussed in Chapter 23.

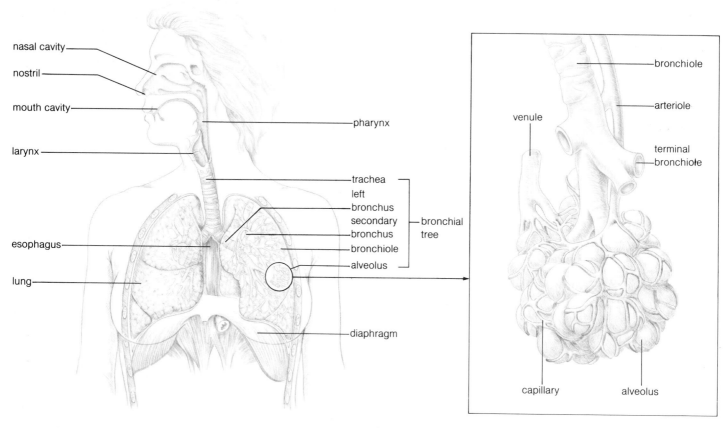

Figure 21.1 The structure of the respiratory system, with an enlarged drawing of alveoli.

The respiratory system consists of a set of passageways through which air enters and leaves the system. From the surface of the body inward, they include the nasal cavity, pharynx, larynx, trachea, bronchi, bronchioles, and alveoli (Figure 21.1). At the lower end of the trachea the passageway branches to form two primary bronchi; each primary bronchus branches to form secondary bronchi, which in turn branch many times, forming bronchioles and alveoli. Thus, the many branches of each primary bronchus resemble an inverted tree. Some of the bronchioles merely conduct air, but others, the respiratory bronchioles, have very thin walls surrounded by capillaries and are able to carry on gas exchange. The thin-walled, saclike alveoli also are surrounded by capillaries and carry on gas exchange. Thus, the respiratory bronchioles and the alveoli comprise the **respiratory portion** of the respiratory system. The remainder of the structures in the respiratory system comprise the **conducting portion** because they carry air to and from the respiratory portion but do not engage in gas exchange.

One primary bronchus enters each of the two lungs, and all subsequent branches form the tissues of the lungs. The lung as an organ is thus a mass of tubes and thin-walled sacs, along with some connective tissues that support the other tissues.

To properly understand the respiratory system and respiration, we must keep in mind the relationship between the respiratory and circulatory systems. Gases are exchanged between the air and the blood in the lungs. The blood vessels then transport the blood to all other tissues, where gases are exchanged between the blood and the cells. Therefore, the role of the circulation of blood in internal respiration is similar to the role of breathing in external respiration.

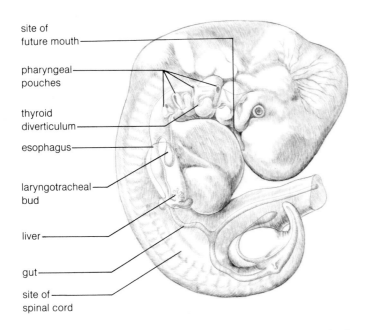

site of
future mouth

pharyngeal
pouches

thyroid
diverticulum

esophagus

laryngotracheal
bud

liver

gut

site of
spinal cord

Figure 21.2 A side view of an embryo early in the second month of development, showing the pharynx and laryngotracheal buds that contribute to the development of the respiratory system.

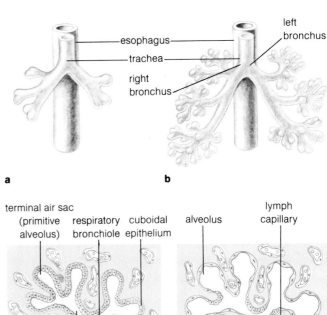

esophagus

left bronchus

trachea

right bronchus

a

b

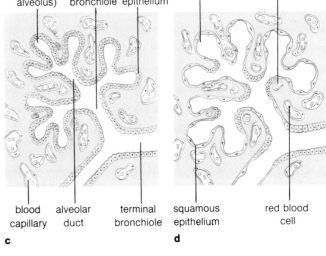

terminal air sac (primitive alveolus) respiratory bronchiole cuboidal epithelium

alveolus

lymph capillary

blood capillary alveolar duct terminal bronchiole squamous epithelium red blood cell

c

d

Figure 21.3 Development of bronchioles and alveoli: (**a**) laryngotracheal buds at five weeks, (**b**) further development of buds at eight weeks, (**c**) cuboidal epithelium in cross-section of alveoli at twenty-four weeks, (**d**) squamous epithelium in cross section of alveoli at full term development.

DEVELOPMENT

Objective 2. Describe the general embryological development of the respiratory system.

The primitive gut of the embryo consists of a tube of endodermal cells that grows both anteriorly and posteriorly. In the anterior portion of the embryo several pouches form that extend outward from the walls of the tube. These **pharyngeal pouches** form in the embryos of all vertebrates. In fish they contribute to the gills. In humans the pharyngeal pouches form such structures as the auditory tube, the fossae in which the tonsils lie, the parathyroid glands, and the thymus gland. A diverticulum (pocket) near one of these pouches gives rise to the thyroid gland (see Figure 21.2).

A **laryngotracheal bud** projects from the pharynx and grows posteriorly. As it grows, it forms the larynx and trachea and then branches to form the left and right bronchi and all of their branches (Figure 21.3).

The entire respiratory system is lined with epithelium of endodermal origin. Up to about twenty-four weeks of development, the lining of the alveoli consists of cuboidal epithelium; gradually in the later weeks of development, the epithelial cells flatten and become squamous in shape. At the time of birth the epithelium of the alveoli has become thin enough to allow gas exchange to occur. Premature infants often experience respiratory difficulties partly because the cells of the alveolar epithelium are still cuboidal in shape.

In the head area of the embryo during the second month of development, several lateral processes grow toward the midline to form the face, including the nose, lips, and palate (Figure 21.4). These lateral processes normally meet and fuse with the nasomedial process; should this fusion fail to occur properly, cleft lip and/or cleft palate result.

TISSUES

Objective 3. Name the tissues of the respiratory system and explain how the epithelial tissues are specialized to perform their particular functions.

The nasal cavity and pharynx are lined with **pseudostratified, ciliated columnar epithelium** (Figure 21.5). The cilia in this part of the respiratory tract beat downward toward the pharynx so that mucus, along with the debris trapped in it, is moved into the pharynx, from which it is ejected or swallowed to enter the digestive tract. The effectiveness of the mucus is in part dependent on its viscosity. Slightly viscous mucus is more effective than very viscous mucus in moving debris. Ultimately, the mucus leaves the body through the digestive tract. A similar epithelium lines the bronchial tubes; here the cilia beat upward toward the pharynx so that mucus and debris are moved away from the lungs. These cilia and the mucus they move are referred to as the **mucociliary escalator**.

The respiratory portion of the tract (the alveoli and smallest bronchioles) is lined with a thin sheet of nonciliated, squamous epithelium. This epithelium is always moist and constitutes the surface membrane across which gas exchange takes place.

Other tissues of the respiratory system include the cartilage that supports all but the smaller respiratory passages, the smooth muscle of the bronchioles, and the connective tissues that support and protect the tract. The characteristics of these tissues were discussed in Chapter 4.

NASAL CAVITIES, PHARYNX, AND LARYNX

Objective 4. Locate and identify the structures of the nasal cavities and explain their respiratory functions.

Objective 5. Locate and identify the anatomical structures of the pharynx and the larynx and explain their respiratory functions.

Nasal Cavities

The structure of the nasal cavity is shown in Figure 21.6. The external openings to the nasal cavity, the **external nares**, or nostrils, are surrounded by the **nose**. The nose consists of bone and cartilage covered with skin. The nasal cavity extends from the nose deep into the facial bones of the skull to the **internal nares**. Between the external and internal nares the **nasal cavity** is bounded by the bones of the cranium superiorly and by the **hard** and **soft palates** inferiorly. The entire nasal cavity is lined with mucous membrane.

The nasal cavity is separated into left and right sides by the **nasal septum**, which is composed of two bones, the vomer and the perpendicular plate of the ethmoid, and some cartilage. Extending from the superior roof of the nasal cavity are three pairs of membrane-covered bones, the **nasal conchae**. The portion of the nasal cavity in front of the conchae is called the **vestibule**.

The upper part of the membrane that covers the nasal conchae contains the olfactory receptor cells. Airborne particles or molecules or odorous substances are swept into contact with the moist membrane as the air swirls through the passageways between the conchae. These substances dissolve in the fluid and then stimulate the olfactory receptor cells.

As air passes through the nasal cavity, it is warmed, moistened, and filtered. Mucus traps large debris and prevents it from passing beyond the pharynx, but it fails to trap fine particles. The fine particles are inhaled deep into the lungs, where they may become lodged in the smaller passageways. If the particles remain suspended, they may be exhaled.

Pharynx

The **pharynx** is a passageway that extends from the internal nares to the larynx and esophagus (Figure 21.6). It consists of a tube of skeletal muscle lined with mucous membrane. This lining is continuous with the lining of the mouth, nasal cavity, larynx, and esophagus. The pharynx is divided into three areas, the nasopharynx, oropharynx, and laryngopharynx. The most superior portion, the **nasopharynx**, lies next to the internal nares. It is connected to each middle ear by the **auditory tube**. Superior and posterior to the auditory tubes are the **pharyngeal tonsils**. When these tonsils become enlarged, usually because of chronic infection, they are called **adenoids**. The nasopharynx, a passageway for the respiratory tract only, joins the **oropharynx** (throat), which is a common passageway for both the respiratory and di-

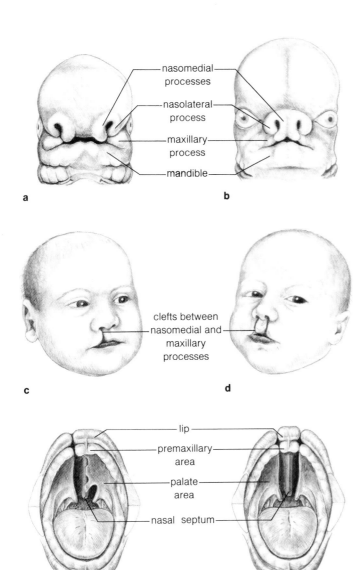

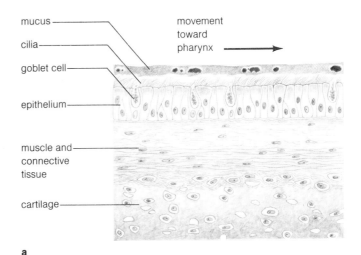

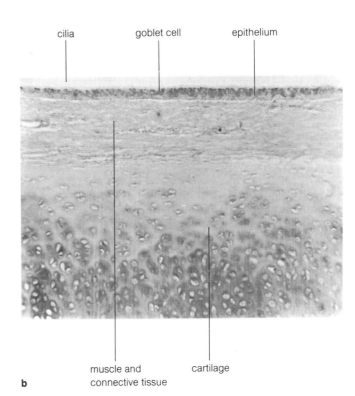

Figure 21.4 Development of face, including nose, lip, and palate: (**a**) location of medial and lateral processes at 5½ weeks, (**b**) normal fusion of processes at 7 weeks, (**c**) unilateral cleft lip, (**d**) bilateral cleft lip, (**e**) unilateral cleft lip and palate, (**f**) bilateral cleft lip and palate.

Figure 21.5 The structure of the pharynx: (**a**) diagram, (**b**) photomicrograph, × 73. (Photograph by author.)

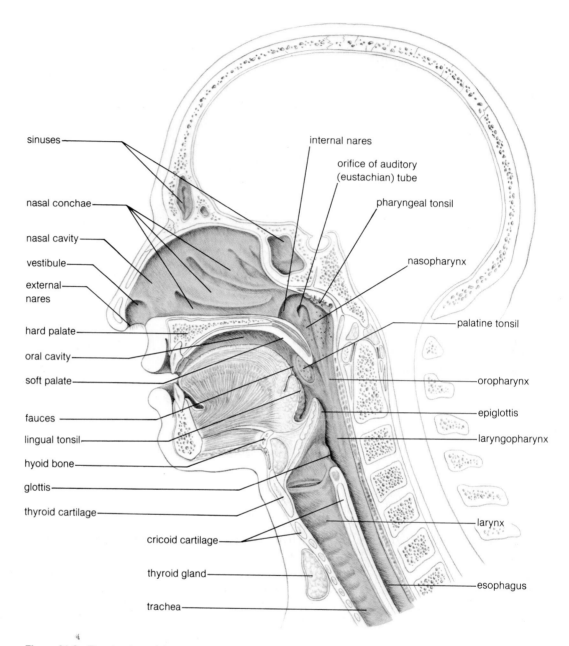

Figure 21.6 The structure of the nasal cavity, pharynx, and larynx in sagittal section.

gestive tracts. Near the **fauces**, the boundary between the mouth and the oropharynx, are the **palatine tonsils**, and beneath the tongue are the **lingual tonsils**. All tonsils are masses of lymphatic tissue, as noted in Chapter 20. The **laryngopharynx**, the most inferior portion of the pharynx, serves as a passageway for both the respiratory and digestive systems.

Larynx

The **larynx**, or voice box, lies between the laryngopharynx and the trachea (Figure 21.6) and connects these two passageways. Like most other respiratory passageways, it is lined with mucous membrane. The larynx has a rigid structure provided by muscles, ligaments, and nine cartilages (Figure 21.7). The largest of these cartilages, the **thy-**

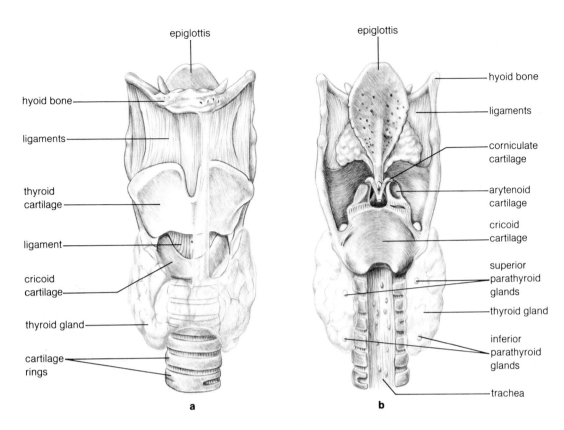

epiglottis

hyoid bone

ligaments

thyroid
cartilage

ligament

cricoid
cartilage

thyroid gland

cartilage
rings

hyoid bone

ligaments

corniculate
cartilage

arytenoid
cartilage

cricoid
cartilage

superior
parathyroid
glands

thyroid gland

inferior
parathyroid
glands

trachea

a   **b**

Figure 21.7   The larynx: (**a**) from the anterior surface, (**b**) from the posterior surface.

roid cartilage, or Adam's apple, forms the anterior surface of the larynx. Below the thyroid cartilage is a complete ring of cartilage, the **cricoid cartilage**. The **epiglottis** is the third unpaired cartilage of the larynx. The paired **arytenoid, corniculate**, and **cuneiform** cartilages complete the structure of the larynx. The cuneiform cartilages lie anterior to the arytenoids and are not seen in the figure.

During swallowing the rest of the larynx is pulled toward the epiglottis, and the **glottis**, the opening from the laryngopharynx to the larynx, is shielded from the esophagus. Normally, food passes from the pharynx to the esophagus without entering the larynx; choking occurs when the epiglottis fails to shield the glottis.

Inside the larynx, supported by the cartilages and stretched across the glottis, are the **vocal cords** (Figure 21.8). The outer pair, the **false vocal cords**, have little to do with sound production. When air passes through the glottis, the inner **true vocal cords** are set into vibration, thereby producing sound. The pitch of a sound is determined by the

tension on the vocal cords—the greater the tension, the higher the pitch. The tension is regulated by intrinsic (within an organ) muscles of the larynx moving the arytenoid cartilage. Voluntary contractions of these muscles allow us to change the pitch of our voice when we speak or sing.

During puberty testosterone causes the male larynx to enlarge and the vocal cords to lengthen. These changes produce the male Adam's apple (the enlarged thyroid cartilage) and the lowered pitch of the male voice.

THE BRONCHIAL TREE, RESPIRATORY BRONCHIOLES, AND ALVEOLI

Objective 6. Locate and identify the anatomical structures of the trachea, bronchi, bronchioles, and alveoli and explain their respiratory functions.

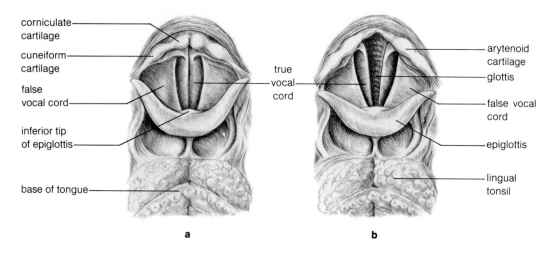

Figure 21.8 A superior view of the larynx, showing the vocal cords. The glottis is closed in (**a**) and open in (**b**).

Labels (left diagram, a):
- corniculate cartilage
- cuneiform cartilage
- false vocal cord
- inferior tip of epiglottis
- base of tongue
- true vocal cord

Labels (right diagram, b):
- arytenoid cartilage
- glottis
- false vocal cord
- epiglottis
- lingual tonsil

Trachea

The **trachea** (Figure 21.9) is an unpaired tube that connects the larynx to the bronchi. Sometimes called the windpipe, it is 2 to 3 centimeters in diameter and 12 to 13 centimeters long. Its walls are composed of an inner ciliated mucous membrane, a middle intermittent layer of hyaline cartilage, and an outer layer of connective tissue. The cartilage is arranged in C-shaped rings extending around the trachea except for a short distance on the posterior side, where there is smooth muscle (Figure 21.10). The cartilage rings keep an airway open in the trachea, and the smooth muscle allows the trachea to be pushed forward and slightly collapsed as food passes through the esophagus.

Bronchi and Bronchioles

The **bronchi** branch from the trachea as the limbs of a tree branch from the trunk, forming what is called the **bronchial tree** (Figure 21.9). One **primary bronchus** goes to each lung: the right bronchus is wider in diameter and lies in a more vertical position than the left bronchus. Each bronchus makes twenty-three subsequent branchings. The first sixteen sets of branches form the bronchi, the bronchioles, and the terminal bronchioles. The last seven sets of branches form the respiratory bronchioles, alveolar ducts, and alveolar sacs—the portion of the respiratory system associated with gas exchange. This complex branching arrangement greatly increases the surface area exposed to air flowing into and out of the lungs. In the primary bronchi air flow is fairly rapid, but due to the great increase in total cross-sectional area, flow is much slower in the smallest branches.

The larger bronchi have rings of cartilage similar to those in the trachea, but the smaller bronchioles have only small plates of cartilage or none at all. Smooth muscle innervated by the autonomic nervous system surrounds the tubes that lack cartilage. The epithelial lining of these tubes also differs from the larger to the smaller tubes. In the large bronchi the epithelium is pseudostratified, ciliated columnar, but in the smaller ones it is cuboidal and lacks cilia.

The bronchioles end in sacs that look a little like a cluster of grapes. Such sacs are called **alveoli**. The walls of the alveoli and the walls of the smallest bronchioles consist primarily of simple squamous epithelium. These smallest branches of the bronchial tree will be discussed in the next section.

The function of the bronchial tree is to conduct fresh air to the thin membranes of the alveoli and to return used air outside the body.

Respiratory Bronchioles, Alveolar Ducts, and Alveoli

The terminal bronchioles branch into **respiratory bronchioles**, which in turn branch into **alveolar ducts** surrounded by alveoli (Figure 21.11). Some alveoli are found on the respiratory bronchioles. Sometimes an alveolar duct

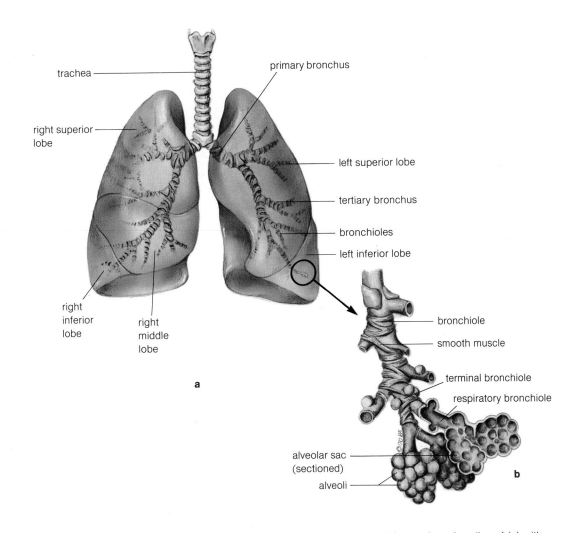

Figure 21.9 The bronchial tree: (**a**) the major branches of the bronchial tree, (**b**) an enlarged portion of (**a**) with smaller branches of the tree.

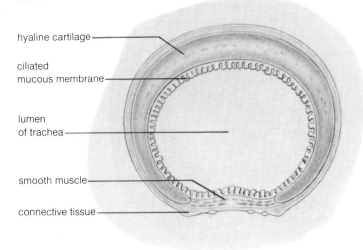

Figure 21.10 A cross section through the trachea, showing the location of cartilage and other tissues.

leads to an **alveolar sac**, which in turn leads to several alveoli. Together, the human lungs contain about 300 million alveoli.

Each cluster of alveoli is surrounded by elastic connective tissue and is supplied with blood and lymphatic vessels. Branches of the pulmonary artery carry blood to the capillaries of the alveoli, and branches of the pulmonary vein carry blood from these capillaries back to the heart. Lymphatic vessels drain interstitial fluid from around the alveoli.

The total surface area of the alveoli amounts to about one square meter per kilogram of body weight. Thus, someone weighing 68 kg (150 lbs) would have 68 square meters of alveolar surface area—about half the surface area of a tennis court. This extensive surface area is well supplied

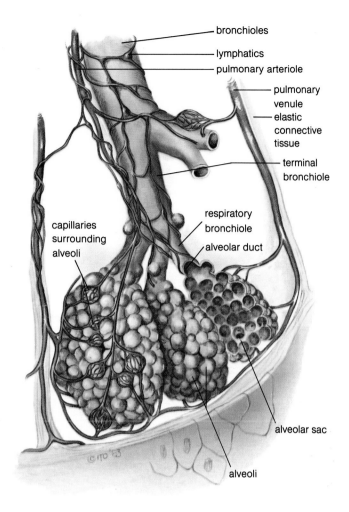

a

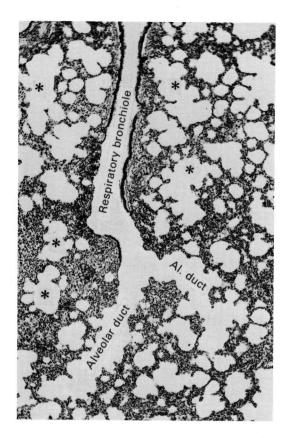

b

Figure 21.11 (a) The branching of terminal bronchioles to form the respiratory membranes and the arrangement of blood and lymph vessels supplying these tissues. (b) A very low-power photomicrograph of the lung of a young child. The respiratory bronchiole is cut longitudinally and may be seen opening into two alveolar ducts. The asterisks indicate alveolar sacs, which open into round sacs called alveoli, (Photomicrograph reproduced with permission from A. W. Ham, *Histology*, J. P. Lippincott, 1979.)

with capillaries, and the walls of both the alveoli and the capillaries are extremely thin. Gas exchange, the diffusion of gases across thin membranes, takes place between the air in the lungs and the blood in the lung capillaries. The oxygen concentration is higher inside the alveoli than in the blood, so oxygen diffuses into the blood. The carbon dioxide concentration is higher in the blood than inside the alveoli, so carbon dioxide diffuses into the alveoli.

LUNGS AND BREATHING

Objective 7. Describe the overall structure and location of the lungs and their surrounding membranes, including their blood supply and innervation.

Objective 8. Explain the process of breathing, including inhalation, exhalation, and volumes of air moving.

Having considered the branching structure of tubules

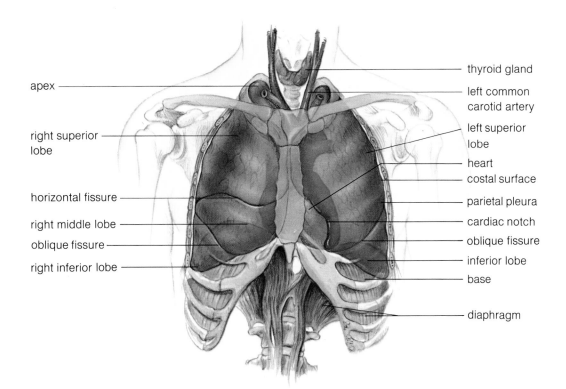

apex

right superior
lobe

horizontal fissure

right middle lobe

oblique fissure

right inferior lobe

thyroid gland

left common
carotid artery

left superior
lobe

heart

costal surface

parietal pleura

cardiac notch

oblique fissure

inferior lobe

base

diaphragm

Figure 21.12 (**a**) The structure
and location of the lungs,
(**b**) a chest X ray. (X ray courtesy
of Alexandria Hospital, Alexandria,
Virginia, Joyce R. Isbel, R.T.)

a

b

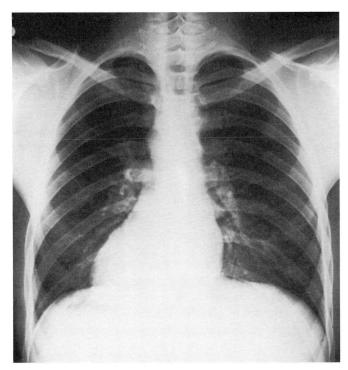

within the lungs, we will now consider the whole lung as an
organ. Though gas exchange occurs in the alveoli, it is ex-
pansions and contractions of the surrounding cavity that
causes air to move into and out of the lungs, constantly
renewing the supply of air within the alveoli. Such ex-
pansions and contractions constitute the movements of
breathing, which will be discussed here. The regulation of
these movements will be considered later with the discussion of the regulation of respiration.

Structure of the Lungs

The **lungs** (Figure 21.12) lie in the **thoracic cavity**, where
they are separated by the heart in the mediastinum. Each
lung is covered by a serous membrane, the **visceral pleura**.
The thoracic cavity surrounding the lungs is lined by another serous membrane, the **parietal pleura**. Between these
two membranes is the **pleural cavity**, only a potential space
because normally the pleura touch one another. Watery
secretions from the serous membranes reduce friction as the
lungs move during respiration.

The thoracic cavity is bounded by the rib cage superiorly and on all sides and by the **diaphragm** inferiorly. The most superior portion of each lung is called the **apex**, and the most inferior portion is called the **base**. The **costal surfaces** of the lungs are so named because they lie next to the ribs. The **medial surfaces** of the lungs lie next to the mediastinum, and it is through a depression in the medial surface of each lung, the **hilum**, that the bronchi, blood vessels, and nerves enter each lung.

The left lung is smaller than the right and has a concavity, the **cardiac notch**, where the heart lies. The **lobes** of the lungs and the fissures that separate them are named in Figure 21.12; the right lung has three lobes, while the left has only two. Each lobe is covered by an elastic connective tissue membrane. Each lung receives a primary bronchus, and each lobe receives a secondary bronchus. The lobes are further subdivided into many **lobules**, each of which receives a tertiary bronchus. Within the lobules tertiary bronchi branch extensively to form the bronchioles and alveoli. Every lobule is supplied with an arteriole, venule, and lymphatic vessel.

The lungs receive blood from two sources. The bronchial arteries nourish the conducting, nonrespiratory portions of the lungs, and the bronchial veins drain them. The pulmonary arteries and veins serve the respiratory portions of the lungs, where gas exchange is carried out.

Nerves important in producing breathing movements are the phrenic nerve and the thoracic spinal nerves. The phrenic nerve supplies the diaphragm, and the thoracic spinal nerves supply the intercostal muscles. The lungs are also supplied with sympathetic and parasympathetic nerve fibers, but their effect on breathing is minimal.

Mechanics of Breathing

Breathing serves to provide a continuous supply of fresh air to the respiratory membranes of the alveoli. It occurs in two phases: **inspiration**, the breathing in of air, and **expiration**, the breathing out of a mixture of gases that result from gas exchange. Both of these phases are dependent on certain characteristics of the lungs and the thoracic cavity. The mechanism of breathing is illustrated in Figure 21.13.

The lungs are suspended within the airtight thoracic cavity, with the moist visceral and parietal pleura adhering to each other. The pleura slide over each other easily but resist separation as two moist sheets of glass slide on each other but resist separation. In addition, an **intrapleural pressure** (the pressure between the lungs and the chest wall) of about –2.5 mm Hg (less than atmospheric pressure) helps the pleura to adhere. The membranes lining the intrapleural cavity constantly absorb fluids as they enter the cavity, thereby maintaining the negative pressure.

The alveoli are in direct communication with the outside air by way of the respiratory passages. Just before inhalation the air pressure inside the alveoli is equal to the atmospheric pressure (760 mm Hg at sea level).

The respiratory muscles are the diaphragm and the intercostals. The diaphragm is a dome-shaped muscle that forms the inferior boundary of the thoracic cavity. When it contracts, it is drawn downward—about 1.5 centimeters during quiet inspiration and up to 7 centimeters during deep inspiration. Contraction of the diaphragm accounts for about three-fourths of the increase in **intrathoracic volume** (the volume of the thoracic cavity) during inspiration. The external and internal intercostal muscles are attached to the ribs—the externals slanting anteriorly and inferiorly, the internals slanting posteriorly and inferiorly. The ribs, which are attached to the vertebrae at joints somewhat like hinges, pivot when these muscles contract. During inspiration the external intercostals contract, pulling the ribs upward and outward and increasing the anterior–posterior dimension of the thoracic cavity. These muscles account for about one-fourth of increase in intrathoracic volume during inspiration. Relaxation of the diaphragm and external intercostals decreases the volume of the thoracic cavity during expiration. During forceful expiration the internal intercostals contract, pulling the ribs inward and downward and decreasing the anterior–posterior dimension of the thoracic cavity.

Inspiration

Because inspiration involves the contraction of muscles and therefore the expenditure of energy, it is an active process. For air to be drawn into the lungs, the pressure inside the lungs must be lower than the atmospheric pressure. This low pressure is created when the diaphragm and the external intercostal muscles contract. The lungs expand, increasing the intrapulmonary volume—the volume of the alveoli and passageways. Thus, the intrapulmonary pres-

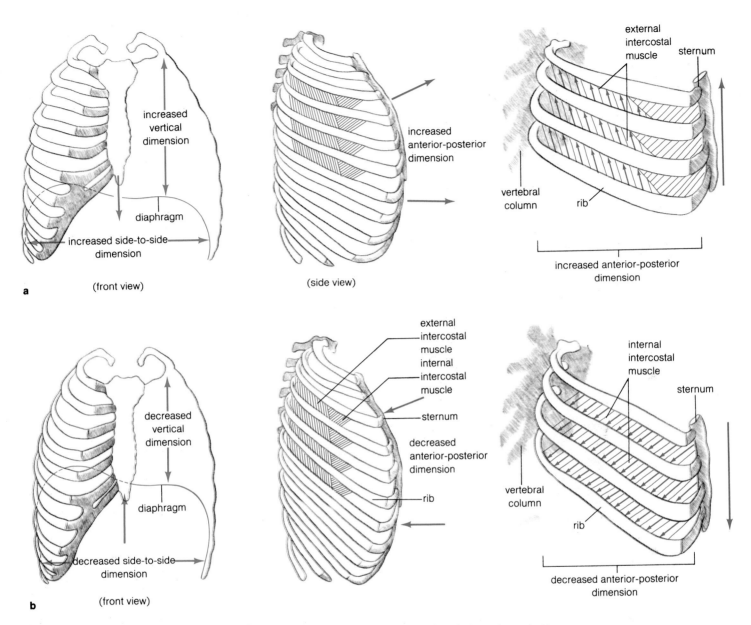

Figure 21.13 The mechanism of breathing: (**a**) In inspiration the diaphragm and external intercostal muscles contract.
(**b**) In expiration those muscles relax, and in forceful expiration the internal intercostal muscles contract.

sure—the pressure inside the alveoli and passageways of the lungs—becomes less than the atmospheric pressure by about 2 mm Hg, or about ¼ of 1% of atmospheric pressure. Because of this negative pressure (relative to atmospheric pressure), air from outside the body moves into the lungs until the intrapulmonary pressure is again equal to the atmospheric pressure.

The lungs and the chest wall each display **compliance**, or stretchability. Compliance of lung tissue is due to the presence of elastic tissue. Chest wall compliance is due to elasticity of the muscles of the chest wall. The degree of compliance is measured by determining the increase in intraalveolar volume per unit increase in intraalveolar pressure.

Expiration

Like inspiration, expiration is caused by a change in the pressure inside the lungs. As the diaphragm and the external intercostal muscles relax, the volume of the thoracic cavity decreases. This decreases the intrapulmonary volume and causes the intrapulmonary pressure to increase to about 2 mm Hg above atmospheric pressure. Air leaves the lungs until the pressure in the lungs again equals atmospheric pressure.

During expiration the lungs and chest wall display **elastic recoil**, in which the volume of both the lungs and the thoracic cavity decreases. The decrease in volume of the lungs is due to surface tension of the moist membranes of the alveoli and to the elastic fibers in the lung tissue. The inner surfaces of the alveoli are coated by a mixture of phospholipids called **surfactant** secreted by certain cells of the alveolar epithelium. Surfactant lowers the surface tension, allowing some elastic recoil but preventing complete collapse of the alveoli. Elasticity of the muscles of the chest wall allows them to recoil during exhalation.

Expiration is essentially a passive process; it results from the relaxation of the muscles that contracted during inspiration. This is a little like what happens when you relax the tension on a stretched rubber band. Forceful expiration can be accomplished by actively contracting the internal intercostals and the abdominal muscles. Like the external intercostals, the internal intercostals lie between the ribs; their fibers are arranged so that they pull the upper ribs down toward the lower ribs and decrease the size of the thoracic cavity. Contraction of the abdominal muscles compresses the abdomen and pushes its contents toward the diaphragm.

The processes of inspiration and expiration are summarized in Figure 21.14.

Volumes of Air Exchanged

During normal breathing at rest the volume of air moved into and out of the lungs in one cycle of inspiration and expiration is about 500 milliliters. This volume, called the **tidal volume**, is composed of alveolar volume and dead space volume. **Alveolar volume**, which amounts to about 350 milliliters, consists of air that reaches the respiratory surfaces of the alveoli and engages in gas exchange. The **dead space volume**, which amounts to about 150 milliliters, consists of air that does not reach the respiratory surfaces. Some of the air in the dead space volume occupies the conductive tubes that do not exchange gases—the **anatomical dead space volume**. The total, or **physiological dead space volume**, includes the anatomical dead space volume and the volume of any alveoli that cannot exchange gases. The physiological dead space volume is increased in diseases that involve damage to the alveoli.

In addition to tidal volume the lungs are able to inhale and exhale larger volumes. If a person inhales the maximum possible amount of air in one very deep breath, about 2000 to 3000 milliliters of air beyond the tidal volume can be inhaled. This additional volume is the **inspiratory reserve volume**. Conversely, if, after a normal exhalation, a person forcefully exhales the maximum amount of air, 800 to 1200 milliliters of air can be exhaled. This volume is the **expiratory reserve volume**. After the expiratory reserve volume is exhaled, 1000 to 1300 milliliters of air remain in the lungs. This is the **residual volume**. The sum of all of the volumes mentioned above is the total lung capacity—a volume of 4300 to 6000 milliliters, depending on the size of the individual.

Several other volumes are defined as combinations of some of the above categories. **Vital capacity** is the total amount of air that can be moved into and out of the lungs with maximum effort in one breath. It equals the total lung capacity minus the residual volume. **Inspiratory capacity**, the total volume of air that can be inhaled after a normal exhalation, includes tidal volume plus the inspiratory reserve volume. **Functional residual capacity** is the sum of expiratory reserve volume and residual volume. These volumes are shown in Figure 21.15.

Another important volume is the **minute respiratory volume**, the product of the tidal volume and the respiratory rate. For example, if an individual has a tidal volume of 500 milliliters and a respiratory rate of 12 breaths per minute, that person's minute respiratory volume would be 6 liters per minute—a typical resting minute volume. However, a large young male forcing himself to breathe as deeply and rapidly as possible (voluntary hyperventilation) might sustain a minute respiratory volume of 150 liters per minute for

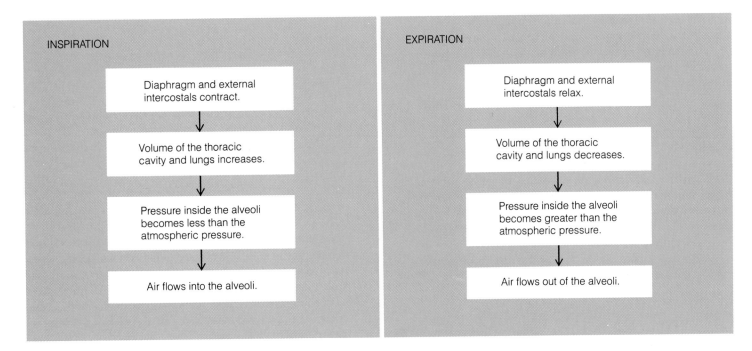

Figure 21.14 Summary of the events in inspiration and expiration.

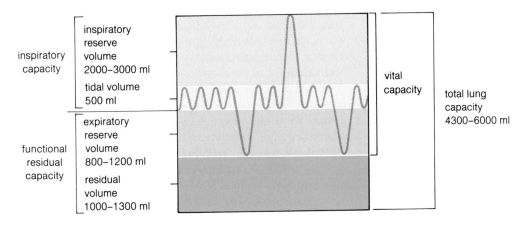

Figure 21.15 Volumes of air in the lungs.

about 15 seconds; such an individual could probably maintain a minute respiratory volume of 100 liters per minute for a few minutes of strenuous exercise. The effect of hyperventilation on blood gases is important and will be discussed later in this chapter.

TRANSPORT AND EXCHANGE OF GASES

Objective 9. Describe the exchange of gases between the respiratory membranes and the blood, and between the blood and the cells.

Objective 10. Describe the transport of gases between the lungs and the cells.

Objective 11. Explain the role of the respiratory system in the regulation of acid–base balance in the body.

Gas Exchange

As we saw earlier, external respiration is the exchange of gases between the lungs and the blood in the capillaries of the pulmonary circulation, whereas internal respiration is the exchange of gases between the blood of the systemic circulation and the cells of the body. Before we can understand how gas exchange takes place, we need to know more about the properties of gases.

Earth's atmosphere is a mixture of gases—primarily nitrogen, oxygen, and carbon dioxide. The total pressure of a gas is equal to the sum of the pressures of the individual component gases. The pressure exerted by a single gas in a mixture is called the **partial pressure** of that gas (P_g). For example, in atmospheric air the concentration of oxygen is about 20.9% and that of carbon dioxide about 0.04%. In dry air at sea level conditions the total atmospheric pressure is 760 mm Hg. Thus, the partial pressure of oxygen is 158 mm Hg (20.9% of 760), and the partial pressure of carbon dioxide is 0.3 mm Hg (0.04% of 760). The partial pressure unaccounted for is due mainly to nitrogen, an inert gas.

Changes occur in the concentrations, and thus in the partial pressures, of oxygen and carbon dioxide during breathing. The partial pressures given above are those found in freshly inhaled air. As this fresh air enters the alveoli, it is mixed with some of the gas that remained in the alveoli after the last expiration. If you review the respiratory volumes described earlier, you will find that only a small portion of the total amount of gas in your lungs is replaced with each respiration. Thus, the **alveolar gas** is a mixture of inhaled (atmospheric) air and the residual gas that was not expelled.

Table 21.1	Composition of Inhaled, Alveolar, and Exhaled Air	
Type of Air	Oxygen Partial Pressure (mm Hg)	Carbon Dioxide Partial Pressure (mm Hg)
Inhaled (atmospheric)	158	0.3
Alveolar	100	40.0
Exhaled	124	26.8

Gas exchange occurs continuously in the alveoli, and alveolar gas is always losing oxygen to the blood and gaining carbon dioxide from the blood. Expired air is a mixture of alveolar gas and the atmospheric air that fills the trachea and bronchioles. Because the air in the trachea and bronchioles at the end of inspiration never reaches the respiratory membranes, it is unchanged. Mixing this gas with alveolar gas during expiration produces a mixed expired gas that is lower in carbon dioxide and higher in oxygen than alveolar air. Nevertheless, this mixed expired gas is higher in carbon dioxide and lower in oxygen than atmospheric air. The differences in the composition of inhaled, alveolar, and exhaled air are summarized in Table 21.1.

Gas exchange takes place across the membranes of the alveoli and the capillary walls that lie adjacent to them. This exchange depends on the difference in the partial pressures of each of the gases—oxygen and carbon dioxide—in the alveoli when compared to the partial pressures in the blood (Figure 21.16). Though gases passing through the respiratory membranes are dissolved in fluid, they continue to exert their partial pressures. In blood entering the capillaries of the lungs, the partial pressure of oxygen, P_{O_2}, is approximately 40 mm Hg, and that of carbon dioxide, P_{CO_2}, is approximately 45 mm Hg. In the alveoli the partial pressure approximately 45 mm Hg. In the alveoli the partial pressure of oxygen is about 100 mm Hg, and that of carbon dioxide is about 40 mm Hg.

Gases diffuse from the region of their higher partial pressure to the region of their lower partial pressure. Thus, in external respiration oxygen diffuses from the alveoli into the blood, and carbon dioxide diffuses from the blood into the alveoli. However, diffusion must take place through the barriers shown in Figure 21.17. As blood passes through the capillaries of the alveoli and diffusion continues to occur, the amount of oxygen in the blood increases, and the amount of carbon dioxide decreases. Thus, blood in the pulmonary veins and in the systemic arteries contains more

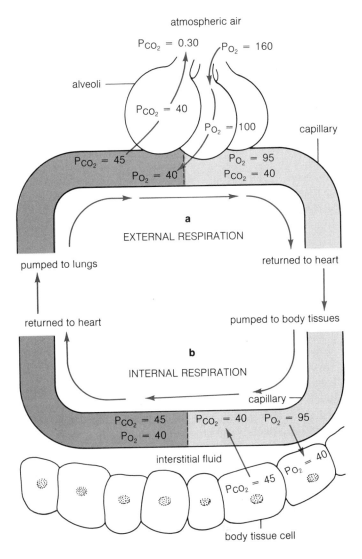

Figure 21.16 The diffusion of gases in external and internal respiration, as determined by the partial pressures of each gas (in mm Hg).

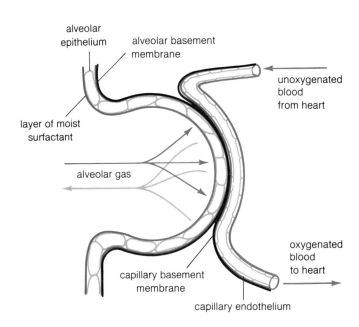

Figure 21.17 Barriers through which gases diffuse in the lungs.

Table 21.2	Partial Pressures of Oxygen and Carbon Dioxide				
Gas	Atmosphere	Alveoli	Arterial Blood	Average Venous Blood	Average Tissue Cells*
P_{O_2}	158	100	95	40	25
P_{CO_2}	0.3	40	40	45	46

*The concentrations of gases with cells vary widely among different kinds of cells.

oxygen and less carbon dioxide than blood entering the pulmonary circulation. In systemic arterial blood prior to its circulation through the tissues, the partial pressure of oxygen is about 95 mm Hg (less than the 100 mm Hg in the alveoli because pressure is not completely equalized during diffusion), and the partial pressure of carbon dioxide is about 40 mm Hg.

When the blood reaches the capillaries of the systemic circulation, the partial pressures of oxygen and carbon dioxide in the tissues are such that oxygen diffuses from the blood into the cells, and carbon dioxide diffuses from the cells into the blood. Though the partial pressures of these gases differ greatly in blood being returned from the various tissues and in accordance with the degree of exercise, the partial pressure of oxygen in blood in the systemic veins entering the heart has decreased to about 40 mm Hg, and the partial pressure of carbon dioxide has increased to about 45 mm Hg. Therefore, during internal respiration, the cells receive oxygen and get rid of carbon dioxide. Figure 21.16 and Table 21.2 summarize the changes in partial pressures as a result of both external and internal respiration.

Transport of Gases

In the foregoing discussion it has been assumed that gases are transported in the blood to and from cells. However, the processes involved in this transport require further explanation.

Transport of oxygen Oxygen diffuses into the blood until its partial pressure in the blood is nearly as great as its partial pressure in the alveoli. However, blood actually carries far more oxygen than it would if the oxygen were only dissolved in it. As much as 99% of the oxygen carried in blood may be carried on molecules of hemoglobin in erythrocytes, though the amount of oxygen carried this way varies greatly, depending on the concentration of hemoglobin.

One hemoglobin molecule carries four molecules of oxygen, and each erythrocyte contains over 200 million molecules of hemoglobin. Consequently, in a person with a normal number of red blood cells, each liter of blood holds 200 cubic centimeters of oxygen when the hemoglobin is fully saturated. Oxygen combines with hemoglobin as shown in the following equation:

$$\text{Hb} + \text{O}_2 \underset{\text{in tissues}}{\overset{\text{in lungs}}{\rightleftharpoons}} \text{HbO}_2$$

deoxygenated hemoglobin   oxygen   oxyhemoglobin

In blood entering the capillaries of the lungs, the hemoglobin molecules of the red cells have lost much of their oxygen to the tissues. Many are carrying carbon dioxide, as we shall see later. In the presence of a high concentration of oxygen and a low concentration of carbon dioxide in the alveoli, hemoglobin easily loses carbon dioxide and combines with available oxygen.

In blood entering the capillaries of the tissues, the reaction is reversed. The oxygen dissolved in the plasma is diffusing into the cells, and as this occurs, oxygen is released from hemoglobin to the plasma. Thus, the lowered concentration of oxygen in the plasma contributes to the release of oxygen from hemoglobin.

Two other factors cause hemoglobin to release even more oxygen: lowered pH (increased H^+ concentration) and increased temperature. Both of these factors decrease the affinity of hemoglobin for oxygen, as shown in Figures 21.18 and 21.19. These properties of hemoglobin account for its ability to supply oxygen to tissues that need an increased supply of oxygen. For example, during exercise muscles contract and give off heat. This increases the temperature of the area around the contracting cells and therefore the temperature of the blood passing through the muscle tissue, causing oxygen to dissociate more readily. As

energy is released for muscle contraction, carbon dioxide and lactic acid are also released. The lactic acid produces some H^+, and in erythrocytes the carbon dioxide produces more H^+, according to the following reaction:

$$\underset{\substack{\text{carbon} \\ \text{dioxide}}}{\text{CO}_2} + \underset{\text{water}}{\text{H}_2\text{O}} \rightleftharpoons \underset{\substack{\text{carbonic} \\ \text{acid}}}{\text{H}_2\text{CO}_3} \rightleftharpoons \underset{\substack{\text{hydrogen} \\ \text{ion}}}{\text{H}^+} + \underset{\substack{\text{bicarbonate} \\ \text{ion}}}{\text{HCO}_3^-}$$

This release of hydrogen ions lowers the blood pH, also causing oxygen to dissociate from hemoglobin more readily. These reactions tend to maintain an adequate supply of dissolved oxygen where it can diffuse into the active cells.

Transport of carbon dioxide About twenty times as much carbon dioxide as oxygen can be transported dissolved in the plasma. Thus, carbon dioxide can be removed from cells under almost all physiological conditions. As we shall see later, the removal of carbon dioxide is important in the regulation of the pH of body fluids as well as in the respiratory process.

Carbon dioxide in gaseous form diffuses out of the cells into the capillaries, where it is transported in several ways. Because of its high solubility some carbon dioxide is transported dissolved in the blood plasma. Much of the carbon dioxide diffuses into the erythrocytes, where the enzyme **carbonic anhydrase** causes it to combine rapidly with water, forming carbonic acid. Most of the carbonic acid rapidly dissociates to form bicarbonate and hydrogen ions. (See reaction above.) The hydrogen ions combine with hemoglobin, and the negatively charged bicarbonate ions are released into the plasma.

The attachment of hydrogen ions to hemoglobin is an example of the buffering capacity of hemoglobin. (Buffers are substances that resist changes in pH, as will be explained in Chapter 26.) The buffering capacity of hemoglobin is enhanced by a decline in its saturation with oxygen, which occurred as oxygen diffused into the cells.

The protein part of hemoglobin also has a number of available amino acids to which molecules of carbon dioxide can attach, forming **carbaminohemoglobin**. The binding sites to which carbon dioxide attaches are different from those used by oxygen. A small amount of carbon dioxide also attaches to other plasma proteins.

About 70% of the bicarbonate ions formed in the erythrocytes diffuses into the plasma. This causes a significant difference in the electrical balance between ions in the plasma and those inside the erythrocytes. Positively charged ions do not readily move out of the erythrocytes, but negatively charged chloride ions move into the ery-

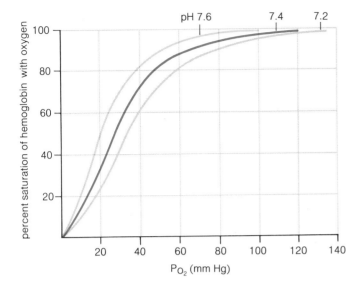

Figure 21.18 The oxyhemoglobin dissociation curve for pH: As pH decreases, hemoglobin releases more of the oxygen it is carrying. At any point in time and for a given pH, the graph can be used to determine the relative amounts of oxygen on hemoglobin and carried in the plasma. The curve for pH = 7.4 is is the normal curve.

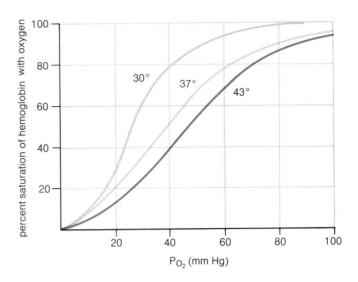

Figure 21.19 The oxyhemoglobin dissociation curve for temperature (Celsius): As the temperature of the blood increases, hemoglobin releases more of the oxygen it is carrying. At any point in time and for a given temperature, the graph can be used to determine the relative amounts of oxygen on hemoglobin and carried in the plasma. The curve for a temperature of 37° C is the normal curve.

throcytes. This phenomenon, called **chloride shift**, maintains electrical balance between erythrocytes and plasma.

When blood reaches the capillaries of the alveoli, these processes are reversed. Carbon dioxide dissolved in the plasma diffuses into the alveoli. Bicarbonate ions and hydrogen ions (carried by hemoglobin) recombine to form carbonic acid, and carbonic acid is broken down into carbon dioxide and water, replacing some of the carbon dioxide that has already diffused into the alveoli. Carbon dioxide carried by hemoglobin enters the plasma, and still more carbon dioxide diffuses into the alveoli until the partial pressure of carbon dioxide in the blood is near that in the alveoli. As these processes occur, hemoglobin also becomes resaturated with oxygen.

Thus, carbon dioxide is carried in three ways: (1) as a gas dissolved in plasma, (2) as bicarbonate ions, and (3) attached to hemoglobin (forming carbaminohemoglobin) and to certain plasma proteins. The relative amounts of carbon dioxide carried by each mechanism are summarized in Table 21.3.

Summary of transport and exchange of gases As blood passes through alveolar capillaries, it loses carbon dioxide and

picks up oxygen. As it passes through other body tissues, the process is reversed. The oxygen-carrying capacity of the blood is greatly increased by the presence of hemoglobin in the erythrocytes. More carbon dioxide than oxygen is dissolved in the plasma. Much of the carbon dioxide is transported as bicarbonate ions, and some is transported attached to the protein part of hemoglobin. These processes are summarized in Figure 21.20.

Table 21.3	**Transport of Carbon Dioxide**
Mechanism	Percent
Dissolved gas	7
Bicarbonate ion	70
Associated with hemoglobin and plasma proteins	23
Total	100

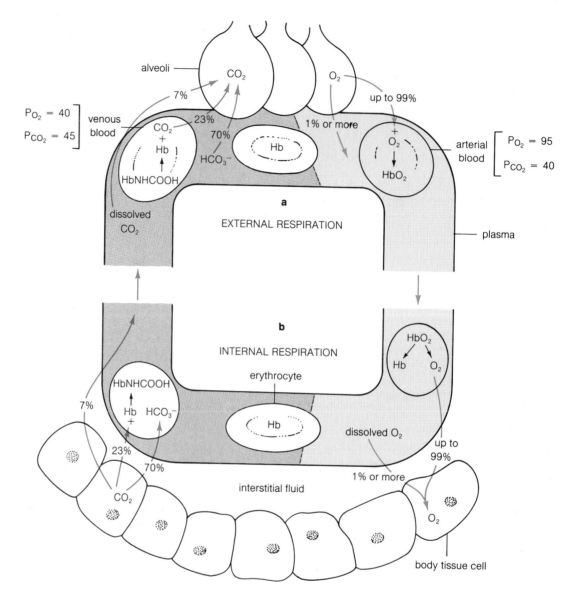

Figure 21.20 A summary of the transport and exchange of gases in external and internal respiration.

Regulation of Acid-Base Balance by the Respiratory System

The pH of arterial blood remains in a narrow range between 7.35 and 7.45, with venous blood having a lower pH than arterial blood. How much the venous blood pH is lowered depends on the amount of carbon dioxide and hydrogen ions it contains. More carbon dioxide (and thus more hydrogen ions) is produced by actively metabolizing tissues, particularly contracting muscles, than by relatively inactive tissues.

As you might expect, the respiratory system is the main system involved in the removal of carbon dioxide from the body. Since carbon dioxide can have an important effect on the hydrogen ion concentration, the rate at which it is removed from the blood or retained in it affects the blood pH. For example, when a person is breathing very slowly or has some pathological condition, such as pneumonia or emphysema, that interferes with gas exchange, carbon dioxide will accumulate in the blood. As carbon dioxide accumulates, some of it combines with water, forming carbonic acid. Carbonic acid ionizes, releasing hydrogen ions. The accumulation of hydrogen ions causes the blood pH to decrease. Such an individual is said to have **respiratory acidosis**, a low blood pH resulting from accumulation of carbon dioxide. This reaction can be summarized as follows:

$$\text{excess } CO_2 + H_2O \rightarrow H_2CO_3 \rightarrow H^+ + HCO_3^-$$

A different situation exists when an individual is breathing very rapidly because of intentional hyperventilation, aspirin poisoning, or anxiety. Instead of carbon dioxide accumulating in the blood, more than the usual amount of carbon dioxide is removed from the blood by the lungs. The above reaction goes in the opposite direction:

$$H^+ + HCO_3^- \rightarrow H_2CO_3 \rightarrow H_2O + \text{excess } CO_2 \text{ removed}$$

Such an individual is said to have **respiratory alkalosis**, an elevated blood pH resulting from a lowering of the blood carbon dioxide.

Within limits the body can correct acidosis or alkalosis. However, if an individual has some kind of impairment of respiratory function, the respiratory system is incapable of completely correcting acidosis or alkalosis; in such cases the kidneys help to correct the blood pH. This process is discussed in more detail in Chapter 26.

Acidosis and alkalosis may be caused by defects in metabolism. For example, untreated diabetes can lead to metabolic acidosis through the accumulation of acids in the blood, and excessive vomiting can lead to metabolic alkalosis through the loss of acid in the vomitus (see Chapter 23). When acidosis or alkalosis occurs in an individual with a normally functioning respiratory system, the respiratory system can help to correct these conditions by adjusting the amount of carbon dioxide that is removed from the blood.

REGULATION OF RESPIRATION

Objective 12. Explain the role of neural and chemical control systems in the regulation of respiration.

Breathing normally occurs at a regular, rhythmic rate. Both the rate and the depth of breathing are regulated in response to physiological changes. The regulation of respiration is a complex process that is not fully understood; however, both neural and chemical factors are known to be involved.

Neural Regulation of Respiration

The muscles that control breathing movements are skeletal muscles; to contract they must receive discharges from motor fibers of spinal nerves. The motor neurons in turn must receive impulses from nerve centers in the brain. Two separate neural mechanisms, both of which involve the brain, regulate respiration. One of these mechanisms regulates voluntary changes in respiration; the other regulates automatic involuntary changes in respiration.

The voluntary mechanism of respiratory control, located in the cerebral cortex, sends signals to the respiratory motor neurons by way of the corticospinal tracts. This mechanism makes it possible for you to vary your rate of breathing and even to "hold your breath," at least for a short time. Should you attempt to hold your breath for a long time, the automatic mechanism overrides the voluntary one, and you are forced to resume breathing.

The automatic mechanism for respiratory control is located in the respiratory centers of the pons and the medulla. These centers send signals to the motor neurons that supply the respiratory muscles by way of the lateral and ventral tracts of the spinal cord. When these signals stimulate inspiratory muscles, they inhibit expiratory muscles and vice versa. This phenomenon is called **reciprocal innervation**.

Several centers in the pons and medulla are involved in automatic respiratory control (Figure 21.21). What has been called the **respiratory center** of the medulla is now known to contain two groups of neurons, the **dorsal group** and the **ventral group**, both of which are present on both sides of the medulla. The dorsal group sends signals through the phrenic nerve to the diaphragm, stimulating its rhythmic contraction. The ventral group sends several kinds of signals, some stimulating inspiration and others stimulating expiration. Though **inspiratory neurons** and **expiratory neurons** are not neatly separated anatomically, it is helpful to think of the respiratory center of the medulla as a center that contains both of these kinds of neurons. Respiratory centers in the pons include the pneumotaxic center, which consists of one nucleus on each side, and the median apneustic center. The **apneustic center** prolongs inspiration by allowing the medullary inspiratory neurons to continue to

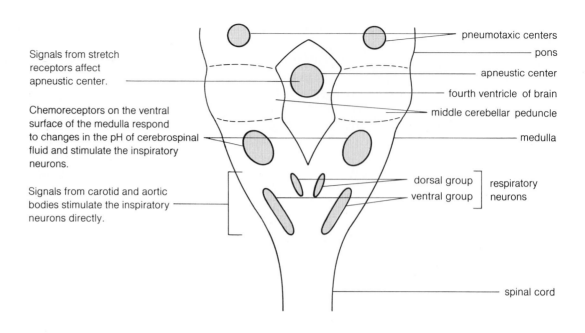

Signals from stretch receptors affect apneustic center.

Chemoreceptors on the ventral surface of the medulla respond to changes in the pH of cerebrospinal fluid and stimulate the inspiratory neurons.

Signals from carotid and aortic bodies stimulate the inspiratory neurons directly.

pneumotaxic centers
pons
apneustic center
fourth ventricle of brain
middle cerebellar peduncle
medulla
dorsal group ⎤ respiratory
ventral group ⎦ neurons
spinal cord

Figure 21.21   The location of neural structures, chemoreceptors, and chemoreceptor effects in the brainstem.

send signals. (**Apneusis** is a prolonging of respiration during inspiration.) The **pneumotaxic center** prevents apneusis by intermittently inhibiting the inspiratory neurons.

In a resting individual breathing normally, impulses from the inspiratory neurons cause the diaphragm and external intercostal muscles to contract, as described earlier. The neurons of the inspiratory center have a self-excitatory capacity by which they initiate inspiration at a fairly regular rate; thus, they are dominant over the expiratory neurons. In the absence of other stimuli normal resting level breathing is maintained at a regular rate by the oscillation between the actions of the inspiratory center and the expiratory center (Figure 21.22a). However, other stimuli are almost never absent—stretch receptors and chemoreceptors participate in the regulation of resting level breathing. Because these stimuli are also important in altering the frequency and depth of breathing, they are discussed separately below.

How depth and frequency of breathing are altered   The primary regulation of the depth and frequency of breathing depends on the duration and frequency of signals sent out by the inspiratory neurons. In resting breathing these neurons

spontaneously send out bursts of signals for several seconds about twelve to fifteen times per minute; however, the frequency and duration of their signals can be altered by several factors. Signals from the apneustic center increase the duration of these bursts. Signals from the pneumotaxic center inhibit the inspiratory neurons directly and also indirectly by inhibiting the apneustic center (Figure 21.22b).

Stretch receptors in the tissues of the lungs also play a role in controlling both the depth and the rhythm of breathing (Figure 21.22c), and they may also help to prevent the lungs from becoming overinflated. Though these receptors have only a small effect on normal resting level breathing, they have a great effect when inspiration is deep. They send signals to the apneustic center in proportion to the degree of stretching of the lung tissue. When inhalation is deep, as might occur during exercise, the stretch receptors are maximally stimulated. Their signals to the apneustic center inhibit it and prevent further prolongation of inhalation. This response to the stimulation of stretch receptors, called the **Hering-Breuer reflex**, is one factor in limiting the amount of air you can inhale in a single very deep breath.

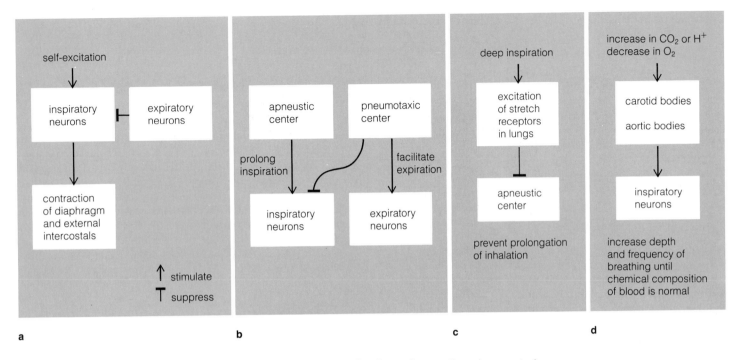

Figure 21.22 The regulation of breathing: (**a**) normal resting breathing, (**b**) effects of apneustic and pneumotaxic centers, (**c**) Hering-Breuer reflex, (**d**) effects of chemoreceptors.

Chemical Regulation of Respiration

When the chemical composition of the blood changes, other respiratory regulating mechanisms come into play. **Chemoreceptors** are found in the carotid bodies, located in the walls of the carotid arteries, and in the aortic bodies, located in the wall of the aorta. These chemoreceptors are stimulated by an increase in the partial pressure of carbon dioxide, by an increase in the concentration of hydrogen ions in arterial blood, and to a lesser extent by a decrease in the partial pressure of oxygen. When stimulated, the chemoreceptors relay signals to the inspiratory neurons of the respiratory center, where the signals stimulate an increase in the frequency of breathing (Figure 21.22d). The effect of this mechanism is to increase the amount of fresh air moving into the lungs and thus increase the rate at which oxygen is taken into the blood and the rate at which carbon dioxide is removed from it. The extreme sensitivity of these chemoreceptors to small changes in the composition of the blood and the rapid response of the inspiratory neurons keep the blood partial pressures of carbon dioxide and oxygen within a narrow range.

Other chemoreceptors in the fourth ventricle (in the medulla) are sensitive to changes in the hydrogen ion concentration of cerebrospinal fluid. These receptors, like other chemoreceptors, relay signals that stimulate the inspiratory neurons.

Regulation of respiration during exercise That the respiratory rate and the depth of breathing increase during exercise is common knowledge, but determining how these changes are regulated has posed a problem to researchers. Studies have shown that the partial pressures of carbon dioxide and oxygen in the blood during exercise remain relatively constant. Many physiologists believe that these chemicals cannot be responsible for regulating respiration during exercise because the body's response is too rapid to be mediated chemically. It is thought instead that the respiratory rate during exercise is controlled by nerve impulses from the cerebrum and from the proprioceptors in the joints and skeletal muscles. Within a few seconds of the beginning of exercise, the frequency and depth of breathing increases; immediately at the end of exercise the frequency and depth of breathing decrease. Such abrupt changes are more likely to be caused by neural rather than chemical means.

CLINICAL APPLICATIONS

Objective 13. Describe the alteration of function that occurs in the following conditions: (a) sinusitis, (b) choking, (c) pharyngitis and laryngitis, (d) bronchitis, (e) asthma, (f) emphysema, (g) pneumonia, (h) hyaline membrane disease, (i) smoking, (j) hypoxia, (k) narcosis, and (l) decompression sickness.

Objective 14. Explain briefly the effects of (a) inhalation anesthesia and (b) cardiopulmonary resuscitation.

Diseases of the Respiratory System

Sinusitis   **Sinusitis**, a common condition, is an inflammation of the mucous membrane lining the paranasal sinuses. These sinuses, described in Chapter 6, open into the nasal cavity and can become infected by microorganisms from the nasal cavity. The resulting inflammation causes the membranes to swell and produce excess mucus. The sinuses become blocked, and mucus and gases trapped within them cause pain and stuffiness. Normally, the sinuses serve as resonating chambers for sound; when they are filled with mucus and gases, this function is impaired, and the quality of the voice changes.

Choking   **Choking** caused by the blockage of the airway by food or other materials is a leading cause of accidental death. The victim cannot breathe or talk and may become cyanotic and die within about five minutes unless the obstructing material is removed. If quick blows on the back do not work, the rescuer stands behind the victim and grasps the victim around the waist with hands overlapping wrists while the victim leans forward. The rescuer then compresses the victim's abdomen forcefully and sharply. This action elevates the diaphragm and forces air out of the lungs. The air under pressure often forces the obstruction from the airway. With an unconscious victim lying on his or her back, the base of the hand (with the other hand overlying the first) can be used to compress the abdomen and elevate the diaphragm.

Pharyngitis and laryngitis   **Pharyngitis** is an inflammation of the pharynx, often called sore throat. It may accompany the common cold, and it usually involves inflammation of the tonsils (tonsillitis). **Laryngitis** is an inflammation of the larynx that often accompanies pharyngitis. In laryngitis inflammation of the larynx impairs the ability of the vocal cords to vibrate, and speaking is difficult or impossible.

Bronchitis   An inflammation of the bronchi, **bronchitis** is caused by an infection or some other form of irritation. The linings of the bronchi swell and produce excess mucus, and the cilia that normally sweep mucus out of the bronchi fail to function adequately. In chronic bronchitis fluid may accumulate in the tissues of the bronchi, further narrowing the air passageways. Treatment includes antibiotics for infection, the removal of irritating agents, and the breathing of humidified air to relieve coughing.

Asthma   **Asthma**, more correctly termed bronchial asthma, is often caused by an allergic reaction to foreign substances that affects the respiratory tract. As noted in Chapter 20, allergens stimulate the release of histamine from the mast cells. Histamine has several effects, one of which is to cause bronchiolar smooth muscle to contract. In asthma this hinders the passage of air to and from the alveoli. Exhaling is more difficult than inhaling. The pressure of the incoming air tends to push the bronchioles open, but the expelling of air tends to compress the already contracted bronchioles. Epinephrine and sympathomimetic drugs are used to control the symptoms of asthma.

Emphysema   **Emphysema** is a respiratory disorder in which many of the septa between the alveoli are destroyed, and much of the elastic tissue of the lungs is replaced by connective tissue (Figure 21.23). Major causes are cigarette smoking and the inhalation of other smoke or toxic substances over a period of time. As the alveolar septa collapse, the surface area for gas exchange is greatly reduced, and as elasticity is lost, exhalation becomes more difficult. The lungs remain inflated, and the individual must work to exhale. Eventually, capillaries around the alveoli are damaged because they are compressed by the inflated alveoli. Pressure increases in the pulmonary arteries, and the right ventricle must work much harder to force blood through the pulmonary circulation. Treatment involves removal of the irritating substances, breathing exercises, and drugs to dilate the air passageways. Some affected individuals use portable oxygen tanks to self-administer oxygen when needed.

Pneumonia   In **pneumonia** alveoli become acutely inflamed, and fluid and white blood cells accumulate in the lung tissues. The alveoli fill with fluid and dead cells, limiting gas exchange. Pneumonia may be caused by bacteria, fungi, viruses, chemical irritants, or other foreign materials. It can affect one lobe (lobar pneumonia), both lungs ("double pneumonia"), or both the alveoli and the bronchi (bronchial pneumonia). Antibiotics are used to treat bacterial infections, and oxygen may be given to increase the partial pressure of oxygen in the blood.

Hyaline membrane disease   **Hyaline membrane disease** (HMD), also called respiratory distress syndrome (RDS) of the newborn, is caused by a deficiency of surfactant. Premature infants born before the twenty-eighth week of development are most frequently affected by HMD because their lungs do not produce sufficient quantities of surfactant. The disease gets its name from the fact that, after a few hours of labored breathing, the lungs fill with a

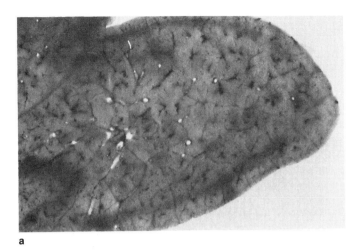

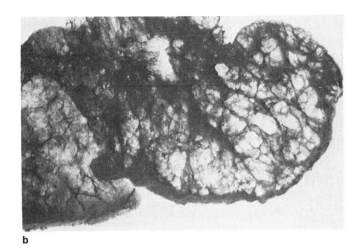

a

b

Figure 21.23 The lung of (**a**) a normal person, (**b**) a person with emphysema. (Webb-Waring Institute for Medical Research, courtesy Environmental Protection Agency.)

high-protein fluid that has a glassy or hyalinelike appearance on autopsy. One of the major problems in treating the disease is to prevent **atelectasis**, the collapse of the alveoli. Currently, this is done by providing gases to the airway under positive pressure so that even during exhalation the alveoli remain expanded. Failure to maintain adequate gas exchange at the alveolar membranes leads to respiratory acidosis. Even with the best available care infants with HMD often do not survive.

Smoking **Smoking**, or even the accidental inhalation of any kind of smoke, causes several abnormalities in the respiratory system. Smoke damages the epithelial lining of the bronchi and alveoli and is a major contributor to the development of emphysema. When smoke comes in contact with the cilia and the mucus-secreting goblet cells, it causes gradual deterioration of the cilia and enlargement of the goblet cells. Thus, particles from smoke are not as effectively removed from the bronchi, and excess mucus leads to smoker's cough. Chemicals in smoke cause changes in the epithelium; sometimes these changes are malignant. Malignant epithelial cells pass through the basement membrane of the epithelium and invade the underlying tissues. Smoke contains carbon monoxide, which diffuses into the blood, combines with hemoglobin, and impairs oxygen-carrying capacity.

Hypoxia **Hypoxia** is an insufficiency of oxygen reaching the tissues of the body. It can be caused by a number of factors, including hypoventilation and disorders of the circulatory system or the blood. Hypoventilation may be due to obstruction of the airways (asthma), destruction of alveoli (emphysema), or a neuromuscular disorder (polio). Heart defects that allow mixing of ar-

terial and venous blood (tetralogy of Fallot, described in Chapter 17) and anemias may also lead to hypoxia. Living at a high altitude may lead to hypoxia, but the bodies of most individuals who remain at high altitudes compensate for the reduced oxygen in the air by enlargement of the lungs and right ventricle of the heart and increased numbers of erythrocytes.

Narcosis **Narcosis** is a depression of the central nervous system, including the respiratory centers. Drugs that cause narcosis may be depressants such as alcohol, nitrogen gas, and a variety of legally controlled substances such as heroin and barbiturates. In narcosis the respiratory centers fail to respond effectively to stimulation from the chemoreceptors. Even when the carbon dioxide level is high or the oxygen level or pH is low, the respiratory centers do not sufficiently increase depth and frequency of breathing.

Nitrogen narcosis occurs in divers and other people who work in locations where the pressure is greater than sea-level atmospheric pressure. Under water pressure doubles for every 33 feet of depth. As pressure increases, nitrogen diffuses into the blood and causes nitrogen narcosis. One of the first symptoms of this disorder is euphoria—sometimes called "rapture of the deep." Impairment of nerve transmission and unconsciousness follow, probably because nitrogen dissolves in the lipids of cell membranes and acts as an anesthetic.

Decompression sickness When a diver who has been in deep water for a period of time ascends too rapidly to the surface, nitrogen dissolved in the blood and tissue fluids comes out of solution and forms bubbles, causing **decompression sickness**, commonly called the bends. Such bubbles accumulate in the blood and in the cells; they have their greatest effect on the joints and the spinal cord. In the blood vessels the bubbles can obstruct the flow of blood and lead to hypoxia in the tissues served by the affected vessels. Bubbles also can disrupt cells and cause permanent nerve damage. Decompression sickness is preventable by carefully determining the depth of a dive and the time spent at that depth, and controlling the ascent so gases diffuse from the blood slowly and obstructive bubbles do not form. Most of the serious cases of decompression sickness are seen in amateur divers who fail to heed the warning about the need for slow decompression.

Medical Techniques Related to the Respiratory System

Inhalation anesthetics **Inhalation anesthetics** are gases administered by inhalation that impair synaptic transmission in the central nervous system. These gases include nitrous oxide, cyclopropane, ether, ethylene, and chloroform. They are absorbed into the blood in the lungs and are transported by the blood to the brain. Here they cross the blood–brain barrier and impair the transmission of signals across snyapses.

Cardiopulmonary resuscitation **Cardiopulmonary resuscitation** (CPR) is a technique for maintaining the circulation of blood and the movement of air into and out of the lungs of a person who has stopped breathing and whose heart has ceased to beat. The three main steps in the procedure are: (1) to make sure that the airway to the lungs is open, (2) to provide air by mouth-to-mouth breathing, and (3) to keep the blood circulating by compressing the heart.

Everyone should become proficient at CPR, but *no one should attempt it without adequate training*. Improperly performed CPR can do more harm than good. Many colleges and several organizations such as the American Heart Association and the American Red Cross offer courses in CPR.

Clinical Terms

anoxia (an-oks'e-ah)   deficiency of oxygen

apnea (ap-ne'ah)   cessation of breathing

asphyxia (as-fiks'e-ah)   suffocation

atelectasis (at-el-ek'tas-is)   partial collapse of the alveoli; imperfect expansion of the alveoli

dyspnea (disp-ne'ah)   difficult or labored breathing

hypercapnea (hi-per-kap'ne-ah)   an excess of carbon dioxide in the blood

hypoxemia (hi-pox-e'me-ah)   a deficiency of oxygen in the blood

rale   an abnormal respiratory sound usually heard through a stethoscope

rhinitis (ri-ni'tis)   an inflammation of the nasal mucous membrane; runny nose

tracheotomy (tra-ke-ot'o-me)   cutting of the trachea, usually to provide an artificial airway

Essay: Sudden Infant Death Syndrome

Sudden infant death syndrome (SIDS) is characterized by sudden cessation of breathing during sleep in infants, usually those less than one year old. Typically, the parents put a perfectly normal-appearing infant to bed at night and in the morning discover that the infant is dead.

About 7000 babies, one in every 500 born, die of this malady each year in the United States. SIDS is the leading cause of infant death in this country and in many other countries as well.

Though the causes of SIDS are not yet completely understood, much has been learned in the past decade. Various researchers have investigated different anatomic and physiological effects of SIDS. Autopsies of victims of the syndrome showed an abnormal increase in the thickness of the muscle layer of the smaller pulmonary arteries in about 60% of the cases. This finding suggested that underventilation of the alveoli had led to the increase in muscle and constriction of the arteries. Underventilation lowers the level of oxygen in arterial blood that supplies the tissues and leads to other physiological changes that were observed in over half of the victims of SIDS: (1) Abnormal retention of brown fat. Brown fat normally surrounds certain vital organs at birth and helps neonates to maintain body temperature. Though the amount of brown fat generally decreases during the first year of life, it apparently persists later into the first year in SIDS infants than in normal infants. (2) Abnormal increase in the release of epinephrine from the adrenal gland. The excessive secretion of epinephrine may be caused by hypoventilation and may in turn stimulate the retention of brown fat. (Brown fat reappears in adults whose adrenal glands produce excessive amounts of epinephrine.) (3) Increased production of erythrocytes. Hypoxemia, lowered oxygen level in the blood, stimulates the kidneys to activate erythropoietin, which stimulates the production of erythrocytes. (4) A lag in growth characteristic of lowered oxygen supply. The growth pattern of SIDS infants resembles that of experimental animals made hypoxemic by being kept in a low oxygen environment.

Though the above alterations in physiology of SIDS infants are related to hypoxemia, they do not explain why the infants become hypoxemic. Abnormalities in the respiratory control centers are thought to be the most likely cause of hypoxemia. These centers apparently do not respond to an excess of carbon dioxide as do the centers in normal infants. In addition, more than half the victims of SIDS studied had underdeveloped carotid bodies. Why the respiratory centers fail to respond and why the carotid bodies are underdeveloped are problems still under study. Some possibilities being considered are the proliferation of glial cells in the respiratory centers and delayed myelination (and therefore maturation) of neurons in the brain stem.

If defects in the respiratory centers or carotid bodies are the direct causes of SIDS, then one might ask how these defects arise. Both genetic factors and factors that might cause damage during pregnancy, labor, or delivery are being investigated. Because the incidence of SIDS among related individuals is not higher than the incidence in the general population, a genetic factor as the direct cause of the defects appears to have been ruled out. However, infants with blood type B have a higher incidence of SIDS than infants with other blood types. Though blood type is a genetically determined characteristic, how it might relate to SIDS is unknown.

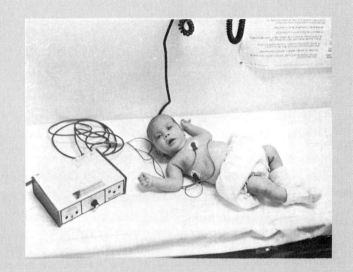

Figure 21.24 This 3½ month old baby girl has in the past experienced respiratory difficulties and is now connected to the monitor shown here whenever she sleeps. Should her breathing rate or her heart rate drop below normal for more than 20 seconds, an alarm sounds to wake her parents. The parents are trained in emergency resuscitation techniques. (Photograph by author; arrangements courtesy of Childrens Hospital National Medical Center, Washington, D.C. Photograph is used with the permission of the parents.)

Other factors correlated with SIDS include: (1) bacterial infection of the amniotic fluid during pregnancy, (2) anemia in the pregnant mother, (3) the mother's use of cigarettes, (4) barbiturates taken by the mother during pregnancy, (5) crowded housing conditions, and (6) a deficiency in the vitamin biotin (see Chapter 24) combined with environmental stress. However, one or more of these factors are present in only about one-third of infant deaths attributed to SIDS.

Though the exact causes of SIDS are not yet understood, some infants who have experienced respiratory difficulties have been kept alive by the use of an electronic monitor that sounds when respiration decreases (Figure 21.24). The parents are trained in techniques to restore breathing in such emergencies, and the monitor is usually used through the first year of life. According to one study, the monitor and the parents' activities apparently have saved the life of all but 4 of over 150 infants who experienced respiratory difficulty while connected to the monitor.

CHAPTER SUMMARY

(Chapter summary points and review questions are numbered to correspond to the numbered objectives in the text of each chapter.)

Organization and General Functions

1. Describe the overall plan of the respiratory system and explain its general functions.
  a. The respiratory system consists of a set of passageways that carry gases to and from the respiratory membranes, through which gases diffuse between the lungs and the blood.
  b. The functions of the respiratory system are to carry oxygen to the blood and to remove carbon dioxide from it.

Development

2. Describe the general embryological development of the respiratory system.
  a. The respiratory system develops from portions of the pharynx and from the laryngotracheal bud.

Tissues

3. Name the tissues of the respiratory system and explain how the epithelial tissues are specialized to perform their particular functions.
  a. The nasal cavity, pharynx, and bronchi are lined with ciliated epithelium in which the cilia beat to move mucus and debris toward the pharynx.
  b. The eipthelium of the alveoli is squamous epithelium, which allows gas exchange.
  c. Cartilage, smooth muscle, and connective tissue are found in most of the walls of passageways of the lungs.

Nasal Cavities, Pharynx, and Larynx

4. Locate and identify the structures of the nasal cavities and explain their respiratory functions.
  a. The nasal cavities are bounded by the external and internal nares, the bones of the cranium, and the hard and soft palates.
  b. The nasal septum separates the left and right halves of the cavity. The nasal conchae within the cavity are covered with membranes that contain the olfactory receptor cells.
  c. The nasal cavity warms, filters, and moistens air and its mucus, and cilia help to remove foreign particles.

5. Locate and identify the anatomical structures of the pharynx and the larynx and explain their respiratory functions.
  a. The pharynx extends from the internal nares to the larynx and is divided into the:

  (1) nasopharynx
  (2) oropharynx
  (3) laryngopharynx
  b. The pharynx conducts air from the nasal cavity to the larynx.
  c. The tonsils, masses of lymphatic tissue, are located in the pharynx.
  d. The larynx, or voice box, lies between the laryngopharynx and the trachea. It is supported by nine cartilages and contains the vocal cords.
  e. One of the cartilages, the epiglottis, helps to prevent food from entering the glottis, the opening from the pharynx to the larynx.
  f. The vocal cords in the larynx vibrate when air passes through the larynx, producing sound.

The Bronchial Tree, Respiratory Bronchioles, and Alveoli

6. Locate and identify the anatomical structures of the trachea, bronchi, bronchioles, and alveoli and explain their respiratory functions.
  a. The bronchial tree consists of the trachea, bronchi, bronchioles, alveolar ducts, alveolar sacs, and alveoli.
  b. These passageways, except for the respiratory bronchioles and the alveoli, are supported by cartilage rings or plates.
  c. The respiratory bronchioles are the most distal of the bronchioles; they branch into the alveolar ducts, which are surrounded by alveoli.
  d. Alveoli consist of thin membranes through which gases diffuse between the lungs and the blood.
  e. Blood from the pulmonary artery passes through the capillaries that surround the respiratory membranes; here the capillaries receive oxygen and get rid of carbon dioxide.

Lungs and Breathing

7. Describe the overall structure and location of the lungs and their surrounding membranes, including their blood supply and innervation.
  a. The lungs lie in the thoracic cavity and are covered by visceral pleura.
  b. The thoracic cavity is lined with parietal pleura. A serous fluid lubricates the parietal and visceral pleura, which slide over one another during breathing movements.
  c. The costal surfaces of the lungs lie next to the ribs, and the medial surfaces lie next to the mediastinum, where bronchi, blood vessels, and nerves enter each lung at the hilum.
  d. The lungs are divided into lobes, two in the left lung and three in the right lung. Each lobe is further divided into lobules; each lobule receives a tertiary bronchus and is covered by elastic tissue.

e. The phrenic nerve innervates the diaphragm, an important muscle in breathing; thoracic spinal nerves innervate the intercostal musles; and autonomic nerves supply the smooth muscle of the lungs.

8. Explain the process of breathing, including inhalation, exhalation, and volumes of air moving.

   a. Breathing, or ventilation, includes inspiration and expiration; it provides a continuous supply of fresh air to the respiratory membranes.

   b. The thoracic cavity is an airtight cavity.

   c. When the muscles of inspiration (the diaphragm and the external intercostals) contract, the volume of the thoracic cavity increases and air is drawn into the lungs because the pressure inside the lungs is less than atmospheric pressure.

   d. When the muscles of inspiration relax, the volume of the thoracic cavity decreases, and air is pushed out of the lungs because the pressure inside them is greater than atmospheric pressure.

   e. The total lung capacity includes:

      (1) tidal volume, the volume of air moved into and out of the lungs during normal breathing, which includes alveolar volume (the volume reaching respiratory membranes) and dead space volume (the volume not reaching respiratory membranes)

      (2) inspiratory reserve, the maximum volume beyond tidal volume that can be inhaled in one very deep breath

      (3) expiratory reserve, the maximum volume beyond tidal volume that can be forcefully exhaled after a normal exhalation

      (4) residual volume, the air that remains in the lungs after forceful exhalation.

Transport and Exchange of Gases

9. Describe the exchange of gases between the respiratory membranes and the blood, and between the blood and the cells.

   a. Gas exchange depends on the different partial pressures of oxygen and carbon dioxide on the two sides of a respiratory membrane.

   b. In the lungs oxygen diffuses into the blood, and carbon dioxide diffuses out of the blood.

   c. In other tissues oxygen diffuses from the blood into the cells, and carbon dioxide diffuses from the cells into the blood.

10. Describe the transport of gases between the lungs and the cells.

    a. While oxygen is being transported in the blood, only a small amount of it is dissolved in the plasma; up to 99% of the oxygen is carried on hemoglobin molecules in the erythrocytes.

    b. While being transported in the blood, carbon dioxide is mostly converted to bicarbonate ions in the erythrocytes and released into the plasma; carbon dioxide is also carried dissolved in the plasma and on hemoglobin molecules and certain plasma proteins.

11. Explain the role of the respiratory system in the regulation of acid–base balance in the body.

    a. Blood pH is maintained within a very narrow range around pH 7.4; it is lowered by an excess of carbon dioxide and elevated if too much carbon dioxide is removed.

    b. The lungs help to maintain blood pH in the normal range by adjusting the amount of carbon dioxide removed from the blood.

    c. Pathological conditions that reduce gas exchange in the lungs lead to accumulation of carbon dioxide and respiratory acidosis; hyperventilation removes too much carbon dioxide from the blood and leads to respiratory alkalosis.

Regulation of Respiration

12. Explain the role of neural and chemical control systems in the regulation of respiration.

    a. Resting rhythmic breathing is maintained by the self-excitatory capacity of the inspiratory neurons of the respiratory center.

    b. Depth and frequency of breathing is altered by:

       (1) the apneustic center, which prolongs inspiration

       (2) the pneumotaxic center, which facilitates expiration directly by stimulating the expiratory neurons and indirectly by inhibiting the apneustic center

       (3) the Hering-Breuer reflex, in which inflation of the lungs stimulates stretch receptors to send signals to inhibit the apneustic center

       (4) chemoreceptors in the carotid and aortic bodies and in the medulla, which respond to changes in hydrogen ion concentration and partial pressures of carbon dioxide and oxygen, and stimulate the inspiratory neurons when carbon dioxide or acidity increase or (to a lesser extent) when oxygen decreases

Clinical Applications

13. Describe the alteration of function that occurs in the following conditions: (a) sinusitis, (b) choking, (c) pharyngitis and laryngitis, (d) bronchitis, (e) asthma, (f) emphysema, (g) pneumonia, (h) hyaline membrane disease, (i) smoking, (j) hypoxia, (k) narcosis, and (l) decompression sickness.

    a. Sinusitis is an inflammation of the paranasal sinuses.

    b. Choking is the prevention of breathing by a blockage of the airway.

    c. Pharyngitis and laryngitis are inflammations of the pharynx and larynx, respectively.

    d. Bronchitis is an inflammation of the bronchi.

    e. Asthma, often caused by an allergic reaction, is a constriction of air passages that interferes with breathing.

    f. Emphysema involves loss of alveolar surface, which impairs gas exchange, and loss of elasticity, which makes exhalation difficult.

    g. Pneumonia is an inflammation of the alveoli in which fluid and dead cells accumulate in the alveoli, hindering gas exchange.

    h. Hyaline membrane disease, caused by a deficiency of surfactant in premature infants, involves the collapse of alveoli and therefore impaired gas exchange.

i. Smoking damages epithelial cells, increases mucus, and may lead to malignant changes in cells. Smoke contains carbon monoxide, which impairs oxygen transport.

j. Hypoxia is an insufficiency of oxygen reaching the tissues of the body.

k. Narcosis is a depression of the central nervous system, including the respiratory centers.

l. Decompression sickness results from rapid release of nitrogen bubbles into the blood as an individual who has been exposed to environmental pressure greater than atmospheric pressure rapidly returns to atmospheric pressure.

14. Explain briefly the effects of (a) inhalation anesthesia and (b) cardiopulmonary resuscitation.

a. Inhalation anesthetics are gases that diffuse into the blood from the lungs, travel to the central nervous system, and impair synaptic transmission.

b. Cardiopulmonary resuscitation is a technique for maintaining the circulation of blood and the movement of air into and out of the lungs in a person who has stopped breathing and whose heart has ceased to beat.

REVIEW

Important Terms

alveoli	intrathoracic volume
apneustic center	larynx
bronchi	minute respiratory volume
carbonic anhydrase	narcosis
cellular respiration	pleura
dead space volume	pneumotaxic center
expiratory reserve volume	residual volume
external respiration	respiration
functional residual capacity	respiratory acidosis
hypoxia	respiratory alkalosis
inspiratory capacity	surfactant
inspiratory reserve volume	tidal volume
internal respiration	trachea
intrapulmonary pressure	vital capacity
intrapulmonary volume	

Questions

1. a. What are the major components of the respiratory system?
   b. What are the major functions of the respiratory system?

2. Briefly describe the development of the respiratory system.

3. What are the characteristics of the lining of the respiratory tract?

4. a. What boundaries define the nasal cavity?
   b. What are the functions of the nasal cavity?

5. a. What are the three regions of the pharynx, and what is one structural characteristic of each region?
   b. Describe the cartilages that form the larynx.
   c. Where are the vocal cords, and what is their function?

6. a. Make a diagram to show the major components of the bronchial tree.
   b. Make another diagram to show the relationships among the respiratory portions of the respiratory tract.
   c. What criteria must a structure meet to be called a respiratory structure?

7. a. Explain the relationship of the pleurae to the lungs.
   b. Describe the gross anatomy of the lungs, including the structure of the lobes.

8. a. Distinguish between respiration and breathing.
   b. What causes inhalation and exhalation?
   c. How does air move into and out of the lungs?
   d. Define the terms that refer to volumes of air in the lungs.

9. How are partial pressures of gases related to gas exchange in the body?

10. a. Compare the transport of oxygen to the transport of carbon dioxide.
    b. How would a deficiency of hemoglobin affect oxygen transport? Carbon dioxide transport?

11. a. What is the role of the lungs in maintaining acid-base balance?
    b. What is respiratory acidosis? Respiratory alkalosis?

12. a. How is normal resting level breathing regulated?
    b. How do the apneustic center and the pneumotaxic center affect the depth and frequency of breathing?
    c. What is the Hering-Breuer reflex?
    d. How do chemoreceptors affect the depth and frequency of breathing?

13. For each of the clinical conditions discussed in the chapter, what is the major alteration in function?

14. What are the effects of inhalation anesthetics? Cardiopulmonary resuscitation?

Problems

1. How could you reassure the parents of children who frequently hold their breath to frighten the parents?

2. Suppose you are working with a person who is breathing rapidly and whose laboratory test shows a blood pH of 7.3. What might be the problem? What treatment is needed? Is there any emergency? Why or why not?

REFERENCES AND READINGS

Anonymous. 1979. Preventing crib deaths. *Science News* 115:57 (January 27).

Baker, T. L., and McGinty, D. J. 1977. Reversal of cardiopulmonary failure during active sleep in hypoxic kittens: Implications for sudden infant death. *Science* 198:419 (October 28).

Bergofsky, E. H. 1980. Humoral control of the pulmonary circulation. *Annual Review of Physiology* 42:221.

Broad, W. J. 1979. High anxiety over flights through ozone. *Science* 205:767 (August 24).

Cohen, M. I. 1981. Central determinants of respiratory rhythm. *Annual Review of Physiology* 43:91.

Culver, B. H., and Butler, J. 1980. Mechanical influences on the pulmonary microcirculation. *Annual Review of Physiology* 42:187.

Downing, S. E., and Lee, J. C. 1980. Nervous control of the pulmonary circulation. *Annual Review of Physiology* 42:199.

Eldridge, F. L., and Millhorn, E. 1981. Central regulation of respiration by endogenous neurotransmitters and neuromodulators. *Annual Review of Physiology* 43:121.

Fardy, R. W. 1979. Hyaline membrane disease: A study in body systems. *The Science Teacher* 46(5):44 (May).

Fishman, A. P. 1980. Vasomotor regulation of the pulmonary circulation. *Annual Review of Physiology* 42:211.

Ganong, W. F. 1981. *Review of medical physiology* (10th ed.). Los Altos, Calif.: Lange Medical Publications.

Gil, J. 1980. Organization of microcirculation in the lung. *Annual Review of Physiology* 42:187.

Kaplan, M. M., and Webster, R. G. 1977. The epidemiology of influenza. *Scientific American* 237(6):88 (December).

Nadel, J. A., Davis, B., and Phipps, R. J. 1979. Control of mucus secretion and ion transport in airways. *Annual Review of Physiology* 41:369.

Naeye, R. L. 1980. Sudden infant death. *Scientific American* 242(4): 56 (April).

Smith, B. T. 1979. Lung maturation in the fetal rat: Acceleration by injection of fibroblast-pneumocyte factor. *Science* 204:1094 (June 8).

Strauss, R. H., and Yount, D. E. 1977. Decompression sickness. *American Scientist* 65:598 (September–October).

Wagner, P. D. 1980. Ventilation-perfusion relationships. *Annual Review of Physiology* 42:235.

West, J. B. 1977. *Pulmonary pathophysiology.* Baltimore, Md.: Williams and Wilkins.

West, J. B. 1977. *Ventilation/blood flow and gas exchange.* Oxford, England: Blackwell Scientific Publications. (Distributed in U.S. by J. B. Lippincott, Philadelphia).

22

DIGESTIVE SYSTEM

ORGANIZATION AND GENERAL FUNCTIONS

Objective 1. Describe the general functions of the digestive system and list its major organs.

The digestive system receives and processes foodstuffs into particles that can cross the membranes of the digestive tract and enter the blood or lymph. This chapter deals with the structures within the digestive system, their functions, and how those functions are regulated. It assumes an understanding of the basic chemistry of foodstuffs and enzymes (presented in Chapter 2). It also provides the background for the study of metabolism and nutrition in Chapters 23 and 24.

Like other systems we have considered, the structures of the digestive system are well designed to carry out their functions. Muscles of the digestive tract are capable of exactly the kinds of motility (movement) needed to mix food with digestive juices and to propel it along the tract. Certain parts of the digestive tract contribute secretions in proper amounts to lubricate the tract and to digest, or break down, food substances into small particles. In addition, certain processes within the digestive tract allow these small particles to be transported across the intestinal membrane and to enter the blood or lymph. Strictly speaking, the contents of the digestive tract have not entered the body; only the particles that cross the membrane enter the body.

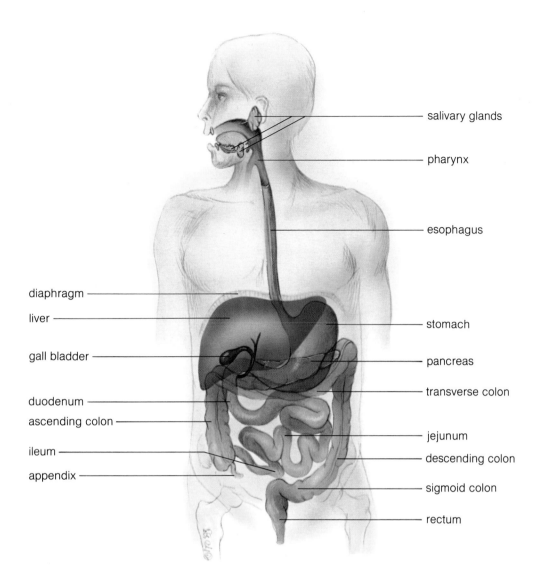

salivary glands

pharynx

esophagus

diaphragm

liver

gall bladder

duodenum

ascending colon

ileum

appendix

stomach

pancreas

transverse colon

jejunum

descending colon

sigmoid colon

rectum

Figure 22.1 Organs of the digestive tract.

All the functions of the digestive system are precisely controlled by a variety of mechanical, chemical, and neural regulators. Therefore, the functioning of the digestive system abounds with examples of homeostatic mechanisms. Hunger and satiety, swallowing, motility, secretion, digestion, transport across membranes, and defecation (the passage of wastes from the digestive tract) are all processes that are closely interrelated and regulated by a complex assortment of homeostatic mechanisms.

The digestive system consists of an elongated tube extending from the lips of the mouth to the anus, with a variety of modifications along that tube to form the various organs. The organs of the digestive tract, in order as the food passes through them, are the mouth, pharynx, esophagus, stomach, small intestine, large intestine, rectum, and anus. Also included in the digestive system are accessory organs, connected by ducts to the organs they assist: salivary glands to the mouth, and the liver, gallbladder, and pancreas to the small intestine (Figure 22.1).

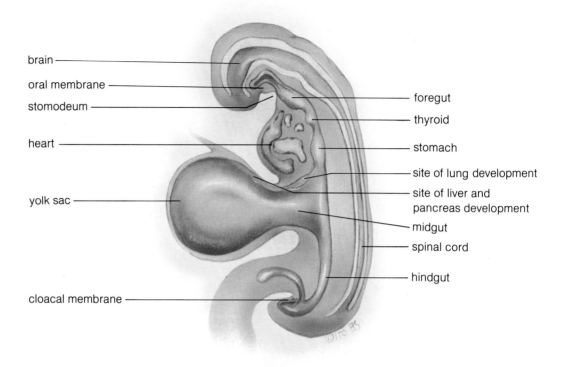

brain
oral membrane
stomodeum
heart
yolk sac
cloacal membrane

foregut
thyroid
stomach
site of lung development
site of liver and
pancreas development
midgut
spinal cord
hindgut

Figure 22.2 The digestive tract at the beginning of the fourth week of development.

DEVELOPMENT

Objective 2. Describe in general the formation of the digestive system and list some common congenital defects of that system.

Shortly after the development of the three germ layers, as described in Chapter 4, the primitive gut cavity forms a tube that is closed off at both ends (Figure 22.2). The ectoderm of the anterior surface of the embryo and the endoderm of the gut meet to form the two-layered oral membrane across the tube. This membrane ruptures at about twenty-four days to form the **stomodeum**, which later differentiates into the mouth. Another double membrane, the cloacal membrane, across the posterior end of the embryo ruptures at about seven weeks to form the anal opening. The body wall (eventual skin and muscles) grows around the primitive gut, and the tube elongates. Outgrowths from the tube form the liver and pancreas. By the eighth week all of the organs of the digestive tract are present in at least rudimentary form.

The face, mouth, and palate develop during the second month from processes of tissue, as described in Chapter 21. Failure of these processes to meet and fuse properly leads to congenital defects such as cleft lip or cleft palate (Figure 21.4).

Other congenital defects associated with the digestive tract include esophageal atresia, pyloric stenosis, and imperforate anus. In the normal development of the esophagus cells proliferate into the lumen, later to be eroded away. If this erosion does not occur, a blocking of the esophagus, **esophageal atresia**, results. In **pyloric stenosis** the muscles of the pyloric end of the stomach near where it joins the small intestine are overdeveloped. An infant having this defect vomits forcibly and becomes malnourished because so little food is allowed to pass from the stomach to the small intestine. **Imperforate anus** results from the failure of the posterior membrane to rupture and must be corrected surgically.

Objective 3. Describe the basic layers of the digestive tract and explain briefly how the structures in those layers carry out the four main functions of the digestive tract.

The Tissues

Throughout most of its length the digestive tract is composed of four basic layers, each of which may be modified to complement the function of a particular region along the tract. From the outer surface inward to the lumen, the layers (Figure 22.3) are as follows: (1) The **serosa** is the outer membranous covering of the digestive tract, so named because it is lubricated by a serous, or watery, fluid. It is continuous with the mesentery. (2) A layer of smooth muscle, the **muscularis**, composed of outer longitudinal fibers and inner circular fibers, accounts for most of the contractions that mix and propel food through the tract. (3) The **submucosa** consists of loose connective tissue richly supplied with blood and lymphatic vessels and in some areas with glands. Both the muscularis and the submucosa are supplied with nerve endings, the **myenteric plexus**, or the **plexus of Auerbach**, and the **submucosal plexus**, or the **plexus of Meissner**, respectively. (4) The **mucosa**, so named because it secretes mucus that lubricates the inner lining of the tract, has within it three layers. The thin **muscularis mucosa** lies next to the submucosa. The **lamina propria**, the middle layer of the mucosa, consists of loose connective tissue, blood vessels, glands, and some lymphoid tissue. The innermost layer, the **epithelium**, comes in contact with food as it passes through the lumen. In the small intestine the mucosa is folded to form villi (singular, villus). Other modifications in various regions of the digestive tract are summarized in Table 22.2, later in this chapter.

In addition to the tissues of the wall of the digestive tract, a set of membranes support and protect the tract. These membranes include the **visceral peritoneum** (the same membrane as the serosa), the **parietal peritoneum**, and the **mesenteries** and omenta (Figure 22.4). Each of these membranes is composed of one or more layers of epithelial cells supported by connective tissue. Together, they form a continuous sheet of tissue. The parietal peritoneum lines the entire abdominal cavity. At the posterior midline the left and right sheets of the membrane come together to form a double membrane called a mesentery. Each of the abdominal organs is suspended by this mesentery. As the sheets separate to surround an organ, they become the visceral peritoneum, or serosa, of the organ. In two places within the abdominal cavity mesenteries extend beyond the or-

gans and form an apron over them. These membranes become folded so as to contain four thicknesses and are called omenta. One of these, the **lesser omentum**, lies between the liver and the stomach; the other, the **greater omentum**, lies between the stomach and the small intestine.

The mesenteries contain many branches of blood vessels that supply the organs of the digestive tract. Omenta serve as depots for the storage of fats and also contain phagocytic cells that help to fight infections of the abdominal cavity. **Peritonitis**, an inflammation of these membranes, may result from infection or chemical irritation.

Functions of the Tissues

As the ingested food passes along the digestive tract, it is digested, and nutrients, water, and electrolytes are delivered to the blood or lymph for eventual transport to all body cells. The four functions of the digestive tract that contribute to this process are **motility, secretion, digestion,** and **absorption**.

Motility Motility of the digestive tract mixes the food in the lumen with the digestive juices and propels the mixture through the tract. Mechanical and chemical receptors in the gut wall are stimulated by the presence of food in the lumen. These receptors relay signals to the submucosal (Meissner's) plexus and to the myenteric (Auerbach's) plexus, and these plexuses in turn relay signals to smooth muscles and secretory cells of the digestive tract. (Their effects on secretory cells will be discussed later.) Signals to the smooth muscle may increase or decrease the muscle tone, increase both the intensity and the rate of rhythmic contractions, and also increase the velocity of nerve signals from one part of the tract to the next. This intrinsic (inside the organ) innervation is capable of executing the functions of the gut without any signals from extrinsic (outside the organ) nerves. However, signals from autonomic (extrinsic) nerves modulate the effects of the intrinsic nerves. In general, stimulation from sympathetic nerves slows down or blocks movement of food, and stimulation from parasympathetic nerves accelerates movement of food. These stimuli act primarily on the myenteric plexus. Together, neural impulses and the contractility of muscle cells account for the motility of the gut.

Of the two kinds of movement mixing movement involves only local contractions, but propulsive movement, or **peristalsis**, involves waves of contraction (Figure 22.5). Contractions occur at adjacent locations in a sequence proceeding toward the anus; their net effect is to push the contents of the lumen toward the anus. Distention in an area

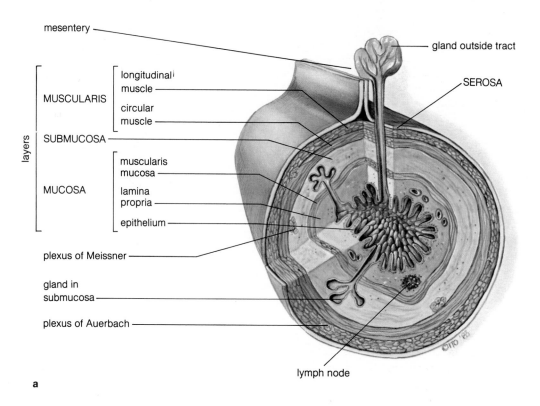

mesentery

gland outside tract

SEROSA

MUSCULARIS
longitudinal muscle
circular muscle

SUBMUCOSA

MUCOSA
muscularis mucosa
lamina propria
epithelium

layers

plexus of Meissner

gland in submucosa

plexus of Auerbach

lymph node

a

Figure 22.3 Layers of the digestive tract: (**a**) diagram, (**b**) photomicrograph of mammalian small intestine, × 25. (Photograph by author.)

of the digestive tract stimulates contraction of the gut wall a few centimeters above the distention and relaxation of the wall below the distention, thereby facilitating movement.

Secretion The digestive tract produces two kinds of secretions. **Mucous secretions**, produced by goblet cells distributed throughout the epithelium of the tract, serve to lubricate and protect the epithelium. **Digestive secretions**, produced by secretory glands within the tract or by accessory organs such as the pancreas, break down food particles into smaller molecules. Digestive secretions are normally released in response to the presence of food in the tract; the kind and amount of secretion is determined by the kind and amount of food present.

Digestion Digestion takes place in the lumen of the digestive tract, particularly in the small intestine and to a limited extent in the stomach. It occurs through the action of enzymes in the digestive secretions. The enzymes digest foodstuffs into their component amino acids, monosaccharides, fatty acids, and other substances. Many of the enzyme-controlled chemical reactions involve hydrolysis, the breaking of a larger molecule into two smaller ones and the addition of water as a hydrogen ion (H^+) to one molecule and a hydroxyl group (OH^-) to the other.

Absorption Absorption is the process of moving digested nutrients from the lumen of the digestive tract into the

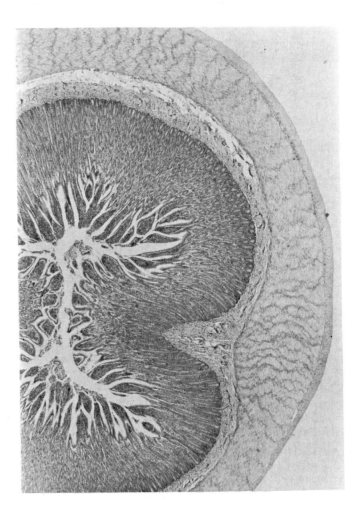

b

MOUTH

Objective 4. Describe the anatomical structure of the mouth, including the salivary glands and teeth.

Objective 5. Explain how each of the following structures functions in digestion: teeth, tongue, taste buds, and salivary glands.

Objective 6. Explain the regulation of hunger and satiety.

Structure of the Mouth

The initial processing of food occurs in the mouth, and the structures found in the mouth are well designed to carry out this initial processing.

The **oral cavity**, buccal cavity, or mouth (Figure 22.6) is bounded by the **teeth**, the **gingivae** or gums, the **hard palate** and **soft palate**, and the **oropharynx**. The **fauces** is the opening between the mouth and the oropharynx. Outside the oral cavity proper is the **oral vestibule**, the space between the gums and the lips. (Several other structures are also shown in Figure 22.6.) Both the oral cavity and the vestibule are lined with mucous membranes.

Lying in the floor of the mouth is the thick, muscular **tongue**, attached to the floor by the **frenulum**. The tongue helps to move food in the processes of chewing and swallowing. On the upper surface of the tongue are several kinds of papillae that are sensitive to touch and that add roughness to the surface. Some of the papillae contain taste buds. (Refer to Chapter 14 for further discussion of the structure and function of taste buds.) In addition to the tongue the salivary glands and teeth are important components of the mouth.

blood or lymph. **Villi**, folds in the epithelium of the small intestine, and **microvilli**, folds in the epithelial cell membranes, greatly increase the surface area of the small intestine and therefore facilitate the process of absorption. Directly beneath the villi in the lamina propria are blood vessels into which most nutrients pass. Fats, however, pass first into **lacteals** (lymph capillaries) and then into lymphatic vessels of the lamina propria. Later, the contents of the lymphatic vessels enter the bloodstream.

Now that we have a general idea of the basic plan of the digestive tract, we will study each of the organs in more detail, seeing how each is modified to carry out its specialized activities. We will also consider some disorders of the digestive tract.

Salivary glands Three pairs of salivary glands secrete saliva into the mouth through ducts (Figure 22.6). The large **parotid glands** are located near the ears; their secretions are carried by **parotid ducts**, which pass over the buccinator muscle on each side of the face and open into the oral vestibule near the upper second molars. The small **sublingual glands** are located beneath the tongue; their ducts open into the floor of the oral cavity. The medium-sized **submandibular glands** are located in the floor of the oral cavity near the angle of each mandible; their secretions pass through **Wharton's ducts** directly under the oral mucosa and open into the oral cavity near the lower central incisors. The disease mumps is a viral infection that may involve one or more of the salivary glands.

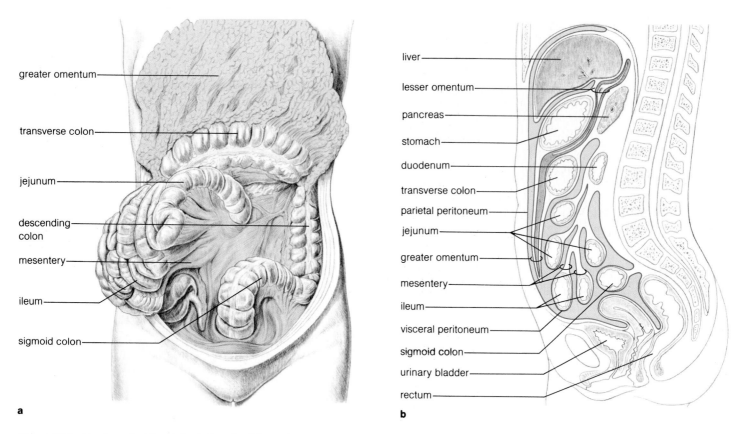

greater omentum

transverse colon

jejunum

descending colon

mesentery

ileum

sigmoid colon

a

liver

lesser omentum

pancreas

stomach

duodenum

transverse colon

parietal peritoneum

jejunum

greater omentum

mesentery

ileum

visceral peritoneum

sigmoid colon

urinary bladder

rectum

b

Figure 22.4 Membranes of the abdominal cavity: (**a**) anterior view with greater omentum reflected (lifted out of the way of other structures), (**b**) lateral view in cross section.

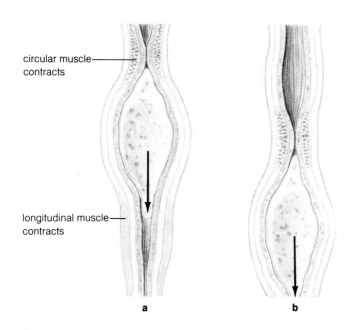

circular muscle contracts

longitudinal muscle contracts

a   b

Figure 22.5 Peristalsis.

Teeth Each jaw of the human adult contains sixteen teeth, making a full adult complement of thirty-two teeth (Figure 22.7a). Starting at the midline of the upper or lower jaw and moving toward the back of the mouth are two **incisors**, one **canine** or **cuspid**, two **bicuspids**, and three **molars**. The posteriormost molars are sometimes called "wisdom teeth." Each kind of tooth is shaped for a particular function: Incisors bite, canines tear, bicuspids and molars grind. The left and right sides of the jaws are symmetrical and have the same configuration of teeth.

In the human infant **deciduous**, or **milk**, **teeth** begin to erupt through the gums at about six months of age and continue to erupt periodically until the child has a set of twenty teeth at about age two (Figure 22.7b). At about age six the first permanent molars erupt posterior to the deciduous teeth, and the deciduous teeth begin to be replaced by the permanent teeth. As each permanent tooth completes its development beneath the gum, it begins to move toward the surface. Permanent teeth destined to replace the deciduous ones exert pressure on the roots of the deciduous

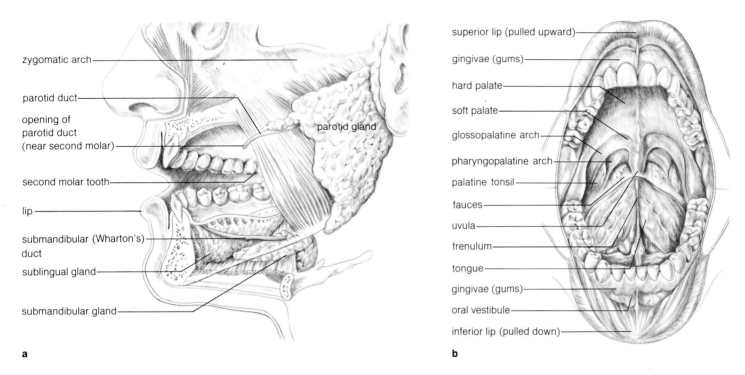

zygomatic arch

parotid duct

opening of
parotid duct
(near second molar)

second molar tooth

lip

submandibular (Wharton's)
duct

sublingual gland

submandibular gland

parotid gland

a

superior lip (pulled upward)

gingivae (gums)

hard palate

soft palate

glossopalatine arch

pharyngopalatine arch

palatine tonsil

fauces

uvula

frenulum

tongue

gingivae (gums)

oral vestibule

inferior lip (pulled down)

b

Figure 22.6 Anatomy of the mouth (**a**) a lateral cut-away view, (**b**) an anterior view of the open mouth.

teeth and stimulate the roots to erode. The deciduous teeth, having lost their roots, loosen and fall out.

Structurally, a tooth consists of two main parts, the **crown**, covered with **enamel**, and the **root**, covered with **cementum** (Figure 22.8). Enamel, the hardest substance in the body, is well designed to withstand the grinding of one tooth against another during chewing. Cementum is similar to bone. The tooth is held in the **alveolus**, or tooth socket, by the **periodontal ligament**, which consists of fibers running from the cementum to the bone of the socket. The **neck** of the tooth, which marks the separation of the root and crown portions, appears as a slight constriction in the tooth at the gum line. Under the hard outer layer of both the crown and the root is the **dentin**, another bonelike substance that forms the bulk of the tooth. The **pulp cavity** occupies the central portion of the tooth and extends down into the roots, forming the **root canals**. Blood and lymph vessels and nerves enter the pulp cavity through the **apical foramina** at the tips of the roots. **Pulp** consists of connective tissue in which vessels and nerves are imbedded.

Digestive Functions of the Mouth

Chewing and the actions of saliva accomplish the digestive functions of the mouth. Though chewing is partially under conscious control, the following reflex pattern also occurs. When food enters the mouth, the presence of a **bolus**, or mass of food, causes reflex inhibition of the chewing muscles, and the lower jaw drops. The drop initiates a stretch reflex and causes the jaw muscles to contract and press on the bolus of food. This cycle results in rhythmic chewing motions, during which the teeth break apart all food—especially the cellulose cell walls in plant materials—create small particles, and increase the surface area within the bolus.

The salivary glands together produce over one liter of saliva a day. The parotids contribute much of the starch-digesting enzyme **salivary amylase**; the sublinguals and submaxillaries contribute both the enzyme and **mucin**, a glycoprotein that lubricates the membrane lining the mouth and causes food particles to adhere to each other. These

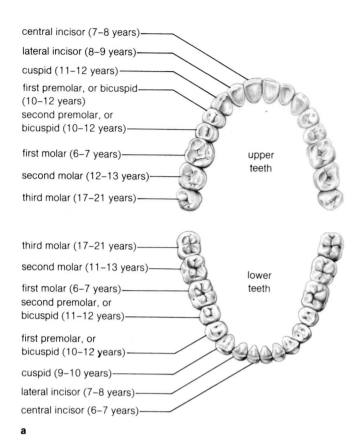

central incisor (7–8 years)
lateral incisor (8–9 years)
cuspid (11–12 years)
first premolar, or bicuspid (10–12 years)
second premolar, or bicuspid (10–12 years)
first molar (6–7 years)
second molar (12–13 years)
third molar (17–21 years)

upper teeth

third molar (17–21 years)
second molar (11–13 years)
first molar (6–7 years)
second premolar, or bicuspid (11–12 years)
first premolar, or bicuspid (10–12 years)
cuspid (9–10 years)
lateral incisor (7–8 years)
central incisor (6–7 years)

lower teeth

a

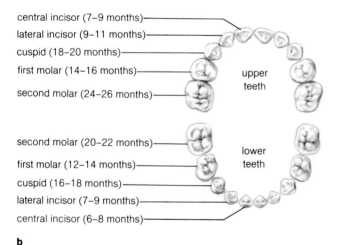

central incisor (7–9 months)
lateral incisor (9–11 months)
cuspid (18–20 months)
first molar (14–16 months)
second molar (24–26 months)

upper teeth

second molar (20–22 months)
first molar (12–14 months)
cuspid (16–18 months)
lateral incisor (7–9 months)
central incisor (6–8 months)

lower teeth

b

Figure 22.7 (**a**) Permanent teeth, (**b**) deciduous teeth.

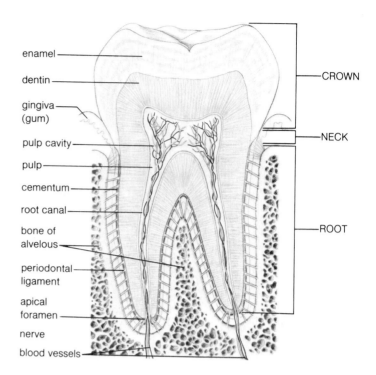

enamel
dentin
gingiva (gum)
pulp cavity
pulp
cementum
root canal
bone of alvelous
periodontal ligament
apical foramen
nerve
blood vessels

CROWN
NECK
ROOT

Figure 22.8 A longitudinal section through a tooth.

chemical constituents of saliva account for only 0.5% of the total volume; most of the remainder is water.

Amylase begins the digestion of starch. To demonstrate to yourself that starch is digested in the mouth, chew a piece of bread thoroughly and try to keep from swallowing it as long as you can. If you succeeded in keeping the bread in your mouth until it began to taste sweet, you have directly observed the effect of salivary amylase as it hydrolyzed the polysaccharide starch to smaller molecules; some disaccharides must be released from the starch for you to perceive sweetness. Though salivary amylase is capable of this degree of digestion, food is usually swallowed before amylase action is complete. In addition to mucin and amylase saliva may contain a fat-digesting enzyme (lingual lipase) and thiocyanate (SCN^-) ions, which may destroy some of the bacteria in food.

Secretion of saliva is entirely under neural control; it can be stimulated by signals from the cerebral cortex or by the presence of food in the mouth. Seeing, smelling, or thinking of food stimulate the appetite area of the hypothalamus and cause it to send efferent impulses to the salivary glands. Even nausea can trigger reflex salivation, an effect that tends to dilute irritating materials in the stomach that may have caused the nausea. Stimulation of taste buds and touch receptors on the surface of the tongue also initiates saliva production—impulses travel along afferent nerve fibers to an area of the brain at the junction of the medulla and pons from which efferent impulses stimulate salivation.

Though absorption is not a primary function of the mouth, some absorption can occur through the thin membrane beneath the tongue. Medication such as nitroglycerine (used to alleviate angina) is often administered by this route.

Hunger

Two centers in the hypothalamus—the **hunger center** and the **satiety center**—appear to regulate appetite for food under normal conditions. Stimulation of the hunger center leads to eating behavior. Stimulation of the satiety center suppresses eating behavior, apparently by inhibiting the hunger center. In experiments with animals, damage to the satiety center causes the animals to gain weight for a period of time, but their food intake eventually levels off. What remains of the hypothalamic centers then appear to maintain the new higher body weight. Such experiments suggest that the hypothalamic centers may control body weight rather than appetite.

After many hours without food stomach contractions sometimes cause painful gnawing sensations called hunger pangs. However, other mechanisms usually come into action before severe hunger pangs are felt.

Glucose concentration in the blood seems to be the most direct factor in the regulation of hunger and satiety, but insulin concentration in the cerebrospinal fluid and cholecystokinin-pancreozymin (**CCK-PZ**) concentration in the brain may also be involved. In animal experiments when the blood glucose concentration drops, feeding increases; when it rises, feeding stops. A rise in glucose is accompanied by an increase in electrical activity in the satiety center and a decrease in that activity in the hunger center. Cells in the satiety center are able to concentrate glucose, suggesting that the amount of glucose they contain may determine their activity in inhibiting the hunger center. Though CCK-PZ is involved in the regulation of digestive functions in the gut (as will be discussed later), this hormone is also found in brain tissue. Studies in mice have shown that normal mice have a higher brain concentration of CCK-PZ than obese mice. This observation suggests that CCK-PZ may also regulate feeding, with high concentrations inhibiting feeding and lower concentrations allowing feeding.

Hypothalamic obesity accounts for a very few cases of obesity. One cause of hypothalamic obesity is a tumor in the ventromedial hypothalamus, where the satiety center is located. When this center is damaged, it fails to send inhibitory signals to the hunger center. Increased food intake and weight gain result.

Certain other factors have some effect on food intake. Blood amino acids have a similar but weaker effect than glucose. Over time an increase in the quantity of adipose tissue tends to decrease feeding. Cold environments increase food intake, and warm ones decrease it. Distention of the digestive tract suppresses hunger, as does food intake itself, even when the food is removed from the digestive tract before it can be absorbed. Such removal is accomplished experimentally in animals by placing a tube from the esophagus to the outside of the body.

PHARYNX AND ESOPHAGUS

Objective 7. Describe the structure of the pharynx and the esophagus.
Objective 8. Explain the processes of swallowing and movement of food through the pharynx and esophagus.

Structure of the Pharynx and Esophagus

The pharynx, located behind the soft palate, is divided into the **nasopharynx**, an air passage from the nasal cavity, the **oropharynx**, posterior to the base of the tongue, and the **laryngopharynx**, near the larynx. These structures were described in Chapter 21. In addition to serving as a passageway for air to and from the lungs, the pharynx is also a passageway for food from the oral cavity to the esophagus.

Extending from the pharynx to the stomach is the **esophagus**, essentially a muscular tube. The walls of the esophagus are similar to the general plan of the digestive tract except that the portion near the pharynx contains skeletal muscle, the middle portion contains both skeletal and smooth muscle, and the lower portion contains only smooth muscle. The entire lining consists of stratified squamous epithelium. Mucus is the only secretion of the esophagus, so no digestion is initiated while the food is in the esophagus. Most of the 25 centimeter length of the esophagus lies behind the trachea, where it is covered by connective tissue

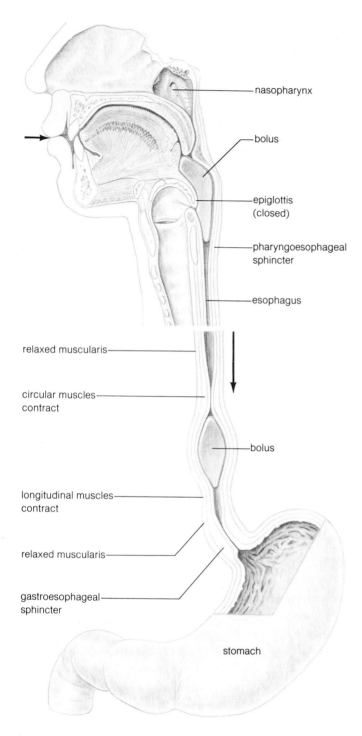

nasopharynx

bolus

epiglottis
(closed)

pharyngoesophageal
sphincter

esophagus

relaxed muscularis

circular muscles
contract

bolus

longitudinal muscles
contract

relaxed muscularis

gastroesophageal
sphincter

stomach

Figure 22.9 The movement of food during swallowing and passage down the esophagus.

called **adventitia**. After the esophagus passes through the diaphragm, it is covered by serosa continuous with the peritoneum. The **pharyngoesophageal** and the **gastroesophageal sphincters** constrict the esophagus at the upper and lower ends, respectively. The latter is a *functional* sphincter; it contains some muscle and can contract to close the esophagus, but it lacks the well-differentiated muscular band seen in *anatomical* sphincters.

Swallowing

Swallowing, or **deglutition**, depends on intact neural mechanisms. It is initiated as the tongue voluntarily forces a bolus of food into the pharynx. The remainder of the swallowing process is essentially involuntary and automatic. In the pharynx the food stimulates swallowing receptors along the inner surface. These receptors send impulses to the swallowing center in the brainstem, which stimulates a series of pharyngeal muscle contractions. The soft palate is elevated to close the nasal passages. The **epiglottis** covers the opening of the larynx, the **glottis**, so food cannot enter the respiratory tract. The pharyngoesophageal sphincter, which normally remains closed to keep air from entering the esophagus during respiration, relaxes, and a wave of peristalsis propels the bolus into the esophagus. This entire process takes only one or two seconds, a fortunate situation because breathing is temporarily arrested while food passes through the pharynx.

Movement of Food in the Esophagus

The esophagus functions solely to conduct food to the stomach. The primary peristaltic wave that propelled the bolus into the esophagus continues all the way to the stomach, pushing the bolus of food along in front of it. The wave of relaxation that precedes a peristaltic contraction relaxes the gastroesophageal sphincter as well as other areas of the esophagus and hastens the movement of the bolus. Passage of the bolus through the esophagus takes less than ten seconds and often requires only the primary peristaltic contraction. Localized secondary contractions within the esophagus can occur if the esophagus becomes distended by the bolus. After the bolus passes through the area of the gastroesophageal sphincter, the sphincter closes again. It normally remains closed except during the passage of food or during vomiting. By remaining closed, it prevents the regurgitation of the highly acid contents of the stomach. Figure 22.9 shows the process of swallowing and subsequent movement of food down the esophagus.

STOMACH

Objective 9. Describe the macroscopic and microscopic anatomy of the stomach.

Objective 10. Describe how the following processes occur in the stomach and explain how each is regulated: (a) storage, mixing, and emptying; (b) secretion; (c) digestion; and (d) absorption.

Anatomy of the Stomach

Macroscopic anatomy   The **stomach** is a hollow, J-shaped organ lying between the esophagus and the small intestine (Figure 22.10). It has a greater and a lesser curvature and several anatomical regions. The **cardiac region** lies adjacent to the point at which the esophagus enters the stomach. The **fundus** extends superiorly from the cardiac region. The main part of the stomach is the **body**, and the narrow portion nearest the small intestine is the **pylorus**. The **pyloric sphincter** separates the stomach from the small intestine. Internally, the mucosa is thrown into folds called **rugae**.

Microscopic anatomy   The layers of the stomach wall follow the general plan of the digestive tract, except as noted later in Table 22.2. The epithelium consists of a single layer of columnar cells interrupted by millions of **gastric pits**, which open into the **gastric glands**. Four kinds of cells are found in the gastric glands (Figure 22.11). In the upper portion of the gland are the **mucous neck cells**, which produce mucus. Deeper in the gland are the **chief cells**, which produce enzymes; the **parietal cells**, which produce hydrochloric acid and intrinsic factor (a substance to be discussed later); and the **argentaffin cells**, which may produce serotonin and histamine. In the pyloric region of the stomach the gastric glands are replaced by pyloric glands that secrete mucus of a particularly viscous and alkaline nature. G-cells in the pyloric region synthesize, store, and secrete the hormone **gastrin**.

Storage, Mixing, and Emptying

The stomach may store as much as 1 liter of food for four to six hours. When food is present, gentle, mixing waves of contraction agitate gastric secretions and food particles lying next to the mucosa. Stronger peristaltic waves propel the mixture toward the pylorus. In the pylorus the mixing contractions are stronger and the food mixture more fluid than in the body, so by the time the mixture reaches the pyloric sphincter, it is semifluid in consistency. This semi-

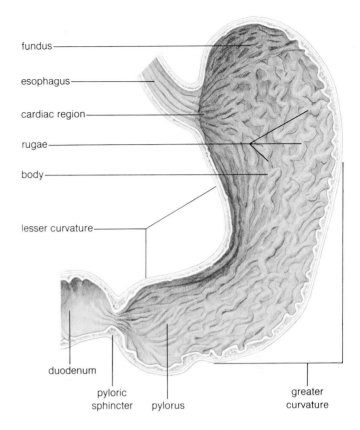

Figure 22.10   Macroscopic anatomy of the stomach.

fluid mixture of food and digestive secretions is called **chyme**.

The pyloric sphincter usually remains closed until the relaxation that precedes a peristaltic contraction causes it to open. Each time the sphincter opens, several milliliters of chyme enter the small intestine.

A variety of factors are involved in regulating the emptying of the stomach. Distention of the stomach stimulates afferent fibers of the vagus nerve, which carry signals to the medulla. Efferent signals from the medulla by way of the vagus nerve stimulate mixing and peristaltic contractions as well as the secretion of digestive juices. Distention of the stomach also stimulates stretch receptors that increase peristaltic movements and cause faster emptying. When protein is present in the stomach, it stimulates the release of gastrin. Though, as will be explained later, this hormone is influential primarily in regulating digestive secretions, it also stimulates peristalsis. Several other hormones—CCK-

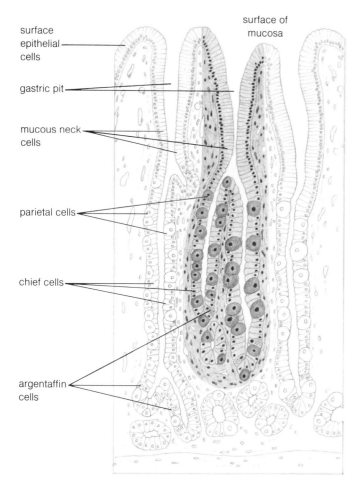

surface
epithelial
cells

gastric pit

mucous neck
cells

parietal cells

chief cells

argentaffin
cells

surface of
mucosa

Figure 22.11 Microscopic anatomy of a gastric gland.

PZ, **secretin**, gastric inhibitory peptide (**GIP**), and vasoactive intestinal peptide (**VIP**)—have been shown to reduce gastric motility. However, their precise physiological role in the regulation of gastric motility remains to be determined.

Other factors are important in slowing stomach emptying. A neural reflex, the **enterogastric reflex**, sends a signal from the duodenum back to the stomach when the chyme in the duodenum is excessively acid (below pH 4) or contains large amounts of fat. This signal slows peristaltic activity of the stomach and slows or even stops the flow of chyme until digestive juices in the duodenum have neutralized the chyme and digested some of the fat. This reflex also operates when the duodenum is distended or irritated or the chyme is excessively hypertonic or hypotonic. It helps to regulate the flow of chyme into the small intestine to allow the intestine to efficiently process its contents.

Secretion

The secretory activities of the stomach are particularly interesting because they create conditions that could digest the stomach itself if they were not properly regulated.

As mentioned above, the gastric glands contain several types of cells, among which are the parietal cells that produce hydrochloric acid (HCl). The mechanism of HCl manufacture is not completely understood, but the following steps are thought to be involved (Figure 22.12). Water ionizes to form H^+ and OH^-. Chloride ions (Cl^-) diffuse from the interstitial fluids into the parietal cells. At the same time, CO_2 enters the parietal cells, where in the presence of carbonic anhydrase it combines with water to form carbonic acid, H_2CO_3. H_2CO_3 partially ionizes, forming bicarbonate ions (HCO_3^-) and H^+. The HCO_3^- returns to the interstitial fluid, correcting the electrical imbalance created by the entry of Cl^-. The H^+ from the ionization of carbonic acid combines with OH^- from the ionization of water and reforms some water molecules. Both the H^+ and Cl^- are actively transported in a coupled reaction across the membrane of the parietal cell into small passageways called canaliculi ("little canals") that extend into the parietal cells. The ions are released from the canaliculi into the lumen of the stomach. Only a small quantity of water is added to the ionized HCl, and it reaches the lumen at a pH of 0.8. The functions of HCl are to activate acid-dependent enzymes and to kill mircroorganisms that have reached the stomach.

The gastric glands also contain chief cells that produce enzymes. Though chief cells produce small quantities of **gastric amylase** and **lipase**, these enzymes contribute little to digestion in the stomach. Amylase action is inhibited by the highly acid condition, and gastric lipase acts only on butterfat. **Pepsin**, the main enzyme secreted by the chief cells, accounts for the major digestive acitvity of the stomach. Pepsin is a proteolytic enzyme that hydrolyzes large protein molecules into smaller molecules. It is produced in an inactive form, **pepsinogen**, and is activated by an acidity of pH 2 or by previously activated pepsin. Once active pepsin is produced, its action must be limited to digesting food proteins—and not the proteins of the stomach cells themselves. To prevent such digestion, the action of pepsin is limited by (1) the presence of mucus, (2) the structure of the mucosa itself, and (3) regulation of the secretion of hydrochloric acid and pepsin, as explained in the following paragraphs.

Mucus is produced by mucous neck cells of the gastric

glands, by the pyloric glands, and by individual cells of the mucosa. Thus, the entire gastric mucosa is protected by a film of mucus. The mucus produced by the pyloric glands is especially viscous and more alkaline than that produced by most other mucus-secreting cells. It provides special protection for the pyloric portion of the stomach, where the most acid chyme accumulates.

The epithelial cells of the mucosa fit together tightly so that it is difficult for acid to seep from the lumen back into the mucosa. Thus, another barrier to digestion of the stomach is created.

Regulation of gastric secretions   Gastric secretions are regulated by a multiplicity of interacting factors. These factors will be considered in three categories: cephalic, gastric, and intestinal.

Cephalic factors affecting gastric secretions are induced by activities of the central nervous system and are mediated by way of signals in the vagus nerve. The presence of food in the mouth or the sight or smell of food stimulates centers in the brain, such as the limbic system and the hypothalamus, ultimately initiating signals in the vagus nerve that stimulate gastric secretions. Anger and excitement tend to amplify these signals; fear and depression tend to inhibit them.

Gastric factors that affect gastric secretions are primarily local, though food in the stomach accelerates the activities of the central nervous system as described above. Food in the stomach also stimulates mechanical and chemical receptors in the stomach wall. These receptors relay signals to the submucosal plexus, which in turn relays signals to the parietal cells, causing them to secrete acid. The presence of **secretagogues** (substances such as partially digested proteins, alcohol, and caffeine) in the stomach stimulates the release of gastrin. Gastrin, being a hormone, is secreted not into the lumen of the stomach but into the blood, where it is carried to the gastric glands. Here, it stimulates the parietal cells to secrete HCl. When the acidity of the stomach contents falls below pH 2, gastrin release is inhibited. This negative feedback mechanism is important in regulating stomach acidity and therefore also in preventing digestion of the stomach itself.

Intestinal factors act from the small intestine and operate by feedback to regulate gastric function. When chyme enters the intestine, it contains acid, fat, and protein breakdown products, and may contain irritating substances or hyperosmotic or hyposmotic fluids. The presence of any of these substances stimulates certain cells of the intestinal mucosa to release the hormones secretin, CCK-PZ, GIP, and possibly others too. CCK-PZ inhibits gastric

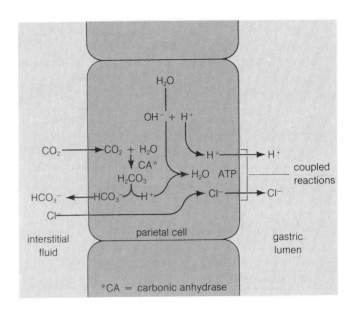

Figure 22.12   The formation of hydrochloric acid in the parietal cells of the gastric mucosa.

motility, and GIP inhibits the secretion of gastric acid. Distention or the presence of acid in the duodenum initiates the enterogastric reflex, which, in addition to suppressing stomach motility as described earlier, also inhibits gastric secretion.

Digestion and Absorption

The main digestive process in the stomach is the hydrolysis of proteins into long chains of amino acids by the action of pepsin. A less significant process is the digestion of butterfat. Even though only a small proportion of the total digestive process occurs in the stomach, the mixing of food particles with digestive juices to produce the semifluid chyme prepares for more digestion in the small intestine.

Like digestion, absorption too is quite limited in the stomach. Only alcohol, aspirin, and some lipid-soluble drugs are passively absorbed in the stomach. The relatively thick mucous coating of the stomach mucosa interferes with absorption. The processes that occur in the stomach and their regulatory mechanisms are summarized in Figure 22.13.

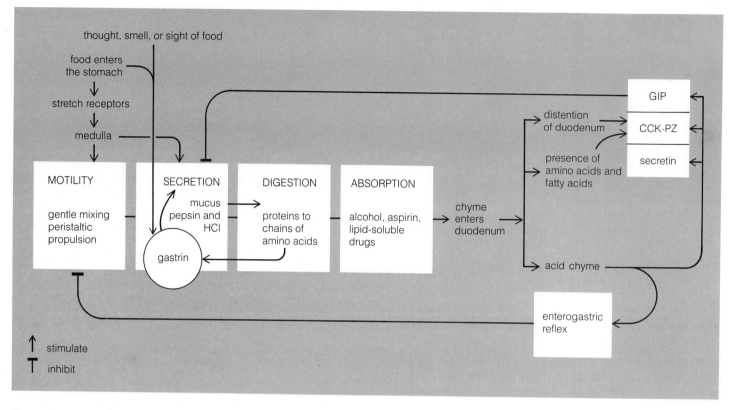

Figure 22.13 Processes that occur in the stomach and how they are regulated.

LIVER AND PANCREAS

Objective 11. Describe the macroscopic and microscopic anatomy of the liver and the gallbladder.

Objective 12. Explain the role of the liver in the digestive process, including the synthesis and functions of bile.

Objective 13. Describe the macroscopic and microscopic anatomy of the pancreas.

Objective 14. Explain how the digestive secretions of the pancreas are produced.

Objective 15. Explain how the functions of the liver and the pancreas are regulated.

Food passes from the stomach directly to the small intestine. However, because the functions of the liver and the pancreas are extremely important in the functioning of the small intestine, these two organs will be discussed first.

Anatomy of the Liver

Macroscopic anatomy The **liver** occupies the upper right quadrant of the abdominal cavity just below the diaphragm (see Figure 22.1). The second largest organ in the body, the liver weighs about 1.4 kilograms and is divided into two main lobes. The **right** and **left lobes** are separated by the **falciform ligament**, a membrane that is continuous with the peritoneum. Attached to the falciform ligament is the **round ligament**, a fibrous cord of connective tissue that extends from the liver to the umbilicus and represents the remains of the fetal umbilical vein. Seen from the inferior side, the right lobe of the liver has two smaller lobes: the posterior **caudate lobe** and the inferior **quadrate lobe**. Also visible on the inferior surface are the gallbladder, common bile duct, hepatic portal vein, hepatic artery, and inferior vena cava (Figure 22.14).

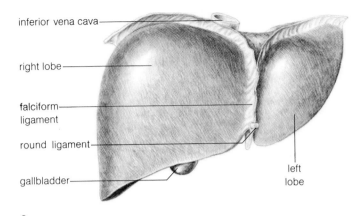

inferior vena cava

right lobe

falciform ligament

round ligament

gallbladder

left lobe

a

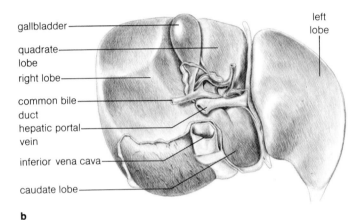

left lobe

gallbladder

quadrate lobe

right lobe

common bile duct

hepatic portal vein

inferior vena cava

caudate lobe

b

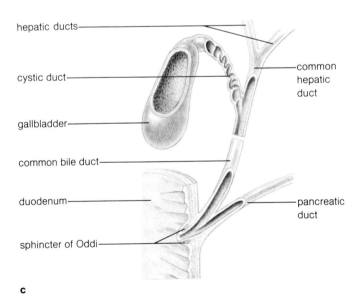

hepatic ducts

cystic duct

gallbladder

common bile duct

duodenum

sphincter of Oddi

common hepatic duct

pancreatic duct

c

Figure 22.14 Macroscopic anatomy of the liver and gallbladder:(**a**) the anterior surface of the liver, (**b**) the inferior surface of the liver and gallbladder, (**c**) the bile ducts.

Microscopic anatomy Within the liver are numerous functional units called **lobules** (Figure 22.15). Each lobule is cylindrical in shape, about 2 millimeters in diameter, and completely surrounded by connective tissue. From the **central vein** in the center of the lobule, cords of liver cells radiate out in all directions. In the spaces between these cords of cells are **sinusoids**, wide capillarylike blood vessels lined with endothelial cells and **Kupffer cells**. Kupffer cells are phagocytic cells that remove bacteria and foreign substances from the blood coming to the liver from the intestine. Around the periphery of each lobule are five to seven clusters of vessels called the **portal triads**. Each triad includes a branch of the **hepatic portal vein**, **hepatic artery**, and **interlobular bile duct**, which receives bile from liver cells by way of bile canaliculi.

Blood enters the liver from two sources, the hepatic artery and the hepatic portal vein. Blood in the hepatic artery, which comes from the aorta, has recently passed through the lungs and heart and carries oxygen to the liver cells. It also carries fats received from the lymphatics. Blood in the hepatic portal vein comes directly from the intestine and carries blood laden with other nutrients. Blood from both the arterial and venous sources passes from vessels in the triads through the sinusoids of the liver and eventually reaches the central vein of each lobule. Blood from the central veins is carried to the hepatic vein and finally to the inferior vena cava.

The cells of the liver secrete small quantities of bile into minute canaliculi that carry the bile to the interlobular bile ducts in the triads. These ducts unite to form the left and right **hepatic ducts**, which in turn unite to form the **common hepatic duct**. The common hepatic duct joins the **cystic duct** from the gallbladder to form the **common bile duct**. This duct, which joins the pancreatic duct, carries bile to the duodenum. When the **sphincter of Oddi** at the end of the common bile duct is closed, some of the bile is conveyed along the cystic duct and stored in the gallbladder. The bile ducts are shown in Figure 22.14c.

Gallbladder

The **gallbladder** is a small pear-shaped organ attached to the ventral surface of the liver. It has an epithelial lining and a muscular wall. As bile enters the gallbladder, some of the water in it is reabsorbed so that the bile becomes five to twelve times as concentrated as when it is secreted. In addition to concentrating bile the main function of the gallbladder is to store bile until it is needed after meals for the emulsification of fats.

Bile and Its Functions

Bile is a solution consisting of water, bile salts, cholesterol, bile pigments, and certain other lipids and electrolytes. Bile salts are synthesized in the liver from cholesterol through a sequence of reactions, forming the primary bile acids cholic and chenodeoxycholic acids. These bile acids are combined with either the amino acid glycine or the amino acid derivative taurine. This combination is called a conjugated bile acid. The terms bile salts and bile acids are used interchangeably; a bile salt is simply a bile acid that has lost a hydrogen ion and gained a sodium or potassium ion.

Bile salts travel with the bile to the small intestine, where they help to emulsify fats. (Emulsification will be explained in the discussion of the small intestine.) In the intestine some bile salts are deconjugated—they lose the glycine or taurine attached to them earlier—and are reabsorbed and returned to the liver. The bile pigments biliverdin and bilirubin are breakdown products of hemoglobin from worn out erythrocytes. They have no digestive function and are merely transported in the bile to the small intestine, where they can be excreted. **Jaundice**, a yellowing of the skin that results from the accumulation of bilirubin in the extracellular fluids, may be caused by excessive destruction of erythrocytes, damage to liver cells, or obstruction of bile ducts. Lipids found in bile include cholesterol, fatty acids, and a phospholipid called lecithin. Lecithin and bile salts help to keep the cholesterol in solution and prevent it from depositing in the gallbladder as a gallstone. Electrolytes found in bile are similar to those found in plasma.

In addition to secreting bile the liver has many other functions. They are summarized in Table 22.1.

Anatomy of the Pancreas

Macroscopic anatomy   The pancreas (Figure 22.16) is a soft, glandular organ about 2.5 centimeters wide and 12 to 15 centimeters long, located posterior to the stomach. The head region of the pancreas fits into the curve of the duodenum just below the stomach. To the left of the head are the body and tail regions of the pancreas. The **pancreatic duct**, or the **duct of Wirsung**, is formed from smaller ducts within the pancreas; it carries **pancreatic juice**, the digestive secretions of the pancreas, to the duodenum. Typically, the pancreatic duct joins the common bile duct, and the two enter the duodenum together at the **ampulla of Vater**.

Microscopic anatomy   Clusters of cells, the **acini**, empty their secretions into tiny tubules, as shown in Figure 15.26

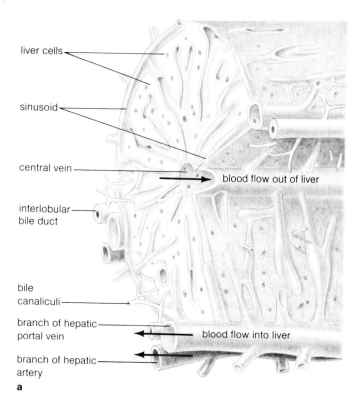

liver cells

sinusoid

central vein

blood flow out of liver

interlobular bile duct

bile canaliculi

branch of hepatic portal vein

blood flow into liver

branch of hepatic artery

a

Figure 22.15   Microscopic anatomy of the liver: (**a**) diagram, (**b**) photomicrograph, × 20. (Photograph by author) (**c**) photomicrograph, × 104. (Reprinted by permission from *Tissues and organs: A text-atlas of scanning electron microscopy* by Richard G. Kessel and Randy H. Kardon. W. H. Freeman and Company. Copyright © 1979.)

(Chapter 15). These tubules join to form larger ducts and eventually unite to form the pancreatic duct. Cells of the acini secrete enzymes, and cells of the tubules secrete water and bicarbonate ions. Other characteristics of the pancreas have been described in Chapter 15.

Pancreatic Secretions

Pancreatic juice contains enzymes capable of digesting each of the major nutrients. Among these enzymes are three **proteolytic enzymes**, each of which is secreted from the acinar cells and transported in an inactive form. These enzymes—**trypsinogen**, **chymotrypsinogen**, and **procarboxypeptidase**—therefore travel through the ducts to the duodenum without digesting the proteins of the ducts. In the duodenum an intestinal enzyme, **enterokinase**, activates trypsinogen to trypsin. Trypsin, in turn, activates chymotrypsinogen to chymotrypsin and procarboxypeptidase to carboxypeptidase. The combined actions of these proteolytic enzymes produce dipeptides and small polypep-

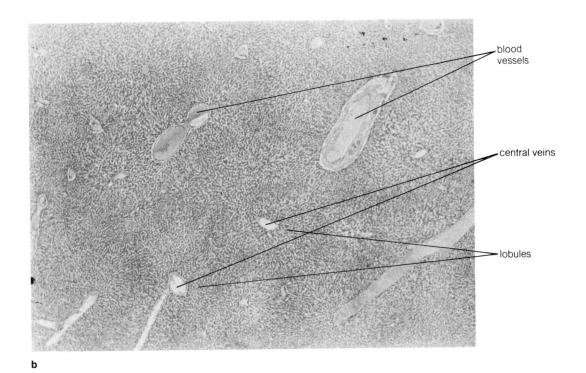

blood vessels

central veins

lobules

b

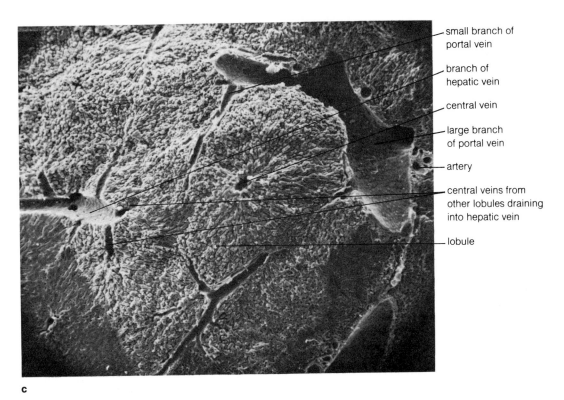

small branch of portal vein

branch of hepatic vein

central vein

large branch of portal vein

artery

central veins from other lobules draining into hepatic vein

lobule

c

Table 22.1   Functions of the Liver
Carbohydrate Metabolism
Glycogenesis—the removal of glucose from the blood after a meal and the storage of glucose in glycogen
Glycogenolysis—the conversion of glycogen back to glucose for release into the blood when the glucose concentration drops between meals
Gluconeogenesis—the synthesis of glucose from noncarbohydrate nutrients as occurs when the glucose and glycogen supplies are depleted
Fat Metabolism
Synthesis of cholesterol, the precursor of all steroids in the body
Synthesis of phospholipids used in growth and repair of cells
Synthesis of lipoproteins, carrier molecules by which lipids are transported to other cells for energy and to adipose cells for storage
Protein Metabolism
Synthesis of plasma proteins
Deamination of amino acids and the production of ammonia
Other Synthetic Functions
Synthesis of urea, a nitrogenous waste product that is formed in part from ammonia released by deamination
Synthesis of several factors that are essential for the clotting of blood
Detoxification of toxic substances, usually by the addition of some chemical substance rendering the toxic substances less harmful
Decomposition of Hemoglobin from Worn-out Erythrocytes
Storage Functions
Storage of a year's supply of vitamin A, several months' supply of vitamin D, and several years' supply of vitamin B_{12}
Combination of iron with the liver protein **apoferritin** for later use in the synthesis of hemoglobin

Individual variations in the pattern of pancreatic ducts are not uncommon; they have no significant effect on function. Some individuals have separate pancreatic and bile ducts entering the duodenum; others may have a second pancreatic duct, the **duct of Santorini**, emptying into the duodenum about 2 centimeters nearer the stomach than the main duct, which enters about 10 centimeters below the pylorus. Some individuals have both these modifications.

tides ready for final digestion by the intracellular enzymes of the intestinal epithelium (Figure 22.17). Other enzymes from the pancreas include pancreatic amylase, pancreatic lipase, cholesterol esterase, ribonuclease, and deoxyribonuclease. The actions of these enzymes will be discussed later.

In addition to the enzymes produced by acinar cells, the tubule cells secrete water and bicarbonate ions in amounts that depend on the degree of stimulation received by the pancreas. Strong stimuli are produced when the acidity of the duodenum drops below a pH of 4. Bicarbonate is released until the acid is neutralized. The actions of the enzymes, water, and bicarbonate are summarized in Figure 22.18.

Regulation of the Function of the Liver and Pancreas

Functions of the liver and pancreas are regulated by nervous and hormonal stimuli. The same parasympathetic stimuli that act on the stomach also stimulate enzyme production in the pancreas. However, hormonal stimulation is necessary for the release of the enzymes.

Two hormones, **secretin** and **CCK-PZ** (*cholecystokinin-pancreozymin*) regulate the functions of the liver and pancreas and coordinate their activities with those of the digestive tract itself. Both hormones are produced by epithelial cells in the duodenum in response to the presence of chyme. They travel through the blood to the liver and pancreas, where they exert their effects.

Secretin stimulates the production of bile in the liver and the production of water and bicarbonate ions in the pancreas. The acidity of chyme is a particularly strong stimulator of secretin release, and the more acid the chyme, the greater the quantity of secretin released. As bicarbonate

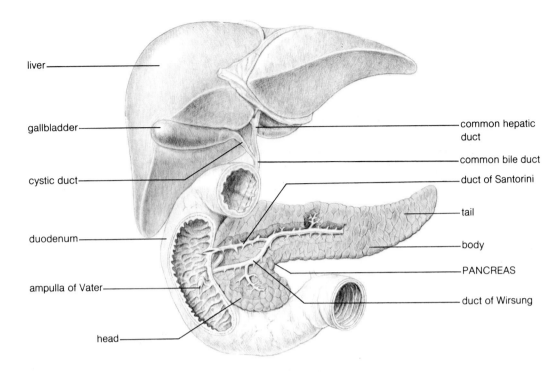

liver

gallbladder

cystic duct

duodenum

ampulla of Vater

head

common hepatic duct

common bile duct

duct of Santorini

tail

body

PANCREAS

duct of Wirsung

Figure 22.16 Macroscopic anatomy of the pancreas and its ducts.

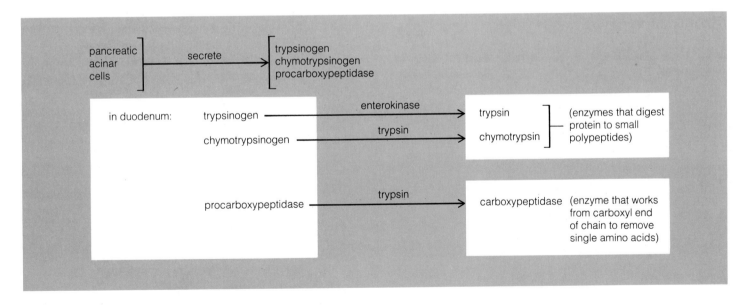

pancreatic acinar cells — secrete → trypsinogen, chymotrypsinogen, procarboxypeptidase

in duodenum:

trypsinogen — enterokinase → trypsin

chymotrypsinogen — trypsin → chymotrypsin

(enzymes that digest protein to small polypeptides)

procarboxypeptidase — trypsin → carboxypeptidase (enzyme that works from carboxyl end of chain to remove single amino acids)

Figure 22.17 Pancreatic proteolytic enzymes.

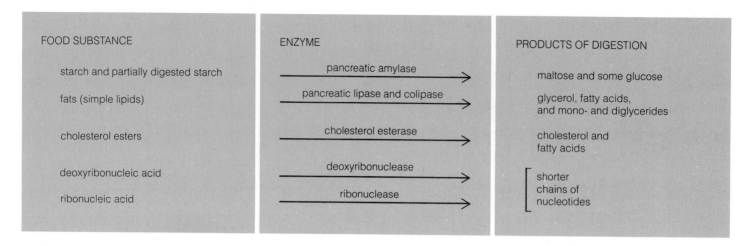

Figure 22.18 Actions of other pancreatic enzymes.

reaches the duodenum, it neutralizes the acid, and because of the reduced acidity secretin release is decreased.

As its name suggests CCK-PZ has two main functions. The word cholecystokinin is derived from three roots: *chol* meaning bile, *cyst* meaning bladder, and *kinin* meaning to move. Thus, cholecystokinin stimulates the movement of bile from the gallbladder. When the hormone reaches the gallbladder, it causes the muscular wall of the gallbladder and its duct to contract rhythmically. Peristaltic waves push bile along the bile duct and relax the sphincter of Oddi, allowing bile to enter the small intestine. The word pancreozymin is derived from pancreas and *zymin*, which means enzyme producer. Thus, pancreozymin stimulates the secretion of pancreatic enzymes. The actions of cholecystokinin and pancreozymin were discovered independently. Subsequently, it was discovered that a single hormone produced both effects.

Both secretin and CCK-PZ augment the effect of the other. Thus, their combined effects are much greater than the effect of either hormone alone.

SMALL INTESTINE

Objective 16. Describe the macroscopic and microscopic anatomy of the small intestine.

Objective 17. Describe how the following processes occur in the small intestine and explain how each is regulated: (a) motility, (b) secretion, (c) digestion, and (d) absorption.

Anatomy of the Small Intestine

Macroscopic anatomy The small intestine is a tubular organ averaging about 2.5 centimeters in diameter and extending from the pyloric end of the stomach to the beginning of the large intestine (see Figure 22.1). The many loops and coils of the small intestine fill a large portion of the abdominal cavity. The length of the small intestine during life is about 3 meters, though in a cadaver it may appear twice as long because of the relaxation of the longitudinal muscle in the intestinal wall.

The small intestine is divided into three regions, the **duodenum**, **jejunum**, and **ileum**. The duodenum, the region nearest the stomach, is about 25 centimeters long. It receives chyme from the stomach and also the secretions from the liver and pancreas. The next two-fifths of the length (about 120 centimeters) of the small intestine is jejunum; the remainder is ileum (about 160 centimeters). Both the jejunum and the ileum are suspended by mesentery.

Microscopic anatomy The layers of the wall of the small intestine follow closely the general plan of the digestive tract. The mucosa contains many **intestinal glands**, the **crypts of Lieberkühn**, that secrete digestive enzymes. In the duodenum the **Brunner's glands** of the submucosa secrete mucus that lubricates the mucosa. In the remainder of the small intestine goblet cells in the mucosa secrete the mucus needed for lubrication.

The entire small intestine is characterized by the presence of **plicae circulares**, circular folds of the submucosa.

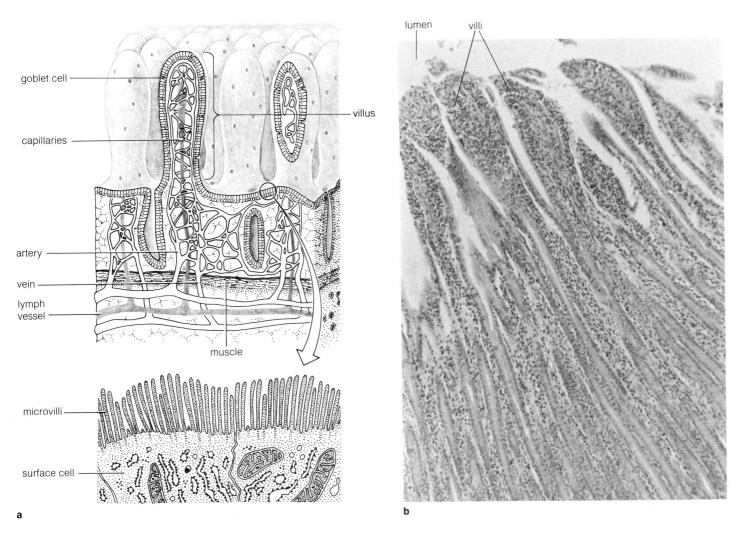

Figure 22.19 Microscopic anatomy of the villi: (**a**) diagram, (**b**) photomicrograph of cross section through villi, × 104. (Photograph by author.)

These folds are most pronounced in the jejunum. **Peyer's patches**, aggregates of lymphatic tissue in the submucosa, are a distinguishing characteristic of the ileum, though less conspicuous lymph nodes are found throughout the small intestine.

The most functionally significant modification of the basic plan of the small intestine is the presence of villi, fingerlike projections of the mucosa that are present throughout the small intestine (Figure 22.19). The villi increase the surface area of the small intestine by about ten times. In addition, each villus is covered with a layer of epithelial cells, each cell of which has about 600 microvilli. The microvilli, which give the cell the appearance of having a brush border, increase the surface area by another twenty times. The plicae circulares account for another threefold increase in the surface area of the small intestine. Because the primary function of the small intestine is the absorption of nutrients, the surface area available for absorption is important. The total absorptive area of the small intestine is about 250 square meters, comparable to the area of three lanes of a 50 meter swimming pool or about one-tenth of the area of a football field.

Within each villus, imbedded in a core of connective tissue, are blood capillaries, a **lacteal** (lymph capillary), and a nerve fiber. The proximity of the blood and lymph capillaries to the epithelial cells of the mucosa is important in the process of absorption.

Motility

Motility in the small intestine serves both to propel and to mix the chyme. Peristaltic contractions, which propel the chyme, are initiated when the wall is stretched. Stretch receptors relay signals to the myenteric plexus and cause the **myenteric reflex**. In this reflex circular smooth muscle contracts behind the point of stimulation and pushes the chyme toward the large intestine at the rate of about 1 centimeter per minute. (Refer back to Figure 22.5.) Relaxation of the smooth muscle in front of the point of stimulation may or may not occur. **Segmentation contractions** mix the chyme and increase its exposure to the surface of the mucosa. These ringlike contractions occur at regular intervals along the gut. As one set of contractions subsides, another set appears at intervals between the first ones, creating a chopping action.

When chyme reaches the terminal ileum, distention of the ileum causes the ileocecal valve (a constriction between the ileum and the cecum) to relax, thereby allowing segmentation contractions and peristaltic movements to push the chyme into the large intestine. The enterogastric reflex can increase both motility and secretion in the small intestine, but it is especially important in moving chyme through the ileocecal valve. This reflex, initiated by the presence of food in the stomach, forces chyme from the previous meal out of the small intestine.

Contraction of the muscularis mucosa, which has fibers extending into the villi, causes the villi to move intermittently. These contractions help to keep the lymph moving in the lacteals and also agitate the fluids around the villi, thereby increasing the rate of absorption. **Villikinin**, a hormone from the mucosa of the small intestine, stimulates motility of the villi.

Secretions

Secretions found in the small intestine come not only from the liver and the pancreas but also from the intestinal epithelium itself. Mucus is secreted by Brunner's glands and goblet cells. The epithelial cells on the surface and in the crypts of Lieberkühn secrete the enzyme enterokinase, which activates trypsin, and also a small amount of a weak amylase. These epithelial cells are constantly being sloughed into the lumen and being replaced by new cells. As the sloughed cells rupture, other enzymes—the mucosal enzymes described below—are also released. Chyme containing a high concentration of solutes causes cells in the crypts of Lieberkühn to secrete about 2000 milliliters per day of a fluid of neutral pH similar to extracellular fluid. This fluid dilutes the chyme and provides a watery medium for the absorption of digested substances. However, more than this amount of fluid is absorbed from the small intestine daily, some coming from the food, so the net movement of fluid is toward the blood and lymph and away from the intestinal lumen.

Mucosal enzymes In addition to the enzymes secreted into the lumen of the small intestine, cells of the intestinal epithelium produce several enzymes that act to digest substances as they pass through the cell in the process of being absorbed. These enzymes include peptidases that digest polypeptides to amino acids; and sucrase, maltase, and lactase, which digest specific disaccharides to monosaccharides.

Regulation of secretion The regulation of secretion in the small intestine is accomplished mostly by the presence of chyme. Its presence creates mechanical and chemical stimuli that cause the crypts of Lieberkühn to produce large volumes of fluid. The presence of chyme also stimulates Brunner's glands to secrete mucus. A hormone, vasoactive intestinal peptide (VIP), stimulates the intestinal secretion of electrolytes (various ions). Water follows the electrolytes by osmosis, allowing more nutrients to dissolve.

Digestion

Digestion in the small intestine is accomplished to a great extent by enzymes produced by the pancreas and is assisted by bile salts. Because of the highly acid quality of the chyme entering the small intestine and the fact that digestive enzymes that act in the small intestine operate at or near neutral pH, the chyme must be neutralized before digestion begins. Bicarbonate contained in the alkaline secretion of the pancreas neutralizes the chyme and stops the action of pepsin. The large quantity of neutral fluid from the crypts of Lieberkühn also dilutes the chyme.

Digestion of carbohydrates in the small intestine begins with the action of enzymes on starch, partially digested starch molecules, and disaccharides that arrive in the small intestine. **Pancreatic amylase**, which is similar to salivary amylase, digests all of the undigested and partially digested

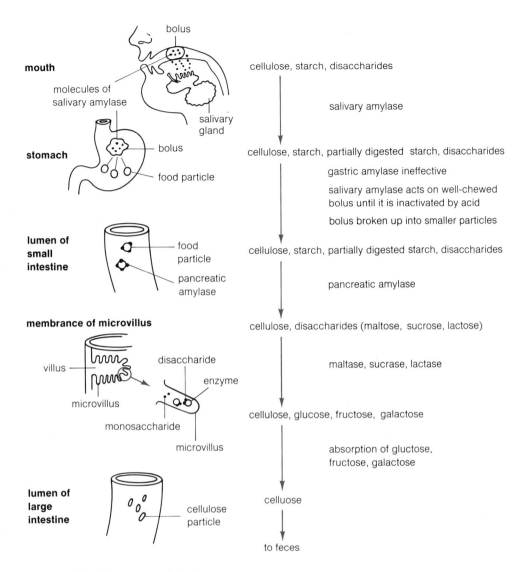

mouth
bolus
molecules of
salivary amylase
salivary
gland

stomach
bolus
food particle

**lumen of
small
intestine**
food
particle
pancreatic
amylase

membrane of microvillus
villus
microvillus
disaccharide
enzyme
monosaccharide
microvillus

**lumen of
large
intestine**
cellulose
particle

cellulose, starch, disaccharides

salivary amylase

cellulose, starch, partially digested starch, disaccharides

gastric amylase ineffective

salivary amylase acts on well-chewed
bolus until it is inactivated by acid

bolus broken up into smaller particles

cellulose, starch, partially digested starch, disaccharides

pancreatic amylase

cellulose, disaccharides (maltose, sucrose, lactose)

maltase, sucrase, lactase

cellulose, glucose, fructose, galactose

absorption of gluctose,
fructose, galactose

celluose

to feces

Figure 22.20   Digestion of carbohydrates.

starch to the disaccharide maltose, completing the digestion begun by the salivary amylase. Cellular enzymes from the intestinal epithelial cells complete the digestion of disaccharides to monosaccharides. These enzymes, located in the microvilli of the epithelial cells, act on the disaccharides as the disaccharides come in contact with the cell membrane. **Maltase** hydrolyzes maltose into two molecules of glucose, **lactase** hydrolyzes lactose into glucose and galactose, and **sucrase** hydrolyzes sucrose into glucose and fructose. Carbohydrates are thus completely broken down into monosaccharides and ready to be absorbed. The digestion of carbohydrates is summarized in Figure 22.20.

Proteins enter the small intestine as long chains of amino acids produced by the action of pepsin in the stomach. After the action of pepsin is stopped by the neutralization of the chyme, other proteolytic enzymes take over. The pancreatic enzymes trypsin, chymotrypsin, and carboxypeptidase digest chains of amino acids to smaller units, some of which are individual amino acids. The **dipeptidases** and **aminopolypeptidases** of the cells of the intestinal epithelium act on the remaining dipeptides and small polypeptides to complete the digestion to individual amino acids. The digestion of proteins is summarized in Figure 22.21.

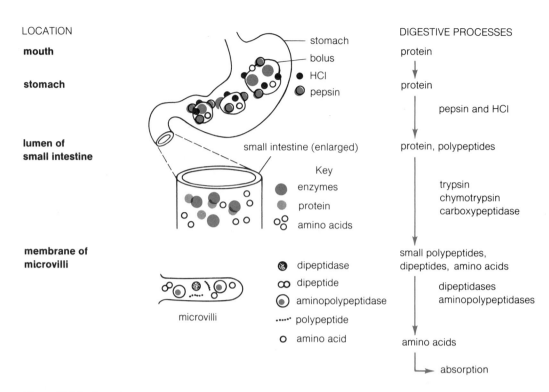

LOCATION

mouth

stomach

**lumen of
small intestine**

**membrane of
microvilli**

microvilli

Key

🔴 enzymes

🟢 protein

∞ amino acids

DIGESTIVE PROCESSES

protein
↓
protein
　　　　pepsin and HCl
↓
protein, polypeptides

　　　　trypsin
　　　　chymotrypsin
　　　　carboxypeptidase
↓
small polypeptides,
dipeptides, amino acids
　　　　dipeptidases
　　　　aminopolypeptidases
↓
amino acids
↓
absorption

🔴 dipeptidase

∞ dipeptide

◉ aminopolypeptidase

····· polypeptide

○ amino acid

Figure 22.21 Digestion of proteins.

Digestion of fats takes place almost entirely in the small intestine. Except for the small amount of butterfat that can be digested in the stomach, fats enter the small intestine in undigested form. Before their digestion can begin, they must be rendered soluble in the watery medium of the

In many humans (and most other animals) lactase activity is high at birth, declines in childhood, and remains low in adulthood. Such low lactase activity is associated with lactose intolerance, the inability to digest lactose (the sugar in milk). However, most Western Europeans and their descendants retain lactase activity in adulthood. In the United States 20% of the white population and 70% of the black population are unable to digest lactose. By avoiding milk and milk products or adding a preparation containing lactase to such foods, diarrhea caused by lactose intolerance can be prevented.

digestive juices. Bile salts from the liver emulsify fats. A bile salt is a steroid molecule with a polar end that is soluble in water and a nonpolar end that is soluble in fat. The fat-soluble part of the molecule attaches to the surface of a globule of fat, and the water-soluble end projects outward into the watery medium. This action of bile salts reduces the surface tension on the fat globule. Agitation of the globules by gentle contractions in the small intestine, along with the action of bile salts and certain phospholipids called lecithins, breaks large fat globules into smaller ones. This process, called **emulsification**, greatly increases the surface area of fat globules so that fat-digesting enzymes can act on more of the fat molecules.

Pancreatic lipase, with the assistance of a protein called colipase, acts on emulsified fats and digests them to glycerol, free fatty acids, monoglycerides, and diglycerides. As this digestion proceeds, smaller particles called **micelles** are formed. Micelles consist of bile salts, fatty acids, diglycerides, and a few other products of digestion. Each of these molecules is oriented with the polar ends toward the surface of the micelle, where they interact with water molecules.

LOCATION

DIGESTIVE PROCESSES

mouth

triglycerides and cholesterol
and cholesteryl esters

stomach

triglycerides and cholesterol
and cholesteryl esters

gastric lipase

**lumen of
small intestine**

triglycerides (except those
from butter fat),
cholesterol, and
cholesteryl esters

bile
pancreatic lipase
calipase
cholesteryl esterase

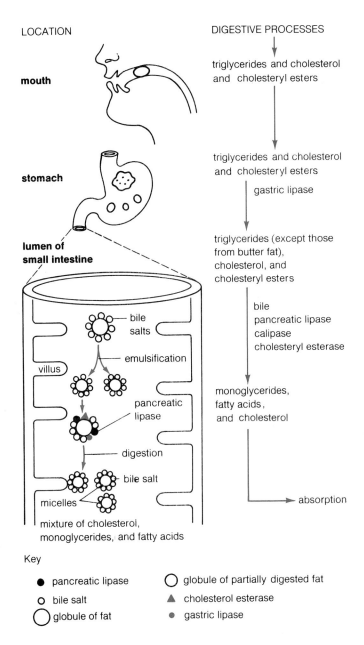

monoglycerides,
fatty acids,
and cholesterol

absorption

mixture of cholesterol,
monoglycerides, and fatty acids

Key

● pancreatic lipase
○ bile salt
◯ globule of fat
◯ globule of partially digested fat
▲ cholesterol esterase
● gastric lipase

Figure 22.22 Digestion of lipids.

Micelles migrate to the microvilli, where the fatty acids and glycerides are absorbed and the bile salts freed for reuse. Bile salts are reabsorbed primarily in the ileum by an active process so efficient that more than 95% of the bile salt molecules are returned to the liver. These bile salts reenter the bile and again participate in emulsification and in the formation of micelles.

In addition to fats the diet, and thus the fat globules, also contains cholesterol, either in the form of cholesterol esters (cholesterol and a fatty acid) or as free cholesterol. The pancreatic enzyme **cholesterol esterase** hydrolyzes the esters into cholesterol and free fatty acids. Both cholesterol and fatty acids are ferried in micelles to the intestinal epithelium, where they are absorbed. The digestion of lipids is summarized in Figure 22.22.

The digestion of nucleic acids makes up only a small part of the digestive process. However, all foods are composed of the cells of previously living things and therefore contain nucleic acids. The pancreatic enzymes ribonuclease and deoxyribonuclease break nucleic acids into components that can be digested by other enzymes.

Absorption

The volume of food entering the digestive tract amounts to about 1.5 liters per day. Gastrointestinal secretions that are added to the food amount to another 7.5 liters. Most of this volume is absorbed in the small intestine. In the average adult the following amounts of nutrients are absorbed daily: 300 to 400 grams of carbohydrate, 50 to 100 grams of amino acids, 100 or more grams of fat, 50 to 100 grams of ions, and 8 or more liters of water—some from the diet and some from digestive secretions.

Absorption takes place across the mucosal cells of the intestinal villi. Immediately adjacent to the mucosal cell membrane is a thin layer of water, the **unstirred water layer**, through which substances diffuse to reach the mucosal membrane. When the substances reach the membrane, they pass through it by a variety of mechanisms, including simple diffusion, facilitated diffusion, and active transport. In addition to passing through the surface membrane of mucosal cells, substances also must pass through the inner membrane of the mucosal cell, the interstitial fluid, and the single layer of cells of walls of blood or lymph capillaries. Because different substances make this journey by different mechanisms, the absorption of each category of nutrients is discussed separately below.

Absorption of carbohydrates Most carbohydrate in the intestinal lumen is in the form of disaccharides—maltose, lactose, and sucrose. These disaccharides are digested to monosaccharides by enzymes in the luminal membrane of mucosal cells. The monosaccharides—glucose, fructose, and galactose—are absorbed as follows: Much of the glucose produced in the membrane enters the mucosal cell on a carrier molecule that also carries sodium ions. Energy from ATP is required to actively transport Na^+. Glucose transport is thus affected by the sodium concentration in the intestinal lu-

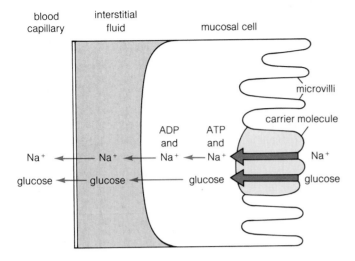

Figure 22.23 The transport of glucose and sodium ions during absorption.

men; a high concentration of Na$^+$ facilitates the movement of glucose, and a low concentration of Na$^+$ slows its movement. After entering the mucosal cell, glucose diffuses into the interstitial space and into the blood capillaries (see Figure 22.23). Galactose is transported by the same mechanism as glucose. However, it is believed that fructose is transported into the mucosal cells by a different carrier molecule that operates independently of the sodium concentration.

Absorption of proteins Proteins are broken down by enzymes into individual amino acids. Like glucose, amino acids are actively transported on carrier molecules that also appear to involve Na$^+$ in some manner. At least three different kinds of amino acid carrier molecules exist; each carries members of a particular group of amino acids with similar chemical properties, but it carries one molecule at a time. Transported amino acids accumulate inside the mucosal cells and apparently move out of these cells across the interstitial fluids and into the blood capillaries by passive diffusion. Of the amino acids absorbed about half come from food and about a fourth each from digested enzyme molecules and from proteins of mucosal cells that have sloughed from the intestinal lining (see Figure 22.24).

Absorption of nucleic acids DNA-ase, RNA-ase, and other enzymes break nucleic acids down into pentose sugars, phosphoric acid, and purine and pyrimidine bases. The pentoses are probably absorbed by diffusion, and the bases are absorbed by active transport. The phosphoric acid ion-

izes; its absorption will be discussed with the absorption of electrolytes and water.

Absorption of lipids Once glycerides, free fatty acids, and cholesterol are produced and incorporated into micelles, the micelles are transported across the unstirred water layer to the mucosal membrane. The processes by which the lipids contained in the micelles enter the mucosal cells are not well understood, but the following events appear to occur. The micelles probably disintegrate near the membrane, releasing fatty acids, monoglycerides, and cholesterol. These lipid-soluble molecules then diffuse through the lipids of the membrane and enter the mucosal cells. Inside the cell monoglycerides and fatty acids recombine to form triglycerides. Small globules of triglycerides and cholesterol form; a protein coat is placed around each small globule, creating a particle called a **chylomicron**. Chylomicrons are extruded from the mucosal cells into the interstitial space, from which they enter the lacteals. After passing through the lymphatic circulation, the chylomicrons enter the blood at the left subclavian vein. Figure 22.25 illustrates the absorption of lipids.

As noted earlier, most bile salt molecules are reabsorbed. As the bile salts repeatedly ferry the products of fat digestion to the mucosa, they are pushed along the intestine, eventually reaching the ileum. Here they are actively transported into the mucosal cells and move by diffusion to the blood capillaries, where they return to the liver and are resecreted in the bile. This process, called enterohepatic circulation of bile salts, is so efficient that some molecules of bile salts may be secreted and reabsorbed as often as five times a day.

Absorption of water, minerals, and electrolytes Large quantities of water from fluids ingested and from digestive juices pass through the small intestine daily, and 90% of this water is absorbed. Water moves freely in both directions across the mucosal membrane of both the small and large intestines, but the net movement is out of the intestine into the blood. Sodium and potassium diffuse in both directions across the mucosal membrane. In addition, sodium is actively transported from the lumen to the mucosal cells. This process is coupled to the movement of glucose, as noted earlier. Potassium also is actively secreted into the intestinal lumen in the jejunum, ileum, and colon. Several other ions, including calcium, iron, magnesium, and phosphate, are actively absorbed in the small intestine. Calcium absorption is enhanced by vitamin D and parathyroid hormone. Iron is actively absorbed and carried in the blood on the plasma protein **transferrin**. Iron absorption is regulated by the amount of iron stored in the protein **ferritin** in intestinal

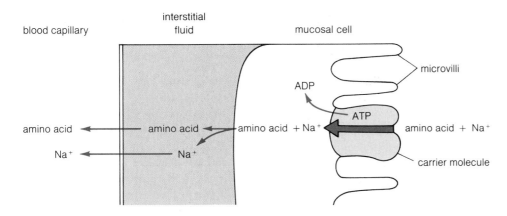

Figure 22.24 The transport of an amino acid during absorption.

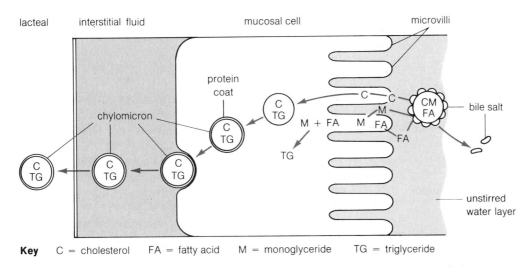

Key   C = cholesterol   FA = fatty acid   M = monoglyceride   TG = triglyceride

Figure 22.25 The absorption of lipids. (C = cholesterol, M = monoglyceride, FA = fatty acid, TG = triglyceride)

mucosal cells and other tissues. When the body's stores of ferritin become depleted, iron absorption increases; when the stores are adequate, absorption decreases. Chloride ions diffuse passively across the mucosa following actively transported sodium ions. Chloride also can be actively transported out of the ileum and colon. Bicarbonate ions, too, can be actively transported into the lumen of the ileum and colon, possibly in response to the accumulation of acid products of bacterial action in the lumen.

Absorption of vitamins   Most vitamins and minerals released by digestion are absorbed in the upper part of the small intestine. Most of the water-soluble vitamins (B complex and C) are rapidly absorbed, but vitamin B_{12} binds to intrinsic factor in the stomach, and the complex is absorbed across the mucosa of the ileum. Fat-soluble vitamins (A, D, E, and K) are absorbed with other fats and therefore require a sufficient supply of pancreatic enzymes and bile salts for optimal absorption.

Summary of processes that occur in the small intestine   The processes of motility, secretion, digestion, and absorption in the small intestine, and their regulation, are summarized in Figure 22.26.

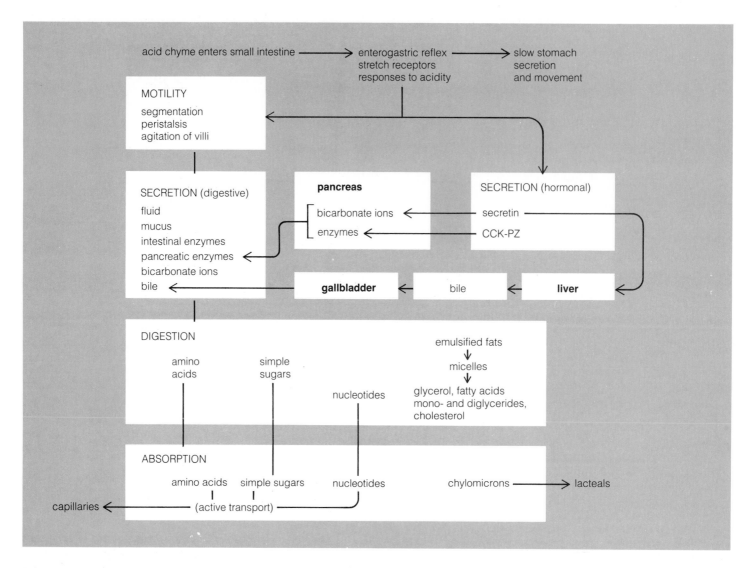

Figure 22.26 Processes that occur in the small intestine and how they are regulated.

LARGE INTESTINE AND RECTUM

Objective 18. Describe the anatomy of the large intestine and rectum.

Objective 19. Describe how the following processes occur in the large intestine and rectum and explain how each is regulated: (a) motility, (b) secretion, (c) absorption, and (d) bacterial action.

Objective 20. Explain the mechanism of defecation.

Anatomy of the Large Intestine and Rectum

The **large intestine**, or **colon**, is about 1.5 meters in length, extending from the **ileocecal valve** to the **rectum** (Figure 22.27). Its diameter varies from one region to another, but it is always larger than that of the small intestine.

The **cecum** is a pouchlike structure extending about 6 centimeters below the ileocecal valve. Attached to the cecum at its blind end is the **vermiform appendix**, a slightly coiled blind tube about 8 centimeters long. Attached to the

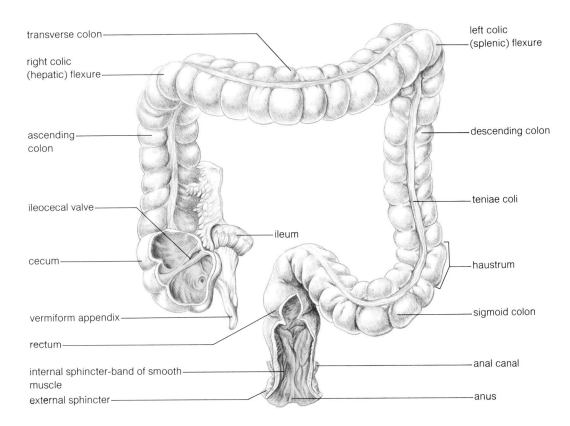

transverse colon

right colic
(hepatic) flexure

ascending
colon

ileocecal valve

ileum

cecum

vermiform appendix

rectum

internal sphincter-band of smooth
muscle

external sphincter

left colic
(splenic) flexure

descending colon

teniae coli

haustrum

sigmoid colon

anal canal

anus

Figure 22.27   Macroscopic anatomy of the large intestine.

cecum at its open end is the **colon**, which is divided into four regions, the **ascending**, **transverse**, **descending**, and **sigmoid colon**. The **right colic**, or **hepatic**, **flexure** marks the boundary between the ascending and transverse colon; the **left colic**, or **splenic**, **flexure** marks the boundary between the transverse and descending colon. The sigmoid colon begins near the left iliac crest and extends in an s-shaped path to the rectum. Mesenteries support the colon.

The rectum comprises the last 20 centimeters of the digestive tract and terminates in the 2 centimeter–long **anal canal**. The **anus**, or opening of the anal canal, has an **internal anal sphincter** comprised of smooth muscle and an **external anal sphincter** composed of skeletal muscle.

The walls of the various regions of the large intestine have certain distinguishing characteristics. The colon has three bands of longitudinal muscle, the **teniae coli**, that contract and draw the remainder of the wall into small pouches, or **haustra**. Deposits of fat in the serosa, the **epiploic appendages**, also are characteristic of the colon. The rectum is firmly attached to the sacrum by the peritoneum and may be distinguished from the colon by the absence of haustra. The anal canal has on the inside a series of **anal columns**, folds in the lining that are well supplied with blood vessels. Enlargement of the anal, or hemorrhoidal, veins and inflammation of the rectum and anal canals results in the condition called **hemorrhoids**.

Motility

Motility in the large intestine is sluggish. As the chyme passes through the ileocecal valve into the cecum and on into the ascending colon, the haustra become distended. In a process called **haustral churning** distention stimulates contraction of the longitudinal muscle bands, and the chyme is pushed ahead into the next haustra. Strong propulsive movements called **mass movements** occur in the large intestine only a few times a day, usually after meals. How contractions of the colon are regulated is not well understood, but intrinsic innervation, CCK-PZ, and probably several other substances are involved. The contractions propel fecal material into the transverse and descending colon and the rectum.

> Studies in which subjects were fed small beads with a meal have shown that about 70% of the beads appear in the feces within seventy-two hours of the meal. As much as a week may be required to recover the remaining beads!

Secretion

In the large intestine goblet cells in the intestinal epithelium and the crypts of Lieberkühn secrete mucus; no enzymes are secreted here. Bicarbonate ions are actively secreted into the lumen by epithelial cells; they serve to neutralize acids produced by bacterial action.

Absorption

Only water, a few electrolytes, and some vitamins are absorbed in the large intestine. Up to 1 liter of chyme enters the large intestine daily. As it passes through the proximal portion of the colon, 100 to 200 milliliters of water are absorbed into the blood vessels of the mucosa. Electrolytes also pass across membranes in this area.

Though the colon may not be called upon to exercise its absorptive capabilities at all times, it can absorb up to 5 liters of water per day. Sodium absorption is efficient and not coupled to glucose transport as it is in the small intestine; it is partially controlled by the hormone aldosterone. Because of the absorptive capacities of the colon, rectal instillation (introduction) of fluids and medications is frequently performed, especially in children.

Bacterial Action

Bacteria (intestinal flora) normally inhabit the large intestine of all humans except newborn infants and individuals who have undergone prolonged antibiotic treatment. Beginning early in life bacteria enter the large intestine in food and are maintained unless temporarily depleted by antibiotics. These bacteria manufacture several vitamins, including thiamine, riboflavin, and vitamins K and B_{12}, and release some amino acids. Absorption of these substances partially fulfills some human nutritional needs, but B_{12} is probably not produced in sufficient quantity to prevent pernicious anemia in individuals on strict vegetarian or other diets without adequate B_{12}.

Mechanism of Defecation

The net result of bacterial action, absorption, and secretion in the part of the colon nearest the small intestine is the conversion of chyme to feces by the time it reaches the distal colon. **Feces** consist of about three-fourths water and one-fourth solids. Bacteria and undigested roughage each account for approximately one-third of the solid volume; the remainder is composed of inorganic material and undigested nutrients. Within the undigested roughage are cellulose, the dried remains of digestive juices, and epithelial cells sloughed from the intestinal lining. The brown color of fecal material is due to the bacterial metabolism of the bile pigment bilirubin.

In **defecation** feces entering the rectum stimulate the **defecation reflex**, and peristaltic waves pass along the descending colon, sigmoid colon, and rectum. The relaxation wave that precedes the peristaltic wave inhibits the internal anal sphincter and allows this portion of the canal to relax. A second, stronger reflex sends signals to the spinal cord and back by way of parasympathetic fibers to the anus, thereby greatly intensifying peristalsis. The external anal sphincter is under voluntary control so that signals that impinge on consciousness may be acted on or ignored and defecation allowed or inhibited, usually at will. Control of this sphincter is learned, as any parent of a toddler is aware.

SUMMARY OF DIGESTIVE TRACT STRUCTURE AND FUNCTION

Early in this chapter we noted that the digestive tract is composed of four layers and that these layers are modified in certain regions in accordance with the function of the region. These modifications are summarized in Table 22.2. As you read that table, try to relate each structural modifi-

Table 22.2   Modifications of Regions of the Digestive Tract

Region	Serosa	Muscularis	Submucosa	Mucosa
Mouth and pharynx	(Do not follow basic plan; consist of outer skin, middle skeletal muscles, and inner stratified, squamous, nonkeratinized epithelium)			
Esophagus	Adventitia, a nonserous connective tissue	Upper third skeletal muscle, middle third mixed skeletal and smooth muscle, and lower third smooth muscle	*	*
Stomach	*	Additional oblique layer of muscle internal to circular layer	*	Rugae apparent in empty stomach; many glands extend into lamina propria
Small intestine	*	*	*	Many glands extend into lamina propria; plicae circularis, villi, and microvilli increase surface area; blood capillaries and lacteals abundant in lamina propria
Large intestine	*	Longitudinal muscle bands, the tenia coli, form haustra	*	Few glands; no modifications to increase surface area
Rectum	Terminal portion surrounded by skeletal muscle	Internal smooth muscle sphincter and external skeletal muscle sphincter	*	Terminal portion contains anal columns

*No major modification of basic plan

cation to the functions of the regions of the digestive tract you have just studied.

Various substances are involved in digestive tract function, including enzymes, hydrochloric acid, bile salts, hormones, and mucus. Mucus binds food particles together in the mouth and lubricates and protects all regions of the digestive tract. Enzymes and other substances involved in digestion are summarized in Table 22.3.

Hormones involved in the regulation of digestion represent one of the most active research fields in physiology today. Several hormones of the digestive tract have been discovered only recently, and their actions are not yet fully understood. All of the gastrointestinal hormones studied so far are peptides, ranging in length from eleven to forty-three amino acids. The current understanding of these hormones is summarized in Table 22.4.

Table 22.3 Summary of Substances Involved in Digestion

Site of Action	Substance	Composition	Source	Action
Mouth				
	Salivary amylase	Enzyme	Salivary glands	Digests starch to intermediate products (and maltose if time permits)
Stomach				
	Hydrochloric acid	Mineral acid	Stomach	Activates pepsin, kills bacteria
	Pepsin	Enzyme	Stomach	Digests proteins to proteoses, peptones, and polypeptides
	Rennin	Enzyme	Child's stomach	Coagulates milk proteins
	Gastric lipase	Enzyme	Stomach	Digests small amounts of butterfat to glycerol and fatty acids
Small Intestine				
	Sodium bicarbonate	Salt	Pancreas	Neutralizes hydrochloric acid
	Amylase	Enzyme	Pancreas	Digests starch and intermediate products to maltose
	Lipases	Enzymes	Pancreas	Digest fats to fatty acids, glycerol, and cholesterol
	Trypsin	Enzyme	Pancreas	Digests proteins and polypeptides to small polypeptides
	Chymotrypsin	Enzyme	Pancreas	Digests proteins and polypeptides to small polypeptides
	Carboxypeptidases	Enzyme	Pancreas	Remove amino acids from the carboxyl end of polypeptides
	Nucleases	Enzymes	Pancreas	Break down DNA and RNA
	Bile salts	Steroids	Liver	Help to form emulsions and micelles
	Enterokinase	Enzyme	Intestinal epithelium	Activates trypsin
	Dipeptidases	Enzyme	Intestinal epithelium	Break dipeptides into amino acids
	Aminopeptidase	Enzymes	Intestinal epithelium	Remove amino acids from the amino end of polypeptides
	Maltase	Enzyme	Intestinal epithelium	Digests maltose to glucose
	Lactase	Enzyme	Intestinal epithelium	Digests lactose to glucose and galactose
	Sucrase	Enzyme	Intestinal epithelium	Digests sucrose to glucose and fructose
	Nucleotide-digesting enzymes	Enzymes	Intestinal epithelium	Break DNA and RNA into purines, pyrimidines, phosphate, ribose, and deoxyribose

Table 22.4   Current Understanding of Gastrointestinal Hormones

Hormone	Site of Production	Main Site of Action	Main Function
Gastrin	G-cells of the pyloric portion of stomach	Stomach	Stimulates secretion of acid
Secretin	Mucosal glands of upper small intestine	Pancreas, stomach	Increases pancreatic secretion of bicarbonate; decreases gastric secretion; augments action of CCK-PZ
Cholecystokinin-pancreozymin (CCK-PZ)	Mucosal glands of upper small intestine	Pancreas, gallbladder	Causes contraction of gallbladder; stimulates secretion of pancreatic enzymes; augments action of secretin; inhibits gastric emptying
Glucagon	Duodenum	Pancreas	Stimulates release of insulin from pancreas when glucose concentration is high in intestine
Gastric inhibitory peptide (GIP)	Duodenum and jejunum	Stomach, pancreas	Inhibits gastric secretion and motility; stimulates insulin secretion
Vasoactive intestinal peptide (VIP)	Small intestine	Small intestine, stomach, blood vessels	Stimulates intestinal secretion of electrolytes (and thus water); inhibits acid secretion; dilates peripheral blood vessels
Motilin	Duodenum	Stomach	Stimulates acid secretion
Substance P	Neurons and endocrine-type cells of gastrointestinal tract	Small intestine	Increases motility of small intestine (not proven to enter blood)
Bombesin	?	Stomach, small intestine, gallbladder	Increases gastrin secretion; increases motility of small intestine and gallbladder
Somatostatin (growth-hormone-inhibiting hormone)	Pyloric mucosa?	?	Same hormone from hypothalamus has several effects on gastrointestinal tract, but effects of locally produced hormone not yet clear

CLINICAL APPLICATIONS

Objective 21. Briefly describe the causes, effects, and treatments of the following conditions: (a) hiatal hernia, (b) heartburn, (c) gastritis, (d) peptic ulcer, (e) pernicious anemia, (f) vomiting, (g) cirrhosis of the liver, (h) hepatitis, (i) gallstones, (j) pancreatitis, (k) sprue, (l) constipation, (m) diarrhea, (n) appendicitis, (o) ulcerative colitis, and (p) obstructions.

Hiatal hernia   In some individuals the muscle tissue of the diaphragm has an area of weakness. The muscle fibers separate, and part of the stomach is pushed into the thoracic cavity. This opening in the diaphragm is called a diaphragmatic, or hiatal, hernia. Pain following meals is the most obvious effect of this condition.

Small frequent meals may allow the affected person to avoid pain, but surgical repair of the hernia may be required.

Heartburn   **Heartburn** has nothing to do with the heart. Though the pain is near the heart, it is caused by the regurgitation of acid from the stomach into the esophagus. The pain may be due to the burning sensation from the acid or to a muscle spasm induced by the acid in the esophagus. Heartburn often occurs after a heavy meal, especially if the person is lying down. Prevention by avoiding heavy meals is a better practice than alleviating symptoms with antacids.

Gastritis   An inflammation of the gastric mucosa, **gastritis** results from the presence of irritating foods, attack of the stomach wall by gastric secretions, bacterial infections, and excessive intake of alcohol. The effects of gastritis include excessive salivation stimulated by the irritation of the stomach, increased permeability of the mucous coating, and increased production of pepsin and hydrochloric acid. Severe, prolonged gastritis may lead to the formation of a peptic ulcer. Gastritis may be prevented by avoiding the things that cause it. It is treated by a bland diet, antacids, and antibiotics if bacterial infection is involved.

Peptic ulcer   **Peptic ulcer**, an erosion of the stomach or intestinal mucosa, affects 10% of all Americans and is increasing in incidence. Predisposing factors may include stress and anxiety and hereditary factors. Two types of peptic ulcers exist: those affecting the stomach mucosa, which probably involve a defect in the normal stomach mucosal defenses against acid, and those affecting the duodenal mucosa, which probably involve excess acid secretion. Gastric peptic ulcer usually occurs when inflammation, aspirin, alcohol, or some other factor disrupts the protective barrier that prevents acid and pepsin from digesting the stomach wall. Though hydrochloric acid secretion may be even less than normal, the acid and the enzyme reach the cells of the mucosa and cause tissue destruction. Duodenal peptic ulcers usually occur in the upper part of the duodenum near the pyloric sphincter. They may be caused by excessive vagal stimulation, especially between meals and at night, which causes the release of gastrin and a subsequent increase in HCl secretion. The excess of HCl leads to ulceration of the duodenal mucosa. The major complication of peptic ulceration (in either the stomach or the duodenum) is hemorrhage, which may be sudden and life threatening. Treatment of ulcers usually involves anticholinergic drugs; frequent, small, high-fat meals; and abstinence from caffeine and alcohol. The high fat content of the ulcer diet inhibits gastric secretions and slows the rate of gastric emptying. A bland diet is often prescribed, but little evidence exists to show that it can alleviate symptoms of the disease.

Pernicious anemia   Pernicious anemia is an anemia caused by a deficiency of vitamin B_{12}. This anemia develops only after several years of the vitamin deficiency. Even with a diet adequate in vitamin B_{12} the deficiency can develop if there is a deficiency of intrinsic factor, a mucopolysaccharide produced by the parietal cells. This factor binds to vitamin B_{12} and protects it from digestion as it passes through the stomach. Intrinsic factor also transports vitamin B_{12} to the ileum and facilitates its absorption. Pernicious anemia may accompany gastritis. If the supply of intrinsic factor is adequate, providing dietary B_{12} will cure the disease; in the absence of intrinsic factor B_{12} injections are needed.

Vomiting   **Vomiting** occurs when impulses from the vagus or sensory nerves reach the vomiting center in the medulla, and motor impulses initiate a complicated sequence of reflexes. These reflexes relax the gastroesophageal sphincter and cause contraction of the diaphragm and muscles of the abdominal wall. Chem-icals and unpleasant sensory and emotional experiences can stimulate the medullary center to cause vomiting, as can nerve impulses from the inner ear via the cerebellum in the case of motion sickness. Treatment involves avoiding food and, if severe, the use of sedatives.

Cirrhosis of the liver   Literally, cirrhosis means orange disease; **cirrhosis of the liver** is so named because it leads to the accumulation of the red pigment bilirubin in the liver. (Because of other substances mixed with the red pigment, the liver appears orange.) Cirrhosis results from damage to liver cells and the subsequent infiltration of connective tissue to repair the damage. Although liver cells are able to divide and regenerate liver tissue, following severe damage the production of connective tissue is often faster than that of liver tissue. As a consequence, some of the sinusoids of the liver may be blocked by connective tissue. Cirrhosis may accompany chemical damage to the liver or may be a consequence of hepatitis or malnutrition. Some animal studies suggest that alcoholism causes cirrhosis directly rather than indirectly through the malnutrition that generally accompanies it. No specific treatment is available. One can only correct the condition that led to it and allow the liver to regenerate to the extent possible.

Hepatitis   By definition **hepatitis** is an inflammation of the liver. It may be caused by infectious agents (viruses, bacteria, and protozoa) or toxic substances (some drugs, carbon tetrachloride, and some anesthetics). Though liver damage may be extensive over a period of several months, the liver can usually repair much of the damage except where extensive infiltration of connective tissue has occurred. Serum hepatitis, caused by a particular strain of virus, can be transmitted on needles and in injectable materials, particularly blood transfused from carriers of the disease. No specific cure exists for this debilitating disease; treatment includes rest, good nutrition, and limited fat intake because normal liver function is required to digest fats.

Gallstones   **Gallstones** form in the gallbladder as a result of the precipitation of cholesterol or other substances. Some gallstones contain large amounts of calcium; they occur when a defect in calcium metabolism exists. When too high a concentration of cholesterol is present in the bile for the amounts of phospholipids and bile acids, cholesterol precipitates and forms gallstones. Inflammation and infection of the gallbladder can also cause gallstones. Individuals with gallstones are advised to limit the fat in their diets; they may require surgical removal of the gallbladder and the enclosed stones (cholecystectomy). Fat digestion usually is not greatly impaired by removal of the gallbladder unless the individual takes in large quantities of fat in a single meal. Stones sometime migrate out of the gallbladder and block ducts along the way to the intestine. If located so as to block the flow of pancreatic juices, the stone may initiate an attack of pancreatitis. In addition, if the stones block the flow out of the gallbladder or the flow from the liver to the gallbladder, bile may back up into the liver, resulting in cholestasis (standing bile). Prolonged cholestasis may

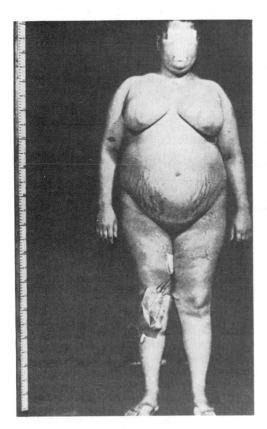 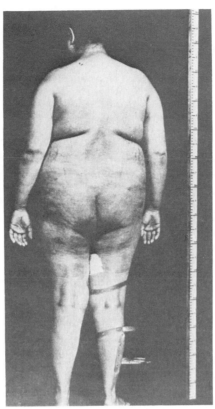

Figure 22.28 A twenty-two-year-old woman with a tumor in the ventromedial hypothalamus. (Courtesy of A. G. Reeves.)

result in cirrhosis and an increase in serum bile acids, which may cause pruritis (itching).

Pancreatitis An inflammation of the pancreas called **pancreatitis** often results from a blocked duct or from chronic alcohol use. Pancreatic secretions accumulate, and, although the pancreas secretes a trypsin inhibitor, α_1 antitrypsin, large accumulations of trypsin can overwhelm the inhibitor and lead to proteolytic digestion of the pancreatic tissue itself. In acute pancreatitis the entire pancreas can be digested in a matter of hours. In chronic pancreatitis blockage may be less complete or secretion less profuse so that destruction is slower. Treatment includes alleviating pain, preventing infection, and replacing lost fluids. Surgery is sometimes attempted to remove obstructions of pancreatic ducts. In spite of treatment, the disease may be fatal.

Sprue **Sprue**, or **celiac disease**, is a disturbance of the absorptive process in which the epithelial cells of the villi fail to be continuously replaced as they are in a normally functioning intestine. One cause of the disease in susceptible individuals is the ingestion of gluten in wheat or rye products. **Gluten** contains **gliadin**, a substance that disrupts the normal development of new cells in the epithelium in susceptible individuals. In severe cases much of the intestinal epithelium is destroyed, and the villi become blunted or disappear entirely. Absorption is greatly impaired, and tissue wasting and vitamin deficiencies occur. If celiac disease is diagnosed before tissue damage is severe, a gluten-free diet prevents further damage and allows intestinal epithelium to regenerate. Another form of this disease known as **tropical sprue** is thought to be due to a bacterial agent because the disease responds to antibiotic treatment.

Constipation   **Constipation** is the infrequent passage of dry, hardened feces. However, individuals vary widely in the normal frequency of defecation—some after each meal and others only once every three days; it is the consistency of the feces and not the frequency of defecation that determines whether a person is constipated. Constipation often results from too little roughage in the diet or from too frequent inhibition of the voluntary defecation reflex. Repeated inhibition leads to reduction in natural reflexes and loss of colon muscle tone. Roughage increases peristaltic movements in the colon and causes the undigested remains of food to be eliminated before they become dehydrated into a hard stool. Though laxatives are used to treat constipation, their excessive use also reduces natural defecation reflexes.

Diarrhea   An infection or inflammation of the mucosa anywhere in the intestinal tract can cause **diarrhea**. More mucus is secreted, the intestine becomes more motile, and more digestive juices are secreted. In severe diarrhea losses of electrolytes and fluids can be life threatening if these are not replaced. (For more information on fluid and electrolyte regulation, see Chapter 26.) Diarrhea is treated by reducing food intake to reduce motility and replacing lost fluids and electrolytes.

Appendicitis   **Appendicitis** is an acute infection of the appendix, the blind tube protruding from the cecum. Cramping pains and vomiting can warn of appendicitis. Swelling of the appendix sometimes blocks the small intestine. Rupture of the appendix can spread infection throughout the peritoneal cavity. Surgical removal of an infected appendix is the usual treatment.

Ulcerative colitis   In ulcerative colitis the mucosal lining of the colon becomes ulcerated. The primary cause of the ulceration is unknown, but possibilities include bacterial action, excoriation or abrasion of the mucosa, and proteolytic digestion of the mucosa. The mucosal lesion is accompanied by abnormal motility of the colon, and strong peristaltic movements occur much of the time. A temporary ileostomy (surgically created external opening from the intestine) is often performed to divert feces from the colon and allow it to heal. If healing does not occur, removal of the colon and construction of a permanent ileostomy may be necessary.

Obstructions   Blocks, or **obstructions**, can occur at several points along the intestinal tract. Causes include congenital defects, malignancy, constrictions formed by fibrotic scar tissue of healing ulcers, and spasms or paralysis of muscles. The effects of an obstruction depend on where the obstruction is located. Pyloric obstruction results in the vomiting of acidic stomach contents and an increase in blood pH (alkalosis) because of the acid loss. Obstructions in the upper small intestine result in neutral vomiting, and those in the lower small intestine result in the vomiting of alkaline intestinal contents and a decrease in blood pH (acidosis). All obstructions that cause vomiting are accompanied by fluid loss and impaired nutrition. Obstructions of the sigmoid colon cause constipation but are less likely to produce vomiting than are obstructions higher in the tract. Surgery is usually required to remove an obstruction.

Clinical Terms

achalasia (ah-kal-a'ze-ah)   failure of the esophageal sphincter to open, and dilation and hypertrophy of the esophagus because of damage to nerve ganglia supplying the esophagus

achlorhydria (ah-klor-hi'dre-ah)   absence of acid secretions in the stomach

aphagia (ah-fa'je-ah)   inability to swallow

cholecystitis (ko''le-sis-ti'tis)   inflammation of the gallbladder

cholelithiasis (ko''le-lith-i'as-is)   presence of gallstones

colostomy (ko-los'to-me)   a surgical procedure to form an artificial opening into the colon

diverticulitis (di-ver-tik''u-li'tis)   formation of small inflamed pouches in the lining of the colon

dumping syndrome   an excessive increase in the rate at which contents of the stomach enter the small intestine, often caused by vagotomy or gastric surgery

flatus (fla'tus)   presence of gas in the stomach or intestines

hemorrhoid (hem'or-oid)   an enlarged vein in the rectal mucous membrane

Hirschsprung's disease   constriction of the lower colon and dilation of the portion above the constriction due to the congenital absence of nerve ganglia that control peristalsis in the colon

mumps   an inflammation of the salivary glands caused by a viral infection

pyloric stenosis (pi-lor'ik sten-o'sis)   hypertrophy of the pyloric opening of the stomach; is usually a congenital condition and usually leads to projectile vomiting

pyorrhea (pi-or-e'ah)   a pussy inflammation of the dental periosteum

Essay: Dental Care

Half of all Americans have lost all of their teeth by age sixty-five. This is in spite of both the much-publicized admonition to "see your dentist twice a year" and the variety of highly advertised toothpastes, dentifrices, and cleaning devices available to consumers. Below we'll investigate some of the causes of tooth loss and look at some of the strategies that help—and don't help—to prevent it.

Periodontal disease is the primary cause of tooth loss in adults. The disease results from the action of bacteria that gather in crevices between the teeth and gums or around bridgework, worn fillings, and sites where teeth have been extracted. The bacteria deposit a white substance called plaque, which hardens on the teeth, especially in areas where teeth and gums meet. Pockets beneath the plaque provide secluded places where bacteria can multiply and do further damage to the gums. When periodontal disease advances, swelling, receding gums, and loose teeth are the result.

The standard treatment for periodontal disease involves oral surgery. The gums are lifted back from the teeth, the plaque and infection cleared away, and the gums restitched in their proper position. Such treatment is expensive (several thousand dollars per patient). Furthermore, little research has been done on the long-term effects of the treatment. Daily or more frequent thorough brushing to remove plaque and periodic removal of plaque by a dentist or dental hygienist will reduce the likelihood of periodontal disease. The need to have plaque removed by a professional varies with the amount of plaque formed and with the degree of removal achieved by brushing.

Dental caries (cavities) begin when oral bacteria lower the pH of the mouth from a normal 6.7 to 5.5 or lower. It is thought that bacteria (probably streptococci) convert carbohydrate to plaque, which deposits on the teeth. Then the bacteria between the plaque and the tooth enamel produce acids that dissolve tooth enamel. In this protected area bacteria are not reached by saliva or by tooth brushing and thus continue to erode enamel. If the enamel is thin or weak to begin with, the process moves very quickly, and bacteria eat through the dentin and may enter the pulp cavity. By this time it may be impossible to save the tooth by drilling and filling.

Prevention of dental caries should start before birth with a nutritious diet during the mother's pregnancy. Vitamin D, calcium, and phosphorus are particularly important in the development of teeth, prenatally and throughout childhood. Strong tooth enamel resists bacterial action.

Sugar, an ingredient in nearly every processed food marketed today, is clearly a causative factor in dental disease. Studies in various countries have shown that consumption of refined sugar and tooth decay are highly correlated; the more sugar consumed, the greater the number of cavities in teeth. This is because sugar in the mouth feeds the acid-producing bacteria. Frequent sugar intake makes matters even worse. The more hours of the day that sugar is present in the mouth, the more opportunity the oral bacteria have to metabolize sugar, produce acid, and erode tooth enamel. Thus, if one must consume sugar, a large amount once a day is far less damaging to the teeth than a small amount several times a day.

The possible role of fluoride in the prevention of tooth decay has been a source of controversy. Evidence now exists that fluoride in the drinking water of young children (those under the age of eight) does increase the hardness of the enamel of forming teeth. Evidence is less convincing that painting fluoride on the teeth or using toothpastes containing fluoride increases the hardness of the enamel. The efficacy of fluoride in any form for adults is debatable.

When periodontal disease or caries are not treated, tooth loss is inevitable. Once a tooth has been extracted, it can be replaced by an artificial tooth (fastened to other teeth) or sometimes by an implant. The implantation of teeth is a relatively new technique, and its success depends primarily on how well fibers between the alveolus and implanted tooth succeed in holding the tooth in the alveolus.

Only scant evidence exists to support the claim that early diagnosis and treatment lead to improved dental health. According to a study done by *Lancet*, a British journal, a group of individuals who had dental examinations at longer intervals than six months did experience a slightly higher incidence of tooth loss than those having more frequent examinations. However, those who had frequent check-ups were sometimes subjected to overtreatment; for example, they may have been subjected to unnecessary X ray. They may also have had caries repaired that would have remineralized without treatment. When a small area of the enamel has been damaged, it is sometimes possible for new minerals to be deposited, thereby repairing the damage.

Given the present state of knowledge regarding dental care, there are several things individuals can do to help to maintain healthy teeth and gums. They include: (1) scraping floss up and down against each tooth as it passes between the teeth, (2) brushing with a soft nylon brush with rounded bristles, making a circular motion with the brush at a 45° angle with the gumline, (3) avoiding tooth whiteners (which erode enamel) and toothpastes or powders with sugar for flavoring, and (4) rinsing of the mouth with water several times a day.

Finally, a part of caring for teeth includes avoiding having them knocked out accidentally. Children, once they have permanent teeth, and anyone else who engages in sports such as football or hockey should wear mouth and face protectors when playing those games.

Keeping teeth cleaned and well protected is worthwhile—except where tooth implantation is successful, once a tooth is lost, it's gone forever.

CHAPTER SUMMARY

(Chapter summary points and review questions are numbered to correspond to the numbered objectives in the text of each chapter.)

Organization and General Functions

1. Describe the general functions of the digestive system and list its major organs.
   a. The general functions of the digestive system are:
      (1) movement of food through the digestive tract
      (2) secretion of digestive juices
      (3) digestion of food into small molecules
      (4) absorption of these small molecules into the blood or lymph
   b. The organs of the digestive system, in order as the food passes through them, are the mouth, pharynx, esophagus, stomach, small intestine, large intestine, rectum, and anus.
   c. The accessory organs of the digestive system are the salivary glands, liver, gallbladder, and pancreas.

Development

2. Describe in general the formation of the digestive tract and list some common congenital defects of that system.
   a. The digestive system develops from the primitive gut into recognizable organs by the eighth week of development.
   b. Common congenital defects include cleft lip and/or palate, pyloric stenosis, and imperforate anus.

Tissues and Their Functions

3. Describe the basic layers of the digestive tract and explain briefly how the structures in those layers carry out the four main functions of the digestive tract.
   a. The basic layers of the digestive tract from the outside in are:
      (1) the serosa, which is continuous with the mesenteries
      (2) the muscularis, which consists of longitudinal and circular muscle fibers
      (3) the submucosa, which contains connective tissue, blood vessels, and lymph vessels
      (4) the mucosa, which contains muscle, connective tissue, blood and lymph vessels, glands, and an innermost epithelium
   b. The functions of the digestive tract are carried out by the following structures:
      (1) Muscles provide for movement of food.
      (2) Glands provide for the secretion of digestive juices.
      (3) The secretions released into the lumen provide for digestion.
      (4) The mucosa provides for absorption.

Mouth

4. Describe the anatomical structure of the mouth, including the salivary glands and teeth.
   a. The mouth, or oral cavity, contains the tongue and teeth and receives secretions from the salivary glands.
   b. Teeth are composed of an enamel-covered crown, a cementum-covered root, and an inner dentin and pulp cavity.
   c. The two sets of human teeth are:
      (1) the deciduous teeth: eight incisors, four canines, and eight molars
      (2) the permanent teeth: eight incisors, four canines, eight premolars, and twelve molars
   d. The salivary glands are located below the ears and in the floor of the oral cavity; their secretions are carried to the mouth by ducts.
5. Explain how each of the following structures functions in digestion: teeth, tongue, taste buds, and salivary glands.
   a. The teeth function to bite, tear, and grind food.
   b. The tongue helps to mix and move food.
   c. The taste buds (mostly on the surface of the tongue) detect the four basic tastes—sweet, salty, sour, and bitter.
   d. The salivary glands produce amylase, which digests starch, and mucin, which binds food particles together and lubricates surfaces.
6. Explain the regulation of hunger and satiety.
   a. Hunger and satiety are regulated by neural centers in the hypothalamus.
   b. These centers may be influenced by blood glucose concentration, insulin, or CCK-PZ.

Pharynx and Esophagus

7. Describe the structure of the pharynx and the esophagus.
   a. The pharynx (described in Chapter 21) is a tube that carries food from the mouth to the esophagus.
   b. The esophagus is a muscular tube containing both skeletal and smooth muscle that carries food from the pharynx to the stomach.
8. Explain the process of swallowing and movement of food through the pharynx and esophagus.
   a. The tongue voluntarily moves food into the pharynx.
   b. Once food is in the pharynx, swallowing is an automatic process involving the closing off of the trachea and contraction of the pharyngeal and esophageal muscles to push food into the stomach.

Stomach

9. Describe the macroscopic and microscopic anatomy of the stomach.

a. Macroscopically, the stomach is a hollow bag with a sphincter at each end and rugae in its inside lining.

b. Microscopically, the stomach contains gastric glands, which consist of:
   (1) mucous neck cells, which secrete mucus
   (2) chief cells, which secrete enzymes, especially pepsin
   (3) parietal cells, which secrete hydrochloric acid and intrinsic factor

10. Describe how the following processes occur in the stomach and explain how each is regulated: (a) storage, mixing, and emptying; (b) secretion; (c) digestion, and (d) absorption.

   a. Storage, mixing, and emptying are accomplished as follows:
      (1) Food enters the stomach, and the stomach serves as a storage bag.
      (2) Peristaltic movements mix the food and propel it to the small intestine.
      (3) Emptying is regulated by distention, the release of gastrin and other hormones, and the enterogastric reflex.

   b. Secretion occurs as follows:
      (1) The gastric glands secrete hydrochloric acid and pepsinogen, which is activated by hydrochloric acid and active pepsin.
      (2) Gastric secretions are regulated by cephalic, gastric, and intestinal factors.

   c. Digestion is limited mainly to the breakdown of protein to polypeptides. It is controlled by the secretion and activation of pepsinogen.

   d. Absorption is limited to alcohol and lipid-soluble drugs because of the thick mucous coating of the stomach lining and the small amount of digestion that has occurred.

   e. These processes are summarized in Figure 22.13.

Liver and Pancreas

11. Describe the macroscopic and microscopic anatomy of the liver and the gallbladder.

   a. Macroscopically, the liver is a large organ in the upper right quadrant of the abdominal cavity. It has several lobes.

   b. Microscopically, the liver consists of lobules, each of which has:
      (1) a central vein, which carries blood to the hepatic vein
      (2) peripheral branches of the hepatic artery, which bring oxygenated blood to the liver
      (3) peripheral branches of the hepatic portal vein, which bring nutrient-laden blood to the liver
      (4) peripheral interlobular bile ducts, which carry bile produced by liver cells to the hepatic ducts, which in turn carry bile to the small intestine or the gallbladder
      (5) sinusoids, which contain phagocytic Kuppfer cells

   c. The gallbladder, which has an epithelial lining and a muscular wall, receives bile by way of the cystic duct and stores and concentrates bile until it is released into the small intestine.

12. Explain the role of the liver in the digestive process, including the synthesis and functions of bile.

   a. Bile, which contains water, bile salts, cholesterol, bile pigments, and certain other lipids and electrolytes, is produced in the liver.

   b. Bile salts in bile emulsify fats in the lumen of the small intestine.

   c. Other functions of the liver are listed in Table 22.1.

13. Describe the macroscopic and microscopic anatomy of the pancreas.

   a. Macroscopically, the pancreas is a soft glandular organ located near the stomach and duodenum and connected to the duodenum by a duct.

   b. Microscopically, the pancreas has acinar tissue that produces digestive juices. (Its other microscopic structures were described in Chapter 15.)

14. Explain how the digestive secretions of the pancreas are produced.

   a. Proteolytic enzymes are produced in inactive form by acinar cells and transported to the duodenum, where they are activated.

   b. Amylase, lipase, cholesterol esterase, and enzymes that digest nucleic acids are produced by acinar cells in active form.

   c. Water and bicarbonate ions are produced by the tubular cells of the pancreas.

15. Explain how the functions of the liver and the pancreas are regulated.

   a. The release of bile from the gallbladder (and liver) is stimulated by CCK-PZ and secretin.

   b. The release of pancreatic enzymes is stimulated by CCK-PZ.

   c. The release of water and bicarbonate ions is stimulated by secretin.

Small Intestine

16. Describe the macroscopic and microscopic anatomy of the small intestine.

   a. Macroscopically, the small intestine is divided into the duodenum, jejunum, and ileum.

   b. Microscopically, its walls contain the same four layers as other digestive organs, and its mucosa contains glands that secrete mucus and enzymes.

   c. Villi and microvilli greatly increase the surface area of the small intestine.

   d. Each villus contains blood and lymph capillaries that receive absorbed nutrients.

17. Describe how the following processes occur in the small intestine and explain how each is regulated: (a) motility, (b) secretion, (c) digestion, and (d) absorption.

   a. Motility in the small intestine:
      (1) includes peristalsis, segmentation contractions, and movements of the villi

(2) is regulated by reflexes, though movements of villi are regulated by villikinin

b. Secretion in the small intestine is limited to mucus and enterokinase, which are regulated by the presence or absence of chyme.

c. Mucosal cells also have membrane-bound enzymes, which digest disaccharides and small peptides.

d. Digestion in the small intestine is accomplished mostly by enzymes from the pancreas and bile from the liver; their release is regulated by factors described above.

e. Most absorption occurs in the small intestine:

  (1) Glucose and other sugars and amino acids are absorbed mainly by active transport across the mucosal membrane. They diffuse out of the mucosal cells, across the interstitial space, and into the blood capillaries.

  (2) Products of fat digestion are transported in micelles across the unstirred water layer to the intestinal mucosa, where they diffuse into mucosal cells, are resynthesized into triglycerides, collected in chylomicrons, and extruded into the intercellular space, where they enter the lymph.

  (3) Water, minerals, electrolytes, and vitamins are also absorbed in the small intestine.

  (4) Absorption is regulated by the availability of ATP and concentration gradients.

f. These processes are summarized in Figure 22.26.

Large Intestine and Rectum

18. Describe the anatomy of the large intestine and rectum.

  a. The large intestine is divided into the cecum and the ascending, transverse, descending, and sigmoid colon.

  b. The colon has longitudinal muscle present in three bands, the teniae coli, which draw the rest of the colon into haustra.

  c. The rectum includes the anal canal and has folds in its inner lining.

19. Describe how the following processes occur in the large intestine and rectum and explain how each is regulated: (a) motility, (b) secretion, (c) absorption, and (d) bacterial action.

  a. Motility, which is sluggish, consists of haustral churning and mass movements, which are controlled by neural and hormonal factors that are not completely understood.

  b. Secretion is limited to mucus and bicarbonate ions.

  c. Absorption includes water, electrolytes, and vitamins produced by intestinal flora.

  d. Bacterial action produces vitamins and amino acids and often leads to the accumulation of acid, which is neutralized by the secretion of bicarbonate.

20. Explain the mechanism of defecation.

  a. Defecation is stimulated by the entry of feces into the rectum.

  b. Strong peristaltic waves propel the feces and inhibit the internal anal sphincter.

  c. Impulses impinging on consciousness allow for voluntary control of the external sphincter.

Clinical Applications

21. Briefly describe the causes, effects, and treatments of the following conditions: (a) hiatal hernia, (b) heartburn, (c) gastritis, (d) peptic ulcer, (e) pernicious anemia, (f) vomiting, (g) cirrhosis of the liver, (h) hepatitis, (i) gallstones, (j) pancreatitis, (k) sprue, (l) constipation, (m) diarrhea, (n) appendicitis, (o) ulcerative colitis, and (p) obstructions.

  a. Hiatal hernia is an opening in the diaphragm.

  b. Heartburn is caused by regurgitation of stomach acid into the esophagus.

  c. Gastritis is an inflammation of the gastric mucosa.

  d. Peptic ulcer is an erosion of the stomach or duodenal mucosa.

  e. Pernicious anemia is caused by a deficiency of vitamin B_{12} that may be produced by dietary deficiency or lack of intrinsic factor.

  f. Vomiting is a sudden reflux of the contents of the digestive tract through the mouth.

  g. Cirrhosis of the liver is the infiltration of the liver by connective tissue and deposition of bilirubin due to liver damage.

  h. Hepatitis is an inflammation of the liver caused by infectious agents or toxic substances.

  i. Gallstones are deposits of cholesterol or other substances in the gallbladder or its ducts.

  j. Pancreatitis is an inflammation of the pancreas.

  k. Sprue is a disturbance of the absorptive process due to the destruction of intestinal epithelium.

  l. Constipation is the infrequent passage of dry, hardened feces.

  m. Diarrhea is the frequent passage of loose, mucus-containing stools due to infection or irritation.

  n. Appendicitis is an inflammation of the appendix.

  o. Ulcerative colitis is the ulceration of the colon.

  p. Obstructions are blocks in the intestinal tract.

REVIEW

Important Terms

absorption	digestion
acini	duodenum
adventitia	enterogastric reflex
apoferritin	gastrin
bolus	gingiva
CCK-PZ	GIP
chief cells	ileum
chylomicron	jejunum
chyme	lacteal
defecation	mesentery

micelle

microvilli

motility

mucin

mucosa

muscularis

omentum

parietal cells

pepsin

peristalsis

proteolytic enzymes

pylorus

rugae

secretagogue

secretin

secretion

segmentation contractions

serosa

sphincter

submucosa

swallowing

villi

villikinin

VIP

Also see Table 22.3.

Questions

1. a. What are the functions of the digestive system?
  b. List the major organs and accessory structures of the digestive system.

2. Briefly describe the development of the digestive system and explain how congenital defects might occur.

3. List the layers of the digestive tract in sequence and describe the structure and function of each layer.

4. Define each boldface term in the discussion of the anatomy of the mouth.

5. a. Describe the structure of a tooth and the variations in structure related to function.
  b. Compare deciduous teeth with permanent teeth in number, shape, and function.
  c. Describe the role of the tongue and taste buds in digestion.
  d. Describe the secretions of each of the salivary glands and their role in digestion.

6. How are hunger and satiety regulated?

7. How does the structure of the esophagus differ from that of the pharynx?

8. List the events that occur during swallowing.

9. a. What are the macroscopic characteristics of the stomach?
  b. Name the secretory cells of the stomach and describe their secretions.

10. a. Describe the movement and mixing of food in the stomach and list the factors that regulate it.
  b. How does the stomach secrete proteolytic enzymes without itself being digested?
  c. How are the stomach secretions regulated?
  d. Write a word equation for proteolytic digestion in the stomach.
  e. Why is absorption limited in the stomach?

11. a. Where is the liver located, and what are its major macroscopic characteristics?

  b. Describe the internal structure of the liver.
  c. Trace the circulation of blood through the liver.
  d. Trace the circulation of bile through the liver and gallbladder.

12. What are the functions of the liver?

13. a. Where is the pancreas located, and what are its major macroscopic characteristics?
  b. Describe the internal structure of the pancreas and the source of its secretions.

14. List the digestive enzymes and other secretions of the pancreas and describe the function of each secretion.

15. How are the secretions of the liver and pancreas regulated?

16. a. Describe the macroscopic characteristics of the small intestine.
  b. What structures increase the absorptive area of the small intestine?

17. a. What kinds of movements occur in the small intestine, and how are they regulated?
  b. What secretions are produced in the small intestine, and what do they do?
  c. What enzymes are found in mucosa cells, and what do they do?
  d. Summarize the digestive actions that take place in the small intestine and how they are regulated.
  e. Describe how each substance absorbed in the small intestine is transported from the lumen to the blood or lymph.

18. What characteristics distinguish the large intestine and rectum?

19. a. What movements occur in the large intestine and rectum, and how are they regulated?
  b. What is secreted and what is absorbed in the large intestine?
  c. What bacterial actions take place in the large intestine?

20. How does defecation occur?

21. Briefly describe each of the disease conditions discussed under clinical applications.

Problems

1. Given that a glass of milk contains lactose, protein, butterfat, vitamins, and minerals, explain what happens to it as it passes through the digestive tract.

2. Suppose you have a patient who complains of abdominal pain. From what you have learned in this chapter, make a list of the clinical conditions that might cause abdominal pain. What questions would you ask the patient to learn more about the condition? Using any additional information you can obtain, what diagnostic tests would you order done on the patient?

3. Select any three clinical conditions mentioned in this chapter. For each condition plan how you would explain the condition to a person suffering from it, how you would explain the treatment, and how you would encourage the person to cooperate in the treatment.

REFERENCES AND READINGS

Davenport, H. W. 1978. *A digest of digestion* (2nd ed.). Chicago: Year Book Medical Publishers.

Dockray, G. 1979. Comparative biochemistry and physiology of gut hormones. *Annual Review of Physiology* 41:83.

Forte, J. G.. Machen, T. E., and Öbrink. 1980. Mechanisms of gastric H^+ and Cl^- transport. *Annual Review of Physiology* 42:111.

Ganong, W. F. 1981. *Review of medical physiology* (10th ed.). Palo Alto, Calif.: Lange Medical Publications.

Grossman, M. I. 1979. Neural and hormonal regulation of gastrointestinal function: An overview. *Annual Review of Physiology* 41:27.

Guyton, A. C. 1981. *Textbook of medical physiology* (6th ed.). Philadelphia: W. B. Saunders.

Jones, A. L., and Schmucker, D. L. 1977. Current concepts of liver structure as related to function. *Gastroenterology* 73:833.

Jones, R. S., and Myers, W. C. 1979. Regulation of hepatic biliary secretion. *Annual Review of Physiology* 41:67.

McDonagh, A. F., Palma, L. A., and Lightner, D. A. 1980. Blue light and bilirubin excretion. *Science* 208:145 (April 11).

Melnick, J. L., Dreesman, G. R., and Hollinger, F. B. 1977. Viral hepatitis. *Scientific American* 237(1):44 (July).

Moog, F. 1981. The lining of the small intestine. *Scientific American* 245(5): 154 (November).

Napoli, M., and Brintzenhofe, D. 1978. Teeth. *Health Facts* 2(10):1 (July–August).

Schulz, I., and Stolze, H. H. 1980. The exocrine pancreas: The role of secretagogues, cyclic nucleotides, and calcium in enzyme secretion. *Annual Review of Physiology* 42:127.

Soll, A., and Walsh, J. H. 1979. Regulation of gastric acid secretion. *Annual Review of Physiology* 41:35.

Weems, W. A. 1981. The intestine as a fluid propelling system. *Annual Review of Physiology* 43:9.

Weisbrodt, N. W. 1981. Patterns of intestinal motility. *Annual Review of Physiology* 43:21.

Wood, J. D. 1981. Intrinsic neural control of intestinal motility. *Annual Review of Physiology* 43:33.

23

METABOLISM

OVERVIEW OF METABOLISM

Objective 1. Describe the overall process of metabolism.

Once nutrients have been absorbed and transported to cells, metabolic processes take place within cells under the control of enzymes. Generally, an enzyme has a particular chemical structure adapted to catalyzing a particular reaction, though a few enzymes catalyze several similar reactions. The enzymes that control particular reactions are not specified in this text, but it should be understood that each reaction is controlled by an enzyme. Because of the specificity of enzymes structure and function are complementary even at the molecular level.

Homeostasis likewise operates at the molecular level. The rates at which reactions occur are determined in part by chemical equilibria. Such reactions provide energy as it is needed by cells; they also provide building blocks for cellular structures. When the products of a reaction accumulate, they shift the chemical equilibrium and slow, stop, or reverse a reaction until some of the product is used in other reactions. This in itself is a kind of negative feedback mechanism—a basic mechanism at the chemical level that helps to maintain homeostasis.

Metabolism includes **anabolic**, or synthetic, reactions in which the substance of cells is produced, and **catabolic**, or degradative, reactions in which nutrients are generally used to produce energy. Three categories of nutrients—**carbohydrates**, **lipids**, and **proteins**—are the substrates, or reactants, of many metabolic reactions. **Water**, of course, is involved in the majority of reactions either directly or as the medium in which the reactions occur. **Vitamins** and **minerals** also are important in metabolism. Vitamins are molecules that the body cannot synthesize and that are needed for normal metabolism. Many vitamins are incorporated into the structure of **coenzymes**, substances that assist enzymes in carrying out certain reactions. Minerals form part of essential molecules (like the iron in hemoglobin) or facilitate reactions (like calcium in the blood-clotting process). Vitamins, minerals, and water will be discussed in Chapter 24, page 633.

The main catabolic reactions can be summarized in the following generalized reaction: glucose + oxygen → carbon dioxide + water + energy. Though the reaction could occur by burning the sugar in the laboratory, inside the cells of the body it takes place in a series of many enzyme-controlled steps. At several of the steps small amounts of energy are converted to a form usable by cells. As mentioned in Chapter 3, the energy is stored in the high-energy bonds of ATP (adenosine triphosphate) or occasionally in other nucleotides that have high-energy bonds.

Representing a high-energy bond by a wavy line, we can write ATP as follows: $A\text{-}P{\sim}P{\sim}P$, where A is adenosine and the Ps are phosphate groups. Energy stored in either of the high-energy bonds is available for use by cells for their many activities. Energy can be used in a controlled manner to permit muscle cells to contract, nerve cells to transmit impulses, gland cells to secrete, or any cells to carry out active transport and to synthesize materials they use for maintenance, growth, or reproduction. Such synthetic processes involve anabolic reactions.

Coenzymes often are responsible for transporting electrons or hydrogen atoms in a way that ultimately leads to the formation of high-energy bonds in ATP. When hydrogen atoms are removed from substrates, they can be transported directly as atoms, or they may ionize into a proton (H^+) and an electron (e^-), after which the electron is transported by the coenzyme and the proton released into the aqueous medium around the enzyme. For example, the coenzyme flavin adenine dinucleotide (**FAD**) can accept two hydrogen atoms to become $FADH_2$ ($FAD + 2H \rightarrow FADH_2$). The coenzyme nicotinamide adenine dinucleotide (**NAD$^+$**) can accept one atom of hydrogen and one electron, becoming NADH. In this reaction the electron of one hydrogen atom neutralizes the charge on NAD^+, and a proton (H^+) is released into the medium ($NAD^+ + 2e^- + 2H^+ \rightarrow NADH + H^+$). The removal of pairs of hydrogen atoms from substrates is an important component of many metabolic reactions. How hydrogen removal relates to the synthesis of ATP will be discussed later.

CARBOHYDRATE METABOLISM

Objective 2. Describe how carbohydrates are temporarily stored and later released to maintain a relatively constant supply of energy for cells.

Objective 3. For each of the following metabolic processes describe the major reactions in proper sequence, where they occur in the cell, and their net effect on energy production: (a) glycolysis, (b) the Krebs, or citric acid, cycle, (c) oxidative phosphorylation, and (d) the phosphogluconate pathway.

Carbohydrate Transport and Storage

As explained in Chapter 22, the primary products of carbohydrate digestion are the monosaccharides—glucose, fructose, and galactose. After crossing the intestinal mucosa, these monosaccharides travel in the blood of the hepatic portal system to the liver, where some are stored, and then to all cells of the body. They are transported across cell membranes by facilitated diffusion, as described in Chapter 3. Except for the transport into brain and liver cells, insulin facilitates the transport of monosaccharides across cell membranes. In the presence of insulin monosaccharides move across the membrane rapidly, but without it they move so slowly that cells can starve even while they are surrounded by extracellular fluids rich in monosaccharides. The role of insulin is best understood in the transport of glucose, but it is thought that insulin also is involved in the transport of other monosaccharides.

After entry into a cell monosaccharides are phosphorylated. In **phosphorylation** energy from ATP is used to attach a phosphate group to one of the carbon atoms of a monosaccharide, forming glucose-6-phosphate, fructose-6-phosphate, or galactose-1-phosphate. (The numbers designate which carbon atom the phosphate group is attached to.) The phosphorylation of a monosaccharide prevents it from moving back across the cell membrane out of the cell and also incorporates enough energy in the molecule to render it capable of undergoing other metabolic reactions.

Galactose and fructose can be converted to glucose and used to make glycogen. All cells can store at least a small amount of carbohydrate in the form of glycogen, but liver and muscle cells store larger amounts. The maximum amount of glycogen stored in muscle cells is about 1% of the weight of the cell and that in liver cells 5 to 8% of the weight of the cell.

Glycogen is stored in the form of granules (undissolved) composed of long chains of glucose units. This is an efficient means of storing readily available energy without disrupting osmotic conditions within the cell. If the same number of glucose molecules were present as individual particles in the cells, the osmotic pressure in the cells would be so greatly increased as to cause eventual rupture of the cell membranes as the cells swelled with water entering by osmosis.

The process of glycogen formation is called **glycogenesis**, and the process of breaking down glycogen into glucose molecules is called **glycogenolysis**. Two separate sets of reactions are involved in these processes, each catalyzed by a particular enzyme (Figure 23.1).

After a meal the glucose concentration in the blood increases as glucose is absorbed through the small intestine. The liver responds to the increased glucose concentration by extracting glucose and other monosaccharides from the blood as it passes through the liver from the hepatic portal circulation. These monosaccharides are converted to glycogen for storage and for later release as needed. As the individual cells of the body use glucose, the blood glucose concentration drops. This stimulates the release of the hormone epinephrine from the adrenal gland. Stimulation by the sympathetic nervous system also can cause the release of epinephrine. A drop in the blood glucose concentration can stimulate the release of the hormone glucagon from the alpha cells of the pancreas. Any of these hormones can activate an enzyme, adenylate cyclase, in the cell membrane of liver cells. This enzyme causes the breakdown of ATP to cyclic-AMP, and the cyclic-AMP activates the enzyme glycogen phosphorylase. This phosphorylase releases phosphorylated glucose from glycogen. Another enzyme, phosphatase, removes the phosphate from the glucose and allows the glucose to be transported out of the liver cells into the blood. (These reactions also occur in kidney and intestinal cells.) Ultimately, the blood carries the glucose to all the cells of the body.

Metabolic Processes

The three basic processes involved in making energy from glucose available to cells are: (1) glycolysis, (2) the Krebs, or citric acid, cycle, and (3) oxidative phosphorylation. Glycol-

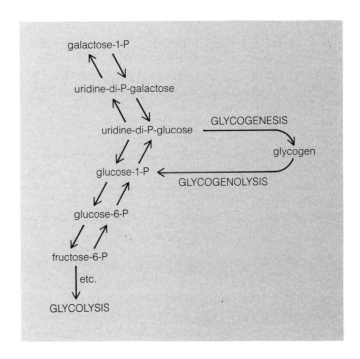

Figure 23.1 Glycogenesis and glycogenolysis. Phosphorylated monosaccharides can be used to synthesize glycogen, but they must first be combined with uridine diphosphate. Glycogen is broken down inro units of glucose-1-phosphate, and these units may go directly into glycolysis, or they may have the phosphate removed to make movement across cell membranes possible. (Energy for phosphorylation is assumed to be available.)

ysis occurs in the cytoplasm and can take place without oxygen; the other processes occur in the mitochondria and require oxygen. The phosphogluconate pathway, which occurs in the cytoplasm, provides an alternate pathway for glucose metabolism.

Glycolysis **Glycolysis** (Figure 23.2) is the process by which a molecule of glucose is broken down into two molecules of pyruvic acid. The pyruvic acid may be converted to lactic acid in the absence of oxygen, as mentioned earlier in the discussion of muscle metabolism (Chapter 8). The process begins with the phosphorylation of glucose, which uses energy from one ATP molecule. Glucose-6-phosphate then rearranges to form fructose-6-phosphate. Another ATP molecule is used to form fructose-1, 6-diphosphate. This six-carbon molecule then splits into two three-carbon molecules, dihydroxyacetone phosphate (DHAP) and 3-phosphoglyceraldehyde (3-PGA). Each DHAP rearranges to form an additional 3-PGA. From this point on in the process

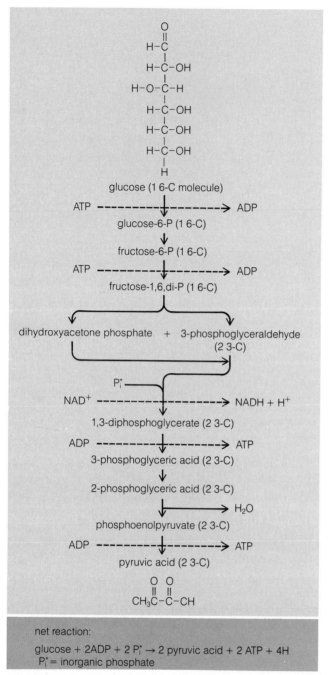

glucose (1 6-C molecule)

ATP - - - - - - - - - - - - - - -> ADP

glucose-6-P (1 6-C)

fructose-6-P (1 6-C)

ATP - - - - - - - - - - - - - - -> ADP

fructose-1,6,di-P (1 6-C)

dihydroxyacetone phosphate + 3-phosphoglyceraldehyde (2 3-C)

P_i^*

NAD^+ - - - - - - - - - - - - - -> $NADH + H^+$

1,3-diphosphoglycerate (2 3-C)

ADP - - - - - - - - - - - - - - -> ATP

3-phosphoglyceric acid (2 3-C)

2-phosphoglyceric acid (2 3-C)

$\longrightarrow H_2O$

phosphoenolpyruvate (2 3-C)

ADP - - - - - - - - - - - - - - -> ATP

pyruvic acid (2 3-C)

net reaction:

glucose + 2ADP + 2 P_i^* → 2 pyruvic acid + 2 ATP + 4H
P_i^* = inorganic phosphate

Figure 23.2 Glycolysis. Two molecules of ATP are required to raise the energy level of glucose so that it can undergo the remainder of the reactions. Fructose-1,6-diphosphate is the compound with the highest energy level. It is broken down into two three-carbon molecules, and the dihydroxyacetone rearranges to form 3-phosphoglyceraldehyde. A molecule of inorganic phosphate is added, and two hydrogen atoms are removed from each three-carbon molecule. The remainder of the sequence involves the formation of two molecules of ATP, the removal of a water molecule, and certain rearrangements of molecules. The direction of the arrows in the diagram indicates the sequence of the reactions when glucose is being broken down.

of glycolysis, two three-carbon molecules must undergo the reactions to account for the fate of one glucose molecule.

To each molecule of 3-PGA one phosphate group is added and two hydrogen atoms are removed, forming 1,3-diphosphoglycerate. The phosphate group comes from the inorganic phosphates within the cell and does not involve the expenditure of energy from an ATP molecule. Of the two hydrogen atoms one is transferred directly to NAD^+; the other ionizes, and its electron neutralizes the charge, forming NADH and a proton (H^+). When 1,3-diphosphoglycerate is converted to 3-phosphoglyceric acid, a phosphate group and energy to form a high-energy bond are transferred to ADP, forming ATP. The 3-phosphoglyceric acid molecule rearranges to form 2-phosphoglyceric acid; a molecule of water is removed from 2-phosphoglyceric acid to form phosphoenolpyruvate (PEP). When PEP is converted to pyruvic acid, the phosphate group and energy to form a high-energy bond are transferred to ADP, forming ATP.

Glycolysis provides cells with a small amount of energy. As shown in Figure 23.2, each three-carbon molecule generates two molecules of ATP, for a total of four ATP molecules per six-carbon glucose molecule. However, two molecules of ATP were used to initiate the reactions, so the net energy produced from glycolysis is two ATP molecules.

Glycolysis takes place in the cytoplasm of a cell and requires a separate enzyme for each of the reactions in the process. Because it is the only energy-producing process that can take place without oxygen, it is responsible for producing the small amount of energy available to oxygen-depleted cells.

The fate of pyruvic acid is determined by the presence or absence of oxygen in the cells. When oxygen is available, pyruvic acid enters the Krebs cycle, as will be explained presently. When oxygen is in short supply, pyruvic acid is converted to lactic acid (Figure 23.3) by the addition of two atoms of hydrogen. The formation of lactic acid allows the cell to temporarily hold hydrogen atoms and allows the hydrogen-removal step of glycolysis to continue. Hydrogen atoms (or electrons from them) previously transferred to NADH are transferred to lactic acid, freeing NAD^+ to accept more hydrogen (or electrons) from 3-PGA. During strenuous exercise lactic acid accumulates in muscle cells and may contribute to the fatigue of muscles before it is carried to the liver. After oxygen becomes available, liver cells convert lactic acid back to pyruvic acid, and the hydrogen atoms and electrons are transferred back to NAD^+, forming $NADH + H^+$. As will be explained in the discussion of oxidative phosphorylation, in the presence of oxygen hydrogen atoms (or electrons) ultimately participate in ATP-producing reactions.

CH_3C—C—C—OH (structure with two C=O groups)

pyruvic acid + NADH + H⁺ ⇌ lactic acid + NAD⁺

CH_3—C—C—OH (structure with OH, O, H)

Figure 23.3 The interconversion between pyruvic and lactic acids.

$$CH_3-C-C-OH$$

$$CH_3-C-CoA$$

pyruvic acid + NAD⁺ + coenzyme A ⟶ acetyl-CoA + NADH + H⁺ + CO_2

Figure 23.4 Pyruvic acid is converted to acetyl-CoA. In the process a molecule of CO_2 and a hydrogen ion are released, and a hydrogen atom and an electron are transferred to NAD⁺.

Krebs cycle Before pyruvic acid can enter the **Krebs cycle**, it must first be converted to **acetyl-coenzyme A**. This conversion occurs in the mitochondria by removal of two hydrogen atoms and one molecule of CO_2 and addition of a molecule of coenzyme A (Figure 23.4). (One H comes from pyruvate and one from coenzyme A.) The hydrogen atoms are transferred to NAD⁺, forming NADH + H⁺. CO_2 ultimately leaves the body in exhaled air, and the two-carbon acetyl group with its attached coenzyme A enters the Krebs cycle.

The Krebs cycle, also called the citric acid cycle or the tricarboxylic acid cycle (Figure 23.5), is a sequence of chemical reactions in which acetyl groups are oxidized to carbon dioxide and hydrogen atoms (or hydrogen ions and electrons). The hydrogen atoms enter the oxidative phosphorylation sequence of reactions, where they combine with oxygen to form water.

Each of the reactions in the Krebs cycle is controlled by a specific enzyme. These enzymes are located inside the mitochrondria, and molecules are passed from one enzyme to the next as they go through the reactions of the Krebs cycle. The sequence of reactions is called a cycle because oxaloacetic acid, which is used in the first step of the cycle, is regenerated at the end of the sequence. As one acetyl group completes the sequence of reactions in the cycle, oxaloacetic acid again becomes available to combine with another acetyl group and go through the same series of reactions.

The steps shown in Figure 23.5 are summarized as follows:

1. Acetyl-CoA combines with oxaloacetic acid, water is added, CoA is removed, and citric acid is formed.

2. Water is removed, and cis-aconitic acid is formed.

3. Water is added, and isocitric acid is formed.

4. Two hydrogen atoms are removed; NADH + H⁺ and α-ketoglutaric acid are formed.

5. Water is added, carbon dioxide is removed, energy is transferred to a high-energy bond in ATP; another two hydrogen atoms are removed, and NADH + H⁺ and succinic acid are formed.

6. Two more hydrogen atoms are removed, and $FADH_2$ and fumaric acid are formed.

7. Water is added, and malic acid is formed.

8. Still another two hydrogen atoms are removed, and NADH + H⁺ is formed; oxaloacetic acid is reformed, ready to receive a new acetyl-CoA.

The above steps illustrate the complexity of the Krebs cycle. At the same time, it is important to identify the significant events in the cycle. Two molecules of CO_2 are produced as the two carbons of the acetyl group are com-

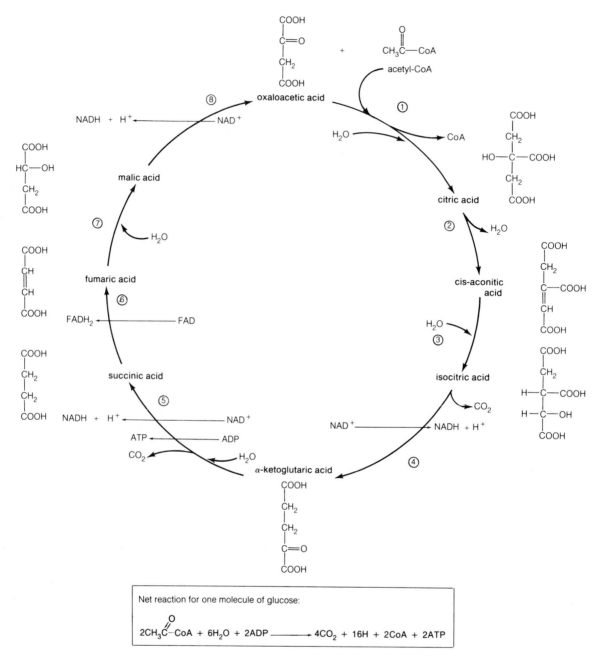

Figure 23.5 The Krebs cycle. In addition to several molecular rearrangements and the addition and removal of water, the important events in the Krebs cycle are the removal of two molecules of CO_2, the transport of eight hydrogen atoms to carriers, NAD^+ and FAD, and the direct formation of one ATP molecule. The circled numbers correspond to the steps listed in the text.

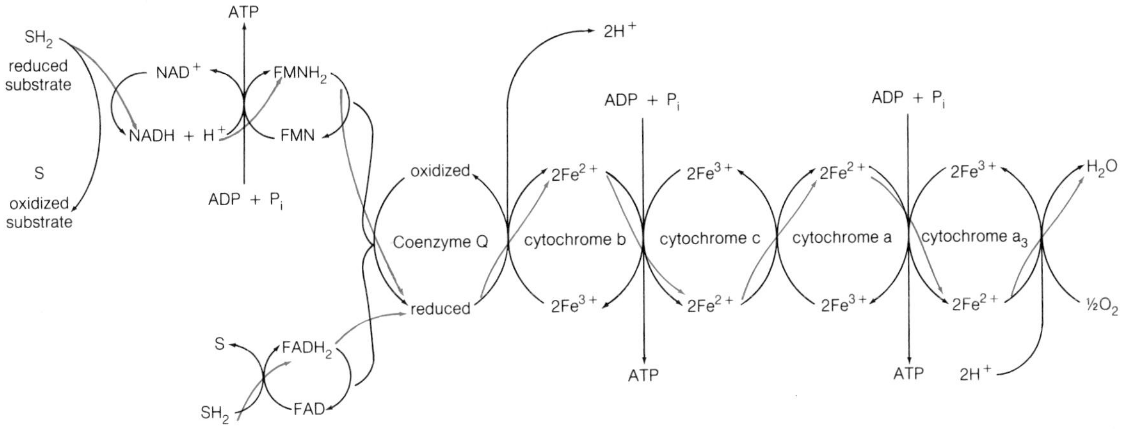

Figure 23.6 Oxidative phosphorylation. See explanation in text.

Net reaction for electrons entering system at NAD$^+$: $SH_2 + \frac{1}{2}O_2 + 3ADP + 3P_i \longrightarrow S + H_2O + 3ATP$.

Net reaction for electrons entering system at FAD: $SH_2 + \frac{1}{2}O_2 + 2ADP + 2P_i \longrightarrow S + H_2O + 2ATP$.

pletely oxidized. Four pairs of hydrogen atoms (or their electrons) are transferred to coenzymes, and significant amounts of energy will be derived from them. Finally, one molecule of ATP is produced directly. Since each molecule of glucose produces *two* molecules of acetyl-CoA, the net energy from a single molecule of glucose is twice that stated above: two molecules of ATP and the energy that will be generated from eight pairs of hydrogen atoms.

Oxidative phosphorylation The process of **oxidative phosphorylation** is closely related to the Krebs cycle and also occurs in the mitochondria. Each step of the process is catalyzed by a specific enzyme. A total of twelve pairs of hydrogen atoms (or their electrons) enter this process from the metabolism of one molecule of glucose: eight pairs from the Krebs cycle, two pairs from glycolysis, and two pairs from conversion of pyruvic acid to acetyl-CoA. The attentive reader will have noted that glucose has only twelve atoms of hydrogen and will wonder how twenty-four atoms are released. The explanation is found in the details of the

Krebs cycle. As indicated in the summary reaction in Figure 23.5, six molecules of water are added to the intermediate molecules for every molecule of glucose (two acetyl groups) that goes through the Krebs cycle. The additional twelve atoms of hydrogen come from these six water molecules.

The sequence of reactions in oxidative phosphorylation is shown in Figure 23.6. Though intact hydrogen atoms are transported by some carrier molecules, the transport of electrons is the significant component of these reactions. Because of the importance of the transport of electrons, the carrier molecules are referred to as **electron carriers** and the system of carrier molecules as the **electron transport system**. The name oxidative phosphorylation implies that both oxidation and phosphorylation occur. Oxidation ultimately results in combining the hydrogen atoms from a substrate (glucose, for example) with oxygen to form water, but as we shall see, this is an oversimplification of the process. Phosphorylation refers to the addition of energy and phosphate to ADP to form ATP. Thus, a combination of oxidative reactions and phosphorylations leads to the formation of water and ATP, two important products of glucose metabolism.

To understand the sequence of reactions that occurs in oxidative phosphorylation, we must first understand what is meant by the terms oxidation and reduction. We have already used the term oxidation to mean combining with oxygen. **Oxidation** can also mean the *removal of hydrogen* or the *loss of an electron*. **Reduction** may be thought of as the opposite of oxidation—the *addition of hydrogen* or the *addition of an electron*. Furthermore, in oxidation-reduction reactions two substances are always involved; one is oxidized, while the other is reduced. For example, in the first step of Figure 23.6 the substrate SH_2 (any substance capable of losing hydrogen) is oxidized by the loss of hydrogen, while the carrier NAD^+ is reduced by the addition of one hydrogen atom and one electron.

Each subsequent step in oxidative phosphorylation involves a similar pair of reactants, one of which is oxidized as the other is reduced. The carrier flavin mononucleotide (FMN) receives two hydrogen atoms as $NADH + H^+$ is reduced. A similar carrier, FAD, receives two hydrogen atoms as a molecule of substrate is oxidized. It should be noted that hydrogen atoms from substrates being metabolized can enter the oxidative phosphorylation process by being transferred to either NAD^+ or FAD. (Recall that most of the hydrogens removed from intermediate products of glucose metabolism are transferred to NAD^+, but hydrogens from succinic acid are transferred to FAD.)

Hydrogen atoms from either $NADH + H^+$ or FADH can be transferred to coenzyme Q, another hydrogen-carrying coenzyme. When the hydrogen atoms are transferred from coenzyme Q, both ionize, and the electrons are transferred to iron ions in the carrier molecules called **cytochromes**. (The protons are released into the medium.) The cytochromes are proteins imbedded in the cristae of mitochondria that contain heme groups like the iron-containing heme of hemoglobin. The iron in the heme has a charge of $+3$ in its oxidized state; when it receives an electron, it is reduced to a charge of $+2$. Because each molecule of cytochrome can carry only one electron, two molecules are required to transfer a pair of electrons. When a pair of electrons reaches the end of the sequence of cytochromes, the electrons combine with an atom of oxygen and two hydrogen ions to form water: $\frac{1}{2}O_2 + 2e^- + 2H^+ \rightarrow H_2O$. Ultimately, twelve pairs of electrons and twelve pairs of H^+ combine with $6O_2$ to form $12H_2O$. Thus, we might think of oxygen as the final electron acceptor.

When oxygen is in short supply in cells, the electron carriers become saturated with electrons and cannot accept any more. When the carriers are saturated, hydrogen atoms cannot be removed from the substrates (the intermediate products of glycolysis and the Krebs cycle). Lactic acid accumulates as the Krebs cycle ceases to operate.

When oxygen is available, electron carriers operate continuously to shuttle electrons from the hydrogen atoms that are removed from the substrates. The efficient operation of the electron transport system allows for the production of large numbers of ATP molecules. At three points along the electron transport system the transfer of electrons releases sufficient energy to create a high-energy bond. As shown by the arrows in Figure 23.6, the transfer of electrons from NADH to FMN allows inorganic phosphate (P_i) to be combined with ADP to form a high-energy bond in ATP. ATP is similarly produced as electrons are transferred from cytochrome b to cytochrome c, and as electrons are transferred from cytochrome a to cytochrome a_3. Therefore, for every pair of electrons first transferred to NAD^+, three molecules of ATP are produced in the process of oxidative phosphorylation. For every pair of electrons first transferred to FAD (rather than NAD^+), only two molecules of ATP are produced because these electrons enter the electron transport system beyond the point at which the first molecule of ATP is produced.

Of the twelve pairs of hydrogen atoms (actually their electrons) transferred to the electron transport system from

Many substances that cause illness or death do so by interfering with metabolic reactions. For example, the poison cyanide exerts its deadly effects by combining with the cytochromes and preventing the production of ATP. Heavy metals, such as lead and mercury, are incorporated into the structure of proteins and disrupt the normal configuration of the molecules. If the molecule happens to be an enzyme, the activity of the enzyme is greatly decreased. Deficiencies of enzymes lead to a slowdown or cessation of the reactions they catalyze. For example, a deficiency of the enzyme glucose-6-phosphate dehydrogenase prevents the phosphogluconate pathway from operating efficiently. Because this pathway is important in making five-carbon sugars such as ribose and deoxyribose, its deficient function leads to a lack of these sugars. A lack of the sugars leads to a deficiency of the building blocks for DNA and RNA and thus to a slowdown in the formation of new cells. Because the most rapidly replaced cells are the erythrocytes, a deficiency in this enzyme leads to anemia.

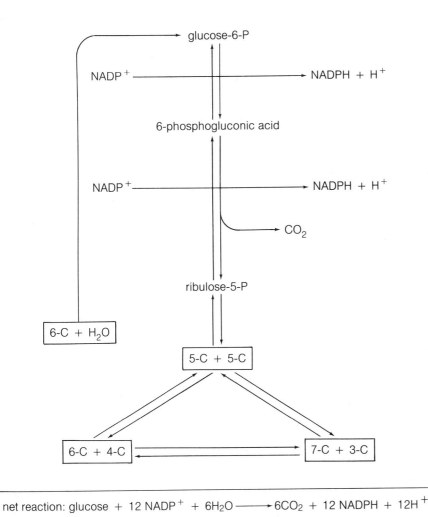

glucose-6-P

$NADP^+$ ⟶ $NADPH + H^+$

6-phosphogluconic acid

$NADP^+$ ⟶ $NADPH + H^+$

⟶ CO_2

ribulose-5-P

6-C + H_2O

5-C + 5-C

6-C + 4-C   7-C + 3-C

net reaction: glucose + 12 $NADP^+$ + 6H_2O ⟶ 6CO_2 + 12 NADPH + 12H^+

Figure 23.7 A summary of the phosphogluconate pathway. The four hydrogens removed from glucose are transferred to the hydrogen carrier, $NADP^+$, forming $NADPH + H^+$. $NADP^+$ is a nucleotide that has one more phosphate than NAD^+ and is essential for the synthesis of fats and many other compounds. Each time a glucose molecule goes through this cycle, one CO_2 is released, and a five-carbon molecule is produced. By various recombinations of three-, four-, five-, six-, and seven-carbon molecules, a new six-carbon molecule is made available for another trip through the cycle. Therefore, six trips through the cycle are necessary to completely metabolize one molecule of glucose.

the metabolism of a molecule of glucose, ten pairs are transferred to NAD^+, and two pairs are transferred to FAD. Thus, oxidative phosphorylation produces thirty-four molecules of ATP for every glucose molecule—three from each of ten pairs of electrons transferred to NAD^+ and two from each of two pairs transferred to FAD. This is seventeen times the amount of ATP produced by glycolysis under anaerobic conditions.

The phosphogluconate pathway Though most carbohydrates are broken down by way of glycolysis and the Krebs cycle, an alternative pathway does exist. As much as 30% of the glucose entering the liver or the fatty tissues of the body is

metabolized by way of the alternate **phosphogluconate pathway**, also called the hexose monophosphate shunt. The phosphogluconate pathway, which occurs in the cytoplasm, is important for three reasons: (1) It can operate when glycolysis is slowed for some reason, (2) it provides a source of five-carbon sugars for making DNA and RNA, and (3) it provides a source of hydrogen bound to a carrier called nicotinamide adenine dinucleotide phosphate ($NADP^+$). Adding hydrogen to $NADP^+$ forms $NADPH + H^+$. This is the only carrier from which hydrogen can be used in the synthesis of fatty acids and several other important compounds. The phosphogluconate pathway is summarized in Figure 23.7. Note that no ATP is produced in this pathway.

LIPID METABOLISM

Objective 4. Describe (a) how lipids are transported across cell membranes, and (b) how they are stored and later released for energy.

Objective 5. Describe the major events in the metabolism of lipids.

Lipid Transport and Storage

After absorption into the lacteals all types of lipids—triglycerides, phospholipids, and cholesterol—are transported in protein-covered chylomicrons, as explained in Chapter 22. Because chylomicrons travel in the lymphatic vessels, they bypass the liver and enter the systemic blood circulation at the left subclavian vein and are then carried to the tissues, particularly the adipose tissues. When chylomicrons are present in the blood, as after a meal, the blood concentrations of glucose and insulin are also elevated. Insulin activates an enzyme, **lipoprotein lipase**, which is bound to the endothelial cells of the blood vessels. As the chylomicrons pass along the endothelial cells, this enzyme digests the triglycerides and phospholipids from the chylomicrons to fatty acids and other molecules that can enter cells, especially the cells of adipose tissue.

Lipids are stored primarily in adipose tissues, the "signet ring" cells of which can store triglycerides in amounts equivalent to 80 to 95% of the cell volume. Glucose also enters adipose cells, being stimulated to do so by the presence of insulin. Inside the cells glucose is converted to α-glycerophosphate and then to glycerol. Glycerol and fatty acids (from the chylomicrons) are combined to form triglycerides. The synthesis and storage of other lipids will be discussed with lipid metabolism.

Stored lipids serve two functions: (1) They act as a store of energy, and (2) they insulate the body against temperature changes. Lipids are an excellent form of energy storage because they are insoluble in water (cannot "wash out" of the body) and because they contain large amounts of hydrogen. As explained in the discussion of carbohydrate metabolism, organic compounds containing large amounts of hydrogen yield significant amounts of ATP through oxidative phosphorylation. Lipids stored in subcutaneous tissues help to prevent heat loss from the body.

Lipid Metabolism

The human diet contains all types of lipids. In fact, half of the energy content of the American diet comes from lipids and as much as half of the carbohydrate energy content is first converted to lipid and only later metabolized for energy. Thus, the metabolism of lipids is an extremely important component of normal metabolism. As explained in Chapter 2, triglycerides are hydrolyzed to glycerol and three fatty acid molecules. The glycerol is metabolized to glyceraldehyde and can then enter either the glycolytic or the phosphogluconate pathway.

Fatty acids are metabolized by the process of **beta oxidation**, so named because fatty acids are broken at the beta carbon—the second carbon from the carboxyl group. The most commonly occurring fatty acids in the human diet are stearic acid (a saturated eighteen-carbon chain), oleic acid (an unsaturated eighteen-carbon chain with a double bond in the middle of the chain), and palmitic acid (a saturated sixteen-carbon chain). These fatty acids and others have an even number of carbons, and each is metabolized by the removal of two-carbon units in beta oxidation (Figure 23.8). In beta oxidation a molecule of ATP is used to energize the fatty acid and to combine it with coenzyme A. A pair of hydrogen atoms transfer to carrier FAD, and a double bond forms in the fatty acid chain between the α- and β- carbons. (The α-carbon is the one next to the acid group, and the β-carbon is the one next to the unaltered carbon chain.) A molecule of water is added to these carbons, removing the double bond and placing the —H on the α-carbon and the —OH on the β-carbon. A pair of hydrogen atoms is removed from the β-carbon, leaving an oxygen atom attached to that carbon. An electron and a hydrogen atom are transferred to NAD⁺. Finally, the acetyl-CoA is split from the molecule, and another CoA is added to the former β-carbon. The fatty acid–CoA complex, having been shortened by two carbons, reenters the cycle. A molecule containing eighteen carbons would therefore go through this cycle eight times to convert it completely to acetyl-CoA groups—one time less than the number of pairs of carbons because the last time through the cycle produces two acetyl-CoA from a four-carbon molecule. A total of sixteen pairs of hydrogen atoms would be removed and eight pairs of electrons transferred to FAD and eight pairs to NAD⁺. The electrons go directly to the oxidative phosphorylation system, and the acetyl-CoA groups are metabolized in the Krebs cycle.

The total energy from beta oxidation of an eighteen-carbon fatty acid includes twenty-four ATPs from the eight pairs of electrons transferred to NAD⁺ and sixteen ATPs from the eight pairs of electrons transferred to FAD. In addition, twelve ATPs are produced from each acetyl-CoA—a total of 108 ATPs as nine acetyl-CoA groups go through the Krebs cycle and oxidative phosphorylation. *Thus, one eighteen-carbon molecule of fatty acid generates a grand total of 148 molecules of ATP!* This is almost 1½ times the

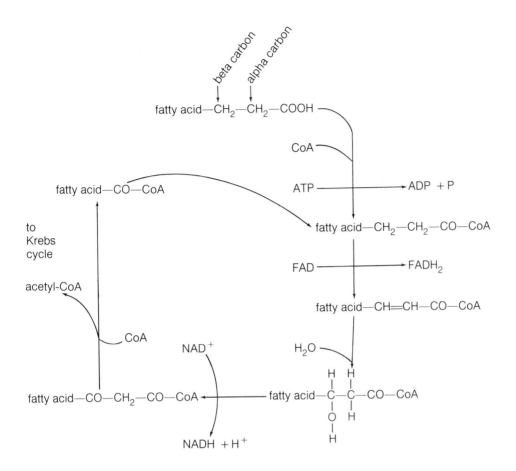

beta carbon

alpha carbon

fatty acid—CH_2—CH_2—COOH

CoA

fatty acid—CO—CoA

ATP ⟶ ADP + P

to
Krebs
cycle

fatty acid—CH_2—CH_2—CO—CoA

acetyl-CoA

FAD ⟶ $FADH_2$

CoA

fatty acid—CH=CH—CO—CoA

NAD^+

H_2O

fatty acid—CO—CH_2—CO—CoA ⟵ fatty acid—$\overset{H}{\underset{O\text{—}H}{C}}$—$\overset{H}{\underset{H}{C}}$—CO—CoA

$NADH + H^+$

Figure 23.8 Beta oxidation of a fatty acid. Each time a molecule of fatty acid goes through this cycle, it loses four hydrogen atoms and an acetyl group with an attached coenzyme A. The fatty acid molecule is shorter by two carbons when it enters the cycle. (See text for further explanation.)

amount of energy produced by oxidation of three glucose molecules (eighteen carbons total), and almost 25 times the amount of energy from glycolysis of three glucose molecules (without oxygen). It's not hard to see the energy advantage of metabolizing lipid.

The role of the liver in lipid metabolism   The liver produces far more acetyl-CoA than it can use for its own energy needs. Liver cells condense two molecules of acetyl-CoA into acetoacetic acid. Much of the acetoacetic acid is converted to β-hydroxybutyric acid, and small quantities are converted to acetone. The production of these molecules, called **ketone bodies**, is shown in Figure 23.9. Both acetoacetic acid and β-hydroxybutyric acid can diffuse freely out of the liver and enter various tissues. Cells in these tissues reconvert these molecules back to acetyl-CoA and use them for energy.

When the body is relying primarily on the metabolism of fat for its energy, excessive amounts of ketone bodies

may build up in the blood and create a condition called **ketosis**. Ketosis occurs when the entry of carbohydrate into cells is greatly reduced. This could result from an absence of carbohydrate in starvation, from a high-fat diet, or from the absence or inactivity of insulin in diabetes mellitus. The accumulation of ketone bodies raises the acid concentration in the blood and can lead to acidosis. The body's mechanisms for compensating for acidosis are discussed in Chapter 26.

In addition to producing ketone bodies the liver can synthesize fatty acids by the process of **beta reduction**. The acetyl-CoA groups are rejoined to form long-chain fatty acids by a sequence of reactions quite different from the reverse of beta oxidation. The hydrogen carrier in this process is NADP, and the source of the hydrogen it carries is the phosphogluconate pathway. Triglycerides can be formed in the liver, or the fatty acids can be transported to adipose cells and the triglycerides formed there. Both fatty acids and triglycerides are carried in lipoprotein particles in the blood.

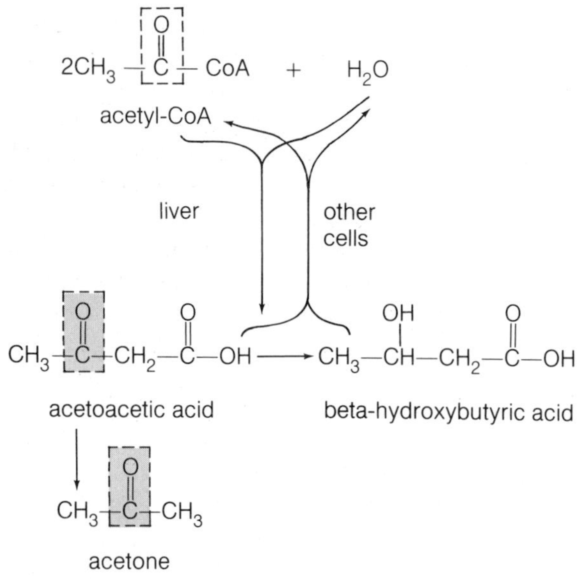

Figure 23.9 The formation and degradation of ketone bodies. A $C = O$ group in a carbon chain is a ketone group. Beta-hydroxybutyric acid has no ketone group but is derived from molecules that do.

the synthesis of vitamin D. Small quantities of cholesterol are also used by the adrenal glands and the gonads (ovaries and testes) to synthesize steroid hormones.

Much research effort is currently focused on factors that contribute to cholesterol deposition. Some studies have provided evidence that maintaining a diet low in cholesterol and saturated fats may minimize the expansion of the body's cholesterol pool. However, when the amount of dietary cholesterol is reduced, the liver responds by synthesizing more. Because the building block of cholesterol synthesis is acetyl-CoA, a component of the metabolism of both lipids and carbohydrates, it is impossible to deprive the body of this raw material. A hereditary condition, hypercholesterolemia, results in an excess of cholesterol carried in the blood in particles called low-density lipoproteins. The effects of atherosclerosis and the possible role of lipoproteins in the disease were discussed in Chapter 19.

Structural lipids Although lipids serve as an important source of energy, some lipids are also important structural components of cell membranes and other structures. All these lipids can be synthesized by available enzymes if the **essential fatty acid** linoleic acid is available from foods that contain vegetable fat. Linoleic acid consists of an eighteen-carbon chain with two double bonds. This essential fatty acid is needed to maintain cell membranes and may also be required for the transport and metabolism of cholesterol.

Cholesterol metabolism Cholesterol, whose structure was described in Chapter 2, is present in any diet containing animal fats. It is slowly absorbed into the lacteals and carried through the lymph and blood in lipoprotein particles. In addition to dietary cholesterol most of the cells of the body can synthesize small quantities of cholesterol; the liver and small intestine can synthesize larger quantities.

The body uses cholesterol in a variety of ways. A significant fraction of the cholesterol is used to synthesize bile acids. (The role of bile acids and their salts in digestion was described in Chapter 22.) Along with other lipids cholesterol is also an important component of cell membranes. It is deposited in large amounts in the stratum corneum of the skin, where it protects against water loss. A derivative, 7-dehydrocholesterol, which is found in the skin, is used in

PROTEIN METABOLISM

Objective 6. Define nitrogen balance and describe how it is maintained.

Objective 7. Describe the major events in the metabolism of proteins.

About three-fourths of the solid portion of the body is composed of protein. The composition of proteins and some of their uses were described in Chapter 2, the mechanism of protein synthesis was described in Chapter 3, and the manner in which proteins are digested was described in Chapter 22.

After proteins are digested into their component amino acids and absorbed into the blood, they are transported into the cells. Absorption from the digestive tract continues for several hours after eating a meal, but when amino acids reach the blood, they are taken up into cells within five to ten minutes.

Nitrogen Balance

Proteins and amino acids, unlike carbohydrates and lipids, are not stored in cells in any significant amounts. Some of the protein components of cells (enzymes and certain structural proteins) are replaced periodically in a process called **protein turnover**. This process occurs continuously and at a fairly rapid rate. When proteins are replaced, the nitrogen they contained is excreted by a process that will be described in Chapter 25. The amount of nitrogen lost in this fashion must be replaced from nitrogen in amino acids in the diet. If the dietary nitrogen equals the nitrogen lost, the body is said to be in **nitrogen balance**. During growth or pregnancy, when more protein is being synthesized than is being degraded, the nitrogen intake exceeds the loss, and the body is in **positive nitrogen balance**. In contrast, during starvation or in certain wasting diseases, the nitrogen intake is less than the nitrogen loss, and the body is in **negative nitrogen balance**.

Protein Metabolism

Of the twenty amino acids normally found in proteins, eight must be supplied from dietary sources because the human body lacks the enzymes to synthesize them. These, the **essential amino acids**, are leucine, isoleucine, lysine, methionine, phenylalanine, threonine, tryptophan, and valine. Two additional amino acids, arginine and histidine, are synthesized in such small quantities in the human body that better nutrition is maintained if these are also included in the diet, especially during periods of rapid growth. How the essential amino acids can be obtained in the diet will be discussed in Chapter 24.

Proteins, long chains of amino acids, form part of the structure of cell membranes, chromosomes, and organelles. Some function as enzymes, and others have specialized functions, such as the contractile proteins of muscle, fibrous proteins of connective tissue, and the various albumins and globulins of blood plasma. As explained in Chapter 3, proper matching with nucleotide bases in RNA molecules is required for correct placement of each amino acid in a protein. A protein molecule can be synthesized only if each of the appropriate amino acids is available to be incorporated into the growing protein chain. Without sufficient quantities of each of the essential amino acids, the cell would be unable to make proteins. The process would stop at the first codon for which the proper amino acid–transfer RNA complex was unavailable.

Some amino acids are important in the synthesis of molecules other than proteins. Tyrosine, for example, is used for the synthesis of both thyroxine and epinephrine. Other amino acids contribute to the formation of the neurotransmitters serotonin and gamma-aminobutyric acid, and the nitrogenous bases of DNA, RNA, ATP, and the carrier molecules in the electron transport system.

Certain amino acids typically undergo chemical reactions called **transamination** and **deamination** (Figure 23.10). In transamination an amino group is transferred from one molecule to another. Some of the nonessential amino acids can be synthesized by transamination from carbohydrate precursors, but this occurs at the expense of removing an amino group from another amino acid.

Deamination is the removal of an amino group from an amino acid, producing an α-keto acid and ammonia. Ammonia is toxic if it accumulates in any significant amount in the blood. As ammonia travels through the liver, it is converted to urea by a complex sequence of reactions called the **urea cycle**. Urea, a much less toxic substance that is easily excreted by the kidneys, is the major form in which nitrogen wastes are removed from the body.

The α-keto acids can enter the Krebs cycle or some other step in carbohydrate metabolism, so deaminated amino acids can be used for energy. The circumstances in which amino acids are used for energy include: (1) starvation, where the supply of carbohydrates and lipids is so depleted that tissue proteins are metabolized for energy; (2) protein turnover, where small amounts of cellular protein are degraded and replaced; and (3) high-protein diets, where more protein than the body needs is taken in.

Gluconeogenesis The synthesis of glucose from other substances such as glycerol and amino acids is known as **gluconeogenesis**. This process is accelerated when the carbohydrate intake is insufficient, and body stores of glycogen have been depleted. About 60% of the amino acids in tissue proteins can be used to synthesize glucose, each by a different chemical process. Many are deaminated and become intermediate three-, four-, or five-carbon compounds that can enter the phosphogluconate pathway.

SUMMARY OF ENERGY-PRODUCING METABOLISM

Objective 8. Summarize the major events in energy-producing metabolism.

The major events in the metabolism of carbohydrates, lipids, and proteins for use as energy are summarized in Figure 23.11. The energy calculations in the figure are based on the metabolism of one molecule of glucose. Glycolysis, the Krebs cycle, and oxidative phosphorylation are each shown in colored blocks. Three bars at the right of the diagram indicate important products of reactions: hydrogen atoms, ATP molecules, and carbon dioxide molecules. Thus, the products of glycolysis are two pyruvic acid mol-

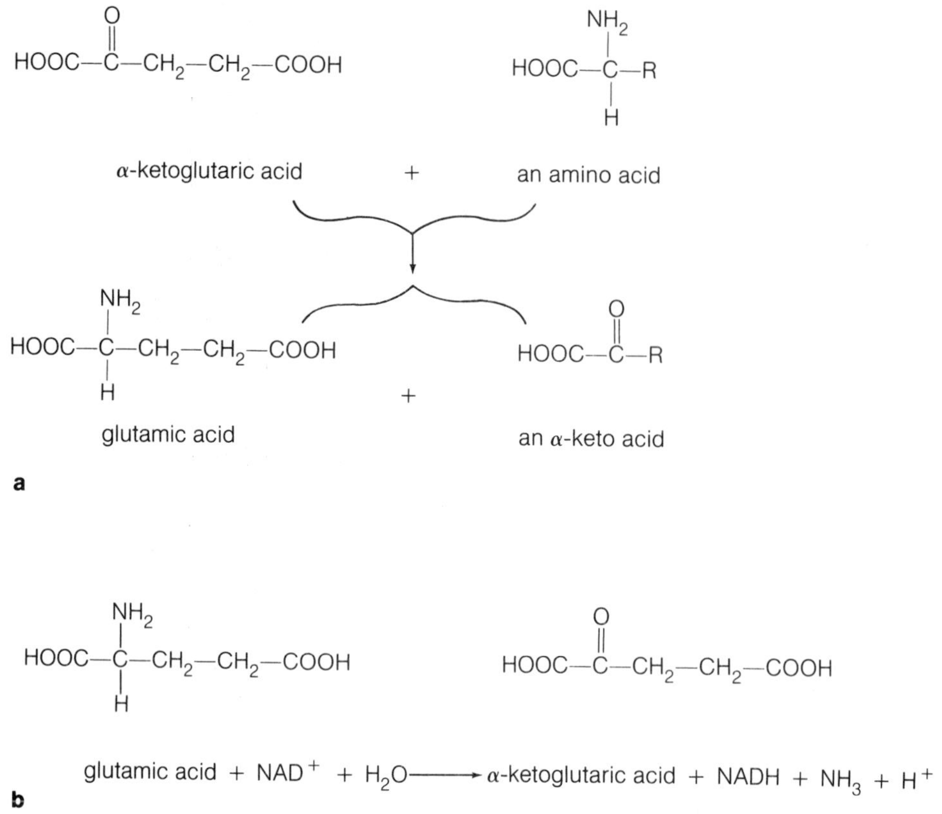

$$HOOC-\underset{\underset{O}{\|}}{C}-CH_2-CH_2-COOH$$

α-ketoglutaric acid   +   an amino acid

$$HOOC-\underset{\underset{H}{|}}{\overset{\overset{NH_2}{|}}{C}}-R$$

$$HOOC-\underset{\underset{H}{|}}{\overset{\overset{NH_2}{|}}{C}}-CH_2-CH_2-COOH$$

glutamic acid

$$HOOC-\underset{\underset{O}{\|}}{C}-R$$

+

an α-keto acid

a

Figure 23.10 Transamination and deamination. (**a**) In transamination the NH$_2$ group from an amino acid is exchanged with the oxygen from a keto group in α-ketoglutaric acid to form glutamic acid and an α-keto acid similar to the amino acid. (**b**) In deamination the amino group is removed from glutamic acid to form the keto acid, and ammonia is released along with two hydrogens.

$$HOOC-\underset{\underset{H}{|}}{\overset{\overset{NH_2}{|}}{C}}-CH_2-CH_2-COOH$$

$$HOOC-\underset{\underset{O}{\|}}{C}-CH_2-CH_2-COOH$$

glutamic acid + NAD$^+$ + H$_2$O ⟶ α-ketoglutaric acid + NADH + NH$_3$ + H$^+$

b

ecules, four hydrogen atoms, and two ATPs. In the conversion of two pyruvic acid molecules to two acetyl-CoAs, four hydrogen atoms and two CO$_2$ molecules are produced. From the processing of two acetyl-CoAs in the Krebs cycle, sixteen hydrogen atoms (or their electrons) are transferred to NAD$^+$, and four are transferred to FAD; two ATPs are produced directly; and four molecules of CO$_2$ are released. Totals at the bottom of each of the three bars show the total number of hydrogen atoms, ATPs, and CO$_2$ molecules produced from one molecule of glucose.

In the summary of oxidative phosphorylation ten ATPs are produced as twenty hydrogen atoms are transferred from NAD$^+$ + H$^+$ to FAD; twelve ATPs are produced from the twenty-four electrons transferred from FAD to the cytochromes, and another twelve from transfers within the cytochrome chain. The twenty-four H$^+$, twenty-four electrons, and six O$_2$ combine to form twelve H$_2$O.

Of the net thirty-eight ATPs produced, four were produced directly—two from glycolysis and two from the Krebs cycle; the other thirty-four came from oxidative phosphorylation.

At the top and left of the figure words in capital letters show where various nutrients enter the metabolic processes. Glycogenolysis and glycogenesis are also related to glycolysis.

REGULATION OF METABOLISM

Objective 9. Distinguish between the absorptive and the postabsorptive metabolic states in terms of (a) processes that occur and (b) how those processes are regulated.

Objective 10. Define metabolic rate and describe the factors that regulate it, including the roles of hunger and satiety and respiratory quotients.

Objective 11. Explain how body temperature is regulated and list the factors that affect it.

Absorptive and Postabsorptive Metabolism

Up to this point in this chapter we have considered the major sequences of chemical reactions involved in the

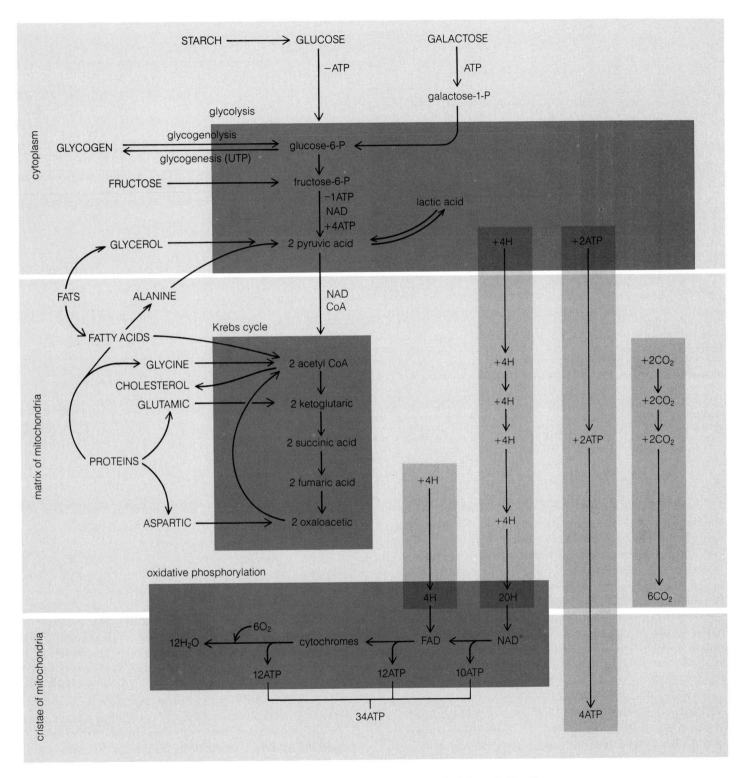

Figure 23.11 Summary of energy-producing metabolism. The total number of ATPs from glycolysis is a net of two; the total number from the Krebs cycle and oxidative phosphorylation is thirty-six. Thus, the major portion of the energy from one molecule of glucose comes from the oxygen-requiring steps. Also shown in the figure are the steps in the process at which the various nutrients enter the process.

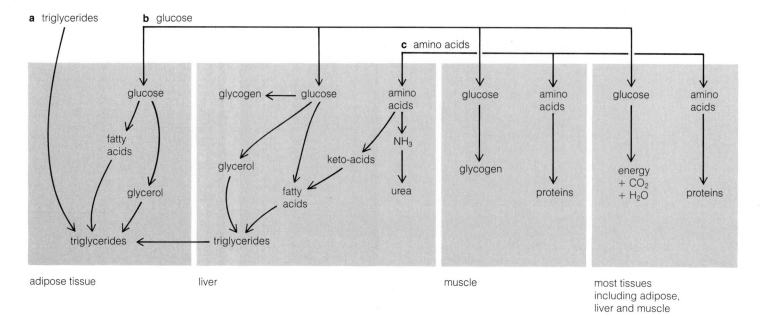

a triglycerides   **b** glucose   **c** amino acids

adipose tissue   liver   muscle   most tissues including adipose, liver and muscle

Figure 23.12 Metabolic events in the absorptive state: (**a**) Triglycerides enter cells of adipose tissue and are stored there. (**b**) In addition to being used to maintain blood glucose concentration, excess glucose enters the liver, where it is converted to glycogen, and the liver or adipose tissue, where it is converted to glycerol and fatty acids, and ultimately to triglycerides. Some glucose also goes to muscle, where it is converted to glycogen, and to most other tissues, where it is used for energy. (**c**) Some amino acids are distributed to all tissues, where they are used to synthesize protein. Some also go to the liver, where they are used to synthesize plasma proteins and can be deaminated and converted to fatty acids and eventually incorporated into triglycerides. Ammonia from deamination is used to synthesize urea, a nitrogenous waste product.

breakdown of nutrients for energy and those involved in the synthesis of the chemical components of cells. Now we are ready to see how these processes are regulated.

To study the regulation of metabolism, it is convenient to consider the absorptive and postabsorptive states separately. The body is in the **absorptive state** for about four hours after a meal while food is being absorbed from the intestine. It is in the **postabsorptive state** for an hour or two before meals and during most of the night when no nutrients are being absorbed from the intestine.

Events in the absorptive state Following absorption glucose (and other monosaccharides) and amino acids first pass through the liver and later go to other tissues of the body. Triglycerides (and some mono- and diglycerides) travel through the lymphatics and blood vessels to enter cells of adipose tissue. The fate of each of these nutrients in the various tissues is summarized in Figure 23.12. The overall effect of absorptive metabolism is to maintain a normal blood glucose concentration and at the same time to conserve energy from all other nutrients by storing that energy

in glycogen or triglycerides. Absorptive metabolism also provides amino acids to cells for protein synthesis.

Events in the postabsorptive state In the postabsorptive state nutrients stored as glycogen and triglycerides are released in a controlled manner. This regulated release maintains a normal blood glucose concentration and provides glucose, fatty acids, or ketones to the cells of all tissues. Under starvation conditions proteins can also be converted to amino acids and metabolized for energy. The use of each of these nutrients in the postabsorptive state is summarized in Figure 23.13. The overall effect of postabsorptive metabolism is to make a source of energy available to all cells when no glucose is being absorbed. The ability of most cells to metabolize fatty acids instead of glucose, a phenomenon called **glucose sparing**, conserves glucose for cells—erythrocytes and neurons—that require it. Though erythrocytes require glucose at all times, after several days of starvation conditions neurons do become able to metabolize ketones, though not fatty acids, for energy.

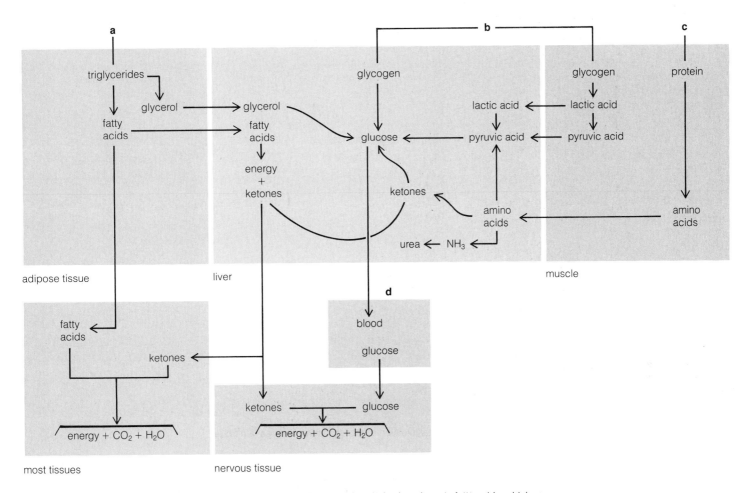

Figure 23.13 Metabolic events in the postabsorptive state: (**a**) Triglycerides are broken down to fatty acids, which are metabolized for energy, and glycerol, which is converted to glucose in the liver and used for energy. (**b**) Glycogen from the liver and from muscles is metabolized to lactic acid or pyruvic acid. These molecules are converted to glucose in the liver. (**c**) When the need for glucose is great, proteins are broken down to amino acids and transported to the liver, where they are deaminated and their keto-acid derivatives used to synthesize glucose. (**d**) The focal event in the postabsorptive state is to maintain a normal blood glucose concentration and a constant supply of glucose for nervous tissue, even though nervous tissue eventually metabolizes ketones under starvation conditions.

Regulatory Processes

The mechanisms that regulate both absorptive and postabsorptive metabolism and that control the shift from one to the other involve hypothalamic centers, hormones, and their interactions with the blood glucose level. Several complex homeostatic mechanisms are in operation. We will examine three of them—the insulin-glucagon mechanism, the epinephrine-hypothalamic mechanism, and the growth hormone–hypothalamic mechanism.

The blood glucose concentration is an important factor in the operation of each of these regulatory mechanisms. In a fasting normal adult the blood glucose concentration is between 80 and 100 milligrams/100 milliliters of blood. For an hour or two following a meal, as glucose is absorbed, the blood glucose concentration rises to a level of 120 to 140 milligrams/100 milliliters of blood. It falls back to normal within two hours after glucose absorption has ceased. With this introduction to normal variation in blood glucose concentration, we are now ready to consider the mechanisms that regulate it.

The insulin-glucagon mechanism   During the absorptive state, as shown in Figure 23.14, blood with a higher than normal glucose concentration flows through the pancreas. The glu-

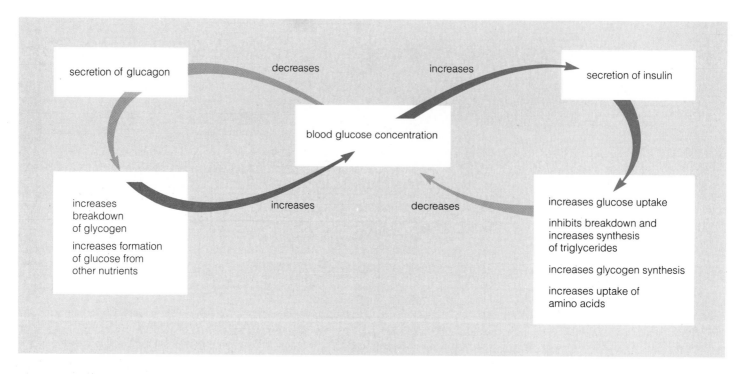

Figure 23.14 The insulin-glucagon mechanism: When the blood glucose concentration increases, insulin is produced, and its action reduces the blood glucose concentration. When the blood glucose concentration is reduced, glucagon (instead of insulin) is produced, and the action of glucagon increases the blood glucose concentration. This system of negative feedback shown by the "figure-8" in the diagram represents one of the homeostatic mechanisms that helps to regulate the blood glucose concentration.

cose stimulates the secretion of the hormone insulin. As insulin is released into the blood, it acts in several ways to reduce the blood glucose concentration. It increases the rate of facilitated diffusion of glucose across cell membranes. When adequate amounts of insulin are available, the presence of glucose in the cells of adipose tissues, in turn, inhibits the breakdown of existing triglycerides and stimulates the synthesis of more triglycerides from the glucose. Insulin also stimulates the synthesis of glycogen in liver and muscle tissue (glycogenesis), and it stimulates both the entry of amino acids into all cells and their use in protein synthesis.

As these actions of insulin occur, the blood glucose concentration drops. As the blood with the lowered glucose content passes through the pancreas, the stimulus for enhanced insulin release is no longer present, and insulin secretion by the pancreas returns to basal levels.

When the blood glucose concentration falls below 70 milligrams/100 milliliters of blood, the pancreas is stimulated to secrete the hormone glucagon. Glucagon stimulates the breakdown of glycogen (glycogenolysis) and the formation of glucose from other nutrients (gluconeogenesis). During strenuous exercise or starvation the secretion of glucagon is increased. Studies of individuals lacking insulin have shown that glucagon secretion can be stimulated even when the blood glucose concentration is high. Apparently, it is the amount of glucose entering the glucagon-secreting cells that regulates their secretion. When too little insulin is available to help move glucose into cells, the glucagon-secreting cells receive little glucose and behave as if the glucose level were low.

Amino acids in the blood provide moderate stimulation of the release of both insulin and glucagon. Thus, a high-protein, low-carbohydrate meal will stimulate the release of both hormones, and they will have a stabilizing effect on the blood glucose concentration. In fact, all hormones are secreted at a certain basal level that maintains homeostasis. Various stimuli enhance or reduce rates of secretion above or below basal levels when these actions are needed to maintain homeostasis.

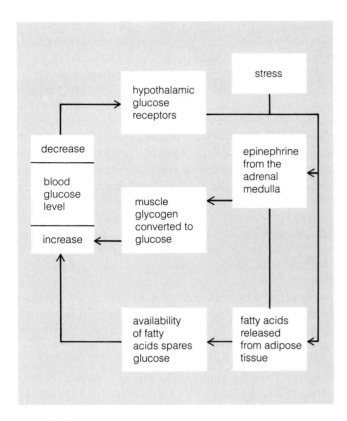

Figure 23.15 The epinephrine-hypothalamic mechanism: A decrease in blood glucose stimulates glucose receptors in the hypothalamus to send nerve signals to adipose tissue and to the adrenal gland. Nerve signals resulting from stress have the same effect. Once stimulated, the adrenal gland releases epinephrine, which stimulates the breakdown of glycogen to glucose in muscles. Fatty acids released from adipose tissue provide an alternative energy source and supplement glucose, thereby increasing the blood glucose concentration.

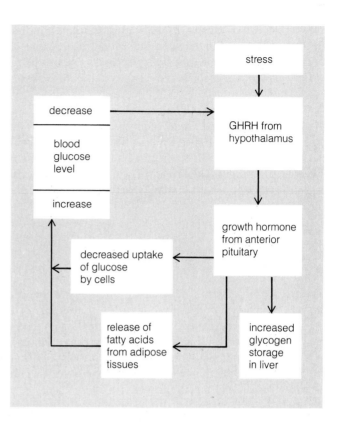

Figure 23.16 The growth hormone–hypothalamic mechanism: When the blood glucose decreases or stress is present, the hypothalamus releases GHRH, which in turn causes the anterior pituitary to release growth hormone. Growth hormone decreases glucose uptake and increases fatty acid release, thereby increasing the blood glucose concentration. The increase in glycogen storage preserves a supply of glycogen, which can later be released to maintain a stable blood glucose concentration over a longer period of time.

The epinephrine-hypothalamic mechanism In addition to the insulin-glucagon mechanism the hormone epinephrine operates in conjunction with the sympathetic nervous system (Figure 23.15). Either as a result of a drop in the blood glucose concentration or because of sympathetic stimuli in response to stress, nerve impulses trigger the direct release of fatty acids from adipose tissues and of epinephrine from the adrenal gland. Epinephrine heightens the effect of nervous stimulation on adipose tissue and also stimulates the breakdown of glycogen to glucose in the muscles (and to some extent in the liver, too). The overall effect of this mechanism is to increase the glucose available in cells and to supplement glucose by providing an alternate source of energy. It operates during the postabsorptive metabolic state and during periods of stress.

The growth hormone–hypothalamic mechanism Although at one time it was believed that growth hormone exerted its influence only during periods of growth, it is now known that growth hormone is secreted throughout adult life, too. Its secretion can be stimulated by changes in the metabolic state produced by stress, starvation, or excitement, all of which create conditions like the postabsorptive metabolic state.

As shown in Figure 23.16, when the blood glucose concentration drops, or during stress, receptors in the hypothalamus respond by stimulating the production of growth-hormone-releasing hormone (GHRH). GHRH, in turn, stimulates the release of growth hormone from the anterior pituitary gland. Finally, growth hormone stimulates the release of fatty acids from adipose tissues, decreases the use of glucose by cells, and stimulates the production of glycogen in the liver. The overall effect of growth hormone is to shift the metabolic processes toward the use of fatty acids and thereby to reduce the rate at which glucose is depleted.

The actions of growth hormone are almost antagonistic to those of insulin, and prolonged hypersecretion of growth hormone may in fact cause diabetes mellitus by exhausting the ability of the B-cells to produce insulin. The hormone somatostatin inhibits the secretion of both insulin and glucagon and therefore has a stabilizing effect on blood glucose concentration.

Metabolic Rate

The **metabolic rate** is usually expressed as the rate of heat liberation from chemical reactions in the body. When energy is transferred to ATP, about 43% of the energy in glucose is captured in the high-energy bonds and the remaining 57% is released as heat. Later, when the ATP is used to carry out cellular activities, heat is again released. Thus, the total heat production over a given period of time can be used as a measure of metabolic rate.

Because of the technical difficulty of directly measuring heat given off from the human body (a body-sized chamber is required), the metabolic rate is usually measured indirectly by determining the amount of oxygen used per unit time and calculating the amount of heat associated with the volume of oxygen used. From studies of controlled oxidation outside the body, the amount of heat liberated per liter of oxygen consumed is known. The unit of energy used to express heat production in metabolic studies is the calorie, c. One calorie is the amount of energy required to raise the temperature of one gram of water one degree Celsius (from 14° to 15°C). Because of the large quantities of energy involved in human energy metabolism, the kilocalorie, C, equal to 1000 c, is generally used to measure it. The energy used by a human can be divided into two components, that used for basal metabolism and that used to carry out various activities.

Basal metabolism The **basal metabolic rate** is the rate at which energy is used for simply carrying on the internal physiological processes necessary to stay alive—breathing, maintaining body temperature, and the like. This rate decreases with age and is slightly higher for males than for females. Expressed in kilocalories (C) per square meter of body surface area per hour, the basal metabolic rate for adult females is about 36 C and for adult males about 38 C. Given that the body surface area varies from 1.4 square meters for a small woman to 2.0 square meters for a large man, the corresponding daily caloric intake to provide energy for basal metabolism ranges from 1200 kilocalories for a small woman to 1800 kilocalories for a large man.

In addition to age and sex other factors that affect the basal metabolic rate include pregnancy, activity of the thyroid gland (thyroxine increases the metabolic rate), growth hormone, and stimulation from the sympathetic nervous system (as explained earlier in this chapter). Glucocorticoids also have some effect on metabolic rate. Moreover, fever can elevate the basal metabolic rate, and prolonged malnutrition and hypothermia can lower it.

Exercise and metabolic rate The level of a person's physical activity is by far the greatest single variable in determining the total daily caloric consumption. Table 23.1 shows the number of kilocalories per hour expended by a 70 kilogram man engaging in different types of activity. If the body weight is to remain constant, the caloric intake must be equal to the sum of the caloric output for basal metabolism and exercise.

Hunger and satiety Hunger and satiety centers in the hypothalamus help to regulate food intake, as explained in Chapter 22. The activities of these centers are important in determining the amount of nutrients available to the body for metabolism.

Respiratory quotients The ratio of carbon dioxide produced to oxygen consumed is the **respiratory quotient** (RQ = CO_2 produced/O_2 consumed). The RQ for carbohydrate is 1.00, for triglycerides 0.71, and for amino acids 0.83. The significance of the RQ is that it can be used to estimate the relative proportion of each type of nutrient being metabolized. For example, shortly after a meal the RQ is very near 1.00 because most energy is being derived from glucose. In untreated diabetes mellitus the RQ is near 0.71 because the body is metabolizing fats rather than carbohydrates.

Regulation of Body Temperature

The regulation of body temperature, like the regulation of several other metabolic processes, is an example of a homeostatic mechanism. Even though the normal human body temperature is said to be 37°C (98.6°F), many people have normal temperatures that are higher or lower by one or two degrees. Body temperature also varies from one part of the body to another; the rectal temperature is generally 1°F higher than the oral temperature. In addition, time of day

Table 23.1 Kilocalories Expended per Hour by a Person Weighing 70 Kilograms* for Various Types of Activity

Activity	Kilocalories/hr	Activity	Kilocalories/hr
Awake lying still	77	Bowling	404
Sitting at rest	100	Horseback riding, trot	410
Standing relaxed	105	Tennis, moderate	420
Dressing and undressing	118	Sawing wood or shoveling snow	480
Typewriting rapidly	140	Swimming, 20 yds/min, sidestroke	506
Walking, 2 mi/hr	200	Jogging 5.3 mi/hr	570
Carpentry, painting, and general housework	240	Skiing downhill	585
Dancing, moderate	250	Tennis, vigorous	590
Sexual intercourse	280	Bicycling, level, 13 mi/hr	650
Swimming, 20 yds/min, crawl	290	Rowing, 20 strokes/min	825
Bicycling, level, 5.5 mi/hr	305	Walking upstairs	1100
Dancing, vigorous	340	Maximal activity (untrained)	1400
Walking, 4 mi/hr	400		

*Persons weighing more or less than 70 kg can estimate their caloric expenditure by finding the proportion of their weight to 70 kg and multiplying the calorie value given by that proportion. For example, a person weighing 77 kg expends 110% of the calories given, and one weighing 56 kg expends 80% of the calories given.

and level of exercise affect body temperature, which can rise above normal by one to several degrees during strenuous exercise and drop below normal by one to several degrees early in the morning. In women of reproductive age early morning body temperature rises about a degree at ovulation and stays elevated for the last half of the menstrual cycle.

The upper range of temperature consistent with life is 41° to 42°C (106°–108°F). At this body temperature most individuals experience convulsions. At 45°C (113°F) proteins are denatured so that enzymes fail to function, and death ensues.

A normal body temperature is maintained primarily by the actions of the thyroid gland in regulating the basal metabolic rate. Excess heat may be produced by muscular activity, by shivering, and by the action of the sympathetic nervous system. Heat loss involves at least four physical processes: (1) radiation of infrared heat waves from the body surface; (2) conduction of heat by transfer from the surface of the body to another surface (cold bed sheets, for instance) or to water or air; (3) convection, in which air movement removes heat from the body; and (4) evaporation by the vaporization of water from sweat. (Sweating has been described in Chapter 5.)

Temperature receptors in the skin (discussed in Chapter 15) and in the spinal cord and abdomen transmit impulses to the hypothalamus. The hypothalamus contains two types of control centers, the **heat-sensitive neurons**, which detect an increase in temperature, and **cold-sensitive neurons**, which detect a decrease in temperature. Because there appear to be too few cold-sensitive neurons to have much effect, temperature regulation is probably accomplished through the action of the heat-sensitive neurons and the peripheral cold receptors in the skin. When the heat-sensitive neurons (referred to as the heat loss center in the simplified discussion of temperature regulation in Chapter 1) are stimulated, they send out impulses to stimulate the sweat glands and inhibit the sympathetic centers that cause shivering and vasoconstriction. Sweating and vasodilation of blood vessels near the skin cause the body temperature to drop. Dilated blood vessels bring the blood closer to the surface of the body so that the heat can be lost. When the peripheral cold receptors are stimulated, they free the inhibition of the sympathetic centers, and shivering and vasoconstriction occur. Cooling also stimulates the contraction of the muscles attached to hair follicles, causing "gooseflesh."

Fever The elevation of body temperature in fever appears to be the result of a resetting of the body's thermostat and not a loss of ability to regulate body temperature. This resetting seems to be accomplished by the release of proteins called **pyrogens** in response to bacterial and other infections and inflammations. For some time it has been known that pyrogens are released by leukocytes and possibly by other types of phagocytic cells, but recent studies have also implicated **prostaglandins** in the production of fever. Prostaglandin synthesis increases in cerebrospinal fluid during fever, and the synthesis of prostaglandins is inhibited by aspirin and other antipyretic (fever-reducing) drugs. However, the mechanism of prostaglandin action is not understood.

By whatever means the thermostat is reset at a higher temperature, the feverish body behaves as if it were hypothermic: the peripheral blood vessels constrict, and the person shivers and wants to cover up with more blankets. When the fever "breaks" and the thermostat returns to its normal setting, the body behaves as if it were hyperthermic: sweating, vasodilation, removal of blankets, and the desire to drink cold liquids occurs.

Though fever usually accompanies an infection, its benefit in fighting the infection is minimal, and its harmful effects may be great. Fever does increase the metabolic rate and thus the rate at which the body can carry out processes to eliminate the infectious organisms. However, fever can damage tissues by interfering with the action of many hormones. It can lead to breakage of blood vessels in the brain (brain hemorrhage), and it can lead to convulsions, especially in young children.

Hypothermia Lengthy exposure to temperatures below 20°C and dampness may lead to hypothermia, excessively low body temperature. Rain-soaked hikers are susceptible to hypothermia even on spring and fall days; failure to realize the danger can lead to death. Because wetness greatly increases the amount of heat lost, an individual immersed in 5°C water has only 20 to 40 minutes before losing so much heat that recovery is unlikely. Early symptoms include numbness, paleness, slurred speech, and uncontrolled shivering. Dizziness, incoherence, and drowsiness follow. The body must be warmed immediately even when the person insists no help is needed; in an incoherent state that person is a poor judge of anything. The direct cause of death when body temperature falls below 32°C (90°F) is heart failure as the heart loses its ability to pump blood.

CLINICAL TERMS

hyperalimentation (hi-per-al-e-men-ta′shun) the intake of an excessive amount of food, sometimes purposely provided for individuals with severe burns or other conditions requiring rapid metabolism

hyperglycemia (hi-per-gli-se′me-ah) excess glucose in the blood

hypoglycemia (hi-po-gli-se′me-ah) deficiency of glucose in the blood

malabsorption (mal″ab-sorp′shun) a disorder leading to the failure of nutrients to enter the blood or lymph from the small intestine

pica (pi′kah) a craving for unnatural foods; eating of nonfood items

Essay: Metabolism of Foreign Substances

The ability of the body to act on toxic or poisonous substances to render them harmless may mean the difference between life and death. Many foreign substances (substances not normally present in the body) enter our bodies when we breathe polluted air, consume foods containing pesticide residues or food preservatives, use alcohol or tobacco, or even take prescribed medications. Any foreign substance is potentially toxic (poisonous); whether it exerts a toxic effect on the body depends on how much of it is present and how well the body can detoxify it.

Most of the chemical reactions that **detoxify** (render harmless) foreign substances take place in the liver. These reactions are carried out by enzymes found in the membranes of the endoplasmic reticulum of liver cells. Four major types of detoxification reactions occur: oxidation, reduction, hydrolysis, and conjugation. Examples of these reactions applied to the inactivation of commonly used drugs are shown in Figure 23.17. The effect of many of these reactions is to convert fat-soluble substances to water-soluble substances that can be excreted by the kidneys.

Combinations of drugs often have unpredictable and sometimes undesirable results because they compete for the same inactivation enzymes. For example, the drug tolbutamide, used to control blood glucose level in non-insulin-dependent diabetics, is metabolized and inactivated more slowly in the presence of any one of several drugs, including phenylbutazone (an antiinflammatory agent), the coagulant dicumarol, and the antibiotic chloramphenicol.

In addition to drugs, other substances such as steroid hormones, dyes, and insecticides are also subject to detoxification in the liver. Many of the detoxification reactions are inducible; that is, the presence of the potentially toxic substance induces activity of the enzymes that detoxify the substance.

When the body is subjected to relatively large amounts of toxic substances, as occurs in alcoholics, the liver becomes adept at producing detoxification enzymes—at least until long-term use of the substances severely impairs liver function. Thus, when an alcoholic abstains from alcohol in a treatment program, the liver produces an overabundance of detoxification enzymes. The person in treatment requires larger than usual doses of any medication because the liver enzymes inactivate the drug very rapidly, and little remains in the blood to reach other tissues.

Although the liver is amazingly successful in detoxifying many substances, it has no effect on some substances. The liver fails to detoxify the pesticide DDT and many other manufactured chemicals because its enzymes have little ability to act on these substances. The liver fails to detoxify heavy metals such

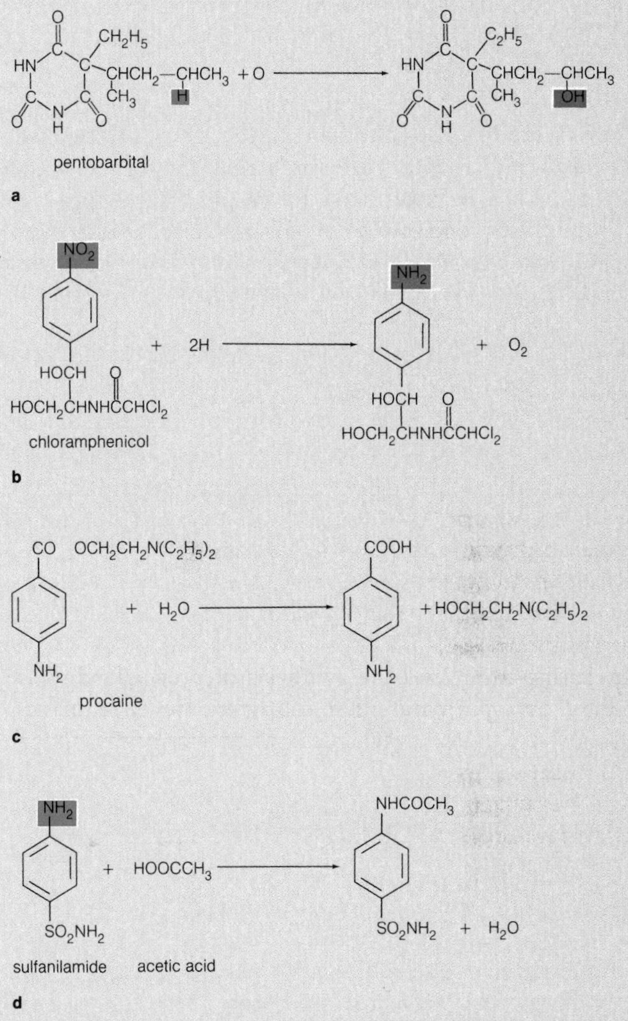

Figure 23.17 The inactivation of foreign substances: (**a**) oxidation of pentobarbital, (**b**) reduction of chloramphenicol, (**c**) hydrolysis of procaine, and (**d**) conjugation of sulfanilamide.

as lead and mercury because heavy metals destroy proteins, including enzymes in the liver and in all other cells.

Wide individual differences in the ability to detoxify drugs and other chemicals are due to variations in the efficiency of liver enzymes in carrying out the detoxification reactions. The high sensitivity of infants to drugs seems to be related to the immaturity of their livers and the consequent ineffectiveness of liver enzymes. Fetuses are particularly susceptible to damage from toxic substances that can cross the placenta. The mother may suffer no adverse effects, but the fetus may be deformed, as has been demonstrated by the absence of limbs in infants whose mothers took thalidomide during pregnancy. When the mother uses excessive amounts of alcohol or is addicted to narcotics, the fetus becomes dependent on these substances and suffers withdrawal symptoms at birth. The elderly also have impaired ability to detoxify substances because of gradual degenerative changes that occur in the liver as a part of the aging process.

Even though the liver successfully detoxifies small to moderate amounts of many foreign substances that enter the body, exposure of the body to potentially toxic substances should be avoided. Thus, it is important that new drugs, food additives, insecticides, and other manufactured chemical substances be carefully tested for possible toxicity to humans before they are marketed.

CHAPTER SUMMARY

(Chapter summary points and review questions are numbered to correspond to the numbered objectives in the text of each chapter.)

Overview of Metabolism

1. Describe the overall process of metabolism.
   a. Metabolism includes all anabolic and catabolic reactions that occur in body cells.
   b. Anabolism is the synthesis of proteins and other cell products.
   c. Catabolism is the breakdown of molecules for energy.

Carbohydrate Metabolism

2. Describe how carbohydrates are temporarily stored and later released to maintain a relatively constant supply of energy for cells.
   a. Carbohydrates are generally transported by facilitated diffusion stimulated by insulin.
   b. Carbohydrates are temporarily stored as glycogen, which can be released to maintain a nearly constant blood glucose concentration.

3. For each of the following metabolic processes describe the major reactions in proper sequence, where they occur in the cell, and their net effect on energy production: (a) glycolysis, (b) the Krebs, or citric acid, cycle, (c) oxidative phosphorylation, and (d) the phosphogluconate pathway.

   a. Glycolysis:
   (1) involves the breakdown of glucose to two molecules of pyruvic acid
   (2) occurs in the cytoplasm
   (3) produces two net ATPs per glucose molecule under anaerobic conditions
   b. The Krebs, or citric acid, cycle:
   (1) involves the breakdown of pyruvic acid to acetyl-CoA, which combines with oxaloacetic acid and undergoes a sequence of reactions that release carbon dioxide, ATP, and hydrogen
   (2) occurs in the matrix of the mitochondria
   (3) produces thirty-six ATPs per original glucose molecule when coupled with oxidative phosphorylation
   c. Oxidative phosphorylation:
   (1) involves the use of oxygen and production of ATP as hydrogen or electrons are transported through the respiratory enzymes, eventually forming water from the hydrogen and oxygen
   (2) occurs in the cristae of the mitochondria
   (3) produces three ATPs for every pair of hydrogen atoms transferred to NAD^+ and two ATPs for every pair of hydrogen atoms transferred to FAD
   d. The phosphogluconate pathway:
   (1) involves the conversion of glucose to five-carbon molecules and the production of $NADPH + H^+$
   (2) occurs in the cytoplasm, especially in liver and adipose tissue
   (3) is not important in the production of energy

Lipid Metabolism

4. Describe (a) how lipids are transported across cell membranes, and (b) how they are stored and later released for energy.

    a. Lipids are transported as chylomicrons and cross membranes by diffusion after being digested to fatty acids and other small molecules.

    b. Lipids are stored as triglycerides, primarily in adipose tissue, and can be broken down into glycerol and fatty acids and released to be used for energy.

5. Describe the major events in the metabolism of lipids.

    a. Triglycerides are broken down into glycerol and fatty acids, and the fatty acids are further broken down by beta oxidation.

    b. Triglycerides can also be resynthesized or converted to ketone bodies in the liver.

    c. Lipids form part of the structure of membranes and other cell components.

Protein Metabolism

6. Define nitrogen balance and describe how it is maintained.

    a. Nitrogen balance is the ratio of nitrogen intake to nitrogen excretion; it is positive during growth and negative during starvation.

    b. Nitrogen balance is maintained by taking in sufficient protein to compensate for the nitrogen excreted.

7. Describe the major events in the metabolism of proteins.

    a. Amino acids are actively transported into cells but are not stored in any appreciable quantity.

    b. Essential amino acids must be obtained from the diet because the human body lacks the enzymes to synthesize these amino acids.

    c. The body uses amino acids to synthesize proteins by the mechanism described in Chapter 3.

    d. Amino acids are also used to synthesize certain neurotransmitters, nitrogenous bases, and carrier molecules in the electron transport system.

    e. Amino acids may undergo transamination or deamination and be used for energy or for the synthesis of glucose.

Summary of Energy-Producing Metabolism

8. Summarize the major events in energy-producing metabolism.

    a. The total net energy from one molecule of glucose is thirty-eight ATPs—thirty-six from the aerobic metabolism and two from glycolysis.

    b. Fats and amino acids can be converted to carbohydratelike substances and metabolized like glucose.

Regulation of Metabolism

9. Distinguish between the absorptive and the postabsorptive metabolic states in terms of (a) processes that occur and (b) how those processes are regulated.

    a. Absorptive metabolism:

        (1) occurs for several hours after a meal when nutrients are being absorbed

        (2) leads to the storage of excess nutrients in glycogen and fats

        (3) is stimulated by insulin

    b. Postabsorptive metabolism:

        (1) occurs before meals and during the night when nutrients are not being absorbed and energy is needed

        (2) leads to the release of glycogen and fatty acids, which are then metabolized for energy

        (3) is stimulated by glucagon, epinephrine, growth hormone, and hypothalamic factors

10. Define metabolic rate and describe the factors that regulate it, including the roles of hunger and satiety and respiratory quotients.

    a. The metabolic rate is determined by measuring heat production in kilocalories and includes energy for basal metabolism and for activity; it is influenced by age, sex, body size, and activity.

    b. Hunger and satiety regulate food intake and therefore the amount of food that is available for producing energy (see Chapter 22).

    c. The respiratory quotient is the ratio of the amount of carbon dioxide produced to the amount of oxygen used; it reflects the composition of the nutrients being metabolized.

11. Explain how body temperature is regulated and list the factors that affect it.

    a. Body temperature varies with the individual, the time of day, and the degree of activity; it is regulated by messages from heat sensors in the hypothalamus.

    b. Fever is triggered by pyrogens (and maybe prostaglandins) and involves a resetting of the body's "thermostat."

    c. Hypothermia results from exposure to low temperature, especially if accompanied by dampness.

REVIEW

Important Terms

absorptive state	essential amino acids
acetyl-CoA	essential fatty acid
basal metabolic rate	FAD
beta oxidation	gluconeogenesis
beta reduction	glucose sparing
cytochrome	glycogenesis
electron transport system	glycogenolysis

glycolysis	oxidation
ketone bodies	oxidative phosphorylation
ketosis	phosphogluconate pathway
Krebs cycle	postabsorptive state
metabolism	protein turnover
NAD^+	pyrogens
$NADP^+$	reduction
nitrogen balance	respiratory quotient

Questions

1. Distinguish between anabolism and catabolism.
2. **a.** How are carbohydrates transported across cell membranes?
   b. Distinguish between glycogenesis and glycogenolysis.
3. **a.** List the major reactions in sequence for glycolysis, the Krebs cycle, oxidative phosphorylation, and the phosphogluconate pathway.
   b. Describe where each process occurs and how much energy it produces.
4. **a.** How are lipids transported in the blood, and how do they cross cell membranes?
   b. Describe the processes by which lipids are stored and released.
5. **a.** Explain beta oxidation.
   b. Discuss the role of the liver in lipid metabolism.
   c. Name the essential fatty acid.
   d. Describe how lipids are used in the structure of cells.
   e. Discuss the role of cholesterol in lipid metabolism.
6. **a.** How do amino acids enter cells?
   b. Define nitrogen balance and list conditions that cause positive and negative balance.
7. **a.** List the essential amino acids and tell why they are needed.
   b. Distinguish between transamination and deamination and explain their significance in protein metabolism.
   c. Define gluconeogenesis.
8. Make your own diagram to summarize metabolism.
9. **a.** Explain how absorptive metabolism differs from postabsorptive metabolism.
   b. How are absorptive metabolism and postabsorptive metabolism regulated?
10. Define basal metabolism, calorie, and respiratory quotient.
11. How is body temperature regulated during normal conditions and during fever?

Problems

1. Explain how a meal consisting mostly of protein, instead of a combination of carbohydrate, fat, and protein, would modify the events in the absorptive metabolic state and in the postabsorptive metabolic state.

2. Repeat problem (1) for a meal consisting mostly of carbohydrates and for a meal consisting mostly of fat.

REFERENCES AND READINGS

Ganog, W. F. 1981. *Review of medical physiology* (10th ed.). Los Altos, Calif.: Lange Medical Publications.

Guyton, A. C. 1981. *Textbook of medical physiology* (6th ed.). Philadelphia: W. B. Saunders.

Harper, H. A., Rodwell, V. W., and Mayes, P. A. 1979. *Review of physiological chemistry* (17th ed.). Los Altos, Calif.: Lange Medical Publications.

Hinkle, P. C., and McCarty, R. E. 1978. How cells make ATP. *Scientific American* 238(3):104 (March).

Holum, J. R. 1978. *Fundamentals of general, organic, and biological chemistry.* New York: John Wiley.

Kluger, M. J. 1978. The evolution and adaptive value of fever. *American Scientist* 66(1):38 (January–February).

Montgomery, R., Dryer, R. L., Conway, T. W., and Spector, A. A. 1980. *Biochemistry: A case-oriented approach.* St. Louis, Mo.: C. V. Mosby.

24

NUTRITION

PRINCIPLES OF NUTRITION

Objective 1. Define nutrition and describe the nutritional needs generally supplied by each of the four basic food groups.

Objective 2. Explain the changes in intake of certain nutrients that may result from adhering to the U.S. Dietary Goals statement and explain the health risks these goals seek to reduce.

Objective 3. Discuss the strengths and weaknesses of the Recommended Dietary Allowances of nutrients.

Nutrition Defined

Nutrition deals with the provision of all the substances necessary for maintaining health through the ingestion of food. These substances include carbohydrates, proteins, fats, vitamins, minerals, and water. The primary role of carbohydrates in nutrition is to provide sufficient calories to meet the body's demands for energy. Likewise, the role of fats is to provide calories for energy, but fats are also important as energy-storage molecules, and some fats, particularly the essential fatty acid linoleic acid, are important in providing the molecules from which cell membranes, prostaglandins, and other substances are synthesized. The role of proteins in nutrition is to provide amino acids for protein synthesis and the synthesis of other cell components. The essential amino acids are particularly important in nutrition since our bodies cannot make them. Protein needs are greatest during growth, repair, pregnancy, and lactation. The metabolic processes by which the body uses carbohydrates, proteins, and fats, including essential amino acids and fatty acid, were described in Chapter 23.

Vitamins, minerals, and water are also essential nutrients in the maintenance of health. Most **vitamins** and **minerals** act in some way to assist enzymes in catalyzing important reactions. Water, which makes up about 60% of the body weight, is important in nearly every chemical reaction as a reactant, a product, or the medium in which a reaction occurs. Vitamins, minerals, and water are discussed in more detail later in this chapter.

As nutritionists learn more about metabolic reactions, they can be more precise about what nutrients are essential and in what quantities they are required. Generally, nutritional needs are determined at the cellular and molecular levels, according to how much energy is being expended, how much protein is being used for growth and repair, and how much of each vitamin and mineral is required to keep enzymes functioning.

Nutrition is not simply a matter of providing essential nutrients and sufficient calories to meet energy needs; it is a social as well as a biological process. Age, sex, and religious and social customs contribute significantly to what people consider to be a suitable diet. For example, some people think hot dogs are "kid" food, soft and bland foods are for the elderly, fancy salads are feminine, and steak and potatoes are masculine. Certain foods have religious significance for some people, and other foods are customarily associated with holidays—like the Thanksgiving turkey. A nutritionist attempting to change an individual's eating habits would be well advised to consider all these factors as well as the individual's attitudes about food.

Basic Four Food Groups

Although you probably have heard about the **basic four food groups** since elementary school, you may not have considered what each group contributes to the body's overall nutritional needs. This is shown in Table 24.1.

When the cells of the body fail to receive the essential nutrients, **malnutrition** is the result. Malnutrition can be caused by the unavailability of proper foods, the failure to eat them, or the inability to absorb them from the intestine. One of the consequences of malnutrition is decreased resistance to infection. When an infection occurs, food intake is reduced, and vomiting and diarrhea may further reduce the availability of food for absorption. Malnutrition then becomes more serious as a vicious cycle is created: The body's ability to produce antibodies and phagocytic cells is decreased and the resistance to infection thus further de-

creased. Other consequences of malnutrition in infants and children are slowed development of the brain and stunted general body growth.

Fad diets, if followed for more than a short period of time, can also lead to malnutrition because they emphasize only a few foods. For example, the so-called macrobiotic diet has as a goal becoming able to exist on a diet of only unpolished rice. A strict vegetarian diet also limits the variety of foods eaten. Serious vitamin and protein deficiencies may result from a diet of only rice; and a vitamin B_{12} deficiency may result from a strictly vegetarian diet. However, the ovo-lacto-vegetarian diet that includes eggs and dairy products can be completely adequate. The best way to guarantee adequate nutrition is to eat a variety of foods, including some from each of the four food groups, daily.

U.S. Dietary Goals

The average diet in the United States has changed significantly in the last seventy years. On a per-person basis we are using more meat, poultry, fish, dairy products, fats and oils, sugars and other sweeteners, and salt. We are using less grain and fewer grain products, eggs, fruits, and vegetables. Because of these changes and their implications for the health of the population, *Dietary Goals for the United States* was prepared in 1977 by the staff of the Select Committee on Nutrition and Human Health Needs of the United States Senate. The following seven **U.S. dietary goals** were set:

1. To avoid overweight, consume only as much energy (calories) as is expended; if overweight, decrease energy intake and increase energy expenditure.

2. Increase the consumption of complex carbohydrates and "naturally occurring" sugars from about 28% of energy intake to about 48% of energy intake.

3. Reduce the consumption of refined and processed sugars by about 45%, to account for about 10% of total energy intake.

4. Reduce overall fat consumption from approximately 40% to about 30% of energy intake.

5. Reduce saturated fat consumption to account for about 10% of total energy intake and balance that with polyunsaturated and monounsaturated fats, each of which should account for about 10% of energy intake.

6. Reduce cholesterol consumption to about 300 milligrams a day.

7. Limit the intake of sodium by reducing the intake of salt to about 5 grams a day.

Table 24.1   The Basic Four Food Groups and Their Contributions to Nutrition

Group	Recommended Daily Amounts	Nutritional Needs Satisfied
Milk group	Serving: 8 oz milk or 1½–2 oz cheese 2 servings for adults 3 servings for children and pregnant women 4 servings for lactating mothers	Each serving provides 8 g protein, 3 g fat, and about 140 calories. Contains vitamins A and riboflavin and provides an especially good supply of calcium, phosphorus, potassium, and magnesium.
Meat group	Serving: 3 oz lean meat or 2 eggs or 1 c cooked legume, or 4 T peanut butter 2 servings	Each serving provides 15–25 g protein, 10–40 g fat, and 150–400 calories. Contains phosphorus, iron, sodium, potassium, riboflavin and other B vitamins. Legumes are very low in fat. Peanut butter is high in fat but also high in niacin. Eggs provide some vitamin A.
Fruit and vegetable group	Serving: ½ cup 4 servings, including one good source of vitamin A and one of vitamin C	Foods that provide vitamin A: spinach and other green leafy vegetables, carrots and other yellow vegetables, and fruits. Foods that provide vitamin C: citrus fruits and juices. Fruits and vegetables also provide some B vitamins and vitamin K, as well as some minerals. Raw foods in this group have larger amounts of vitamins than cooked foods.
Bread and cereal group	Serving: 1 slice of bread or 1 oz of prepared cereal or ½ cup of cooked cereal, rice, pasta, or noodles 4 servings	Each serving provides energy, some protein, and, if made of whole grain, a good supply of B vitamins. Eating food from this group with a legume increases the protein value of both foods.

In Figure 24.1 the American diet at the time of the report is contrasted with the diet that would satisfy the goals. Recommended changes in the diet to accomplish these goals include increasing the consumption of fruits, vegetables, and whole-grain products, and decreasing consumption of meats, saturated fats, eggs, sugar and presweetened foods, and salt and salted foods. Substitutions of poultry and fish for red meat, unsaturated fats for saturated, and nonfat milk for whole milk were also recommended. Of these recommendations perhaps the hardest to follow is the substitution of unsaturated fats for saturated fats. It may be helpful to know that all animal fats have a higher proportion of saturated fats than fats from vegetable sources. However, among animal products poultry and fish have much lower total fat content than beef or pork. Another recommendation that requires special knowledge is the limitation of cholesterol. Foods that are high in cholesterol include organ meats and eggs, an average serving of which exceeds the 300 milligram/day limit. Shrimp, lobster, and tuna are also rel-

atively high in cholesterol. To keep one's diet within the cholesterol limits it would be necessary to eat a serving of these foods no more than two or three times per week. However, as we saw in Chapter 22, because the body can synthesize cholesterol, limiting dietary intake may have only a modest effect.

The health risks these dietary goals attempt to reduce include heart disease and atherosclerosis, diabetes, tooth decay, and hypertension. Other disorders that may be diet induced include migraine headaches from excessive salt intake; excessive gastric secretions and stomach cancer; allergies to specific foods; and obesity.

Recommended Dietary Allowances of Nutrients

For many years the **recommended dietary allowances** of nutrients published by the National Academy of Sciences–National Research Council has been the standard

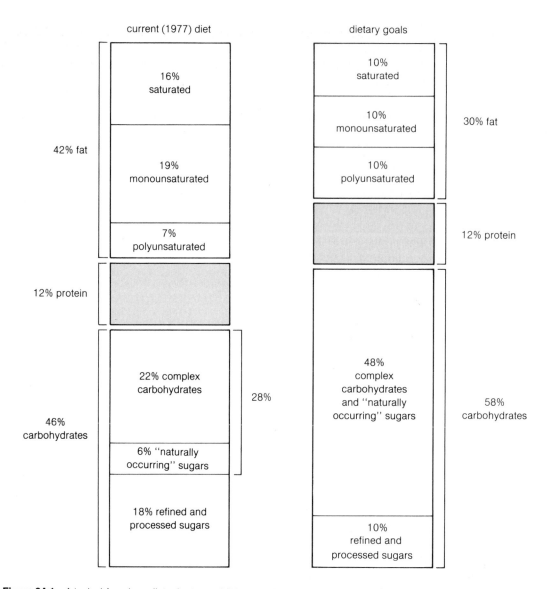

current (1977) diet

42% fat
- 16% saturated
- 19% monounsaturated
- 7% polyunsaturated

12% protein

46% carbohydrates
- 22% complex carbohydrates
- 6% "naturally occurring" sugars
- 18% refined and processed sugars

28%

dietary goals

30% fat
- 10% saturated
- 10% monounsaturated
- 10% polyunsaturated

12% protein

58% carbohydrates
- 48% complex carbohydrates and "naturally occurring" sugars
- 10% refined and processed sugars

Figure 24.1 A typical American diet prior to establishment of dietary goals compared with a diet consistent with those goals. (From *Dietary Goals for the United States*, U.S. Government Printing Office.)

for nutritional planning. Though recommended dietary allowances (RDAs) may be useful as general guidelines for the nutrients they cover, their use has a number of pitfalls. First, they do not cover all known essential nutrients. Second, studies on humans are often impossible, so recommendations are frequently extrapolated from animal studies. Third, historically, the RDAs were established by using the amount thought to satisfy the requirements of 97.5% of the population. However, the average amount thought to be required and a range of values above and below the average would have been more useful. Finally,

the most devastating criticism of the RDAs is that they lull people into a false sense of security. They tend to assume that, if they have consumed the proper quantities of every nutrient listed, they have a nutritionally adequate diet, even though many nutrients are not included in the RDAs. In fairness, if one obtains a diet adequate according to RDAs, then other nutrients might also be present in adequate quantities. However, this principle also works in reverse. Some manufacturers of highly processed and enriched foods have made a point of listing contents of packages in RDAs. When they place vitamins and minerals in a product like presweetened cereals, the consumer may get a large amount of refined sugar along with the vitamins. Nevertheless, with all their pitfalls RDAs remain the *only* scientific measure of nutritional needs. The most recent edition of RDAs is presented in Table 24.2.

In connection with RDAs for vitamins the so-called megavitamin therapy deserves mention. While many far-reaching claims have been made for massive doses of vitamin C to combat the common cold and for large doses of certain vitamins for the treatment of schizophrenia, too little carefully controlled data are available to evaluate such treatments objectively. The data on vitamin-responsive metabolic disorders reported later in this chapter suggest that individual variations in vitamin needs may be far greater than is indicated by a table of RDAs. Carefully designed research studies are greatly needed to determine vitamin needs as well as a number of other nutritional standards.

VITAMINS, MINERALS, AND WATER

Objective 4. Describe the biochemical action, dietary sources, and effects of excesses and deficiencies of the vitamins and minerals needed by the body.

Objective 5. Briefly discuss the role of water in metabolism.

Vitamins and Minerals

The biochemical action, common dietary sources, and effects of excesses and deficiencies of vitamins and minerals are summarized in Table 24.3. Water-soluble vitamins are listed first, fat-soluble vitamins second, and minerals last. The minerals are listed in order from those needed in greatest quantities to those needed in smallest quantities.

In summary, it can be said that most vitamins and minerals act as cofactors in enzyme reactions. A few are structural components of essential molecules, such as riboflavin in the flavin coenzymes FMN and FAD, and carotene in the light-sensitive cells of the eye. All are required in relatively small quantities, but they must be present nonetheless. Excesses are generally excreted with no harm to the body, except for the fat-soluble vitamins, which are stored in the liver and can become toxic. Some minerals have deleterious effects if consumed in excess.

Water

Most metabolic reactions take place in an aqueous medium, and many metabolic reactions actually involve water mol-

ecules. Both solid foods and beverages contain water; in addition, the oxidation of nutrients produces an additional supply of water, the **metabolic water**. Metabolic water is derived primarily from the passage of hydrogen to oxygen in oxidative phosphorylation. The role of water in physiological processes is discussed in more detail in Chapter 26.

METABOLIC DISORDERS

Objective 6. Discuss the possible causes and effects of the following metabolic disorders: (a) genetic defects, (b) diabetes mellitus, (c) obesity, (d) anorexia nervosa, and (e) alcoholism.

The causes and effects of **metabolic disorders** are extremely varied. All interfere in some way with metabolism, and they usually alter nutritional requirements. The disorders discussed here provide a sampling of the great diversity of such disorders and the complexity of their causes.

Genetic Defects

Some metabolic disorders are caused by the presence of defective genes, often located at a single gene locus. (The basic concepts of genetics are presented in Chapter 27.) Disorders that fall in the category of genetic defects include cystic fibrosis, phenylketonuria and some related disorders, and several vitamin-responsive inherited disorders.

Cystic fibrosis **Cystic fibrosis**, inherited as an autosomal recessive trait, occurs in one of every 2000 live births among Caucasians. Ducts of glands, particularly the pancreas, become blocked, and the reduced flow of digestive enzymes from the pancreas leads to poor digestion and malnutrition even when the affected person eats well. Nondigestive effects of the disease include obstructive mucous secretions in the respiratory tract and excessive secretion of salt from the sweat glands. Recent research efforts have shown that individuals with cystic fibrosis have a lowered level of lipoproteins, the substances that transport lipids in the plasma during the postabsorptive period. The lack of cholesterol, linoleic acid, and other lipids may lead to inadequate synthesis of cell membranes. The lowered transport of fat-soluble vitamins may lead to deficiencies in those vitamins. Treatment of cystic fibrosis involves administering vitamins, salt, and digestive enzymes and removing mucus from the respiratory tract by postural drainage, a technique using certain body positions to keep mucus flow from passageways in the lungs.

Table 24.2 Food and Nutrition Board, National Academy of Sciences—National Research Council Recommended Daily Dietary Allowances[1]
Revised 1980
(Designed for the maintenance of good nutrition of practically all healthy people in the U.S.A.)

	Age (years)	Weight (kg)	Weight (lb)	Height (cm)	Height (in)	Protein (g)	Fat-Soluble Vitamins Vitamin A (μg RE)[2]	Vitamin D (μg)[3]	Vitamin E (mg α-TE)[4]
Infants	0.0–0.5	6	13	60	24	kg × 2.2	420	10	3
	0.5–1.0	9	20	71	28	kg × 2.0	400	10	4
Children	1–3	13	29	90	35	23	400	10	5
	4–6	20	44	112	44	30	500	10	6
	7–10	28	62	132	52	34	700	10	7
Males	11–14	45	99	157	62	45	1000	10	8
	15–18	66	145	176	69	56	1000	10	10
	19–22	70	154	177	70	56	1000	7.5	10
	23–50	70	154	178	70	56	1000	5	10
	51 +	70	154	178	70	56	1000	5	10
Females	11–14	46	101	157	62	46	800	10	8
	15–18	55	120	163	64	46	800	10	8
	19–22	55	120	163	64	44	800	7.5	8
	23–50	55	120	163	64	44	800	5	8
	51 +	55	120	163	64	44	800	5	8
Pregnant						+ 30	+ 200	+ 5	+ 2
Lactating						+ 20	+ 400	+ 5	+ 3

Phenylketonuria and related disorders In normal individuals the amino acid phenylalanine is metabolized to another amino acid, tyrosine; in individuals with **phenylketonuria** the enzyme that catalyzes the synthesis of tyrosine is missing. Phenylketonuria is caused by the presence of a pair of recessive genes, neither of which carries the correct information for the synthesis of the enzyme. In people who have *one* dominant gene capable of directing the synthesis of the enzyme, the metabolism of phenylalanine is normal. But such people also have *one* recessive gene, which they can transmit to their offspring. The consequences of the disease, if untreated, are mental retardation and other impairments of normal development. Infants who are diagnosed early and placed on a low phenylalanine diet may be spared these very severe consequences.

Many other missing enzyme disorders have been identified. Some involve the absence of enzymes that are needed for the proper metabolism of other amino acids.

Table 24.2 Food and Nutrition Board, National Academy of Sciences—National Research Council Recommended Daily Dietary Allowances[1]
Revised 1980 (continued)
(Designed for the maintenance of good nutrition of practically all healthy people in the U.S.A.)

Water-Soluble Vitamins							Minerals					
Vitamin C (mg)	Thiamin (mg)	Riboflavin (mg)	Niacin (mg NE)[5]	Vitamin B_6 (mg)	Folacin[6] (μg)	Vitamin B_{12} (μg)	Calcium (mg)	Phosphorus (mg)	Magnesium (mg)	Iron (mg)	Zinc (mg)	Iodine (μg)
35	0.3	0.4	6	0.3	30	0.5[7]	360	240	50	10	3	40
35	0.5	0.6	8	0.6	45	1.5	540	360	70	15	5	50
45	0.7	0.8	9	0.9	100	2.0	800	800	150	15	10	70
45	0.9	1.0	11	1.3	200	2.5	800	800	200	10	10	90
45	1.2	1.4	16	1.6	300	3.0	800	800	250	10	10	120
50	1.4	1.6	18	1.8	400	3.0	1200	1200	350	18	15	150
60	1.4	1.7	18	2.0	400	3.0	1200	1200	400	18	15	150
60	1.5	1.7	19	2.2	400	3.0	800	800	350	10	15	150
60	1.4	1.6	18	2.2	400	3.0	800	800	350	10	15	150
60	1.2	1.4	16	2.2	400	3.0	800	800	350	10	15	150
50	1.1	1.3	15	1.8	400	3.0	1200	1200	300	18	15	150
60	1.1	1.3	14	2.0	400	3.0	1200	1200	300	18	15	150
60	1.1	1.3	14	2.0	400	3.0	800	800	300	18	15	150
60	1.0	1.2	13	2.0	400	3.0	800	800	300	18	15	150
60	1.0	1.2	13	2.0	400	3.0	800	800	300	10	15	150
+20	+0.4	+0.3	+2	+0.6	+400	+1.0	+400	+400	+150	[8]	+5	+25
+40	+0.5	+0.5	+5	+0.5	+100	+1.0	+400	+400	+150	[8]	+10	+50

Reproduced from *Recommended Dietary Allowances*, 1980, with the permission of the National Academy of Sciences, Washington, D.C.

[1]The allowances are intended to provide for individual variations among most normal persons as they live in the United States under usual environmental stresses. Diets should be based on a variety of common foods in order to provide other nutrients for which human requirements have been less well defined.

[2]Retinol equivalents. 1 retinol equivalent (RE) = 1 μg retinol or 6 μg β carotene.

[3]As cholecalciferol. 10 μg cholecalciferol = 400 IU of vitamin D.

[4]α-toeopherol equivalents. 1 mg d-α tocopherol = 1 α-TE.

[5]1 NE (niacin equivalent) is equal to 1 mg of niacin or 60 mg of dietary tryptophan.

[6]The folacin allowances refer to dietary sources as determined by *Lactobacillus casei* assay after treatment with enzymes (conjugases) to make polyglutamyl forms of the vitamin available to the test organism.

[7]The recommended dietary allowance for vitamin B_{12} in infants is based on average concentration of the vitamin in human milk. The allowances after weaning are based on energy intake (as recommended by the American Academy of Pediatrics) and consideration of other factors, such as intestinal absorption.

[8]The increased requirement during pregnancy cannot be met by the iron content of habitual American diets nor by the existing iron stores of many women; therefore the use of 30–60 mg of supplemental iron is recommended. Iron needs during lactation are not substantially different from those of nonpregnant women, but continued supplementation of the mother for 2–3 months after parturition is advisable in order to replenish stores depleted by pregnancy.

Table 24.3 Vitamins and Minerals

	Biochemical Actions	Dietary Sources	Effects of Excess	Effects of Deficiency
Water-Soluble Vitamins				
B_1-thiamine	Part of decarboxylation enzyme in Krebs cycle	Organ meats, whole grains, and legumes	None known	Arrests metabolism at pyruvate; beriberi (neurological impairment, heart failure)
B_2-riboflavin	Part of FAD	Dairy products, eggs, and whole grains	None known	Sensitivity to light, eye lesions, and cracks in corners of mouth
Niacin	Part of NAD and NADP	Whole grains, meats and legumes; can be formed from tryptophan	Flushing of skin in sensitive people	Pellagra (skin and digestive lesions, mental disorders)
Pantothenic acid	Part of coenzyme A	Widely distributed	None known	Fatigue, nervous and motor impairment (rare in humans)
B_6-pyridoxine	Coenzyme for metabolism of amino acids and fats	Whole grains, meats, and vegetables	None known	Dermatitis, nervous disorders, kidney stones
Folacin (folic acid)	Coenzyme for metabolism of amino acids and nucleic acids	Meats, legumes, green vegetables, and wheat	None known	Impairs production of erythrocytes, intestinal disturbances
B_{12}-cyanocobalamin	Coenzyme in nucleic acid metabolism	Meats, eggs, and dairy products	None known	Pernicious anemia, nervous disorders
Biotin	Coenzyme in fat and glycogen synthesis, amino acid metabolism	Egg whites, legumes, vegetables, and meats	None known	Dermatitis, muscle pains, weakness, and depression
Choline (may not be a vitamin	Form phospholipids and acetylcholine	Egg yolk, liver, grains, and legumes	None known	None known in humans
C-ascorbic acid	Acts in synthesis of collagen and matrix of connective tissue	Citrus fruits	Possibly kidney stones	Scurvy (degeneration of teeth, skin, and blood vessels)
Fat-Soluble Vitamins				
A-carotene	Forms visual pigments; maintains epithelia	Green and yellow vegetables, fruits, milk, and egg yolks	Headache, loss of appetite, elevated blood calcium, and peeling of skin	Night blindness, excess keratin in tissues of eye
D-calciferol	Acts in absorption of calcium and bone growth	Fish oils, liver, and fortified dairy products	Kidney damage, vomiting, diarrhea, and weight loss	Bone softness and deformity (rickets in children and osteomalacia in adults)
E-tocopherol	Maintains integrity of erythrocytes	Green leafy vegetables, seeds, and oils	None known	Anemia because of fragility of erythrocytes
K-phylloquinone	Acts in synthesis of prothrombin	Liver, green leafy vegetables, gut bacteria	May cause jaundice in high doses	Failure of blood coagulation, hemorrhage

Table 24.3 Vitamins and Minerals (continued)

	Biochemical Actions	Dietary Sources	Effects of Excess	Effects of Deficiency
Minerals				
Calcium	Bone formation, muscle contraction, nerve impulse transmission, blood clotting	Eggs, fish, dairy products, and legumes	Renal damage	Tetany, softening of bones, hemorrhage
Phosphorus	Bone formation, buffers, phosphates in lipids and nucleotides	Dairy products, legumes, meats, and grains	Hypocalcemia	Probably loss of minerals in bones
Magnesium	Cofactor for enzymes, regulates nerve and muscle function	Green vegetables, meat, and milk	Respiratory depression if renal excretion depressed	Tetany
Sodium	Excitability of cells, maintenance of ionic and osmotic balance	Table salt and most foods	Hypertension and edema	Dehydration, renal failure, and cramps in muscles
Potassium	Excitability of membranes in nerve and muscle function	Most foods	Heart arrhythmias	Alteration in muscle contraction and in ECG patterns
Sulfur	Part of certain amino acids and other important compounds	Foods containing proteins	None known	None known; deficiency may never have been observed
Chlorine	Osmotic and acid–base balance	Table salt and most foods	Edema	Cramps in muscles and alkalosis
Iron	Part of heme of hemoglobin and cytochromes	Liver, eggs, nuts, legumes, and raisins	Hemochromatosis	Lack of hemoglobin in erythrocytes, anemia
Copper	Acts in hemoglobin formation	Liver and meats	Tachycardia, hypertension, and coma	Anemia
Cobalt	Acts in hemoglobin formation	Meats	Cardiomyopathy	Anemia
Iodine	Part of thyroxine	Fish, iodized salt	None	Cretinism, goiter
Manganese	Cofactor in enzymes	Leafy vegetables and whole grains	Muscle weakness, nervous disturbances	Decrease in rate of cellular respiration
Zinc	Part of insulin and some enzymes	Many foods	None known	Growth inhibition, testicular atrophy, skin lesions
Fluorine	Suppresses action of oral bacteria	Milk, dentrifices	Mottling of teeth	Dental caries

Table 24.4   Vitamin-Responsive Inherited Metabolic Disorders

Vitamin	Biochemical Defect	Disorder	Manner of Inheritance*	Therapeutic Dose/Day
B_1-thiamine	Pyruvate decarboxylase	Pyruvicacidemia	Unknown	5–20 mg
B_6-pyridoxine	Glutamate decarboxylase?	Infantile convulsions	Autosomal recessive	10–50mg
	Unknown	Hypochromic anemia	Sex-linked recessive	>10mg
B_{12}-cyanocobalamin	Intrinsic factor deficiency, inactive intrinsic factor, transport deficiency	Megaloblastic anemia	All autosomal recessives	5–100 µg
Folic acid	Intestinal folate absorption	Megaloblastic anemia	Unknown	<0.05 mg
	A folate reductase enzyme	Mental retardation, schizophrenic psychosis	Autosomal recessive	>10 mg
Biotin	Propionyl-CoA carboxylase	Propionicacidemia ketoacidosis and retardation	Autosomal recessive	10 mg
Niacin	Intestinal and renal transport of tryptophan	Hartnup disease, cerebellar ataxia	Autosomal recessive	>40 mg
D-calciferol	Unknown	Hypophosphatemic rickets	Sex-linked dominant	>100,000 units (>4 g cholecalciferol)
	An enzyme in calciferol synthesis	Vitamin D–dependent rickets	Autosomal recessive	>25,000 units (>1 g cholecalciferol)

*See Chapter 27 for an explanation of inheritance.

Other disorders lead to the excessive storage of glycogen because the body lacks enzymes to break down glycogen once it is stored.

Vitamin-responsive inherited disorders   A number of disorders have been discovered that involve the ineffectiveness of a coenzyme rather than the absence of an enzyme. It is possible that an enzyme that activates the coenzyme may be missing because of a genetic defect. A genetic defect is likely as these disorders appear to be inherited. The affected individual displays symptoms of a vitamin deficiency, although the problem actually may be in the absorption of the vitamin, its entry into the cells, its conversion from a vitamin to a coenzyme, or its union with the enzyme it assists. In some disorders therapeutic large doses of specific vitamins may be helpful. Table 24.4 provides some examples of **vitamin-responsive inherited disorders**.

Other Metabolic Disorders

Diabetes mellitus   Though **diabetes mellitus** (sugar diabetes) was discussed briefly in Chapter 15, the causes and metabolic effects of the disorder will be described in more detail here.

Once thought to be a single disease characterized by excessive amounts of glucose in the blood, diabetes mellitus is now recognized as having several forms. We will consider the two most clinically distinct forms. In **insulin-dependent** (juvenile-onset) diabetes the individual requires insulin injections to compensate for the decreased number or complete lack of functional B-cells in the pancreas and the consequent decreased output of insulin. In **non-insulin-dependent** (maturity-onset) diabetes the individual may have normal amounts of insulin in the blood, but it somehow fails to act effectively on the target cells. Other differences between these two forms of diabetes are summarized in Table 24.5.

A substantial amount of evidence now supports the idea that insulin-dependent diabetes is caused by a viral infection in individuals who are susceptible to certain viruses. The most convincing evidence is that a virus known as the coxsackie B4 virus was isolated from the pancreas of a child who suddenly developed diabetes and died within a few days. This virus was successfully used to induce diabetes in susceptible laboratory animals. Other evidence that supports the view that insulin-dependent diabetes may be due to an infection is as follows: (1) Symptoms appear suddenly, often in the fall and winter, and (2) the pancreas becomes inflamed, and some of the B-cells are destroyed.

Though a family history of insulin-dependent diabetes is uncommon, the disease does appear frequently in individuals who have a particular configuration of HLA histocompatibility antigens. These antigens, usually labeled A, B, C, and D, are coded on chromosome 6 of the set of twenty-three pairs of human chromosomes. They are the antigens that determine whether donor and recipient tissues are compatible in organ transplants. (We discussed them briefly in Chapter 20.) Recently, some combinations of these antigens have been associated with the high incidence of certain diseases. Insulin-dependent diabetes appears with an unusually high frequency in individuals who have B8 and B15 antigens; certain other HLA antigens seem to confer resistance to this type of diabetes. If an individual is genetically susceptible to insulin-dependent diabetes, any of several viruses may trigger the disease, including mumps and rubella viruses and various other members of the coxsackie family of viruses.

Insulin-dependent diabetes is difficult to control, and the affected individual must receive insulin injections. Metabolic acidosis is a frequent complication because much of the body's energy is derived from fats instead of glucose, and acids accumulate in the blood. Acidosis is discussed in more detail in Chapter 26.

Non-insulin-dependent diabetes, though apparently not associated with a viral infection, does tend to run in families, where it seems to involve several inherited factors. In studies of identical twins if one twin developed this form of diabetes after age fifty, the other twin was extremely likely to develop it within a few years. The probability of a person developing non-insulin-dependent diabetes doubles with each decade of life and with every 20% increase above ideal body weight.

Non-insulin-dependent diabetes can usually be controlled by dietary restriction of carbohydrate, especially sugar, weight reduction in the obese, and the use of oral

Table 24.5	Differences between Insulin-dependent and Non-insulin-dependent Diabetes	
Characteristic	Insulin-Dependent (juvenile-onset)	Non-insulin-dependent (maturity-onset)
Age at onset	Usually under 20	Usually over 40
Percent of all diabetics	About 10%	About 90%
Time of year of onset	Fall and winter	No seasonal trend
Appearance of symptoms	Sudden and usually acute	Gradual and slow to develop
Metabolic acidosis	Frequent	Rare
Obesity at onset	Uncommon	Common
B-cells	Decreased	Variable
Insulin	Decreased	Variable
Inflammation of pancreas	Present at onset	Absent
Family history of diabetes	Uncommon	Common
Association with HLA antigens	Yes	No

hypoglycemic drugs if necessary to maintain a normal blood glucose concentration.

Compared to nondiabetic individuals, diabetic individuals (of both types) have an incidence of blindness twenty-five times as high, kidney disease seventeen times as high, gangrene five times as high, and heart disease twice as high. Complications of atherosclerosis are the leading cause of death in diabetic individuals.

Though excess glucose in the blood is characteristic of both forms of diabetes mellitus, the reasons for its accumulation appear to be quite different in the two forms. In insulin-dependent diabetes there is a deficiency of insulin. In non-insulin-dependent diabetes the affected individual may have adequate insulin production, but the number of insulin receptors on the cells may be reduced. Studies of obese individuals have shown that the number of insulin receptors is markedly reduced at the onset of the disease. If these individuals reduce their weight by 10 to 15%, the number of receptors often returns to normal. One explanation of this mechanism is that, as food intake leads to excess glucose in the blood, insulin production increases. In cells exposed to an excess of insulin, the insulin receptors become inactive or reduced in number. Thus, a kind of negative feedback that would seem to protect cells against excess glucose actually leads to symptoms of diabetes.

The major effects of diabetes are due in some way to inadequate amount or action of insulin. They include: (1) decreased entrance of glucose into most cells (insulin is not required for glucose to enter brain cells, except for certain hypothalamic cells); (2) increased mobilization of fats from adipose tissue; and (3) depletion of proteins. Because of the inability of cells to use glucose, the concentration of blood glucose builds to high levels—300 to 500 milligrams/100 milliliters blood—and even higher in some cases. When the blood glucose concentration reaches about 180 milligrams/100 milliliters of blood, glucose begins to be excreted by the kidneys. Excess amounts of glucose in the blood (**hyperglycemia**) and in the urine (**glucosuria**) create changes in osmotic pressures. The high blood glucose concentration draws fluids from the cells, and the high concentration in the urine causes the volume of the urine to increase. Loss of fluid leads to thirst. Thus, the main symptoms of diabetes mellitus are often referred to as the three "polys"—polyuria, or large volume of urine; polyphagia, or excessive eating; and polydipsia, or excessive thirst.

In addition to affecting osmotic pressures, diabetes also creates acid-base balance problems. Metabolism of fatty acids (instead of glucose) leads to release of ketone bodies into the blood (**ketosis**), which increase the acidity of the blood, causing acidosis. (Ketone bodies are shown in Figure 23.9, Chapter 23, and compensation for acidosis is discussed in Chapter 26.) Finally, as the kidney excretes excessive amounts of urine, thereby ridding the body of some of the excess glucose and some of the ketone bodies, large quantities of sodium are also excreted. This depletes the sodium in extracellular fluids and also reduces the blood volume as water follows the sodium into the urine.

Several theories have been proposed to explain the long-term effects of diabetes. One is that a thickening of the basement membrane surrounding the capillaries contributes to the poor peripheral circulation of the patient and thus to tissue damage throughout the body. Another theory is that intermediates of glucose metabolism, such as sorbitol, accumulate in the tissues, especially in the nervous system and lenses of the eyes. These metabolites increase the osmotic pressure in the cells and lead to edema and tissue damage. A third theory proposes that excess glucose becomes chemically bonded to the amino acids of proteins and that these chemical complexes somehow lead to tissue damage.

In the treatment of both forms of diabetes it has been standard practice to limit the amount of mono- and disaccharides in the diet and to supply only sufficient insulin or oral antidiabetic medication to keep the blood glucose concentration in the normal range. Since it has been observed that, when obese individuals with non-insulin-dependent diabetes reduce their weight, the number of insulin receptors returns to normal, weight reduction for such persons has become an important goal of treatment. One of the problems of monitoring the effectiveness of treatment by measuring blood glucose concentration alone is that the concentration of lipids in the blood may be continuously elevated. Therefore, current treatment in some clinics consists of supplying sufficient glucose and insulin to keep both the lipid and glucose levels in the blood in the normal range.

Obesity **Obesity** is an excess of body fat, usually making up more than 10% of the body weight. In contrast, overweight without obesity may be due to excessively large muscles or a large skeleton. Thus, to determine acceptable body weight, the weight of bones, muscles, and other organs must be considered. Fat should not exceed 10% of the weight of other structures. When energy input from nutrients is greater than energy output, weight gain (in the form of fat) occurs at the rate of 1 gram of fat for every 9.3 kilocalories not expended. Once excess fat has been acquired, it is maintained by balancing the energy input and output. Weight loss will occur only if the energy output exceeds the input.

The causes of obesity are not well understood, and much research is currently focused on improving that understanding. Behavioral, physiological, genetic, and developmental factors have been implicated.

Behavioral factors include psychogenic factors and habits of exercise. Psychogenic factors may cause people to eat to reduce tension or to satisfy oversolicitous parents as a child. Exercise is implicated in obesity in two ways: (1) Exercise is important in maintaining energy balance, and (2) it may inhibit feeding. If the latter is true, sedentary people eat more because they get too little exercise to take advantage of its appetite-inhibiting action.

Physiological factors include malfunction of the hunger–satiety centers and decreased activity of the cellular sodium-potassium pumps. Malfunction of the hunger-satiety centers may, on rare occasions, be due to a hypothalamic tumor or, more frequently, to a hyperactive hunger center or an impaired or nonfunctional satiety center.

As noted in Chapter 22, CCK-PZ may be involved in regulating the hunger–satiety centers, and a deficiency in CCK-PZ may lead to obesity. Experimental evidence to support the malfunction of the hunger–satiety centers in obesity comes from the observation that some formerly obese individuals who have succeeded in achieving normal weight continue to have far greater than normal hunger stimuli (conscious desire to eat). In individuals whose cells have fewer than the normal number of sodium-potassium pumps, far less than the normal amount of energy is expended in the operation of the pumps. The reduced basal metabolism in such individuals may lead to excess food intake, which in turn may lead to obesity.

An important genetic factor in some cases is the so-called fat-storage defect, in which a deficiency in the cellular fat-hydrolyzing enzyme prevents the breakdown of fat once it has been stored in adipose tissue. Defects in the hunger–satiety centers and psychogenic factors also may be genetically determined. However, the mechanisms of inheritance in these factors are not understood.

A developmental factor that may lead to obesity is triggered by the overfeeding of infants. Such overfeeding may stimulate the development of excessive numbers of fat cells early in life when they are still capable of rapid division. Later in life these large numbers of cells can fill with fat and lead to obesity.

The adipose tissue in obese people is qualitatively no different from the adipose tissue in thin people. However, individuals who are obese do sometimes metabolize glucose more slowly than normal, and their metabolic processes tend to lead to fat deposition. On reducing diets obese people do not develop ketosis to the extent that normal people on the same diets do.

The complications of obesity are so numerous that one might expect greater efforts to control it. Not only are obese people often unhappy with their appearance, they suffer a variety of mechanical problems due to their weight (osteoarthritis, varicose veins, hernias, flat feet, and lack of agility that leads to accident proneness). They are predisposed toward diabetes, hypercholesterolemia, gallstones, hypertension, and increased peripheral resistance in the blood vessels so the heart must work much harder than normal. If fat deposits increase the effort required for breathing, carbon dioxide may be retained, and this can lead to sleepiness and reduced activity. Life expectancy is greatly reduced by obesity.

Treatment of obesity has been less than successful over the long term. Reducing the caloric intake and increasing the energy expenditure has been the standard treatment, although psychomotor-stimulating drugs such as amphetamines have been used. These drugs suppress the appetite for a short period of time but lose their effectiveness rapidly and may have undesirable side effects. Better methods for treating obesity must await a more complete understanding of its causes.

Anorexia nervosa A syndrome seen primarily in adolescent females, but not limited to them, **anorexia nervosa** is characterized by a persistent desire to avoid gaining weight or even to reduce an already subnormal weight (Figure 24.2). Anorexic individuals become extremely emaciated, lose hair, and cease menstruating—all symptoms of starvation. They may refuse to eat or gorge themselves and then induce vomiting. The cause of this disorder is unknown, but it is thought to involve some psychological factors or some abnormality of the hypothalamus. Unless new eating habits can be established, the condition may be fatal.

Alcoholism **Alcoholism** is a disorder in which the individual regularly consumes substantial quantities of alcohol and is unable to control the urge to drink. The causes of alcoholism include possible multiple genetic factors and assorted environmental factors. Studies of offspring of alcoholics, even those raised away from and without knowledge of the alcoholic parent, have shown four times as high an incidence of alcoholism as that in the general population. In another study, volunteer subjects with a family history of alcoholism and control subjects lacking such a history were given ethanol (0.5 ml/kg body weight), and blood samples were taken at 15–30 minute intervals. The blood level of acetaldehyde, a metabolite of alcohol, rose much more sharply in subjects with a family history of alcoholism than in the controls. This finding suggests that acetaldehyde production might be used to detect individuals at high risk for becoming alcoholic. Environmental stresses seem to contribute to the development of alcoholism in genetically susceptible individuals. Because in the United States alcoholism has become the third leading cause of death in the twenty-five to sixty-five age range, the disease deserves serious study.

Alcohol is quickly absorbed from the stomach and small intestine and can be metabolized only in the liver. Hydrogen is removed and transferred to NAD^+, leaving acetaldehyde as the product. Acetaldehyde is then converted to acetate and metabolized to carbon dioxide and water. When large quantities of alcohol are consumed, toxic levels of acetaldehyde may accumulate in the blood. Within the liver of many alcoholics alcohol (or acetaldehyde) leads to excessive synthesis of fat and the release of excessive lipids into the blood. Liver cells become engorged

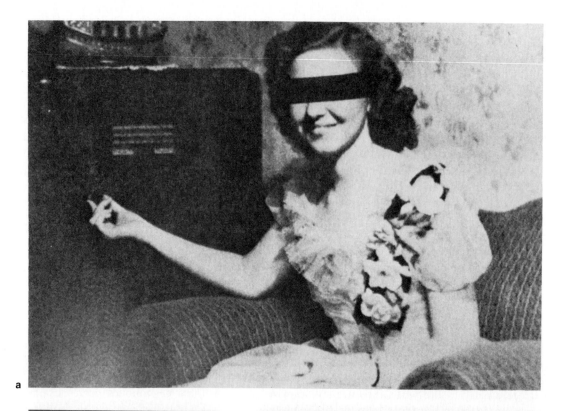

a

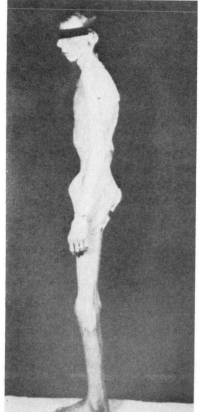

b

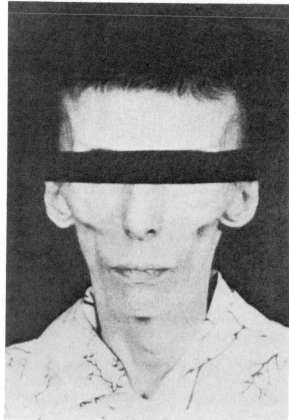

c

Figure 24.2 (**a**) An eighteen-year-old girl, weight 55 kg; (**b**) and (**c**) same girl at age twenty-one, suffering from anorexia nervosa. (Reproduced with permission from A. J. Bachrach, W. J. Erwin, and J. P. Mohr, ''The Control of Eating Behavior in an Anorexic by Operant Conditioning Techniques,'' in L. P. Ullmann and L. Krasner (eds.), *Case Studies in Behavior Modification* (New York: Holt, Rinehart and Winston, 1965), pp. 153–163.)

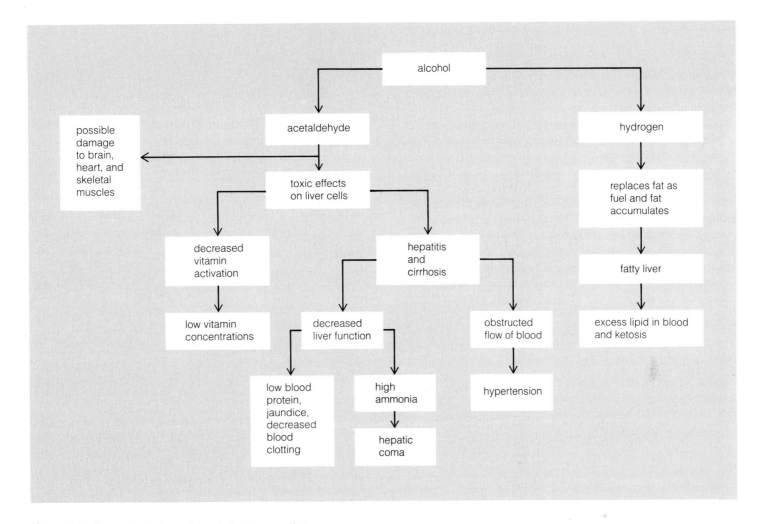

Figure 24.3 Some effects of excessive alcohol consumption.

with fat and fail to function efficiently. Eventually, as liver cells become inflamed, the patient suffers from alcoholic hepatitis. Finally, cirrhosis of the liver occurs as fibrous scars severely disrupt liver function.

The broad effects of alcoholism include malnutrition and vitamin deficiencies because too much of the diet consists of alcohol instead of nutritious foods and because alcohol specifically interferes with the absorption of nutrients. Acetaldehyde interferes with the activation of some vitamins. In addition to intoxication, alcoholism also causes increased susceptibility to infections, gastritis, liver damage, and damage to brain tissue. The alcoholic individual may develop increased dependence and social and financial problems. Of these effects the effects on the liver and the brain are of greatest physiological significance (see Figure 24.3).

Impaired liver function interferes with the liver's ability to detoxify substances, but in the early stages of alcoholism the **detoxification** mechanisms are stimulated to work at high efficiency. As we saw in Chapter 23, drugs administered when an alcoholic is sober are inactivated much more rapidly than in nonalcoholics because of the amplified detoxification. The taking of drugs *with* alcohol, however, can lead to serious complications because the alcohol may tie up detoxification sites and slow the rate of inactivation of the other drugs.

Effects of alcohol on the nervous system are thought to be due to acetaldehyde, but none of the proposed mechanisms of its action have been confirmed. One mechanism may be that acetaldehyde competes with an enzyme that normally inactivates some brain neurotransmitters. When acetaldehyde (instead of the enzyme) combines with a neurotransmitter, it forms a compound strikingly similar to morphine; this substance may account for the development of dependence on alcohol. Individuals genetically predisposed to accumulate acetaldehyde, presumably because of a metabolic defect, may be especially susceptible to developing dependence on alcohol.

The treatment of alcoholism presents a difficult problem because the available methods require the cooperation of the alcoholic individual, who may deny the problem and refuse treatment. Most alcoholic treatment programs make use of psychotherapy to help the alcoholic discover the unconscious psychological problems that led to the uncontrollable desire to drink. The organization Alcoholics Anonymous has helped to keep many of its members from backsliding into their former habits through mutual support among the members. The drug antabuse, which induces vomiting and palpitations when alcohol is consumed, helps some alcoholics to avoid yielding to their temptations. Unfortunately, none of these treatment methods focuses on the physiological problems of alcoholism.

CLINICAL TERMS

kwashiorkor (kwash-e-or'kor) protein-calorie malnutrition; in Ghandian, literally the disease that comes after the second child, as the first child no longer receives breast milk, and the available diet is deficient in protein and calories

marasmus (mar-az'mus) wasting and emaciation characteristic of deprivation of all nutrients, often applied to children under two years of age

Essay: Vegetable Proteins

The idea that large quantities of meat, especially beef, are essential to well-being is a culturally defined attitude; it is not substantiated by nutritional studies. Protein is essential in the human diet, but it need not come from meat. What humans really need is a supply of the essential amino acids plus enough additional amino acids to provide the proper proportions for protein synthesis. This need can be met with plant proteins, primarily grains, if care is taken to eat them in the right combinations.

Most plants are deficient in specific essential amino acids, but not all plants are lacking in the same ones. Generally, plant proteins lack one or more of the following amino acids: lysine, isoleucine, tryptophan, and the sulfur-containing amino acids cysteine and methionine. Some examples of plant and animal (nonmeat) foods and estimates of their amino acid content are given in Table 24.6. By learning which plants or non-animal-muscle foods are good sources of various essential amino acids, you can plan meal combinations that will provide adequate supplies of protein. Some complementary combinations are shown in Figure 24.4. Specific combinations that could be substituted for meat in the diet are listed in Table 24.7.

Because human tissues are similar to the tissues of other animals, particularly other mammals, meat and other animal products provide amino acids in a proportion that is close to the ideal for human nutrition. Even so, our bodies can use only about 90% of the amino acids in an egg, 80% of those in milk, and 70% of those in meat, poultry, and fish. These percentages, called the **net protein utilization**, represent the proportion of amino acids that can be converted to human proteins. Plants generally have lower net protein utilization values—they range from 70% for rice to 40% for kidney beans. This indicates that in some cases a somewhat larger amount of plant foods must be eaten to provide sufficient quantities of protein. For example, 4 ounces of cooked hamburger (one large burger) provides 30 grams of protein, 67%, or 20 grams, of which your body can use. A meal containing 1 cup of rice and ¾ cup of soybeans contains 32 grams of protein, 61%, or 20 grams, of which your body can use.

Eating less meat has some important advantages, both nutritional ones and ecological ones. Nutritionally, increased consumption of foods from plant sources can greatly increase the amounts of vitamins, minerals, and roughage in the diet. Consuming plant proteins also reduces the amount of pesticide residues taken into the body. Pesticides do not accumulate appreciably inside plant tissues, and they can be washed off. When grazing animals such as cattle eat plants with pesticides

Table 24.6	Availability of Selected Essential Amino Acids			
Food	Tryptophan	Isoleucine	Lysine	Sulfur-Containing Amino Acids
Soybeans	+ + +	+ +	+ + +	+
Peas, beans, and other legumes	+	+ +	+ + +	+
Nuts and seeds	+ + +	+	+ + +	+
Grains and whole-grain foods	+ +	+	+	+ +
Corn	0	+	+	+ +
Green vegetables	+ +	+	+ +	+
Dairy products	+ +	+ + +	+ + +	+ +
Eggs	+ + +	+ + +	+ + +	+ + +
Seafoods	+ +	+ +	+ + +	+ +
Meat and poultry	+ +	+ +	+ + +	+ +

+ + + = excellent source, + + = good source, + = poor source,
0 = very poor source

Table 24.7	Some Sample Vegetable Protein Combinations and Some Vegetable-Dairy Protein Combinations and Their Protein Content	
Combination		Protein Content
1 oz cheese and 4 slices whole grain bread or 1½ c macaroni		15 g
1 c beans and 2 c milk or ⅔ c grated cheese		15 g
⅓ c beans and ½ c sesame seeds		15 g
1 potato and ⅓ c cheese or 1 c milk		12 g
1 c rice and ¾ c soybeans		32 g
1 c rice and ⅓ c sesame seeds		18 g
1 c rice and 1⅓ c milk		30 g
½ c peanut butter and ¾ c milk		36 g

on them, however, the pesticides accumulate in their tissues, which carry a concentrated dose when the animals are eaten by humans. In addition, plant foods eaten in an unprocessed or natural state help people avoid intake of food additives, the effects of which are not well understood. Finally, meat often contains large amounts of saturated fats and cholesterol, while plants contain mostly unsaturated fats and *no* cholesterol.

In terms of biological economics consider this: It takes about 20 pounds of plant proteins to produce 1 pound of edible beef protein. Thus, raising a single animal for human consumption requires a large mass of plant material, and consequently a large area of land devoted exclusively to grazing. That same land, assuming it is suitable for cultivation, could produce grain to feed far more people than can be fed from butchering that single animal. Furthermore, cattle are also fed grain themselves for a certain period of time before slaughter to produce higher (usually fatter) grades of meat—grain that otherwise could be used for human consumption.

We have been considering only protein here; as mentioned earlier, some vitamins, notably B_{12}, are lacking in strictly vegetarian diets. Therefore, some consumption of animal products—such as eggs, milk, and milk products—seems essential. Still, muscle meat does not appear to be necessary to maintain an adequate diet.

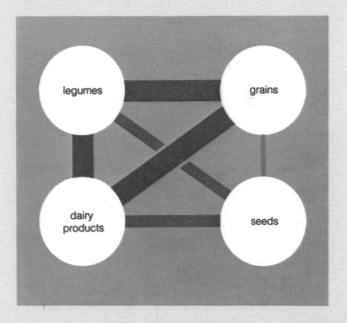

Figure 24.4 Summary of complementary protein relationships. Thickness of arrows indicates relative value of protein combination.

CHAPTER SUMMARY

(Chapter summary points and review questions are numbered to correspond to the numbered objectives in the text of each chapter.)

Principles of Nutrition

1. Define nutrition and describe the nutritional needs generally supplied by each of the four basic food groups.
  a. Nutrition deals with provision, through the intake of food, of all the nutrients necessary for maintaining health.
  b. The nutritional needs of healthy individuals are generally met by consuming the recommended amounts of the basic four food groups:
   (1) The milk group provides calories, protein, fat, vitamin A and riboflavin, calcium, phosphorus, potassium, and magnesium.
   (2) The meat group provides calories, protein, fat, phosphorus, iron, sodium, potassium, and B vitamins.
   (3) The fruit and vegetable group provides vitamins A, B, C, and K, and certain minerals; sweet fruits and starchy vegetables provide more calories than green leafy vegetables.
   (4) The bread and cereal group provides calories, some protein, and, if whole grain, a good supply of B vitamins.

2. Explain the changes in intake of certain nutrients that may result from adhering to the U.S. Dietary Goals statement and explain the health risks those goals seek to reduce.
  a. U.S. Dietary Goals seek to reduce the amount of fat (especially saturated fat and cholesterol), sugar, and salt in the diet and to increase the amount of complex carbohydrate in the diet.
  b. These recommendations are intended to reduce the risk of heart disease, atherosclerosis, diabetes, tooth decay, and hypertension.

3. Discuss the strengths and weaknesses of the Recommended Dietary Allowances of nutrients.
  a. Recommended dietary allowances have been established for some nutrients, but the methods used to determine RDAs are open to some question.
  b. Despite their pitfalls, RDAs are the only scientific measure of nutritional needs.

Vitamins, Minerals, and Water

4. Describe the biochemical action, dietary sources, and effects of excesses and deficiencies of the vitamins and minerals needed by the body.
  a. Vitamins and minerals generally assist enzymes in catalyzing metabolic reactions.
  b. Their biochemical actions, dietary sources, and effects of excesses and deficiencies are summarized in Table 24.3.

5. Briefly discuss the role of water in metabolism.
  a. Most metabolic reactions take place in an aqueous medium, and many reactions involve water molecules.
  b. In addition to water consumed in foods and beverages, metabolic water is produced as food substances are oxidized.

Metabolic Disorders

6. Discuss the possible causes and effects of the following metabolic disorders: (a) genetic defects, (b) diabetes mellitus, (c) obesity, (d) anorexia nervosa, and (e) alcoholism.
  a. Genetic defects discussed include:
   (1) cystic fibrosis, a condition in which excessive mucus causes digestive and respiratory malfunctions
   (2) phenylketonuria and related disorders, in which an enzyme to metabolize a particular amino acid is missing, and development is disturbed
   (3) vitamin-responsive inherited disorders, in which a cofactor for an enzyme is impaired in function and anemia or other effects are seen
  b. Diabetes mellitus is a set of disorders, two of which were considered:
   (1) Insulin-dependent diabetes usually occurs before the age of twenty, may be caused by a viral infection, involves decreased function or absence of B-cells, and is treated with insulin and diet.
   (2) Non-insulin-dependent diabetes usually occurs after forty years of age, may be inherited, involves ineffective insulin action, and is usually treated with diet and drugs that stimulate insulin action.
  c. Obesity is an excess of body fat, the causes of which are poorly understood. Its effects include psychological problems, mechanical problems, physiological disturbances, and reduced life expectancy. Its treatment is not usually successful.
  d. Anorexia nervosa occurs primarily in adolescent females and involves a persistent desire to lose weight. Causes are probably psychogenic, and treatment requires establishing new eating habits.
  e. Alcoholism is the consumption of substantial quantities of alcohol and an uncontrollable desire for alcohol; it may be caused by genetic or environmental factors. The effects of alcoholism include malnutrition, impaired liver and brain function, and various social consequences; its treatment, which involves changes in behavior, requires the cooperation of the alcoholic.

REVIEW

Important Terms

alcoholism	nutrition
anorexia nervosa	obesity
basic four food groups	phenylketonuria
cystic fibrosis	recommended dietary allowance (RDA)
detoxification	
diabetes mellitus	U.S. dietary goals
malnutrition	vitamin
metabolic disorders	vitamin-responsive inherited disorders
mineral	

Questions

1. Keep a record of everything you eat for a day. Compare your diet with the recommendations from the basic four food groups and plan a menu for a day that corrects any deficiencies in your diet.

2. Compare your diet with the recommendations from U.S. Dietary Goals and plan a menu that corrects any deficiencies in your diet.

3. How could the recommended dietary allowances of nutrients be improved?

4. What vitamin and mineral deficiencies or excesses might develop on the following diets? (a) milk-free diet, (b) animal protein–free diet, (c) a diet lacking whole-grain cereals, (d) a diet lacking citrus fruits, (e) a diet consisting primarily of carrots and other yellow vegetables, and (f) a diet of sugar and other "junk" foods.

5. a. What is metabolic water?
   b. Why is water important in the diet?

6. Discuss the causes and effects of cystic fibrosis, phenylketonuria, diabetes, obesity, anorexia nervosa, and alcoholism.

Problems

1. Apply your knowledge of nutrition and obesity to plan a diet and exercise program that an obese person might be likely to follow. (Make reasonable assumptions about the preferences and habits of the person.)

2. Plan a menu for a week following the guidelines for a vegetable-protein diet.

3. Suppose you are working with a person who has just been diagnosed as having insulin-dependent diabetes. What complications would you watch for, and how would you help the person to adjust to the disease?

4. How would you change your strategies if the person were obese and had non-insulin-dependent diabetes?

REFERENCES AND READINGS

Chafetz, M. E. 1979. Alcohol and alcoholism. *American Scientist* 61:293 (May–June).

Davidson, S., Passmore, R., Brock, J. F., and Truswell, A. S. 1975. *Human nutrition and dietetics.* New York: Longman.

DeLuca, H. F. 1981. Recent advances in the metabolism of vitamin D. *Annual Review of Physiology* 43:199.

Fleck, H. C. 1976. *Introduction to nutrition* (3rd ed.). New York: Macmillan.

Food and Nutrition Board. 1980. *Recommended dietary allowances* (9th ed.). Washington: National Academy of Sciences.

Greenberg, D. 1979. Nutrition hype. *Omni* 1(5):101 (February).

Kolata, G. B. 1979. Blood sugar and the complications of diabetes. *Science* 203:1098 (March 16).

Lappé, F. M. 1971. *Diet for a small planet.* New York: Ballantine Books.

Lieber, C. S. 1976. The metabolism of alcohol. *Scientific American* 234(3):25 (March).

Mann, J. I. 1980. Diet and diabetes. *Diabetologia* 18:80.

Maugh, T. M. 1979. Virus isolated from juvenile diabetic. *Science* 204:1187 (June 15).

Maurer, A. C. 1979. The therapy of diabetes. *American Scientist* 67:422 (July–August).

Notkins, A. L. 1979. The causes of diabetes. *Scientific American* 241(5):62 (November).

Oscar-Berman, M. 1980. Neuropsychological consequences of long-term chronic alcoholism. *American Scientist* 68:410 (July–August).

Page, L., and Friend, B. 1978. The changing United States diet. *BioScience* 28(3):192 (March).

Rose, R. C. 1980. Water-soluble vitamin absorption in intestine. *Annual Review of Physiology* 42:157.

Rosenberg, L. E. 1976. Vitamin-responsive inherited metabolic disorders. *Advances in Human Genetics* 6:1.

Schuckit, M. A., and Rayses, V. 1979. Ethanol ingestion: Differences in blood acetaldehyde concentrations in relatives of alcoholics and controls. *Science* 203:54 (5 January).

Select Committee on Nutrition and Human Needs, United States Senate. 1977. *Dietary goals for the United States.* Washington, D.C.: U.S. Government Printing Office.

Thiele, V. F. 1980. *Clinical nutrition* (2nd ed.). St. Louis, Mo.: C. V. Mosby.

25

URINARY SYSTEM

ORGANIZATION AND GENERAL FUNCTIONS

Objective 1. Describe the overall plan of the urinary system and name its major functions.

The urinary system consists of the kidneys, ureters, urinary bladder, and urethra (Figure 25.1). Though we often think of this system as a waste-removal system, it does much more than that. The kidneys filter a volume equivalent to all of the blood plasma in the body about every five minutes, and they regulate the blood concentration of many different substances. In addition to removing wastes, they help to regulate the pH of the blood and to maintain electrolytes (ionized particles) in proper concentrations. Thus, the kidneys are extremely important in the maintenance of homeostasis. Materials filtered from the blood by the kidneys go into the urine. The ureters carry urine from the kidneys to the urinary bladder, where urine is stored until it is voluntarily released through the urethra.

The kidneys have a remarkable ability to regenerate functional tissue. They may sustain a loss of 90% of their nephrons (the functional units of the kidney) and recover without any apparent loss of function.

DEVELOPMENT

Objective 2. Describe the general development of the urinary system.

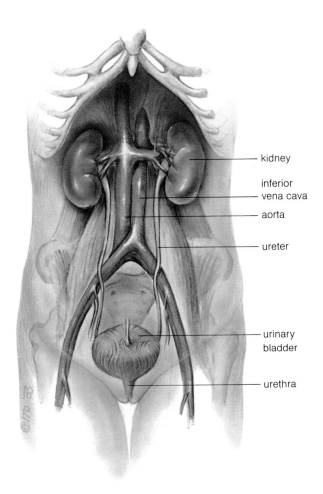

	kidney
	inferior vena cava
	aorta
	ureter
	urinary bladder
	urethra

Figure 25.1   The urinary system.

That organs such as the pronephros and mesonephros should develop and then be reabsorbed as a part of normal embryonic development seems to be a wasteful process. Though an explanation of why these changes occur may not make the process appear less wasteful, it will make it more understandable. Kidneys of the pronephros type appear in all vertebrate embryos and were probably the functional kidneys of the ancestors of primitive vertebrates. As vertebrates evolved, kidneys of the mesonephros type developed slightly posteriorly to the degenerating pronephric kidneys in the embryos. Such kidneys became the functional kidneys of adult fishes and amphibians. As evolution proceded, some vertebrate embryos came to have metanephric kidneys. These kidneys persist as the functional excretory organs in reptiles, birds, and mammals. Thus, as a human embryo develops, it seems to recapitulate some of the changes that occurred in the evolution of its distant ancestors.

The **ureteric bud** gives rise to the ureter and certain parts of the metanephros, including the renal pelvis, the calyces, and the collecting ducts. We will learn more about these parts later. Tissue from the metanephric portion of the urogenital ridge gives rise to the nephrons. The bladder forms from the cloaca and opens to the exterior through the urethra The allantois has little significance in mammals; it collects wastes in reptiles and birds during embryonic development. Some of these structures are shown in Figure 25.2.

Of all the body systems the urinary system is most susceptible to developmental defects. Kidneys may be absent, undersized, filled with cysts, or displaced. In some cases a person is born with only one kidney, with more than two, or with a ''horseshoe'' kidney resulting from the fusion of the kidneys across the midline of the body. Many abnormalities are also seen in the arrangement of the ureters. Unless urinary function is impaired, these abnormalities usually go undetected.

Before the end of the first month of development, a ridge of mesoderm called the urogenital ridge develops on the left and right sides of the back. The superior ends of each ridge develop into a rudimentary kidney, the **pronephros**. Ducts from these kidneys grow inferiorly to the cloaca, a common sac that forms the end of both the urogenital system and the digestive system in the embryo. By the end of the fourth week of development, the pronephros has degenerated, and the **mesonephros**, or second kidney, has begun to form on each side of the body. The mesonephros also degenerates by the end of the second month of development, except for portions that become part of the reproductive system. By the fifth week of development the third and final kidney, the **metanephros**, has begun to develop on each side of the body.

ANATOMY OF THE KIDNEY

Objective 3. Locate and identify the anatomical structures of the kidneys, including the blood supply and cortical and juxtamedullary nephrons.

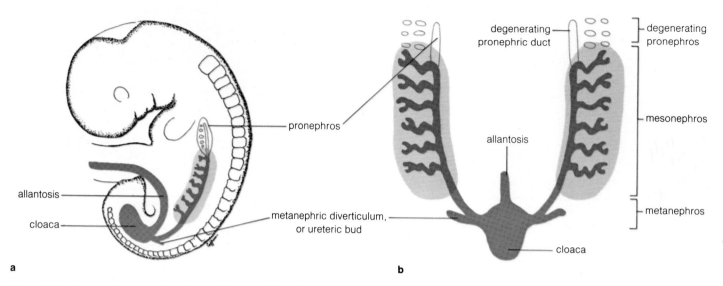

Figure 25.2 The development of the kidney: (**a**) a lateral view, (**b**) an enlarged anterior view.

Gross Anatomy

Each kidney is a bean-shaped organ that lies behind the parietal peritoneum next to the abdominal wall; this location is said to be **retroperitoneal**. The kidneys are located in the region of the upper three lumbar vertebrae, with the right kidney being slightly lower than the left (see Figure 25.1). Because the liver takes a large amount of space in the right abdomen, the right kidney is pushed downward.

In an adult the kidney is about 11 centimeters long, 5 to 7 centimeters wide, and about 2.5 centimeters thick. It is covered by a layer of fibrous connective tissue, the **renal capsule**, which protects it from infection and trauma. Around the capsule is a layer of fat, the **adipose capsule**, and an outer fibrous membrane, the **renal fascia**. Both the fat and the fascia help to protect the kidney, and the fascia anchors it to the abdominal wall. On the medial surface of each kidney is the **hilum**, a notchlike depression where blood and lymph vessels enter and leave the kidney and where the ureter attaches to the kidney (Figure 25.3).

Internally, the kidney consists of an outer **cortex** and an inner **medulla**. Between the cortex and the medulla is the **juxtamedullary zone**. The cortex contains 80% of the microscopic **nephrons**. The medulla contains only 20% of the nephrons and consists mainly of **collecting ducts** that drain urine from the nephrons to the calyces. Blood vessels are interspersed among the ducts. Cone-shaped aggregations of collecting ducts form the **pyramids** of the medulla. All of the ducts of a pyramid terminate in a structure called a **papilla**. Between the pyramids the substance of the cortex extends into the medulla and forms the **renal columns**. The ducts in each of the pyramids drain into a **minor calyx**, and several minor calyces drain into a **major calyx**. The two or three major calyces drain into the **renal pelvis**, which in turn drains into the **ureter**.

Blood Supply

Blood enters each kidney through a renal artery (Figure 25.4 and Table 25.1). Compared to the size of the organs they serve, the renal arteries are very large vessels. Each renal artery branches into the **interlobar arteries**, which pass between the pyramids. When they reach the boundary between the medulla and the cortex, the interlobar arteries branch into the **arcuate arteries**. Anastomoses among these vessels assure that blood will circulate to functional areas of the kidney even when some areas have been damaged. Branches from the arcuate arteries, the **interlobular arteries**, extend into the cortex. The latter branch into arterioles, with one afferent arteriole going to each nephron. (The circulation of blood through the nephron will be described later.) Blood leaving the capillaries of the nephron enters venules and then flows through veins that parallel the arteries described above and that have the same names.

The major blood vessels of the kidneys are supplied

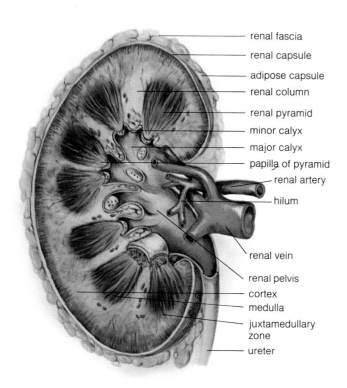

Figure 25.3 A longitudinal section through the kidney, showing its gross anatomy.

renal fascia
renal capsule
adipose capsule
renal column
renal pyramid
minor calyx
major calyx
papilla of pyramid
renal artery
hilum
renal vein
renal pelvis
cortex
medulla
juxtamedullary zone
ureter

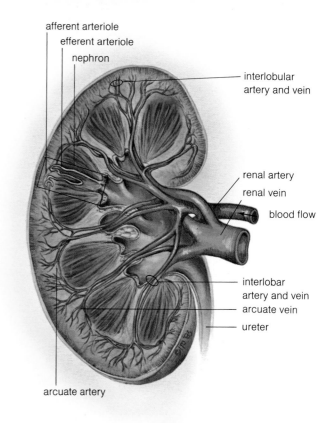

Figure 25.4 The blood vessels of the kidney.

afferent arteriole
efferent arteriole
nephron
interlobular artery and vein
renal artery
renal vein
blood flow
interlobar artery and vein
arcuate vein
ureter
arcuate artery

with nerves from the autonomic nervous system. These nerves help to regulate the size of the small blood vessels and thus the flow of blood through the kidneys.

Nephrons

The **nephron** (Figure 25.5) is the functional unit of the kidney. Each kidney contains about one million nephrons, some of which—the **cortical nephrons**—are located primarily in the cortex, and some of which—the **juxtamedullary nephrons**—extend into the medulla. Each nephron consists of a tubule and its associated blood vessels. The structure of the juxtamedullary nephron will be described first, followed by the variations in the cortical nephron.

Juxtamedullary nephron The tubule of a nephron is a long, coiled, hollow structure that is unattached at one end and attached to a collecting duct at the other end. The unattached portion consists of the **glomerular capsule**, or **Bowman's capsule**, a cuplike structure in which a tuft of capillaries, the glomerulus, is found. (The glomerulus will be described in more detail later.) The capsule contains two

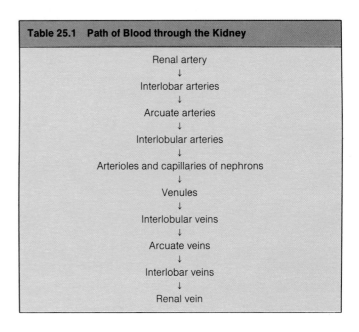

Table 25.1 Path of Blood through the Kidney

Renal artery
↓
Interlobar arteries
↓
Arcuate arteries
↓
Interlobular arteries
↓
Arterioles and capillaries of nephrons
↓
Venules
↓
Interlobular veins
↓
Arcuate veins
↓
Interlobar veins
↓
Renal vein

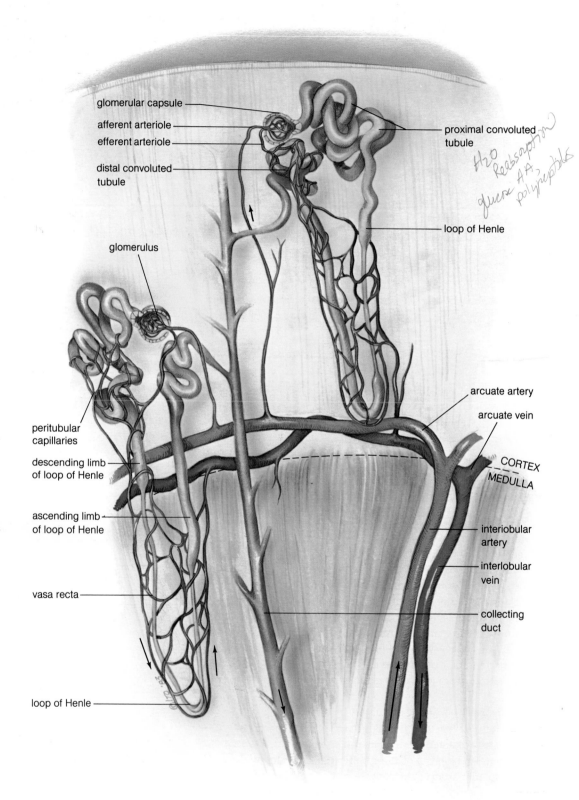

glomerular capsule

afferent arteriole

efferent arteriole

distal convoluted tubule

proximal convoluted tubule

loop of Henle

glomerulus

peritubular capillaries

descending limb of loop of Henle

ascending limb of loop of Henle

vasa recta

loop of Henle

arcuate artery

arcuate vein

CORTEX

MEDULLA

interiobular artery

interlobular vein

collecting duct

H2O Reabsorption glucose AA, polypeptids

Figure 25.5 The structure and blood supply of nephrons.

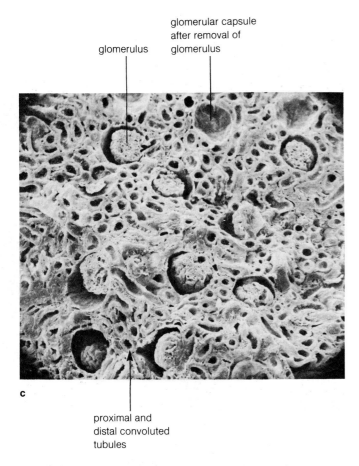

glomerulus

glomerular capsule
after removal of
glomerulus

proximal and
distal convoluted
tubules

c

Figure 25.5c The renal cortex. Photomicrograph × 162. (Reprinted by permission from *Tissues and organs: A text-atlas of scanning electron microscopy* by Richard G. Kessel and Randy H. Kardon. W. H. Freeman and Company. Copyright © 1979.)

layers of cells, an inner layer of epithelial cells called **podocytes** and an outer layer of squamous epithelium. Between the two layers of cells is a space in which the fluid filtered from the blood enters the tubule.

From the capsule the continuous renal tubule is differentiated into several areas: the **proximal convoluted tubule**, the **descending limb of the loop of Henle**, the **loop of Henle** proper, the **ascending limb of the loop of Henle**, and the **distal convoluted tubule**, which leads to a collecting duct. Anatomically, the collecting duct is not part of the nephron, but it receives urine from several nephrons. Even though different segments of the tubule are recognized, the lumen of all of the segments is continuous from the Bowman's capsule to the collecting duct. By tracing the path of the tubule in Figure 25.5, you can see that the capsule and the proximal convoluted tubule are located in the cortex and that the parts of the loop of Henle extend into the medulla. The tubule then returns to the cortex, where it is called the distal convoluted tubule.

The blood vessels surrounding the tubule are also part of the nephron, and each nephron has two sets of capillaries, the **glomerulus** and the **peritubular capillaries**. (The presence of two sets of capillaries between an artery and a vein is an unusual arrangement.) Many **afferent arterioles** branch from each interlobular artery; each carries blood to one glomerulus, where many substances are filtered out of the blood. From the glomerulus blood enters the **efferent arteriole** and is carried to the peritubular capillaries. Peritubular capillaries surround the proximal and distal convoluted tubules and the loop of Henle. The capillaries around the loop of Henle are called **vasa recta**. Many substances move between the fluid in the tubule and the blood in the peritubular capillaries. Blood leaving the peritubular capillaries enters **venules** that lead to the interlobular veins.

Cortical nephron   Like the juxtamedullary nephron, the cortical nephron begins with a glomerular capsule and its associated glomerulus. From the capsule the tubule continues as the proximal convoluted tubule. However, the loop of Henle is very short and barely extends into the medulla. From the loop of Henle the tubule continues as the distal convoluted tubule. Table 25.2 summarizes the structure of the tubules and their blood supply.

The juxtaglomerular apparatus   Each nephron also has a specialized structure called the **juxtaglomerular apparatus** (Figure 25.6). This apparatus consists of **juxtaglomerular cells** in the wall of the afferent arteriole near where it enters the

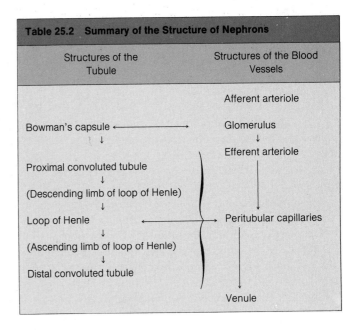

Table 25.2 Summary of the Structure of Nephrons	
Structures of the Tubule	Structures of the Blood Vessels
	Afferent arteriole
Bowman's capsule ⟷	Glomerulus
↓	↓
Proximal convoluted tubule	Efferent arteriole
↓	
(Descending limb of loop of Henle)	
↓	
Loop of Henle ⟷	Peritubular capillaries
↓	
(Ascending limb of loop of Henle)	
↓	
Distal convoluted tubule	
	Venule

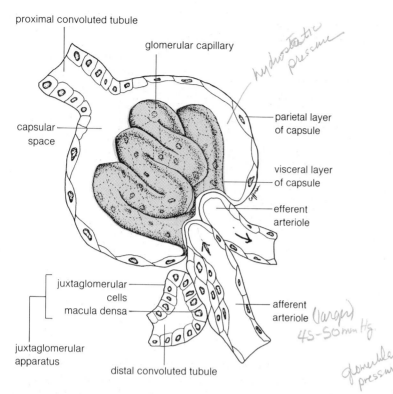

proximal convoluted tubule

glomerular capillary

hydrostatic pressure

capsular space

parietal layer of capsule

visceral layer of capsule

efferent arteriole

juxtaglomerular cells

macula densa

afferent arteriole *(larger)* *45–50 mm Hg*

glomerular pressure

juxtaglomerular apparatus

distal convoluted tubule

Figure 25.6 Juxtaglomerular apparatus, and its relationship to the glomerulus and glomerular capsule.

glomerulus, and large cells, the **macula densa** of the distal convoluted tubule. As we shall see later, this apparatus helps to regulate blood pressure.

PHYSIOLOGY OF THE KIDNEY

Objective 4. Explain how the processes of filtration, reabsorption, and secretion occur in the nephron and how they regulate the concentration of substances in the blood.

Objective 5. Describe the processes that regulate kidney function.

As mentioned earlier, the nephron is the basic functional unit of the kidney. The overall function of the nephron is to regulate the concentration of various substances in the blood so that blood leaving the capillaries of a nephron has had wastes removed and the concentration of electrolytes, acids, and bases adjusted within the normal range. To understand this overall process, we need to consider what happens in each portion of the nephron.

Glomerular Filtration

Glomerular **filtration** occurs when blood passes through the capillaries of a glomerulus. The special way these capillaries are associated with the podocytes of the capsule determines which substances pass from the blood to the lumen of the glomerular capsule (Figure 25.7). The capillary consists of a **fenestrated endothelium**. (Fenestrated means having many openings, or windows.) The podocytes of the capsule have many small processes called **pedicles**, with **filtration slits** between them. A **basement membrane** lies between the endothelium and the podocytes. About 20% of the plasma volume flowing through the kidney is filtered from the glomeruli to the capsular space, and all substances in the filtrate have the same concentration as in the plasma.

The hydrostatic pressure of the blood as it enters the glomerulus is between 45 and 50 mm Hg. This pressure is due in part to the different diameters of the afferent and efferent arterioles. Because the efferent arteriole carrying blood away from the glomerulus is smaller in diameter than the afferent arteriole that carries blood toward it, blood in the glomerulus is under fairly high pressure. However, two forces oppose this pressure. One force is the osmotic pressure created by the plasma proteins, as in any other capillary; the other is the hydrostatic pressure within the glomerular capsule itself. Together, these forces exert a pressure of about 30 mm Hg against filtration. Thus, the **net filtration pressure** pushing substances out of the glomerulus is between 15 and 20 mm Hg⁻ higher than in an ordinary capillary.

The walls of the capillaries, though subject to the above pressure, are constructed so that only certain substances pass through. As shown in Figure 25.7b, the sievelike endothelial layer allows most substances in the blood to pass through; only the blood cells are held back by this layer. The basement membrane prevents large protein molecules from leaving the capillary, and the epithelial cells of the glomerular capsule prevent other protein molecules from leaving. Thus, plasma containing all solutes smaller than protein molecules passes from the capillary into the lumen of the glomerular capsule.

In addition to filtration pressure and properties of the capillary wall, other factors affect the movement of substances from the blood to the renal tubule. Sympathetic stimulation, for example, causes constriction of both afferent and efferent arterioles. If the stimulation is intense, the afferent arterioles become more constricted than the efferent ones. The effects of such stimulation are to reduce the blood pressure in blood entering the glomerulus and to decrease the amount of blood entering the kidney. Because these arterioles can be stimulated independently of the rest of the blood vessels in the body, filtration pressure can

glomerular Capillary

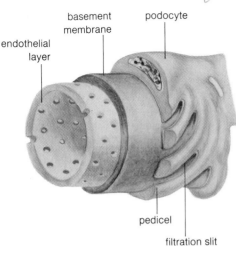

endothelial
layer

basement
membrane

podocyte

pedicel

filtration slit

a

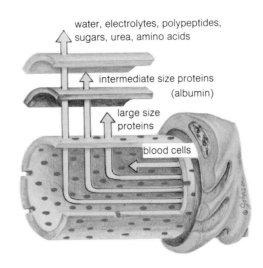

water, electrolytes, polypeptides,
sugars, urea, amino acids

intermediate size proteins
(albumin)

large size
proteins

blood cells

b

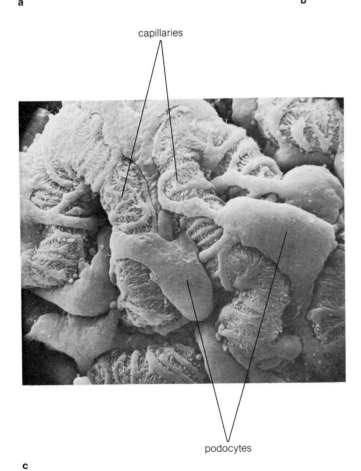

capillaries

podocytes

c

Figure 25.7 (a) The structure of a glomerular capillary and associated podocyte, (b) the nature of substances that pass through the various layers, (c) photomicrograph × 3643. (Reprinted by permission from *Tissues and organs: A text-atlas of scanning electron microscopy* by Richard G. Kessel and Randy H. Kardon. W. H. Freeman and Company. Copyright © 1979.)

decrease without the systemic blood pressure changing. The end result is decreased urine formation. Epinephrine has effects similar to sympathetic stimulation. As we shall see later, other chemicals can also affect glomerular filtration.

In a normal pair of kidneys about 125 milliliters of fluid enter the glomerular capsules every minute. This is the **glomerular filtration rate** (GFR), a rate determined primarily by the net filtration pressure described earlier. Over a twenty-four-hour period glomerular filtration produces about 180 liters of filtrate, from which only about 1 liter of urine will be formed. Obviously, only a small amount of the filtrate is excreted as urine. As we shall see, the functions of other parts of the nephron account for the selective return of certain components of the filtrate to the blood (Table 25.3).

Tubular Reabsorption

The filtrate received by the glomerular capsule passes into the proximal convoluted tubule and on through the remaining segments of the renal tubule. As the filtrate passes through these segments, many substances are returned to the blood by the process of tubular **reabsorption**. In the proximal tubule approximately 70% of the water is reabsorbed. Nutrients such as glucose, amino acids, and polypeptides are nearly all returned to the plasma from the proximal tubule. Certain ions are reabsorbed, especially in the proximal tubule: Na^+, K^+, Ca^{2+}, Cl^-, and HCO_3^-. The rapid reabsorption in the proximal tubule is related to its particular structural and functional characteristics. The

Table 25.3	The Relative Concentrations of Selected Substances in the Plasma, Glomerular Filtrate, and Urine of Normal Adults		
	Concentrations (mg/100 ml)		
Substance	Plasma	Glomerular Filtrate	Urine
Glucose	100	100	0
Urea	26	26	1820
Uric acid	4	4	50
Creatinine	1	1	190
	Concentrations (mEq/l)		
Substance	Plasma	Glomerular Filtrate	Urine
Sodium (Na^+)	142	142	125
Potassium (K^+)	5	5	60
Calcium (Ca^{2+})	4	4	5
Magnesium (Mg^{2+})	3	3	15
Chlorine (Cl^-)	103	103	130
Bicarbonate (HCO_3^-)	27	27	14
Sulfate (SO_4^{2-})	1	1	33
Phosphate (PO_4^{3-})	2	2	40

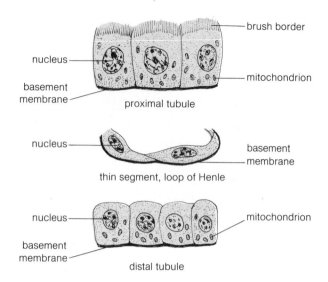

Figure 25.8 The characteristics of tubular epithelium in different regions of the renal tubule.

epithelium of the proximal tubule has a brush border composed of many tiny microvilli (Figure 25.8). Microvilli increase the surface area across which reabsorption takes place. As shown in the figure, other areas of the tubule are less well suited to reabsorption.

Of the substances that are reabsorbed some move passively, and others move by active transport. Examples of actively transported substances are glucose, amino acids, and ions such as phosphate, calcium, and sodium, though some sodium moves passively. Sodium will be used to illustrate the process.

To reach the blood plasma from the lumen of the tubule, sodium must first pass through the membrane of a tubular epithelial cell and enter the cell. It does this by passive diffusion. Then sodium is actively transported out of the epithelial cell into the interstitial fluid. Finally, it diffuses through the endothelium of the capillary at a rate that depends on the concentration gradient. The process as a whole is considered to be active because at least one step requires active transport.

Because active transport requires ATP and carrier substances, the process can occur only as rapidly as carriers are freed and energy is available. Therefore, active tubular reabsorption of any particular substance has a maximum rate.

The maximum concentration of a substance that can be returned to the plasma is called the **renal threshold**. For example, all the glucose in the filtrate is normally returned to the plasma. However, in untreated diabetes mellitus the glucose concentration in the plasma becomes very high. It likewise becomes elevated in the glomerular filtrate. If the amount of glucose in the filtrate exceeds what the active transport system can remove from the filtrate, some of the glucose remains in the filtrate. It is because the active transport system of the renal tubule is overloaded that diabetics sometimes have glucose in their urine. Additionally, the glucose increases the osmotic pressure in the urine, thereby preventing reabsorption of water and causing dehydration.

Other substances that are transported out of the lumen include chloride ions and water. However, their passive transport is controlled by the active movement of sodium.

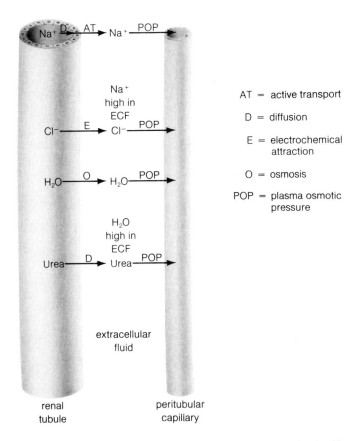

AT = active transport

D = diffusion

E = electrochemical
attraction

O = osmosis

POP = plasma osmotic
pressure

Figure 25.9 A summary of the active and passive processes involved in tubular reabsorption.

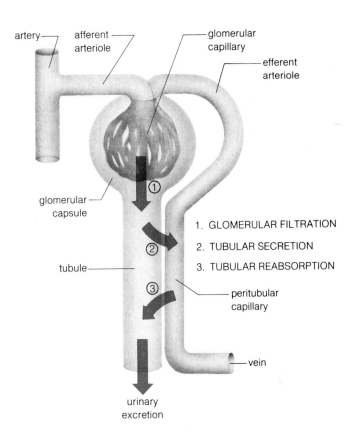

1. GLOMERULAR FILTRATION

2. TUBULAR SECRETION

3. TUBULAR REABSORPTION

Figure 25.10 The three processes by which substances enter or leave the renal tubule are glomerular filtration, tubular reabsorption, and tubular secretion.

As sodium is transported out of the tubular lumen, it causes a slight negativity inside the tubule and a slight positivity in the extracellular fluids outside the lumen. This electrochemical force causes the negatively charged chloride ions to follow the sodium ions until the charge is equalized. Sodium also affects the movement of water. As the sodium ions (and the chloride ions) move out of the lumen, they cause the osmotic pressure to increase in the extracellular fluids outside the tubule. Water is then drawn out of the tubule by osmosis. A small amount of the waste substance, urea, also is passively transported back into the plasma. As the water moves out of the tubule, the concentration of urea in the tubule increases because it is dissolved in a smaller amount of water. Thus, urea diffuses from its area of high concentration in the tubule to its area of lower concentration in the extracellular fluids. All of these substances are returned to the capillary by the concentration gradient between the renal tubule and the capillary. The processes of

active and passive tubular reabsorption are summarized in Figure 25.9.

The overall rate of reabsorption in a normal pair of kidneys is 124 milliliters per minute. Since the glomerular filtration rate is 125 milliliters per minute, the rate of urine formation is normally 1 milliliter per minute.

Tubular Secretion

In addition to entering by glomerular filtration substances enter the renal tubule by tubular **secretion**. The main functions of tubular secretion are to remove waste substances from the blood, regulate the concentrations of electrolytes (ions) in body fluids, and regulate the pH of the blood and extracellular fluids. Tubular secretion may be thought of as the opposite of tubular reabsorption in that the substances are moving in opposite directions in the two processes. Figure 25.10 summarizes these processes.

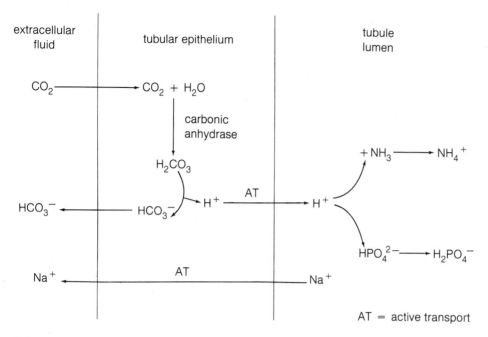

Figure 25.11 Tubular secretion of hydrogen ions.

Hydrogen ions are actively secreted into the tubule to maintain the pH of the blood in the normal range of 7.35 to 7.45. Because most foods produce acids rather than bases when they are metabolized, hydrogen ions accumulate in the blood. The removal of hydrogen ions actually begins with the passage of carbon dioxide from the extracellular fluids into the epithelial cells of the tubule wall (Figure 25.11). Inside the epithelial cell carbonic anhydrase causes the carbon dioxide to combine with water to form carbonic acid. The acid ionizes into a bicarbonate ion and a hydrogen ion. The hydrogen ion is actively transported from the epithelial cell to the lumen of the tubule, and the bicarbonate ion is returned to the extracellular fluid accompanied by a sodium ion. Bicarbonate in the extracellular fluid and the blood acts as a buffer; that is, it contributes to keeping the pH of blood and extracellular fluids in a normal range (see Chapter 21).

Once inside the lumen of the renal tubule, the hydrogen ions can combine with ammonia (from the deamination of amino acids) or with phosphate ions (of the phosphate buffer system, which maintains normal pH in the same way that bicarbonate does). When hydrogen ions are combined with these substances, they do not contribute to the acidity of urine. Thus, acid is removed from the blood, yet the acidity of the urine is kept within the physiological range.

Though potassium ions enter the filtrate from the glomerulus and are almost totally reabsorbed, they also are secreted into the lumen of the distal tubule and collecting duct. The active secretion of K^+ is coupled with the active reabsorption of Na^+ in an Na^+–K^+ pump mechanism. Aldosterone helps to regulate this process, as will be explained in Chapter 26.

Most other substances that enter the tubule by tubular secretion move by active transport. Tubular secretion removes a number of end products of normal metabolism, penicillin and certain other drugs, and some toxic substances from the body. (Tubule function is summarized later in Table 25.4.)

Role of the Kidneys in Acid–Base Balance

As was mentioned in Chapter 21, both the lungs and the kidneys help to compensate for acidosis or alkalosis in the blood and body fluids. Referring again to Figure 25.11, when a person is in acidosis, the amount of CO_2 in the blood increases. This accelerates the formation of H_2CO_3 in the tubular cells, and some of the H_2CO_3 ionizes. The active transport of H^+ into the tubule lumen increases, and the diffusion of HCO_3^- from the tubular cells into the blood increases. Thus, the blood comes to contain more HCO_3^- and less CO_2, and the blood pH becomes more normal. Conversely, when a person is in alkalosis, the tubule cells secrete less H^+, and again the blood pH becomes more normal.

Table 25.4 Summary of Movements of Substances in the Renal Tubule

Segment	Process	Substances Moved
Glomerulus to capsule	Filtration	Water, electrolytes, glucose, urea, amino acids, polypeptides
Proximal tubule	Reabsorption	70% of water and NaCl; nearly all glucose, amino acids, and polypeptides; several electrolytes (K^+, Ca^{2+}, HCO_3^-)
	Secretion	H^+, NH_3, organic acids and bases
Loop of Henle	Reabsorption	NaCl in excess of H_2O by countercurrent mechanism
Distal tubule	Reabsorption	Small fraction of NaCl and H_2O
	Secretion	H^+, K^+, NH_3
Collecting ducts	Reabsorption	NaCl; H_2O, depending on ADH concentration; K^+, depending on aldosterone concentration; urea
	Secretion	NH_3; H^+; and K^+, depending on aldosterone concentration

Clearance

In studying kidney function it is often useful to have a quantitative measure of how fast substances are removed from the plasma. **Clearance**, one such measure, is the volume of blood that can be cleared, or freed, of a substance in one minute. It can be expressed as follows:

$$\text{clearance} = \frac{UV}{P}$$

where U = concentration of substance in urine (mg/ml)

V = volume of urine produced (ml/min)

P = concentration of substance in arterial plasma (mg/ml)

Thus, UV = amount of substance added to the urine per minute (mg/min)

and clearance = volume of plasma cleared of substance (ml/min)

When all of a substance that is filtered out of the blood by the glomeruli is excreted and none is reabsorbed or secreted by the tubules, the clearance of that substance equals the glomerular filtration rate (GFR). A substance that is both *filtered* and *secreted* should have a clearance greater than the GFR; a substance that is *filtered* and *reabsorbed* should have a clearance less than the GFR. Variations in

For example, U = concentration of urea in urine = 12 mg/ml

V = volume of urine produced per minute = 1 ml/min

P = concentration of urea in arterial plasma = 0.2 mg/ml

$$\text{clearance of urea} = \frac{12 \text{ mg/ml} \times 1 \text{ ml/min}}{0.2 \text{ mg/ml}} = 60 \text{ ml/min}$$

Thus, 60 milliliters of plasma is freed of urea per minute.

clearance and GFR from normal values often indicate kidney disease.

Countercurrent Mechanism

So far we have considered how the kidney filters, reabsorbs, and secretes substances and thereby helps to maintain normal concentrations of various substances in the blood. The kidney also regulates the amount of water that remains in the blood. When very little fluid has been taken in, the kidney must get rid of wastes and at the same time conserve water. Under such conditions a small amount of concentrated urine is excreted. On the other hand, when large quantities of fluid have been taken in, the kidney must get rid of excess fluid along with the wastes. The **countercurrent mechanism** regulates the amount of water excreted in the urine. Let us see how it works.

The countercurrent mechanism involves the loop of Henle of the juxtamedullary nephrons, the vasa recta, nearby collecting ducts, and the extracellular fluids between these structures (see Figure 25.5). To illustrate how this mechanism works, let us begin with a hypothetical situation in which the concentration of sodium ions is uniform throughout the loop of Henle (Figure 25.12a). As the mechanism begins to function, the ascending loop of Henle actively transports chloride ions out of the tubule into the extracellular fluid. Sodium ions passively follow the chloride ions due to their electrical attraction. Both ions move into the fluid between the ascending and descending parts of the loop, and some diffuse into the descending part (Figure 25.12b). The mechanism is said to be a countercurrent mechanism because the outflow (in the ascending loop) runs parallel to and in the opposite direction of the inflow (in the descending loop). As a result of the countercurrent movement of NaCl, the extracellular fluids around the loop of Henle come to contain large quantities of NaCl, the highest concentration being found near the tip of the loop of Henle. Because the ascending loop has a very effective active transport system for moving NaCl out of its lumen, most of the NaCl that reaches the ascending loop is actively transported out of it.

The filtrate passes from the ascending loop of Henle through the distal convoluted tubule and enters a collecting duct. The collecting duct passes adjacent to the loop of Henle and therefore runs through an area where the extracellular fluids contain large amounts of NaCl. The high osmotic pressure created by the NaCl causes water to diffuse out of the collecting duct into the extracellular fluid and eventually to the blood. This process constitutes the body's primary means of conserving water. The result is that the filtrate, now called urine, has been greatly concentrated (Figure 25.13).

A similar mechanism, the **countercurrent exchanger**, operates between the extracellular fluids and the blood passing through the vasa recta, also shown in Figure 25.13. As the capillary passes along the ascending loop of Henle, NaCl diffuses into the blood, and water diffuses out of the blood. This process is reversed as the capillary passes along the descending loop of Henle. Recall that the blood flows around the loop of Henle from the ascending to the descending side, while the fluid passing through the loop of Henle goes in the opposite direction. This arrangement

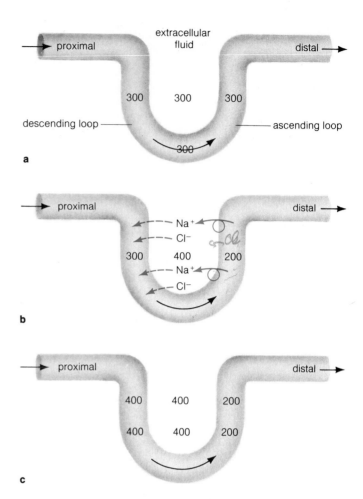

Figure 25.12 The movement of NaCl and fluid in the countercurrent mechanism. Because the ascending loop of Henle actively transports chloride ions out (with sodium ions following them) and is relatively impermeable to the return of the ions, NaCl is concentrated in the extracellular fluids. (The numbers in the diagrams refer to concentrations of Na$^+$ in mEq/l. The solid arrows pertaining to movement of ions indicate the movement of many ions; the dotted arrows indicate the movement of relatively few ions.)

helps to maintain the concentration gradient of NaCl. By the time the blood has reached the region near the upper portion of the descending loop of Henle, it has lost the excess NaCl and enters the interlobular vein having a concentration of NaCl appropriate for blood reentering the general systemic circulation. The overall effect of the movement of NaCl into and out of the vasa recta has little to do with the blood itself. The main function of this movement is to

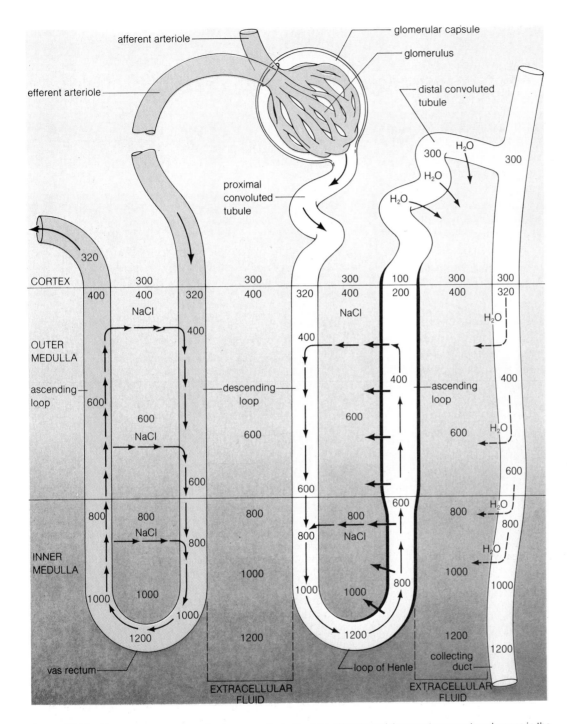

afferent arteriole

efferent arteriole

glomerular capsule

glomerulus

distal convoluted tubule

proximal convoluted tubule

H_2O

H_2O

H_2O

300

300

320

CORTEX

300 400 NaCl 320

300 400

320 400 NaCl 100 200

300 400

300 320 H_2O

OUTER MEDULLA

400

400

400

H_2O

ascending loop

600 600 NaCl 600

descending loop 600

600 600 800 600

ascending loop 600

400 H_2O 600

600

INNER MEDULLA

800 800 NaCl 800

800

800 NaCl 800

800

800 H_2O 800 H_2O

1000

1000 1000 1000

1000 1000

600 1000 1000

1000 1000

1200

1200 1200 1200

1200 1200

800 1200

collecting duct 1200

vas rectum

loop of Henle

EXTRACELLULAR FLUID

EXTRACELLULAR FLUID

Figure 25.13 The countercurrent mechanism operates in the loop of Henle and the countercurrent exchanges in the vasa recta (singular, vasa rectum). Their overall function is to concentrate sodium chloride in the extracellular fluids and thereby cause water to diffuse out of the collecting ducts and concentrate the urine.

help keep the NaCl concentrated in the extracellular fluids around the tip of the loop of Henle.

In fact, the main function of countercurrents in both the loops of Henle and the vasa recta is to concentrate NaCl in the extracellular fluids. In turn, the high concentration of NaCl in these fluids creates osmotic pressure that causes water to leave the tubules. This entire process is regulated by antidiuretic hormone, as described below.

Summary of Tubule Function

Filtration, reabsorption, and secretion occur at various points in the renal tubule. The functions of each segment are summarized in Table 25.4.

Antidiuretic Hormone

As noted in Chapter 15, **antidiuretic hormone** (ADH) is released from the posterior pituitary gland when osmoreceptors in the hypothalamus detect that the blood has become too concentrated—that is, it has become hyperosmotic. ADH is also released when there is a drop in blood pressure, as in hemorrhage. ADH affects the epithelial cells of the distal convoluted tubules and collecting ducts, causing them to become more permeable to water. Water moves passively by osmosis out of the ducts because of the hyperosmotic extracellular fluid.

When the blood becomes too dilute, as might occur after the intake of large quantities of fluid, the hypothalamic receptors are not stimulated, and ADH is not released. In the absence of ADH the junctions between the cells of the distal tubules and collecting ducts remain tight and are impermeable to water. As a result the water in the tubule cannot be reabsorbed, and more water is excreted in the urine. Thus, the turning on and off of ADH is a homeostatic mechanism that regulates blood volume (Figure 25.14).

The disease **diabetes insipidus** (not to be confused with diabetes mellitus) is due to a deficiency of ADH. When this hormone is lacking or in short supply, the kidneys produce a very dilute urine, and a large volume of fluid is lost—up to 15 liters per day. This condition is treated by administering ADH.

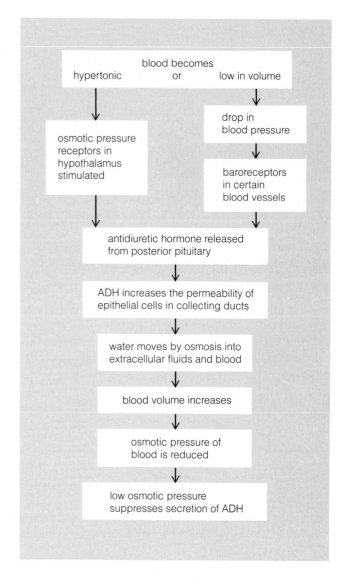

Figure 25.14 The role of ADH in regulating blood volume and, to some extent, blood pressure.

The Juxtaglomerular Apparatus

The **juxtaglomerular apparatus** (see Figure 25.6) helps to regulate blood pressure. As blood passes through the afferent arterioles on its way to the glomerulus, it passes by the cells of the juxtaglomerular apparatus. These cells are sensitive to changes in the renal blood pressure. When the blood pressure drops below normal, the cells release the enzyme **renin** into the blood. Renin acts on a protein normally found in plasma, **angiotensinogen**, converting it to **angiotensin** I. Another enzyme converts angiotensin I to

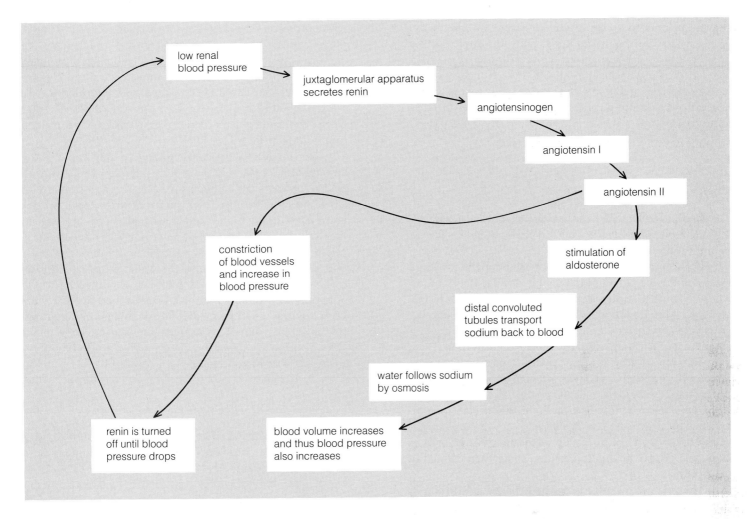

Figure 25.15 The effects of the juxtaglomerular apparatus on blood pressure. Low blood pressure turns on this system, and high blood pressure turns it off.

angiotensin II. Angiotensin II has several effects that help to elevate blood pressure, two of which are described here. First, it directly affects the smooth muscle of the arterioles, causing general vasoconstriction. Second, it stimulates the adrenal cortex to secrete aldosterone. Aldosterone in turn stimulates the distal convoluted tubules to transport sodium back into the blood and potassium into the lumen. As sodium is reabsorbed, water follows it by osmosis, and the blood volume increases, thereby increasing blood pressure. The amount of urine excreted is reduced as a by-product of this action. The overall effect of the action of the juxtaglomerular apparatus is to maintain the blood pressure in the blood entering the glomeruli at a high enough level to insure filtration of substances from the glomeruli to the renal tubules (Figure 25.15).

When the blood pressure is above normal, renin is not released. In its absence the mechanisms that increase blood pressure are not stimulated, and the blood pressure drops. Thus, the turning on and off of renin is a homeostatic mechanism that regulates the blood pressure in the renal circulation and to some extent elsewhere in the body. The presence of excess fluid in the body also increases the blood pressure and suppresses the secretion of renin until some of the fluid has been removed. A malfunction of the juxtaglomerular apparatus leading to release of renin when blood pressure is *not* low is one of the causes of **renal hypertension**.

URINE

Objective 6. Describe the normal characteristics of urine and explain how its volume and contents can be altered naturally and in disease states.

The volume and composition of urine depend to a large extent on the amount of fluid taken in and the kind of food eaten. Typically, urine is a transparent, light yellow or amber-colored liquid with a slightly acid pH and a specific gravity greater than water. It can become turbid (cloudy) on standing because of the oxidation of substances in it.

The color of urine is caused by the pigment urochrome, which is a breakdown product of hemoglobin from worn-out red blood cells. The intensity of the color is determined in part by the concentration of the urine. It also may be affected by foods such as beets, by vitamin supplements such as the B group, or by certain medications. A dark red or brown color may be due to bleeding somewhere along the urinary tract.

The pH range of urine is normally between 5.0 and 7.8, depending on the amount of acidic and basic foods in the diet. Fruits increase the acidity, and vegetables increase the alkalinity of the urine. A high-protein diet also produces an acid urine because of acidic products from amino acid metabolism.

The specific gravity of urine is usually between 1.008 and 1.030. Specific gravity is a relative measure determined by comparing the weight of a given volume of a substance to the weight of the same volume of water. For example, 100 milliliters of water weighs 100 grams by definition. The specific gravity of pure water is thus always 1.000. If 100 milliliters of a sample of urine weighs 101.2 grams, its specific gravity would be 1.012. The specific gravity of urine is greater than 1.000 because of the substances dissolved in it. Following an excessive intake of fluid the specific gravity of urine will be only slightly greater than 1.000. During a fever or after profuse sweating or reduced fluid intake, the specific gravity will be higher.

The chemical composition of urine was compared to plasma and glomerular filtrate in Table 25.3. At least 95% of the volume of urine is water; the remainder is composed of

waste products from metabolism and electrolytes that were present in the blood in excess of normal quantities. Urea and uric acid are the products of the metabolism of proteins and nucleic acids; creatinine is produced from muscle metabolism. Large quantities of sodium and chloride ions are normally found in urine, and smaller quantities of other electrolytes are present. Notice that no glucose is normally found in the urine.

The volume of urine is influenced not only by the amount of fluid taken into the body but also by the function of the nephrons. If the nephrons lack filtration pressure or for some other reason fail to produce urine, toxic wastes accumulate in the blood, and tissues and fluids are pushed into the extracellular spaces. The failure to produce urine is called **anuria**; a slightly less serious condition, the production of only small quantities of urine, is called **oliguria** (*oligo* = few or little). Both anuria and oliguria lead to the accumulation of wastes in the blood. At the other extreme, when there is a deficiency of ADH or some other malfunction interferes with the concentration of urine, large quantities of urine are produced. This condition is called **polyuria** (*poly* = many or much).

Certain substances have a **diuretic effect**; that is, they cause the body to excrete fluids. Beverages containing alcohol or caffeine have such an effect.

Under certain circumstances some abnormal substances may be found in the urine, or some substances may be found in abnormal quantities. The laboratory technique of **urinalysis** yields many important facts about the composition of urine that can be useful in the diagnosis and management of diseases. Urinalysis is discussed in more detail in the essay at the end of this chapter.

ANATOMY OF THE URETERS, BLADDER, AND URETHRA

Objective 7. Describe the anatomy of the ureters, bladder, and urethra, including their innervation.

In addition to the kidneys the urinary system includes the paired ureters, the urinary bladder, and the urethra.

The **ureters**, which lie behind the peritoneum, extend from the hilum of the kidney to the bladder. Each ureter, attached to the renal pelvis of the kidney, collects urine from the kidney, transporting it to the bladder. The ureter is about 25 centimeters long and varies in diameter, increasing to about 1.5 centimeters at its widest point near the bladder. The wall of the ureter is composed of three layers—an inner mucous membrane containing transitional epithelium, a middle muscular layer, and an outer fibrous layer (Figure 25.16). The **mucous membrane** consists of several layers of epithelial cells and is continuous with the epithelium of the nephrons and collecting ducts of the kidney. The **muscular layer** contains circular and longitudinal bundles of smooth muscle that help to propel fluid through the ureter. The outer **fibrous layer** helps to protect the ureter and hold it in place.

The **urinary bladder** (Figure 25.17) is located in the pelvic cavity inferior to the peritoneum and posterior to the pubic bone. It is anterior to the vagina and uterus in the female and anterior to the rectum in the male. The urinary bladder is a hollow bag with a wall that can be easily stretched (Figure 25.18). The wall of the bladder consists of an inner transitional epithelium and a middle thick muscular layer. Externally, a fibrous layer surrounds the inferior portion, and parietal peritoneum overlies the superior portion. As mentioned in Chapter 4, the epithelium is called a transitional epithelium because its cells are flattened when the bladder is stretched and filled with urine and rounded up when the bladder is empty (Figure 25.19).

The muscular layer of the bladder, the **detrusor muscle**, consists of inner and outer longitudinal fibers with a middle layer of circular fibers. Interspersed among the muscle fibers are stretch receptors that respond to distension of the bladder. Nerves of the parasympathetic nervous system innervate the smooth muscle of the bladder. In the area where the bladder and urethra join some of the circular smooth muscle is modified to form the **internal sphincter**. Inferior to the internal sphincter is an **external sphincter**, made of skeletal muscle.

Internally, the bladder has a triangular anatomical landmark, the **trigone**, shown in Figure 25.18. The bounds of the trigone are defined by the posterolateral openings through which the ureters enter the bladder and the anteromedial opening through which the urethra leaves the bladder.

The **urethra** conveys urine from the urinary bladder to the outside of the body. In the female it is only about 4 centimeters long, but in the male it passes through the penis and is about 20 centimeters long. The long male urethra is divided into three regions: the **prostatic urethra**, the first 2.5 centimeters of which passes through the prostate gland; the **membranous urethra**, which passes through the pelvic wall; and the **penile urethra** in the penis. The urethra terminates

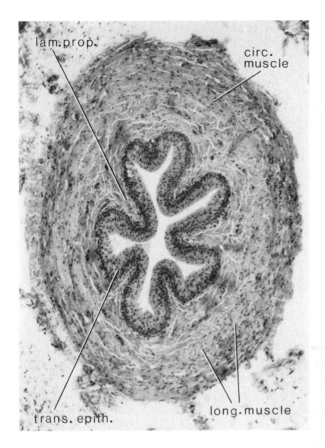

Figure 25.16 A low-power photomicrograph of a ureter, showing the layers of its wall. Note, from the lumen outward, the transitional layer, the longitudinal and circular smooth muscle layers, and the fibrous outer layer. (The lamina propria is a thin layer of connective tissue between the epithelium and the muscle layer.) (Reproduced with permission from A. W. Ham, *Histology*, J. P. Lippincott, 1979.)

in the **external urethral orifice** in both sexes. In the male it is in the glans penis and in the female it is anterior to the vagina and posterior to the clitoris. (Structures of the reproductive system mentioned here are described in more detail in Chapter 28.)

In both the male and female the lining of the urethra consists of a mucous membrane that is continuous with the lining of the bladder and other parts of the urinary tract. Underlying the mucous membrane in the male is another membrane that attaches the urethra to surrounding tissues. In the female a plexus of veins underlies the mucous membrane, and smooth muscle continuous with the bladder surrounds this venous layer.

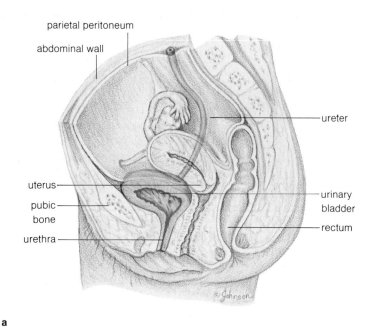

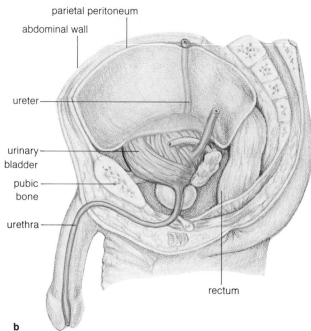

Figure 25.17 The location of the urinary bladder in (**a**) a female, (**b**) a male.

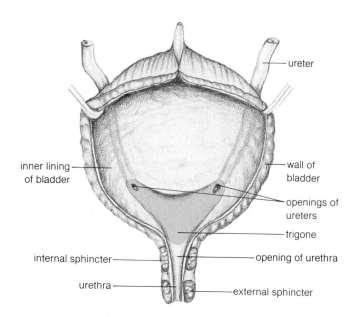

Figure 25.18 The wall and internal structure of the urinary bladder.

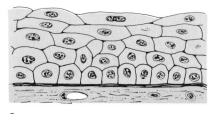

a

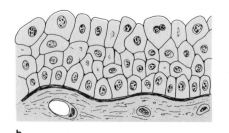

b

wall of bladder in distended condition

wall of bladder in collapsed condition

Figure 25.19 The epithelial lining of the urinary bladder has (**a**) flattened, almost squamous cells when it is distended and (**b**) rounded-up, almost cuboidal cells when it is empty.

PHYSIOLOGY OF THE URETERS, BLADDER, AND URETHRA

Objective 8. Describe the functions of the ureters, bladder, and urethra.

Objective 9. Explain how micturition is controlled.

Functions

The ureters are capable of producing peristaltic waves of contraction. Such contractions, which occur as frequently as five times per minute or as infrequently as once every two minutes, are initiated by the presence of urine in the renal pelvis—the more rapidly the pelvis fills, the more frequently a peristaltic wave occurs. The function of these waves is to move urine from the kidney to the bladder.

The function of the bladder is to store urine. Its capacity is about 750 milliliters, but it rarely fills completely. Micturition, or emptying of the bladder, occurs before the bladder is completely full. The control of micturition is described below.

The function of the urethra is to serve as a passageway for urine to the outside of the body after it has been released from the bladder. In the male it also serves as a passageway for sperm during ejaculation.

Micturition

Micturition, or urination, is the release of urine. It is initiated when the stretch receptors in the wall of the bladder are stimulated. Such stimulation begins when the bladder is about half full. Sensory nerves carry impulses from the stretch receptors to the spinal cord. Motor impulses go from the spinal cord through parasympathetic nerves to the muscle cells of the bladder, causing the bladder to contract. Once initiated, this sequence of impulses is self-perpetuating and constitutes an example of positive feedback. As the bladder contracts, the stretch receptors are further stimulated, and another cycle of impulses occurs. The process is repeated until the system fatigues. Thus, the **micturition reflex** consists of a cycle in which there is rapid increase in the contraction of the bladder, sustained contraction, and finally relaxation of the bladder back to its prereflex muscle tone. If this reflex fails to result in micturition, it fatigues and is suppressed for several minutes to one hour, after which it is reinitiated. Each subsequent cycle of the reflex is stronger than the one before, and inhibition between cycles is of shorter duration until micturition finally occurs.

When impulses from the stretch receptors arrive in the spinal cord, they are transmitted to the brainstem and to the cerebrum, though the exact pathways are not well understood. These impulses reach both the facilitatory and the inhibitory centers in the brainstem and the centers in the cerebral cortex. Generally, the cerebral centers inhibit micturition even in the presence of the micturition reflex until the time and place are appropriate. Then the cortical centers allow the action of parasympathetic fibers to initiate micturition and relax the external urinary sphincter. Except during micturition this sphincter is contracted and prevents constant dribbling of urine. During micturition it is voluntarily relaxed. The internal sphincter relaxes when the tone of the smooth muscle decreases with the stretching of the bladder. Thus, it contributes little to the control of micturition.

CLINICAL APPLICATIONS

Objective 10. Describe the alterations in normal kidney function that occur in pyelonephritis and glomerulonephritis.

Objective 11. Explain how the artificial kidney works and discuss some of the problems of individuals on kidney dialysis.

Objective 12. Describe the alteration of normal function that occurs in (a) cystitis, (b) urine retention, and (c) incontinence.

Pyelonephritis

Pyelonephritis is an inflammation of the renal pelvis and the medullary tissue of the kidney. This disease is usually caused by bacteria that reach the kidney by way of the urethra and ureter. Such bacteria sometimes enter the urinary tract from fecal material, so proper hygiene can help to prevent infection. Partial obstruction of the ureters may also contribute to the development of pyelonephritis because movement of urine is impeded. Sluggish flow allows bacterial growth to occur in the urine and may lead to the backup of urine into the kidney. Although pyelonephritis can affect the cortex of the kidney, it usually affects mainly the countercurrent mechanism in the medulla. Affected individuals have reasonably normal renal function except for their inability to concentrate urine. Signs and symptoms include frequent and painful urination, fever, and pain in the lumbar area. Prompt antibiotic treatment of urinary tract infections can prevent permanent inability to concentrate urine.

Glomerulonephritis

Glomerulonephritis can be caused by the advance of pyelonephritis, by trauma to the kidney, by congenital kidney defects, or by an allergic reaction to the toxins of bacteria such as streptococci. The glomeruli become inflamed and engorged with blood, the products of antigen–antibody reactions accumulate, and the permeability of the capillaries is greatly increased so that proteins and red blood cells enter the filtrate. Sometimes the disease progresses to a chronic state in which the permeability of the membranes is permanently altered. The walls of the capillaries may be replaced by fibrous tissue and thus become nonfunctional. If a sufficiently large number of the glomeruli become nonfunctional, the individual will die from renal failure unless an artificial kidney is used. Prompt antibiotic treatment may prevent permanent damage from an infection.

The Artificial Kidney

Though the kidneys are capable of significant repair of damage caused by various disorders, sometimes this damage is extensive enough to prevent adequate function. People suffering from such kidney damage often receive **hemodialysis**, or treatment with an artificial kidney (Figure 25.20). Hemodialysis is the separation of certain substances from blood by the use of a selectively permeable membrane. The pores in the membrane allow some substances to pass through while holding others back.

The patient is connected to the machine by a tube attached to an artery, often the radial artery. Blood from the artery is pumped into a tube that runs through the dialyzer. The dialyzer is filled with dialysis fluid, which contains the same quantities of electrolytes and nutrients as normal plasma but contains no waste products. The pores in the cellophanelike tubing inside the dialyzer are small enough to prevent blood cells and proteins from entering the dialysis fluid but large enough to allow smaller molecules to diffuse into the fluid. Molecules of waste substances such as urea, ammonia, and water diffuse into the dialysis fluid. Net diffusion of other substances such as glucose, amino acids, and electrolytes is prevented by the presence of these substances in the dialysis fluid in the same concentration as in normal plasma. Only excesses of such substances leave the blood and enter the dialysis fluid. Diffusion in the dialyzer operates on the same principle as diffusion in any other situation: Substances diffuse from their area of higher concentration to their area of lower concentration. This property of dialysis can also be used to cause substances to enter the blood. For example, a malnourished patient can receive glucose from the dialysis fluid simply by the placement of an excess of glucose in that fluid. Following dialysis blood is returned to the person's body, usually through the radial vein. Chronic dialysis patients have surgical shunts to avoid damage to arteries and veins.

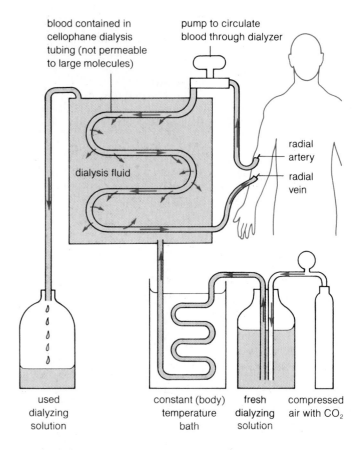

Figure 25.20 A schematic diagram to illustrate the operation of an artificial kidney (hemodialysis unit). In dialyzer large arrows show direction of blood flow; small arrows show removal of wastes from blood.

Although hemodialysis is a life-saving process for patients with serious kidney impairment, it is not without its problems. The removal and replacement of blood in a person's body always presents a risk of infection, although careful use of sterile techniques can minimize this risk. Furthermore, the blood must be prevented from clotting while it is in the dialyzer. An anticoagulant is added to the blood as it leaves the body, and it must be counteracted before the blood is returned to the body. The person with kidney disease must often seriously curtail fluid intake even when thirsty to prevent the accumulation of fluids in the tissues (edema). Urine production is scanty, and both wastes and fluids accumulate in the body. As most individuals do not undergo dialysis more than a few times per week, their blood accumulates wastes between treatments, and these wastes have physiological and psychological effects; dependence on a machine can be psychologically stressful. Finally, hemodialysis over a long period of time is both time consuming and expensive.

Hemodialysis is an extremely useful technique for short-term use during renal failure or while a person is waiting for a suitable kidney for transplant. It has limitations as a lifetime replacement for normal kidney function; however, it may be the only option available to many persons.

Cystitis, Urine Retention, and Incontinence

Cystitis is an inflammation of the urinary bladder that may be caused by an infection that has spread from the urethra or, in males, by pressure exerted by an enlarged prostate gland. If the nerves that stimulate emptying of the bladder are damaged or the bladder sags downward from its normal position (cystocele), incomplete emptying may lead to chronic cystitis. Symptoms include frequent, painful, burning urination and sometimes a sense of pressure in the pelvic area. Because of the shorter urethra infectious organisms can reach the bladder more easily in females than in males, making the incidence of cystitis higher in females than in males. Most such infections can be cured by sulfa drugs or antibiotics.

Urine retention is the failure to urinate, even though the nephrons are producing urine. It may be caused by a lack of stimuli from the nerves of the bladder or by an obstruction. Another condition, **atonic bladder**, leads to urine retention. The bladder becomes completely filled, and, instead of micturition occurring, the overflow continuously dribbles out of the bladder. Obstructions may be removed surgically; catheterization is the usual treatment for nerve and muscle disorders.

Incontinence is the inability to control the release of urine. In children under the age of two it is due to immaturity of the neural pathways to the external sphincter. In adults it may be due to nerve damage as might be done in prostate surgery, bladder injury, irritating substances in the urine, or emotional stresses. Exercises to strengthen the sphincter or gradual reestablishment of neural pathways may correct the condition; the use of plastic-covered absorbent clothing may be necessary.

In the past few years a new technique called **continuous ambulatory peritoneal dialysis** (CAPD) has become available. An individual whose kidneys have failed has a valve surgically implanted in the abdomen. One to two liters of sterile dialysis fluid from a plastic bag are introduced into the abdominal cavity through the valve. The fluid is left in the cavity for about two hours and then drained back into the plastic bag. While the fluid is in the abdominal cavity, waste materials diffuse out of capillaries of the peritoneal membranes into the dialysis fluid. Removal of the dialysis fluid then removes the wastes from the body. The advantages of this technique over hemodialysis are that the individual can carry out the technique unassisted; greater mobility is possible (CAPD is usually performed four times per day and can even be done during the work day); and CAPD is much less expensive than hemodialysis. Individuals on CAPD can have somewhat more fluid by mouth than those on hemodialysis, and they are not subject to alterations in blood pressure and other problems involved in the removal and return of blood to the body. However, the use of CAPD does lead to a high risk of peritonitis (inflammation of the peritoneum). To minimize this risk, the user must strictly adhere to the sterile techniques learned at the time CAPD is first used.

Clinical Terms

albuminuria (al″bu-min-u′re-ah)   the presence of albumin in the urine

azotemia (az-o-te′me-ah)   the presence of excess urea and other nitrogenous waste products in the urine

cystoscope (sis′to-skōp)   an instrument for examining the inside of the bladder

diuresis (di-u-re′sis)   increased production of urine

enuresis (en-u-re′sis)   involuntary release of urine

gout (gowt)   a metabolic disorder in which an excess of uric acid accumulates in the body and is deposited in joints

nephrosis (nef-ro′sis)   any disease of the kidney, usually leading to degeneration of kidney tissue

proteinuria (pro″te-in-u′re-ah)   the presence of protein in the urine

renal calculus (kal′ku-lus)   an abnormal aggregation of mineral salts or other substances in the kidney; kidney stone

uremia (u-re′me-ah)   the presence of urinary waste products in the blood

ureteritis (u″re-ter-i′tis)   inflammation of a ureter

urethritis (u-re-thri′tis)   inflammation of the urethra

Wilm's tumor   an embryonic malignancy of the kidney

Essay: The Role of Urine in Diagnosis

Most of us have had the experience of going to a physician and being asked to "donate" a urine sample, often without blood or any other samples being taken. It may have seemed odd that urine could be used to assess health. However, urine contains all the substances that have been removed from the blood—including a variety of products of metabolism, hormones, acids, bases, electrolytes, and nitrogenous waste materials—so the examination of urine can provide valuable information about the physiological status of the body. Below, we'll investigate how urine is used in medical diagnosis.

Urine to be analyzed should be taken as a "clean catch" (midstream flow) preferably in the morning when the individual has had no fluids for 12 hours. This technique insures the collection of a concentrated urine. Urine should be placed in a clean, dry bottle and examined within 2 hours.

The standard urinalysis includes the determination of specific gravity; pH; presence or absence of glucose, ketones, and proteins; and the microscopic examination of urinary sediment. Electrolyte concentrations may also be determined (Figure 25.21). When the specific gravity of an early morning specimen falls below 1.025, the individual may have distal renal tubule disease or a deficiency of antidiuretic hormone. An excessively low pH (below 4.6) indicates acidosis; a high pH (above 8.0) indicates alkalosis. The conditions associated with these and other findings are listed in Table 25.5.

Glucose in the urine is often associated with diabetes mellitus. However, in an early morning specimen glucose may not be found in the urine even if the person has diabetes. This is probably because the bladder was emptied at bedtime, and the blood glucose concentration at night is low enough to prevent its appearance in the urine. The blood glucose concentration must be about 140 milligrams/100 milliliter for glucose to "spill over" into the urine. The blood concentration at which a substance appears in the urine is called the renal threshold. At the renal threshold the blood concentration of a substance is so high that the kidney cannot return any more of that substance to the blood. In a few individuals who have an especially low renal threshold for glucose, glucose may be found in the urine even when the blood glucose is not elevated.

Protein in the urine can be associated with a variety of pathological conditions. Though glomerulonephritis is most commonly detected through protein in the urine, it and other conditions can be diagnosed by additional laboratory tests. For example, in glomerulonephritis the urine also contains blood and casts (hardened masses of epithelial cells, fat cells, and red and white blood cells). Casts can be observed in microscopic

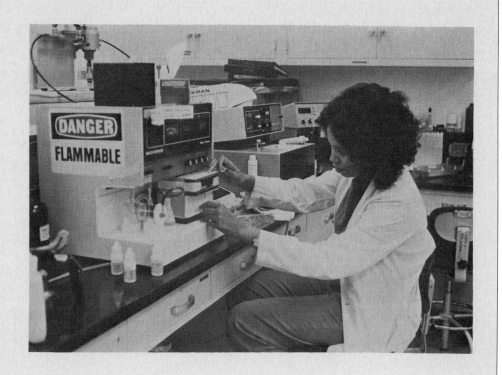

Figure 25.21 The equipment shown here is used to measure electrolytes in either blood or urine. Sodium, potassium, and chloride ions are being measured in a urine specimen, and the technician is adjusting the machine to obtain the desired analyses. (Photograph by author; arrangements courtesy of Childrens Hospital National Medical Center, Washington, D.C.)

studies of urine sediment. The blood of a person with glomerulonephritis also contains excess amounts of urea and creatinine (a waste product from muscle metabolism). Individuals with the malignant disease multiple myeloma have a characteristic protein in both their blood and their urine. Called Bence-Jones protein, it is an abnormal antibodylike protein thought to be made by the malignant cells.

Ketones, which result from the metabolism of fats, are found in the urine of patients who have acidosis or an abnormality in the metabolism of glucose. The presence of ketones is often associated with diabetes mellitus, but a number of other conditions also lead to ketones in the urine. Low-carbohydrate weight-reduction diets cause the body to metabolize fats and thus lead to the production of ketones.

The presence of bilirubin, a breakdown product of heme, in the urine indicates that the liver is unable to metabolize the heme properly. Likewise, urobilinogen in the urine indicates either liver disease or one of several blood diseases. This metabolic product of bilirubin is normally excreted in the feces, but when it is present in excess, it may be reabsorbed into the blood and excreted in the urine.

In addition to the chemical characteristics of urine that can be used to diagnose diseases, calculi and casts may also be present in urine. Calculi, or so-called kidney stones, may form anywhere along the urinary tract. These stones are composed of minerals such as calcium phosphate, calcium oxalate, and uric acid. Excessive secretion of parathyroid hormone often leads to the formation of calculi. Alkaline diets foster their formation because the calcium salts are less soluble in alkaline conditions, so patients who have a tendency to form calcium calculi are often placed on acidic diets.

Hormones present in the urine also can be used in diagnostic tests. For instance, chorionic gonadotropin, a hormone produced only by the early placenta and present in the urine of pregnant women, is the basis of many pregnancy tests. Though a variety of endocrine abnormalities can be detected by urinalysis, a discussion of these tests is beyond the scope of this essay.

As we have emphasized throughout this book, health can be thought of as the body's successful maintenance of homeostasis. The kidneys help to maintain homeostatic balance by removing substances that are present in potentially harmful amounts. Thus, the composition of urine can indicate homeostatic imbalances in pH or water concentration, as well as problems in the function of other organs. Health professionals can use this information to aid the body in restoring its healthy balance.

Table 25.5 Some Abnormal Characteristics of Urine and the Conditions Associated with Them

Urine Abnormality	Associated Conditions
Red blood cells	Glomerulonephritis, congenital defects, malignancies, chronic infection, sickle cell anemia, drugs such as phenacetin and sulfonamide, bacterial endocarditis
Hemoglobin	Renal hypertension, hemolytic anemia, transfusion reactions, allergic reactions, severe burns, eclampsia (a complication of pregnancy)
Excessive acidity	Acidosis, diarrhea, dehydration, starvation, emphysema
Excessive alkalinity	Renal failure, bacterial infections, vomiting, alkalosis, low-carbohydrate diets
Protein	Glomerulonephritis, pyelonephritis, hypertension, congestive heart failure, bacterial endocarditis, gout, toxemia of pregnancy, potassium depletion, high fever
Glucose	Diabetes mellitus, pancreatitis, lowered renal threshold, coronary thrombosis, hyperthyroidism, shock, pain, excitement
Ketones	Acidosis, vomiting, diarrhea, glycogen-storage disease, starvation, low-carbohydrate diets, hyperthyroidism, eclampsia, trauma, chloroform or ether anesthesia
Bilirubin	Hepatitis, obstructive jaundice, cirrhosis of the liver, carcinoma of the pancreas, noxious fumes, chlorpromazine hepatitis
Urobilinogen	Some of same conditions as bilirubin, hemolytic anemias, pernicious anemia, thalassemia, hepatitis associated with infectious mononucleosis

Data based on urine profile prepared by Ames Division, Miles Laboratories, Inc., Elkhart, IN 46515 (1975).

CHAPTER SUMMARY

(Chapter summary points and review questions are numbered to correspond to the numbered objectives in the text of each chapter.)

Organization and General Functions

1. Describe the overall plan of the urinary system and name its major functions.
   a. The urinary system consists of the kidneys, ureters, urinary bladder, and urethra.
   b. The functions of the urinary system are:
      (1) to remove wastes from the plasma
      (2) to adjust the concentrations of electrolytes in the plasma
      (3) to adjust the pH of the plasma

Development

2. Describe the general development of the urinary system.
   a. The urinary system develops from mesoderm of the urogenital ridge.
   b. The kidneys go through three stages of development, the final one being the metanephric kidneys.
   c. The ureter and parts of the kidney develop from the ureteric bud.
   d. The bladder and urethra develop from the cloaca.

Anatomy of the Kidney

3. Locate and identify the anatomical structures of the kidneys, including the blood supply and cortical and juxtamedullary nephrons.
   a. The kidneys are located near the upper lumbar vertebrae behind the peritoneum.
   b. Each kidney is bean-shaped and has a medial hilum, where blood vessels and the ureter enter.
   c. Internally, the kidney consists of cortical and juxtamedullary nephrons. Collecting ducts, which run through an area called a pyramid, end in structures called papillae and drain into minor calyces, major calyces, and finally the renal pelvis.
   d. Blood flows in the kidney through the renal artery, interlobar arteries, arcuate arteries, interlobular arteries, afferent arterioles, glomerulus, efferent arterioles, and peritubular capillaries; it returns to the renal vein through veins that parallel the above-named arteries.
   e. Each nephron consists of a glomerular (Bowman's) capsule, proximal convoluted tubule, loop of Henle, and distal convoluted tubule, which drains into a collecting duct.
   f. The loop of Henle is much longer in juxtamedullary nephrons than in cortical nephrons.
   g. The juxtaglomerular apparatus consists of specialized cells in the afferent arteriole and the distal convoluted tubule.

Physiology of the Kidney

4. Explain how the processes of filtration, reabsorption, and secretion occur in the nephron and how they regulate the concentration of substances in the blood.
   a. When blood passes through the glomerulus, substances filter out of the blood into the glomerular capsule by glomerular filtration. These substances include water, electrolytes, glucose, urea, amino acids, and polypeptides.
   b. Except for wastes and excesses of electrolytes, most of these substances are reabsorbed from the tubule back into the plasma:
      (1) Glucose, amino acids, and some of the sodium are actively transported to the plasma.
      (2) Chloride ions follow the sodium ions.
      (3) Water and most electrolytes move passively by diffusion.
   c. Some substances, such as hydrogen and potassium ions, are actively secreted into the lumen of the tubule. The active secretion of hydrogen ions helps to maintain the pH of the blood within a normal range.
   d. The countercurrent mechanism concentrates sodium in extracellular fluids around the loop of Henle and the collecting ducts. It thus can draw water out of the collecting ducts by osmosis, thereby concentrating the urine.

5. Describe the processes that regulate kidney function.
   a. Kidney function is regulated by the juxtaglomerular apparatus:
      (1) When blood pressure drops below normal, the juxtaglomerular cells secrete renin, which causes angiotensin II to be produced in the blood.
      (2) Angiotensin II constricts blood vessels and stimulates the production of aldosterone.
      (3) Aldosterone stimulates the transport of sodium into the blood, and water follows the sodium passively.
      (4) Constriction of blood vessels and increased blood volume both serve to increase blood pressure.
      (5) When the blood pressure goes above normal, this mechanism ceases operating until the pressure again goes below normal.
   b. Kidney function also is regulated by antidiuretic hormone:
      (1) When the osmoreceptors in the hypothalamus detect an increase in the blood osmotic pressure, antidiuretic hormone (ADH) is released.
      (2) ADH causes more water to be returned to the blood by causing epithelial cells in the distal convoluted tubules and collecting ducts to become more permeable to water.

(3) ADH is released until the blood osmotic pressure returns to normal.

   c. Together, the juxtaglomerular apparatus and ADH are important in maintaining normal blood pressure and blood volume.

Urine

6. Describe the normal characteristics of urine and explain how its volume and contents can be altered naturally and in disease states.

   a. The volume and composition of urine depend on the fluid intake and the kind of food eaten.

   b. The color of urine is normally determined by a pigment called urochrome from the breakdown of hemoglobin; a darker color may be due to certain foods, vitamins, or medications or to bleeding within the urinary tract.

   c. The pH of the urine, determined by the composition of the diet, is usually between 5.0 and 7.8.

   d. The specific gravity of urine, determined by the amount of solids dissolved in the fluid, is normally between 1.008 and 1.030.

   e. Urine, usually 95% water and 5% solids, contains urea, uric acid, creatinine, and a variety of electrolytes. The presence of red blood cells, hemoglobin, protein, glucose, ketones, bilirubin, or urobilinogen is abnormal.

Anatomy of the Ureters, Bladder, and Urethra

7. Describe the anatomy of the ureters, bladder, and urethra, including their innervation.

   a. The ureters, tubes that carry urine from the renal pelvis to the urinary bladder, consist of:
   (1) an inner transitional epithelium
   (2) a middle muscle layer
   (3) an outer fibrous layer

   b. The bladder, a hollow bag that stores urine, consists of:
   (1) an inner transitional epithelium
   (2) a thick muscle layer, the detrusor muscle
   (3) an inferior fibrous layer and the superior parietal peritoneum

   c. The bladder smooth muscle is innervated by parasympathetic fibers.

   d. The urethra, which conveys urine from the bladder to the outside of the body, is lined with epithelium. Its underlying structures attach it to adjacent tissues.

Physiology of the Ureters, Bladder, and Urethra

8. Describe the functions of the ureters, bladder, and urethra.

   a. The ureters carry on peristaltic contraction when they are stimulated by the presence of urine in the renal pelvis, thereby propelling urine to the bladder.

   b. The bladder has stretch receptors that send impulses to the spinal cord when the bladder becomes distended.

   c. Parasympathetic nerves and consciously controlled motor nerves stimulate the bladder sphincters.

   d. The urethra serves passively as a passageway from the bladder to the outside of the body.

9. Explain how micturition is controlled.

   a. When the stretch receptors of the bladder are stimulated, they initiate the micturition reflex.

   b. Conscious motor impulses relax the external sphincter and allow micturition to occur.

Clinical Applications

10. Describe the alterations in normal kidney functions that occur in pyelonephritis and glomerulonephritis.

   a. In pyelonephritis, the kidney becomes inflamed, usually by the presence of a bacterial infection; the cortical nephrons are not generally affected.

   b. In glomerular nephritis the glomeruli become inflamed and engorged with blood, and their permeability is greatly increased. Glomerulonephritis may be caused by advancing pyelonephritis, trauma, congenital defects, or allergic reactions to toxins.

11. Explain how the artificial kidney works and discuss some of the problems of individuals on kidney dialysis.

   a. An artificial kidney, or hemodialysis unit, operates on the principle of diffusion to remove wastes from the blood without removing normal constituents.

   b. Individuals on kidney dialysis are always subject to infection, limits on fluid intake, and other physiological and psychological stresses.

12. Describe the alteration of normal function that occurs in (a) cystitis, (b) urine retention, and (c) incontinence.

   a. In cystitis the urinary bladder is inflamed, usually from an infection.

   b. Urine retention, an inability to empty the bladder, may be due to lack of nerve stimuli, obstruction, or atonic bladder.

   c. Incontinence, the inability to control the release of urine, may be caused by immaturity, or in adults by damage to sphincter innervation, bladder injury, irritating substances in the urine, or emotional stress.

REVIEW

Important Terms

afferent arteriole	clearance
angiotensins	collecting duct
antidiuretic hormone	cortex
calyx	countercurrent mechanism

distal convoluted tubule

efferent arteriole

filtration

glomerular capsule

glomerulus

hemodialysis

hilum

juxtaglomerular apparatus

loop of Henle

medulla

metanephros

nephron

papilla

peritubular capillary

proximal convoluted tubule

pyramids

reabsorption

renal pelvis

retroperitoneal

secretion

ureter

urethra

urinalysis

vasa recta

Questions

1. **a.** What are the major organs of the urinary system?
   b. What are the major functions of the urinary system?

2. **a.** Of what embryonic tissue is the urinary system made?
   b. What are the three types of kidneys found in the embryo?

3. **a.** Describe the location and size of the kidney.
   b. Relate the gross anatomical structures inside the kidney to the flow of urine through it.
   c. Trace the flow of blood through the kidney.
   d. Describe the structure of the juxtamedullary nephron.
   e. How is a cortical nephron different from a juxtamedullary nephron?
   f. What is the juxtaglomerular apparatus?

4. **a.** What happens during glomerular filtration?
   b. What is tubular reabsorption, and how does it occur?
   c. How does tubular secretion differ from tubular reabsorption?
   d. List all the mechanisms by which things move in and out of the renal tubule and give an example of where each occurs.
   e. What is the role of the kidneys in acid-base balance?
   f. What is the countercurrent mechanism, and what does it do?

5. **a.** What is the role of ADH in regulating kidney function?
   b. How is the release of ADH regulated?
   c. What is the role of the juxtaglomerular apparatus in regulating kidney function?
   d. How is the release of renin regulated?

6. **a.** Describe the normal constituents of urine.
   b. What might cause the urine to change in color? Volume? pH? Specific gravity?
   c. What is the difference between a calculus and a cast?

7. **a.** How are the walls of the ureters, bladder, and urethra alike, and how are they different?
   b. How do the internal and external sphincters differ?

8. What are the main function of the ureters, the bladder, and the urethra?

9. What is micturition, and how is it controlled?

10. **a.** What is pyelonephritis, and how is it caused?
    b. What is glomerulonephritis, and how is it caused?

11. Suppose you are working in a hemodialysis unit. How would you explain to a patient what is being done? What special precautions would you take in operating the machine? Why is the artificial kidney not an ideal solution to the problem of renal insufficiency?

12. How is function altered in (a) cystitis, (b) urine retention, (c) incontinence?

Problems

1. Suppose you are reading the report of a urinalysis. What diseases might you suspect if the following substances were found in the urine? (a) glucose, (b) protein, (c) red blood cells, (d) hemoglobin, (e) ketones.

2. What is the nature of the defect in each of the conditions in problem (1)?

3. How would you explain to the parents of a toddler why they should not expect to toilet train the child before the age of two?

4. List at least ten substances whose presence in the blood is regulated in some way by the kidney. Explain the role of the kidney in regulating each of these substances.

REFERENCES AND READINGS

Aukland, K. 1980. Methods for measuring renal blood flow: Total flow and regional distribution. *Annual Review of Physiology* 42:543.

Baer, P. G., and McGiff, J. C. 1980. Hormonal systems and renal hemodynamics. *Annual Review of Physiology* 42:589.

Beeuwkes, R., III. 1980. The vascular organization of the kidney. *Annual Review of Physiology* 42:531.

Conger, J. D., and Schrier, R. W. 1980. Renal hemodynamics in acute renal failure. *Annual Review of Physiology* 42:603.

Fanestil, D. D., and Park, C. S. 1981. Steroid hormones and the kidney. *Annual Review of Physiology* 43:637.

Fayemi, A. O., Ali, M., and Braun, E. V. 1979. Oxalosis in hemodialysis patients. *Archives of Pathological Laboratory Medicine* 103:58 (February).

Free, A. H., and Free, H. M. 1976. *Urodynamics.* Elkhart, Ind.: Ames Company.

Giebisch, G., and Stanton, B. 1979. Potassium transport in the nephron. *Annual Review of Physiology* 41:241.

Gottschalk, C. W. 1979. Renal nerves and sodium excretion. *Annual Review of Physiology* 41:229.

Guyton, A. C. 1981. *Textbook of medical physiology* (6th ed.). Philadelphia: W. B. Saunders.

Handler, J. S., and Orloff, J. 1981. Antidiuretic hormone. *Annual Review of Physiology* 43:611.

Insel, P. A., and Snavely, M. D. 1981. Catecholamines and the kidney: Receptors and renal function. *Annual Review of Physiology* 43:625.

Katz, A. I., and Emmanuel, D. S. 1978. Metabolism of polypeptide hormones by the normal kidney and uremia. *Nephron* 22:69.

McManus, J. F. A., and Hughson, M. D. 1979. New therapies and new pathologies: End-stage-dialysis kidneys. *Archives of Pathological Laboratory Medicine* 103:53 (February).

Quayum, A. 1978. Pharmacology of ureter. *Life Sciences* 23:2349.

Schafer, J. A., and Andreoli, T. E. 1979. Rheogenic and passive Na^+ absorption by the proximal nephron. *Annual Review of Physiology* 41:211.

Tilkian, S. M., Conover, M. B., and Tilkian, A. G. 1979. *Clinical implications of laboratory tests.* St. Louis, Mo.: C. V. Mosby.

Ullrich, K. J. 1979. Sugar, amino acid, and Na^+ cotransport in the proximal tubule. *Annual Review of Physiology* 41:181.

Vogel, C. H. 1979. Keeping patients alive in spite of postobstruction diuresis. *Nursing* 9:50.

Warnock, D., and Rector, F. 1979. Proton secretion by the kidney. *Annual Review of Physiology* 41:197.

26

FLUID, ELECTROLYTE, AND ACID-BASE BALANCE; HOMEOSTASIS; AND STRESS

INTERNAL BALANCE AT THE CELLULAR LEVEL

Objective 1. Summarize the movement of substances into and out of cells and explain why cells need a nearly constant environment.

For the last several chapters we have been considering various body systems and how they contribute to supporting life. Now we can look at these systems according to their roles in maintaining a nearly constant internal environment for the millions of individual cells of the body.

In a large, complex multicellular organism such as a human being, each of the several body systems is highly specialized to carry out particular functions—functions that in one way or another involve the individual cells of the body. The cell is the basic functional unit of any living thing. No matter how complex an organism is as a whole, the metabolic functions that maintain its life take place at the cellular level.

For a cell to function normally, it must receive all the things it needs, and it must have its waste products removed. Consequently, substances are always moving into and out of cells (Figure 26.1). Nutrients and oxygen entering cells provide the raw materials for the production of energy and for growth and repair. Carbon dioxide and other wastes leave cells. Electrolytes and water constantly move in and out of cells. Cells receive chemical stimuli from hormones and neural stimuli from neurons. Some cells synthesize products and release them.

As we have noted in earlier chapters, each cell contains **intracellular fluid** and is surrounded by **interstitial fluid**. The interstitial fluid forms the external environment of a

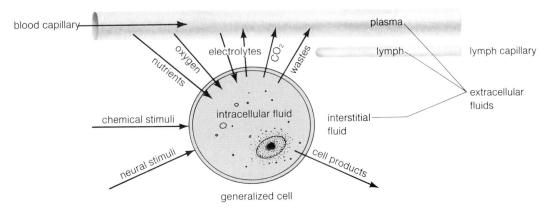

Figure 26.1 A summary of the movement of substances into and out of a generalized cell.

cell; all the substances that enter and leave cells pass through the interstitial fluid. The interstitial fluid must be maintained so that the concentrations of substances in it vary only within a narrow range. Blood plasma and lymph transport substances to and from the interstitial fluid and, along with the mechanisms that move them, help to maintain the nearly constant environment of each cell.

When we speak of a nearly *constant* environment, we do not mean an *unchanging* environment. As you already know, the environment is constantly changing as substances are delivered to and removed from cells. The environment is said to be in **dynamic equilibrium**: Dynamic means active; equilibrium is a state of balance between opposing actions. As fast as nutrients arrive in the interstitial fluid, they enter the cell. As fast as wastes are excreted into the interstitial fluid, they are transported away by the plasma or lymph. Although things are constantly changing in the environment of the cell, the changes are small, and the variations are held within a narrow range. Thus, a dynamic equilibrium exists between cells and their environment, and homeostasis is maintained.

Cells normally cannot survive sudden changes in the temperature, pH, pressure, or volume of the fluid that surrounds them. Nor can they tolerate sudden changes in the concentration of various chemicals in that fluid. Dynamic equilibrium is essential to the survival of cells.

WATER AND FLUID COMPARTMENTS

Objective 2. Describe the fluid compartments of the body and explain how disturbances in water balance can lead to dehydration, water intoxication, or edema.

Every cell in the body contains some water, and cells are generally surrounded by water. Body water ranges from 40 to 65% of total body weight; the average water content is 55% for adult males and 47% for adult females. Of the total water about two-thirds is found within cells in the **intracellular fluid**. The remaining third is in the **extracellular fluid**, which includes the interstitial fluid that occupies small spaces between the cells of a tissue and the plasma of the blood. Lymph, cerebrospinal fluid, and fluid in the joint cavities and eyes are also included in the extracellular fluid.

Physiologists often speak of plasma, interstitial fluid, and intracellular fluid as each occupying a different **fluid compartment**. Membranes are the "walls" of the fluid compartments; for water to move from the intercellular compartment to the plasma, for example, it must cross at least one cell membrane. Each of these fluids contains, in addition to water, a variety of inorganic ions and other substances that affect the osmotic pressure in each compartment. Water moves from one compartment to another, depending on osmotic and other pressures exerted. Factors

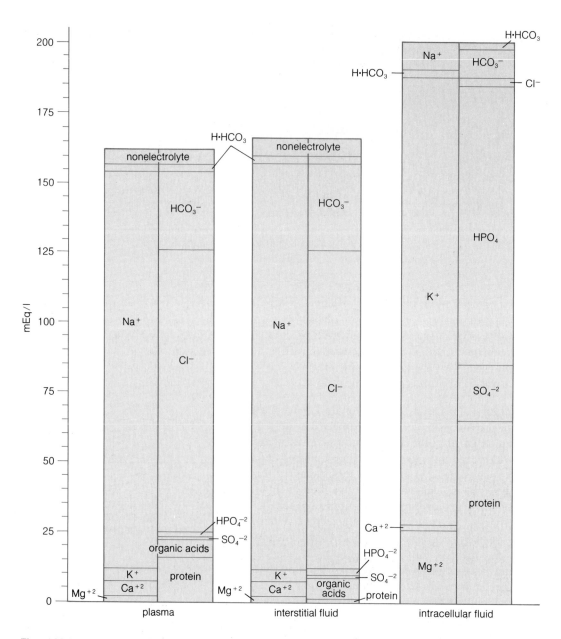

Figure 26.2 Composition of plasma, interstitial fluids, and intracellular fluids.

affecting such movements have already been discussed in Chapter 3.

The composition of the fluid in each compartment is shown in Figure 26.2. Concentrations are expressed in milliequivalents per liter. (One milliequivalent (mEq) is equal to the number of charges in 1/1000 of a mole of hydrogen ions.) Note the similarity of the fluids in the two extracel-lular compartments, plasma and interstitial fluid. Except for the higher concentration of proteins in plasma than in interstitial fluids, the two are much alike. Both contain approximately the same proportions of various electrolytes (ions) and nonelectrolytes (nonionized substances). However, the composition of intracellular fluid differs significantly from that of extracellular fluids; the intracellular

Table 26.1	Typical Water Input and Output in Normal Water Balance			
Water Input	ml/day	Water Output	ml/day
Liquids imbibed	1000	Urine	1300
Water from solid food	1000	Feces	100
Metabolic water	500	Sweat	650
		Water vapor in exhaled air	450
Total input	2500	Total output	2500

fluids have a lower concentration of sodium ions, bicarbonate ions, and chloride ions and a higher concentration of potassium ions, magnesium ions, phosphates, sulfates, and proteins. Of these differences the high extracellular concentration of sodium ions and the high intracellular concentration of potassium ions are of great importance in the permeability and excitability of cell membranes, particularly those of nerve and muscle cells. The role of sodium and potassium in these phenomena has been described in Chapter 3.

Water is essential to the normal operation of metabolic cycles, as discussed in Chapter 24. Water is ingested in food and beverages and produced in metabolism. Daily water loss generally equals daily water intake. Water is lost through urine, feces, sweat, and as water vapor in exhaled air. Table 26.1 shows the amounts of water gained and lost by a typical adult on a normal diet in a temperate climate. When water intake equals water output, the body is said to be in **water balance**. Several factors can disturb the normal water balance.

Dehydration **Dehydration**, the condition in which the body is in **negative water balance**, occurs when more water is lost than is taken in over a period of time. Hemorrhage, burns that leak plasma from the surface of the body, vomiting, diarrhea, and excessive sweating can lead to dehydration. Infants, because of their immature kidneys, cannot concentrate urine as efficiently as adults and thus are more likely than adults to become dehydrated. When the cause of dehydration leads to either the excessive loss of electrolytes or the concentration of electrolytes in the body fluids, electrolyte imbalances can also occur.

Water intoxication An excess of ADH or the intake of an extremely large volume of water (as might occur in psy-

chiatric compulsive water drinking or on water diets to create fullness) can lead to **water intoxication**. As the water enters extracellular fluids, it decreases the osmotic pressure of those fluids; water then enters the cells and can cause the cells to swell. In rare instances the resulting cellular damage can lead to death.

Edema **Edema** is an increase in the volume of extracellular fluids without a change in their osmolality. It is usually caused by an excess of sodium ions, which in turn causes water retention. The amount of water retained is in proportion to the excess of sodium; hence, there is no change in the osmotic balance of the fluid.

FLUID AND ELECTROLYTE REGULATION

Objective 3. Summarize the factors that regulate the fluids and electrolytes in cells and their environment.

The distribution of water in the fluid compartments of the body is described above. The role of the kidney in regulating both the total body water and the concentration of electrolytes in body fluid was described in Chapter 25. Some typical values for the concentrations of electrolytes were given in Figure 26.2. In Table 26.2 concentrations of electrolytes in fluid compartments, glomerular filtrate, and urine are compared. Notice that sodium ions are much more concentrated in all extracellular fluids than in intracellular fluid. This concentration difference is maintained by active transport of sodium out of cells. The concentration of sodium in urine varies considerably, depending on the amount ingested in the diet. Sodium concentration in the urine is also influenced by antidiuretic hormone, aldosterone, and the countercurrent mechanism, as explained in Chapter 25.

The concentration of potassium is much higher in intracellular fluids than in extracellular fluids. (Recall that potassium moves into a cell as sodium moves out during the excitation of the membrane, and that the sodium-potassium pump maintains a concentration gradient with regard to these ions.) The excretion of potassium is determined by chemical equilibria. Virtually all the potassium in the glomerular filtrate is returned to the plasma, and excess potassium is secreted into the kidney tubule. Like sodium, the amount of potassium excreted depends in part on the amount ingested. Normal kidney function is essential for maintaining proper potassium concentrations in cells and body fluids.

Aldosterone plays an important role in the regulation of extracellular fluid volume and of the sodium and potassium concentrations in extracellular fluids. As we have al-

Table 26.2	Concentrations of Selected Electrolytes in Body Fluids (in mEq/l)				
Electrolyte	Intracellular Fluid	Interstitial Fluid	Plasma	Glomerular Filtrate	Urine
Na^+	10	145	142	142	128
K^+	160	4	4	4	60
Cl^-	3	114	103	103	134
HCO_3^-	10	31	27	27	14

ready noted, aldosterone causes sodium to be reabsorbed from the kidney tubules. Aldosterone also causes potassium to be secreted into the kidney tubules. Furthermore, as the extracellular potassium concentration increases, more aldosterone is released, and as the aldosterone concentration increases, more potassium is excreted. Then as the potassium concentration drops, less aldosterone is released. Thus, the concentration of extracellular potassium is homeostatically controlled primarily by aldosterone through a negative feedback mechanism (Figure 26.3).

The movement of chloride ions may be active or passive. In the ascending loop of Henle chloride ions are actively transported out of the tubule into the interstitial fluids. In most other sites chloride ions passively follow sodium ions as the sodium ions move across a membrane. The latter phenomenon, called **chloride shift**, prevents a change in the electrical charges on the two sides of a membrane, which would occur if more positive (sodium) ions than negative (chloride) ions were to cross the membrane.

The movement of bicarbonate (HCO_3^-) is closely associated with the regulation of pH. It will be discussed in the next section of this chapter.

Overall, the electrolyte balance in body fluids is regulated by a combination of chemical equilibria, hormones, and active transport.

Thirst

In addition to the above-mentioned factors the sensation of thirst plays an important role in the regulation of fluids. **Thirst** is defined as the conscious desire for water. Whenever fluid is lost from the extracellular compartment, the remaining extracellular fluid becomes more concentrated and exerts a greater osmotic pressure. Fluid is drawn out of

cells. The **thirst center** in the hypothalamus helps to regulate fluid intake. The cells of the thirst center are osmoreceptors and thus are stimulated by an increase in the osmotic pressure of plasma or extracellular fluid. They send impulses to the cerebrum, and we experience the sensation of thirst. Decreased salivary secretion also stimulates thirst indirectly.

Curiously, we experience relief of thirst immediately after drinking—before the fluid has reached the cells of the thirst center and even before the fluid has been absorbed from the digestive tract. Though the mechanism by which thirst is so suddenly quenched is not fully understood, it seems that distension of the stomach by the fluid is partly responsible. If thirst continued for the 30 minutes it takes for the cells of the thirst center to become fully hydrated, far more fluid than needed would be taken in and the body would be overhydrated. The immediate quenching of thirst is a homeostatic mechanism that helps to maintain adequate hydration without overhydration.

ACID–BASE REGULATION

Objective 4. Define the term buffer and explain how buffer systems help to regulate the pH of body fluids.

Objective 5. Summarize the factors that regulate pH of body fluids and maintain acid–base balance in the body.

The pH of intracellular fluids ranges from 6.7 to 7.0; this slightly acidic pH is due to acid-producing metabolism within cells. As cells carry on their metabolic activities, they release carbon dioxide and waste materials into the interstitial fluid compartment. Even though the fluid inside cells is slightly acidic, the fluids that surround the cells and the blood plasma normally have a pH of 7.35 to 7.45. If the interstitial fluids and the plasma become more acidic or more basic, the body's acid–base regulating mechanisms must correct or compensate for these changes quickly in order to prevent a life-threatening condition resulting from damage to cellular proteins.

The maintenance of acid–base balance is primarily a matter of regulating the concentration of hydrogen ions. Failure to regulate hydrogen ion concentration may lead to **acidosis** (an excess of hydrogen ions) or **alkalosis** (a deficiency of hydrogen ions). The roles of the lungs and kidneys in maintaining acid–base balance have been discussed briefly in Chapters 21 and 25, respectively. Here, the mechanisms of acid–base balance will be discussed in more detail and the roles of the lungs and kidneys integrated into the overall process.

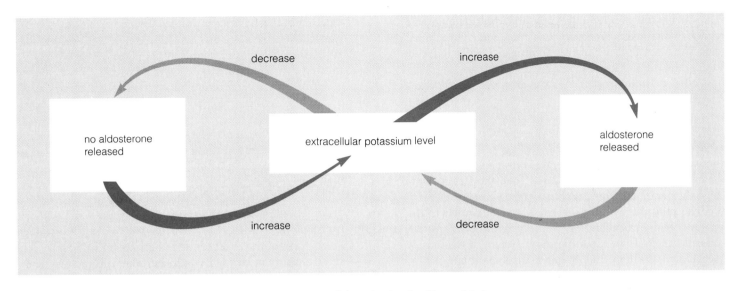

Figure 26.3 The negative feedback mechanism by which the extracellular potassium level is regulated.

Buffers

A **buffer** (sometimes called a buffer system) consists of one or more substances that resist change in the acidity or basicity (alkalinity) of a solution, usually by taking up or releasing hydrogen ions. Hemoglobin and plasma proteins are important buffers because of their ability to take up or release hydrogen ions. Another important buffer is the **carbonic acid–bicarbonate buffer system**, which consists of the weak acid carbonic acid (H_2CO_3) and its salt, sodium bicarbonate ($NaHCO_3$). This buffer system along with hemoglobin and plasma proteins exerts buffering effects primarily in the blood. A fourth buffer, the **phosphate buffer system**, consists of a weak acid, sodium dihydrogen phosphate (NaH_2PO_4), and a weak base, sodium monohydrogen phosphate (Na_2HPO_4). It is of greater importance in urine than in blood. In buffer systems involving a weak acid and one of its salts, the salt acts to neutralize strong acids by accepting hydrogen ions; the weak acid neutralizes strong bases by donating hydrogen ions to them.

The action of a buffer system can be illustrated by showing what happens when a strong acid or strong base is present. For example, hydrochloric acid (HCl) is a strong acid—almost all of its molecules ionize into H^+ and Cl^-. In contrast, carbonic acid is a weak acid—only a small proportion of its molecules ionize to form H^+ and HCO_3^-. Sodium hydroxide (NaOH) behaves like a strong base—almost all of its molecules ionize to form Na^+ and OH^-. The OH^- greatly increases the pH of a solution because it acts as a H^+ acceptor; that is, it removes H^+ from solution. In contrast, the salt sodium bicarbonate acts as a weak base. It ionizes in solution to form Na^+ and HCO_3^-. Na^+ does not affect the pH. (Recall that, by definition, pH is a measure only of H^+ concentration.) The bicarbonate ion is a weak acceptor of H^+. These reactions are summarized below; the size of the arrows are in approximate proportion to the concentration of the substance(s) at the point of the arrow. For example, most of the HCl exists as H^+ and Cl^-, whereas only a little of the H_2CO_3 ionizes and much remains nonionized.

Strong acid: HCl $\rightleftharpoons$ $H^+ + Cl^-$

Weak acid: H_2CO_3 $\rightleftharpoons$ $H^+ + HCO_3^-$

Strong base: NaOH $\rightleftharpoons$ $Na^+ + OH^-$

Salt: $NaHCO_3$ $\Longrightarrow$ $Na^+ + HCO_3^-$

Now let us see how the carbonic acid–bicarbonate system reduces the effects of the strong acids and bases on pH. When a strong acid and a weak base react, a new salt and a weak acid are formed:

$$HCl + NaHCO_3 \rightarrow NaCl + H_2CO_3$$

The salt has no effect on the pH, and the carbonic acid produces far fewer hydrogen ions than the hydrochloric acid. Thus, the number of free hydrogen ions is reduced, holding the pH in a narrow range.

When a strong base and a weak acid react, water and a weak base are formed:

$$NaOH + H_2CO_3 \rightarrow H_2O + NaHCO_3$$

The water has no effect on the pH, and the sodium bicarbonate is far less able to accept H^+ than the strong base. Thus, the pH is again held within a narrow range.

The phosphate buffer system, a system similar to the carbonic acid–bicarbonate system, operates primarily in intracellular fluids and in the urinary system. It consists of a weak acid—sodium dihydrogen phosphate (NaH_2PO_4)—and a weak base—sodium monohydrogen phosphate (Na_2HPO_4). The effects of this system on strong acids and bases are shown in the following reactions:

$$HCl + Na_2HPO_4 \rightleftharpoons NaCl + NaH_2PO_4$$
$$\text{(weak base)} \qquad \text{(weak acid)}$$
$$NaOH + NaH_2PO_4 \rightleftharpoons H_2O + Na_2HPO_4$$
$$\text{(weak acid)} \qquad \text{(weak base)}$$

Hemoglobin and plasma proteins, being composed of amino acids, can combine with or release H^+ and thus also act as buffers. The carboxyl group of an amino acid can gain or lose a hydrogen ion:

$$NH_2-CH_2-COO^- + H^+ \rightleftharpoons NH_2-CH_2-COOH$$

The amino group of an amino acid can gain or lose a hydrogen ion, or it can gain or lose a hydroxyl ion:

$$NH_2-CH_2-COOH + H^+ \rightleftharpoons NH_3^+-CH_2-COOH$$

$$NH_3-CH_2-COOH + OH^- \rightleftharpoons \overset{OH^-}{\underset{}{NH_3^+}}-CH_2-COOH$$

Notice that all these reactions are easily reversible; that is, they can go in either direction. Plasma proteins can therefore hold or release either H^+ or OH^-, and by doing so they act as a powerful buffer system in the blood.

As should be clear from the above examples, buffers are extremely important in the regulation of acid–base balance. The actions of buffers are summarized in Table 26.3.

Table 26.3	The Actions of Buffer Systems
System	**Actions**
Bicarbonate/ carbonic acid	Bicarbonate reacts with a strong acid to form a salt and a weak acid: $HCl + NaHCO_3 \longrightarrow NaCl + H_2CO_3$ Carbonic acid reacts with a strong base to form water and a weak base: $NaOH + H_2CO_3 \longrightarrow H_2O + NaHCO3$
Phosphate	Sodium monohydrogen phosphate reacts with a strong acid to form a salt and a weak acid: $HCl + Na_2HPO_4 \longrightarrow NaCl + NaH_2PO_4$ Sodium dihydrogen phosphate reacts with a strong base to form water and a weak base: $NaOH + NaH_2PO_4 \longrightarrow H_2O + Na_2HPO_4$
Hemoglobin	Hemoglobin can gain or lose a hydrogen ion: $Hb + H^+ \rightleftharpoons H\text{-}Hb^+$ (a weak acid)
Amino acids of plasma proteins	The carboxyl group of an amino acid can gain or lose a hydrogen ion: $NH_2-CH_2-COO^- + H^+ \rightleftharpoons NH_2CH_2COOH$ The amino group of an amino acid can gain or lose a hydrogen ion: $NH_2CH_2COOH + H^+ \rightleftharpoons NH_3^+ CH_2COOH$

Mechanisms of Maintaining Acid–Base Balance

With an understanding of buffer systems we can now consider the mechanisms by which acid–base balance is maintained. We can start with carbon dioxide, which is continuously produced by cells. It might be thought of as the substance most likely to upset acid–base balance because, when it dissolves in the plasma, it produces carbonic acid as the following reaction goes to the right:

$$CO_2 + H_2O \rightleftharpoons H_2CO_3 \rightleftharpoons H^+ + HCO_3^-$$

To prevent the pH of the plasma from becoming more acid, carbon dioxide must be constantly removed to cause the reaction to go to the left.

In the lungs large amounts of carbon dioxide are removed from the plasma, as described in Chapter 21. In the kidney small amounts of carbon dioxide from the extracellular fluid around the kidney tubules enter the epithelial cells of the tubules. In those cells bicarbonate and hydrogen ions are produced according to the above reaction. Hydrogen ions are then actively secreted into the lumen of the tubule, from which they are excreted in the urine.

In blood carbon dioxide is transported mainly in the form of bicarbonate ions, but some carbon dioxide is dissolved directly in the plasma. As the dissolved carbon dioxide is removed from the plasma during gas exchange, hydrogen ions combine with bicarbonate ions, forming carbonic acid, which dissociates (when the above reaction goes to the left). Removal of free hydrogen ions from the plasma in this manner prevents lowering of the blood pH.

Thus, the pH of extracellular fluids is maintained within a narrow range by the action of buffers and by the actions of the lungs and kidneys. The speed with which these three regulatory mechanisms operate varies significantly. The buffer systems react most rapidly but are limited by the accumulation of products that slow the reactions. For example, accumulation of CO_2 reduces the ability of the bicarbonate–carbonic acid buffer system to prevent the accumulation of acid. The lungs can respond relatively rapidly to the accumulation of CO_2 and reduce the accumulation of acid by increasing the rate at which CO_2 is removed from the blood. The kidneys are least rapid in their response to the accumulation of acid, primarily because the removal of acid by the kidney requires the active transport of H^+ into the lumen of the kidney tubules. Though these three mechanisms—buffers, lungs, and kidneys—vary in the speed with which they regulate acid–base balance, all three are extremely important in the process.

Disturbance of Acid-Base Balance

If the acid–base balance is disturbed, acidosis (excess H^+) or alkalosis (deficient H^+) may be produced. Furthermore, each of these conditions may be caused by either respiratory or metabolic disturbances. Thus, there are four abnormal conditions to be concerned with: respiratory acidosis, respiratory alkalosis, metabolic acidosis, and metabolic alkalosis.

In **respiratory acidosis** the ability of the lungs to remove CO_2 from the body is impaired by such conditions as pneumonia or emphysema. CO_2 accumulates in the blood, some of it forming H_2CO_3 which partially ionizes, releasing H^+.

In **respiratory alkalosis** the lungs remove more CO_2 than is required to maintain acid–base balance. Hyperventilation (prolonged rapid, deep breathing) is one cause of

respiratory alkalosis. As CO_2 is removed, more H^+ is combined with HCO_3^- to form H_2CO_3, and the H^+ concentration is reduced.

In **metabolic acidosis** an excess of acid is produced as cells carry on their metabolic activities. This condition frequently accompanies inadequately treated diabetes mellitus, when energy is produced mainly from fat metabolism and acidic ketone bodies are produced. Much of the HCO_3^- in the blood is combined with these acids; HCO_3^- reserves are depleted, and an excess of H^+ develops.

In **metabolic alkalosis** a deficiency of metabolic acids exists. Such a condition might result from excessive vomiting, which removes acid from the stomach and causes the gastric mucosa to produce more acid, thereby depleting the supply of H^+ and also creating an excess of HCO_3^-.

Further Details of Acid–Base Regulation

For a more complete explanation of the regulation of acid–base balance, an understanding of the chemical properties of weak acids and bases is needed. Of particular importance is carbonic acid, which partially ionizes or dissociates as follows:

$$H_2CO_3 \rightleftharpoons H^+ + HCO_3^-$$

For a particular quantity of H_2CO_3 a predictable concentration of both H^+ and HCO_3^- exists. For a weak acid the ionic concentrations are small compared to the concentration of the nonionized acid. All acids dissociate to a degree that is characteristic and constant for the particular acid. The degree of dissociation of such an acid is called its **dissociation constant**, K. Using brackets to represent concentrations, this idea can be expressed as follows:

$$K = \frac{[H^+] \times [HCO_3^-]}{H_2CO_3}$$

For weak acids such as carbonic acid the concentrations of H^+ and HCO_3^- are very small numbers compared to the concentration of H_2CO_3. Thus, the dissociation constant, K, for carbonic acid is a small number, usually expressed in logarithmic form. For example, if

$$K = \frac{1 \times 1}{1,000,000} \text{ or } \frac{1}{10^6},$$

the logarithm (log) is –6. (The 6 is the exponent; the minus shows that the 10^6 is the denominator of a fraction.) To avoid the minus sign, this number is converted to the negative log by multiplying it by -1: $(-1) \times (-6) = +6$. Chemists call the negative log of the dissociation constant the **pK**. (Note that this concept is analogous to pH, the negative log of the hydrogen ion concentration, as explained in Chapter 2.)

The pK of an acid is related to its pH, as expressed in an equation called the Henderson-Hasselbalch equation. For carbonic acid that equation is written:

$$pH = pK + \log \frac{[HCO_3^-]}{[H_2CO_3]}$$

Substituting pH 7.4 for normal blood and pK 6.1, the pK for carbonic acid, we find the log of the ratio of concentrations of bicarbonate to carbonic acid is 1.3:

$$7.4 = 6.1 + \log \frac{[HCO_3^-]}{[H_2CO_3]}$$

$$1.3 = \log \frac{[HCO_3^-]}{[H_2CO_3]}$$

From a table of logarithms we find that the antilog of $1.3 = 20$. Hence, in blood at normal pH the ratio of bicarbonate to carbonic acid is 20:1.

$$\frac{[HCO_3^-]}{[H_2CO_3]} = \frac{20}{1}$$

Because the H_2CO_3 can be thought of as CO_2 dissolved in H_2O, we can approximate the above equation with:

$$\frac{[HCO_3^-]}{[CO_2]} = \frac{20}{1}$$

Thus, at a normal blood pH of 7.4 the ratio of the concentrations of HCO_3 to CO_2 is 20 to 1. Under normal circumstances the combined actions of the buffer, lungs, and kidneys maintain the blood pH between 7.35 and 7.45. However, in conditions of acidosis or alkalosis, either respiratory or metabolic, the pH is altered, as shown in Table 26.4.

When the body is able to completely compensate the imbalance, the pH and the concentrations of bicarbonate and carbonic acid (carbon dioxide) are restored to normal. More often, the condition that caused the acidosis or alkalosis prevents complete correction, and incomplete compensation occurs. In incomplete compensation the pH is returned to normal (the ratio of HCO_3^-:CO_2 is 20:1), but the concentrations of bicarbonate and carbonic acid (carbon dioxide) may be above or below normal (as shown in the table). Because the most specific change in the blood during

acidosis or alkalosis is a change in the concentration of HCO_3^- or dissolved CO_2, these conditions and their compensation are illustrated using the bicarbonate–carbonic acid buffer system and the pK of 6.1 of the dissociation of carbonic acid. Since the pK remains constant, changes in pH involve changes in the concentrations of HCO_3^- and CO_2.

To summarize the information presented in the table, acidosis involves a decrease in the ratio of HCO_3^- to CO_2, and alkalosis involves an increase in that ratio. Incomplete compensation restores the ratio and the normal pH but changes the concentration of both HCO_3^- and CO_2. Complete compensation restores the pH and the concentrations of HCO_3^- and CO_2 to the normal range.

INTEGRATED FUNCTION OF BODY SYSTEMS

Objective 6. Explain how homeostatic mechanisms regulate internal processes so as to maintain dynamic equilibrium between cells and their extracellular fluids.

In the chapters of this unit we have considered many different internal processes and the ways they are regulated. In most cases the process accomplishes something that ultimately helps to maintain dynamic equilibrium between cells and their surrounding fluids. For example, when the tissue cells of the kidney become oxygen deficient, certain cells in the kidney produce erythropoietin. Erythropoietin stimulates the production of new erythrocytes. Larger numbers of erythrocytes in the blood help in the transport of larger quantities of oxygen to the tissues. By this somewhat complex and round-about process, a shortage of oxygen at the cellular level is detected, and action is taken to increase the supply.

This process and a number of other internal processes are listed in Table 26.5. Notice that the table includes a brief description of the homeostatic mechanism that regulates each process and provides examples of clinical conditions that result from the inability of the homeostatic mechanism to completely restore normal conditions. Although the table is not an exhaustive list of all internal processes that are homeostatically regulated, it does provide an overview of the integration of body system functions. A careful study of the table will show that several internal processes are closely related. For example, when there is an injury, the production of leukocytes, hemostasis (stoppage of bleeding), and nonspecific and specific immunity all contribute to returning internal conditions to their normal equilibrium. Similarly, the regulation of the heart beat, stroke volume, blood pressure, and flow of blood to various organs are all integrated to provide adequate supplies of materials to individual cells and to remove wastes from them.

Table 26.4 Acidosis, Alkalosis, and Compensation

	Acidosis	Alkalosis
General		
	Assume pH = 7.1 Given pK = 6.1, then $\log \dfrac{[HCO_3^-]}{[CO_2]} = 1.0$ antilog of 1.0 = 10 $\dfrac{[HCO_3^-]}{[CO_2]} = \dfrac{10}{1}$ (half the normal ratio)	Assume pH = 7.7 Given pK = 6.1, then $\log \dfrac{[HCO_3^-]}{[CO_2]} = 1.6$ antilog of 1.6 = 40 $\dfrac{[HCO_3^-]}{[CO_2]} = \dfrac{40}{1}$ (twice the normal ratio)
Respiratory		
	Caused by impaired ability of lungs to rid the body of CO_2. *Problem: excess CO_2 and thus excess H^+.*	Caused by excessive removal of CO_2 as in hyperventilation. *Problem: deficiency of CO_2 and thus deficient H^+.*
Compensation	Accomplished by kidney because respiratory system malfunction caused the condition and is incapable of correcting it.	
	Kidney excretes more H^+ than normal and returns more HCO_3^- to blood until a blood pH of 7.4 is restored. The HCO_3^- is retained in blood until its concentration is 20 times the CO_2 concentration. Both HCO_3^- and CO_2 are present in excess in incomplete compensation.	Kidney excretes less H^+ than normal and returns less HCO_3^- to blood until a blood pH of 7.4 is restored. Only enough HCO_3^- is present in the blood to restore the ratio of 20:1 with CO_2. Because the CO_2 concentration is below normal, so is the concentration of HCO_3^- below normal in incomplete compensation.
Metabolic		
	Caused by any of several metabolic disorders, such as excesses of metabolic acids, but results in a decrease in bicarbonate. *Problem: deficiency of HCO_3^- and thus excess H^+.*	Caused by any of several metabolic disorders, such as loss of acids, but results in an increase in bicarbonate. Problem: *excess of HCO_3^- and thus deficient H^+*
Compensation	Accomplished by the respiratory system because it is not impaired in metabolic disorders and can compensate the condition more rapidly than the kidney.	
	Lungs release more CO_2 into exhaled air until the blood pH is returned to 7.4 and the ratio of HCO_3^- to CO_2 is restored to 20:1. Because of the original deficiency of HCO_3^-, the concentrations of both HCO_3^- and CO_2 are below normal in incomplete compensation.	Lungs release smaller amounts of CO_2 into exhaled air until the blood pH is returned to 7.4 and the ratio of HCO_3^- to CO_2 is restored to 20:1. Because of the excess of HCO_3^-, the concentrations of both HCO_3^- and CO_2 are above normal in incomplete compensation.

Table 26.5 Internal Processes and Homeostatic Mechanisms

Internal Processes	Homeostatic Mechanisms	Clinical Condition Related to Imbalance
Production of erythrocytes	Cells of kidney produce erythropoietin when they become oxygen deficient.	Anemias, polycythemia
Production of leukocytes	Inflammatory reaction stimulates production of leukocytes.	Infections
Hemostasis	Injury to blood vessel causes vessel spasm and formation of platelet plug, and initiates clotting mechanism.	Hemophilia, other clotting disorders
Regulation of heart beat	Spontaneous depolarization of S-A node maintains rhythmic contractions. Hormones and nerve impulses regulate rate.	Arrhythmias, heart block
Stroke volume	Law of the heart, nerve impulses, and hormones increase strength of contraction. Venous inflow helps to determine filling of ventricles.	Myocardial infarction, heart failure
Blood pressure	Nerve impulses and hormones control size of arterioles. Baroreceptors detect and transmit changes to heart muscle.	Hypertension, postural hypotension, shock, hemorrhage
Flow of blood to various organs	Exercise increases flow of blood to muscles, increase in body temperature increases flow of blood to skin, food in digestive tract increases flow of blood to digestive organs. Effects are mediated by chemoreceptors, heat sensors, and nerve impulses.	Heat stroke, heat exhaustion, frostbite
Nonspecific immunity	Invasion of microorganisms initiates inflammatory response.	Inflammatory response sometimes without invasion
Specific immunity	Antigen elicits the production of antibodies or T-cells, which destroy antigen. (Antigen is usually on invading microorganism.)	Allergy and autoimmune diseases
Breathing rate	Nerve impulses and chemoreceptors regulate rate in accordance with CO_2 and O_2 in blood.	Sudden infant death syndrome, narcosis
Gas exchange	Hemoglobin, concentrations of chemicals in blood regulate rate of gas exchange in lungs and tissues.	Emphysema, pneumonia, hypoxia, decompression sickness, hyaline membrane disease
Maintenance of pH of extracellular fluids in normal range	Buffers reduce the amount of H^+ or OH^- that is free in the fluid. When fluids become too acidic, the lungs remove more CO_2 and shift the equilibrium of the carbonic anhydrase reaction so less H^+ is produced; the kidneys actively secrete H^+ and return HCO_3^- to the blood. These reactions decrease the acidity of the extracellular fluids. When the fluids become too alkaline, the lungs remove less CO_2 and the kidneys secrete less H^+ and return less HCO_3^- to the blood until the fluids return to the normal pH range.	Acidosis, alkalosis
Maintenance of electrolyte balance	Kidneys remove excesses of such electrolytes as sodium, potassium, ammonium, chloride, bicarbonate, sulfate, and phosphate.	Edema from an excess of sodium, potassium depletion from the use of certain diuretics.
Maintenance of fluid balance	When osmoreceptors detect that blood is too concentrated, antidiuretic hormone is released and causes kidneys to return more water to extracellular fluids. Thirst is also stimulated, and fluids are taken in. When baroreceptors detect a decrease in blood pressure (because blood volume is lowered in this case), aldosterone is released by adrenal cortex, and more sodium is reabsorbed. Water follows sodium by osmosis. When the blood volume or blood pressure is above normal, these processes are reversed.	Edema, dehydration, water intoxication
Maintenance of blood glucose level	When blood glucose level rises, insulin and other hormones are released. Glucose is taken into cells and stored as glycogen in the liver. When blood glucose level decreases, glucagon is released. Glycogen is broken down into glucose.	Diabetes mellitus, hypoglycemia

Table 26.5 Internal Processes and Homeostatic Mechanisms (continued)

Internal Processes	Homeostatic Mechanisms	Clinical Condition Related to Imbalance
Maintenance of constant body temperature	Heat gain and heat loss centers in the hypothalamus detect changes in body temperature and stimulate sweating and dilation of surface blood vessels or constriction of blood vessels and shivering.	Fever, chills
Metabolic rate	Metabolic rate is maintained within a narrow range consistent with the energy expenditures of the body by thyroxine and other hormones, exercise, and responses of hunger and satiety centers.	Hypothyroidism, hyperthyroidism
Waste removal	Chemical processes in the kidney remove nitrogenous wastes such as urea from the blood and determine the excesses of electrolytes to be excreted. The liver also produces urea and renders most toxic substances relatively harmless.	Renal failure, hepatitis

RESPONSE TO STRESS

Objective 7. Define stress and describe some of the factors that contribute to stress.

Objective 8. Describe the body's mechanisms for responding to stress.

It is appropriate that we should consider stress in this chapter on homeostasis because stress provides a variety of challenges to the body's homeostatic mechanisms.

What Is Stress?

The concept of physiological stress was first developed by Hans Selye, a physician and physiologist at McGill University. In 1935, while studying the effects of various injected hormone preparations on rats, Selye discovered that the animals responded with the *same* changes to a number of quite *different* substances he injected, including extracts from organs not known to produce hormones and various chemicals including formaldehyde. The three changes that appeared in all animals were: (1) enlargement of the adrenal glands, (2) bleeding ulcers, and (3) atrophy of lymphatic tissues.

From these observations Selye developed the following definitions: (1) **Stress** is a condition of the body produced by a variety of injurious agents. (2) **Stressors** are the agents that produce stress. (3) The **general adaptation syndrome** is the name for the group of changes that appear in animals under stress. In selecting this name Selye chose the words carefully. By general, he meant that the response was the same for many different stressors. By adaptation, he meant that the animal's response made it possible for the body to cope

with the stress—to adapt. By syndrome, he referred to the set of signs and symptoms that occurred together.

It is now known that the severe stress Selye observed in animals is due to excess secretion of ACTH, which in turn causes excess secretion of cortisol. However, it is not necessarily true that all stressors to which humans may be subjected will result in excess cortisol secretion.

What Are Stressors?

Any stimulus that produces stress is by definition a stressor. However, many stressors are mild enough or of sufficiently short duration that the body's homeostatic mechanisms can adjust the internal environment to cope with the effects of the stressor before serious damage occurs. Stressors may be pleasant as well as unpleasant stimuli. Winning a prize in keen competition can be as physiologically stressful as failing to win. Being around people all the time in social situations can be as stressful as social isolation. The birth of a new baby can be as stressful as the death of a loved one.

It is impossible, and even undesirable, to remove all stress from our lives. A certain amount of stress makes life interesting and helps us to meet challenges. Selye makes a distinction between stress that is productive and stress that is harmful. The former he called **eustress**; the latter he called **distress**. Distress is continual stress that causes us to constantly readjust to a situation. Caring for a seriously ill relative, working at a job that is frustrating and unsatisfying, or even having so little to do that one is bored most of the time can all be distressing situations. In fact, mental or emotional stress (distress) is more likely to lead to health problems than physical stress from hard muscular work.

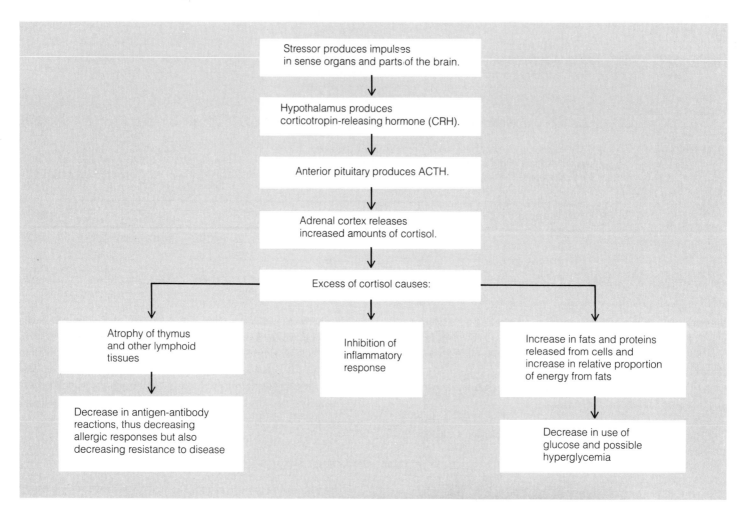

Figure 26.4 Mechanism for the release of cortisol in the alarm reaction and the nature of its effects.

Finally, what constitutes a stressor is different among different individuals or even in the same individual at different times. A job that is distressful to one person may be exactly the right level of stress to cause another to perform best. An event that we find tolerable one day may be almost intolerable on another. How much sleep we have had, what we have or have not eaten, our heredity, our relationships with other people, our past experiences, and many other factors help to determine whether stimuli will produce manageable stress or distress.

How the Body Responds to Stress

Selye also characterized three stages in the body's mechanism of responding to stress. He called these the **alarm reaction**, the **resistance stage**, and the **exhaustion stage**.

Alarm reaction The initial response to a stressor occurs when stimuli from the brain and sense organs arrive in the hypothalamus. The hypothalamus produces corticotropin-releasing hormone (CRH), which stimulates the anterior pituitary to release ACTH. ACTH, in turn, stimulates the adrenal cortex to release increased amounts of cortisol. As shown in Figure 26.4, stressors cause the release of increased amounts of cortisol (and other glucocorticoids). These hormones produce a number of general effects, including decreased allergic reaction, decreased resistance to disease, and increased metabolism of fats.

In addition to its effects on the adrenal gland, a stressor also stimulates the sympathetic nervous system (Figure 26.5). The effects of this kind of stimulation, described in Chapter 15 as the fight-or-flight reaction, include increased blood volume and blood pressure, decreased digestion with

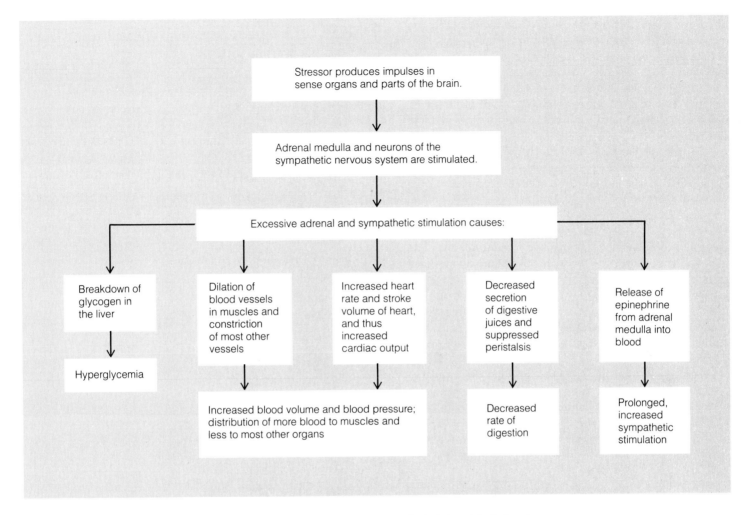

Figure 26.5 Mechanism for the stimulation of the sympathetic nervous system and adrenal medulla in the alarm reaction, and the nature of its effects.

distribution of blood away from the digestive tract to muscles and active organs, and increased blood glucose. The sympathetic stimulation of the adrenal medulla causes the release of excess quantities of epinephrine. The circulation of epinephrine in the blood may prolong the effects of sympathetic stimulation, as explained in Chapter 13.

Resistance stage When the body has been successful through the alarm reaction in adjusting to the effects of the stressor, there is no further response to a given stress. During the resistance stage the body repairs the damages of the stressor; the cortisol production and the sympathetic stimulation return to normal. The body has developed resistance to the stressor.

We experience the alarm and resistance stages of stress many times in our lives; some of us experience these stages daily. We adjust to one stress or another. However, when we encounter a stressor that our bodies cannot adjust to, stress proceeds to the exhaustion stage.

The use of hydrocortisone in promoting healing and in treating allergy and autoimmune diseases is based on effects that are part of the body's alarm reaction. Prolonged use of hydrocortisone can lead to atrophy of the adrenal gland, atrophy of lymphoid tissues, and decreased resistance to infections.

Exhaustion stage In the exhaustion stage cortisol secretion increases to often higher levels than in the alarm stage. It is in the exhaustion stage that the diseases of stress are likely to appear. Such disorders as ulcers, migraine headaches, heart irregularities, and some mental illnesses are often included among the diseases produced by stress. However, it should be noted that stress is not always the cause of these diseases.

In spite of the high level of cortisol secretion at the exhaustion stage, the body is unable to cope with the effects of the stressor. Unless the effects of the stressor can be reversed, ultimately the result is death.

Extensions of Selye's ideas Since the original development of Selye's ideas others have contributed to our understanding of stress. For example, it is now believed that in emotional stress the limbic system of the brain is involved in mediating the stressor response to the hypothalamus. In addition, it appears that the hypothalamus, along with stimulating both the cortex and medulla of the adrenal gland, also stimulates the posterior pituitary to release antidiuretic hormone.

Although originally Selye thought that the release of cortisol helped an organism to resist stress, some physiologists today are debating whether the cortisol helps the body to resist stress or whether its release is simply a symptom of the stress. Further research is needed to answer this question.

CLINICAL TERMS

antacid (an-tas′id) a substance that neutralizes an acid

hyperkalemia (hi-per-kal-em′e-ah) an excess of potassium in the blood

hypernatremia (hi-per-nat-re′me-ah) an excess of sodium in the blood

hypervolemia (hi-per-vol-e′me-ah) increased blood volume

hypokalemia (hi-po-kal-e′me-ah) a deficiency of potassium in the blood

hyponatremia (hi-po-nat-re′me-ah) a deficiency of sodium in the blood

hypovolemia (hi-po-vol-e′me-ah) decreased blood volume

Essay: Stress and Illness

The fact that stress can lead to illness has already been demonstrated in this chapter. As a stressor can be a physical, chemical, or emotional factor and can cause bodily or mental tension (or both), the relationship of body and mind is important in considering stress-related illness.

In general, we think of our "body" as the sum total of all its anatomical parts; we think of "mind" as the thoughts, feelings, perceptions, and desires we experience. These events of the mind occur in the cerebrum, but their effects extend to many other parts of the body, as we have seen in our study of neural and endocrine regulatory mechanisms. Thus, we know that mind and body are integrated both structurally and functionally.

Eastern cultures have historically considered mind and body to be integrated. Consequently, Eastern views about health and illness are generally holistic; that is, they emphasize the structural and functional relationships between parts of the body and the whole body.

In contrast, Western cultures have historically viewed mind and body separately. To the extent that these ideas have been incorporated into our views about health and illness, they have tended to create a separation between physical illness (a specific malfunction of the body) and psychosomatic illness (bodily symptoms caused by, or at least related to, events of the mind). A common error in thinking leads to regarding psychosomatic illness as being "in one's head"—somehow under control so that one could choose to get rid of the illness.

Increased understanding of the biochemistry of disease processes has led to a new view of the mind–body relationship among many health professionals. For example, many new hormones and neurotransmitters have been discovered; some chemicals have been found to serve both functions. New links between physiological and psychological effects of biochemical substances are being discovered with great frequency. Mind and body have come to be viewed as closely related. This change in viewpoint has led many health professionals to consider both the physiological and the psychological aspects of many diseases. In short, Western medicine has become more holistic.

The increasingly holistic viewpoint has suggested relationships between stress and illness. Stress may be involved in such diverse disorders as asthma, rheumatoid arthritis, ulcerative colitis, migraine headaches, and peptic ulcers. In peptic ulcers stress can cause excessive stimulation of the stomach mucosa by way of fibers of the vagus nerve. This stimulation increases the secretion of hydrochloric acid, especially at times when there is no food in the stomach. In asthma, rheumatoid arthritis, and ulcerative colitis, some kind of immunological reaction (allergy, autoimmune response, or other response) may be involved in the disease process, though the mechanism by which stress might cause an immunological reaction is not known.

Stress may be a precipitating factor in anxiety or depression. Once such a mental condition exists, the condition itself leads to bodily changes. People suffering from anxiety are especially sensitive to bodily sensations and usually have a decreased tolerance for pain. Pain and other disease symptoms seem to have two components: (1) the peripheral sensation, and (2) the elaboration of the sensation in the brain. Some people suffering from anxiety tend to amplify their symptoms—focus their thoughts on the symptoms, react to them with intense alarm and worry, and suffer extreme disability—whereas others tend to minimize symptoms—ignore them, deny that they are ill, fail to seek medical attention, and fail to adhere to a prescribed regimen when they finally do seek medical advice. At the present time too little is known about how sensations are elaborated in the brain to explain the observed differences in physiological terms, but it does seem clear that the differences are real (not "just in the head" or under the conscious control of the individual). A further understanding of these differences is likely to come from studies of the actions of various neurotransmitters.

Studies of biochemical changes are already underway on individuals suffering from depression. Such individuals often exhibit behavioral symptoms—insomnia, loss of appetite, decreased sex drive—with a particular periodicity that appears to be associated with variations in the concentrations of biochemical substances (probably neurotransmitters). Studies of the blood and cerebrospinal fluid of affected individuals are being done to determine correlations between biochemical and behavioral changes. Positive findings would add to the accumulating evidence that the functions of the body and the mind are integrated.

The relationship between stress and illness is further demonstrated by the preliminary findings of G. E. Vaillant's long-term study of the psychological health of over 200 men from the sophomore classes of 1942 and 1944 at Harvard University. In this study 185 of the men have been followed for nearly four decades through the use of physical and psychological tests, interviews, and questionnaires. The men who developed chronic mental-health problems generally reported several of the following situations: job dissatisfaction, little occupational progress, visits to a psychiatrist, unhappy marriage, little recreation time, and little vacation time. After grouping the men into several categories, Vaillant observed that, of the 59 with the best mental health, only 2 became chronically ill or died; and of the 48 with the worst mental health, 18 became chronically ill or died. These results seem to confirm that a link between mind and body exists, and that individuals under stress or having chronic mental-health problems run a far greater risk of developing chronic illness or dying at an early age.

Knowing what constitutes stress and the kinds of things that are stressors for us can help us to avoid the distressful kinds of stressors. The National Institute of Mental Health offers the following ten suggestions to help people cope with stress:

1. Work off stress.
2. Talk out your worries.
3. Learn to accept what you cannot change.
4. Avoid self-medication.
5. Get enough sleep and rest.
6. Balance work and recreation.
7. Do something for others.
8. Take one thing at a time.
9. Give in once in a while.
10. Make yourself available—find something interesting to do.

Perhaps by learning to recognize stressful situations and applying these methods of coping with stress, we can maintain better mental and physical health.

CHAPTER SUMMARY

(Chapter summary points and review questions are numbered to correspond to the numbered objectives in the text of each chapter.)

Internal Balance at the Cellular Level

1. Summarize the movement of substances into and out of cells and explain why cells need a nearly constant environment.
   a. Substances move into and out of cells in a variety of ways, which are summarized in Figure 26.1.
   b. A dynamic equilibrium between cells (the functional units of living organisms) and their environment (the extracellular fluids) is essential to life. Serious disturbances in this equilibrium lead to cellular death and eventual death of the organism.

Water and Fluid Compartments

2. Describe the fluid compartments of the body and explain how disturbances in water balance can lead to dehydration, water intoxication, or edema.
   a. The fluid compartments of the body include:
      (1) intracellular fluid, which is inside cells
      (2) extracellular fluid, which includes interstitial fluid, plasma, lymph, cerebrospinal fluid, and the fluid in the joint cavities and eyes
   b. Water balance exists when the fluid intake equals the fluid output.
   c. Disturbances in fluid balance include the following:
      (1) Dehydration occurs when more fluid is lost than is taken in following hemorrhage, vomiting, diarrhea, and excessive sweating.
      (2) Water intoxication occurs when much more fluid is taken in than is lost.
      (3) Edema results from an excess of sodium.

Fluid and Electrolyte Regulation

3. Summarize the factors that regulate the fluids and electrolytes in cells and their environment.
   a. Electrolyte balance is regulated by a combination of chemical equilibria, hormones, and active transport mechanisms.
   b. Total fluid volume in the body is determined by intake and excretion and is regulated by antidiuretic hormone, aldosterone, and neural factors, including the thirst mechanism.

Acid–Base Regulation

4. Define the term buffer and explain how buffer systems help to regulate the pH of body fluids.

   a. A buffer is a substance that resists change in pH; body buffer systems include:
      (1) carbonic acid–bicarbonate system
      (2) phosphate buffer system
      (3) hemoglobin
      (4) plasma protein buffers
   b. Buffer systems help to maintain the normal pH of body fluids by:
      (1) taking up hydrogen ions when the pH becomes acidic
      (2) releasing hydrogen ions when the pH becomes alkaline
5. Summarize the factors that regulate pH of body fluids and maintain acid–base balance in the body.
   a. The lungs and kidneys are the primary organs involved in regulating acid–base balance:
      (1) The lungs remove carbon dioxide from the blood when the pH becomes acidic and allow carbon dioxide to remain in the blood when the pH becomes alkaline.
      (2) The kidneys excrete hydrogen ions and reabsorb bicarbonate ions when the pH becomes acidic and retain hydrogen ions when the pH becomes alkaline.
   b. Conditions of acidosis and alkalosis can be caused by respiratory or metabolic abnormalities; these conditions and the body's mechanisms of compensation are summarized in Table 26.4.

Integrated Function of Body Systems

6. Explain how homeostatic mechanisms regulate internal processes so as to maintain dynamic equilibrium between cells and their extracellular fluids.
   a. The internal processes carried out by the cells of many different organs of the body contribute to maintaining dynamic equilibrium between cells and their environment.
   b. These processes and the homeostatic mechanisms that regulate them are summarized in Table 26.5.

Response to Stress

7. Define stress and describe some of the factors that contribute to stress.
   a. Stress is a condition produced by an injurious agent called a stressor, according to Selye's original definition.
   b. A wide variety of stimuli can be stressors, depending on their intensity and frequency and the body's ability to tolerate them.
8. Describe the body's mechanisms for responding to stress.
   a. The body's response to stress includes:
      (1) the alarm reaction, during which cortisol and sympathetic stimulation produce the general adaptation syndrome

(2) the resistance stage, during which resistance to the stressor develops

(3) the exhaustion stage, during which the body's ability to cope with the stressor is lost

b. In many situations the body succeeds in resisting the stress, and the condition does not proceed to the exhaustion stage.

REVIEW

Important Terms

acidosis

alarm reaction

alkalosis

buffer

chloride shift

dehydration

distress

dynamic equilibrium

edema

eustress

exhaustion stage

extracellular fluid

general adaptation syndrome

interstitial fluid

intracellular fluid

pK

resistance stage

stress

stressor

thirst center

water balance

water intoxication

Questions

1. a. List the materials that normally move into and out of cells and, reviewing other chapters, explain how each moves.
  b. What is dynamic equilibrium in a multicellular organism?
  c. Why is dynamic equilibrium essential to life?

2. a. What are the fluid compartments of the body?
  b. What is water balance, and how is it regulated?
  c. What causes dehydration?
  d. What causes water intoxication?
  e. What causes edema?

3. a. What are the factors that regulate fluid volume?
  b. What are the factors that regulate electrolyte balance?
  c. Review other chapters and explain what happens when fluid volume or electrolytes are not properly regulated.

4. a. What is a buffer?
  b. What are the four major buffer systems in the human body?

5. a. What happens in the lungs and in the kidneys when the acidity of extracellular fluids becomes too great?

b. How is the action of the lungs and the kidneys modified when the extracellular fluids become too alkaline?
  c. What is the role of buffers in acid–base balance?

6. a. What is the relationship of many internal processes to dynamic equilibrium at the cellular level?
  b. How do homeostatic mechanisms help to maintain dynamic equilibrium at the cellular level?
  c. Select three effects of imbalance in homeostatic mechanisms and explain how they occur.

7. a. Define stress, stressor, and general adaptation syndrome.
  b. Discuss the nature of stressors and some factors that contribute to their effects.
  c. What is Selye's distinction between eustress and distress?
  d. What are some actions that help people improve their ability to cope with stress?

8. a. Describe the events in the alarm reaction.
  b. What are the effects of excess cortisol production?
  c. What are the effects of excess sympathetic stimulation?
  d. Evaluate the effects in (a) and (b) according to their contribution to the body's response to stress and their interference with other processes.
  e. Describe the resistance stage of response to stress.
  f. Compare the exhaustion stage of response to stress with the resistance stage.
  g. What are some recent extensions of Selye's ideas about stress?

Problems

1. Use your knowledge of homeostatic mechanisms to explain how a person's body would cope with being lost in the hot desert without water.

2. Explain the homeostatic responses to drinking fairly large amounts of alcohol at a party. To eating nuts and potato chips in excess.

3. Do some research on therapeutic methods that are used to correct fluid, electrolyte, or acid–base imbalances and prepare a report on a currently used therapy.

4. Make a list of things you believe to be stressors in your life. Devise a plan for taking advantage of factors that lead to eustress and lessening the effects of those that lead to distress.

REFERENCES AND READINGS

Anonymous. 1970. Fluid and electrolytes. Chicago: Abbot Laboratories.

Antelman, S. M., Eichler, A. J., Black, C. A., and Kocan, D. 1980. Interchangeability of stress and amphetamine in sensitization. *Science* 207:329 (January 18).

Bricker, N. S. 1975. *The sea within us*. San Juan, Puerto Rico: Searle and Co.

Dennis, V. W., Stead, W. W., and Myers, J. L. 1979. Renal handling of phosphate and calcium. *Annual Review of Physiology* 41:257.

Kurtzman, N. A., Arruda, J. A. L., and Westenfelder, C. 1978. Renal regulation of acid–base homeostasis. *Contributions to Nephrology* 14:1.

Lee, C. A., Stroot, V. R., and Schaper, C. A. 1975. What to do when acid–base problems hang in the balance. *Nursing* 75:32 (August).

Matuchansky, C., and Coutrot, S. 1978. The role of prostaglandins in the study of intestinal water and electrolyte transport in man. *Biomedicine* 28:143.

National Institute of Mental Health. 1977. *Plain talk about stress*. Washington, D.C.: Department of Health, Education and Welfare Publication No. (ADM) 78–502.

Selye, H. 1973. The evolution of the stress concept. *American Scientist* 61:692 (November–December).

Soyka, F., with Edmonds, A. 1977. *The ion effect*. Toronto: McClelland and Stewart-Bantam.

Thomson, R. 1977. *Natural medicine*. New York: McGraw-Hill.

Vaillant, G. E. 1979. Natural history of male psychologic health: Effect of mental health on physical health. *New England Journal of Medicine* 301(23):1249 (December 6).

Walton, S. 1979. Holistic medicine. *Science News* 116:410 (December 15).

UNIT FIVE

CONTINUITY OF LIFE

In the first four units we considered the day-to-day functioning of the human body at all levels from the chemical to the whole system level. We also looked at how these functions are regulated to maintain homeostasis. In this unit we will examine some important questions: How is life maintained from generation to generation? How is genetic information transmitted from parents to offspring? And, what are the stages of human life?

Beginning with meiosis, gametogenesis, and human genetics, we will see how information is transmitted from parents to their offspring, consider a variety of genetic defects and their effects, and conclude Chapter 27 with a brief consideration of genetic screening and counseling and genetic engineering.

In Chapter 28 we will study the human reproductive systems, first the male and then the female. Along with these systems we will consider fertilization and contraception.

In the final chapter of this unit and of the book, we will look at the human life stages from conception to death. Some aspects of the female reproductive system—pregnancy, breast development, labor, and delivery—will be considered in this chapter. We will also discuss embryonic development, infancy, childhood, adolescence, adulthood, aging, and death. Emphasis will be on the anatomical and physiological characteristics of various stages of life.

27

MEIOSIS, GAMETOGENESIS, AND GENETICS

OVERVIEW OF CHAPTER

Objective 1. Define meiosis, gametogenesis, and genetics; describe the relation of these processes to the production of a new individual.

Each person begins life as a single cell. How that single cell arises is an interesting process in itself; how it comes to have all the information needed to direct the development and functioning of a new human being is even more fascinating. In this chapter we will be concerned with the process by which the first cell of a new human being is produced and how that cell acquires information from the parents that produced the individual.

The first cell of a new individual is produced by the union of an egg and a sperm, each of which has only one of each pair of chromosomes that are found in body cells. The process by which cells with half the normal number of chromosomes are produced is called **meiosis**. The process of **gametogenesis** leads to the formation of functional **gametes**—eggs and sperm. Gametogenesis includes, in addition to meiosis, the process by which an ovum, or egg, with a large supply of cytoplasm is produced in a female and the process by which sperm capable of fertilizing the egg are produced in a male. In the next chapter we will consider the details of fertilization; here, it is sufficient to know that, when a sperm fertilizes or combines with an egg, the first cell of a new individual is produced.

Genetics, the study of the transmission of inherited characteristics, is related to meiosis and gametogenesis. During meiosis and gametogenesis half the chromosomes of each parent are transferred to each gamete. When an egg and a sperm unite, the combination of the genetic material from the gametes provides the information to direct the development and functioning of the new individual.

Broadly defined, genetics includes the study of mutations and chromosomal abnormalities, as well as the principles of classical genetics—how specific genes are transmitted. In this chapter we will consider mutations and chromosomal abnormalities directly after the consideration of meiosis and gametogenesis. Then we will consider the principles of genetics. We will conclude our study with a brief consideration of some applications of genetics to genetic screening and counseling and to genetic engineering.

MEIOSIS AND GAMETOGENESIS

Objective 2. Describe the major stages in the process of meiosis.

Objective 3. Contrast the stages in spermatogenesis and oogenesis and describe the outcome of each process.

Objective 4. Explain the significance of meiosis.

Meiosis

In contrast to mitosis (discussed in Chapter 3), meiosis produces cells that are *not* identical to the parent cell. Meiosis leads to the production of gametes. If eggs and sperm contained the same number of chromosomes as body cells, the union of an egg and a sperm would create a cell with twice as many chromosomes as the parent cells had. One of the functions of meiosis, then, is to reduce the number of chromosomes in an orderly manner so that, when an egg and sperm unite, the original complement of chromosomes will be restored. As we shall see later, meiosis also functions to introduce genetic variability into the gametes produced.

Before considering the process of meiosis, it is important to understand what is a normal complement of chromosomes in a human body cell. Normal human body cells contain forty-six chromosomes—twenty-two pairs of homologous chromosomes (carrying information for the same traits) and two sex chromosomes. Females have homologous sex chromosomes, arbitrarily called X chromosomes; males have one X chromosome and one of a different chromosome, called the Y chromosome. A set of human chromosomes is shown in Figure 27.1.

Body cells are said to be **diploid**, or 2n, because they contain pairs of homologous chromosomes and two sex

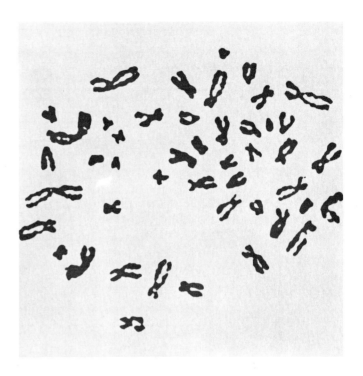

Figure 27.1 Chromosomes of a normal human cell, × 3200. (Courtesy of Dr. Joe Hin Tjio and the National Institute of General Medical Studies, National Institutes of Health.)

chromosomes, XX or XY. Gametes have only twenty-three chromosomes—one of each of the twenty-two paired chromosomes and one sex chromosome, either X or Y. They are said to be **haploid**, or 1n, cells.

Each new individual is formed from two haploid gametes—an egg and a sperm—so each inherits half of his or her chromosomes from each parent. More precisely, each individual receives one member of each pair of chromosomes from the father and one member of each pair from the mother. Therefore, the members of a pair of homologous chromosomes can be designated as maternal and paternal chromosomes.

In the process of meiosis gametes come to have twenty-three chromosomes, and the chromosomes are separated so that one member of each pair goes to each gamete. Two successive cell divisions occur in meiosis: the **first meiotic division** and the **second meiotic division** (Figure 27.2). For ease in following the diagram only two pairs of homologous chromosomes are illustrated, beginning with the **premeiotic interphase** (a). Here, the chromosomes look like long, thin threads. In (b) the threadlike chromosomes have replicated so that each chromosome now consists of two **chromatids**. Each chromatid—a molecule of DNA and

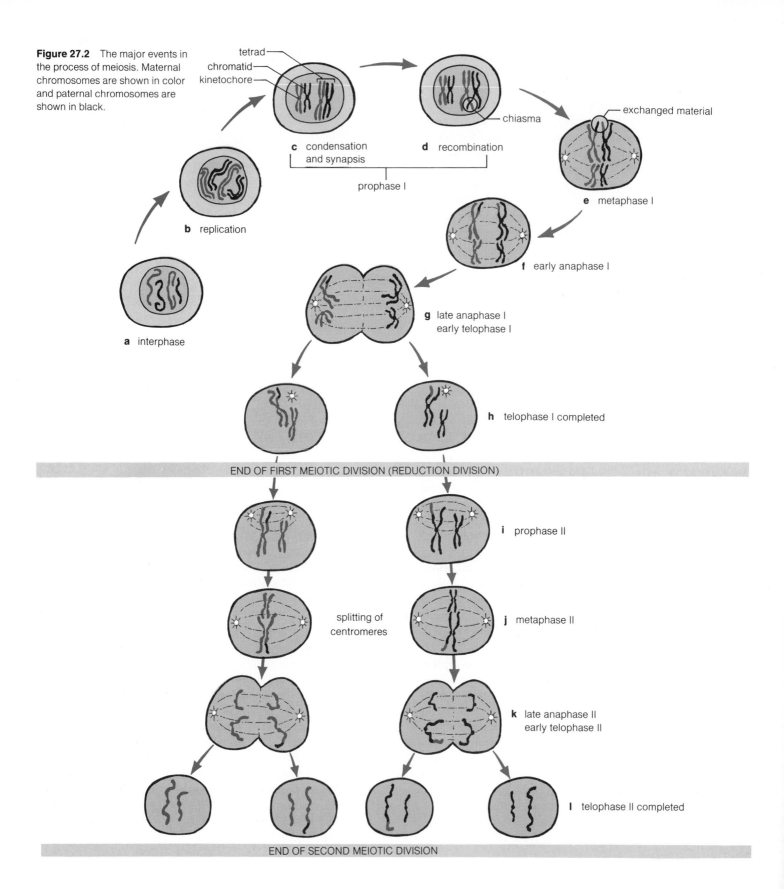

Figure 27.2 The major events in the process of meiosis. Maternal chromosomes are shown in color and paternal chromosomes are shown in black.

tetrad
chromatid
kinetochore

c condensation and synapsis

d recombination

chiasma

prophase I

exchanged material

e metaphase I

b replication

f early anaphase I

a interphase

g late anaphase I early telophase I

h telophase I completed

END OF FIRST MEIOTIC DIVISION (REDUCTION DIVISION)

i prophase II

splitting of centromeres

j metaphase II

k late anaphase II early telophase II

l telophase II completed

END OF SECOND MEIOTIC DIVISION

associated protein—contains all the information in the original chromosome.

In **prophase I**, the prophase of the first meiotic division, the chromosomes condense, or shorten and thicken (c). Though not shown in the figure, spindle fibers appear and the nuclear membrane disappears, as in mitosis. In an event unique to meiosis called **synapsis**, homologous chromosomes come together in pairs. Since each member of the pair has replicated itself before pairing, a total of four chromatids are present in each set of paired or synapsed chromosomes. The four chromatids together are called a **tetrad**. Each chromatid has a **kinetochore**, which replicated with the rest of the chromosome; however the chromatids remain attached to each other at their centromeres.

In another event unique to meiosis, adjacent strands (chromatids) of the paired chromosomes may cross over one another, forming a **chiasma** (d). At a chiasma portions of the chromosomes are exchanged in a process called **crossing-over**. As a result of crossing-over one chromatid is exactly like the original paternal chromosome, one is exactly like the maternal chromosome, and the two that have exchanged material now have a mixture of some maternal and some paternal DNA. The phenomenon of crossing-over introduces genetic variability because it allows new combinations of genetic information to be carried on a single chromatid. This stage of prophase I is appropriately called the **recombination stage**.

In **metaphase I** the paired chromosomes line up in the center of the cell (e). The members of each pair separate from each other in **anaphase I** (f), but the chromatids that are attached by kinetochores remain attached. **Telophase I** (g) and **cytokinesis** (division of the cytoplasm) complete the first meiotic division (h). This division is called the **reduction division** because the number of chromosomes in each of the resulting cells has been reduced from the diploid number to the haploid number: Each cell now contains only one member of each pair of the original homologous chromosomes. However, each of these chromosomes consists of two chromatids—two molecules of DNA from the replication in the premeiotic stage.

No further replication of DNA occurs between the two meiotic divisions, and the second division proceeds in the same way as mitosis. Individual chromosomes appear in **prophase II** (i), align in the center of the cell in **metaphase II** (j), and separate in **anaphase II** (k). No pairing of homologous chromosomes can occur as the cell now contains only one member of each homologous pair of chromosomes. **Telophase II** and **cytokinesis** follow. The result, at the end of the second meiotic division, is four haploid cells from the original single diploid cell (l).

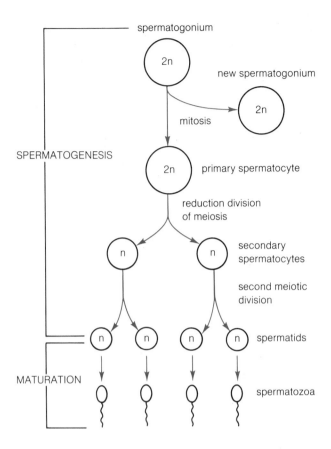

Figure 27.3 Spermatogenesis and maturation of spermatozoa.

Spermatogenesis

Through the process of **spermatogenesis**, which includes the meiotic divisions just described, a cell called a **spermatogonium** produces four **spermatids**. Spermatids then undergo maturation to produce **spermatozoa**, or functional sperm (Figure 27.3). Spermatogenesis begins in the cells adjacent to the walls of the seminiferous tubules, small tubules inside the testes. These spermatogonia continuously divide by mitosis throughout the reproductive years of the male, thereby providing a constant supply of new spermatogonia. Some spermatogonia migrate away from the wall of the tubule, increase in size, and become **primary spermatocytes**. In the reduction division of meiosis the primary spermatocytes each divide to form two **secondary spermatocytes**. Each of the two secondary spermatocytes divides again in the second meiotic division, forming a total of four spermatids. Spermatids continue to migrate toward the lumen of the tubule and undergo changes to become mature spermatozoa. More will be said about the role of the testes in this process in Chapter 28.

Oogenesis

Like spermatogenesis, **oogenesis** also involves meiosis and results in the production of haploid cells. However, in oogenesis only one of the four meiotic products becomes a functional gamete, the ovum. Figure 27.4 shows how this occurs. At the time a human female is born, her ovaries contain many **primary oocytes** within small spherical bodies called primordial follicles. The development of the primary oocytes is arrested at the prophase of the first meiotic division until the female reaches sexual maturity, at which time primary oocytes become capable of completing the reduction division. In this division a **secondary oocyte** and a **first polar body** are formed. Half the nuclear material goes to each of these cells, but nearly all the cytoplasm remains with the secondary oocyte. The first polar body divides again and produces two nonfunctional haploid cells. The secondary oocyte is released from the ovary and enters the uterine tube, where it may be fertilized by a sperm introduced into the female reproductive tract during sexual intercourse. If fertilization occurs, the secondary oocyte undergoes the second meiotic division, forming an **ootid** and a **second polar body**, each containing twenty-three chromosomes. The ootid becomes the functional ovum, its nucleus being capable of uniting with the nucleus of the sperm that fertilized it. It should be noted that together the secondary oocyte and the polar bodies contain enough chromosomal material to form four gametes. However, the polar bodies that are formed in oogenesis eventually disintegrate. They consist almost entirely of nuclear material and serve to dispose of unneeded chromosomes while the bulk of the cytoplasm remains with the single functional ovum. Nutrients in this cytoplasm maintain the ovum until it reaches the uterus.

Significance of Meiosis

The significance of meiosis, regardless of whether it occurs in oogenesis or spermatogenesis, is that haploid cells with increased genetic variability are produced. As noted earlier, the phenomenon of crossing-over accounts for some genetic variability. Because in any one primary spermatocyte or primary oocyte, one member of each pair of homologous chromosomes comes from that individual's mother and one member from the father, the particular combination of chromosomes that end up in a particular gamete also contributes to the genetic variability.

To see that chromosomes can be distributed in many different ways, let us select three pairs of homologous chromosomes and one gene out of the many genes carried on each chromosome. Ignoring crossing-over, the chromo-

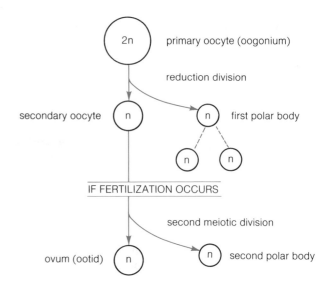

Figure 27.4 Oogenesis.

somes available to enter the gametes can be designated A, B, and C for the maternal chromosomes and a, b, and c for the paternal chromosomes. The letters A', B', C', a', b', and c' designate a particular gene on the designated chromosome. As shown in Figure 27.5, a gamete can receive any combination of maternal and paternal chromosomes, as long as one member of each pair is present. The total number of possible combinations is 2^n, where n is the haploid number of chromosomes found in the gamete. For example, in Figure 27.5 the total possible combinations is 2^3, or 8. In humans the number of combinations is 2^{23}, or more than 8 million. Thus, reassortment of chromosomes during meiosis can result in new combinations of maternal and paternal genes and produces recombination of genetic information on *different* chromosomes. (In addition, crossing-over results in new combinations of genetic information *within* a chromosome.)

MUTATIONS AND CHROMOSOMAL ABNORMALITIES

Objective 5. Define the term mutation and explain how mutations might affect the structure and function of the body.

Objective 6. Explain how abnormal kinds or numbers of chromosomes might be produced; describe the chromo-

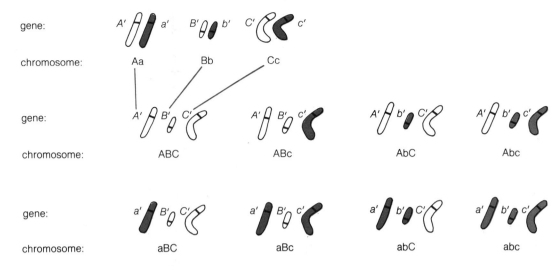

gene:

chromosome: Aa   Bb   Cc

gene:

chromosome: ABC   ABc   AbC   Abc

gene:

chromosome: aBC   aBc   abC   abc

Figure 27.5 The possible combinations of maternal and paternal chromosomes (and particular genes) that can enter a gamete (n = 3). The bar on each chromosome indicates the locus of the gene on the chromosome.

somal abnormality and its effects in (a) Down's syndrome, (b) Klinefelter's syndrome, and (c) Turner's syndrome.

Mutations

Besides reassortment and crossing-over, yet another source of genetic variability is **mutation**, a change in the sequence of the nucleotides in a gene. (A gene, as explained in Chapter 3, is a functional unit of a chromosome usually responsible for determining the structure of a single protein or polypeptide.) Mutations can occur in any cell. If they occur in cells other than gamete-producing cells, they are called somatic, or body cell, mutations, and they affect the function of the mutated cell and its progeny. Some forms of cancer may result from somatic mutations. If mutations occur in gametes or gamete-producing cells, the modified DNA may be transmitted to a new individual in the next generation, and all the cells of the new individual will contain the modified DNA. When that individual forms gametes, the modified DNA will be transmitted to half the gametes, and the mutation can be transmitted to yet another generation.

Mutations that affect a single base in the DNA are called **point mutations**. In a point mutation the sequence of the nucleotide bases in the DNA is altered by the **substitution** of a single wrong base at one point along the DNA molecule. When messenger RNA is later synthesized using this modified template, one of the codons is changed. (Re-

call from Chapter 3 that in protein synthesis the message in RNA is read in codons—sequences of three bases.) This may or may not lead to a protein in which one of the amino acids is different from the normal protein. Even if one amino acid

Genetic variability is important for several reasons. From an evolutionary point of view great variability among individuals in a population means that some individuals are likely to have a selective advantage in any new environment. Certain individuals will have a combination of genes that will help them to survive a given change in the environment; others might survive in another changed environment—variability improves the chances that some individuals will survive no matter what environmental changes occur. From a more personal viewpoint our genes are what give us our unique characteristics. Except for identical twins (those that develop from the same fertilized egg), each human has a different set of genes from any other human. Finally, variability is important from a medical point of view. When we realize, for example, that humans are genetically highly variable, we can understand how individual responses to diseases and treatments can be so variable.

is different, the functioning of the protein product may or may not be altered.

Mutations that involve the addition or deletion of one or more bases are called **frameshift mutations**. (Frameshift mutations are sometimes considered a kind of point mutation.) In a frameshift mutation the sequence of the bases beyond the addition or deletion is altered. For example, if the normal sequence of bases is A-T-T-C-G-C-G-A-C-T, deleting the first C causes the triplets to read A-T-T, G-C-G, A-C-T, instead of A-T-T, C-G-C, and G-A-C. Adding a third T following the first two T's changes the triplets to read A-T-T, T-C-G, C-G-A. Clearly, the sequence of amino acids in the resulting protein would be vastly different from the sequence in the normal protein. Frameshift mutations are almost always deleterious.

The most common causes of mutations are chemicals and radiation, such as X rays and ultraviolet light. These agents, called mutagens, may cause substitution, addition, or deletion of bases, affecting the triplets as described above. They also may alter the charges on the bases or their molecular structure and thus their chemical properties. Some chemical mutagens slip between the bases in DNA and deform the helix so that errors are introduced into the pairing process.

The effects of mutations on the structure and function of the body are varied. Most, however, involve modifications in the structural proteins or enzymes of the affected cells. Such changes can be small, such as a change in a single amino acid in protein, but most are more extensive. Sickle cell anemia, for example, results from the substitution of one amino acid in the protein portion of hemoglobin, causing the coiled structure of hemoglobin to change. This greatly reduces the oxygen-carrying capacity of the erythrocytes. Many metabolic diseases result from the absence of a single enzyme, as will be explained later in this chapter. More extensive alterations may lead to some of the chromosomal abnormalities described below.

Chromosomal Abnormalities

Chromosomal abnormalities include a variety of alterations in either the configuration or the number of chromosomes. All of these abnormalities are more extensive than the mutations discussed earlier, and many are lethal. Each of the twenty-two pairs of homologous human chromosomes, as well as chromosomes X and Y, have distinguishing structural characteristics, and each homologous pair is designated by a number from 1 to 22. A photograph of the chromosomes arranged in numerical order is called a **karyotype**. The karyotype of a female child (2X chromosomes

and no Y chromosome) with Down's syndrome is shown in Figure 27.6. (Down's syndrome is discussed below.) Through special cell culture techniques scientists can determine the nature of chromosomal alterations in abnormal conditions. Such abnormalities can be classified into two general categories, chromosomal aberrations and changes in chromosome number.

Many kinds of **chromosomal aberrations** can occur; two—deletion and translocation—will be discussed here.

A **deletion** occurs when a segment of a chromosome is lost. Using letters of the alphabet to represent whole genes, a chromosome can be represented as follows: A-B-C-D-E-F-G-H-I-J-K. (Of course, a chromosome contains many more genes than represented here, but for simplicity we will look only at a few genes.) In a deletion some of the genes are lost so our hypothetical chromosome could be represented as: A-B-C-D-E-F-G-H, where I-J-K is the lost segment. The "cat cry" syndrome (*cri du chat*) in which an infant has a mewing, catlike cry, is an example of a deletion defect; part of chromosome 5 is missing. Individuals with this syndrome survive but are seriously mentally retarded and have a number of other defects.

A **translocation** occurs when a segment of one chromosome breaks away from its normal location and attaches to another nonhomologous chromosome. Again, the altered configuration may interfere with the pairing of homologous chromosomes, and some information may be lost at the break points. Translocation of parts of chromosomes 14 and 21 can lead to Down's syndrome.

Changes in chromosome number result in the creation of individuals with more or less than the normal forty-six chromosomes. Two of the several ways such an event can occur are as follows: (1) The chromatids of a chromosome fail to separate during meiosis so that one gamete receives two chromosomes, and the other gamete receives none. This event is called **nondisjunction**. (2) One of a pair of chromatids lags behind in the spindle formation, and one gamete is formed lacking a chromosome while the other gamete is normal. (The lagging chromosome is simply lost; it fails to become incorporated in either of the gametes.)

Most individuals with Down's symdrome have the normal complement of chromosomes plus all or most of an extra chromosome 21 (Figure 27.6). This condition, called trisomy 21, results from an error in oogenesis or spermatogenesis, so that one of the gametes has an extra chromosome 21, or from a translocation. Until recently it was thought that the error usually occurred in the ovum, though evidence now exists that in about one-fourth of the cases the error is in the sperm. Analyses of the frequency of infants with Down's syndrome by age of the parents indicates that older women, older men, extremely young women, and

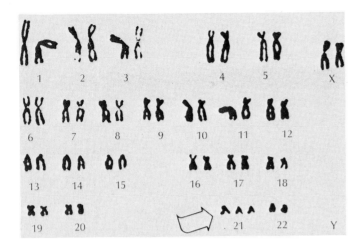

Figure 27.6 A karyotype of a female child with Down's syndrome. (Courtesy of Dr. Joe Hin Tjio and the National Institute of General Medical Studies, National Institutes of Health.)

extremely young men run a higher than normal risk of producing a child with Down's syndrome. When parents have had a child affected by Down's syndrome, they are often concerned about the likelihood of having another such child. Data show that in families where the syndrome was caused by translocation a high risk of recurrence exists, but in families where the syndrome was caused by nondisjunction the risk of recurrence is no greater than in families where the syndrome has not appeared.

Individuals affected by Down's syndrome are usually severely mentally retarded and have a number of other physical abnormalities; 60% do not survive beyond ten years of age. They also have a propensity toward developing cataracts and leukemia. In the past most affected children were institutionalized, but many are now cared for at home because of the greater mental and physical development they can achieve.

Several chromosomal abnormalities result from defective transmission of the sex chromosomes. Individuals with **Klinefelter's syndrome** (Figure 27.7) have an extra X chromosome (XXY), which may be received from either parent through nondisjunction. Such people have male genitals but are usually sterile. They may develop breasts, their limbs may be elongated, and their mental development may be slightly or significantly below normal. Individuals with **Turner's syndrome** (Figure 27.8) have a single X chromosome and no Y chromosome, usually designated XO. The X chromosome may be received from either the mother or the father. These individuals are female but are sterile. They

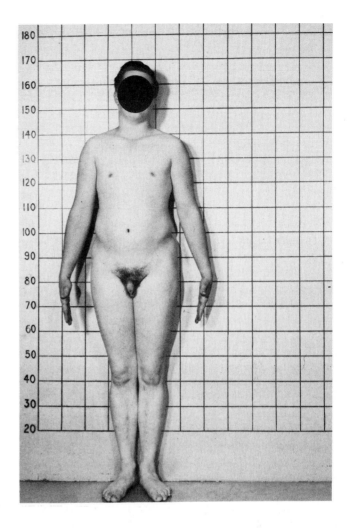

Figure 27.7 Nineteen-year-old boy with Klinefelter's syndrome. (Reproduced with permission from John Money, *Sex Errors of the Human Body*, The Johns Hopkins University Press, 1968.)

often have poor spatial visualization ability and may be below normal in intelligence.

PRINCIPLES OF GENETICS

Objective 7. Define the major terms used in genetics.

Objective 8. Explain the principles of segregation and independent assortment.

Objective 9. Explain how probability is involved in determining inheritance and use a Punnett square to illustrate selected probabilities.

Objective 10. Interpret a pedigree diagram.

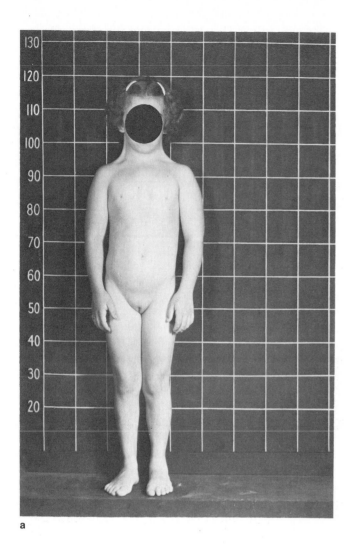

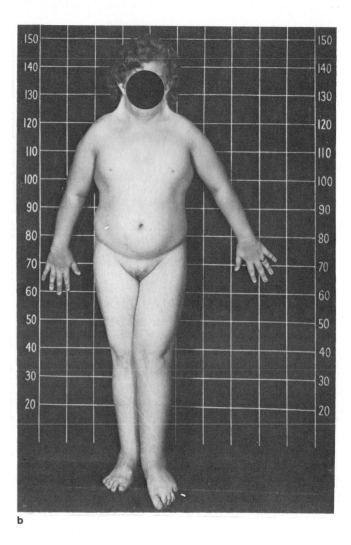

Figure 27.8 Girls with Turner's syndrome: (**a**) a 10½-year-old, (**b**) a 15-year-old. (Reproduced with permission from John Money, *Sex Errors of the Body*, The Johns Hopkins University Press, 1968.)

Genetic Terminology

The basic terminology of genetics is summarized in Table 27.1. Use of the terms is illustrated in the following example of the action of genes that carry information about the presence or absence of skin pigmentation.

Pairs of homologous chromosomes having different forms of the same gene on them were shown in Figure 27.5. For example, form *A* of the gene is present on one member of a pair of chromosomes, and form *a* is present on the other member of the pair. The alternate forms—*A* and *a*—of the gene are called **alleles**. Let us suppose that allele *A* carries information that is essential for the development of normal skin pigmentation and that allele *a* is modified so that it

fails to allow normal pigment development. If the homologous chromosomes both carry the same allele, *AA* or *aa*, the individual is said to be **homozygous** for the characteristic. If the homologous chromosomes carry different alleles, *Aa*, the individual is said to be **heterozygous** for the characteristic.

The terms genotype and phenotype can be applied to a particular inherited characteristic or to all of the inherited characteristics of an individual. The combination of alleles present for a particular characteristic, *AA*, *Aa*, or *aa*, is the **genotype** for that characteristic. The entire genotype is the combination of all the alleles on all the chromosomes that determine the inherited characteristics of the individual.

Table 27.1 Basic Terminology of Genetics

Term	Definition
Allele	One of two or more alternate forms of a gene that occupies a particular locus or site on a particular chromosome
Homozygous	A condition in which the alleles of a gene on the two homologous chromosomes are alike
Heterozygous	A condition in which the alleles of a gene on the two homologous chromosomes are not alike
Genotype	The combination of the alleles at a given locus carried by an individual; for all genes together the genetic make-up of the individual
Phenotype	The outward appearance of the individual with respect to a particular characteristic (or all characteristics) determined by the genotype
Dominant	An allele that is expressed in the phenotype when it is carried either homozygously or heterozygously
Recessive	An allele that is expressed in the phenotype only when carried homozygously
Carrier	A heterozygous individual of normal phenotype who has in his or her genotype a hidden recessive allele and can thus transmit the recessive allele to offspring
Autosomal inheritance	Inheritance of characteristics that are carried on one of the twenty-two pairs (in humans) of autosomal, not sex, chromosomes
Sex-linked inheritance	Inheritance of characteristics carried on the X chromosome

The **phenotype** is the appearance of the individual with respect to a particular inherited characteristic or the overall appearance with respect to all inherited characteristics. For the characteristics in our example the phenotype might be either normal skin color or albinism (lack of pigment). Phenotypically albino individuals will have the genotype aa for that characteristic. Individuals with normal skin color will have a genotype of either AA or Aa (and you could not tell which by looking at them).

To understand more about how the genotype determines the phenotype, we need to distinguish between dominant and recessive alleles. A **dominant** allele (symbolized by a capital letter, such as A in our example) is expressed in

the phenotype whenever it appears in the genotype. A **recessive** allele (symbolized by a lowercase letter, such as a in our example) is expressed in the phenotype when it is carried homozygously and the dominant allele is absent. Individuals with genotype either AA or Aa will have normal skin pigment because of the presence of the A allele; only individuals with the genotype aa will lack pigment and have the recessive phenotype of albinism.

Heterozygous individuals are **carriers** of an unexpressed recessive gene. In our example an individual with genotype Aa has normal skin color but is a carrier of an allele for albinism, which may be transmitted to offspring.

Of the twenty-three pairs of chromosomes in the human genetic makeup, twenty-two pairs are said to be **autosomes**: They are normally present in homologous pairs so that two alleles for each characteristic are present. These alleles may be identical, as in homozygous individuals, or different, as in heterozygous individuals. The inheritance of genes on these chromosomes is called **autosomal inheritance**. The other (twenty-third) pair of chromosomes are the sex chromosomes, X and Y, which are not homologous. As we saw earlier, males have one of each of these chromosomes, but females have two X chromosomes. In addition to carrying genes that code for sexual characteristics, the X chromosome carries a number of genes that code for characteristics unrelated to sex, such as color blindness (discussed later in this chapter). In females the homologous X chromosomes behave in much the same way as the autosomes because two alleles of each gene are present for each characteristic. The Y chromosome carries little genetic information, but it does cause the reproductive system to develop male structures (see Chapter 28). None of the genes on the Y chromosome is homologous to any one of the genes on the X chromosome. A male has only one X chromosome and thus only one of each of the genes on the X chromosome; any recessive alleles present are not masked by the presence of a dominant allele. The inheritance of genes on the X chromosome is called **sex-linked inheritance**.

Principle of Segregation

The **principle of segregation** states that the alleles on homologous chromosomes are segregated, or separated, in the production of gametes. Recall that in meiosis one member of each pair of homologous chromosomes is distributed to each gamete. For example, an individual who is a carrier of albinism (genotype Aa) has normal allele A on one member of a pair of homologous chromosomes and allele a on the other chromosome of that pair. When the individual with genotype Aa forms gametes, half the gametes will receive a copy of the chromosome with allele *A* and half will receive a copy of the chromosome with allele *a*. Thus, the alleles of homologous chromosomes are separated, or segregated, into different gametes during the process of meiosis. A gamete contains *either* allele *A* or allele *a* and *never* a mixture of that information; a gamete can never be heterozygous.

> The observation originally noted by Gregor Mendel that characteristics are inherited through the transmission of discrete units of information, now called genes, was a significant step in our understanding of inheritance. Prior to the acceptance of Mendel's work, some scientists thought different tissues—muscle, skin, nerve—contributed particles to eggs or sperm, and that the particles blended together in the new individual to determine its characteristics.

The principle of segregation also applies to genes with more than two alleles. As explained in Chapter 16, there are three alleles of the gene for ABO blood types. However, any one individual carries only two of these—one on each of a pair of homologous chromosomes.

Principle of Independent Assortment

The **principle of independent assortment**, which applies to the inheritance of two or more traits, states that the genetic information for each trait is distributed to the gametes independently of the distribution for the other traits; that is, the assortment or distribution of the alleles for trait A occurs separately or independently of the alleles for trait B. Gregor Mendel first proposed this principle in 1866, though the significance of his work was not recognized until 1900. Following the characteristics of garden peas, he based his principle on the observation that seed shape and seed color, for example, were each inherited independently of one another. We now know that it is chromosomes and not individual genes that assort independently. Refer to Figure 27.2 and note that whole chromosomes and not individual genes separate during meiosis, and all of the genes on a single chromosome go to the same gamete. This generalization about independent assortment of chromosomes always holds true. However, some genetic variability of the chromosomes is produced when chromosome segments are exchanged during crossing-over.

To illustrate independent assortment, two characteristics must be followed simultaneously. Suppose each member of a couple carries recessive alleles for both albinism and phenylketonuria. Let us assume that the genes for these two characteristics are carried on separate chromosomes. In addition to the symbols *A* and *a*, already defined for albinism, we will use *P* to denote the normal gene for metabolism of phenylalanine and *p* to denote the defective gene. (See Chapter 24 for a discussion of phenylketonuria.) The genotypes of both the mother and the father are *Aa Pp*; members of one pair of homologous chromosomes carry genes *A* and *a*, and members of another pair carry genes *P* and *p*. Each parent will produce four different kinds of gametes in equal numbers, depending on which gene for skin pigment and which gene for phenylalanine metabolism appear in the same gamete. The possible gametes of each parent and the genotypes and phenotypes that can be produced from the union of gametes are shown in Figure 27.9. Notice that 9/16 (9 out of 16) of the hypothetical offspring in the figure have at least one dominant gene for each characteristic. Thus, the probability is 9/16 that any particular child of this couple will be normal, *A-P-*. (The dashes indicate that either a dominant or a recessive gene may be present as the other member of the gene pair.) As long as one dominant gene is present for each characteristic, the child will be normal with regard to the two characteristics being considered. The couple also has a 3/16 probability of producing a child with normal skin color but affected with phenylketonuria, *A-pp*. Likewise, they have a 3/16 probability of producing an albino child who is normal with respect to phenylketonuria, *aaP-*. Finally, they have a 1/16 probability of having a child affected by both defects, *aapp*.

Probability and Punnett Squares

Figure 27.9, called a **Punnett square**, is a way of diagramming the assortment of alleles in the parents' gametes to see the **probability** that particular genotypes and phenotypes will be produced. All of the possible gametes (with respect to the alleles being studied) that the mother can produce are placed along the top columns of the square. All of the possible gametes that the father can produce are placed along the left side of the rows of the square. Each cell of the square is filled in with the genes from the appropriate row and column.

Probabilities are determined by counting the total number of squares and expressing the number with a given characteristic as a fraction of the total. It is essential to understand that the probability of a second child having a certain characteristic is independent of the probability of a

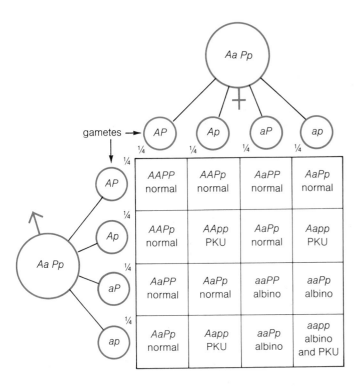

Figure 27.9 A Punnett square showing the parents' gametes, and the genotypes and phenotypes possible among their offspring, for the albinism–phenylketonuria example.

first child having the same characteristic. In the example above the probability of the couple having a child with both defects is 1/16. Even if the first child has the defects (or does not have the defects), the probability of the second child having both defects is still 1/16.

Pedigrees

A **pedigree** is a tracing of the phenotypic characteristics through several generations of a family. As explained below, genotypes can often be inferred by studying the phenotypes of several generations. In a pedigree squares are used to represent males and circles to represent females. A horizontal line between a male and a female symbol indicates a mating. The offspring of a mating are shown as symbols suspended from a long horizontal line below but connected to the symbols for the parents. Each row of symbols in a pedigree represents a generation—parents at the top, their children and the spouses of the children in the second row, and the grandchildren (and spouses) in the third row. Individuals having the phenotypic characteristic under study are designated by shaded symbols.

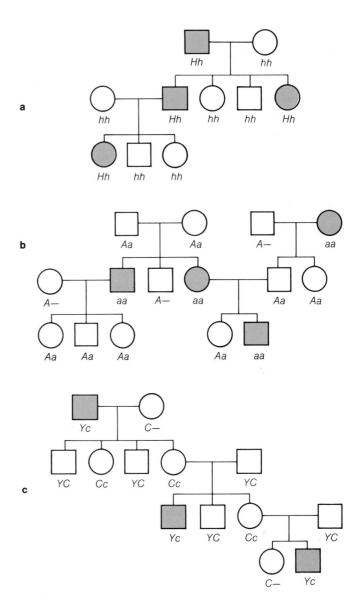

Figure 27.10 Pedigrees illustrating three different forms of inheritance: (**a**) an autosomal dominant characteristic, (**b**) an autosomal recessive characteristic, (**c**) a sex-linked recessive characteristic.

Figure 27.10 shows the pedigrees of three different types of inheritance. The properties seen in a pedigree illustrating the inheritance of an autosomal dominant characteristic (a) are that (1) all affected individuals have at least one affected parent, (2) about half the progeny of an affected individual are also affected, and (3) both sexes are affected with equal frequency.

Let us suppose that the particular disorder in this pedigree is Huntington's disease, a genetic defect that leads to degeneration of the nervous system. All normal individuals have the genotype *hh*; affected individuals may have the genotype *Hh* or *HH*. (Incidentally, this example illustrates that recessive genes may be normal, though dominant genes more often are normal.) The disorder usually does not appear until after an individual has had children and has possibly passed the defective gene on to them. However, if a geneticist can study several members of a family who are past the typical age of onset of the disease (thirty-five to fifty), a fairly reliable determination of genotypes can be made. In the figure we can determine that the affected children and grandchildren are heterozygous because each has one normal parent past the onset age. The normal parent must have been homozygous and must have passed to all offspring the normal recessive allele.

Pedigrees can often be useful in determining the exact genotype of an individual and thus the probability of that particular individual transmitting a gene to offspring. Any heterozygous individual who has Huntington's disease has a 50:50 chance of transmitting it to each offspring. The difficulty of making predictions about Huntington's disease is that the disease often does not appear until after the reproductive years.

The properties seen in a pedigree illustrating the inheritance of an autosomal recessive characteristic (b) are that (1) parents lacking the characteristic in their phenotypes can produce offspring displaying the characteristic, (2) the characteristic often skips a generation, and (3) both sexes are affected with equal frequency.

Let us suppose that the characteristic in the pedigree is albinism, the inability to produce melanin pigment. All affected individuals have the genotype *aa*, and normal individuals may have the genotype *AA* or *Aa*. An albino must be homozygous and thus always transmits an allele for albinism to all offspring. Therefore, normal offspring of an albino and a normal parent are always heterozygous *Aa*. If two normal parents produce albino offspring, both must be heterozygous *Aa*. The pedigree shows that all the individuals in the third generation are heterozygous except for the affected individual. Should one of these heterozygous individuals marry another heterozygous individual, the couple would have a 25% chance of having an albino child. (Prepare a Punnett square to demonstrate that this is so.)

The properties seen in a pedigree illustrating the inheritance of a sex-linked recessive characteristic (c) are that (1) parents lacking the characteristic in their phenotypes can produce offspring with the characteristic, (2) the characteristic often skips a generation, and (3) more males than females are affected. (Sex-linked dominant characteristics do exist, but they are rare and will not be discussed here.)

Suppose the characteristic being studied in the pedigree is color blindness. The gene for color blindness is carried on the X chromosome; hence, males have a single allele for color blindness or a single allele for normal color vision. The Y chromosome carries no information for color vision. We will use the symbol Y for the Y chromosome, *C* for an allele for normal vision on the X chromosome, and *c* for an allele for color blindness on the X chromosome. Thus, the genotype of a color-blind male is Y*c* and the genotype for a male with normal color vision is Y*C*. Females with normal color vision may have genotypes *CC* or *Cc*. Those with *Cc* are carriers of the color blindness allele and may transmit it to their offspring. In the rare instances that a woman is color blind, she has the genotype *cc*.

Punnett squares can be used to illustrate the inheritance of color blindness. A normal father and a carrier mother (Figure 27.11a) have a ¼ probability of producing each of the following offspring: normal (noncarrier) female, carrier female, normal male, and color-blind male. Among the offspring of a normal (noncarrier) mother and a color-blind father (Figure 27.11b) all the females will be carriers, and all the males will be normal. A carrier mother and a color-blind father (Figure 27.11c) have a ¼ probability of producing each of the following offspring: carrier female, color-blind female, normal male, and color-blind male.

Several generalizations about the inheritance of color blindness (and other sex-linked recessive characteristics) can be made. Color-blind males always transmit an allele for color blindness to their daughters (on the X chromosome) and a Y chromosome to their sons. Daughters of color-blind males are always carriers of at least one allele for color blindness; should they also receive a recessive gene for color blindness from their mothers, they will be color blind. Color blindness appears more frequently in males than in females because males require only one color blindness allele to display the condition, whereas females require two such alleles. Color blindness often skips a generation—grandfather is color blind, mother is a carrier, and her son is color blind.

Pedigrees also can be used to illustrate the effects of deleterious (harmful) genes. Deleterious alleles arise as mutations that are most often recessive. Estimates are that every human being carries between one and ten deleterious recessive alleles. However, these genes do no harm un-

	C	c
C	CC normal female	Cc carrier female
Y	YC normal male	Yc color-blind male

	C	C
c	Cc carrier female	Cc carrier female
Y	YC normal male	YC normal male

	C	c
c	Cc carrier female	cc color-blind female
Y	YC normal male	Yc color-blind male

a   b   c

Figure 27.11 Punnett squares showing the inheritance of color blindness: (**a**) a normal father and a carrier mother, (**b**) color-blind father and normal (noncarrier) mother, (**c**) color-blind father and carrier mother.

less an individual receives the deleterious allele from both parents, in which case the recessive deleterious characteristic will be expressed. The recessive genetic defects listed in Table 27.2 in the next section are examples of alleles that arose as mutations many generations previously.

The likelihood of both parents carrying the same recessive allele is greatly increased through inbreeding. The pedigree of a first cousin marriage (Figure 27.12) illustrates how such transmission might occur. All of us receive half our chromosomes (and thus half our genes) from each parent. The genes from each parent in turn came from our grandparents—half of each parent's genes from each grandparent. Thus, we receive about one-fourth of our genes from each grandparent. However, because of independent assortment (and to a lesser degree because of crossing-over) the parents' gametes may contain somewhat more or less than equal numbers of the grandparents' genes. Because first cousins have common grandparents, approximately one-fourth of their genes come from each of the two common grandparents. Because of these common genes first cousins run a high risk of receiving the same harmful gene from one of the grandparents. Thus, matings between cousins increase the likelihood that the offspring will receive two copies of the same recessive harmful gene and thus express the defect.

In most cultures marriage between closely related individuals is discouraged or even forbidden by law. The origin of such customs is obscure, but it is known that the incidence of spontaneous abortions and stillbirths is much higher among related mates than among unrelated ones.

Spontaneous abortions and stillbirths can be caused by the presence of **lethal genes**—extremely deleterious genes that cause death. Though some lethal genes may have arisen as new mutations, most are carried in the population in the heterozygous condition. When an individual receives two such alleles and is homozygous for the lethal characteristic, death is inevitable.

Other Mechanisms of Inheritance

The various mechanisms of inheritance discussed here—dominant versus recessive and autosomal versus sex-linked—account for the inheritance of many characteristics. Other mechanisms do exist, however. Often a dominant gene does not completely mask the presence of a recessive gene, and both the dominant and the recessive characteristic will be present to some degree in the phenotype. For example, in sickle cell anemia the normal individual has the genotype SS, the individual with sickle cell anemia has the genotype ss, and the individual with sickle cell trait has the genotype Ss. The heterozygous individual has two kinds of hemoglobin—some synthesized by the S gene and some by the s gene; the dominant gene does not completely mask the recessive one.

Another mechanism of inheritance is **polygenic inheritance**, in which several genes at different locations on the chromosomes operate together to determine a characteristic. Examples of characteristics inherited in this manner include height; intelligence; color of skin, hair, and eyes (other than albinism); and many other human traits.

A third mechanism involves penetrance or the lack of it. The **penetrance** of a gene is the degree to which it is expressed when present. For example, some dominant genes (which theoretically should be expressed if present)

Table 27.2 Selected Human Genetic Diseases

Name of Disease and Inheritance Pattern	Description
Achondroplasia (autosomal dominant)	Dwarfism, with especially short limbs and adult height of about 4 feet. Defect has a high mutation rate and can appear in families never before affected.
Albinism (autosomal recessive)	Lack of an enzyme to convert amino acid tyrosine to the pigment melanin. Individuals have white hair and very fair skin; the iris of the eye appears pink due to blood vessels unobscured by normal pigmentation.
Brachydactyly (autosomal dominant)	Individuals have very short, stubby fingers.
Bruton agammaglobulinemia (X-linked recessive)	Almost complete inability to form antibodies to infectious agents. Affected individuals require lifelong gamma globulin treatment and remain susceptible to infections.
Cystic fibrosis (autosomal recessive)	Excess mucus blocks respiratory passages and impairs release of digestive enzymes. Affected individuals receiving intensive therapy sometimes live to adulthood.
Duchenne muscular dystrophy (X-linked recessive)	Muscle wasting usually begins by age six and leads to paralysis and death by early adulthood. Frequent appearance of new cases in previously unaffected families due to high rate of new mutations. Research to detect carriers is in progress.
Huntington's disease (autosomal dominant)	Onset from ten to sixty years of age but often not until after affected individual has had children. Progressive deterioration of nervous system leads to uncontrollable movements, personality changes, mental impairment, and, ultimately, death. Research to detect carriers is in progress.
Lesch-Nyhan syndrome (X-linked recessive)	Enzyme defect causes overproduction of uric acid. The affected individual is mentally retarded and engages in self-mutilation. Uric acid accumulation leads to kidney damage, but this effect can now be minimized by drug treatment. Tests are available to detect carriers.
Marfan's syndrome (autosomal dominant)	Produces long spidery appendages, eye defects, and aortic disease. It has been speculated that Abraham Lincoln was mildly affected by the disease.
Phenylketonuria (PKU) (autosomal recessive)	Enzyme defect causes inability to metabolize the amino acid phenylalanine. Mental retardation results unless the patient is placed on a diet that is low in phenylalanine in the first few weeks of life. Tests are available to detect this defect in neonates.
Sickle cell anemia (autosomal recessive)	Enzyme defect causes abnormal hemoglobin production. Results in chronic anemia and crises with extreme pain in joints, blockage of blood vessels by sickle-shaped red blood cells, and need for transfusions. Research looks promising to find a chemical to prevent abnormal behavior of hemoglobin. Heterozygous individuals are resistant to the disease malaria.
Tay-Sachs disease (autosomal recessive)	Defect in lipid metabolism. Results in progressive deterioration of nervous tissue in an apparently normal infant until death at about age three or four. Tests are available to identify carriers and to detect affected fetuses prenatally.

may be incompletely expressed; that is, the characteristic they produce in the phenotype is not as clearly defined as might be expected. This is called incomplete penetrance. Marfan's syndrome, mentioned in Table 27.2, is caused by a dominant gene that may show incomplete penetrance. An individual affected by the syndrome may have severe effects if the gene achieves complete penetrance but only mild symptoms if the gene achieves only incomplete penetrance.

HUMAN GENETIC DISORDERS

Objective 11. For the human disorders presented in this section, describe the inheritance pattern and the effects of the disease.

The inheritance pattern and effects of selected human genetic disorders are given in Table 27.2. Additional information on a few of those disorders is given below.

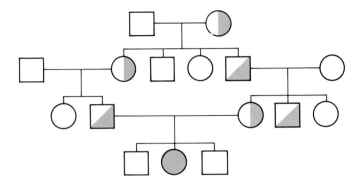

Figure 27.12 Pedigree of a cousin marriage. Half-shaded symbols indicate carriers of a deleterious gene; fully shaded symbol indicates an individual affected by the defect.

Cystic Fibrosis

Cystic fibrosis is an autosomal recessive disorder more common among Caucasians than other races. It causes the mucous glands of the digestive and respiratory systems to produce excessive amounts of a thick mucus that block the ducts of the glands. The enzyme NADH dehydrogenase may be involved in producing cystic fibrosis as it appears to be overactive in some individuals with cystic fibrosis and in some carriers of the disease. If further research confirms the relationship between cystic fibrosis and the enzyme, the properties of the enzyme may be usable in developing a screening test for carriers of the defective gene.

> One characteristic of cystic fibrosis is that fibroblasts from the skin of affected individuals show greater resistance to the toxic effects of the chemical dexamethasone than do normal cells. The cells of carriers are intermediate in their resistance to toxicity. This fact is potentially useful in detecting carriers and for determining whether a developing embryo is affected by the disease.

Huntington's Disease

The nature of the defect produced by the presence of the gene for **Huntington's disease** is unknown, but the disease is characterized by progressive degeneration of nervous tissue. One recent study has shown that lymphocytes from people with Huntington's disease react with brain tissue from others who also have the disease. The reaction is similar to the cellular immune response and suggests that some immunologically active substance may be produced, which may be the cause or the effect of brain degeneration. Although this does not prove that Huntington's disease is an autoimmune disease, it does offer a possible avenue of investigation that might further understanding of the disease.

Lesch-Nyhan Syndrome

Lesch-Nyhan syndrome is an incurable sex-linked recessive disease caused by the absence of an enzyme needed to metabolize uric acid. An affected child produces excessive amounts of uric acid and engages in self-mutilation—chewing away parts of the lips and fingers. Efforts to determine why this occurs have led to the finding that victims of Lesch-Nyhan syndrome produce smaller quantities of norepinephrine during stress than normal individuals. The relatively diminished response of the sympathetic nervous system to stress may provide clues to the further clarification of the mechanism of this disease.

Sickle Cell Anemia

Sickle cell anemia was the first inherited disease to be understood at the molecular level. When an individual receives two alleles for sickle cell anemia, these alleles cause the synthesis of hemoglobin in which the protein globin differs from normal by a single amino acid. With one normal and one sickle cell allele, some normal and some abnormal globin is produced. Therefore, a seemingly minor error in the gene, and therefore in the hemoglobin, causes many physiological effects in the person suffering from the disease. Some of these effects were described in Chapter 16.

GENETIC SCREENING AND GENETIC COUNSELING

Objective 12. Define genetic screening; explain the different purposes of neonatal and adult screening; list several factors that enter into the development and operation of genetic screening programs.

Objective 13. Define genetic counseling and describe the major components of the counseling process.

Genetic Screening

Various estimates of the prevalence of genetic disease in the United States indicate that between 5 and 10% of the population are affected in some way by an inherited disease and that about one-fourth of all hospital beds are occupied by individuals who are suffering from some effect of genetic disorders. In pediatric wards the proportion of occupants with genetic diseases is even higher. Genetic screening can help to identify affected infants so that any available treatment may be initiated. It can also help to identify prospective parents who are at risk of producing genetically defective infants. Thus, screening offers opportunities to reduce the suffering and the cost of treatment now associated with genetic diseases.

Genetic screening is a process for identifying individuals with genotypes that produce disease or carriers who can transmit the disease-producing allele to descendants. The intent of genetic screening is both to improve the care received by those with genetic diseases and to provide information to those who might transmit a harmful gene so they can make informed decisions about reproduction (see Figure 27.13).

Neonatal screening is used to detect the presence of genetic-metabolic diseases at an early age. Screening tests are available to identify about thirty different inborn metabolic errors; a number of chromosomal disorders also can be detected. Perhaps the most widely used screening test is directed toward the detection of phenylketonuria (PKU). The test involves discovering the abnormal metabolic product of phenylalanine in blood or urine. If the condition is identified in the first few weeks of life, the infant can be placed on a diet low in phenylalanine, and the usual effects of mental retardation can be prevented or greatly reduced.

PKU screening is an example of a program that meets most of the criteria for a good screening program. First, the screening test is sufficiently reliable to be used with only a small risk of error. Second, the cost of performing the test is low enough to make mass screening feasible. Third, effective therapy exists to treat the disease when it is detected. Fourth, economic benefits of detection and treatment clearly exist because the alternative is years of institutional care. Finally, legal and ethical issues are minimal.

One of the aims of **screening for adult carriers** of harmful genes is to give carriers an informed choice of reproductive options. One of the most effective screening programs for carrier detection has been developed for Tay-Sachs disease, a lipid storage disorder caused by an abnormal enzyme. The disease leads to progressive neurological deterioration and ends in death at about four years of age. The disorder is rare except in the descendants of Ashkenazi (of eastern European ancestry) Jews, where it occurs with a frequency of 1:3600 births. The factors that have contributed to the success of Tay-Sachs screening programs are the following:

1. The allele is most common in a small, defined population.

2. Simple, reliable, and relatively inexpensive testing can detect the carriers of the autosomal recessive allele.

3. Mated carriers are the only couples at risk of producing an affected child.

4. Prenatal diagnosis through amniocentesis and cell culturing can be used to determine whether the fetus is affected early enough in the pregnancy for the pregnancy to be safely terminated if that option is chosen.

5. The at-risk population is generally well educated and interested in avoiding the disease.

6. Prescreening educational efforts have made voluntary screening known to many potential carriers and reduced resistance to the discovery that one is a carrier of a harmful gene.

Amniocentesis **Amniocentesis** (Figure 27.14) is a procedure for withdrawing amniotic fluid (the fluid that surrounds a developing fetus) from inside the uterus. The sample of fluid is usually taken about the fourteenth or fifteenth week after conception when the total volume of fluid is about 200 milliliters. As much as 25 milliliters can be withdrawn without danger of collapsing the amniotic cavity. Sonography, a technique involving high-frequency sound waves to locate tissues of different densities within the body, is used to determine the location of the fetus and placenta just prior to performing amniocentesis, thus preventing accidental damage to the fetus and placenta.

Amniotic fluid contains cells from the skin of the fetus and other sources. These cells can be used to determine the sex of the infant, to detect certain biochemical and enzymatic abnormalities, and to identify some abnormalities in the number of chromosomes.

Other screening methods Blood samples taken from adult prospective carriers of genetic diseases can reveal a number of inborn errors of metabolism. The list of detectable errors is growing rapidly, particularly for conditions involving an abnormality in a single enzyme. Improved techniques for measuring enzyme activity have led to the ability to detect carriers of some abnormal recessive alleles. A typical

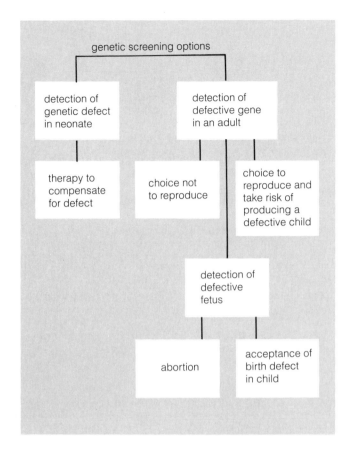

Figure 27.13 Flow chart describing genetic screening options.

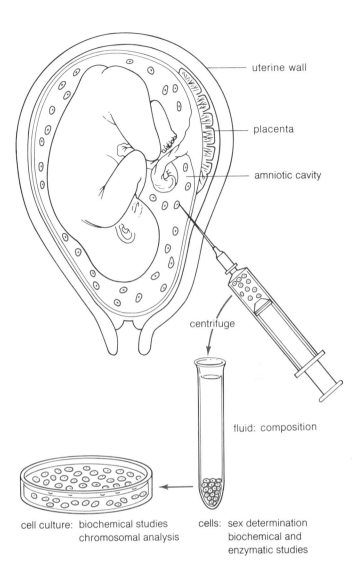

Figure 27.14 The procedure for amniocentesis.

screening test for carriers depends on the carrier's enzyme activity being sufficiently high to allow adequate function but significantly lower than the activity found in normal noncarrier individuals.

Factors to be considered in screening programs   Improved opportunities for screening and increased responsibility to use the procedures will go hand in hand with other current trends in health care. These trends will probably include more emphasis on health maintenance and disease prevention, technological advances in the detection and treatment of genetic defects, improved education, and the emerging expectation that people take greater personal responsibility for their own health. Both health professionals and those they serve will be involved in determining the nature and extent of genetic screening programs. Some of the factors that must be considered in the development and operation of screening programs are summarized in Table 27.3.

Genetic Counseling

As screening techniques improve, there is greater need for people to use counseling services to help them make informed decisions. Thus, genetic counseling is becoming a significant component of total medical services.

Genetic counseling is the provision to counselees of information about a genetic disease. It also includes assistance in coping with the problem the disease has caused or may cause for the counselees and their relatives. Most counseling sessions are arranged after it has been determined that the counselee or a family member may be affected by a harmful gene, a chromosomal abnormality, or a birth defect.

Table 27.3 Factors Considered in Screening Programs

Factor	Comments
Incidence of affected individuals and carriers	The greater the frequency of a defect, the more likely it is that screening will reduce its frequency if affected individuals choose not to have children. Screening is also effective when a portion of the population has a much higher incidence of a defective gene than the general population (Tay-Sachs in Ashkenazi Jews, for example).
Severity of disease and prognosis	Genetic traits range from slight inconveniences (left-handedness) to serious disease (hemophilia) and may even cause death (muscular dystrophy and Huntington's disease). The more serious the defect and the less available any treatment, the greater is the need for screening programs.
Screening of carriers versus fetuses	Detecting carriers allows the carriers to make choices about whether to conceive children. Prenatal screening of fetuses offers only the option of abortion or having the child if the fetus is found to be affected.
Cost of screening	Neonatal screening for PKU costs only a few dollars per infant; the cost of screening 11,500 infants to detect one case is relatively high. Screening adults in a population known to have a high number of carriers of a particular gene detects such carriers at reasonable cost. Amniocentesis is generally performed only in high-risk pregnancies because of the expense (and also the small risk of the procedure itself).
Economic aspects of screening	Cost-benefit analysis can be used to compare the cost of institutional care of a PKU child versus the cost of screening and treatment. Similar analyses could be applied to other genetic diseases for which differences in costs depend on whether the disease is detected.
Reliability of tests	Even when tests are performed by experienced technicians, the possibility of false positives and false negatives must be considered.
Legal aspects of screening	Though most legal decisions rest on precedent, precedent may not be available for legal decisions about screening. Furthermore, precedent may not be appropriate unless the earlier decision made use of currently available genetic information. Problems usually involve consent (whether or not it was informed consent), mandatory testing, and access to the results of the test by employers, insurance companies, prospective spouses, and family members.
Ethical aspects of screening	Decisions can be more ethical if all relevant facts are available, feelings of involved parties are considered, and the decision is free from self-interest and strong feelings. (See the essay on ethical decision making at the end of this chapter.)
Social aspects of screening	All the above factors that enter into decisions about genetic screening operate in a social context. Society pays the cost (through taxes) for much of the hospital and other institutional care of those with genetic disease. Thus, society must make some decisions regarding allocation of resources for screening, treatment, and custodial care.

Components of the counseling process During a typical counseling session the counselor would first verify the diagnosis and then explain in detail the effects of the disease or defect and its prognosis, including available therapy if it exists. Next, the counselor assesses the risk to the client or family members. Assuming an accurate diagnosis, risk is determined by applying knowledge of the genetic mechanism involved in transmitting the disease to data from a complete family history. Risk should be interpreted in terms that are practical and meaningful to the counselee.

Most individuals facing a genetic problem come to the counseling session with a burden of misinformation about the disease and a poor understanding of probability. Unless the counselor overcomes these barriers to effective counseling, the client is unlikely to receive much benefit from the session. Thus, the counselor must be sure that misinformation is replaced with correct information and that probabilities are clearly and simply explained. For example, few prospective parents realize that in any pregnancy there exists a 1 to 2% probability of giving birth to a fetus with some defect. Another concept that is often difficult to explain is that the probability of a given defect appearing in later births is the same as it was for the first birth. As we saw earlier, if the probability of a defect is ¼ for the couple's first child, the probability of that defect appearing in a second, third, or later child is still ¼, regardless of whether any previous children were affected.

Counselors should also be prepared to explain reproductive options that are available. If the client is already pregnant, the choices may be limited to aborting the fetus or taking the risk of giving birth to a defective child. If prenatal diagnosis for the defect is possible, the client may be able to know with certainty whether the fetus is affected. If counseling is obtained before conception, choices can include refraining from conception, adopting, using artificial insemination (by a donor), planning for prenatal diagnosis and deferring the decision of whether to bear a child until then, or taking the risk of delivering a child with a genetic defect.

In addition to providing information, counselors also assist their clients in weighing risks, choosing among alternatives, and finally planning how they will cope with their problem. Even after the nature of the disease and the risk of its occurrence are understood, the counselee is confronted with the difficult problem of determining what is a personally acceptable risk.

A significant number of individuals who seek counseling find it difficult to acknowledge that the genetic problem really affects them. It is painful to accept the idea that, though they themselves may be healthy, they carry a harmful gene that can be transmitted to a child. Feelings of denial, guilt, and anger often accompany the realization that one carries a harmful gene. Counselors can alleviate this problem to some degree by explaining the randomness of gene assortment and indicating that every individual carries some abnormal genes. Counselors also can serve as concerned listeners as the client works through these problems.

Ultimately, the decision about how to deal with the problem must be made by the counselees. It must be a decision that they can live with. Clients vary in the kinds of risks they are willing to take; the observations of counselors seem to indicate that the seriousness of the impairment and the likely duration of the physical, emotional, and financial stresses receive greater weight than the probability that the defect exists.

GENETIC ENGINEERING

Objective 14. Define genetic engineering and list examples of different kinds of genetic engineering.

Definition

Genetic engineering is the manipulation of reproduction and heredity. Though the goal of such manipulations is to correct genetic defects or to make it possible for couples to

have children who would not be able to do so otherwise, very few techniques are currently applicable to humans.

Kinds of Genetic Engineering

Artificial insemination by a donor The first kind of genetic engineering to become available was **artificial insemination by a donor** (AID). The idea of artificial insemination is not new; it is recorded in the Talmud and has been in continuous use since the end of the eighteenth century. This technique is useful in cases in which the male partner does not ejaculate or in which he carries a harmful allele he does not wish to transmit to offspring. For example, in rare instances males ejaculate sperm into the bladder instead of through the penis. Techniques are available to flush urine from the bladder, collect sperm, and introduce them into the female's vagina, allowing such males to have their own sperm used instead of those from a donor. In cases where males carry defective genes, a sample of semen is collected from an anonymous donor. Although the father who raises the child did not contribute genes to the child, he did avoid transmitting a known defective allele.

In vitro fertilization Many women who are unable to conceive produce normal ova that never reach the uterine tubes and therefore fail to be fertilized. In England on July 25, 1978, the first infant known to have developed from in vitro ("test tube") fertilization was born. An ovum was removed from her mother's ovary and transferred to a carefully prepared sterile medium outside the mother's body. Here, the ovum was fertilized by sperm from the child's father and allowed to develop for a short period of time. The developing embryo was then transplanted to the mother's uterus, where it developed normally and was born naturally.

This technique offers hope for many infertile couples to have natural children, but it also presents various ethical questions. Although the infant that developed from in vitro fertilization (and a number of others born since) was born without apparent genetic or birth defects, it is possible that manipulation of the ovum through in vitro fertilization and transplantation could result in the creation of such defects. In a world already overpopulated the allocation of resources to develop in vitro fertilization techniques is another difficult issue.

Donating and removing alleles Although the technologies required to add or to remove an allele from a human cell are not yet available, such technologies have been developed in some other forms of life. In theory, such procedures could be developed so that a defective allele could be removed from the cells of an embryo in the early stages of development or a new allele added to the cells of the embryo. A whole chromosome might be added or removed. Even a whole nucleus might be removed and replaced with another nucleus. As with other techniques of genetic engineering, ethical issues are numerous; many have not even been considered let alone resolved.

The capability of DNA to undergo rearrangement and recombination of segments of the molecule and the universality of the genetic code in virtually all organisms have allowed the development of a controversial research area of genetic engineering called **recombinant DNA technology**. In such research parts of the DNA molecules from two different species are combined, creating new, recombinant DNA. Such research is controversial because it has the potential for creating new species, some of which might produce disease in humans or other organisms. At the same time, it has the potential for benefiting humans. For example, genetic information for the synthesis of an antibiotic, hormone, or other biologically active compound could be attached to the DNA of a bacterium, and the bacterium could then synthesize the product. Many such bacteria could be used to produce large quantities of the compound for use in the treatment of disease. As noted in Chapter 20, interferon has been produced in this manner.

Cloning   **Cloning** is the development of many identical cells from a single cell. (Produced by mitosis, such cells are genetically identical.) Originally used to describe culture techniques for single-celled organisms, the term is now used for techniques that could produce genetically identical copies of higher forms of life. Many lower organisms have been cloned, but no reputable scientist has demonstrated

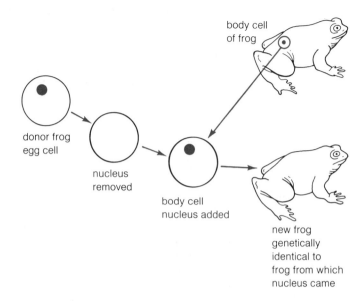

Figure 27.15   One method by which cloning can be used to produce a new individual.

the cloning of a human being, and most would have serious reservations about doing so.

The technique of cloning usually involves taking an unfertilized ovum of some particular species of organism, removing its nucleus, and replacing it with the nucleus of a diploid body cell such as a skin cell of another organism of the same species (Figure 27.15). The new individual that develops from the resulting cell is genetically identical to the individual from which the nucleus came.

Since it is now possible to remove an ovum from a human female, fertilize it in vitro, and transplant it to the uterus, the next step of replacing the nucleus of the ovum with the nucleus of a body cell is not entirely beyond the realm of possibility. The cloning of humans is an awesome thing to consider, and the ethical questions raised by such a possibility certainly have not been answered.

CLINICAL TERMS

dizygotic (di-zi-got'ik)   derived from two separate zygotes, pertaining to fraternal twins

hermaphroditism (her-maf'rod-īt-izm)   the presence of reproductive organs of both sexes; a condition in which the sex of the individual is unclear

lethal (le'thal) *gene*   a gene that causes death

monozygotic (mon-o-zi-got'ik)   derived from a single zygote, pertaining to identical twins

Essay: Ethical Decision Making

The availability of genetic engineering techniques, life-support systems for the critically ill, birth control, abortion, the possibility of euthanasia (the act of killing hopelessly ill individuals) and other choices about life and death create difficult ethical problems. Health professionals and others in the community will be faced with making decisions about such ethical issues.

Ethical decision-making techniques have been developed to help people deal with the social and ethical implications of such problems. Various techniques are available; those presented here are based on the idea that value judgments can be made in a rational manner, even though the decision makers may have strong feelings about an issue. Too often we are not consciously aware of the values we hold, and we often make judgments at the emotional level without carefully considering all of the alternatives open to us. The purpose of considering ethical decision making in this text is to help you learn to identify your own values more clearly and to apply those values to decisons involving social and ethical issues.

A Procedure for Ethical Decision Making

The procedure presented here is based on the work of Raths, Harmin, and Simon (1966) and that of Kieffer (1979), which are listed in the end-of-chapter references.

Stating the problem   The first step in this procedure is to identify the problem clearly. For example, let us assume that a couple has a male child with Duchenne muscular dystrophy. They have decided that their problem is how to avoid having another child similarly affected.

Determining possible courses of action   The second step is to identify all possible courses of action. It is known that the disease is inherited as a sex-linked recessive characteristic. Because neither parent has the disease, it can be assumed that the mother carries one normal and one defective gene. The possible courses of action include the following:

1. Refraining from having another child.

2. Having a fetal blood sample taken after conception and having enzyme studies done on the blood to determine whether the fetus is affected.

3. Having amniocentesis performed and the sex of the fetus determined (only a male child can be affected).

4. Doing nothing and accepting the 25% risk of having another affected child. (The chance of having a male child is 50% and the chance of a male being affected is 50%; the chance of both occurring simultaneously is the product of the probabilities: $.50 \times .50 = .25$.)

Can you think of other courses of action?

Determining the consequences of each course of action   After identifying the various courses of action, it is necessary to list all the consequences of each, regardless of whether the consequence might be considered as positive, negative, or neutral. In fact, in itemizing consequences it is desirable to avoid making any value judgment about any particular consequence.

In this example some of the consequences are as follows:

1. Refraining from having another child (a) completely avoids the possibility of having an affected child; (b) deprives the parents of the experience of having another child of their own; (c) prevents the possibility of transmitting the gene to a female child who would be normal but would eventually be faced with the possibility of having an affected child of her own.

2. Having a fetal blood sample used for enzyme studies (a) subjects the fetus and the mother to a potentially dangerous procedure; (b) runs the risk of obtaining erroneous results from the enzyme studies; (c) if the fetus appears to be affected, leaves the parents faced with the decision of whether to abort the fetus; (d) if the fetus appears to be normal, leaves the parents to face the possibility that the test was in error and the child is affected; and (e) incurs significant medical expense.

3. Having amniocentesis and sex determination (a) if the fetus is female, assures parents that the child will be normal (except for the same degree of risk of other defects that exists in any pregnancy); (b) if the fetus is male, creates the need to decide whether to abort a fetus that has a 50% chance of being affected; (c) subjects the fetus and the mother to a small risk from amniocentesis; and (d) incurs moderate medical expense.

4. Doing nothing and accepting the 25% risk of having an affected child (a) does not really solve the stated problem; (b) avoids extra expense during the pregnancy but may incur significant expense if the child is affected; (c) avoids the risk of prenatal diagnostic procedures; and (d) may result in the birth of a second affected child.

Can you think of other consequences? If you proposed other courses of action, list the consequences of these.

Stating values involved in each course of action   As an individual with your own particular set of values, you probably have a positive or negative attitude about each of the courses of action proposed in this example. You may have an attitude about the original problem. The reason for your attitude can be expressed in a value statement. Examples of possible values pertaining to the courses of action are given below.

One who accepts the parents' problem as legitimate expresses the value that parents have the right to attempt to avoid having a child with this genetic disease. One who rejects the legitimacy of the problem expresses the value that parents should accept any children conceived by them.

Several values might be expressed about refraining from having another child. The possibility of having a child with a genetic disease ought—or ought not—to influence one's actions. The possibility of passing a defective gene to future generations should—or should not—be considered. Human rights may—or may not—include the right to procreate.

Other values that might be expressed pertain to fetal blood sampling, amniocentesis, and abortion. Here are some examples:

1. Prenatal diagnosis is the right of every pregnant woman.

2. No one should be allowed to subject a fetus to prenatal testing.

3. Abortion is unacceptable under any conditions.

4. Abortion is acceptable if the fetus is known to be defective but not if it has a 50% chance of being normal.

5. Abortion is the right of any parents—of any woman.

6. Every child deserves to be a wanted child.

7. Nothing should be done to a developing fetus.

These examples by no means exhaust all the possible values that might be involved in the choice of action; they simply illustrate what a value statement is. Prepare your own list of value statements for each course of action in this example.

Rank ordering values Among the values an individual holds some are more important than others. For example, almost every one of us values money, but few of us would choose a course of action in this example solely on the basis of how much it costs. Priorities can be assigned to values according to how important each value is in arriving at an acceptable solution.

Rank order your entire list of values, regardless of which course of action they concern. First, find the one value you feel most strongly about—for example, that a defective gene should not be passed on under any circumstances, or that an abortion is wrong under any conditions. Then find the second most important and the third until you have ranked all the value statements on your list. If you have fewer than ten value statements, you probably have not considered the situation carefully enough. Go back to the sample courses of action and consider them further until you have at least ten value statements on your list. Continue ranking these statements until you have them ranked from one (most important) to ten (least important).

Deciding on a personal course of action The most important values are used to select a course of action. By evaluating each according to how well it satisfies the needs expressed in your most important values, you should be able to decide on a course of action. The validity of such a decision can be evaluated by asking yourself if you could live with the decision. If you find that you cannot, try to determine which of your values is in conflict with the decision and modify the decision accordingly.

Decide what course of action you would choose if you were one of the parents in the example.

Participating in social policy decisions Though some biological decisions are individual, many involve larger groups; some decisions involve the entire population of a country. In addition to emotional comfort (the criterion of whether you could live with the decision you reached), two other criteria can be used to assess the validity of a decision—universality and proportionate good. The criterion of universality asks whether the result would be acceptable if everyone made the same decision in a similar situation. The criterion of proportionate good asks whether the decision results in the greatest good for the most people.

Suppose that you are faced with the problem of what services should be made available to all parents who already have a child with a genetic disease rather than the problem of a single couple making a decision. Is amniocentesis to be available to all? What about the technique of obtaining a fetal blood sample? Under what circumstances will abortions be made available? Who will pay for the services? Should any services be mandatory?

As in any situation that requires a group consensus, you may find that you will be unable to persuade other members of the group to accept your solution. Identify trade-offs you would be willing to make. For example, if your solution is compatible with all the values in your rank-ordered list, you may be able to accept a solution that is not consistent with the ninth or tenth place values on your list. Be prepared to accept solutions that sacrifice the values that are least important to you in order to retain the values that are most important to you.

Application of these ethical decision-making techniques should be of help to you in coping with the increasing number of ethical issues facing health professionals—and all citizens—in today's complex world.

CHAPTER SUMMARY

(Chapter summary points and review questions are numbered to correspond to the numbered objectives in the text of each chapter.)

Overview of Chapter

1. Define meiosis, gametogenesis, and genetics; describe the relation of these processes to the production of a new individual.
   a. Meiosis is the process by which sex cells with half the normal number of chromosomes are produced.
   b. Gametogenesis is the production of gametes—eggs in females and sperm in males.
   c. Genetics is the study of the transmission of inherited characteristics.
   d. Meiosis and gametogenesis contribute to the production of new individuals by producing the male and female gametes that can unite to form the first cell of a new individual.
   e. Inherited genes in the cells of the new individual determine the characteristics of that individual.

Meiosis and Gametogenesis

2. Describe the major stages in the process of meiosis.
   a. Meiosis involves two divisions of the nucleus of a gamete-producing cell:
      (1) Chromosomes are replicated prior to the initiation of the first division.
      (2) The first division, the reduction division, reduces the number of chromosomes in each cell from 2n to n.
      (3) The second division separates the chromatids of each chromosome.
      (4) Each division goes through the stages of prophase, metaphase, anaphase, and telophase; no replication of chromosomes occurs between divisions.
3. Contrast the stages in spermatogenesis and oogenesis and describe the outcome of each process.
   a. In spermatogenesis each spermatogonium goes through the stages of a primary spermatocyte, secondary spermatocytes, spermatids, and mature spermatozoa.
   b. In oogenesis each oogonium goes through the stages of a primary oocyte, a secondary oocyte, an ootid, and a mature ovum.
   c. In spermatogenesis four functional spermatozoa are produced; in oogenesis one functional ovum is produced, and the other cells in the process become polar bodies.
4. Explain the significance of meiosis.
   a. Meiosis provides haploid cells capable of uniting to form the first diploid cell of a new individual.
   b. Meiosis also increases the genetic diversity of the gametes.

Mutations and Chromosomal Abnormalities

5. Define the term mutation and explain how mutations might affect the structure and function of the body.
   a. A mutation is a change in the sequence of nucleotides in a gene:
      (1) Point mutations involve the substitution of an incorrect base for the correct one.
      (2) Frameshift mutations involve the addition or deletion of bases and may seriously disturb the information in the code.
   b. Mutations are often caused by chemicals or radiation that affect the cell's DNA and thus the kinds of proteins it can make and how it functions.
6. Explain how abnormal kinds or numbers of chromosomes might be produced; describe the chromosomal abnormality and its effects in (a) Down's syndrome, (b) Klinefelter's syndrome, and (c) Turner's syndrome.
   a. Abnormal kinds of chromosomes are produced by deletion, inversion, or translocation of portions of chromosomes.
   b. Abnormal numbers of chromosomes are produced by errors in the distribution of chromosomes to the cells that arise from meiosis.
   c. Specific abnormalities include the following:
      (1) Down's syndrome, which results from the presence of a third chromosome number 21, leads to mental retardation and a variety of other symptoms.
      (2) Klinefelter's syndrome, which results from the presence of an extra X chromosome (XXY), leads to sterility in phenotypically male individuals.
      (3) Turner's syndrome, which results from the presence of a single X chromosome (XO), leads to sterility in phenotypically female individuals.

Principles of Genetics

7. Define the major terms used in genetics.
   a. Definitions of major genetic terms are given in Table 27.1.
8. Explain the principles of segregation and independent assortment.
   a. The principle of segregation states that alleles on homologous chromosomes are segregated, or separated from each other, in the production of haploid gametes.
   b. The principle of independent assortment states that the alleles for one trait separate independently of the alleles for another trait, provided the genes are on different chromosomes.
9. Explain how probability is involved in determining inheritance and use a Punnett square to illustrate selected probabilities.

a. Probability is used in genetics to determine the likelihood of a particular genotype (or phenotype) appearing among the offspring of parents with particular genotypes.
b. The use of a Punnett square is illustrated in Figure 27.9.

10. Interpret a pedigree diagram.
   a. In a pedigree diagram squares represent males, and circles represent females; horizontal lines represent matings, and vertical lines indicate offspring of a mating.
   b. Pedigree diagrams can help to determine whether a particular characteristic is dominant, recessive, or sex linked.

Human Genetic Disorders

11. For the human disorders presented in this section, describe the inheritance pattern and the effects of the disease.
   a. Selected human genetic disorders are summarized in Table 27.2.

Genetic Screening and Genetic Counseling

12. Define genetic screening; explain the different purposes of neonatal and adult screening; list several factors that enter into the development and operation of genetic screening programs.
   a. Genetic screening is a process for identifying individuals with genotypes that produce disease or that are capable of transmitting a disease to descendants.
   b. Neonatal screening is used to detect the presence of genetic-metabolic diseases; adult screening is usually used to detect carriers of harmful alleles in order to give such adults an informed choice of reproductive options.
   c. Factors to be considered in screening programs are summarized in Table 27.3.

13. Define genetic counseling and describe the major components of the counseling process.
   a. Genetic counseling is the provision to counselees of information about a genetic disease. It also includes assistance in coping with the problems the disease has caused or might cause for the counselees and their relatives.
   b. The components of the counseling process include:
      (1) verification of diagnosis
      (2) explanation of the effects of the disease
      (3) assessment of risks to the counselees and family
      (4) interpretation of risks to the counselee
      (5) correction of misinformation
      (6) explanation of reproductive options
      (7) assistance in dealing with the problem
      (8) serving as a concerned listener without making decisions for the counselee

Genetic Engineering

14. Define genetic engineering and list examples of different kinds of genetic engineering.

a. Genetic engineering is the manipulation of reproduction and heredity.
b. Kinds of genetic engineering include:
   (1) artificial insemination
   (2) in vitro fertilization
   (3) donation and removal of genes
   (4) recombinant DNA technology
   (5) cloning of nonhuman organisms

REVIEW

Important Terms

allele	independent assortment
amniocentesis	karyotype
autosomal inheritance	meiosis
carrier	oogenesis
chromatid	pedigree
cloning	phenotype
crossing-over	point mutation
diploid	probability
dominant	Punnett square
frameshift mutation	recessive
gamete	segregation
genotype	sex-linked inheritance
haploid	spermatogenesis
heterozygous	tetrad
homozygous	

Questions

1. Define meiosis, gametogenesis, and genetics and describe how each is related to the development of a new individual.

2. a. What are the steps in meiosis?
   b. What is reduction division?
   c. What happens during crossing-over?

3. How do oogenesis and spermatogenesis differ?

4. What is the significance of meiosis?

5. What is the effect of a point mutation? A frameshift mutation?

6. What are the two main kinds of chromosomal abnormalities?

7. Without looking at the definitions, define the terms in Table 27.1.

8. a. What is the principle of independent assortment?
   b. What is the principle of segregation?

9. Make a Punnett square with alleles for any two inherited characteristics.

10. Select an inherited characteristic and draw a pedigree showing how the characteristic might be transmitted from one generation to the next.

11. a. Though neither of them is affected with cystic fibrosis, the Smiths have a child who has this disease. What are their chances of having another child similarly affected?

b. What is the probability that a couple, both of whom are achondroplastic dwarfs, could have a normal child?

c. What proportion of infants receive an X chromosome from their fathers? What proportion receive a Y chromosome from their fathers? What proportion receive an X chromosome from their mothers?

d. If a woman with normal vision whose father was color blind marries a man who is color blind, what is the probability of their having a son who is color blind? A daughter who is color blind? A normal daughter who is a carrier of the color-blind gene?

e. A woman with brachydactyly married a man with Marfan's syndrome. Assuming that both are heterozygous for the specified diseases, determine the probability of their having a child with either of the diseases and with both of the diseases.

f. Three infants were mixed up in the hospital nursery. One of the nurses decided to determine the blood types of the babies and their parents to match the infants to the proper parents. The results she received from the laboratory were as follows: Baby 1 had blood type O, baby 2 had blood type B, and baby 3 had blood type AB. One set of parents had blood types A and B, another set had blood types B and O, and the third set of parents both had blood type O. The nurse was successful in solving the problem. Can you solve it?

g. For the pedigree shown in Figure 27.16 determine the genotypes and phenotypes for blood type and color vision for as many individuals in the pedigree as possible.

12. a. What is genetic screening?

b. How does the purpose of genetic screening of neonates differ from screening of adults?

c. What are the factors to be considered in the development and operation of a genetic screening program?

13. a What is genetic counseling?

b. What are the major components of the counseling process?

14. a. What is genetic engineering?

b. Give examples of at least three kinds of genetic engineering.

Problems

1. A woman whose father had Duchenne muscular dystrophy is married to a man who thinks his grandfather might have had it. What are the couple's chances of having an affected child if the father's grandfather did in fact have the disease?

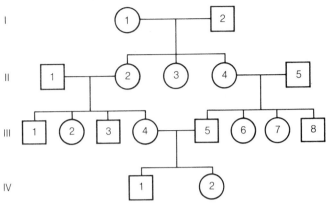

Individual	Blood Type	Color Vision
II-1	B	
II-3	O	normal
II-4		color blind
II-5	B	
III-1	A	normal
III-2	B	
III-3	AB	
III-4	O	color blind
III-5	AB	
III-6	A	
III-7	B	color blind
III-8	O	

Figure 27.16 Pedigree of blood types and color vision.

2. The Jones family has just learned that their son has Duchenne muscular dystrophy. They are surprised because there has **never** been a case of the disease in either of their families. How can you explain this event?

3. A couple has discovered that their son has Bruton agammaglobulinemia. His care will be expensive and will create a serious strain on the emotional as well as financial resources of the family. Nevertheless, they would like to have another child, especially a little girl. What is the probability that a female fetus would be affected by the disease? Would this family be justified in aborting a male fetus? Give reasons for your answer.

4. Suppose that the couple described in problem 3 had discovered instead that their son has Lesch-Nyhan syndrome. How would your answers to the questions in that problem differ? Why?

5. Suppose that you are the person affected by one of the above problems. Apply the ethical decision-making techniques to deciding how you would handle the problem.

6. Suppose that you are a genetic counselor. Show how you could use the counseling procedures and ethical decision-making techniques to help a client decide how to handle one of the above problems.

7. Evaluate the decisions that were made in problem 6 according to the following criteria:
   a. Did you have all the relevant facts?
   b. Did you consider the consequences of all alternatives before making a decision?
   c. Did you rank order values associated with each action?
   d. Did you consider the feelings of all parties involved?
   e. Were your decisions free from self-interest and strong emotions?
   f. Were your decisions consistent with other decisions you have made about similar problems?

REFERENCES AND READINGS

Arehart-Treichel, J. 1979. Questioning the new genetics. *Science News* 116:154 (September 1).

Arehart-Treichel, J. 1979. Down's syndrome: The father's role. *Science News* 116:381 (December 1).

Bank, A., Mears, J. G., and Ramirez, F. 1980. Disorders of human hemoglobin. *Science* 207:486 (February 1).

Breslow, J. L., Epstein, J., Fontaine, J. H., and Forbes, G. B. 1978. Enhanced dexamethasone resistance in cystic fibrosis cells: Potential use for heterozygote detection and prenatal diagnosis. *Science* 201:180 (July 14).

Cohen, S. M. 1975. The manipulation of genes. *Scientific American* 233(1):25 (July).

DeRobertis, E. M., and Gurdon, J. B. 1979. Gene transplantation and the analysis of development. *Scientific American* 241(6):74 (December).

Fuchs, F. 1980. Genetic amniocentesis. *Scientific American* 242(6):47 (June).

German, J., Simpson, J. L., Chaganti, R. S. K., Summitt, R. L., Reid, L. B., and Merkatz, I. R. 1978. Genetically determined sex-reversal in 46,XY humans. *Science* 202:53 (October 6).

Kieffer, G. H. 1979. Can bioethics be taught? *American Biology Teacher* 41(3):176 (March).

Kormondy, E. J., Sherman, T. F., Salisbury, F. B., Spratt, N. T., Jr., and McCain, G. 1977. *Biology*. Belmont, Calif.: Wadsworth.

Lake, C. R., and Ziegler, M. G. 1977. Lesch-Nyhan syndrome: Low dopamine-beta-hydroxylase activity and diminished sympathetic response to stress and posture. *Science* 196:905 (May 20).

Marx, J. L. 1978. Successful transplant of a functioning mammalian gene. *Science* 202:610 (November 10).

McKusick, V. A. 1975. *Mendelian inheritance in man. Catalogs of autosomal dominant, autosomal recessive, and X-linked phenotypes* (4th ed.). Baltimore, Md.: Johns Hopkins University Press.

McKusick, V. A., and Ruddle, F. H. 1977. The status of the gene map of human chromosomes. *Science* 196:391.

Mertens, T. R. 1975. *Human genetics: Readings on the implications of genetic engineering*. New York: Wiley.

Miller, J. A. 1979. A tumor in the family. *Science News* 115:60 (January 27).

Miller, J. A. 1980. Spliced genes get down to business. *Science News* 117:202 (March 29).

Milunsky, A. 1977. *Know your genes*. Boston: Houghton Mifflin.

Murray, R. F., Jr. 1974. Genetic disease and human health. *Hastings Center Report* (September):4.

Murray, R.F., Jr. 1972. Problems behind the promise: Ethical issues in mass genetic screening. *Hastings Center Report* (April):10.

National Institute of General Medical Sciences. 1975. *What are the facts about genetic disease?* Bethesda, Md.: National Institutes of Health.

National Research Council. 1975. *Genetic Screening: Programs, principles, and research*. Washington, D.C.: National Academy of Sciences.

Novitski, E. 1977. *Human genetics*. New York: Macmillan.

Pines, M. 1976. *The new human genetics*. Bethesda, Md.: The National Institute of General Medical Sciences, DHEW Publication No. (NIH) 76–662.

Raths, L. E., Harmin, M., and Simon, S. B. 1966. *Values and teaching*. Columbus, Ohio: Charles E. Merrill.

Starr, C. (ed.). 1975. *Biology today* (2nd ed.). New York: Random House.

Stine, G. J. 1977. *Biosocial genetics*. New York: Macmillan.

Wallace, B. 1972. *Genetics, evolution, race, radiation biology* (Essays in Social Biology, Vol. II). Englewood Cliffs, N.J.: Prentice-Hall.

28

REPRODUCTIVE SYSTEM

ORGANIZATION AND GENERAL FUNCTIONS

Objective 1. Describe the overall organization of the male and female reproductive systems and list their major functions.

The organs of the reproductive system produce gametes (eggs or sperm) and provide for the transport of these gametes. In the human female the reproductive system also provides a place for the embryo to develop—the uterus. Both the male and female reproductive systems also produce hormones that help to regulate the reproductive process and to stimulate the development of secondary sex characteristics.

The male reproductive system consists of testes in which the sperm and hormones are produced, a set of ducts that deliver the sperm to the outside of the body, and several glands that contribute their secretions to the fluid in which the sperm are carried.

The female reproductive system consists of ovaries in which the ova and hormones are produced, the uterine ducts that transport the ova, the uterus in which the embryo develops, and the vagina through which sperm are deposited and the birth of the fetus takes place.

DEVELOPMENT

Objective 2. Compare the development of the male and female reproductive systems.

Though the genetic sex of an infant is determined at the time of conception, the reproductive organs begin to develop in the same way in both sexes (Figure 28.1). In fact,

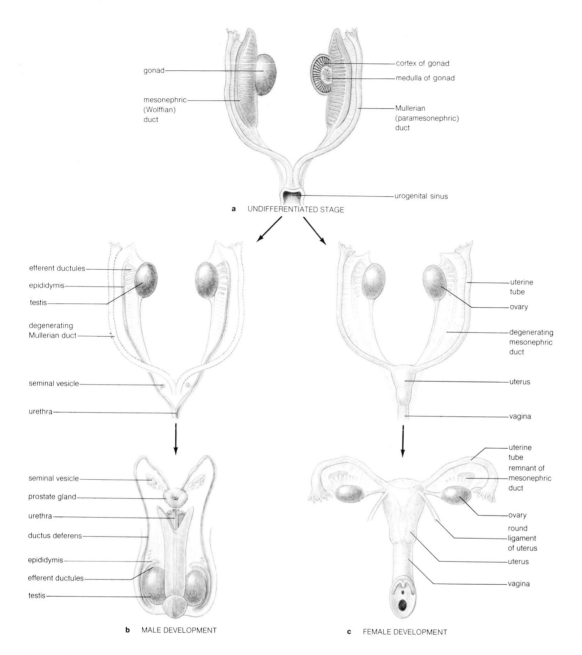

Figure 28.1 The development of the internal reproductive systems.

the ducts of both male and female systems begin to develop in every early embryo. How an individual ultimately comes to have either a male or a female reproductive system is discussed below.

The gonads (ovaries or testes) begin to develop from mesoderm just medial to the kidneys. Whether the gonads are ovaries or testes cannot be determined prior to about the eighth week of development. The medulla of each undif-

ferentiated gonad is destined to become a testis in males and the cortex an ovary in females. Ducts of both the male and female systems are present. This stage of development corresponds to the undifferentiated stage shown in Figure 28.1. As development proceeds in the female, the ovaries develop, the mesonephric duct degenerates, and the Mullerian duct becomes the uterine duct. The uterine ducts fuse in the midline to form the uterus and vagina. (Several

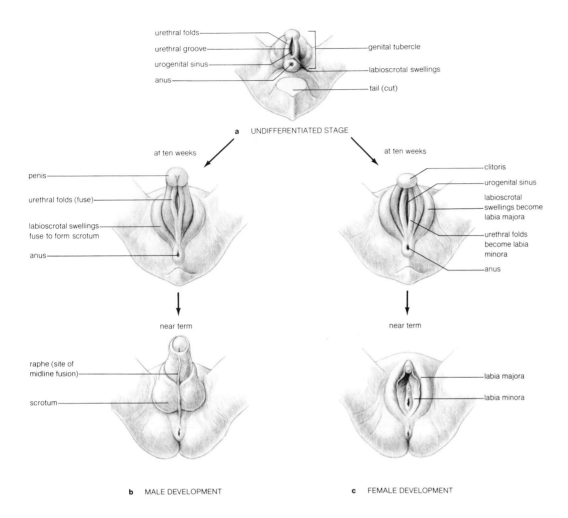

urethral folds
urethral groove
urogenital sinus
anus

genital tubercle
labioscrotal swellings
tail (cut)

a   UNDIFFERENTIATED STAGE

at ten weeks

penis
urethral folds (fuse)
labioscrotal swellings fuse to form scrotum
anus

at ten weeks

clitoris
urogenital sinus
labioscrotal swellings become labia majora
urethral folds become labia minora
anus

near term

raphe (site of midline fusion)
scrotum

near term

labia majora
labia minora

b   MALE DEVELOPMENT

c   FEMALE DEVELOPMENT

Figure 28.2   The development of the external reproductive structures.

other structures are also labeled in the figure.)

The development of the male genital ducts is influenced by hormones from the developing testes. Normally, in an embryo that is genetically male (has XY chromosomes), the testes will develop and begin to secrete testosterone. The development of the testes and their secretion of testosterone is stimulated by chorionic gonadotropin, a hormone produced by the placenta. Testosterone stimulates the development of the male genital ducts, especially the external ducts. If the testes are experimentally removed from an animal with XY chromosomes, the animal develops female genital ducts, thus showing that testosterone is necessary to cause the male genital ducts to develop even in embryos that are genetically male. Conversely, in an embryo that is genetically female (has XX chromosomes), the ovaries and female ducts develop in the absence of

testosterone. If a female embryo is injected with testosterone, the testes and male ducts develop, and the female organs degenerate. In other words, though sex is determined genetically, it is through the production of testosterone by male embryos that the male reproductive system develops and through the absence of this hormone in female embryos that the female reproductive system develops.

The development of the external reproductive structures follows a similar pattern, also beginning with an undifferentiated stage (Figure 28.2). Like the internal organs, the external organs of both males and females are identical until about the eighth week of development and consist primarily of a **genital tubercle**. When the male begins to produce hormones, the anterior portion of the genital tubercle develops into the **penis**. The urethral folds close around the urethra at the raphe, leaving an opening only at the tip of the penis. The labioscrotal swellings enlarge, fuse, and develop into pouches that become the scrotum. Later in development, usually a month or two before birth, the testes descend from the abdominal cavity through the inguinal canal into the scrotum. In females, in the absence of testosterone, the anterior part of the genital tubercle becomes the **clitoris**. The urethral folds remain around the urogenital sinus and become the **labia minora**. The labioscrotal swellings fail to fuse as they do in the male and become the **labia majora**, which surround the other genital organs. Both the urethra and the vagina open to the surface between the labia minora.

THE MALE REPRODUCTIVE SYSTEM

Objective 3. Describe the structure and function of the testes and scrotum.

Objective 4. Describe the structure and function of the ducts and glands of the male reproductive system.

Objective 5. Explain how the function of the male reproductive system is regulated.

Objective 6. Describe the alterations of function that occur in (a) prostatitis, (b) prostate cancer, (c) impotence, and (d) sterility.

Structure and Function of the Testes and Scrotum

The adult **testes** are oval organs about 5 centimeters long and 2.5 centimeters in diameter, surrounded by a connective tissue capsule, the **tunica albuginea** (Figure 28.3). Inside each testis septa form several hundred compartments called lobules. Each lobule usually contains one to three convoluted (folded and coiled) **seminiferous tubules**. A cross section through the wall of a seminiferous tubule (Figure 28.4) shows two kinds of cells: (a) Sertoli cells, and (b) interstitial cells of Leydig.

Germinal epithelium The **spermatogonia**, as discussed in Chapter 27, are the cells that give rise to the sperm. Spermatogonia form the germinal epithelium and are located near the walls of the tubule, where they undergo mitosis throughout the reproductive years of the male. Some of these cells migrate inward toward the lumen, increase in size, and become primary spermatocytes. As a result of meiosis secondary spermatocytes and spermatids are

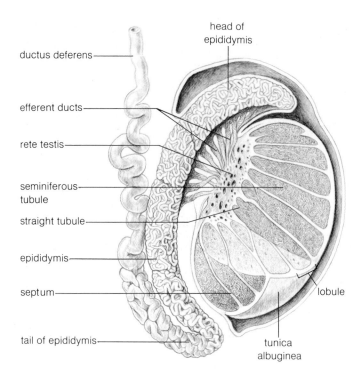

Figure 28.3   A sagittal section through the testis.

formed. The cells continue their migration toward the lumen as they undergo meiosis. Finally, the spermatids attach to Sertoli cells and mature into spermatozoa.

A mature spermatozoan, or sperm cell (Figure 28.5), has a rounded **head** that is filled by the nucleus of the cell. The tip of the head of the sperm consists of the **acrosome**, a protective caplike structure that contains proteins. One of those proteins is the enzyme hyaluronidase, which helps the sperm to penetrate the ovum. The **neck** of the sperm separates the head from the **middle piece**, which contains helically arranged mitochondria that are presumed to provide energy for the movement of the sperm. The **tail** consists of a flagellum containing actinlike protein filaments that are responsible for the movement of the sperm.

Sertoli cells The **Sertoli cells** are found interspersed among the spermatids. The cytoplasm of these large cells extends from the basement membrane to the lumen. Because the spermatids undergo maturation while attached to Sertoli cells, it is believed that the Sertoli cells provide nutrients, enzymes, and perhaps hormones that are needed by the spermatids in the maturation process.

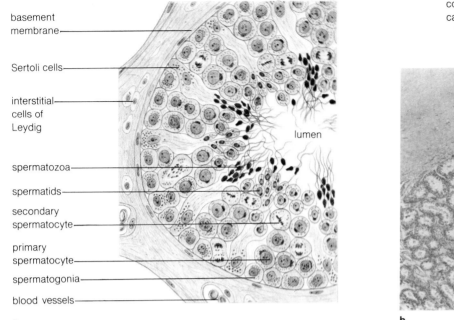

basement
membrane

Sertoli cells

interstitial
cells of
Leydig

lumen

spermatozoa

spermatids

secondary
spermatocyte

primary
spermatocyte

spermatogonia

blood vessels

a

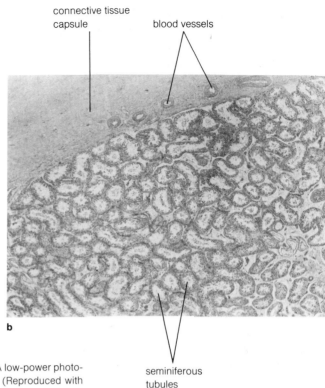

connective tissue
capsule

blood vessels

seminiferous
tubules

b

Figure 28.4 (**a**) A diagram of the cell types found within a seminiferous tubule. (**b**) A low-power photomicrograph of the human testis, showing seminiferous tubules and interstitial cells. (Reproduced with permission from A. W. Ham, *Histology*, J. B. Lippincott, 1979.)

Interstitial cells and testosterone The **interstitial cells of Leydig** are located in the supporting tissues between the coils of the seminiferous tubules. These cells produce the hormones called androgens, the most important of which is testosterone.

Testosterone has several effects on the male body. We have already noted its effect on the development of the male reproductive ducts. Testosterone also stimulates the descent of the testes into the scrotum one to two months before birth. During puberty testosterone stimulates and controls the growth and development of the male sex organs and the development of secondary sex characteristics. These characteristics include male body hair pattern, muscular development and skeletal growth that lead to broader shoulders than hips, and the enlargement of the thyroid cartilage that produces a deepening of the voice.

After puberty testosterone is important in maintenance of the male sex organs and the secondary sex characteristics. It is also important in the production of sperm. After about age twenty-five the production of testosterone slowly decreases, but it is produced in small amounts throughout the life of the male. In the late forties or fifties males experience a somewhat greater decline in testosterone production, sometimes accompanied by slowly decreasing sexual function.

Transport of sperm through the testis After the mature spermatozoa reach the lumen of the convoluted seminiferous tubules and pass through the coiled portion, they pass into the **straight tubules** (see Figure 28.3). From the straight tubules the sperm pass through a network of tubes, the **rete testis**, and on through the **efferent ducts** to the epididymis, which joins the testis with the ductus deferens. As the sperm pass through these tubules of the testis, they continue to mature, so that by the time they have passed through the epididymis they are fully functional.

Descent of the testes As we noted in discussing the development of the reproductive systems, the testes develop in the abdominal cavity and descend into the scrotum during the last month or two of development. As the testes descend (Figure 28.6), they carry with them the blood vessels and nerves that supply them and push along in front of them the **tunica vaginalis**, a membrane that surrounds the testes

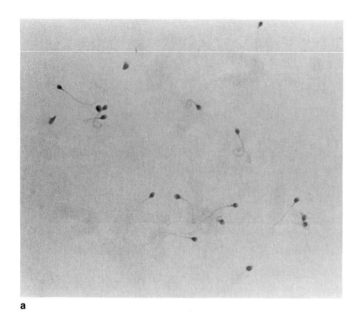

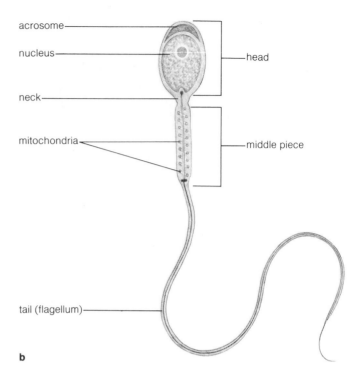

acrosome

nucleus

neck

mitochondria

tail (flagellum)

head

middle piece

b

a

Figure 28.5 (**a**) Photomicrograph of sperm, × 340. (Photograph by author.) (**b**) The structure of a mature sperm.

when they reach the scrotum. The **gubernaculum**, a structure consisting of connective tissue and smooth muscle, connects each testis and epididymis to the scrotal sac. It shortens as the body grows and helps to guide the testis into the scrotum.

The scrotum As described in the discussion of development, the **scrotum** develops from the labioscrotal swellings. Its walls consist of a layer of skin, beneath which is superficial fascia. Some of the fascia and associated smooth muscle form a median septum, which divides the scrotum internally into two separate sacs. Each sac contains one testis. The walls of the scrotum also contain fascia and smooth muscle, together called the **dartos**.

The normal temperature of the testes in the scrotum is about 2°C lower than the internal body temperature—the ideal temperature for developing sperm. When the body is chilled, the smooth muscle contracts and brings the testes closer to the pelvic cavity. The cremaster muscle of the spermatic cord also contracts during chilling. Movement toward the pelvic cavity when the temperature drops allows the testes to absorb heat from the rest of the body so that the sperm cells do not become chilled. A spermatic cord passes between each testis and the abdominal cavity and contains,

In about 3% of males one or both testes fail to descend into the scrotum before birth. In this condition, called **cryptorchidism**, spontaneous descent occurs during the first year of life in about 80% of the cases and by puberty in another 10% of the cases. When descent does not occur spontaneously prior to puberty, the condition may be treated with hormones or by surgery. Untreated cryptorchidism leads to sterility because the developing sperm are destroyed by the high temperature of the abdominal cavity.

in addition to the cremaster muscle, the ductus deferens and the nerves and blood vessels of the testes and scrotum.

Ducts of the Male Reproductive System

The ducts of the male reproductive system carry the sperm from the testes to the outside of the body or, during intercourse, to the reproductive tract of the female. These ducts include the epididymis, the ductus deferens, and the ejacu-

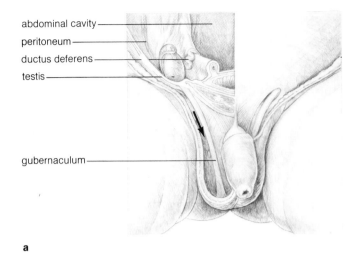

abdominal cavity

peritoneum

ductus deferens

testis

gubernaculum

a

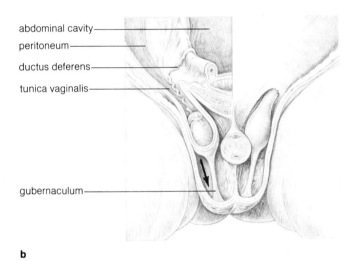

abdominal cavity

peritoneum

ductus deferens

tunica vaginalis

gubernaculum

b

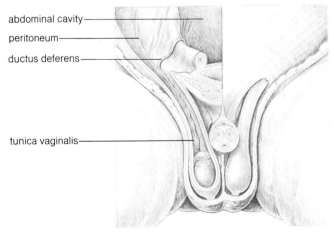

abdominal cavity

peritoneum

ductus deferens

tunica vaginalis

c

Figure 28.6 The descent of the testes into the scrotum: (**a**) testis beginning descent, (**b**) tunica vaginalis being pushed ahead of testes as gubernaculum guides movement, (**c**) testes arriving in scrotum.

latory duct (each of which is paired), and the urethra (an unpaired structure), which is also part of the urinary system (see Figure 28.7).

Epididymis   The **epididymis** consists of a coiled tubule that extends from the efferent ductules of the testis to the ductus deferens. Its **head** is on the superior surface of the testis; it extends along the posterior surface of the testis to its **tail**, where it joins the ductus deferens. (Refer back to Figure 28.3) The coiled duct of the epididymis is about 4 centimeters long; uncoiled, it is about 6 meters long. While stored in the epididymis, sperm become capable of motility as the neck of each sperm becomes flexible. During ejaculation smooth muscle in the wall of the epididymis contracts and pushes the sperm into the ductus deferens.

Ductus deferens   The **ductus deferens**, also called the **vas deferens**, is about 45 centimeters long. Its diameter is slightly larger than the epididymis, and its wall contains three layers of smooth muscle. Continuous with the tail of the epididymis, the ductus deferens carries sperm from the epididymis to the ejaculatory duct. Along its path from the scrotum it becomes part of the spermatic cord and passes through the inguinal canal and over the pubic bone to the pelvic cavity. Other structures found in the **spermatic cord** include arteries, veins, lymphatics, nerves, and the cremaster muscle. Inside the pelvic cavity the ductus deferens passes over and behind the urinary bladder, where it joins the duct from the seminal vesicle. It is then called the **ejaculatory duct**. Peristaltic contractions of the ductus deferens move the sperm through the lumen of the duct.

Ejaculatory duct   The **ejaculatory duct** is continuous with the ductus deferens and lies inferior to the bladder. Each of the paired ejaculatory ducts receives sperm from one of the testes and is capable of ejecting them into the urethra. In addition to the sperm, each ejaculatory duct receives secretions from the seminal vesicle, as discussed below.

Urethra   The **urethra**, the common passageway for both urine and sperm, consists of three parts. The **prostatic urethra** passes from the bladder through the prostate gland to the membranous urethra. The ejaculatory ducts join it as it passes through the prostate gland. The **membranous**

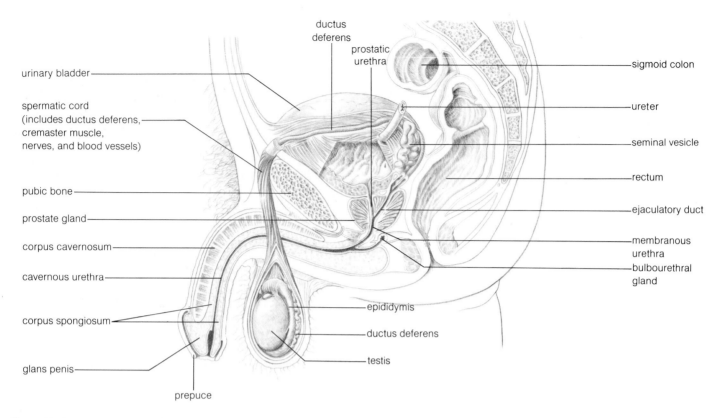

ductus deferens

prostatic urethra

urinary bladder

spermatic cord
(includes ductus deferens,
cremaster muscle,
nerves, and blood vessels)

pubic bone

prostate gland

corpus cavernosum

cavernous urethra

corpus spongiosum

glans penis

prepuce

sigmoid colon

ureter

seminal vesicle

rectum

ejaculatory duct

membranous urethra

bulbourethral gland

epididymis

ductus deferens

testis

Figure 28.7   The male reproductive system.

urethra passes from the prostatic portion through the **urogenital diaphragm**, the muscular floor of the pelvic cavity, and becomes the **spongy**, or **cavernous**, **urethra**. The cavernous urethra passes through the penis.

Penis   The penis, in addition to conducting urine from the body, is the male copulatory organ; it deposits sperm into the reproductive tract of the female during sexual intercourse. The penis contains three cylindrical masses of erectile tissue (Figure 28.8)—two dorsal **corpora cavernosa** and one ventral **corpus spongiosum**. These bodies are surrounded by fibrous tissue. The corpus spongiosum, which contains the urethra, is enlarged at the distal end of the penis to form the **glans penis**. The penis is covered with smooth skin; the skin extending over the glans is called the **prepuce**, or **foreskin**. During sexual arousal the three bundles of tissue in the penis become engorged with blood. One explanation for this engorgement is that the arterioles dilate and fill with blood, thereby compressing the venules so that little blood can leave the penis. Thus, the penis enlarges and stiffens, and an **erection** is produced.

In some male infants the foreskin is removed in an operation called circumcision. Jewish males are nearly always circumcised for both religious and hygienic reasons. Some evidence exists to show that the incidence of cervical cancer is lower in Jewish women than in non-Jewish women, but the relationship between circumcision and the low incidence of cervical cancer may not be a direct one. The practice of circumcision among non-Jewish as well as Jewish males is much more common in the United States than in many European countries, but physicians in this country are beginning to question whether the operation is necessary.

**Glands of the Male Reproductive System
and Production of Semen**

Glands   Three kinds of glands contribute their secretions to the fluid that is ejaculated with the sperm. These glands are

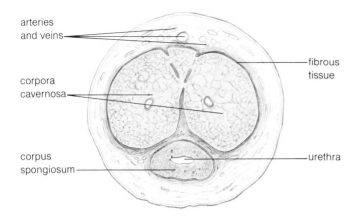

arteries and veins

corpora cavernosa

corpus spongiosum

fibrous tissue

urethra

Figure 28.8 A cross-section through the penis.

the seminal vesicles, the prostate gland, and the bulbourethral glands. The ductus deferens also contributes some fluid.

The **seminal vesicles** are saclike structures near the base of the bladder; their ducts join the ductus deferens to form the ejaculatory ducts. The viscous secretions of the seminal vesicles contain fructose and prostaglandins. The fructose is a source of energy for the sperm; the prostaglandins stimulate uterine contractions and thus may help the sperm to be moved to the female's uterine tubes, where fertilization takes place.

The **prostate gland** is a single large gland that surrounds the urethra. It secretes a milky fluid that aids in sperm motility. This fluid contains a small amount of citric acid, some lipids, and a few enzymes; as well as significant numbers of bicarbonate ions, which give the semen its alkaline pH. A number of small ducts carry fluid from the prostate to the urethra.

A pair of **bulbourethral glands**, or **Cowper's glands**, are located in the floor of the pelvic cavity. Their secretions, which contain mucus for lubrication, enter the semen through ducts attached to the membranous portion of the urethra.

Semen The **semen** contains the secretions of the above glands and the sperm from the testes. When the penis is erect, semen is ejected from the penis during ejaculation. Each ejaculate contains about 400 million sperm in 2 to 6 milliliters of fluid. Semen has a pH of 7.35 to 7.50; its alkalinity helps to neutralize the acidity of the urethra left from the passage of urine and protects the sperm from the acidity of the vagina.

Regulation of the Male Reproductive System

Before puberty the testes produce little testosterone and no sperm. Exactly what triggers the onset of puberty is not known, but it is thought that prior to puberty some mechanism inhibits the hypothalamus from stimulating the pituitary gland. At the onset of puberty the hormone LH-RH probably stimulates the pituitary, which in turn stimulates the gonads.

After puberty two important regulatory processes operate to control the male reproductive system. The secretion of testosterone and the production of sperm are controlled by hormones, and the erection of the penis is controlled by the nervous system.

Regulation of testosterone and spermatogenesis At the onset of puberty the anterior pituitary gland secretes follicle-stimulating hormone (FSH) and luteinizing hormone (LH), sometimes called interstitial-cell-stimulating hormone (ICSH) in males. Release of these hormones is stimulated by LH-RH, as explained in Chapter 15.

FSH plays a role in stimulating the seminiferous tubules to produce sperm. LH contributes to the development of mature sperm, but its main function is to stimulate the interstitial cells of Leydig to secrete testosterone.

When the testosterone concentration in the blood becomes elevated, the testosterone inhibits the release of LH-RH; in the absence of LH-RH, LH is not released. No further stimulation of the interstitial cells occurs until the testosterone concentration in the blood drops. As it drops, its inhibitory effect is lost, and LH-RH is again secreted. This system of regulating testosterone secretion is another example of a negative feedback mechanism.

Though the mechanism by which FSH release is regulated is not fully understood, it appears that LH-RH is involved, as is a substance called inhibin. Inhibin is released from the Sertoli cells when sperm are being produced; as its concentration increases, it inhibits release of FSH. It is also thought that FSH exerts its stimulatory effect on spermatogenesis through the Sertoli cells. These regulatory mechanisms are summarized in Figure 28.9.

Regulation of erection The most direct stimulus that leads to the erection of the penis is mechanical stimulation of the glans. Impulses from the penis travel to the spinal cord, where they stimulate the parasympathetic nerve fibers and inhibit the sympathetic fibers that control the arterioles and cavernous tissue of the penis. The arterioles dilate, and blood enters the cavernous spaces of the erectile tissue. The parasympathetic nerves also stimulate the bulbourethral glands to secrete mucus, which plays a role in lubricating the glans.

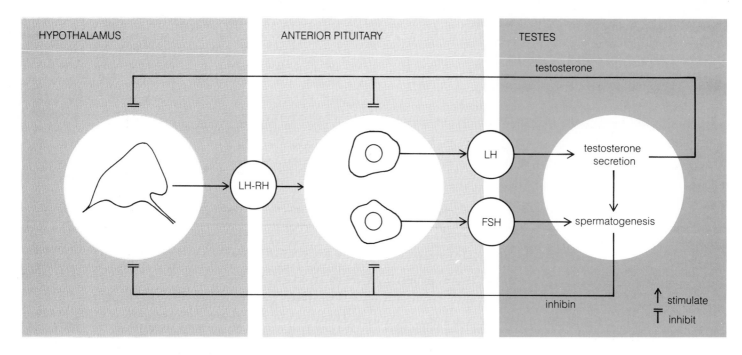

Figure 28.9 The regulation of testosterone secretion and sperm production.

In addition to this direct stimulation of an erection, the central nervous system can also cause or inhibit an erection. Psychological factors have a significant effect on the erectile tissue of the penis, sometimes stimulating and sometimes inhibiting erection. Alcohol can promote or interfere with erection, probably by obliterating inhibitions or by blocking some central nervous impulses, respectively. The regulation of erection is summarized in Figure 28.10.

Emission and ejaculation When sexual stimulation becomes extremely intense, spinal reflex centers send impulses to the genital organs and initiate emission. During **emission** it is thought that the epididymis and the ductus deferens contract, forcing sperm into the urethra. Contractions of the seminal vesicles and the muscular coat surrounding the prostate gland expel fluids from these glands. The sperm and these glandular fluids mix with the mucus from the bulbourethral glands, forming the semen. This collection of fluids and sperm in the urethra constitutes emission.

The presence of semen in the urethra causes nerve impulses to travel to the sacral region of the spinal cord, where they elicit rhythmic nerve impulses to the muscle surrounding the erectile tissue. Thus, rhythmic contractions cause **ejaculation**, or release of semen from the urethra. Ejaculation is accompanied by pleasurable sensations called **orgasm**.

Applications

Prostatitis **Prostatitis** is an inflammation of the prostate gland. When the prostate gland swells, it frequently blocks the urethra and makes urination painful or difficult. Untreated prostatitis can lead to kidney damage. When urine is blocked from passing out of the bladder, back pressure builds up in the kidneys and damages nephrons. The failure of the bladder to drain properly also increases the risk of recurrent infections.

After age sixty the prostate gland often becomes enlarged due to unknown causes. Such benign hypertrophy of the prostate is usually treated by surgical removal of the prostate, after which the man is sterile but not necessarily impotent. If left untreated, this condition can also cause kidney damage.

Prostate cancer **Cancer of the prostate gland** is an extremely common malignancy, accounting for 2 to 3% of male deaths. Malignant prostate cells are usually stimulated by testosterone, so treatment often involves removal of the testes, thereby preventing production of the hormone. Another treatment is the administration of estrogens, which seem to counteract the effects of testosterone. Because metastasis of malignant prostate cells to bone and other tissues is common, this form of cancer is difficult to cure. However, these treatments arrest metastases and allow at least temporary healing of the bones.

Impotence **Impotence** is the inability to achieve or hold an erection long enough to complete sexual intercourse. Psychological factors are most often cited as causes, but neurological disorders, vascular disorders, and syphilis can also cause impotence.

Sterility In males **sterility** is the inability to fertilize an ovum. Though factors such as gonorrhea and other infections or inadequate nutrition may cause degenerative changes in the ducts, inadequate numbers of sperm or abnormal sperm are more common causes of sterility. A sperm count of less than 20 million per milliliter of semen frequently leads to sterility. If more than 20 percent of the sperm are abnormal or reduced in motility, as shown in laboratory tests, sterility is very likely.

THE FEMALE REPRODUCTIVE SYSTEM

Objective 7. Describe the structure and function of the ovaries.

Objective 8. Describe the structure and function of the uterine tubes, uterus, vagina, and external genitalia.

Objective 9. Describe the structure of the mammary glands (breasts).

Objective 10. Summarize the regulation of function of the female reproductive system, including the menstrual cycle and the way it is altered in pregnancy and menopause.

Objective 11. Explain how the normal functioning of the female reproductive system is altered in cancer of the breast or cervix, ovarian cysts, menstrual disorders, and infertility.

The female reproductive system (Figure 28.11) consists of the ovaries, uterine tubes, uterus, vagina, and the external genitalia. Other structures labeled in the figure will be discussed later. Because of their role in nourishing the offspring, the breasts or mammary glands are considered part of the female reproductive system.

Ovaries

Structure The ovaries are paired structures located in the upper pelvic cavity. Each ovary, shaped like an unshelled almond, is about 3.5 centimeters long, 2 centimeters wide, and 1 centimeter thick. As we shall see later, the ovaries are responsible for producing female sex hormones and ova.

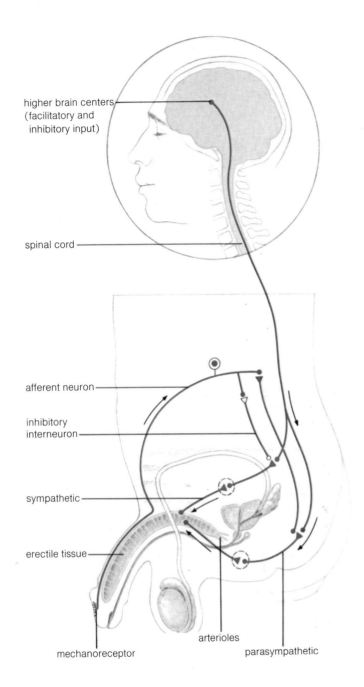

Figure 28.10 The regulation of penile erection.

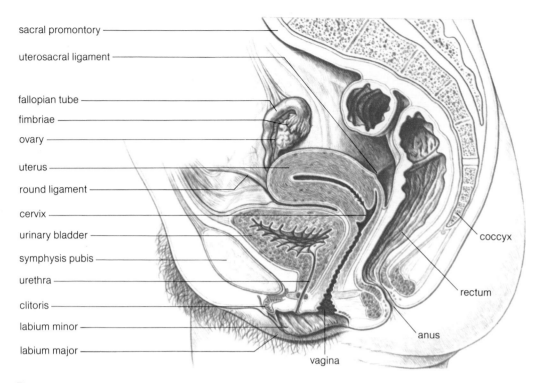

sacral promontory

uterosacral ligament

fallopian tube
fimbriae
ovary
uterus
round ligament
cervix
urinary bladder
symphysis pubis
urethra
clitoris
labium minor
labium major

coccyx

rectum

anus

vagina

Figure 28.11 The female reproductive system.

The ovary (Figure 28.12) is covered by a layer of cuboidal epithelium called the **germinal epithelium**. Beneath the epithelium is the **tunica albuginea**—a layer of connective tissue—and underlying it is the stroma. The **stroma** consists of a dense outer layer called the **cortex** and a less dense inner portion called the **medulla**. Interspersed throughout the cortex are many **ovarian follicles** in different stages of development.

Maturation of follicles During embryonic development several million oogonia (potential ova) migrate from the yolk sac to the germinal epithelium, where their development is arrested at prophase I of meiosis. Many of these primary oocytes undergo **atresia**, a kind of degeneration. At birth about 2 million primary oocytes remain, and by puberty about 400,000 remain, 200,000 in each ovary. A human female is thus born with all the oocytes she will ever have.

Oocytes migrate from the germinal epithelium into the cortex, where they become surrounded by **granulosa**, or **follicular cells**. These follicular cells eventually produce estrogens, which stimulate the development of secondary sexual characteristics and carry out other functions to be described later. An oocyte and the single layer of follicular

cells that surround it form a **primary follicle**. All the follicles remain in this primordial condition until, at puberty, a few follicles begin to mature each month, but usually only one reaches maturity. What causes a single follicle to reach maturity and the other partially developed follicles to degenerate is not known.

When a primary follicle matures, it goes through several stages. As soon as it begins to develop, it is called a **secondary follicle**. First, the oocyte enlarges and is called a **primary oocyte**, and the follicular cells increase in number. Next a thick membrane, the **zona pellucida**, develops between the primary oocyte and the follicle cells. Connective tissue from the stroma forms a covering, or **theca**, around the follicle. Eventually, a space called the **antrum** becomes hollowed out inside the follicle, and the oocyte protrudes into this space. The follicular cells produce a fluid that fills the antrum. As the antrum increases in size, the follicle protrudes from the surface of the ovary. The now-mature follicle, sometimes called a **Graafian follicle**, will soon be released from the ovary.

In the meantime, the primary oocyte has undergone its first meiotic division and is called a **secondary oocyte**. The release of the secondary oocyte from the ovary when the

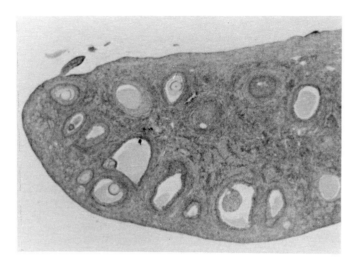

a

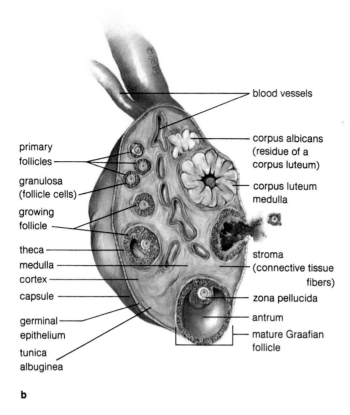

blood vessels

primary
follicles

corpus albicans
(residue of a
corpus luteum)

granulosa
(follicle cells)

corpus luteum
medulla

growing
follicle

theca

stroma
(connective tissue
fibers)

medulla

cortex

capsule

zona pellucida

antrum

germinal
epithelium

mature Graafian
follicle

tunica
albuginea

b

Follicular fluid

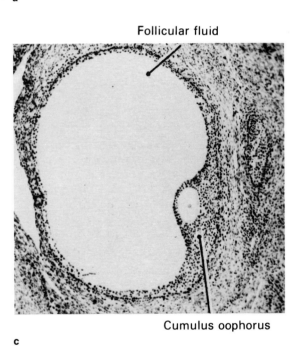

Cumulus oophorus

c

Theca externa

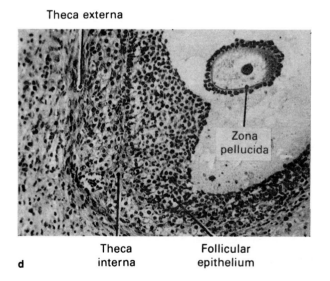

Zona
pellucida

Theca
interna

Follicular
epithelium

d

Figure 28.12 (**a**) Photomicrograph of a cat ovary, × 25. (Photograph by author.) (**b**) Diagram of a cross section through an ovary, showing maturation of follicles. (**c**) A very low-power photomicrograph of a developing follicle distended with follicular fluid. The primary oocyte is surrounded by follicular cells collectively called the cumulus oophorus. (**d**) A low-power photomicrograph of a more mature follicle containing a secondary oocyte, surrounded by a thick membrane called the zona pellucida. The oocyte and its associated cells are still attached to the wall of the follicle, even though the attachment is not apparent in this particular microscopic section through the follicle. (**c** and **d** reproduced with permission from A. W. Ham, *Histology*, J. P. Lippincott, 1979.)

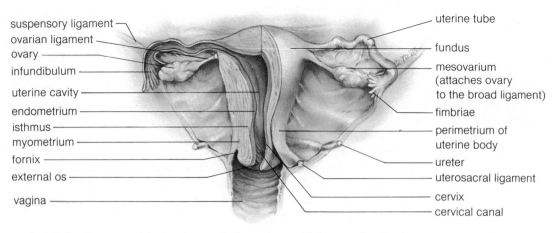

suspensory ligament
ovarian ligament
ovary
infundibulum
uterine cavity
endometrium
isthmus
myometrium
fornix
external os
vagina

uterine tube
fundus
mesovarium
(attaches ovary
to the broad ligament)
fimbriae
perimetrium of
uterine body
ureter
uterosacral ligament
cervix
cervical canal

Figure 28.13   The organs of the female reproductive system and their supporting structures.

follicle ruptures is called **ovulation**. If the secondary oocyte is fertilized after it enters the uterine tube, it completes the second meiotic division to form an **ootid**. The ootid matures and becomes a functional ovum.

Secretions   In addition to releasing an oocyte, the follicle also produces hormones. While the follicle is maturing, some of the follicular cells produce **estrogens**, mainly **estradiol**. After ovulation many of the follicular cells remain in the collapsed follicle on the surface of the ovary. The antrum fills with a partially clotted fluid. The follicular cells enlarge and fill with a yellow pigment, **lutein**. Such a follicle is called a **corpus luteum**—literally, yellow body. The luteal cells secrete small amounts of estradiol and significant amounts of the hormone **progesterone**. If the ovum is not fertilized, the corpus luteum persists for about ten days and then degenerates, leaving a white scarlike area, the **corpus albicans**—literally, white body. If the ovum is fertilized, the corpus luteum enlarges and persists as an endocrine gland, producing small amounts of estradiol and large amounts of progesterone. The secretions of the corpus luteum are essential to maintain pregnancy during the first six weeks, after which the placenta supplies these secretions. (Pregnancy will be discussed in Chapter 29.)

Supporting structures   The ovary is anchored in close proximity to the rest of the organs of the female reproductive

system (Figure 28.13). The **ovarian ligament** attaches the ovary to the uterus and to the **suspensory ligament**. Each ovary is also supported by the **mesovarium**, a membrane that attaches the ovary to the **broad ligament**.

Uterine Tubes, Uterus, Vagina, and External Genitalia

Also shown in Figure 28.13 are the uterine tubes, uterus, and vagina. The paired uterine tubes extend from the ovaries to the uterus. In fact, the uterus is formed from the fusion during development of the paired tubes. The vagina is a muscular tube that leads from the uterus to the outside of the body.

Uterine tubes   The **uterine tubes** (also known as Fallopian tubes or oviducts) are not directly connected to the ovaries. The distal end of the uterine tube, the **infundibulum**, is funnel shaped and has fingerlike projections called **fimbriae**. When an ovum is released at ovulation, the ciliated epithelium of the fimbriae help to direct it into the uterine tube. Should the ovum fail to enter the uterine tube, it would go into the abdominal cavity and degenerate. The proximal ends of the uterine tubes are directly attached to the uterus.

The uterine tubes, which are supported by a portion of the **broad ligament**, are about 10 centimeters long. Their walls consist of three layers of tissue—an outer serous membrane that is continuous with the peritoneum, a middle layer of smooth muscle, and an inner epithelium. Some of the cells of the epithelium are ciliated, and it is thought that their cilia help to sweep the ovum through the tube. The ovum is also propelled by peristaltic contractions of the smooth muscle. Fertilization normally occurs in the uterine tube within twenty-four hours after ovulation.

Uterus The uterus is a pear-shaped organ that lies between the urinary bladder and the rectum. Before the first pregnancy the uterus is about the size of a clenched fist. It is held in place by three pairs of ligaments and two single ligaments. All of these ligaments except for the round ligaments arise from folds in the peritoneum. The paired **broad ligaments** suspend the uterus and form a partition across the pelvic cavity. The paired **round ligaments**, which consist of fibrous bands of connective tissue imbedded in the broad ligaments, contain nerves and blood vessels and attach the uterus to the external genitalia. The paired **uterosacral ligaments** attach the uterus to the sacrum on either side of the rectum. The single **posterior ligament** attaches the uterus to the rectum, and the single **anterior ligament** attaches the uterus to the bladder. The posterior ligament forms the deep **rectouterine pouch** (pouch of Douglas), where pus sometimes collects during pelvic infections. The anterior ligament forms the shallow **vesicouterine pouch**.

The uterus is divided into a rounded superior portion called the **fundus**, a central portion called the **body**, a constricted area called the **isthmus** and the most inferior portion, called the **cervix**. The **internal os** of the isthmus divides the cavity inside the uterus into the superior **uterine cavity** and the inferior **cervical canal**. The **external os** marks the transition from cervix to vagina.

The walls of the uterus consist of three layers. The outer serous layer, the **perimetrium**, consists of parietal peritoneum and is continuous with the broad ligament. It covers most of the surface of the uterus except for the area near 'he cervix. The middle layer, the **myometrium**, is composed of smooth muscle and accounts for most of the bulk of the uterus. The inner layer, the **endometrium**, is a mucous membrane. It is the surface portion of this layer, the **functionalis**, that is sloughed during menstrion, leaving the basal layer, the **basalis**, intact.

Vagina The **vagina** is a tube about 10 centimeters long that extends from the cervix to the outside of the body. It provides a passageway for the menstrual flow, serves as the receptacle for sperm during intercourse, and forms part of the birth canal during labor. It is lined with mucous membrane and has thick, easily stretched transverse rugae (folds) in its muscular walls. A recess called the **fornix** surrounds the area where the cervix projects into the vagina. The posterior fornix is deeper than the anterior and lateral fornices. The opening of the vagina, called the **vaginal orifice**, is partially covered by a membrane called the **hymen**. If the hymen completely closes off the vaginal orifice, a condition called imperforate hymen, it must be removed to allow menstrual flow.

External genitalia The female **external genitalia** are also referred to as the vulva or pudendum (Figure 28.14). The anterior-most portion of the external genitalia is the **mons pubis**, a fatty area covered with skin and pubic hair. Posterior to the mons pubis is the **clitoris**, which terminates in the **glans clitoris** and is surrounded by the **prepuce**. These structures are homologous to the penis and are capable of erection. The glans clitoris is sensitive to stimulation just as is the glans penis. Because of this sensitivity sexual intercourse is accompanied by pleasurable sensations called **orgasm**.

Posterior to these structures in the midline are the urethral opening and the vaginal orifice. Two pairs of skin folds surround the midline structures. Closest to the vaginal orifice are the **labia minora**, which are covered with stratified squamous epithelium. The space beween the labia minora and the vagina is called the **vestibule** of the vagina. A pair of **Bartholin's glands** secrete mucus into the vestibule. The **labia majora** are thicker, more lateral folds that are partly covered by pubic hair and are homologous to the scrotum. The **perineum** comprises the external area from the pubic symphysis to the coccyx; the clinical perineum is the area between the vagina and the anus.

> When the birth canal is too small to allow the birth of a child without tearing, an incision in the clinical perineum, called an **episiotomy**, is made. This purposeful incision prevents more traumatic tearing.

Mammary Glands

The **mammary glands**, or breasts, (Figure 28.15) are modified sweat glands that lie over the pectoral muscles. These glands are undeveloped in children and in postpubertal males. At puberty in females the mammary glands begin to develop under the stimulation of estradiol and other hormones. Externally, the breast is covered with skin and has a nipple surrounded by a pigmented area called the **areola**.

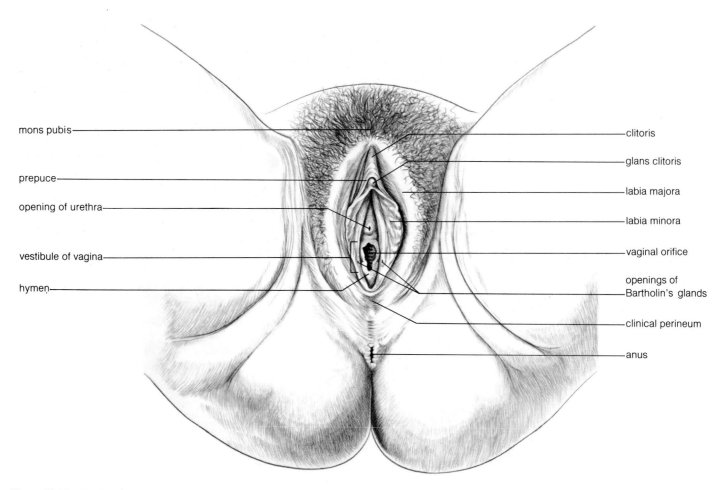

Figure 28.14 The female external genitalia.

mons pubis

prepuce

opening of urethra

vestibule of vagina

hymen

clitoris

glans clitoris

labia majora

labia minora

vaginal orifice

openings of Bartholin's glands

clinical perineum

anus

The surface of the areola is rough because of the presence of modified sebaceous glands beneath the surface. Internally, the mammary gland contains fifteen to twenty **lobes**, each containing many lobules of glandular tissue imbedded in adipose tissue, the **fatty stroma**. Variation in the size of the mammary glands is due to the amount of fatty stroma present and has no relation to the milk-producing capability of the glands. Within each lobe are many small alveoli, which contain the secretory cells. As milk is secreted from these cells, it enters the **secondary tubules**. Several secondary tubules come together to form a **mammary duct**. Just beneath the nipple the mammary ducts become expanded to form the **ampullae**. The **lactiferous ducts** carry the milk from the ampullae to the nipple. Each breast has approximately the same number of lactiferous ducts as it has lobes, except that sometimes a lactiferous duct may drain two lobes. The preparation of the breasts for lactation will be discussed in Chapter 29.

Regulation of Function of the Female Reproductive System

The functions of the ovaries and the uterus are regulated and coordinated by several hormones in a sequence of events called the **menstrual cycle**.

The initiation of the menstrual cycle During puberty **menarche**, the first menstrual cycle, is initiated by the anterior pituitary secreting FSH and LH. LH-RH from the hypothalamus appears to play a role in maintaining the responsiveness of the anterior pituitary but may not directly stimulate the release of FSH and LH. All subsequent cycles are initiated in the same way. The presence of FSH in the blood stimulates the development of several ovarian follicles and the oocyte within each of them. One of these follicles will eventually mature each month. FSH also helps to stimulate the secretion of estradiol from the follicular cells. The presence of LH in the blood likewise stimulates the secretion of

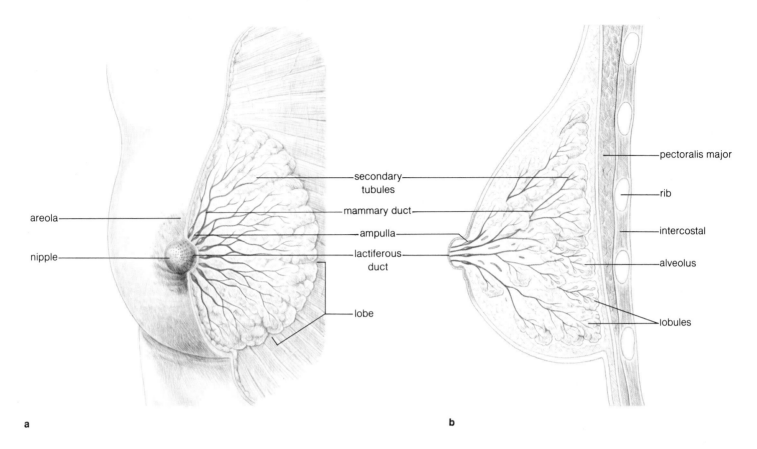

Figure 28.15 The mammary gland: (**a**) anterior view, (**b**) lateral view.

estradiol from the follicular cells and also helps to stimulate the development of the follicle and oocyte. As estradiol is produced, it too stimulates the development of the follicle and acts by negative feedback to suppress the release of both LH-RH and LH. These processes occur over a period of about fourteen days—the preovulatory portion of the cycle, summarized in Figure 28.16. This corresponds to the period during which the menstrual flow occurs and about ten days thereafter. However, wide variations that occur in the length of the menstrual cycle are due to variations in the length of the preovulatory portion of the cycle.

Ovulation On about the fourteenth day of a normal menstrual cycle, there is a midcycle surge of LH and FSH. How this can occur when the estradiol concentration in the blood is increasing has been a topic of much research. The mechanism by which LH causes ovulation is not fully understood, but it is thought that it probably stimulates the

Variation in the length of the menstrual cycle occurs in the preovulatory phase; the length of the postovulatory phase is fourteen days. Hence, abstaining from intercourse around the fourteenth day of the cycle (the rhythm method) is a very unreliable method of birth control.

production of enzymes that digest the thin membrane covering the surface of the bulging follicle. The regulation of ovulation and the postovulatory portion of the cycle are summarized in Figure 28.17.

Postovulatory portion of the cycle Following ovulation the ovum enters the uterine tube and travels to the uterus.

Meanwhile, the remaining follicular cells become the **corpus luteum**. The corpus luteum is maintained by the presence of LH; while it is functional, the corpus luteum secretes the hormone progesterone in additon to estradiol. The functions of progesterone are to stimulate the endometrium, which has previously been stimulated by estradiol to become ready for the implantation of a fertilized ovum, and the mammary glands to prepare to secrete milk. Progesterone also stimulates the secretion of viscous mucus in the cervix and during pregnancy maintains the endometrium and inhibits uterine contractions. **Human chorionic gonadotropin** (HCG), which is released by the placenta during pregnancy, plays an important role in stimulating continued production of progesterone and thus in maintaining pregnancy.

If fertilization does not occur, the corpus luteum degenerates after about ten days. What causes this degeneration is not fully understood, but it appears that a decrease in LH is not necessarily the cause, as some have supposed. Measures of blood concentrations of LH indicate that it decreases only slightly during the postovulatory phase of the menstrual cycle.

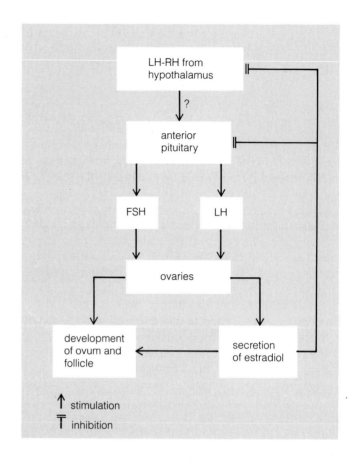

Figure 28.16 (right) Summary of the regulation of ovarian function in the preovulatory portion of the menstrual cycle.

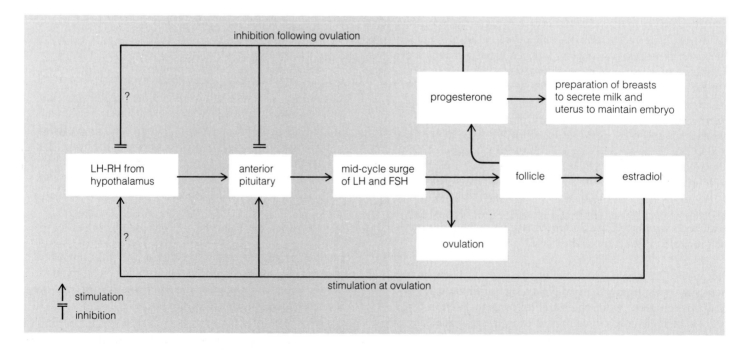

Figure 28.17 Summary of the regulation of ovulation and events in the postovulatory portion of the menstrual cycle.

Figure 28.18 summarizes the changes in the concentrations of pituitary and ovarian hormones throughout the menstrual cycle. It also summarizes the changes in the uterine lining that are discussed below.

Duration of the cycle The duration of one menstrual cycle is arbitrarily said to extend from the beginning of one menstrual flow to the beginning of the next menstrual flow. A typical cycle is about twenty-eight days in duration, but variations from twenty-four to thirty-five days are very common.

Uterine changes during the cycle Changes in the uterine lining during the menstrual cycle are under the direct control of estradiol and progesterone. During the first five days of the cycle, when pituitary stimulation is at its lowest level, estradiol and progesterone drop to their lowest concentrations. The functionalis portion of the endometrium (the layer nearest the uterine lumen) that has built up since the last menstrual flow is sloughed and passes through the vagina and out of the body. The total volume of blood lost ranges from 25 milliliters to 65 milliliters. As the cycle proceeds, small quantities of estradiol that are present through most of the preovulatory phase of the cycle stimulate the smooth muscle cells of the uterus to grow and the endometrium to proliferate large numbers of new cells. These changes, which begin to prepare the uterus for pregnancy, constitute the **proliferative phase** of uterine development.

Following ovulation the concentration of progesterone increases. Progesterone stimulates the further development of the endometrium. The glands of the endometrium are stimulated to secrete fluid, and the endometrium becomes extensively vascularized, thus completing the preparation of the uterus to receive a fertilized ovum. This portion of the uterine cycle is called the **secretory phase**. If no fertilized ovum arrives, the lining is sloughed, and the cycle begins again. The actions of the various hormones in the female reproductive cycle are summarized in Table 28.1.

Effects of pregnancy Should a fertilized ovum arrive and implant in the uterus, the lining is retained, and part of it contributes to the formation of the placenta. Cells associated with the embryo produce human chorionic gonadotropin (HCG), which causes the corpus luteum to continue to secrete estradiol and progesterone for about two months. These cells later become part of the placenta and continue to produce HCG. HCG and the hormones it stimulates maintain the uterine lining and prevent menstruation during pregnancy. After about the third month of pregnancy, the placenta begins to produce estradiol and progesterone itself,

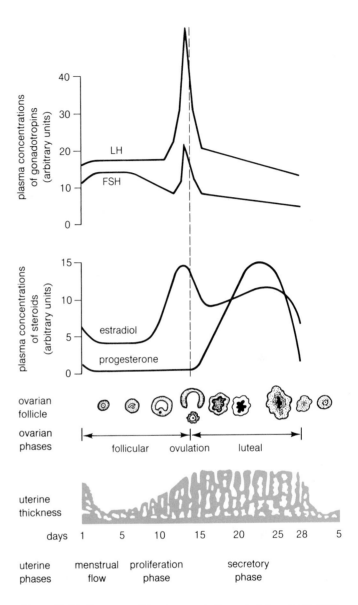

Figure 28.18 Summary of blood concentrations of pituitary and ovarian hormones correlated with phases of the uterine cycle.

and after that time only small amounts of HCG are produced. Thus, the placenta stimulates the corpus luteum to produce hormones until the placenta is able to take over that task itself.

The concentrations of HCG and other hormones during pregnancy can be monitored by measuring the amounts excreted in the urine (Figure 28.19) because some of each of the hormones is removed from the blood as it passes through the kidneys. The presence of large amounts of

Table 28.1 Actions of Hormones Involved in the Female Reproductive Cycle	
Hormone	Actions
Follicle-stimulating Hormone (FSH)	Stimulation of follicle growth
	Stimulation of estradiol production
Estradiol (low level)	Increase in sensitivity of anterior pituitary to LH-RH/FSH-RH
	Stimulation of anterior pituitary to emphasize LH production over FSH production
	Inhibition of LH release
	Proliferation of cells of uterine lining
Estradiol (high level)	Inhibition of FSH release
	Stimulation of LH release
	Cause of LH surge
Luteinizing Hormone (LH)	Induction of ovulation
	Stimulation of follicle growth
	Formation and maintenance of corpus luteum (source of more estradiol and progesterone)
	Stimulation of progesterone production
Progesterone (high level)	Further development of uterus in preparation for implantation
	Increase in size and sensitivity of breasts (with estradiol)
	Inhibition of LH release
	Inhibition of further follicle development
Progesterone (low level)	Degeneration of corpus luteum
	Increase in production of FSH (thus cycle begins again)

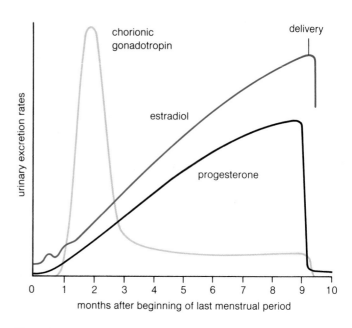

Figure 28.19 Urinary excretion of hormones that maintain pregnancy.

HCG in the urine in the early months of pregnancy forms the basis for most pregnancy tests, though some new techniques to measure HCG in blood are now available.

Menopause The menstrual cycles continue at more or less regular intervals from puberty to **menopause**, except during pregnancy and sometimes during lactation. During menopause the menstrual periods become irregular, and eventually they cease altogether. Estradiol production decreases markedly, usually throughout much of the fifth decade of a woman's life. This decrease occurs in spite of the fact that

Hot flashes—periods of sweating and feeling intense warmth—result from the dilation of arterioles in the skin. Although the reduction in estradiol certainly contributes to the hot flashes of menopause, recent studies have shown a correlation between the experience of a hot flash and a sudden increase in the amount of LH being released. Hot flashes have also been observed in women whose pituitary glands have been removed, suggesting that LH-RH may be the ultimate cause of hot flashes. In the absence of the pituitary hormones, LH-RH continues to be released, probably because no feedback is received to suppress it.

the pituitary gonadotropins are secreted in much larger than normal amounts.

Applications

Breast and cervical cancer Breast and cervical cancer are the leading causes of death from cancer among women. **Breast cancer**, rarely seen before the age of thirty, increases in incidence after menopause. Because breast cancer is difficult to detect and can go unnoticed until it has metastasized or spread to other organs, regular self-examination of the breasts is an essential activity that all women should carry out monthly. Though most lumps are not malignant, if a lump is found, it should be examined by a physician immediately. The standard treatment for breast cancer is a mastectomy. Radical mastectomies in which the entire breast, underlying pectoral muscles, and axillary lymph nodes are removed have been the most common treatment, but in recent years there has been a trend toward modified mastectomies, in which only the breast or a portion of it is removed. Radiation therapy, chemotherapy, or both may be used following a mastectomy to minimize the likelihood of metastasis.

Cervical cancer is a relatively slow-growing cancer; its main risk is that it will go unnoticed until it has invaded other tissues. Cervical cancer may be treated by radiation or surgery. Until recently most physicians recommended an annual Papanicolaou test, or **Pap smear**. In this test cells removed by a swab from the cervix are examined for malignant changes.

Ovarian cysts **Ovarian cysts** are fluid-filled tumors of the ovary. Such cysts sometimes rupture and regress (get smaller) during pregnancy, but in older women they sometimes must be removed surgically. Cysts can arise from follicular tissue, corpus luteum, or even cells of the endometrium that have migrated out of the uterine tubes to the surface of the ovary or the abdominal cavity.

> Controversy now exists as to whether all women or only those at high risk of developing cervical cancer should receive regular Pap smears. Statistically, women at high risk seem to be those who have had a history of genital herpes (to be discussed later), who began to have sexual intercourse early, or who have had many different sexual partners. It has been suggested that the herpes virus may be the actual cause of cervical cancer.

Endometriosis Cysts of endometrial tissue often slough and cause premenstrual or menstrual pain; if these cysts migrate outside the uterus (by way of the uterine tubes), a condition called **endometriosis** exists. Endometrial tissue in any location is subject to stimulation of the same hormones that stimulate it within the uterus. Consequently, the tissue grows and is sloughed into the abdominal cavity, frequently causing extreme discomfort. If this condition does not respond to hormone therapy, surgical removal of the ovaries may be necessary in premenopausal women. Endometriosis disappears following menopause, when the tissue is no longer stimulated by estradiol.

Menstrual disorders **Menstrual disorders** include amenorrhea, or the absence of menstruation; excessive or abnormal bleeding of the uterus; and dysmenorrhea, or painful menstruation. **Primary amenorrhea**, the complete absence of menstruation, is usually due to a genetic or birth defect and sometimes due to an endocrine disorder. **Secondary amenorrhea**, the lack of menstruation in a woman who has previously menstruated, is usually caused by an endocrine disorder or anorexia nervosa (see Chapter 24), but pregnancy should be ruled out before other causes are considered. Excessive bleeding or bleeding between menstrual periods or after menopause also may be caused by endocrine disorders, but other factors including cancer may be involved.

Dysmenorrhea affects from 30 to 50% of all women of childbearing age. This disorder, often called cramps, may be caused by fibroid tumors of the uterus, endometriosis, or some other identifiable cause. However, until recently no known cause had been found in the majority of cases. It is now believed that excessive production of prostaglandins by the uterus is responsible for dysmenorrhea. These prostaglandins appear to be important in initiating both menstruation and labor, causing the uterus to contract in both cases. The pain seems to result from reduced blood flow through the uterine muscle because of sustained partial contraction. Women with severe dysmenorrhea have been shown to have much higher than normal concentrations of prostaglandins in the menstrual fluid than women not bothered by the disorder. Prostaglandin inhibitors are now being tested to determine their effects on dysmenorrhea. Some of these drugs are already on the market as antiinflammatory drugs, and experimental studies show that they are usually effective in alleviating dysmenorrhea. So far, the only conditions that appear to be aggravated by prostaglandin-inhibitors are asthma and gastrointestinal ulcers.

Birth control pills are also effective in controlling dysmenorrhea, possibly by reducing the development of the uterine lining. When the uterine lining fails to reach its normal thickness, the amount of prostaglandin it can produce is greatly reduced. A problem with this therapy is that it requires the woman to take doses of hormones for twenty-one days to control a condition that lasts only one or two days.

Infertility **Infertility** in women is the inability to become pregnant. It may be due to failure to ovulate or to some anatomical factor that prevents the union of egg and sperm. Certain drugs, often called fertility drugs, are used in the treatment of infertility due to failure to ovulate. One such drug, Clomiphene, appears to release the hypothalamic-anterior pituitary system from inhibition by estradiol. The effect is to stimulate ovulation. Some drugs used to stimulate ovulation occasionally cause the release of an unusually large number of ova. If these ova are fertilized and become implanted in the uterus, a multiple pregnancy of as many as five or six fetuses may occur. Infertility caused by blockage of the uterine tubes is treated surgically. In some though not all, cases the uterine tubes can be opened so that an ovum can pass along a tube normally.

FERTILIZATION

Objective 12. Describe the process of fertilization and the factors that may affect it.

Fertilization

Fertilization occurs in the upper end of the uterine tube, about one-third of the way between the ovary and the uterus. Sperm are introduced into the vagina through sexual intercourse. Rhythmic contractions of perineal muscles in both the male and female during intercourse help to propel the sperm part way through the uterus. Peristaltic movements of the uterus and uterine tubes likewise help to propel the sperm, as do movements of the flagella of the sperm themselves. Cilia in the uterine tube and contractions of the tube move the ovum toward the sperm.

Fertilization usually occurs within 24 hours after ovulation and 4 to 6 hours after intercourse, but it may occur in as little as 30 minutes. The sperm must be in the genital tract for this length of time to allow the enzyme hyaluronidase of the acrosome to become sufficiently active to dissolve the membrane around the ovum. The hyaluronidase of many sperm is needed to dissolve the membrane, though only one sperm enters the ovum. When the sperm has gained entry

In some instances a fertilized ovum fails to move out of the uterine tube to implant in the uterus. In other instances an ovum may enter the abdominal cavity instead of the uterine tube, and a sperm may fertilize it there. Implantation of a fertilized ovum in a site other than the uterus is called an **ectopic pregnancy**. Such pregnancies usually have to be aborted surgically to prevent damage to the uterine tube or abdominal organs.

into the ovum, a fertilization membrane develops around the ovum and prevents the entry of additional sperm. The fertilized egg then completes the second meiotic division. After entering the ovum, the sperm becomes the **male pronucleus**. Similarly, the nucleus of the ovum becomes the **female pronucleus**. The fusion of these two nuclei to form a single nucleus constitutes fertilization. The resulting cell is called a zygote, the first cell of the developing embryo. (We will consider the further development of the embryo in Chapter 29.)

SEXUALLY TRANSMITTED DISEASES

Objective 13. Summarize the causes and effects of sexually transmitted diseases.

Sexually transmitted diseases, or venereal diseases, are spread primarily through sexual intercourse or other sexual contact. Many different sexually transmitted diseases (STDs) exist, and about 10 million people per year in the United States are infected by one of these diseases; two-thirds of the victims are under twenty-five years of age. Gonorrhea is by far the most common of all STDs; it is even more common than chickenpox. Syphilis is the next most common STD, but genital herpes is becoming increasingly common. Other diseases that may be transmitted sexually include cytomegalovirus infection, nongonococcal urethritis, group B streptococcal infection, trichomoniasis, candidiasis, hepatitis B, pediculosis pubis, and venereal warts. Of these diseases only the three most common will be considered here.

Gonorrhea **Gonorrhea** has 3 million known victims in the United States; some health officials believe that additional unreported cases might boost that figure to more than 20 million! Caused by a bacterium, *Neisseria gonorrhoeae*, gonorrhea may be asymptomatic and go undetected until complications appear. When there are symptoms, a discharge of pus from the penis or excessive vaginal secretion may be seen. However, signs are less apparent in women than in men, and vaginal secretion may be ignored as only slightly greater than normal. Burning on urination and pain around the genitals are also frequent symptoms. Most cases of gonorrhea are curable with antibiotics, but a penicillin-resistant strain does exist in the United States. When such a strain is encountered, other more expensive antibiotics must be used.

The victim can spread the disease to others at any stage of the disease, and transmission is generally through sexual contact. However, because cases of gonorrhea have been reported in young children who show no signs of sexual molestation, the organism may survive on bathroom fixtures or bed linens long enough to be transmitted, or nonsexual intimacy with infected adults may provide an avenue for transmission. Because having the disease does not confer immunity, individuals who have been infected can easily be reinfected, especially if they continue to have contact with those who have the disease and have not been treated. Because of the lack of immunity and because of the almost epidemic extent of the disease, it is imperative that all who are exposed be checked for the disease and, if infected, treated until completely cured.

The complications of gonorrhea can be severe. Pelvic inflammatory disease is a common complication, and the bacterium can invade the urinary tract and other organs. Fever, severe abdominal cramps, and vomiting may occur as the disease spreads. Permanent damage to the uterine tubes frequently leads to sterility. If gonorrhea is contracted during pregnancy, the organism will not be transmitted across the placenta to the fetus. However, the eyes of the infant may become infected as it passes through the birth canal. Silver nitrate or an antibiotic is routinely placed in the eyes of newborns to prevent transmission of the infection in this way.

Syphilis **Syphilis** is caused by the spirochete (spiral bacterium) *Treponema pallidum*. Because of its long incubation period—from ten to ninety days—individuals who have had several sexual contacts during the incubation period may find it difficult to determine the source of the infection. Regardless of the difficulty, all people who may be infected should be checked and treated if necessary. Though the incidence of syphilis in the United States is less than that of gonorrhea, it is nonetheless a serious problem because the long-term consequences of untreated syphilis are far more severe than those of gonorrhea.

The symptoms of syphilis occur in three stages. The first stage usually consists of a painless lesion called a **chancre** at the organism's site of entry. The chancre is usually on the external genitals, but in women it may be inside the vagina. The chancre heals quickly even without treatment, and the victim is likely to think that the disease is gone. Nothing could be further from the truth; the organism is simply invading other tissues. The second stage begins as the organism enters the blood. Symptoms such as fever, a flulike illness, a skin rash, hair loss, and swollen joints may come and go over a period of several years. After these symptoms finally disappear, the disease may be quiescent for years, with the third stage appearing up to forty years after the initial exposure. In this third stage permanent brain damage, heart disease, and blindness often occur.

Syphilis can be cured with large doses of antibiotics. However, if it is left untreated, syphilis proceeds through the above stages, and the victim is infectious when lesions are present. Even with treatment immunity does not develop, so reinfection is likely unless all of the victim's sexual partners are also treated.

Unlike gonorrhea, syphilis can be transmitted across the placenta to a fetus. The organisms enter the fetus's bloodstream and invade all the tissues of the body. This disease, congenital syphilis, may cause brain damage and even death of the fetus, or the child can be born and die later.

Genital herpes **Genital herpes** is caused by a virus, herpes virus hominis, type 2. It begins with a genital rash and itching within two to twenty days of exposure. Painful fluid-filled blisters develop and are accompanied by a flulike illness and swollen lymph nodes. The disease subsides and reoccurs periodically throughout life; it is contagious whenever the lesions are present. The incidence of cervical cancer is much higher in individuals infected with genital herpes than in those not known to have been infected. In women the disease can account for spontaneous abortions, premature births, and stillbirths. The infant may acquire meningitis during birth.

Until recently there was no effective treatment for genital herpes. Now two treatments have been tried with somewhat promising results. The injection under the skin of flu vaccine and the topical application of a sugar called 2-deoxy-D-glucose have both been shown to alleviate the symptoms of the disease. In the few patients who have been treated with the sugar and followed for two years, only two out of eighteen have had recurrences of the disease, and they have had milder symptoms on recurrence.

CLINICAL TERMS

laparoscopy (lap-ar-os'ko-pe)   visual examination of the interior of the abdomen by the use of a lighted instrument inserted through a small incision

leukorrhea (lu-ko-re'ah)   a viscid, whitish discharge from the uterine cavity and vagina

salpingitis (sal-pin-ji'tis)   inflammation of a uterine tube

smegma (smeg'mah)   cheesy secretion found under the prepuce or labia minora

vaginitis (vaj-in-i'tis)   inflammation of the vagina

Essay: Birth Control

Human beings have attempted to control their own fertility for as long as there is recorded history of any human activity. Yet, historically, there has been strong opposition to the distribution of information on birth control.

The modern birth control movement was launched in England in 1822 by Francis Place, who recommended that the working people control their numbers so they would have no more children than they could care for and so the numbers of working people would be small enough that they could command living wages. In the United States the Comstock Law, passed by Congress in 1873, made it a criminal offense for anyone, even a physician, to transport in interstate commerce "any article of medicine for the prevention of conception or for causing abortion." This law stayed in force until the middle of the twentieth century. Margaret Sanger, who worked in the New York City tenements, is credited with leading the crusade to destroy this law and make birth control information available. Though today we take for granted the availability of contraceptive devices, the battle that made them available was a long and difficult one.

Birth control can be defined as the intentional prevention of fertilization of an ovum or the prevention of implantation of a fertilized ovum. Methods of birth control vary in their effectiveness and in the advantages and disadvantages of their use. Side effects, other health factors, and the long-term effects on the ability to have children also vary among the different methods. These attributes of a number of contraceptives are summarized in Table 28.2. The use of various methods is illustrated in Figure 28.20.

The mechanisms by which contraceptives prevent child-

birth are varied. Vasectomy prevents the sperm from leaving the testes; tubal ligation prevents the ovum and sperm from meeting in the uterine tube. Oral contraceptives, or birth control pills, manipulate the production of hormones so that ovulation does not occur. One type of pill, the combination pill, contains both estradiol and progesterone and keeps the levels of these hormones high enough to prevent the preovulation surge of LH, thereby preventing ovulation. Another type of pill that contains only progesterone is effective for unknown reasons. The exact effect of the IUD is not well understood, but it probably causes changes in the endometrium that prevent implantation of a fertilized ovum should one arrive in the uterus. Both the diaphragm and the condom serve as mechanical barriers to prevent sperm from entering the uterus. Spermicidal foam, cream, and jelly kill sperm. The rhythm method of abstinence from intercourse during fertile periods relies on the rise in body temperature or on changes in the amount of vaginal secretion that occur at ovulation. Because these changes are not always detectable, the method has serious drawbacks.

Research is underway to develop other kinds of contraceptives. These include a "morning-after pill" and injectable and implantable materials. The "morning-after pill," which consists of diethylstilbesterol (DES), probably acts by preventing implantation. The injectable substance is a progesterone derivative called Depo-Provera, which inhibits follicle development; it must be injected about once every three months. Implantable materials that are being developed for both males and females contain hormones that are released slowly and interfere with the production of sperm or ova.

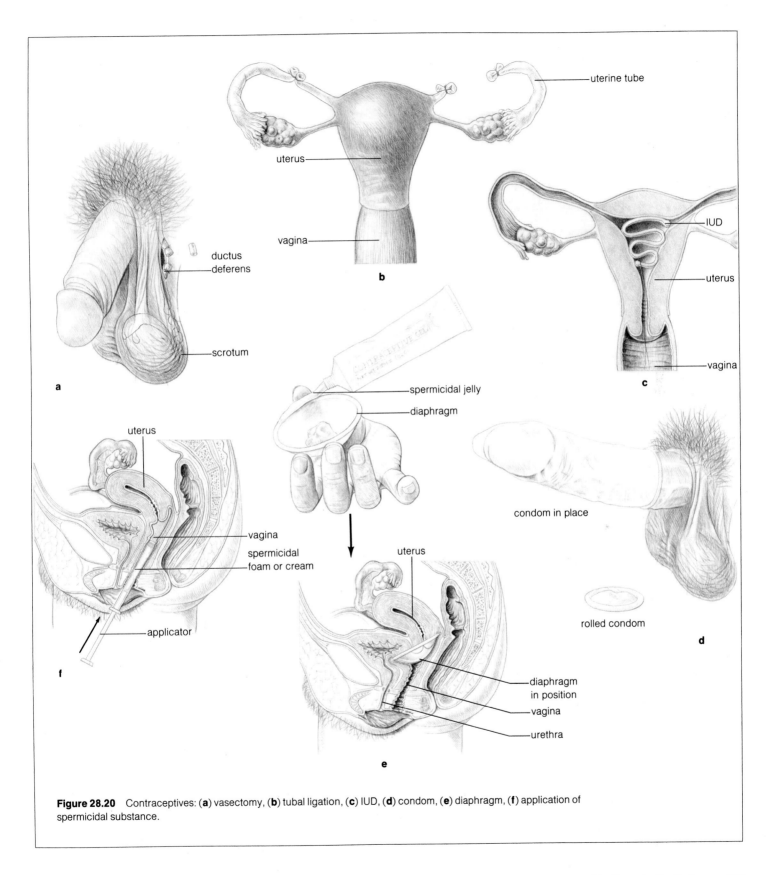

Figure 28.20 Contraceptives: (**a**) vasectomy, (**b**) tubal ligation, (**c**) IUD, (**d**) condom, (**e**) diaphragm, (**f**) application of spermicidal substance.

Table 28.2 Characteristics of Birth Control Methods

Method	Effectiveness	Advantages and Disadvantages	Side Effects	Health Factors to Consider	Long-Term Effect on Ability to Have Children
Vasectomy	Virtually 100%	One time procedure for male; does not require hospitalization; should be considered permanent; other contraceptive must be used for a few months until all sperm are out of reproductive tract.	Complications in less than 4% of cases can include infection and inflammatory reaction.	Autoimmune reactions, testicular cysts.	Procedure is not generally reversible.
Tubal ligation	Virtually 100%	One time procedure for female; does require hospitalization, usually in outpatient facility; should be considered permanent.	Complications are rare but include infection, bleeding, and injury to other organs.	Surgery carries some risk and varies with the general health of the patient.	Procedure is not generally reversible.
Oral contraceptives	Less than 1 pregnancy in 100 woman-years* with the estrogen–progesterone pill; 2–3 pregnancies in 100 woman-years with progesterone only pill.	No action needed except to take pill, which must be taken regularly; combination is taken for 21 days each month, and progesterone is taken continuously.	Tender breasts, nausea, loss or gain of weight; can cause blood clots; increases risk of heart attack, especially in smokers; high blood pressure and gallbladder disease in a few users.	Women who smoke should not use the pill, nor should those who already have heart disease, blood clots, or breast cancer. Migraine headaches, depression, fibroids of the uterus, kidney disease, asthma, high blood pressure, diabetes, and epilepsy may be made worse by the pill.	Using the pill does not seem to prevent later pregnancy, but user should wait a few months after stopping the pill before becoming pregnant; after childbirth nursing mothers should not use the pill because the drugs appear in the milk and long-range effects on the infant are not known.
Intrauterine device (IUD)	Effectiveness depends on whether IUD stays in place; 1–6 pregnancies per 100 woman-years.	Must be inserted by a physician and checked annually, though woman can check for strings extending into vagina; may cause discomfort when inserted; may cause cramps and heavier flow; can be expelled without woman knowing.	Complications are relatively infrequent but include anemia, pregnancy outside uterus, infection, and perforation of the uterus.	Women who have or have had the following conditions should discuss them with a physician before deciding to use the IUD; cancer of cervix or uterus, heavy or irregular bleeding, pelvic infection, abortion, miscarriage, VD, severe cramps, anemia, fainting, vaginal discharge, or suspicious or abnormal Pap smear.	Pelvic infection in some IUD users may result in future inability to have children.
Diaphragm (with spermicidal cream, foam, or jelly)	Effectiveness depends on how correctly the method is used; 2–20 pregnancies in 100 woman-years.	Diaphragm and spermicide must be inserted no more than 2 hours before intercourse; no effect on chemical or physical processes of the body; must be left in place for 6 hours after intercourse; must be fitted by a physician and refitted after childbirth or abortion; requires instruction in insertion technique; some women whose cervix protrudes abnormally into the vagina cannot use a diaphragm.	A few women are allergic to the rubber of the diaphragm or to the spermicidal jelly.	None	None

Table 28.2 Characteristics of Birth Control Methods (continued)

Method	Effectiveness	Advantages and Disadvantages	Side Effects	Health Factors to Consider	Long-Term Effect on Ability to Have Children
Condom	Effectiveness depends on how correctly the method is used; 3–36 pregnancies in 100 woman-years.	Easily available, requires no long-term planning; also protects against VD; some users feel the condom reduces the pleasure of intercourse; male must interrupt foreplay and fit condom in place before sexual entry into the woman; condom can slip or tear and release sperm into the vagina.	A few men are allergic to rubber condoms, but can use those made of lamb cecum.	None	None
Spermicidal foam, cream, or jelly used alone	Effectiveness depends on how correctly the method is used; 2–36 pregnancies in 100 woman-years.	Easy to obtain and use; must be used 1 hour or less before intercourse; must be left in vagina 6–8 hours after intercourse.	Allergic reaction may cause irritation of penis or vagina; can be corrected by changing brands.	None	None
Rhythm method	Effectiveness depends on how correctly the method is used; 11–25 pregnancies in 100 woman-years using temperature or vaginal secretion with calendar.	No drugs or devices needed; careful record must be kept to predict approximate time of ovulation; temperature must be taken on arising to determine when ovulation occurs (temperature rises), or record of mucus in vaginal secretions must be kept (mucus increases after ovulation); method is difficult to use if cycles are irregular.	No physical effects, but because couple must abstain from intercourse for a long time prior to and shortly after ovulation, the method can create pressures on a couple's relationship.	None	None

*A woman-year refers to one woman for one year. Pregnancies per 100 woman-years usually means that a certain number of pregnancies occurred among 100 women over a period of one year.

CHAPTER SUMMARY

(Chapter summary points and review questions are numbered to correspond to the numbered objectives in the text of each chapter.)

Organization and General Functions

1. Describe the overall organization of the male and female reproductive systems and list their major functions.
   a. The organs of the male reproductive system include the testes, a system of ducts, and several glands.
   b. The organs of the female reproductive system include the ovaries, uterine ducts, uterus, and vagina.
   c. Both systems produce gametes and provide for their transport to the point of union in fertilization. In addition, the female reproductive system provides a place for the embryo to develop.
   d. Both systems produce hormones that initiate and regulate the reproductive processes; these hormones are in turn regulated by other hormones.

Development

2. Compare the development of the male and female reproductive systems.

a. The gonads begin development as undifferentiated organs.

b. In the presence of a Y chromosome the external male ducts are stimulated to develop by the production of testosterone in the male fetus.

c. In the absence of a Y chromosome the female organs develop.

d. The external genitalia likewise begin as undifferentiated structures, with male and female homologous structures becoming differentiated during development.

The Male Reproductive System

3. Describe the structure and function of the testes and scrotum.

a. The testes, located in the scrotum, produce sperm and the hormone testosterone:

(1) Sperm are produced by a process called spermatogenesis.

(2) Sertoli cells nourish the sperm.

(3) Interstitial cells of Leydig produce testosterone.

(4) Mature sperm are released into the lumen of the convoluted seminiferous tubules. They pass through the straight tubules to the rete testis and on to the efferent ductules before leaving the testis and entering the epididymis.

b. Testes normally descend into the scrotum, a baglike structure covered with skin, prior to birth.

c. The temperature of the scrotum, a few degrees below the abdominal temperature, is the optimum temperature for developing sperm.

4. Describe the structure and function of the ducts and glands of the male reproductive system.

a. The ducts of the male reproductive system include:

(1) the epididymis, a coiled tube that extends along the posterior side of the testis

(2) the ductus deferens, a straight tube that extends from the epididymis to the ejaculatory duct

(3) the ejaculatory duct, a short tube that carries sperm from the ductus deferens to the urethra

(4) the urethra, a common passageway for both semen and urine, which runs from the ejaculatory duct through the penis to the outside of the body

b. The penis contains tissues that fill with blood and make an erection possible.

c. The glands of the male reproductive system include:

(1) the seminal vesicles, which secrete a viscous fluid containing fructose and prostaglandins

(2) the prostate gland, which secretes a milky fluid that makes up most of the volume of semen

(3) the bulbourethral, or Cowper's, glands, which also contribute secretions to the semen

5. Explain how the function of the male reproductive system is regulated.

a. In the regulation of the male reproductive system, testosterone and sperm production are regulated by hormones from the pituitary gland:

(1) FSH (follicle-stimulating hormone) stimulates sperm production.

(2) LH stimulates the interstitial cells of Leydig to produce testosterone and also contributes to the development of sperm.

b. LH-RH may stimulate the release of the pituitary hormones.

c. Neural factors regulate the erection of the penis during sexual activity.

6. Describe the alterations of function that occur in (a) prostatitis, (b) prostate cancer, (c) impotence, and (d) sterility.

a. Prostatitis is an inflammation of the prostate gland in which the gland enlarges and sometimes blocks the flow of urine.

b. Prostate cancer, an extremely common malignancy in males, is often stimulated by testosterone. It may be treated with estrogens that counteract the effects of testosterone or by removal of the testes.

c. Impotence, the inability to achieve and hold an erection long enough to complete sexual intercourse, may be caused by psychological or physiological factors.

d. Sterility, the inability to fertilize an ovum, is caused by factors that reduce the number or cause abnormality of sperm.

The Female Reproductive System

7. Describe the structure and function of the ovaries.

a. The ovaries are small glands that produce ova and the hormones estradiol and progesterone.

b. The ovaries contain primary follicles, which develop into mature Graafian follicles ready to release an ovum.

c. At ovulation the ovum is released, and the remaining follicle cells become the corpus luteum. The copus luteum persists through the first two months of pregnancy and secretes progesterone, which helps to maintain pregnancy.

d. If the ovum is not fertilized, the corpus luteum degenerates and becomes the corpus albicans.

e. The ovary is supported by the ovarian and suspensory ligaments.

8. Describe the structure and function of the uterine tubes, uterus, vagina, and external genitalia.

a. The uterine tubes have fimbriated ends, which receive the ovum from the ovary and transport it to the uterus.

b. When fertilization takes place, it occurs in the uterine tube.

c. The uterine tubes, supported by a portion of the broad ligament, consist of three layers of tissue—an outer serous layer, a middle muscular layer, and an inner ciliated epithelium.

d. The uterus, supported by the broad and round ligaments, also consists of three layers—serous, muscular, and epithelial. The epithelial layer, called the endometrium, is partly shed during menstruation.

e. The uterine cavity is separated from the vagina by the cervix and the cervical canal.

f. The vagina is a muscular tube extending from the cervix to the vaginal orifice. It is lined with mucous membrane and is partially closed by the hymen.

    g. The external genitalia include the mons pubis, the clitoris, and the labia minora and labia majora.

9. Describe the structure of the mammary glands (breasts).

    a. The mammary glands are modified sweat glands that develop in females at puberty.

    b. Lobes of secretory tissue produce milk, which is carried to the nipple by a set of ducts.

10. Summarize the regulation of function of the female reproductive system, including the menstrual cycle and the way it is altered in pregnancy and menopause.

    a. The function of the female reproductive system is regulated by hormones from the anterior pituitary gland and a releasing factor from the hypothalamus.

    b. The menstrual cycle consists of a sequence of events in the ovaries and uterus. This process delivers an ovum to the uterine cavity once each month and provides conditions for its development if it has been fertilized.

        (1) In a typical cycle the first fourteen days are devoted to the development of a mature ovum, which is then released.

        (2) During the preovulatory phase the endometrium of the uterus has also undergone proliferation.

        (3) After ovulation the ovum travels along the uterine tube, where it may be fertilized.

        (4) Also after ovulation the uterine lining completes its development and is ready to receive a fertilized ovum; if a fertilized ovum is received, it implants, and pregnancy ensues.

        (5) If the ovum is not fertilized, the uterine lining begins to degenerate and is shed after the twenty-eighth day of the cycle.

        (6) The menstrual flow marks the beginning of the next cycle.

    c. Menopause occurs in the fifth decade of life and is marked by the cessation of menstruation and the reduced production of estradiol by the ovaries.

11. Explain how the normal functioning of the female reproductive system is altered in cancer of the breast or cervix, ovarian cysts, menstrual disorders, and infertility.

    a. Cancer of the breast and cervix are common kinds of malignancies of the female reproductive system. Breast self-examination and Pap smears of cervical tissue are useful methods for early detection of these malignancies.

    b. Ovarian cysts, fluid-filled tumors of the ovary, can arise from various tissues, including endometrium. The presence of endometrial cysts outside the uterus is called endometriosis.

    c. Menstrual disorders include:

        (1) amenorrhea, the absence of menstruation

        (2) dysmenorrhea, painful menstruation

        (3) excessive or abnormal bleeding of the uterus

    d. Infertility is the inability to conceive.

Fertilization

12. Describe the process of fertilization and the factors that may affect it.

    a. Fertilization is the union of the male and female pronuclei of the sperm and ovum, respectively.

    b. Factors that facilitate fertilization are muscular contractions during intercourse, contractions of the uterine tubes, beating of flagella of sperm, and beating of cilia of the uterine tubes.

Sexually Transmitted Diseases

13. Summarize the causes and effects of sexually transmitted diseases.

    a. Sexually transmitted diseases include gonorrhea, syphilis, genital herpes, and many other less common or less serious diseases.

    b. Gonorrhea is caused by a bacterium and is treatable with antibiotics.

    c. Syphilis is also caused by a bacterium and is treatable with antibiotics if diagnosed in the early stages.

    d. Genital herpes is caused by a virus and has recently been treated effectively with the sugar 2-deoxy-D-glucose.

REVIEW

Important Terms

acrosome	interstitial cells of Leydig
Bartholin's glands	lactiferous duct
bulbourethral glands	menarche
clitoris	menstrual cycle
corpus albicans	myometrium
corpus luteum	ovulation
ductus deferens	perimetrium
ejaculatory duct	perineum
endometrium	prepuce
epididymis	proliferative phase
erection	prostate gland
fertilization	secretory phase
fimbriae	semen
follicular cells	seminal vesicles
Graafian follicle	seminiferous tubules
infundibulum	Sertoli cells

Questions

1. **a.** What are the functions of the male and female reproductive systems?
   b. Name the major organs of the male reproductive system and of the female reproductive system.

2. **a.** Describe the differentiation of the male and female reproductive systems, noting homologies between the two.
   b. What are the roles of the Y chromosome and testosterone in the development of the reproductive system?

3. **a.** How are sperm produced?
   b. What are the functions of testosterone?

4. **a.** Trace the pathway of sperm from where they are produced to their release from the male reproductive system during ejaculation.
   b. Name the glands of the male reproductive system and describe their secretions that help to make up semen.

5. **a.** How is the production of testosterone regulated?
   b. How is the production of sperm regulated?
   c. How is an erection created?

6. How is the function of the body altered in (a) prostatitis, (b) prostate cancer, (c) impotence, and (d) sterility?

7. **a.** Describe the structure of an ovary and explain how a primary follicle becomes a Graafian follicle.
   b. What hormones are produced by the ovary, where are they produced, and what are their functions?

8. **a.** How is the structure of the uterine tube well suited for the site of fertilization?
   b. How is the structure of the uterus well suited for the implantation of an embryo?
   c. Describe the structure of the vagina.
   d. Describe the structure of the female external genitalia.

9. **a.** Where in the mammary gland is milk produced?
   b. How does the milk get to the nipple?

10. **a.** Describe the events in the ovary during the menstrual cycle.
    b. What happens to the uterine lining at the various stages of the menstrual cycle?
    c. What is the role of the hypothalamus and the anterior pituitary gland in regulating the menstrual cycle?
    d. Compare the events that follow ovulation when an ovum is fertilized to those when an ovum is not fertilized.
    e. What happens to the ovaries and the menstrual cycle during menopause?

11. **a.** What is breast cancer, and how is it treated?
    b. What is a possible cause of cervical cancer?
    c. What are the symptoms of an ovarian cyst? Of endometriosis?
    d. Name three kinds of menstrual disorders and distinguish among them.
    e. What is infertility, and how might it be treated?

12. **a.** What is fertilization?
    b. What factors contribute to the movement of the sperm and the movement of the ovum?

13. Describe the cause and effects of (a) gonorrhea, (b) syphilis, and (c) genital herpes.

Problems

1. Suppose a couple came to you for help with their problem of infertility. What steps would you take to determine the cause of the problem? For at least three different kinds of problems, what treatment would you recommend and why?

2. Suggest some ways that the incidence of sexually transmitted diseases might be decreased.

REFERENCES AND READINGS

Anonymous. 1979. A promising treatment for herpes. *Science News* 115:5 (July 7).

Behrman, H. R. 1979. Prostaglandins in hypothalamo-pituitary and ovarian function. *Annual Review of Physiology* 41:685.

Casper, R. F., Yen, S. S. C., and Wilkes, M. M. 1979. Menopausal flushes: A neuroendocrine link with pulsatile luteinizing hormone secretion. *Science* 205:823 (August 24).

Epel, D. 1977. The program of fertilization. *Scientific American* 237(5):129 (November).

Food and Drug Administration. 1978. *Contraception: Comparing the options.* Rockville, Md.: U.S. Department of Health, Education and Welfare Publication No. (FDA) 78–3069.

Grobstein, C. 1979. External human fertilization. *Scientific American* 240(6):57 (June).

Hardin, G., ed. 1964. *Population, evolution, and birth control.* San Francisco: W. H. Freeman.

Heber, D., and Swerdloff, R. S. 1980. Male contraception: Synergism of gonadotropin-releasing hormone analog and testosterone in suppressing gonadotropin. *Science* 209:936 (August 22).

Leung, P. C. K., and Armstrong, D. T. 1980. Interactions of steroids and gonadotropins in the control of steroidogenesis in the ovarian follicle. *Annual Review of Physiology* 42:71.

Marx, J. L. 1978. The mating game: What happens when sperm meets egg. *Science* 200:1256 (June 16).

Marx, J. L. 1978. Contraception: An antipregnancy vaccine. *Science* 200:1258 (June 16).

Marx, J. L. 1979. Dysmenorrhea: Basic research leads to a rational therapy. *Science* 205:175 (July 13).

Marx, J. L. 1979. The annual Pap smear: An idea whose time has gone? *Science* 205:177 (July 13).

Means, A. R., Dedman, J. R., Tash, J. S., Tindall, D. J., van Sickle, M., and Welsh, M. J. 1980. Regulation of the testis Sertoli cell by follicle stimulating hormone. *Annual Review of Physiology* 42:59.

Miller, J. A. 1980. Unisex birth control chemical. *Science News* 117:331 (May 24).

Sanborn, B. M., Heindel, J. J., and Robison, G. A. 1980. The role of cyclic nucleotides in reproductive processes. *Annual Review of Physiology* 42:37.

Schally, A. V. 1978. Aspects of hypothalamic regulation of the pituitary gland. *Science* 202:18 (October 6).

Wills, M. S. 1979. Cervical caps: Old and yet too new. *Science News* 116:431 (December 22 and 29).

Yarber, W. L. 1978. Waging war on VD. *The Science Teacher* 45(5):38 (May).

29

LIFE STAGES

OVERVIEW OF LIFE STAGES

Objective 1. List the stages of human life from conception to death.

From conception to death the stages of human life are prenatal development, birth, the neonatal period, infancy, childhood, adolescence, adulthood, and old age. Most of the information presented so far in this text has concerned the anatomy and physiology of the adult; in this chapter we will consider the anatomical and physiological conditions that distinguish the other stages of life. We will also discuss the physiology of pregnancy.

PRENATAL DEVELOPMENT

Objective 2. Describe the major events in prenatal development.

Objective 3. Define the term teratogen and describe the effects of selected teratogens.

Major Events in Prenatal Development

After fertilization occurs in the uterine tube, the fertilized ovum, or **zygote**, undergoes several mitotic divisions known as **cleavage**. To review the process described in Chapter 4, a single cell becomes two; each of the two divides, making four; each of the four divides, making eight cells; and so on,

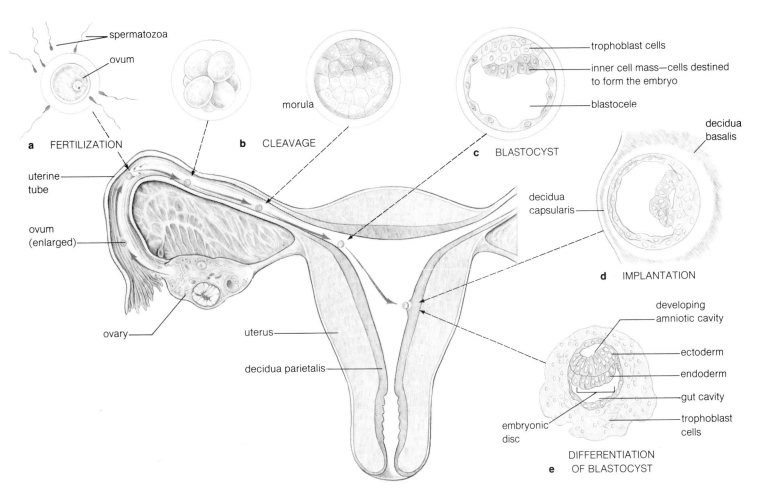

Figure 29.1 An overview of the developmental stages of an embryo from fertilization to early differentiation following implantation.

until a solid ball of cells, the **morula**, is formed. These changes take place as the embryo travels along the uterine tube toward the uterus (Figure 29.1). About three days after fertilization the morula arrives in the uterine cavity, where its cells undergo a rearrangement to form a hollow ball, the **blastocyst**. At the end of the first week the blastocyst consists of an outer layer of cells called the **trophoblast**, an **inner cell mass**, and a cavity called the **blastocele**.

During the second week the blastocyst undergoes further changes before it implants in the wall of the uterus. The cells of the inner cell mass continue to divide by mitosis, and two cavities—the **gut cavity** and the **amniotic cavity**—form. Between these two cavities is the **embryonic disc**, from which the developing embryo will form. In a process called **gastrulation** the layer of cells nearest the amniotic cavity becomes **ectoderm**, and the layer of cells nearest the gut cavity becomes **endoderm**. These tissues, mentioned in Chapter 4, are the first of the embryonic germ layers to appear.

Toward the end of the second week of development, the blastocyst enzymatically digests its way into the **decidua basalis**, the deepest layer of the endometrium, and is covered by other uterine tissue called the **decidua capsularis**. This process is called **implantation**.

During the third week of development, after implantation, the third embryonic tissue, the **mesoderm**, appears between the other two layers. The tissues derived from each of the embryonic layers were listed in Chapter 4.

During the fourth week of development, in a process called **neurulation**, the **neural tube** sinks below the sur-

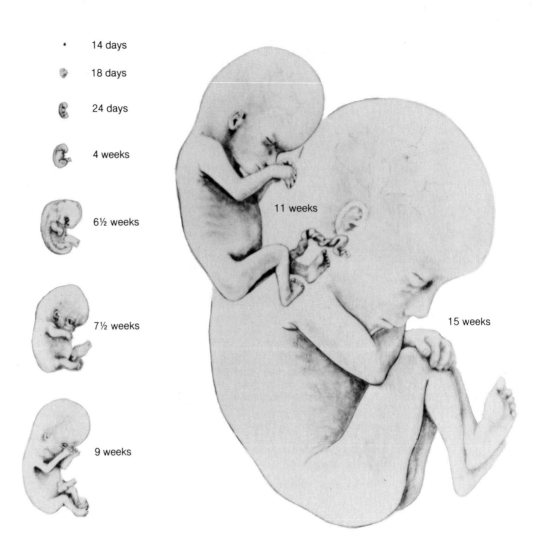

Figure 29.2 Changes in body size from implantation to the fifteenth week of development. (Embryos are shown at approximately natural size.) (Reproduced with permission from Jensen et al., *Biology*, Wadsworth, 1979, p. 237.)

14 days

18 days

24 days

4 weeks

6½ weeks

7½ weeks

9 weeks

11 weeks

15 weeks

Differentiation is the process by which genetically identical embryonic cells give rise to the different tissues of the body. One explanation of how differentiation could occur is that some genes become functional in some cells but not in others. For example, the gene for epinephrine production is "turned on" in cells of the adrenal medulla but not in muscle cells, bone cells, or others. What regulates the differentiation process is the subject of much interest and research.

face on the posterior side of the embryo, as explained in Chapter 10. In addition, the somites form, eventually giving rise to bones, muscles, and dermis, as described in Chapter 5.

As the embryo continues to develop in the second month, it takes on a clearly human form; before this it would be hard to distinguish from other mammalian embryos. The brain is the first organ to differentiate, and the heart is the first organ to become functional. By the end of the second month the basic structure of all the organs and systems is laid down. The embryo is now called a **fetus**.

In the fetal period (from the beginning of the third month of development to birth) the structure of organs is refined during the third month; growth is the primary process that takes place during the remaining six months. Changes in body size from implantation to the fifteenth week of development are shown in Figure 29.2. The events of early development are summarized in Table 29.1 and

Table 29.1 Events of Early Human Development

Age in Weeks	Length in Millimeters	Description
2.5	1.5	Neural groove indicated; blood islands formed; embryonic disc flat
4	5.0	All somites present; limb buds indicated; heart prominent; eye, jaws, thyroid present; gut tube differentiated; liver, pancreas, lungs, kidney, nerves forming
5	8.0	Tail prominent; umbilical cord organized; mouth and pharyngeal glands form; intestine elongates; genital ridge forms
6	12.0	Head becomes dominant in size; limbs recognizable; gonads form; heart has general definitive form; cartilage formation begins
8	23.0	Nose forms; digits recognizable; tongue muscles well formed; gut structure further differentiates; liver large; testis or ovary recognizable as such; main blood vessels have typical plan; first indication of bone formation; definitive muscles of head, trunk, limbs formed
12	56.0	Sex readily determined by external inspection; tooth primordia formed; fusion of palate complete; blood formation in bone marrow begins, blood vessels well formed; ossification spreading, with many bones outlined; brain and spinal cord attain general structural form
16	112.0	Face looks human; head hair appears; muscles become spontaneously active; gastric glands formed; kidney has typical form; skin glands form; eye, ear, nose approach typical appearance
20–40 (5–9 months)	160.0– 350.0	Body lean but has "baby" proportions (month 6); eyelids open (7); testes descend into scrotum (8); fat collects (8–9); tooth formation continues; tonsils, appendix, spleen acquire typical structure; fingernails form (8); spinal cord myelinization begins (5); brain myelinization begins (9); retina of eye complete and light-sensitive (7); taste sense present (8)

Reproduced with permission from Jensen et al., *Biology*, Wadsworth, 1979, p. 239.)

illustrated in Figure 29.3. Some of the labeled structures were discussed in Chapters 4, 5, and 10; others will be discussed later in this chapter.

The first three months of development are especially critical to the production of a normal fetus. Diseases contracted and drugs taken by the mother during these early months are most likely to damage the fetus because these are the months during which the organ structures are formed.

In addition to the embryo itself, the embryonic membranes also develop during the first two months (Figure 29.4). Each of four membranes surrounds a specific cavity. The **amnion** forms the amniotic cavity, which contains the embryo and is filled with **amniotic fluid**. Amniotic fluid acts as a kind of shock absorber for the developing fetus. The amnion, sometimes called the "bag of waters," often ruptures just before the birth of the infant. The **yolk sac** surrounds the gut cavity in human embryos. (In reptiles and birds it surrounds a large yolk that nourishes the developing embryo.) In humans the yolk sac is of little importance in nourishing the embryo; it does supply the cells that later give rise to gametes before it becomes a nonfunctional part of the umbilical cord. The **allantois** surrounds the **allantoic sac**, which collects nitrogenous wastes in reptiles and birds. In humans the allantois provides the blood vessels that connect the fetus with the placenta. As we shall see, the placenta provides nutrients and removes wastes from human embryos, so the yolk sac and allantois are of less significance in humans (and other mammals) than in reptiles and birds. The **chorion** develops from the trophoblast and surrounds the entire developing structure—embryo, amnion, and all other membranes. Eventually, it becomes the embryonic portion of the placenta and attaches to the decidua basalis, which forms the maternal portion of

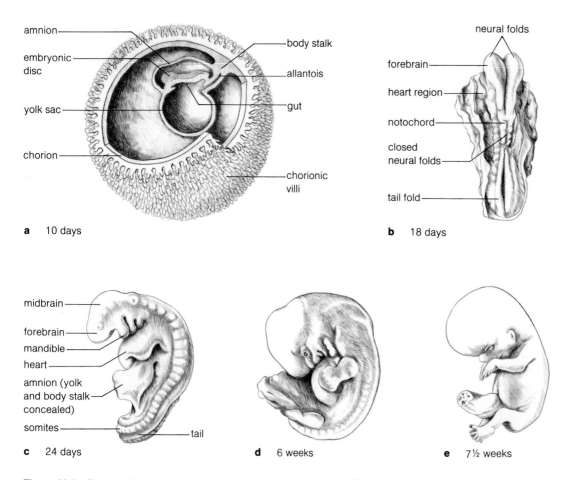

amnion
embryonic disc
yolk sac
chorion
body stalk
allantois
gut
chorionic villi

a 10 days

neural folds
forebrain
heart region
notochord
closed neural folds
tail fold

b 18 days

midbrain
forebrain
mandible
heart
amnion (yolk and body stalk concealed)
somites
tail

c 24 days

d 6 weeks

e 7½ weeks

Figure 29.3 Events in the development of an embryo from 10 days to 7½ weeks. (These drawings can be equated to the earlier stages shown in Figure 29.2.) (Reproduced with permission from Jensen et al., *Biology*, Wadsworth, 1979, p. 238–239.)

the placenta. The chorion and its precursor trophoblast cells secrete human chorionic gonadotropin (HCG).

By the end of the third month of development the **placenta** and the **umbilical cord** are complete and fully functional (Figure 29.5). In the functional placenta maternal blood vessels extend from the decidua basalis into the chorion, where they open into sinuses. The fetal blood vessels also extend into the chorion as **chorionic villi**. Materials such as nutrients, oxygen, carbon dioxide, and wastes are exchanged across the thin walls of the chorionic villi

between the fetal blood in the villi and the maternal blood in the sinuses. No mixing of blood occurs during normal development. However, at the time of delivery some fetal blood may enter the maternal sinuses and travel to the maternal blood vessels when the placenta detaches from the rest of the endometrium.

The umbilical cord, surrounded by a layer of amnion, contains two umbilical arteries and a single umbilical vein. A connective tissue containing much mucus lies around the blood vessels; this mucus, called **Wharton's jelly**, is pro-

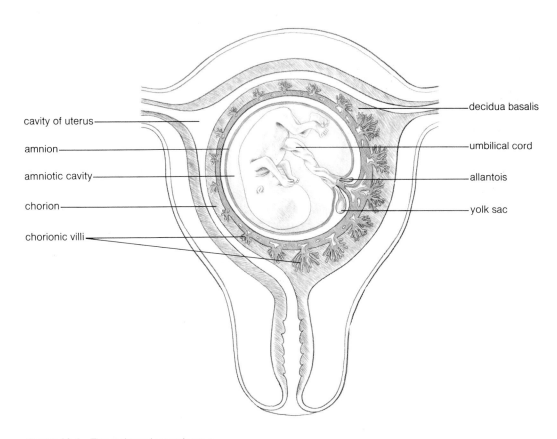

cavity of uterus

amnion

amniotic cavity

chorion

chorionic villi

decidua basalis

umbilical cord

allantois

yolk sac

Figure 29.4 The embryonic membranes.

duced by the allantois. At birth the placenta detaches from the uterus and is delivered as the "afterbirth." The umbilical cord is cut, and the mark left by the degeneration of the stub of the umbilical cord is called the **umbilicus**, or navel.

Multiple Births

Of all multiple births twins are of course most common, occurring about once in 80 births. Triplets occur less than once in 5000 births and quadruplets only about once in 500,000 births. However, as we saw in Chapter 28, the use of fertility drugs in recent years to stimulate ovulation has led to an increased frequency of multiple births because the drugs cause the release of several ova at the same time.

Twins may be monozygotic (identical) or dizygotic (fraternal). **Monozygotic** twins arise from a single fertilized egg and therefore have the same genetic makeup. Cells of the two-cell stage separate and give rise to two separate embryos. **Dizygotic** twins develop from two separate eggs, each of which is fertilized by a different sperm. Thus, dizygotic twins are no more alike than other siblings except that they are born at the same time. Monozygotic twins are always of the same sex; dizygotic twins may be of the same sex or different in sex. Triplets and other multiple births may be a combination of monozygotic twins and separately fertilized eggs.

The causes of twinning and other multiple births are not completely understood. It can be said that the occurrence of monozygotic twins is a random event. The rate of such twinning is much the same in all populations and it does not appear to run in families; a woman who has had

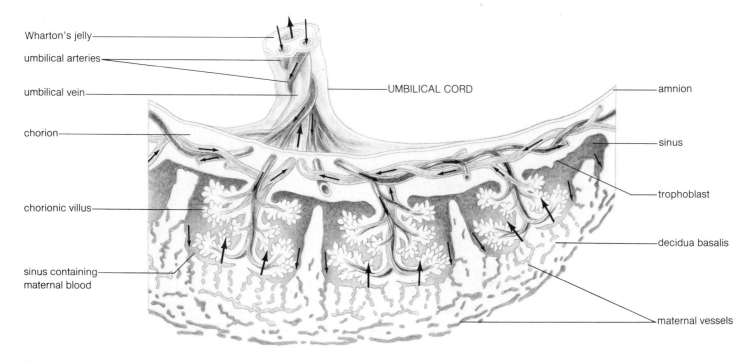

Wharton's jelly
umbilical arteries
umbilical vein

chorion

chorionic villus

sinus containing
maternal blood

UMBILICAL CORD

amnion

sinus

trophoblast

decidua basalis

maternal vessels

Figure 29.5   The structure of the placenta and umbilical cord.

identical twins has no greater likelihood of having other multiple births than one who has not had twins. However, the rate of dizygotic twinning does appear to be influenced by genetic factors. Women who come from families with a history of dizygotic twins are more likely to have such twins. Older women and women who have had several children are also more likely to have dizygotic twins than other women.

When more than one embryo implants in the uterus, it is likely that each will have its own amnion and placenta. This seems reasonable when we consider that fertilization and several cell divisions take place prior to implantation. The separate placentas account for differences in the size of twins since one may receive a more substantial blood supply than the other.

Effects of Teratogens on Development

A **teratogen** is any substance or agent that can cause malformations in the developing embryo or fetus. How a tera-

togen affects an embryo depends on what part of the embryo was most susceptible to damage when the teratogen was present. Many teratogens interfere with cell division or with the differentiation of tissues. Often a teratogen causes several different abnormalities because several systems are vulnerable to the effects of the teratogen at the same time.

Certain kinds of infections contracted by the mother during pregnancy are especially likely to cause defects in her offspring. Rubella (German measles) causes congenital heart disease, blindness, and deafness, and produces an inflammatory reaction in many of the body organs of the fetus. Syphilis, if untreated, causes many of the same defects. The herpes virus causes defects in the nervous system.

Hormones taken by the mother also can cause birth defects. Ingestion of hydrocortisone by the mother is related to cleft palate in the fetus. Diethylstilbesterol (DES) causes masculinization of the female fetus, abnormalities of the genital organs in male fetuses, and possibly vaginal cancer later in life in female offspring. DES is fed to cattle, and the metabolism of the drug in animal tissue is not well understood. It is possible that humans can ingest quantities of the drug in the meat they eat and fetuses could thereby be affected; whether this occurs is at present unknown. Other drugs used to maintain pregnancy during the threat of a spontaneous abortion may also cause fetal defects.

Various kinds of commonly used medications are now known to contribute to the development of birth defects. Salicylates (aspirin, for example) and dicumarol (an anticoagulant) cause bleeding in the fetus and sometimes anatomical malformations. Some antibiotics, such as tetracycline and streptomyosin, can cause retardation of the growth of the fetus, deafness, and hemolysis of fetal blood cells. Thiouracil, sometimes used to treat hyperthyroidism, can cause goiter in the fetus.

Psychotropic drugs seem to be especially likely to cause defects in offspring. Thalidomide, the tranquilizer used some years ago, led to the birth of many infants with malformed or missing limbs. Several psychotropic drugs affect the behavior of the newborn. Such drugs, classified as behavioral teratogens, include alcohol, heroin, methadone, and certain drugs commonly used during labor and delivery. Infants born to mothers who have used alcohol, heroin, or methadone are often born addicted to these drugs and go through withdrawal symptoms after birth.

Smoking by the mother during her pregnancy leads to reduced birth weight of the infant and can sometimes cause other serious defects, including microcephaly, a significantly reduced head and brain size.

PHYSIOLOGY OF PREGNANCY

Objective 4. Describe the normal changes that occur in the mother's body during pregnancy and explain how they are regulated.

Objective 5. Explain how the breasts develop to prepare for lactation and how this process is regulated.

Objective 6. Describe the nature of the abnormal function that occurs in (a) toxemia, (b) eclampsia, and (c) spontaneous abortion.

From conception to birth the duration of pregnancy is about 280 days, or forty weeks. However, one week longer or shorter duration is not uncommon. Infants born before the twenty-eighth week generally have little chance of survival.

Normal Changes in the Mother's Body

In addition to the cessation of menstruation, one of the first signs of pregnancy for some women is severe nausea called hyperemesis gravidarum, or the less severe "morning sickness." The cause of morning sickness is unknown, but the large amount of chorionic gonadotropin present early in pregnancy may be responsible.

Weight changes are characteristic of pregnancy. Most women lose a few pounds during the first few months of pregnancy, possibly because of the nausea. The normal weight gain over the duration of a pregnancy is about 24 pounds, distributed as follows: fetus—7 pounds (3.2 kg); amniotic fluid, placenta, and fetal membranes—4 pounds (1.8 kg); increased weight of the uterus—2 pounds (0.9 kg) and the breasts—3 pounds (1.4 kg); accumulation of fluid—6 pounds (2.7 kg); and fat—2 pounds (0.9 kg). When weight gain exceeds this amount, most of it is due to deposition of fat.

As was mentioned in Chapter 28, estradiol and progesterone are important in maintaining pregnancy because they prevent the uterine lining from being shed. During the first three months of pregnancy the corpus luteum that formed after ovulation produces these hormones in large quantities. Chorionic gonadotropin from the placenta stimulates this hormone production.

By the end of the third month of development, the production of chorionic gonadotropin has dropped to a very low level, and the placenta itself has begun to secrete large quantities of estradiol and progesterone. During pregnancy the estradiol concentration reaches a peak that is fifty times the peak concentration during the normal menstrual cycle; the progesterone level becomes ten times as great as it is in the monthly cycle. These hormones act to maintain pregnancy until the time of delivery.

The placenta also produces a hormone—human placental lactogen—that has some of the same effects on the mother's body as growth hormone and prolactin from the anterior pituitary. This hormone is thought to be important to the mother's body in several ways: (1) It helps to maintain positive protein balance; that is, it somehow stimulates the mother to take in sufficient protein to supply the fetus without using protein from the mother's tissues. (2) It helps to mobilize fats for energy. (3) It helps to regulate the blood glucose level so that the needs of both the fetus and the mother are met.

In addition to the hormonal changes several other changes occur in the mother's body during pregnancy. Her metabolic rate increases significantly (5 to 10%). Increased appetite provides protein and energy for her needs and nutrients for the growth and development of the fetus. The tissues of a pregnant woman retain more sodium and therefore more water than those of a nonpregnant woman. This phenomenon is probably due to increased production of renin, aldosterone, and antidiuretic hormone, although what causes those increases is not known. This fluid contributes to a 1 liter increase in blood volume and a 2 liter increase in tissue fluids.

The relationship of the fetus to the body of the mother is an interesting one. As each fetus receives half of its genes from its father, and only a small proportion of these genes are likely to be the same as those it receives from its mother, one would expect that the tissues of the fetus would be histologically incompatible with those of the mother. And, in fact, in animal studies tissue grafts from offspring to mother are rejected. Yet tissue incompatibility is not normally seen between the fetus and the mother. Apparently, the trophoblast has certain properties that prevent an immunological reaction in either the mother or the fetus during pregnancy. Recent studies indicate, however, that some cases of spontaneous abortion or stillbirth may be due to immunological reactions. Some of these reactions involve the AB blood antigens.

Breast Development for Lactation

The structure and development of the breasts at puberty has been discussed in Chapter 28. The development of the breasts, or mammary glands, is under the influence of several hormones. Estradiol and progesterone from the newly functional ovaries stimulate the development of both the ducts and the secretory portions of the mammary glands. Prolactin and growth hormone are also important in the development of the mammary glands.

During pregnancy progesterone and estradiol cause further development of the tissues of the mammary glands in preparation for milk secretion. Though milk can be expressed from the nipples of some women late in pregnancy, no significant amount of milk is produced during pregnancy. The hormone prolactin, the primary hormone in the initiation of milk secretion, is released in ever-increasing amounts throughout pregnancy. However, its effects are inhibited by the presence of estradiol and progesterone in the tissues of the breasts. When the placenta is removed from the uterus as the afterbirth, the hormones it secretes are no longer present to interfere with the action of prolactin, and the prolactin can then stimulate milk production.

The sucking of the infant is the primary stimulus for the release of prolactin and thus **lactation**, the production of

milk. The sucking of the infant stimulates mechanoreceptors in the nipples; impulses from these mechanoreceptors go to the hypothalamus and prevent the release of prolactin-inhibiting hormone; the anterior pituitary is then free to release prolactin. Prolactin reaches the secretory portion of the breasts, and milk is produced. As long as sucking continues, milk production also continues, unless it is interrupted by pregnancy. In some instances infants are born with some milk being produced by their own mammary glands. The production of this milk, called "witches' milk," is due to the high concentration of hormones that stimulate breast development and lactation in the mother. Shortly after birth, when the infant is removed from the influence of the hormones, the milk production ceases, and the breast development regresses.

The factors described above account for the release of milk into the ducts between the alveoli and the ampullae. However, milk must be moved into the ampullae and the ducts within the nipple. Such movement is also stimulated by the sucking of the infant, which causes the release of oxytocin from where it is stored in the posterior pituitary gland. Oxytocin causes the contraction of specialized cells, the **myoepithelial cells**, surrounding the alveoli. The contraction pushes milk into the ampullae and ducts of the nipple; this movement is called **milk let-down**. Oxytocin also causes uterine muscle to contract. Consequently, many lactating mothers can also feel uterine contractions while their infants are nursing. The uterus returns to normal size quickly in a nursing mother, at least in part because of such contractions.

The reflexes from stimulation of the mechanoreceptors affect the hypothalamus, but psychological factors can also affect the hypothalamus and contribute to or interfere with the production of prolactin and oxytocin and thus with the production and release of milk.

The factors that regulate lactation are summarized in Figure 29.6.

Sucking also sometimes causes the suppression of the release of FSH and LH from the hypothalamus. When these hormones are suppressed, ovulation does not occur. Lactation can then be a means of birth control in women who do not ovulate while they are nursing an infant. However, in many women the effect of sucking is not sufficient to suppress FSH and LH, and ovulation occurs. Therefore, lactation is not a reliable means of birth control.

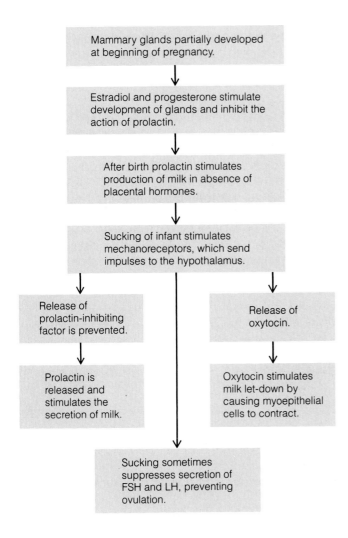

Mammary glands partially developed at beginning of pregnancy.

↓

Estradiol and progesterone stimulate development of glands and inhibit the action of prolactin.

↓

After birth prolactin stimulates production of milk in absence of placental hormones.

↓

Sucking of infant stimulates mechanoreceptors, which send impulses to the hypothalamus.

Release of prolactin-inhibiting factor is prevented.

↓

Prolactin is released and stimulates the secretion of milk.

Release of oxytocin.

↓

Oxytocin stimulates milk let-down by causing myoepithelial cells to contract.

Sucking sometimes suppresses secretion of FSH and LH, preventing ovulation.

Figure 29.6 Summary of factors that regulate lactation. Psychological factors also can contribute to or interfere with the production of milk.

Applications

Toxemia and eclampsia Under normal circumstances the amount of sodium and water retained in the tissues is greater during pregnancy than at other times. In **toxemia** excessive amounts of fluid are retained. Protein is excreted in the urine, and hypertension may be severe. Though the cause of toxemia is unknown, it may be due to some kind of immunological reaction to the presence of the fetus. The fluid retention may be part of an inflammatory response or may have to do with some alteration in kidney function. Perhaps the best evidence that toxemia is related to the presence of the fetus is that the symptoms usually disappear within a few days after delivery. The most common treat-ment for the symptoms of toxemia is to limit the mother's intake of salt. Though the relationship between salt and the immunological reaction is not clear, in many cases the treatment seems to be sufficient to prevent the accumulation of fluids and the other symptoms that follow fluid retention.

Eclampsia is a severe form of toxemia that occurs in less than 1% of pregnancies. It strikes shortly before or within a day or two after delivery. In eclampsia the blood vessels throughout the mother's body undergo spasmodic contraction. Kidney function is greatly reduced, hypertension is severe, the functioning of the liver is impaired, and convulsions may occur, followed by coma. Eclampsia is treated by the use of vasodilator drugs and diuretics. If these efforts are successful, the vascular spasm is reversed and the blood pressure lowered. However, about one in twenty individuals with severe eclampsia dies in spite of these treatments.

One of the important reasons for a pregnant woman to receive good prenatal care is to detect symptoms of toxemia when they first appear and to prevent them from worsening. Eclampsia generally occurs in women who have had symptoms of toxemia prior to delivery.

Spontaneous abortion Miscarriage, or **spontaneous abortion**, occurs in about 10% of all pregnancies, usually during the first four months. In most spontaneous abortions the embryo or fetus has some defect that is incompatible with life. Abnormalities in the uterus or deficiencies in the production of hormones by the mother's body may also lead to spontaneous abortions. Spontaneous abortion, as distinguished from induced abortion, occurs naturally without any intervention. It seems to be nature's way of preventing further development of defective fetuses.

LABOR AND DELIVERY

Objective 7. Describe the events in normal labor and delivery and explain how they are controlled.

Objective 8. Explain the effects on the fetus of breech birth and prolonged labor.

Normal Labor and Delivery

Labor is initiated by both hormonal and mechanical factors that lead to contractions of the uterus and the eventual expulsion of the fetus. The progesterone level drops a few weeks before birth; because progesterone normally inhibits uterine contractions, the decrease may allow the contractions to occur. When the fetus is fully developed, the muscle of the uterus becomes progressively more excitable until it finally begins to contract rhythmically. Although the exact causes of the onset of labor are not completely understood, the **positive feedback theory** provides a plausible explanation. According to this theory, the normal periodic episodes of weak uterine contraction that are a property of uterine muscle and occur throughout pregnancy become progressively stronger toward the end of pregnancy as the excitability of the uterus increases. These contractions push the head of the fetus (or the amnion prior to its rupture) against the cervix and stretch the cervix. The stretching of the cervix initiates a reflex that causes a wave of contraction in the body of the uterus. Each contraction stretches the cervix further and initiates another stronger uterine contraction.

The hormonal factors involved in labor include estradiol and oxytocin. Although both estradiol and progesterone are secreted throughout pregnancy, during the last two months estradiol is secreted in much greater quantities than progesterone. When the amount of estradiol present exceeds the amount of progesterone, estradiol can stimulate uterine contractions. Furthermore, oxytocin seems to be secreted in greater quantities toward the end of pregnancy than at other times, and the responsiveness of the uterus to it also increases at that time. The stretching of the cervix also appears to create reflex stimulation of the posterior pituitary and cause the release of oxytocin.

Mechanical factors that are involved in labor include stretching of the uterine muscle itself and stretching of the cervix. As the size of the fetus increases, it causes stretching of the uterus; intermittent movements of the fetus cause additional stretching. The observation that twins are usually born about two or three weeks earlier than single infants suggests that mechanical pressure within the uterus contributes to the onset of labor. Stretching of the cervix also, as noted above, probably contributes to the onset and acceleration of the labor process. As the uterine contractions accelerate, reflexes from the birth canal to the spinal cord and thence to the abdominal muscles cause strong abdominal contractions, which work with the uterine contractions to push the fetus through the cervix.

Uterine contractions begin in the fundus and spread through the body of the uterus to the cervix, forcing the baby down toward the cervix. In most cases uterine contractions at the beginning of labor occur only about once every 30 minutes and increase in intensity and frequency. In the final stages of labor strong contractions occur once every one to three minutes. It is important that there be a period of relaxation between contractions for two reasons: (1) The circulation of blood through the placenta to nourish the fetus occurs only during relaxation, and (2) the circulation of blood through the uterine muscle itself occurs only during relaxation. If the uterine muscle remained contracted, it would become ischemic, and the fetus would become anoxic (lacking in oxygen).

Labor is divided into three stages. The **first stage** is the dilation of the cervix to a diameter equal to the diameter of the fetus's head. This is the longest stage of labor; it lasts eight to twenty-four hours in the first pregnancy but is much shorter in subsequent pregnancies. The **second stage** of labor, delivery of the fetus, consists of the movement of the fetus through the birth canal and its entry into the outer world. This stage lasts about thirty minutes in a first pregnancy but may be only a few minutes in subsequent pregnancies. The positions of the fetus during labor are shown in Figure 29.7. The **third stage** of delivery is the separation and expulsion of the placenta. As the placenta separates from the rest of the uterine wall, the uterine muscle contracts strongly, closing off blood vessels in the endometrium that had supplied the placenta. In a normal delivery the amount of blood lost does not exceed 350 milliliters.

Relaxin, a hormone that is produced by the corpus luteum, may be involved in the preparation of the mother's body for labor and delivery. It has been implicated in the softening of the cervix in preparation for dilation, in the inhibition of uterine motility, and in the softening of the ligaments of the pubic symphysis. It now seems likely that these effects may be more pronounced in guinea pigs, rats, and other animals than they are in humans. The functions ascribed to relaxin may in fact be carried out by estradiol and progesterone, but further research is needed to clarify this issue.

Applications

Breech births are births in which the buttocks are the presenting part of the infant. Only about 5% of births are breech. The main problem created by a breech presentation is that passage through the birth canal is made much more difficult, and labor may be prolonged. Attempts to change the position of the baby—by the use of forceps, for example—can lead to injuries to the infant. Some infants in breech position cannot be delivered vaginally; a caesarean section must be performed.

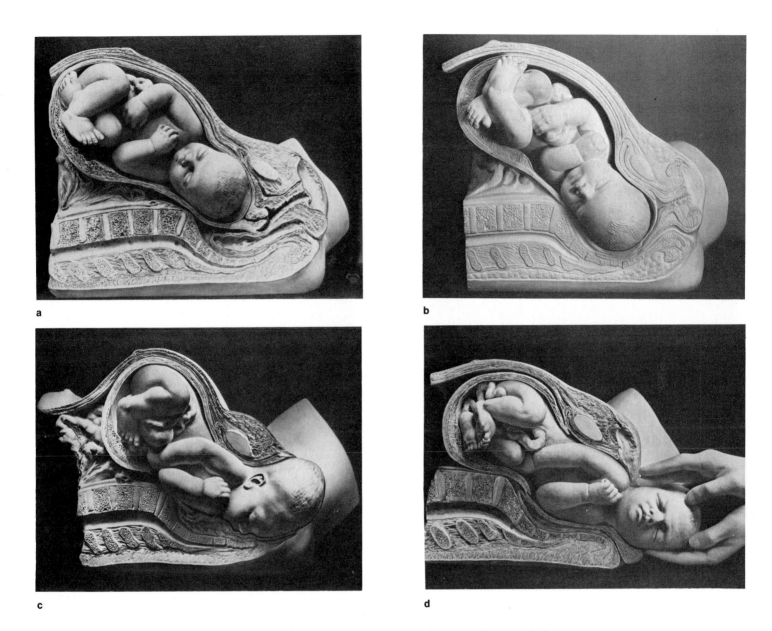

a

b

c

d

Figure 29.7 Positions of the fetus during labor: (**a**) normal position of a full-term fetus just prior to the onset of labor, (**b**) position of fetus during the first stage of labor (cervix partially dilated), (**c**) position of fetus during the early part of the second stage of labor, (**d**) rotation of the head during a later part of the second stage of labor. (Reproduced from the *Birth Atlas* with permission of The Maternity Center Association.)

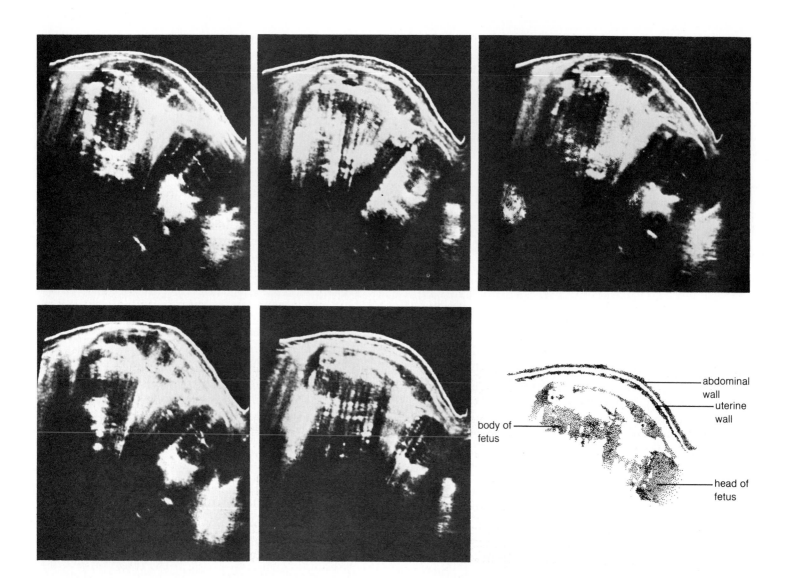

Figure 29.8 Sonograms of a near-term fetus in utero, with a diagram showing the orientation of the fetus. The head circumference is measured to be between 25.5 centimeters and 25.8 centimeters. (Sonograms courtesy Alexandria Hospital, Alexandria, Virginia, Joyce R. Isbel, R.T.)

Sonograms (Figure 29.8) are photographs of internal structures made by subjecting the structures to ultrasound—very high-frequency sound waves in the inaudible range. Sonograms are frequently used to study developing fetuses. They can determine whether more than one infant is developing within the uterus, determine the size of the head and other body parts, ascertain the position of the fetus, and sometimes detect fetal abnormalities. Ultrasound is much safer than X ray for studying a fetus because the sound waves apparently do not harm the fetus, whereas X ray subjects the whole body of the fetus to radiation.

Prolonged labor poses a threat to the infant because the placenta may separate from the uterine wall before the infant has been expelled. Such an event can result in asphyxiation of the infant because its supply of oxygen is cut off. Compression of the umbilical cord during labor can have the same effect. The heart rate of the fetus is often monitored electronically or by stethoscope in difficult deliveries. The normal heart rate of an infant at delivery is between 120 and 160 beats per minute. A higher or lower rate indicates that the infant may be experiencing oxygen deprivation.

THE NEONATAL PERIOD

Objective 9. Explain how the APGAR rating is used to assess the condition of a newborn infant.

Objective 10. Compare the physiology of a neonate with that of an adult.

The APGAR Rating

The newborn infant, or **neonate**, has just experienced birth, one of the most traumatic experiences of a lifetime. As noted in Chapter 19, significant changes in blood flow occur, and the lungs are used for the first time. The APGAR rating scale is used to assess the physiological condition of the neonate immediately after birth and again five minutes later. APGAR is an acronym for five physiological characteristics: **a**ppearance, **p**ulse, **g**rimace, **a**ctivity, and **r**espiratory effort. Each of these characteristics is assessed on a scale of 0 to 2, where 2 denotes normal function, 1 denotes somewhat impaired function, and 0 denotes seriously impaired function. These ratings are summarized in Table 29.2. The APGAR rating is the sum of the ratings of each characteristic and can range from 0 to 10. Although the APGAR rating is only a general indication of the physiological status of the neonate, it can be used to determine whether more careful assessment is needed and whether the neonate may need special assistance to stay alive.

Table 29.2 The APGAR Rating Scale for Neonates			
		Rating	
Characteristic	0	1	2
A Appearance (skin)	Pale or blue	Body pink, limbs blue	Whole body pink
P Pulse (heart rate)	None	Less than 100	More than 100
G Grimace (reflex response to stimulation of sole of foot)	No response	Facial grimace and some movement	Facial grimace and extensive movement
A Activity (muscle tone)	Flaccid	Extremities partially flexed	Good muscle tone and active movement
R Respiratory effort	None	Irregular and slow, no crying	Rapid and generally regular, strong cry

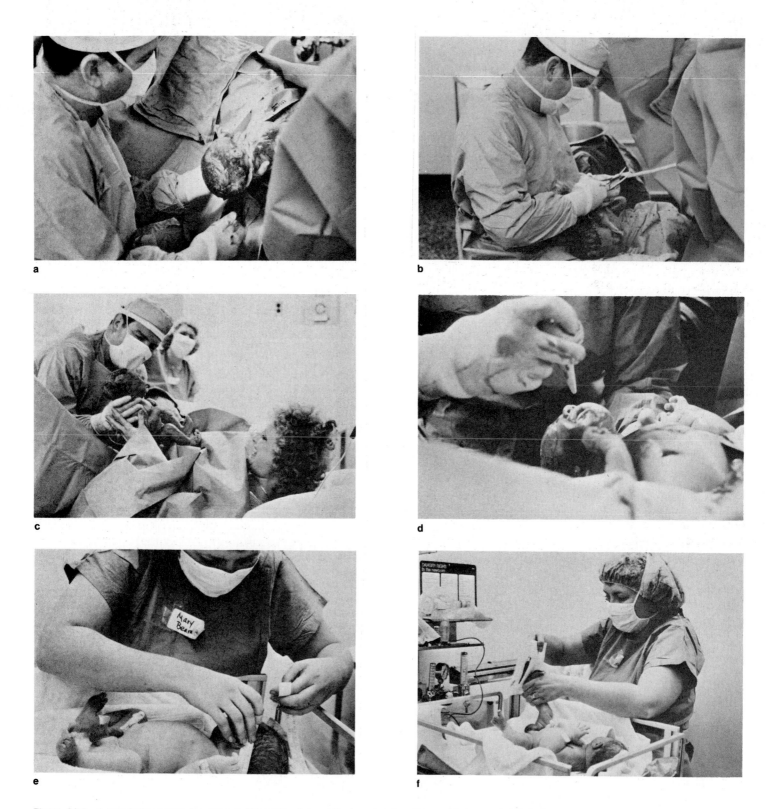

Figure 29.9 A new baby arrives: (**a**) delivery, (**b**) cutting the umbilical cord, (**c**) mother and baby meet, (**d**) doctor aspirates mucus from baby's nose and throat, (**e**) baby is measured, (**f**) footprints are made. (Courtesy of Susan and Arty Trivers.)

Physiology of the Neonate

The neonatal period is the first four weeks after birth. During a normal delivery the neonate has usually been deprived of optimum gas exchange and thus at birth is suffering from a slight acidosis due to the accumulation of carbon dioxide in the blood. Neonates also show characteristic kinds of immaturity. For example, their bodies are less able to regulate temperature than the bodies of adults, their kidneys are unable to concentrate urine as well as they will later, and their immunity to disease is lower than it will be later in life. Their breathing rates (30 to 50 breaths per minute) and their heart rates (120 to 140 beats per minute) are much faster than those of adults. Neonatal blood pressure (75/40) is lower than adult blood pressure.

There are several consequences of these physiological differences. Because the neonate has poor temperature regulating ability, it needs an environment that has a stable temperature to minimize the demands on the regulatory mechanism. Because the kidneys are unable to concentrate urine to any great degree, the neonate is subject to dehydration and problems with electrolyte balance. The urine excreted by a neonate daily accounts for 3 to 6% of its body weight, whereas that of an adult is less than 2% of the body weight. The antibody-producing mechanism is not functional at birth, so it is important to prevent exposure of a neonate to infectious agents. However, it receives some protection from passive antibodies received through placental transfer from the mother and additional protection from breast milk if it is breast fed. The rapid and irregular respirations of a neonate are not always cause for concern, but the neural mechanism, explained in Chapter 21, that regulate respiration is immature, so neonates are more subject to respiratory failure than normal adults.

Rapid growth is one of the most obvious characteristics of the neonate. Although increase in size occurs more rapidly during prenatal development than ever again, the neonatal period is the period of most rapid postnatal growth. A full-term infant weighs between 3 and 3½ kilograms and is 48 to 52 centimeters in length. Although 5 to 10% of the birth weight is lost as water in the first two days of life, this weight is quickly regained. An additional 800 to 1000 grams of weight gain occurs in the first month of life, and about 3 centimeters are added to the length in the first month. The head circumference is between 33 and 36 centimeters at birth and increases about 1 centimeter in the first month.

Behavior during the neonatal period is limited to reflexes and activities controlled by the lower brain centers. Movements are mostly random. Though sensory stimuli are received, the infant has yet to learn to localize and respond to stimuli. Circadian rhythms, the twenty-four-hour daily rhythms, are not yet established (as any parent of a neonate knows).

INFANCY AND CHILDHOOD

Objective 11. Summarize the anatomical and physiological development that occurs during infancy and childhood.

The transition from the neonatal period to infancy occurs at four weeks of age. Infancy extends from four weeks to two years of age, and childhood extends from infancy to puberty.

Growth is a characteristic of infancy and childhood, although the rate of growth decreases through this period. Weight gain, increase in height, and increase in head circumference are measures of growth that can be used to assess normal development.

In early infancy weight gain averages 200 grams per week. At one year a typical infant weighs about 10 kilograms and at two years about 12½ kilograms. In childhood weight gain averages about 2 kilograms per year until puberty.

Height increases by about 2–3 centimeters per month during the first year and about 1 centimeter per month during the second year. During childhood height continues to increase but at a slower rate of about 5–6 centimeters per year in the years just prior to puberty.

In infants increase in head circumference is a measure of brain development. During the second month of life an increase of 2 centimeters is typical, and an increase of 1 centimeter is typical during subsequent months. Greater increases may indicate the presence of hydrocephalus (an accumulation of excess cerebrospinal fluid). By six months of age the brain has reached half its adult size and by two years three-fourths of its adult size.

Each individual has a characteristic growth rate; infants and children show a wide range of variation in size and rate of growth. Genetic endowment, nutritional status of the infant (or the mother prenatally), and a number of other factors including hormones influence growth.

The physiology of the infant and child differs from that of an adult in several ways. The heart rate decreases with age from the range of 120–140 beats per minute in infancy to 80–90 beats per minute in adolescence. Blood pressure increases from typical infant pressures of 80/50 to typical adolescent pressures of 110/70. Respiratory rate gradually decreases from 20–30 breaths per minute in infants to 14–16

Table 29.3 Summary of Development During Preschool Years

Abilities Seen in 75% of Infants and Children at Age:	Gross Motor	Fine Motor	Language and Social
2 months	Lifts head when placed on stomach	Follows objects with eyes	Makes noncrying sounds Smiles responsively
4 months	Holds head steady when placed in sitting position Rolls over	Grasps objects placed in hand	Laughs and squeals Smiles spontaneously
6 months	Bears some weight on legs	Reaches for objects	Makes speechlike sounds
9 months	Sits without support Stands holding on	Passes objects hand to hand Uses thumb and finger to pick up small objects	Imitates speech sounds Feeds self crackers Plays peek-a-boo Works to get to toy that is out of reach
1 year	Walks holding on to furniture Stands momentarily	Bangs two cubes together	Says dada or mama Plays pat-a-cake
1½ years	Walks well Stoops and regains standing position without falling	Stacks two cubes Scribbles spontaneously Imitates movements of others	Says three words other than mama and dada Drinks from cup Uses spoon fairly well
2 years	Walks up stairs Can walk backward Kicks ball and throws ball overhand	Stacks four cubes	Combines two different words Follows simple directions Removes garments
3 years	Jumps in place Pedals tricycle	Stacks eight cubes Copies ''o'' Makes vertical line	Uses plurals Washes and dries hands Puts on clothing
4 years	Does broad jump Balances on one foot for 5 seconds	Copies '' + '' Picks longer line of two presented	Plays simple games Gives name Recognizes colors Comprehends prepositions Dresses without supervision
5 years	Hops on one foot Catches bounced ball most times	Copies cubes Draws three part human figure	Defines words sometimes Comprehends simple opposite analogies

in adolescence. The urine volume increases but at a rate slower than the growth rate. The slow rate of increase in urine volume occurs partly because of increased ability to concentrate urine.

Motor and mental development are characteristic of infancy and childhood. Although it is beyond the scope of this book to consider these factors in detail, some of the highlights of such developments are summarized in Table 29.3.

ADOLESCENCE

Objective 12. Summarize the major changes in males and in females during puberty.

Changes during Puberty

A growth spurt normally marks the beginning of puberty. In females it begins somewhere between ages 10½ and 13

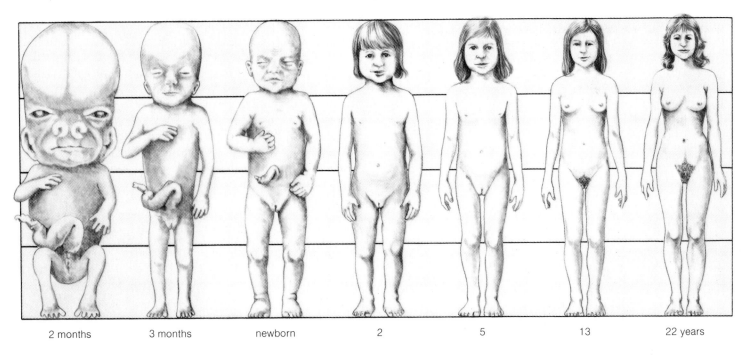

| 2 months | 3 months | newborn | 2 | 5 | 13 | 22 years |

Figure 29.10 Changing proportions of the human body during prenatal and postnatal growth. All stages are drawn to the same total height. (Reproduced with permission from Jensen et al., *Biology*, Wadsworth, 1979, p. 233.)

and in males somewhere between ages 12½ and 15. During the growth spurt females grow at rates of about 8 centimeters per year and males at rates of 9 to 10 centimeters per year. The growth spurt is followed by several years of slower growth until adult stature is reached. Females generally reach adult stature at 17–18 years and males at 19–20 years, but a wide range of individual differences is seen in rate of growth, total height, and age at which growth ceases.

Maturation of reproductive organs and development of secondary sex characteristics also occur during puberty. A sudden drop in the amount of melanin from the pineal gland may be responsible for triggering the onset of puberty. In a typical female the changes occur in the following order after the growth spurt: Breasts and nipples enlarge, and the areolae become pigmented; the pelvis widens; pubic hair begins to grow, and apocrine glands develop in the axillae; menstruation begins about two years after the growth spurt.

In a typical male changes occur after the growth spurt in the following order: the penis and testicles enlarge; hair begins to grow first in the pubic area, then the axillae, upper lip, thighs, chest, and finally other parts of the face about two years after the appearance of pubic hair; the larynx increases in size, and the voice deepens. The first ejaculation

occurs spontaneously as a nocturnal emission usually a few months after the appearance of the pubic hair.

In addition to changes occurring in the reproductive organs, physiological changes occur in other systems of the body. As the rate of growth decreases, the metabolic rate also decreases. As in earlier stages of development, the heart rate continues to decline until the adult rate is reached, and the blood pressure continues to increase until the adult level is reached. The respiratory rate reaches the adult level. Although much of the development of the brain and other parts of the nervous system occur during prenatal development and in the first year of life, some parts of the brain such as the reticular formation and some cortical association areas do not become fully myelinated until the teen years or even later in life.

From the above considerations of growth at various stages in human development, it should be clear that body proportion changes as growth occurs. As shown in Figure 29.10, the length of the head accounts for nearly half the total body length at two months of prenatal development; at adulthood the length of the head is only about one-eighth of the total height. Also, the brain and the reproductive organs show different rates of growth than the body in general (Figure 29.11), the brain growing rapidly in infancy and

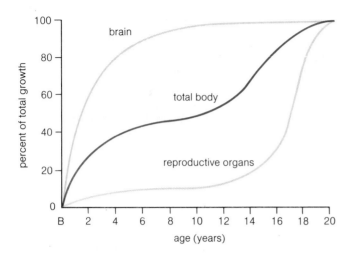

Figure 29.11 Relative growth rates of different parts of the body.

early childhood and the reproductive organs growing rapidly in adolescence.

When all the body systems have reached their adult levels, the individual is considered to have reached physiological maturity. Such maturity is usually reached at about twenty-five years of age, even though some cortical myelination occurs after that time.

AGING

Objective 13. Describe the process of aging and the factors that affect the aging process.

Objective 14. Summarize the major theories of aging.

The Aging Process and Factors That Affect It

Aging is variously defined as (1) progressive decline in cellular efficiency that occurs after maturation, (2) the sum total of all changes that occur in a living organism with the passage of time, or (3) the sum total of the above changes that lead to functional impairment and death.

One of the principal events in aging is the *decreased ability to adapt to a changing environment*—in other words, the decreased ability to maintain homeostasis. With the passage of time all living organisms, including humans, experience increasing difficulty in adjusting to change, and any given change creates greater stress on an older organism than it does on a younger one. The elderly maintain a precarious homeostatic balance; eventually a stress is encountered in

which the capacity of the body to adjust is surpassed, and death ensues.

Various parts of the body show signs of aging at different times in the life cycle. For example, accommodation of the eye to near objects begins to diminish in early adulthood and has generally reached a minimum by age fifty. Ability to adapt to the dark also begins to decrease at age twenty and continues to decline throughout the remainder of life. Auditory acuity begins to decrease in adolescence and declines steadily until about age fifty, after which the rate of decline is much slower.

> Environmental and other factors affect aging. For example, auditory acuity appears to decline later in life in populations that live in relatively noise-free environments. Some effects of aging become apparent long after the aging process has begun. In atherosclerosis, for instance, vascular function may not be impaired until middle or old age even though the vascular lesions began in infancy. One might even argue that atherosclerosis is not a normal part of aging and occurs only as a result of other factors—genetics, diet, or lifestyle.

Physiological processes that are regulated by a number of control mechanisms are less susceptible to aging than those that have only a few control mechanisms. For example, acid–base balance and regulation of blood sugar level each have multiple control mechanisms. Thus, they generally remain stable into old age. Other processes—locomotion, cardiovascular function, kidney function, respiratory function, brain function, and immunological competence—seem to be especially susceptible to degenerative changes.

Peak muscular strength occurs in the third decade of life and decreases at an accelerating rate with age. The reduction in strength seems to be due to biochemical changes in muscle fibers themselves as well as in the neuromuscular junctions. As muscle tissue undergoes degeneration, it is replaced by connective tissue and fat. The bones lose minerals and become less dense with aging, and the cartilage and other parts of the joints are subject to degenerative and inflammatory changes.

Cardiovascular function declines with aging. The total cardiac output during rest decreases, as does the cardiac reserve. In a young athlete cardiac output during exercise can increase from 5 liters per minute to 35 liters per minute.

In an older person, even though the heart rate and blood pressure increase, these changes are not sufficient to increase the cardiac output enough to meet the demands of extreme exertion. The atherosclerotic process also contributes to the decline in cardiovascular function. Aging of the heart muscle itself is a third factor in diminished cardiovascular function. Studies directed toward determining how an aging heart differs from a younger heart have shown that the heart's response to some neurotransmitters decreases with age, either because smaller amounts of the transmitters are produced or because the heart becomes less responsive to them. Reduced responsiveness may be due to a decrease in the number of active receptor sites. The aging heart muscle is also slower to relax between contractions than a young heart, its walls are thicker, and the electrical activity of the pacemaker system decreases with age.

Predictors of heart disease in the elderly seem to be hypertension, abnormal findings in electrocardiograms, and diabetes. Low blood pressure seems to predict resistance to heart disease, especially in women.

Kidney function becomes irreversibly impaired in advanced age. Although part of this decrease in function is undoubtedly due to impaired renal blood flow, the functioning of the glomeruli and the tubules also is impaired.

Effects of aging on the respiratory system are seen as decreased elasticity of the lung tissue and increased rigidity of the chest wall. Although the total lung volume does not decrease significantly, ability to move air in and out of the lungs does decrease. Furthermore, the ability of the lung tissue to absorb oxygen decreases, mostly because of rupture of membranes between alveoli. At twenty years of age the amount of oxygen entering the blood is about 4 liters per minute, but at seventy-five years of age only about 1.5 liters of oxygen enter the blood each minute. This decline in availability of oxygen undoubtedly affects the functioning of the heart and skeletal muscles and the central nervous system.

Research on aging in brain tissue is largely limited to animal studies, in which brain cell loss seems to occur at the greatest rate early in life. For example, studies of the brains of rats have shown that the greatest decline in the number of brain cells occurred during the first 108 days of life. After that time to 650 days (old age in a rat) only small decreases in the number of cells were noted. Furthermore, it has been shown that a stimulating environment leads to thickening of the cortex of the brain in young rats. If one can generalize from rats to people, it would seem that a stimulating environment (along with good nutrition) helps to maximize the development of the brain and to minimize the degree of structural change during aging.

An interesting aspect of aging brains (as seen in autopsy specimens) indicates that the senile plaques found in aged human brains resemble the degenerative changes called amyloidosis seen in the islets of Langerhans of the pancreas. Amyloidosis is thought to be the result of immunological disturbances in the pancreas, and it has been suggested that similar changes may occur in the brain.

Changes in the immune system may be important in the initiation of other events in the aging process. During aging the immune system loses its ability to react to antigens from outside the body and at the same time tends to increase its reactivity to antigens within the body. Thus, resistance to disease is reduced, and the tendency toward development of autoimmune diseases is increased. T-lymphocytes decrease in function with aging and fail to destroy abnormal cells, probably contributing to an increased rate of cancer in older people. Exactly how these changes take place is not well understood, but further investigation of the problem may lead to a better understanding of both the function of the immune system and the aging process.

Theories of Aging

It might be said that there are as many theories of aging as there are investigators studying the question. Some theories have become better known than others; a few of the most widely publicized theories will be summarized here.

The theory of **cytologic aging** states that the body is progressively damaged by the cumulative effects of injuries to individual cells or macromolecules within them. Possible causes of aging according to this theory would include ionizing radiation, liberation of "free radicals"—ions that damage various structures in the cells—and the accumulation of lipofuscin, a so-called age pigment found in cells that have lost their ability to divide. Evidence to support this theory is found in observations of cells in tissue cultures. Generally, these cells divide a finite number of times, and eventually the culture dies.

The **fat metabolism** theory suggests that aging may be due to a decreasing ability to metabolize fats and that excessive food intake early in life may lead to a later reduction in fat metabolism. In food-restricted rats the rate at which ability to metabolize fats is lost is greatly reduced, and these rats far outlive animals permitted to eat freely. The hormones glucagon and adrenalin normally promote fat metabolism, but during aging the fat cells become less responsive to these hormones. Fats accumulate in the body, and serum lipid levels increase. If these observations can be generalized to humans, they might account for tendencies toward both heart disease and obesity as age increases. Another finding was that rats acquire additional fat cells, especially in the fat around the kidney, as a part of the aging process. Although it had been thought that the total number of fat cells in the body remains constant throughout adulthood, with only the amount of fat stored in them changing, it now appears that this is not the case, at least in rats.

Many investigators think that aging is caused primarily by **intrinsic factors**. These intrinsic factors include alteration of proteins and other molecules by the formation of irreversible chemical bonds or by the insertion of incorrect amino acids in certain proteins. Thus, some of the essential proteins of cells are rendered inoperable because of the bonds or because of the genetic error. These changes are thought to accumulate throughout life, eventually culminating in a sufficiently large accumulation of errors that the cells can no longer function and therefore die.

A number of investigators are beginning to believe that there may be some kind of **brain–endocrine master plan** that is genetically encoded in the brain and expressed as a scheduled sequence of events in the life cycle. Because certain phenomena have been shown to be governed by a kind of biological clock, it seems reasonable to suppose that a biological clock of aging might exist. It is also hypothesized that environmental factors might influence the intrinsic genetic factors and introduce variability in the basic genetic plan.

The brain–endocrine theory of programmed aging is summarized in Figure 29.12. One interpretation of this theory is that programmed alterations in the brain, pituitary, and target organs would lead to the many alterations and declines in function that are characteristic of aging. These deficits would lead to a failure of homeostatic mechanisms and to the loss of the ability to adapt to changes in the environment such as large temperature variations. Another interpretation of the theory is that the brain–endocrine systems constitute a program to activate target tissues and that the tissues depend on the program for optimum function. Part of the program is the direction of age-related changes. The pacemaker center might have certain stimulatory effects during development and early adulthood. With aging, imbalances in the effects of the pacemaker might lead to the production of abnormal or incomplete hormones in the pituitary. These hormones would result in impaired control of other endocrine glands and target tissues.

Future Possibilities

As biologists learn more about the aging process, it is possible that an antiaging drug might be developed. In fact, such a drug is currently being evaluated by the Food and Drug Administration. The possibility of having a drug that extends the normal life span by a number of years poses several ethical and social questions. For example, would the drug prolong the productive years or prolong life after chronic debilitating changes had occurred? Would the drug be available to everyone or to only a few who could afford it? Should there be research on the effects of the drug with human subjects? Should any research of any kind on such a drug be prohibited? If such a drug became available, what kinds of changes would occur in lifestyles, education, use of leisure, employment, quality of life for the elderly, and other societal conditions?

DEATH AND DYING

Objective 15. Define death and describe the physiological processes that occur during dying.

Objective 16. Evaluate the effects of hospices and other services for the dying and the effects of the use of life-support systems for the terminally ill.

The subject of death and dying is enveloped in emotion, myth, and ritual. In recent years, however, it has become more acceptable in our society to discuss death openly and to help people who are dying talk about their feelings. Much could be written about the psychological aspects of death and dying, but emphasis here will be on the physiological aspects.

Definition of Death

The simplest definition of death is the loss of spontaneous heartbeat and respiration. However, since these functions can be maintained by mechanical means, other definitions of death have been devised. They include permanent cessation of all life functions and absence for at least twenty-four hours of any cerebral function (as shown by a "flat" electroencephalogram).

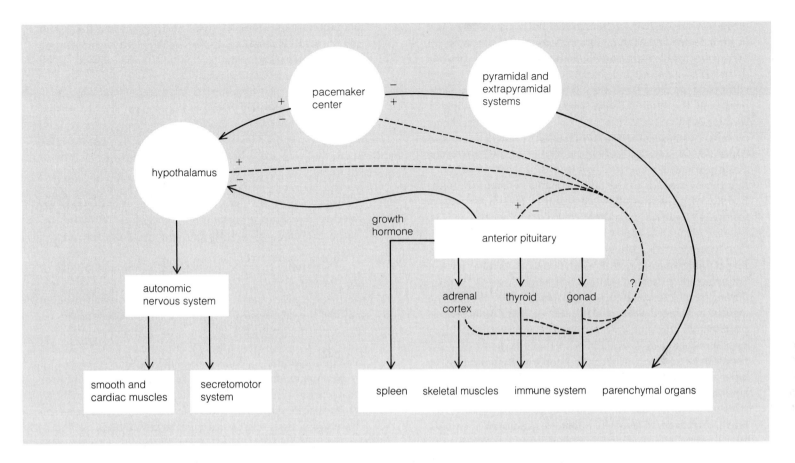

Figure 29.12 The brain–endocrine theory of programmed aging postulates that neurons in the higher brain centers are the "pacemakers" that regulate the biologic clock controlling growth, development, aging, and death. Pacemaker neurons may stimulate (+) or inhibit (−) the neurosecretory cells of the hypothalamus, which controls the anterior pituitary secretions. Pituitary secretions, in turn, regulate other endocrine secretions or act directly on target tissues. Hormones determine metabolic activity and function of responsive tissues and modulate neuroendocrine interactions by positive stimulation or negative feedback (dashed lines) on the pituitary, hypothalamus, and other brain structures. The hypothalamus, through the autonomic nervous system, also regulates secretomotor functions and smooth and cardiac muscles. The pacemaker neurons also influence the rate of stimulation of the pyramidal and extrapyramidal systems, which control skeletal muscle tone and movement. (Reproduced with permission from P. S. Timiras, "Biological Perspectives on Aging," *American Scientist*, September 1978.)

Physiological Processes during Dying

Even when the vital functions of heartbeat, respiration, and urine formation have stopped or are showing signs of stopping, many of the cells in the body remain alive. As long as cells can get some oxygen and nutrients, they can carry on metabolism sufficient to stay alive. Consequently, cellular death does not take place in all the cells of the body until an hour or more after the vital functions have ceased.

When death comes to an aged person, it often results from the failure of a particular organ such as the heart or the

It is during the time shortly after death that organs can be removed from the body to be transplanted to another person. When a patient has had a "flat" EEG for twenty-four hours, the person is pronounced dead. Life-support systems used until the transplantable organs can be removed keep the tissues of these organs alive, greatly increasing the likelihood that they will function in the recipient's body.

kidneys. Even so, many other parts of the body are impaired in their function as the effects of the failure of one organ spread to other organs, and soon none of the vital functions occur. For example, in a patient dying of kidney failure (assuming an artificial kidney is not in use), wastes accumulate in the blood. These wastes cause tissue ischemia throughout the body. Because of the ischemia the heart muscle becomes less able to function and brain cells are also damaged. Eventually, consciousness is lost, and the heart stops beating.

Applications

Hospices and other services for the dying   A **hospice** is a home for dying patients. More common in countries such as Switzerland, Austria, and England than in the United States, hospices are increasing in number here. A hospice differs from a hospital in several ways. First, the staff is mainly concerned with making the person's last days as comfortable and pain free as possible and with providing opportunities to discuss death and the fear of it that most people have. Second, the dying people are encouraged to have family members around them, and the family members are helped to accept the inevitable death. Third, the atmosphere of a hospice is relaxed and casual. The furniture is arranged to make it homelike, and staff members take time to talk at length with the patients and are honest with them. Patients know that they are dying and that there will be every effort to make them as comfortable as possible and to provide them emotional support.

Even when a hospice is not available for a dying patient, many of the same services can be provided by a sensitive family that has the strength to care for a dying relative at home. In some communities nurses and social workers are available to counsel dying patients and their families. Courses are available in some locations for people who want to learn to assist dying patients. Even the recent trend toward discussing death and dying in a more open way helps to make people more able to cope with the death of a relative or their own death.

Life-support systems and ethical issues in their use   Now that respirators, heart–lung machines, artificial kidneys, and other life-support devices are available, many people can be kept alive who would otherwise have died. Such kinds of equipment are of unquestioned benefit in helping a person who has a chance to recover over a crisis. However, in those who have very little chance of recovering, the life-support systems may simply prolong the process of dying and increase the emotional stress and financial burden on the family.

Many ethical issues are created by the availability of life-support systems. Who should decide which patients will receive such services? What criteria will be used in making the decision? If a patient who is dependent on life-support systems for survival appears to have no chance of recovery, can the machines be disconnected? Who should decide? What criteria will be used? What legal action might be taken against the persons or institution responsible for the decision? If more people need life-support systems than are available, how will those to receive the service be chosen? Because the use of such equipment is generally extremely expensive, who will pay for such services? And most important, what concern should there be for the wishes of the patient?

In the minds of many people death with dignity is quite different from being placed in a hospital room surrounded with machines that keep failing organs functioning. Developing answers to these and other ethical questions concerning dying and the use of life-support systems will be one of the major challenges facing the medical profession and all of society in the years to come.

CLINICAL TERMS

abortion (ab-or'shun)   the premature expulsion of a fetus from the uterus

abruptio placentae (ah-brup'te-o pla-sen'ta-e)   premature detachment of the placenta from the uterine wall

curettage (ku-ret-ahzh')   the removal of tissue from a cavity (such as the uterus) by the use of a scraping instrument

hydatidiform (hi-dat'id-if-orm) mole   a benign tumor of the placenta

hydramnios (hi-dram'ne-os)   an excess of amniotic fluid

lochia (lo'ke-ah)   the vaginal discharge that occurs for a week or two following childbirth

meconium (me-ko'ne-um)   a dark green substance in the intestine of a full-term fetus

placenta previa (pla-sen'tah pre've-ah)   a condition in which the placenta is attached near the cervix and subject to rupture

puerpera (pu-er'per-ah)   a woman who has just given birth

Essay: Natural Childbirth

"In sorrow thou shalt bring forth thy children." This statement from Genesis 3:16 has been used for centuries to support the idea that it was God's will for women to suffer during childbirth. Though Queen Victoria consented to receive chloroform as an anesthetic during the delivery of her eighth child in 1853, the clergy continued to object to a practice that so clearly ran counter to their understanding of the will of God.

In the 1930s an English physician, Grantly Dick-Read, published his views that women experienced pain during childbirth because they had been socially conditioned to expect to suffer. He described a "fear-tension-pain" cycle to account for pain. According to Dick-Read, women learned to fear labor and in their fear tensed the muscle of the lower uterus and other muscles. The muscle tension resulted in the perception of pain. By explaining to women that they need not fear labor and by teaching them relaxation exercises, he was able to guide many through labor and delivery without anesthesia and with little pain.

Later, Velvovsky, a Russian researcher, and his associates used the work of Pavlov to design conditioning exercises for pregnant women. These methods spread to the western world in the 1940s, mainly through the writings of the French physician Fernand Lamaze, and have become known as the Lamaze method of natural childbirth.

Numerous subsequent studies of the effectiveness of natural childbirth methods have been made. Many of the studies lacked control groups, and some that had controls failed to assign patients at random to treatment or control groups. Thus, it is possible that the women with the least fear of labor volunteered for the treatment—that is, participated in the exercise and conditioning classes. The control group, when it existed, included those women who were not aware of the availability of classes or who were invited but declined to participate.

The conclusions from these uncontrolled studies amount to reports of the observations of attending physicians whose basis for comparison was their previous experience with patients who had had no exposure to training for natural childbirth. Some of the claims for the training are as follows: decreased perception of pain, increased cooperation of the mother during labor, a lowered incidence of postpartum de-pression, a better attitude about future pregnancies, reduced use of anesthetics and analgesics, decreased blood loss during delivery, shortened labor, and less need for forceps, episiotomies, and caesarean sections. Furthermore, it was claimed that the neonates delivered by natural childbirth begin to breathe more quickly, had a higher oxygen level in their blood at birth, were better adjusted in the nursery, and had a reduced risk of sickness or death in the neonatal period.

Some of these claims have been more or less substantiated in a study that included some degree of experimental control. For example, among 400 primiparas (women having their first babies), 200 received training in what to expect during delivery and how to prepare for the event psychologically and through exercise and breathing activities. The other 200 were untrained. Follow-up showed that 45 (22%) of the trained women but only 2 (1%) of the untrained women withstood labor without drugs. No forceps were needed in the deliveries of 116 of the trained women and 82 of the untrained women. The duration of labor averaged 13.5 hours in the trained group and 15.5 hours in the untrained group (Van Auken and Tomlinson, 1953).

Some recent studies have made use of biofeedback techniques to assist mothers in natural childbirth. Two groups of thirty women each were used, and all but one mother in each group had had Lamaze training during the current pregnancy or a previous one. The treatment group received at least two sessions of biofeedback-aided relaxation training supplemented with home practice. Most of the mothers in the study were multiparas (experiencing their second or subsequent pregnancy), so results are not available for primiparas. The biofeedback-trained multiparas had significantly shorter labors and required less analgesia and anesthetic. There was no significant difference in the APGAR scores of the infants born to the two groups (Gregg, Frazier, and Nesbit, 1975).

Though the available studies of natural childbirth leave much to be desired with respect to experimental design, the evidence is clearly in favor of natural childbirth, at least for women who elect that method. How much of the difference is due to the attributes of the women who choose natural childbirth remains to be determined.

CHAPTER SUMMARY

(Chapter summary points and review questions are numbered to correspond to the numbered objectives in the text of each chapter.)

Overview of Life Stages

1. List the stages of human life from conception to death.
   a. The stages of human life are prenatal development, birth, the neonatal period, infancy, childhood, adolescence, adulthood, and old age.

Prenatal Development

2. Describe the major events in prenatal development.
   a. The major events in prenatal development include:
      (1) formation of the zygote
      (2) cleavage
      (3) formation of the morula
      (4) formation of the blastocyst
      (5) formation of the embryonic disc, gut cavity, and amniotic cavity
      (6) development of the primary germ layers, ectoderm, mesoderm, and endoderm
      (7) formation of all the organs and systems from the germ layers
3. Define the term teratogen and describe the effects of selected teratogens.
   a. A teratogen is any substance or agent that can cause malformations in the developing embryo or fetus.
   b. Infectious agents, hormones, and certain kinds of medications frequently act as teratogens.
   c. Teratogens often cause congenital heart defects, abnormalities of the reproductive system and limbs, deafness, mental retardation, and a variety of other defects.

Physiology of Pregnancy

4. Describe the normal changes that occur in the mother's body during pregnancy and explain how they are regulated.
   a. The duration of pregnancy is about 280 days.
   b. Pregnancy is maintained in the following ways:
      (1) Estradiol and progesterone are produced by the corpus luteum during the first three months of pregnancy and from the placenta during the remainder of pregnancy.
      (2) Chorionic gonadotropins regulate the production of estradiol and progesterone.
   c. The placenta also produces human placental lactogen, which is thought to help to maintain positive protein balance, mobilize fats for energy, and regulate the blood glucose concentration.

   d. In addition to hormonal changes, the mother's body undergoes other changes:
      (1) Her metabolic rate increases.
      (2) Her tissues retain sodium and fluids in greater quantities than in the nonpregnant state.
      (3) Her body adapts to the presence of the fetus, usually without an immunological response.
5. Explain how the breasts develop to prepare for lactation and how this process is regulated.
   a. During pregnancy the mammary glands increase in size, and the glandular portion is prepared to secrete milk under the influence of prolactin.
   b. The sucking of the infant stimulates mechanoreceptors in the nipples. Signals from these receptors prevent the release of prolactin-inhibiting hormone and also stimulate the release of oxytocin, which stimulates the let-down of milk and uterine contractions.
6. Describe the nature of the abnormal function that occurs in (a) toxemia, (b) eclampsia, and (c) spontaneous abortion.
   a. Toxemia is characterized by the accumulation of fluids in the tissues of a pregnant woman, hypertension, and the excretion of protein. Regulation of sodium intake is usually an effective treatment.
   b. Eclampsia, a severe form of toxemia that may occur shortly before, during, or within a few days after delivery, leads to greatly reduced kidney function, severe hypertension, convulsions and coma, and sometimes death.
   c. Spontaneous abortion or miscarriage is the sudden expulsion of the fetus. It occurs in about 10% of pregnancies and usually involves a defective fetus.

Labor and Delivery

7. Describe the events in normal labor and delivery and explain how they are controlled.
   a. Labor is initiated by hormonal and mechanical factors. It is thought to involve positive feedback, with each contraction leading to a stronger contraction.
   b. Estradiol and oxytocin and the mechanical pressure of the fetus stimulate uterine contractions.
   c. The stages of labor are:
      (1) the first stage, in which the cervix is dilated to accommodate the head of the fetus
      (2) the second stage, in which the infant is delivered
      (3) the third stage, in which the placenta detaches from the uterus and passes through the birth canal
   d. Relaxin may be involved in preparing the mother's body for birth.
8. Explain the effects on the fetus of breech birth and prolonged labor.

a. Breech births, in which the buttocks is the presenting part of the fetus, prolong labor and increase the risk of birth injuries.

b. Prolonged labor increases the likelihood that the fetus will become anoxic.

The Neonatal Period

9. Explain how the APGAR rating is used to assess the condition of a newborn infant.

    a. The APGAR rating assesses the condition of the fetus with respect to appearance, pulse, grimace, activity, and respiratory effort.

    b. Low ratings indicate that the neonate may require special care.

10. Compare the physiology of a neonate with that of an adult.

    a. The neonate differs from the adult in that it:

        (1) is less able to regulate body temperature

        (2) is less able to concentrate urine

        (3) has less immunological competence

        (4) has a higher respiratory rate

        (5) has a higher pulse rate

        (6) has a lower blood pressure

        (7) grows rapidly

Infancy and Childhood

11. Summarize the anatomical and physiological development that occurs during infancy and childhood.

    a. Infancy extends from four weeks to two years of age, and childhood extends from two years to puberty.

    b. Growth is characteristic of both stages but is more rapid in infancy than in childhood.

    c. The heart rate and respiratory rates decrease, and the blood pressure increases through these stages.

    d. Motor and mental development proceed along a fairly fixed sequence of stages, though much individual variation is seen among normal children in the rate of these developments.

Adolescence

12. Summarize the major changes in males and in females during puberty.

    a. The changes that occur in puberty include rapid growth, maturation of reproductive organs, and development of secondary sex characteristics.

    b. The heart rate, respiratory rate, and blood pressure reach adult values during late adolescence.

Aging

13. Describe the process of aging and the factors that affect the aging process.

    a. Aging may be defined as a decreased ability to adapt to a changing environment. It occurs at different rates in different organs:

        (1) Accommodation of the eye and auditory acuity diminish much earlier than cardiovascular, respiratory, kidney, and brain functions.

        (2) Locomotion and immune response are also impaired with age.

    b. Factors that affect the aging process include:

        (1) degenerative changes in regulatory mechanisms

        (2) biochemical changes within organs

14. Summarize the major theories of aging.

    a. Theories of aging include:

        (1) the cytologic theory, which asserts that aging is caused by cumulative effects of cellular injury

        (2) the fat metabolism theory, which asserts that aging may be due to a decreased ability to metabolize fats

        (3) the theory of intrinsic factors, which asserts that formation of irreversible chemical bonds and errors in protein synthesis accumulate and cause cells to die

        (4) the brain–endocrine theory, which asserts that a master plan is encoded in the brain and expressed as a schedule of events in the life cycle

Death and Dying

15. Define death and describe the physiological processes that occur during dying.

    a. Death is the loss of all life functions; when life-support systems are in use, it may be defined as the absence of cerebral function for at least twenty-four hours.

    b. When all life functions have ceased, the individual cells take several hours to die.

    c. Death is usually precipitated by the failure of one organ, and the effects of its failure create conditions that cause other organs to fail.

16. Evaluate the effects of hospices and other services for the dying and the effects of life-support systems for the terminally ill.

    a. Hospices, counselors for the dying, and more openness about discussing death and dying are contributing to reducing pain and increasing emotional support for a dying person.

    b. The availability of life-support systems creates many ethical issues concerning their use.

REVIEW

Important Terms

allantois

amnion

amniotic cavity

blastocyst

chorion

chorionic villi

cleavage

cytologic aging

eclampsia

fetus

gastrulation

hospice

implantation

lactation

neonate

neurulation

placenta

relaxin

teratogen

toxemia

umbilicus

yolk sac

zygote

Questions

1. What are the stages in the human life cycle?

2. **a.** What are the events in embryological development from fertilization to implantation?

   b. What are the three germ layers in the embryo, and what tissues are derived from each?

   c. What are the four embryonic membranes, and what structures do they form in the developing embryo?

   d. What is the placenta, and how does it form?

   e. What is the difference between an embryo and a fetus?

3. **a.** What is a teratogen?

   b. What are some agents that can act as teratogens, and what are their likely effects on the embryo or fetus?

4. **a.** What is the role of the ovaries in producing the hormones of pregnancy?

   b. What is the role of the placenta in producing hormones and in regulating the production of hormones?

   c. What changes besides hormonal changes occur in the body of a pregnant woman?

   d. Explain the statement that the fetus is a kind of transplant or graft on the body of the mother.

5. **a.** What developments take place in the mammary glands during pregnancy?

   b. What hormones control these developments?

   c. What changes occur at birth to allow milk production to begin soon after birth?

   d. How does the sucking of an infant stimulate milk production?

6. **a.** What are the symptoms of toxemia, and how is it treated?

   b. What is eclampsia, and how is it treated?

   c. What is a spontaneous abortion?

7. **a.** How does the positive feedback theory explain the onset and acceleration of labor?

   b. Name the three stages of labor and explain what happens in each.

   c. What might be the role of relaxin in preparing the body for delivery?

8. **a.** What is a breech birth, and what hazards does it create?

   b. How does prolonged labor create a risk to the fetus?

9. What is the APGAR rating, and how is it used?

10. **a.** How does the physiology of a neonate differ from that of an adult?

    b. What kinds of special care does a neonate require because of its physiology?

11. **a.** Summarize the changes in the rate of growth through infancy and childhood.

    b. How does the physiology of an infant or child differ from that of an adult?

12. **a.** Explain how the growth of females differs from that of males during adolescence.

    b. What is the usual sequence of changes in the female body during puberty?

    c. What is the usual sequence of changes in the male body during puberty?

    d. What physiological changes other than those associated with the reproductive system occur during adolescence?

13. **a.** What is aging?

    b. What are some typical changes that occur in the body during the aging process?

    c. What factors may affect the aging process?

14. Distinguish among the theories of aging.

15. **a.** Define death.

    b. What is the difference between cessation of life functions and cellular death?

    c. What is the effect of the failure of a vital organ on the process of dying?

16. What is a hospice, and what services does it provide?

Problems

1. Suppose you are working in a prenatal care clinic and you encounter pregnant women with the following conditions:

   a. Weight gain of 3 pounds in two weeks

   b. Blood pressure of 145/85

   c. Glucose in the urine

   d. Protein in the urine

What is the significance of each of these conditions? What treatment is indicated?

2. What ethical questions are raised by the use of life-support systems for dying patients? Use the ethical decision-making technique from Chapter 27 to answer some of these questions.

REFERENCES AND READINGS

Anonymous. 1979. Melatonin: a puberty switch. *Science News* 116:373 (December 1).

Beaconsfield, P., Birdwood, G., and Beaconsfield, R. 1980. The placenta. *Scientific American* 243(2):95 (August).

Beck, N. C., and Hall, D. 1978. Natural childbirth. *Obstetrics and Gynecology* 52(3):371 (September).

Beer, A. E., and Billingham, R. E. 1974. The embryo as a transplant. *Scientific American* 230(4):36 (April).

Bongaarts, J. 1980. Does malnutrition affect fecundity? A summary of evidence. *Science* 208:564 (May 9).

Bower, T. G. R. 1976. Repetitive processes in child development. *Scientific American* 235(5):38 (November).

Callahan, S., and Childress, J. F. 1978. Regulating an anti-aging drug. *Hastings Center Report* 8(3):19 (June).

Caplan, A. I., and Ordahl, C. P. 1978. Irreversible gene repression model for control of development. *Science* 201:120 (July 14).

Diamond, M. C. 1978. The aging brain: Some enlightening and optimistic results. *American Scientist* 66:66 (January–February).

Dickman, Z., Gupta, J. S., and Dey, S. K. 1977. Does "blastocyst estrogen" initiate implantation? *Science* 195:687 (February 18).

Fowles, J. 1978. The impending society of immortals. *The Futurist* 12(3):175 (June).

General Clinical Research Centers Branch, Division of Research Resources, National Institutes of Health. 1977. *How children grow.* Bethesda, Md.: DHEW Publication No. (NIH) 77–166.

Gintzler, A. R. 1980. Endorphin-mediated increases in pain threshold during pregnancy. *Science* 210:193 (October 10).

Greenberg, J. 1979. Old age: What is normal? *Science News* 115:284 (April 28).

Gregg, R. H., Frazier, L. M., and Nesbit, R. A. 1975. Relaxation training effects on childbirth. Outline of exhibit presented at clinical meeting of the American College of Obstetricians and Gynecologists, Boston (May).

Harley, C. B., and Goldstein, S. 1980. Retesting the commitment theory of cellular aging. *Science* 207:191 (January 11).

Hayflick, L. 1980. The cell biology of human aging. *Scientific American* 242(1):58 (January).

Kolata, G. B. 1977. The aging heart: Changes in function and response to drugs. *Science* 195:166 (January 14).

Kolata, G. B. 1979. Scientists attack report that obstetrical medications endanger children. *Science* 204:391 (April 27).

Kolata, G. B. 1979. Sex hormones and brain development. *Science* 205:985 (September 7).

Landfield, P. W., Waymire, J. C., and Lynch, G. 1978. Hippocampal aging and adrenocorticoids: Quantitative correlations. *Science* 202:1098 (December 8).

Marx, J. L. 1979. Hormones and their effects in the aging body. *Science* 206:805 (November 16).

Masoro, E. J. 1979. Decline in fat metabolism may be cause of shortened life. Paper presented at the annual meeting of the American Association for the Advancement of Science, January 3–8, Houston, Texas.

Moskowitz, B. A. 1978. The acquisition of language. *Scientific American* 239(5):92 (November).

Raisz, L. G., and Kream, B. E. 1981. Hormonal control of skeletal growth. *Annual Review of Physiology* 43:225.

Reinisch, J. M., Simon, N. G., Karow, W. G., and Gandelman, R. 1978. Prenatal exposure to prednisone in humans and animals retards intrauterine growth. *Science* 202:436 (October 27).

Sabath, L. D., Philipson, A., and Charles, D. 1978. Ethics and the use of drugs during pregnancy. *Science* 202:540 (November 3).

Serón-Ferré, M., and Jaffe, R. B. 1981. The fetal adrenal gland. *Annual Review of Physiology* 43:141.

Shiu, P. C., and Friesen, H. G. 1980. Mechanism of action of prolactin in the control of mammary gland function. *Annual Review of Physiology* 42:83.

Simpson, E. R., and MacDonald, P. C. 1981. Endocrine physiology of the placenta. *Annual Review of Physiology* 43:163.

Soloff, M. S., Alexandrova, M., and Fernstrom, M. J. 1979. Oxytocin receptors: Triggers for parturition and lactation. *Science* 204:1313 (June 22).

Streissguth, A. P., Landesman-Dwyer, S., Martin, J. C., and Smith, D. W. 1980. Teratogenic effects of alcohol in humans and laboratory animals. *Science* 209:353 (July 18).

Tietze, C., and Lewit, S. 1977. Legal abortion. *Scientific American* 236(1):21 (January).

Timiras, P. S. 1978. Biological perspectives on aging. *American Scientist* 66:605 (September–October).

Trotter, R. J. 1980. Born too soon. *Science News* 118:234 (October 11).

Van-Auken, W. B. D., and Tomlinson, D. R. 1953. An appraisal of patient training for childbirth. *American Journal of Obstetrics and Gynecology* 66:100.

Vorhees, C. V., Brunner, R. L., and Butcher, R. E. 1979. Psychotropic drugs as behavioral teratogens. *Science* 205:1220 (September 21).

Wolpert, L. 1978. Pattern formation in biological development. *Scientific American* 239(4):154 (October).

Some of the less familiar words in this Glossary are followed by a phonetic guide to pronunciation. Such phonetic spellings are interpreted as follows: (1) An unmarked vowel not followed by a consonant in the syllable has a long sound. (2) An unmarked vowel that is followed by a consonant in the syllable has a short sound. (3) A macron (ˉ) indicates a long vowel. (4) A breve (˘) indicates a short vowel. (5) Strongly accented syllables are marked with a single accent ('). (6) Less strongly accented syllables are marked with a double accent (").

Names of specific bones, muscles, nerves, and blood vessels are not included in the Glossary; see tables in relevant chapters. Prefixes, suffixes, and combining forms are listed on the inside front and back covers.

GLOSSARY

abdomen (ab'do-men) Portion of the body between the diaphragm and the pelvis.

abduction (ab-duk'shun) Movement of a body part away from the midline.

absorption (ab-sorp'shun) Taking in of substances by membranes or cells.

absorptive state State of absorbing nutrients from the intestinal tract.

acceleratory reflexes Reflexes that maintain balance and coordination during starting, stopping, or turning movements.

accommodation Adjustment of focal distance of the eye.

acetabulum Cuplike depression in the os coxa.

acetoacetic acid A ketone body from fatty acid oxidation.

acetone A ketone body from fatty acid oxidation.

acetylcholine (as"ĕ-til-ko'lēn) Substance secreted at the axon end of many neurons that transmits a signal across a synapse.

acetyl-coenzyme A, acetyl-CoA A molecule consisting of a two-carbon fragment and coenzyme A; product of fatty acid oxidation and carbohydrate degradation.

Achilles (ah-kil'-ēz) **tendon** Tendon that attaches gastrocnemius and soleus muscles to calcaneus.

acid A substance that releases hydrogen ions when dissolved in water.

acidosis (as"ĭ-do'sis) A condition in which the pH of body fluids is below normal.

acinus (plural, **acini**) Grapelike cluster of cells found in the secretory portion of many glands.

acne (ak'ne) An inflammatory disease of the sebaceous glands.

acromegaly (ak"ro-meg'al-e) Enlargement of face, hands, and feet caused by excessive secretion of growth hormone.

acromion (ak-ro'me-on) Lateral end of the spine of the scapula; forms part of shoulder joint.

acrosome (ak'ro-sōm) Dense cover on anterior head of sperm; contains enzymes that help sperm to penetrate ovum.

ACTH adrenocorticotropic hormone.

actin (ak′tin) Protein molecule found in thin filaments of sarcomeres.

action (ak′shun) A movement—flexion, adduction, rotation—produced by a muscle.

action potential An altered electrical potential across the membrane of a muscle or nerve cell when it is stimulated.

activation energy Energy needed to initiate a chemical reaction.

active site A portion of an enzyme molecule that combines with a substrate and causes a reaction.

active transport Transport of a substance (usually against a gradient) using an enzyme, a carrier, and ATP.

adaptation (ad″ap-ta′shun) A decrease in the excitability of sensory receptors in response to repeated stimuli of constant intensity.

Addison's disease Deficiency of adrenocortical hormones.

adduction (ah-duk′shun) Movement toward a midline.

adenine A nitrogenous base found in nucleotides.

adenohypophysis (ad″en-oh-hi-pof′eh-sis) Anterior portion of pituitary gland.

adenoids Enlarged pharyngeal tonsils.

adenosine diphosphate, ADP (ah-den′o-sēn di-fos′fāt) A molecule that can form a high-energy bond with another phosphate.

adenosine triphosphate, ATP The main energy-carrying molecule in living organisms; consists of adenine, ribose, and three phosphates and contains high-energy bonds.

adenylate cyclase (ah-den-ēl-ate′ sī′klās) Enzyme acting on ATP to form cyclic AMP.

ADH Antidiuretic hormone.

adipose (ad′eh-pōs″) Related to fat.

ADP Adenosine diphosphate.

adrenal Above the kidney.

adrenaline Epinephrine.

adrenergic Relating to an axon that releases epinephrine or norepinephrine.

adrenocorticotropic (ah-dre″no-kor″ti-ko-trōp′ik) **hormone, ACTH** A hormone from the anterior pituitary that stimulates growth and secretion of adrenal cortex.

adrenogenital (ah-dre″no-gen′eh-tal) **syndrome** A condition in which male sexual characteristics appear in a female infant because of excessive secretion of male hormones from the adrenal gland during development.

adventitia (ad″ven-tish′ah) Outermost connective-tissue covering of an organ or a blood vessel.

aerobic (ār″ob′ik) Pertaining to the presence of oxygen.

afferent Pertaining to movement toward an organ.

afterbirth Placenta and membranes expelled after the fetus.

after-discharge A response to stimulation of a sensory nerve that persists after stimulation has ceased.

agglutination (ah-gloo″ti-na′shun) Sticking together.

agglutinin (ag-lu′tin-in) Antibody in an agglutination reaction.

agglutinogen (ag-lu-tin′o-jen) Antigen in an agglutination reaction.

agonist The prime mover in a group of muscles; opposed by the antagonist.

albino Lacking pigment.

albumin (al-bu′min) Protein found mainly in blood; small amounts found in many tissues.

aldosterone (al-dos′ter-ōn) An adrenocortical hormone that increases sodium reabsorption.

alkaline Basic; having higher than neutral pH.

alkalosis (al″kah-lō′sis) A condition in which the pH of body fluids is above normal.

allantois (al-an′to-is) A fetal membrane that contributes to the formation of the placenta.

alleles (ah-lēls′) Genes that occupy corresponding positions on homologous chromosomes.

allergen (al′er-jen) A substance capable of producing allergy or hypersensitivity.

allergy (al′er-je) Unusual sensitivity to a substance that is harmless to most people in the same concentration.

all-or-none law Principle that, when a nerve is stimulated, it conducts an impulse of maximum strength.

alveolus (al-ve′ol-us) (plural, **alveoli**) Saclike structure in lungs and secretory portion of glands; tooth socket.

amenorrhea (am-en-or-e′ah) Absence or abnormal stoppage of menstruation.

amine (am′in) A molecule containing an NH_2 group.

amino (am′in-o) **acid** A molecule containing an organic acid (COOH) and an NH_2 group.

aminopeptidase (am″in-o-pep′tīd-ās) An enzyme that cleaves amino acids from the amino end of a peptide.

amniocentesis (am″nē-oh-sen-te′sis) A procedure for removing a sample of amniotic fluid from around a developing fetus.

amnion (am′ne-on) Membrane that encloses an embryo.

amniotic cavity Cavity formed by amnion; contains amniotic fluid and embryo.

amphiarthrosis (am″fe-ar-thro′sis) A joint in which the surfaces are connected by cartilage; permits little movement.

ampulla (am-pul′ah) **of Vater** A dilation at the entrance of the common bile duct and pancreatic duct into the duodenum.

amygdaloid (am-ig′dal-oid) Almond-shaped.

amylase (am′i-lās) An enzyme that breaks down starch and some other polysaccharides.

anabolism (an-ab′oh-lis″m) Energy-requiring synthetic processes by which cell substances are made.

anaerobic (an″ār-ōb′ik) Pertaining to the absence of oxygen.

anaphase (an′ah-fāz) A stage in mitosis during which chromosomes move apart.

anaphylactic (an″ah-fī-lak′tik) Pertaining to severe reaction to second exposure to an antigenic substance.

anastomosis (an-as″to-mo′sis) A communication between two blood vessels or nerves.

anatomical position Position of the body standing erect with palms of hands parallel with the anterior surface of the body.

anatomy The study of the structure of organisms.

androgen (an′dro-jen) A molecule having male sex hormone activity.

anemia A hemoglobin deficiency.

anesthesia Loss of sensation.

aneurysm (an'u-riz"m)   A saclike dilation in the wall of an artery.

angina (an-jīn'ah)   Severe, suffocating, constrictive pain, usually associated with heart disease.

angiotensins (an-je-o-ten'sins)   Vasoconstrictor substances derived from angiogensionogen; when antiogensin II is produced from antiogensin I, it causes constriction of blood vessels and release of aldosterone.

anion (an'i-on)   A negatively charged ion.

annulus fibrosus (an'nu-lus fi-bro'sis)   The outer fibrous ring of an intervertebral disc.

anorexia nervosa (an-o-rek'se-ah ner-vo'sah)   A serious nervous condition in which the individual takes in little food and becomes emaciated.

ANS   Autonomic nervous system.

antagonist   A muscle that opposes an agonist.

anterior   Ventral, front.

antibody   A protein produced in response to the presence of an antigen.

anticoagulant (an'te-ko-ag'u-lant)   A substance that prevents blood clotting.

anticodon (an"tĭ-ko'don)   A sequence of three bases in tRNA that attach by base pairing with a codon in mRNA.

antidiuretic (an"tĭ-di"u-ret'ik) **hormone, ADH**   A hormone from the posterior pituitary that increases reabsorption of water in the kidney. (See also vasopressin.)

antigen (an'tĭ-jen)   A substance that stimulates the immune system to produce antibodies.

antihistamine (an"tĭ-his'ta-meen)   A substance that counteracts the effects of histamine.

anuria (an-u're-ah)   Inability to produce urine.

aortic sinus   Region of aorta that contains baroreceptors.

apex   The top or pointed extremity of an organ.

apical (ap'ik-al)   Pertaining to the apex.

apnea (ap-ne'ah)   Temporary cessation of breathing.

apneusis (ap-nu'sis)   Prolongation of inspiration.

apocrine (ap'o-krīn)   A gland that loses part of its protoplasm while secreting; the secretion of such a gland.

apoferritin (ap"o-fer'rĭ-tin)   An iron-storing protein.

aponeurosis (ap"o-nu-ro'sis)   A fibrous sheet of connective tissue to which muscles attach.

appendicular (ap"en-dik'u-lar)   Pertaining to the appendages.

appendix   Worm-shaped sac attached to the cecum.

aqueous   Watery.

arachnoid (ar-ak'noid)   A cobweblike membrane; root means pertaining to a spider.

arbor vitae (ar'bor ve'ta)   Treelike pattern of white matter seen in a section of the cerebellum.

arcuate (ar'ku-āt)   Arched or bowed.

areola (ah-re'o-lah)   Pigmented region surrounding the nipple of the mammary gland.

areolar (ah-re'o-lar)   Loosely organized; having openings or spaces.

arrector pili (ah-rek'tor pil'i)   Smooth muscles that pull hairs up away from skin.

arrhythmia (ah-rith'me-ah)   Loss of rhythm.

arteriole (ar-te're-ōl)   Small artery; connects larger artery to capillaries.

arteriosclerosis (ar-te"re-o-sklĕ-ro'sis)   Hardening of the arteries.

artery   Vessel carrying blood from the heart.

arthritis   Joint inflammation.

arthrosis (ar-thro'sis)   A joint.

articular (ar-tik'u-lar) **cartilage**   Hyaline cartilage that covers the ends of bones in synovial joints.

articulation (ar-tic"u-la'shun)   A connecting together.

ascorbic (as-kor'bik) **acid**   Vitamin C.

association area   An area of the cerebral cortex concerned with memory, reasoning, emotions, and other mental processes.

association fiber   A neural tract within the cerebrum that carries signals from one association area to another.

asthma (az'mah)   A condition in which bronchioles constrict and cause difficulty in breathing.

astigmatism (ah-stig'mah-tiz-m)   A condition in which refractile surfaces of the eye have unequal curvatures.

astrocyte (as'tro-sīt)   A star-shaped cell; found in the central nervous system.

atelectasis (at-el-ek'tas-is)   Collapse (or failure to expand) of alveoli of lungs.

atherosclerosis (ath"er-o-sklĕ-ro'sis)   Hardening and obstruction of arteries due to deposition of lipids and other substances.

atom   Smallest particle of an element having all the properties of the element.

atomic number   The number of protons in an atom.

atomic weight   Number approximately equal to the number of protons plus the number of neutrons in an atom.

atonic (at-on'ik)   Lacking normal tone.

ATP   Adenosine triphosphate.

atresia (ah-tre'ze-ah)   Absence of an opening; degeneration of an ovarian follicle.

atrioventricular (a"tre-o-ven-trik'u-lar), **AV**   Pertaining to the atrium and ventricle of the heart.

atrium (a'tre-um)   A chamber or opening.

atrophy (at'ro-fe)   A decrease in size.

auditory (aw'di-to"re)   Pertaining to hearing.

auricle (aw'ri-kl)   An earlike appendage.

auscultation (aws"kul-ta'shun)   The act of listening for sounds within the body.

autoimmune (aw"to-im-mūn') **disease**   A condition caused by the body reacting to some of its own substance.

autonomic (aw"to-nom'ik)   Independent, not under voluntary control.

autonomic (aw-to-nom'ik) **nervous system**   A self-regulating component of the nervous system that controls visceral functions.

autosomal (aw'to-som-al) **inheritance**   Transmission of heritable characteristics on one of the twenty-two paired chromosomes.

axial   Pertaining to the head and trunk.

axilla (ak-sil'ah)   Armpit.

axon A process of a neuron that carries impulses away from the cell body.

axon hillock Enlarged area of a neuron cell body where the axon arises.

azygos (az'ig-os) An unpaired structure in the body.

Babinski (ba-bin'ske) **reflex** The reflexive spreading of the toes when the sole of the foot is stroked; normal in infants but indicates damage to neural tracts in older individuals.

baroreceptor (ba''ro-re-sep'tor) A receptor that responds to pressure.

Barr body A mass of chromatin near the nuclear membrane in females that represents an X chromosome.

Bartholin's glands Vulvovaginal glands.

basal metabolic rate Amount of energy used to maintain life in an awake, resting individual.

basal nuclei Distinct masses of gray matter (cell bodies) within the cerebral hemispheres.

base A chemical substance that can combine with an acid to form a salt.

basement membrane A layer of extracellular material beneath the deep surface of epithelium.

basophil (ba'so-fil) A leukocyte having granular cytoplasm and able to be stained with a basophilic dye.

B-cells Antibody-producing cells.

beta-hydroxybutyric acid A ketone body produced from the oxidation of fatty acids.

beta-lipotropin (ba'tah-lip'o-trop-in) A substance produced by the anterior pituitary gland that mobilizes fats in some animals.

beta oxidation Breakdown of a fatty acid for energy.

beta particles Electrons derived from the disintegration of a neutron.

beta reduction The process by which fat is synthesized from other substances.

biaxial joint A joint in which movement occurs in two planes.

biceps Having two heads.

bicuspid Having two points, or cusps.

bifid Split into two parts.

bilateral Pertaining to both sides of the body; having two sides.

bile Fluid secreted by the liver that aids in the digestion of fats.

bilirubin (bil-e-roo'bin) A red bile pigment from the breakdown of hemoglobin.

biliverdin (bil-e-ver'din) A green bile pigment from the breakdown of hemoglobin.

binocular vision Vision with two eyes; because each eye views an object from a slightly different angle, a three-dimensional effect is created.

biofeedback (bi''o-feed'bak) A process in which signals indicating levels of autonomic processes are made perceptible so the person perceiving the signals can learn to control the autonomic processes.

biological clock The regulatory mechanism for biorhythms.

bipolar cells Neurons that have two processes.

blastocele (blas'to-sēl) The cavity of a blastula.

blastocyst (blas'to-sist) Hollow ball of cells comprising an early stage in embryonic development.

blind spot Region of retina where optic nerve fibers leave the eye and where light-sensitive cells are absent.

blood Fluid circulating in the heart and blood vessels.

blood–brain barrier Specialized capillary structure that limits passage of substances from the blood into the tissues of the brain.

B lymphocyte A lymphocyte that gives rise to plasma cells, which in turn give rise to antibodies.

BMR Basal metabolic rate.

bolus (bo'lus) A mass.

Bowman's capsule Glomerular capsule; end of nephron where substances filter from blood.

brachial (bra-ke'al) Pertaining to the arm.

bradycardia (brad-e-kar'de-ah) Abnormal slowness of the heart rate.

bradykinin (brad'e-ki'nin) A polypeptide having potent vaso-dilation action.

brain asymmetries (a-sim'me-trēs) Variations in the shape and size of brain parts such that the left and right halves of the brain are different.

brainstem All of the brain except the cerebrum, cerebellum, and the white matter that connects those parts; the internal core of the brain.

brain waves Electrical signals, detectable from the scalp, that represent various types of brain activity.

Broca's motor speech area A functional area of the cerebrum in which thoughts are translated into speech.

Brodmann's area 17 An area of the brain where visual signals are processed.

bronchiole (bron'ke-ōl) Branch of airway leading to alveoli.

bronchitis (bron-ki'tis) Inflammation of the bronchi.

bronchus (bron'kus) (plural, **bronchi**) A tube leading from the trachea to a lung.

Brown-Sequard syndrome Specific impairment resulting from hemisection of the spinal cord.

Brunner's glands Mucous glands in the duodenum.

buffer A substance that decreases changes in the pH of a solution.

bulk flow Streaming flow of molecules, more rapid than diffusion.

bursa (plural, **bursae**) A sac filled with synovial fluid found at pressure points at or near joints.

bursitis (bur-si'tis) Inflammation of a bursa.

calcification (kal''sĭ-fĭ-ka'shun) Deposition of calcium salts in an organic matrix.

calcitonin (kal''sĭ-to'nin) A hormone that lowers blood calcium.

callus A thickened area.

calorie The amount of energy required to raise the temperature of 1 gram of water 1°C.

calyx (ka'liks) (plural, **calyces**) A cup-shaped organ or cavity.

cAMP Cyclic adenosine monophosphate.

canaliculus (kan''ah-lik'u-lus) (plural, **canaliculi**) A small canal.

cancellous (kan'sel-us) Having a spongy, latticelike structure.

capillary (kap'ĭ-ler''e) A small blood vessel that connects an arteriole and a venule.

capitulum (kap-it'u-lum) A small bony eminence.

capsule A fibrous or membranous sac that covers an organ.

carbaminohemoglobin (kar''bah-me'no-he''mo-glo'bin) Hemoglobin carrying carbon dioxide.

carbohydrate An organic compound containing several alcohol groups and at least one aldehyde or ketone group.

carbon monoxide CO, a poisonous gas.

carbonic anhydrase (an-hi'drās) An enzyme that catalyzes the conversion of carbonic acid to carbon dioxide and water or the reverse.

carboxyl (kar-box'l) A functional group giving a molecule acid properties; COOH.

carboxypeptidase (kar-box''e-pep'tīd-ās) An enzyme that cleaves amino acids from the carboxyl end of a peptide.

carcinogenic (kar''sin-o-gen'ik) A substance that induces cancer.

cardiac (kar'de-ak) Pertaining to the heart.

cardiac center A nucleus in the medulla that regulates heartbeat and force of contraction.

cardiac cycle A repetitive sequence of events involving systole and diastole in the heart's pumping of blood.

cardiac output The volume of blood leaving the heart; the product of the volume of blood pumped with each beat times the number of beats per minute.

cardiac tamponade (tam''pon-ād') Compression of the heart due to the collection of fluid or blood in the pericardial sac.

cardioinhibitory area Area of the brain that sends signals to the heart, causing the heart rate to decrease.

cardiovascular center Center in the medulla that regulates both heart rate and diameter of blood vessels.

carotene (kār'o-teen) An orange pigment found in such foods as carrots; precursor to vitamin A.

carotid (kah-rot'id) **body** Structure at the branching of the carotid arteries that contains chemoreceptors.

carotid sinus Structure at the branching of the carotid arteries that contains baroreceptors.

carpal Pertaining to the wrist.

carrier (1) Substance that transfers electrons, atoms, or molecules in a metabolic pathway or in a membrane transport system; (2) an individual who carries an unexpressed allele of a gene.

cartilage (kar'tĭ-laj) A firm, resilient connective tissue.

catabolism (ka-tab'o-liz-m) The breakdown of molecules, usually for obtaining energy.

catalyst (kat'ă-list) A substance that increases the rate of a chemical reaction without being changed by the reaction.

cataract (kat'ah-rakt) An opacity of the lens of the eye.

catecholamine (kat''ĕ-kol-am'in) A group of similar amines that act as neurotransmitters; dopamine, epinephrine, and norepinephrine.

cation (kat'i-un) A positively charged ion.

cauda equina (kaw'da ek'win-a) The bundle of spinal nerve roots that extend below the end of the spinal cord; root meaning, horse's tail.

caudal Toward the tail; in humans, inferior.

CCK-PZ Cholecystokinin-pancreozymin.

cecum (se'kum) Blind pouch; usually refers to digestive tract.

cell The functional unit of a living organism.

cell-mediated immunity Destruction of microorganisms or other foreign cells by a reaction involving T-cells.

cementum The covering of the root of a tooth.

central nervous system, CNS The brain and spinal cord.

centriole (sen'tre-ōl) One of a pair of structures that participate in forming the mitotic spindle.

centromere (sen'tro-meer) A constricted region of a chromosome to which spindle fibers attach during mitosis.

cephalic (seh-fal'ik) Toward the head; in humans, superior.

cerebellum (ser-e-bel'um) A portion of the brain behind the cerebrum and above the pons concerned with the coordination of movements.

cerebral aqueduct A narrow canal connecting the third and fourth ventricles of the brain; contains cerebrospinal fluid.

cerebral cortex The outermost layer of the cerebrum.

cerebral palsy (ser'e-bral pawl'ze) Paralysis caused by a brain lesion.

cerebrospinal (ser'e-bro-spi'nal) **fluid, CSF** The fluid produced in the ventricles of the brain; also surrounds the central nervous system.

cerebrovascular accident, CVA The blockage or rupture of a blood vessel in the cerebrum.

cerebrum (ser'e-brum) Upper main portion of human brain, concerned with receiving and responding to sensory signals and carrying out mental processes; includes the cerebral hemispheres and basal nuclei.

cerumen (sĕ-roo'men) Waxy substance produced by cells that line the external ear canal.

cervix (ser'vix) Neck; narrow end of uterus, where it joins the vagina.

chemoreceptor (ke''mo-re-sep'tor) A sensory receptor that responds to a chemical change.

chemotaxis (ke''mo-tax'is) The process by which chemical stimuli attract or repel; responsible for some migrations of leukocytes.

chiasma (ki-az'mah) A crossing; occurs in some fibers of the optic nerves.

chief cells Cells of the gastric glands of the stomach that secrete enzymes.

chloride shift The movement of chloride ions to equalize the electrical charge in a body fluid.

cholecystectomy (ko''le-sis-tek'-to-me) Surgical removal of the gallbladder.

cholecystokinin-pancreozymin, CCK-PZ (ko''le-sis-to-kin'in pan''kre-o-zi'min) A hormone from the intestinal mucosa that causes the gallbladder to release bile and the pancreas to release enzymes.

cholesterol (ko-les′ter-ol) A steroid found in bile and used by the body to make a variety of hormones.

cholesterol esterase (es′ter-ās) An enzyme that removes a fatty acid attached to cholesterol.

cholinergic (ko″lin-er′jik) Describes a nerve fiber whose terminals release acetylcholine.

cholinesterase (ko″lin-es′ter-ās) An enzyme that breaks down acetylcholine.

chondroblast (kon′dro-blast) A cell that forms cartilage.

chondrocyte (kon′dro-sīt) A cartilage cell.

chordae tendinae (kor′de ten′din-e) Strands of connective tissue that attach the cusps of the A-V valves to papillary muscles in the heart's ventricles.

chorion (ko′re-on) The outermost fetal membrane.

chorionic villi (ko′re-on-ik vil′le) Tufts of fetal blood vessels that exchange substances with maternal blood.

choroid (ko′roid) Skinlike; highly vascular middle layer of eyeball.

choroid plexus Vascular projections into the ventricles of the brain that produce cerebrospinal fluid.

chromatid (kro′mah-tid) A member of a duplicate pair of chromosomes.

chromatin (kro′mah-tin) Nuclear material that gives rise to chromosomes during cell division.

chromosomal (kro″mah-so′mal) **aberration** The deletion, inversion, or translocation of a segment of DNA of a chromosome.

chromosomal abnormality Any modification of the configuration of DNA in a chromosome.

chromosome (kro′mo-sōm) A strand of DNA and protein found in the nucleus of a cell; carries genetic information.

chylomicron (ki″lo-mi′kron) A very small droplet of fat coated with protein found in lymphatic vessels.

chyme (kīm) Semiliquid food mass leaving the stomach.

chymotrypsin (ki″mo-trip′sin) A proteolytic enzyme from the pancreas.

cilia (sil′e-ah) Tiny hairlike projections found on some epithelial cells.

ciliary (sil′e-er″e) **body** Anterior-most portion of choroid layer of the eye; contains ciliary muscles that participate in accommodation.

circadian (ser″kah-de′an) **rhythm** Daily rhythmic variations in physiological processes and behavior.

circle of Willis A group of arteries forming a circle around the pituitary gland and allowing blood to take alternate pathways through the brain.

circumduction (ser″kum-duk′shun) Circular movement.

cirrhosis (sir-o′sis) A liver disease in which liver cells are replaced with connective tissue; root means orange.

cisterna (sis-ter′nah) Cavity or reservoir.

citric acid cycle Major pathway for the oxidation of carbohydrate and other nutrients; Krebs cycle.

clearance The rate at which a substance is removed from the blood by the kidney.

cleavage (kle′vāj) Division into two equal parts; the process by which a zygote becomes a multicellular ball of cells.

climacteric (kli-mak-ter′ik) Normal age-related decrease in sexual function.

clitoris (klit′o-ris) Small erectile organ located in the anterior part of the vulva; homologous to the penis.

clonal (klo′nal) **selection theory** A theory proposing that specific cells respond to antigens by producing a clone, the cells of which produce antibodies or "remember" the antigen to which they were sensitized.

clone (klōn) A group of cells derived from a single cell.

cloning (klōn′ing) The process by which a multicellular organism identical to another organism is produced.

closed reduction The realignment of the ends of a fractured bone without opening the skin over the fracture.

CNS Central nervous system.

coarctation (ko-ark-ta′shun) A straightening, pressing together, or constriction.

cochlea (kok′le-ah) Snail-shaped bony portion of inner ear; contains sound receptors.

codon (ko′don) A sequence of three bases in messenger RNA that specifies the placement of an amino acid in a protein.

coenzyme (ko-en′zīm) A nonprotein substance that is required for the action of an enzyme.

collagen (kol′ah-jen) A major protein of connective tissue.

collateral (kol-at′er-al) **circulation** Accessory to; secondary pathways in the blood vessels created by branching of the vessels.

colliculi (kol-ik′u-li) Small elevations.

colloid (kol′loid) Resembling glue; a state of matter in which small particles are suspended in a medium.

colloid osmotic pressure Pressure due to presence of colloidal particles in a medium; proteins in blood plasma exert such pressure.

colon (ko′lun) Large intestine from cecum to rectum.

color blindness Lack of ability to distinguish certain colors.

comminuted (kom′in-u-ted) Broken into small pieces, as in a bone fracture.

commissure (kom′is-ūr) A bundle of nerve fibers that connect the left and right sides of the brain or spinal cord.

communicating ramus (ra′mus) A branch of a spinal nerve that carries fibers to the sympathtic chain.

compensation (1) Process by which the body counterbalances any defect; (2) the returning of the blood pH to the normal range without complete correction of electrolyte concentrations.

competitive inhibition Prevention of the action of an enzyme by a substance attaching to the active sites without undergoing a reaction; the relative concentrations of the normal substrate and the competing substance determine the degree of inhibition.

complement A group of enzymes that are involved in certain antigen–antibody reactions.

compliance The ability of a structure to be distended or deformed, especially the lung.

compound A substance that consists of two or more elements combined in a definite proportion.

compound lipid A fatty substance that contains some other substance in addition to the fatty material.

concave Having a hollowed-out curved surface.

concentration gradient A graded difference in the amount of a substance dissolved in a fluid.

conception Fertilization.

concha (kong'kah) A shell-shaped structure, such as any of the bones of the nasal cavity.

conduction (1) The transfer of heat by direct contact; (2) the transmission of energy, as in the conduction of nerve impulses.

conduction deafness An impairment of hearing due to the failure of the bones of the middle ear to conduct vibrations to the inner ear.

condyle A large, rounded surface at the end of a bone.

cones Receptor cells in the eye capable of detecting color.

congenital (kon-jen'ĭ-tal) Present at birth.

conjunctiva (kon"junk-tĭ'vah) The mucous membrane lining the eyelids and covering the anterior surface of the eyeball.

connective tissue A tissue consisting of scattered cells, such as fibroblasts, in large amounts of intercellular substance.

consciousness Awareness of signals from the sense organs.

contact inhibition The prevention of further cell division by the touching of cell surfaces.

contraceptive (kon"trah-sep'tiv) An agent or device that prevents conception.

contractility The ability to develop tension or to shorten.

contraction The production of tension; shortening.

contraction cycle Repetitive reactions of actin and myosin in a muscle filament that increase the degree of shortening of the filament.

contracture Permanent shortening of a muscle.

contralateral On the opposite side.

conus medullaris (ko'nus med"u-lar'is) Termination of spinal cord.

convection Transfer of heat through a medium such as air or water.

convergence Coming together.

convex Having a bulging curved surface.

copulation Sexual intercourse, coitus.

coracoid (kor'ak-oid) Like a crow's beak; refers to sharp processes on bones.

corium (ko're-um) Dermis.

cornea (kor'ne-ah) Transparent surface of anterior portion of the eye.

cornified Horny; hard, dry tissue.

cornu (kor'nu) Any hornlike projection.

coronal (kor'o-nal) Crownlike; pertaining to the crown of the head.

coronal plane Frontal plane that divides anterior and posterior parts of an object.

coronary (kor'o-na-re) Circling like a crown, especially blood vessels of the heart.

coronoid (kor'o-noid) Like a crow's beak; refers to sharp processes on bones.

corpus (kor'pus) Body or mass.

corpus albicans (kor'pus al'bih-kanz) White body; scar that remains after degeneration of a corpus luteum.

corpus callosum (kor'pus kah-lo'sum) A mass of myelinated nerve fibers connecting the right and left cerebral hemispheres.

corpus luteum (lu'te-um) Yellow body; cells that remain after an ovum has been released and that serve to produce hormones.

cortex (kor'tex) Outer portion of an organ; root means bark.

corticosteroid (kor"tih-ko-ster'oid) A steroid hormone from the cortex of the adrenal gland.

corticotropin An anterior pituitary hormone that stimulates the adrenal cortex; ACTH.

cortisol (kor'tĭ-sol) An adrenocortical hormone that regulates carbohydrate metabolism.

costal (kos'tal) Pertaining to a rib.

countercurrent mechanism A mechanism involving fluids flowing in opposite directions.

covalent (ko-va'lent) **bond** A chemical bond in which two atoms share electrons.

CPR Cardiopulmonary resuscitation; a technique for maintaining air and blood flow in an individual whose heartbeat and breathing have stopped.

cramp A painful spasmodic muscular contraction.

cranial Pertaining to the head.

craniosacral (kra"ne-o-sa'kral) Pertaining to the cranium and sacrum; pertaining to the parasympathetic division of the autonomic nervous system, the neurons of which originate in these regions.

cranium Skull bones that encase the brain.

creatine phosphate (kre'ah-tin fos'fāt) A high-energy compound found in muscle.

creatinine (kre-at'in-in) A product of the breakdown of creatine found in the urine.

crenation (kre-na'shun) Shrinking or shriveling of a cell due to loss of fluid.

cretinism (kre'tĭ-nizm) Decreased physical and mental development due to a deficiency of thyroid hormone in infancy.

cribriform (krib'rif-orm) Perforated like a sieve.

cricoid (kri'koid) Ring shaped.

crista Ridge or crest.

cross-bridge The attachment between filaments during the contraction of a muscle.

crossing-over An interchange of segments between homologous chromosomes.

cross section A transverse slice through the body or a body part.

crown Portion of a tooth extending above the gum.

cruciate (kru'she-āt) Crossing; shaped like a cross.

cryptorchidism (krip-tor'kid-izm) Failure of testes to descend into the scrotum.

crypts of Lieberkühn (kriptz of Le'ber-kuhn) Tubular mucous glands in the intestine.

CSF Cerebrospinal fluid.

cupula (ku"pu-lah) A domelike, cup-shaped structure.

curare (koo-rah're) A drug that causes paralysis by blocking transmission of signals at neuromuscular junctions.

Cushing's disease A disorder caused by excessive secretion of

ACTH or of adrenocortical hormones.

cusp A tapering projection.

cutaneous (ku-ta′ne-us) Pertaining to the skin.

cuticle (ku′tik-l) outer layer of skin, especially around nails.

cyanosis (si″ah-no′sis) Bluishness of skin and mucous membranes due to lack of oxygen in blood.

cyclic adenosine monophosphate, cAMP A derivative of ATP that acts as a mediator of certain hormone actions.

cyclic center A brain center that regulates the menstrual cycle.

cystic (sis′tik) **duct** The duct leading from the gallbladder to the common bile duct.

cystic fibrosis (sis′tik fi-bro′sis) A disease in which excessive mucous is produced, and pancreatic and respiratory function are disturbed.

cystitis (sis-ti′tis) Inflammation of the urinary bladder.

cytochrome (si′to-krōm) A hemelike substance responsible for transporting electrons in cellular respiration.

cytokinesis (si″to-kin-e′sis) The division of the cytoplasm following the division of the nucleus.

cytologic (si″to-log′ik) **aging** A theory that aging is due to changes in cells.

cytology (si-tol′o-ge) The study of cells.

cytoplasm (si′to-plazm) The substance of the cell excluding the nucleus.

cytosine (si′to-seen) A nitrogenous base found in DNA and RNA.

dead space volume The volume of the respiratory passageways in which no gas exchange occurs.

deamination (de-am-in-a′shun) The removal of amino groups from an amino acid.

decidua (de-sid′u-ah) Falling off.

deciduous (de-sid′u-us) **teeth** Teeth that are not permanent; "baby" teeth.

decompression sickness A disorder caused by nitrogen bubbles in the tissues due to too rapid a decrease in barometric pressure; the bends.

decubitus (de-ku-bī′tus) Lying down.

decussation (de-kus-a′shun) Crossing the median plane of the body.

deep Below the surface of the body.

defecation The passage of the contents of the rectum out of the body.

defibrillation (de-fi-bril-a′shun) The use of an electrical current to terminate an extremely rapid heart rate.

deglutition (de-glu-ti′shun) The act of swallowing.

dehydration (de-hi-dra′shun) Removal of water from the body; the condition that results from excessive water loss.

deletion The loss of one or more bases from a strand of DNA.

denaturation (de-na-tūr-a′shun) A change in the shape of a protein molecule that causes it to lose some of its characteristics and often its function.

dendrite (den′drīt) A cytoplasmic process of a neuron that receives signals from other neurons.

denervate (de-ner′vāt) Destroy the nerve supply.

dens (denz) A toothlike structure.

dentin (den′tin) Bonelike substance of a tooth beneath the surface enamel.

deoxyhemoglobin (de-ox″e-hēm″o-glo′bin) Hemoglobin that is not carrying oxygen.

deoxyribonucleic (de-ox″e-ri′bo-nu-kle′ik) **acid, DNA** The nucleic acid of chromosomes; carries genetic information.

depolarization (de-po″lar-ĭ-za′shun) Reduction of the negative charge inside the cell membrane in excitable tissue.

depression A lowering movement.

depressor An agent that slows or inhibits a process.

dermal papilla (der′mal pa-pil′lă) An upward projection of the dermis into the epidermis.

dermatome (derm′a-tōm) A region of the skin supplied by sensory fibers of a single spinal nerve.

dermis (der′mis) The thick layer of the skin lying under the epidermis.

desmosome (des′mo-sōm) A site at which dense material causes two cells to adhere.

detoxification (de-toks-if-ik-a′shun) Reduction of the toxic properties of a substance.

dextrin (dex′trin) An intermediate breakdown product of starch.

diabetes insipidus (di″a-be′tez in-sip′ĭ-dus) A disorder caused by a deficiency of antidiuretic hormone in which large quantities of dilute urine are produced.

diabetes mellitus (di″a-be′tez mel-li′tus) A disorder caused by a deficiency of insulin activity in which glucose accumulates in the blood and urine.

diabetogenic (di-a-be′to-gen″ik) An agent that elicits symptoms of diabetes mellitus.

dialysis (di-al′ĭ-sis) The separation of small particles from larger ones by causing the smaller ones to pass through a selectively permeable membrane.

diapedesis (di″ah-pē-de′sis) Process by which leukocytes squeeze between the cells of blood vessel walls.

diaphragm (di′ah-fram) A thin wall or partition, as between the abdominal and thoracic cavities.

diaphysis (di-af′ĭ-sis) (plural, **diaphyses**) The shaft of a long bone.

diarthrosis (di-ar-thro′sis) A freely movable joint.

diastole (di-as′to-le) Dilation; period between contractions in the heart.

diastolic (di-as-tol′ik) Pertaining to diastole.

diastolic pressure The blood pressure during relaxation of the ventricles.

differentiation (dif″er-en″she-ā′shun) The specialization of structures in the process of development.

diffusion (dif-fu′shun) The random movement by which particles eventually become equally distributed through an available volume.

digestion The breakdown of food substances into particles that can be absorbed from the digestive tract.

digit A finger or toe.

diglyceride (di-glis′er-īd) A molecule containing glycerol and two fatty acids.

dipeptide (di-pep'tīd)   A compound consisting of two amino acids joined by a peptide bond.

diploe (dip'lo-e)   The loose osseous tissue between the two outer plates of cranial bones.

diploid (dip'loid)   Having the normal paired chromosomes of body cells.

disaccharide (di-sak'ah-rīd)   A sugar produced by the union of two monosaccharides.

dislocation (dis-lo-ka'shun)   The displacement of a body part, especially a bone.

dissociation constant (K)   A measure of the degree to which a chemical compound separates into components (usually ions).

distal (dis'tal)   Farthest from the midline.

diuresis (di"ur-e'sis)   Increased urine production.

diurnal (di-ur'nal)   Daily.

divergence   Movement spreading in different directions.

DNA   Deoxyribonucleic acid.

DNA polymerase (pol-im'er-ās)   An enzyme involved in the synthesis of DNA.

dominant   In genetics, a characteristic that appears in the phenotype whenever the allele for it is present in the genotype.

dopamine (dop'ă-meen)   A neurotransmitter and a precursor of norepinephrine.

dorsal (dor'sal)   Pertaining to the back; in humans, posterior.

dorsiflexion (dor"sĭ-flek'shun)   Movement of the toes and foot upward at the ankle joint.

Down's syndrome   A congenital disorder associated with the presence of a third chromosome 21; characterized by mental retardation.

duct   A passage or canal.

duct of Santorini   An accessory pancreatic duct.

duct of Wirsung   The main pancreatic duct.

ductus arteriosus (duk'tus ar-ter'e-o"-sus)   Blood vessel in the fetus that connects the left pulmonary artery with the aorta; closes and becomes the ligamentum arteriosum a few weeks after birth.

ductus deferens (def'er-enz)   Duct carrying sperm from the epididymis to the ejaculatory duct.

ductus venosus (ven-o'sus)   A fetal vessel carrying blood from the umbilical vein to the inferior vena cava.

duodenum (du"o-de'num)   Portion of the small intestine nearest the stomach; receives secretions from the liver and pancreas.

dural sinus (dur'al si'nus)   A space containing venous blood that lies below the two layers of the dura mater.

dura mater (du'rah ma'ter)   Outermost meningis of brain and spinal cord; in Latin, tough mother.

dynamic equilibrium   (1) The maintenance of balance when the head and body are suddenly rotated; (2) the maintenance of nearly constant internal conditions within the body even though substances are constantly entering and leaving.

dysmenorrhea (dis"men-or-e'ah)   Painful menstruation.

dyspnea (disp-ne'ah)   Labored breathing; shortness of breath.

ECF   Extracellular fluid.

ECG, EKG   Electrocardiogram.

eclampsia (ek-lamp'se-ah)   A severe complication of pregnancy or delivery involving fluid and electrolyte imbalances and often convulsions.

ectoderm (ek'to-derm)   The outermost embryonic germ layer.

ectopic (ek-top'ik)   Not in the normal place, such as a pregnancy outside the uterus or a heartbeat originating somewhere besides the sinoatrial node.

ectopic foci (ek-top'ik fo'si)   Regions of heart muscle not part of the conduction system that establish rhythmic contractions.

eczema (ek'zĕ-mah)   An inflammatory skin disease.

edema (ĕ-de'mah)   Accumulation of excessive fluids in tissues.

EEG   Electroencephalogram.

effector   A structure that responds to a stimulus; muscle or gland.

efferent (ef'er-ent)   Carrying away from.

efferent ductules   Small ducts that carry sperm from the testis to the epididymis.

ejaculation (e-jak"u-la'shun)   Ejection; the release of seminal fluid.

ejaculatory (e-jak'u-lă-to"re) **duct**   The passageway from the vas deferens to the urethra.

elasticity   The ability to be stretched and return to the original shape.

elastin (e-las'tin)   A major protein in elastic connective tissue.

electrocardiogram, ECG, EKG (e-lek"tro-kar'de-o-gram")   A record of electrical changes associated with heart action.

electrode (e-lek'trōd)   A terminal in an electrical circuit.

electroencephalogram (e-lek"tro-en-sef'ah-lo-gram")   A record of electrical changes associated with brain function.

electrolyte (e-lek'tro-līt)   Any substance that ionizes and conducts electricity.

electron (e-lek'tron)   A negatively charged particle in or from an atom.

electron transport system   A series of interconnected chemical reactions in which electrons (or hydrogen atoms) are transported to oxygen, and energy is normally released.

eleidin (el-e'ĭ-din)   A precursor of keratin found in the stratum lucidum of the skin.

element   A substance that cannot be changed into two or more substances by chemical means; a fundamental unit of matter.

elevation   A raising movement.

ellipsoid (el-ips'oid)   Oval.

embolism (em'bo-liz"m)   An obstruction of a blood vessel caused by a moving blood clot or other substance.

embryo (em'bre-o)   An early stage in the development of a living organism; in humans applies to the first two months of development.

embryonic (em-bre-on'ik) **disc**   The cells that give rise to the new individual.

emission (e-mis'shun)   A discharge, especially of semen.

emmetropia (em-met-ro'pe-ah)   The normal condition of the eye; neither nearsighted nor farsighted.

emotion   A state of feeling; the affective aspect of consciousness.

emphysema (em"fĭ-se'mah)   A disorder in which the alveoli are enlarged by destruction or dilation of their walls.

emulsification (e-mul-sĭ-fĭ-ka'shun)   Process by which fat droplets are caused to break up into smaller particles by the action of bile salts.

enamel Hard covering of the exposed part of a tooth.

end-feet Small terminal enlargements of the presynaptic endings of axons.

endocardium (en″do-kar′de-um) Innermost endothelial layer of heart.

endochondral (en-do-kon′dral) Developed within cartilage.

endocrine (en′do-krin) Pertaining to glands that secrete into the blood, or their hormones.

endocytosis (en″do-sit′o-sis) Movement of large particles into cells.

endoderm (en′do-derm) Innermost embryonic germ layer.

endolymph (en′do-limf) Fluid within the membranous labyrinth of the inner ear.

endometriosis (en″do-me-tre-o′sis) Presence of endometrial tissue in abnormal places.

endometrium (en″do-me′tre-um) Epithelial and connective tissue lining of uterus.

endomysium (en″do-mis′e-um) Connective tissue covering individual muscle fibers.

endoneurium (en″do-new′re-um) Connective tissue covering individual nerve fibers.

endoplasmic reticulum (en″do-plaz′mik re-tik′u-lum), **ER** Network of membranous vesicles within a cell.

endorphin (en-dor′fin) A peptide of the brain that alleviates pain; a natural opiatelike substance.

endosteum (en-dos′te-um) Membrane that lines the marrow cavities of bones.

endothelium (en″do-the′le-um) Epithelial lining of blood and lymph vessels.

endothermic (en-do-ther′mik) Requiring energy, as a chemical reaction.

end-plate Junction of a somatic motor neuron and a skeletal muscle fiber.

energy The capacity to do work.

engram (en′gram) A trace left by a stimulus that may account for some memory.

enkephalin (en-kef′ah-lin) A substance, usually derived from beta-lipotropin, having opiatelike properties.

enteric (en-ter′ik) Pertaining to the intestine.

enterogastric (en″ter-o-gas′trik) **reflex** A neural signal activated by the presence of chyme containing excessive acid or fat in the small intestine; it slows stomach peristalsis and reduces the flow of chyme.

enterohepatic (en-ter″o-hĕ-pat′ik) **circulation** Movement by which constituents of bile in the intestine are returned to the liver.

enterokinase (en″ter-o-kīn′āz) A proteolytic enzyme from the intestinal mucosa.

enzyme (en′zīm) A protein capable of catalyzing a chemical reaction.

eosinophil (e″o-sin′o-fil) A granular leukocyte capable of being stained with the dye eosin.

ependyma (ep-en′dim-ah) Membrane made of neuroglial cells that lines the brain ventricles and the central canal of the spinal cord.

epicardium (ep″e-kar′de-um) Visceral pericardium; covering of the heart.

epicondyle (ep″e-kon′dīl) A projection near a condyle on a bone.

epidermis (ep-id-er′mis) Outer epithelium of the skin.

epididymis (ep-id-id′im-is) Coiled tube near testis where sperm are stored.

epigastric (ep-e-gas′trik) Pertaining to the upper middle portion of the abdomen.

epiglottis (ep-e-glot′is) Elastic cartilage that closes the glottis.

epimysium (ep-e-mīs′e-um) Connective tissue covering an entire muscle.

epinephrine (ep-e-nef′rin) Main hormone secreted by adrenal medulla; transmitter substance of adrenegic fibers.

epineurium (ep-e-new′re-um) Connective tissue covering a whole nerve.

epiphyseal (ep-if-iz′e-al) **plate** A cartilaginous area between the epiphysis and diaphysis of a bone where growth occurs.

epiphysis (ep-if′is-is) (plural, **epiphyses**) The end of a long bone.

episiotomy (ep-iz-e-ot′om-e) Surgical incision of the vulvar orifice to prevent tearing during delivery of an infant.

epithelium (ep-ith-e′le-um) A tissue that lines organs or covers surfaces.

eponychium (ep-o-nik′e-um) Skin fold over the root of a nail.

EPSP Excitatory postsynaptic potential.

equilibrium Balance, as when opposing events are occurring at equal rates.

equivalent The weight in grams of an element that replaces or combines with 1 gram of hydrogen.

ER Endoplasmic reticulum.

erection Rigid state of the penis.

erythroblastosis fetalis (er-ith′ro-blas-to′sis fe-tal′is) Disorder of the newborn in which anti-Rh antibodies from an Rh-negative mother destroy erythrocytes of an Rh-positive fetus.

erythrocyte (er-ith′ro-sīt) Red blood cell; RBC.

erythropoiesis (er-ith″ro-po-e′sis) The production of erythrocytes.

erythropoietin (er-ith″ro-po-e′tin) Substance from kidney that stimulates erythropoiesis.

esophagus (e-sof′ă-gus) Tube leading from the pharynx to the stomach.

essential amino acid An amino acid needed for protein synthesis but not made in the body, hence must be present in the diet.

essential fatty acid A fatty acid needed for normal body function but not made in the body, hence must be present in the diet.

essential hypertension (hi″per-ten′shun) Elevated arterial blood pressure of unknown cause.

estradiol (est-ra′de-ol) The major human estrogen.

estrogen (es′tro-jen) A female sex hormone that stimulates sex organs and the development of secondary sex characteristics.

eustachian (u-sta′-ke-an) **tube** Tube connecting middle ear with pharynx.

eustress (u'stress) A form of stress that is productive for the body.

evagination (e-vaj"in-a'shun) An outpocketing or protrusion.

evaporation Change from liquid to gaseous form.

eversion (e-ver'zhun) Turning outward.

excitability Ability to respond to a stimulus.

excitation Stimulation.

excitatory postsynaptic potential (ex-si'ta-to-re post"sin-ap'tik po-ten'shal), EPSP Partial depolarization of a postsynaptic membrane.

excretion Elimination of a waste product; the product being eliminated.

exocrine (ex'o-krin) Pertaining to a gland that releases its secretions to the body surface; the secretion of such a gland.

exocytosis (ex"o-sīt'o-sis) Movement of large particles out of a cell.

exophthalmia (ex-of-thal'me-ah) Protrusion of the eyeballs.

exothermic (ex-o-ther'mik) Giving off heat, as a chemical reaction.

expiration (ex-pi-ra'shun) Exhalation, breathing out.

expiratory reserve Air that can be exhaled after normal exhalation.

extensibility (ex-ten"sĕ-bil'eh-te) The capability of being extended.

extension Movement that increases the angle between two bones.

extensor A muscle that produces extension when it contracts.

external On the outside.

exteroceptor (ex"ter-o-sep'tor) A sensory receptor that detects changes in the environment.

extracellular Outside a cell but within the body.

extracellular fluid compartment, ECF All of the fluid-containing spaces outside cells; consists mainly of interstitial fluids and blood plasma.

extrafusal (ex"tra-fus'al) Outside a muscle spindle.

extrapyramidal tracts Nerve tracts from the brain that fail to pass through the pyramids of the medulla.

extremity An arm or a leg.

extrinsic (ex-trin'sik) Coming from or originating outside the body.

facet A small, smooth articular surface on a bone.

facilitated diffusion Diffusion with a gradient aided by a carrier molecule but requiring no expenditure of energy.

facilitation Increased excitability of a neuron, usually by an excitatory postsynaptic potential.

FAD Flavin adenine dinucleotide.

falciform (fal'sī-form) Shaped like a sickle.

Fallopian (fal-o'pe-an) **tube** Uterine tube; oviduct; tube that transports ovum to uterus.

falx (falks) Structure having a sickle shape.

fascia (fash'e-ah) Fibrous connective tissue sheet beneath the skin or around muscles.

fascicle (fas'ik-l) A bundle of fibers.

fasciculation (fas-ik-u-la'shun) Involuntary twitching of a fasciculus of muscle fibers.

fat Triglyceride; compound containing glycerol and three fatty acids.

fatigue (fah-tēg') Temporary loss of power, as in a muscle that has repeatedly contracted or been held in sustained contraction.

fatty acid A long hydrocarbon chain with an organic acid (COOH) at one end.

feces Material expelled from the digestive tract.

feedback The return of part of a process to the input; effects of a process on a preceding stage of that process.

fenestrated (fen'es-tra-ted) Pierced with one or more openings.

ferritin (fer'e-tin) Molecule consisting of apoferritin (a protein) and iron.

fertilization The penetration of an ovum by a sperm.

fetus An unborn organism within the uterus; in humans an unborn child from the second month of development to birth.

fever An above-normal body temperature.

fibril (fi'bril) A minute fiber, such as actin and myosin of muscle cells.

fibrillation (fi"brĭ-la'shun) Uncoordinated contraction of some of the fibers of a muscle.

fibrin (fi'brin) Protein found in a blood clot.

fibrinogen (fi-brin'o-jen) Plasma protein that is converted to fibrin when blood clots.

fibroblast (fi'bro-blast) Cell that produces fibers and ground substance of connective tissue.

filament Fine threadlike structure.

filtration (fil-tra'shun) Passage of a fluid through a membrane because of a mechanical pressure.

filum terminale (fi'lum ter-min-al'e) Fiber attaching spinal cord to coccyx.

fimbria (fim'bre-ah) Fringelike structure.

fissure A slit or furrow.

flaccid Lacking tone, flabby.

flagellum (flă-gel'lum) Hairlike process on a cell that can cause movement.

flavin adenine dinucleotide (fla'vin ad'ĕ-neen di-nu'kle-o-tīd) A hydrogen-carrying coenzyme.

flexion (flek'shun) A movement that decreases the angle between two bones.

flexor A muscle that produces flexion when it contracts.

follicle (fol'ĭ-kl) A small sac.

follicle-stimulating hormone, FSH An anterior pituitary hormone that stimulates development of ova in females and sperm in males.

fontanel (fon"tah-nel') A membranous area between cranial bones in infants.

foramen (fo-ra'men) Opening or hole.

fornix (for'niks) A vaultlike space.

fossa (fos'ah) A hollow depression.

fovea (fo've-ah) A cup-shaped depression.

fovea centralis A pit in the retina having only cone receptors; region of greatest visual acuity.

fracture (frak'tūr) Breaking of a part, especially a bone.

frameshift mutation A change in the sequence of DNA caused by the addition or deletion of bases, thereby altering the sequence of the coded information.

free-running rhythms Biological rhythms that occur under constant conditions and are not affected by changes in light or dark.

frenulum (fren'u-lum) A small fold in a membrane that limits the movement of an organ or part.

frontal plane A plane dividing anterior and posterior parts of the body.

fructose (fruk'tōs) A ketone sugar.

FSH Follicle-stimulating hormone.

fulcrum (ful'crum) The fixed point about which a lever turns.

functional group The part of a molecule that participates in a chemical reaction.

fundus (fun'dus) The base of an organ farthest from its outlet.

GABA Gamma-aminobutyric acid.

galactose (gah-lak'tōs) A hexose sugar produced by degradation of lactose.

gallbladder A sac on the underside of the liver where bile is stored.

gametes (gam'ētz) Ova and sperm.

gamma-aminobutyric (gam'ah am''in-o-bu-tir'ik) **acid** A substance thought to be a central nervous system neurotransmitter.

gamma rays Electromagentic radiations of short wave length.

ganglion (gang'le-on) An aggregation of nerve cell bodies outside the central nervous system.

gap junction A coupling of adjacent cells having low electrical resistance.

gastric (gas'trik) Pertaining to the stomach.

gastrin (gas'trin) A hormone from the gastric mucosa that stimulates release of hydrochloric acid.

gastroenteric (gas'tro-en-ter''ik) **reflex** A nerve signal from the duodenum that slows stomach peristalsis when chyme entering the intestine is excessively acid or contains large amounts of fat.

gastrointestinal (gas''tro-in-tes'tin-al), **GI** Pertaining to the stomach and intestines; sometimes refers to the whole digestive tract.

gastrulation (gas-tru-la'shun) The process by which the gastrula of an embryo is formed; involves the formation of mesoderm, the third germ layer.

gating theory The theory that nonpain signals may block pain signals and thereby affect pain perception.

gene Functional unit of heredity; the part of a chromosome that transmits a particular hereditary characteristic.

general adaptation syndrome A group of changes that appear in animals under stress.

generator potential The initial depolarization of a sensory receptor.

genetic code The sequence of bases in DNA that determines the structure of various proteins and thus various structures of the body.

genetics (jen-et'iks) The study of heredity.

genitalia (jen-it-a'le-ah) The organs of the reproductive system.

genotype (jen'o-tīp) The combination of alleles at a given locus carried by an individual; for all genes together the genetic make-up of the individual.

germinal (jer'mĭ-nal) **epithelium** The epithelial cells that give rise to the gametes.

gestation (jes-ta'shun) Pregnancy.

giantism (ji'ant-izm) Excessive size due to excessive secretion of growth hormone.

gingiva (jin-ji'vah) The gums.

gland An organ that produces a secretion.

glans A conical structure forming the tip of the penis or capping the clitoris.

glaucoma (glaw-ko'mah) A disorder in which an excessive intraocular pressure develops.

glenoid (gle'noid) Like a socket.

glia (gli'ah) Connective tissue of the nervous system; glue.

gliadin (gli'ah-din) A protein found in wheat and some other grains.

globin (glo'bin) A protein associated with hemoglobin and some other biologically active molecules.

globulin (glob'u-lin) A protein found in blood plasma; some globulins are antibodies.

glomerulonephritis (glo-mer''u-lo-ne-fri'tis) Inflammation of the glomeruli of the kidneys.

glomerulus (glo-mer'u-lus) (plural, **glomeruli**) A tuft of capillaries in the glomerular capsule.

glossal (glos'sal) Pertaining to the tongue.

glottis (glot'tis) A slitlike opening into the trachea.

glucagon (gloo'kah-gon) A hormone from the pancreas that raises blood sugar.

glucocorticoid (gloo'ko-kor'tĭ-koid) A hormone from the adrenal cortex that regulates carbohydrate metabolism.

gluconeogenesis (gloo'ko-ne''o-jen'ĕ-sis) The synthesis of glucose from protein or other substances.

glucose (gloo'kōs) A hexose monosaccharide; the main sugar in the blood.

glucose sparing The use of fatty acids for energy by many cells in the postabsorptive state, leaving glucose for the tissues that cannot use fatty acids.

glucosuria (gloo'ko-su're-ah) Glucose in the urine.

gluten (glu'ten) A protein found in wheat and other grains.

glycerol (glis'er-ol) A three-carbon alcohol found in fats.

glycolysis (gli-kol'is-is) The breaking down of glucose to pyruvic or lactic acid.

glycogen (gli'ko-jen) A glucose-containing polysaccharide stored by animals.

glycogenesis (gli'ko-jen'e-sis) The synthesis of glycogen from glucose.

glycogenolysis (gli''ko-jen-ol'ĕ-sis) The breakdown of glycogen to glucose.

glycoprotein A substance composed of carbohydrate and protein.

goblet cell   A mucus-secreting cell found in some epithelial tissues.

goiter (goy′ter)   Enlargement of the thyroid gland.

Golgi (gol′je) **apparatus**   A cluster of membranous vesicles found in cells; an organelle thought to be active in synthesizing secretions.

gonad (go′nad)   An organ that produces gametes.

gonadotropin (go-nad″o-trōp′in)   A hormone that stimulates development or function of a gonad.

Graafian (grah′fe-an) **follicle**   A fluid-filled ovarian follicle ready to release an ovum.

gradient (gra′de-ent)   The rate of increase or decrease of a variable.

gram molecular weight   An amount of a substance in grams equal to the sum of the atomic weights of the atoms in the molecule.

Grave's disease   Hyperthyroidism, including goiter and protruding eyeballs.

gray matter   Portions of the central nervous system that contain cell bodies and lack myelin.

greater omentum (o-men′tum)   A fold of mesentery suspended from the stomach and colon.

ground substance   Intercellular substance consisting of a protein-polysaccharide and containing intercellular fluid.

growth hormone, GH   An anterior pituitary hormone that stimulates growth; somatotropin.

guanine (gwan′in)   A nitrogenous base found in DNA and RNA.

gyrus (ji′rus)   A fold, such as a convolution of the cerebrum.

habituation   The gradual adaptation to a stimulus.

hair   A filament growing from an epidermal follicle.

half-life   The amount of time required for half the atoms of a radioactive substance to disintegrate.

hallux (hal′uks)   The first digit of the foot; the big toe.

hamstrings   Tendons of the posterior thigh muscles; so named because they are used to suspend hams during the curing process.

haploid (hap′loid)   Having half the normal number of chromosomes, one of each pair.

haustra (haws′trah)   Saclike protrusions of the colon.

haversian (hă-ver′se-an) **system**   Concentric lamellae surrounding a canal in compact bone.

HCG   Human chorionic gonadotropin.

heart block   A condition in which the conduction system of the heart is disrupted, and the atria and ventricles contract independently.

heart failure   The inability of the heart to pump sufficient blood to supply the tissues of the body with oxygen and nutrients.

helicotrema (hel-ik-o-tre′mah)   Helix; the passage that connects the scala tympani and the scala vestibuli at the apex of the cochlea.

hematocrit (he-mat′o-krit)   The proportion of a volume of blood occupied by red blood cells.

heme   The iron-containing pigment responsible for carrying oxygen that forms part of a hemoglobin molecule.

hemisection   Cutting through half a structure such as the spinal cord.

hemodialysis (he″mo-di-al′ĕ-sis)   The removal of substances from the blood by dialysis.

hemoglobin (he″mo-glo′bin), **Hb**   The oxygen-carrying protein in red blood cells.

hemolysis (he-mol′ĕ-sis)   Breakdown of red blood cells and the release of hemoglobin.

hemophilia (he-mo-fil′e-ah)   A hereditary disorder causing defective blood clotting because of the absence of a clotting factor.

hemopoiesis (he″mo-po-e′sis)   Formation of blood cells and platelets.

hemorrhage (hem′o-rij)   Loss of blood.

hemorrhoids (hem′or-oids)   Enlarged blood vessels of the rectal mucosa.

hemostasis (he″mo-sta′sis)   The stoppage of bleeding.

heparin (hep′ah-rin)   An anticoagulant produced by several tissues of the body.

hepatic (hĕ-pat′ik)   Pertaining to the liver.

hepatitis (hep″at-i′tis)   Inflammation of the liver.

Hering-Breuer reflex   A mechanism that limits inspiration.

hernia (her′ne-ah)   Protrusion of an organ or part of an organ through an abnormal opening.

herpes (her′pēz)   A viral inflammatory disease.

heterozygous (het″er-o-zi′gus)   Having unlike alleles at corresponding loci of a pair of chromosomes.

hexose   A six-carbon monosaccharide.

hilus (hi′lus)   Region of an organ where blood vessels and nerves enter and leave.

hippocampus (hip-o-kam′pus)   A portion of the limbic system found in the temporal lobe of the cerebrum.

histamine (his′tah-min)   A substance released from cells when they are injured, causing vasodilation and bronchiolar constriction.

histiocyte (his′te-o-sīt)   A large phagocytic cell found in many connective tissues.

histocompatibility (his″to-kom-pat′ah-bil″eh-te) **antigen**   Substance on the surfaces of cells that may elicit antibody production when introduced into another individual.

histology (his-tol′o-ge)   The study of tissues.

holocrine (ho′lo-krin)   A gland that loses whole cells in its secretions; the secretion of such a gland.

homeostasis (ho″me-o-sta′sis)   A state of dynamic equilibrium in the body's internal environment.

homozygous (ho″mo-zi′gus)   Having like alleles at corresponding loci of an pair of chromosomes.

hormone (hor′mōn)   A substance produced by an endocrine structure and transported in the blood to its target organ(s).

human chorionic gonadotropin (ko″re-on′ik go-nad″-o-trōp′in), **HCG**   Hormone produced by placental cells that stimulates secretion of estradiol and progesterone by the corpus luteum.

humoral (hu′mor-al) **immunity**   Resistance to disease produced by antibodies.

Huntington's disease   A dominanant hereditary disorder that leads to degeneration of the nervous system.

hyaline (hi′ah-lin) Glassy, translucent.

hyaline membrane disease A disorder of newborns in which the lungs lack surfactant and the alveoli collapse, causing respiratory distress.

hyaluronic (hi″al-ur-on′ik) **acid** A component of the ground substance of most connective tissue.

hydrocephalus (hi″dro-sef′ah-lus) Excessive fluid in the brain ventricles.

hydrogen bond A chemical bond that loosely binds hydrogen atoms to other atoms.

hydrolysis (hi-drol′ī-sis) The splitting of large molecules with the addition of water.

hydrostatic (hi-dro-stat′ik) **pressure** Pressure exerted by a fluid such as blood; filtration pressure.

hymen (hi′men) Easily ruptured membrane over the opening to the vagina.

hyperaldosteronism (hi″per-al-dos′ter-on-izm) Excessive secretion of aldosterone.

hyperemesis gravidarum (hi-per-em′ĕ-sis grav-ī-dar′um) Excessive vomiting during pregnancy.

hyperextension Extension of a joint beyond normal range of movement.

hyperglycemia (hi-per-gli-sem′e-ah) Excess of glucose in the blood.

hypermetropia (hi-per-me-tro′pe-ah) Farsightedness.

hyperosmotic (hi-per-os-mot′ik) Producing rapid osmosis.

hyperparathyroidism (hi-per-par″ah-thy′roid-izm) Excessive secretion of parathyroid hormone.

hyperphagia (hi-per-fa′je-ah) Excessive eating.

hyperplasia (hi-per-pla′ze-ah) Increase in the number of cells in a tissue or organ.

hyperpnea (hi-perp-ne′ah) Increased rate of breathing.

hyperpolarization An excessive charge on the membrane of a nerve or muscle cell that makes it more difficult to stimulate.

hypertension High arterial blood pressure.

hyperthermia Above-normal body temperature.

hyperthyroidism (hi-per-thy′roid-izm) Excessive secretion of thyroid hormone.

hypertonic Having a greater than normal osmotic pressure.

hypertrophy (hi-per′trōf-e) Increase in the size of an organ, usually by an increase in the size of its cells.

hyperventilation Increased rate of respiration that usually leads to the loss of excessive amounts of carbon dioxide.

hypochondriac (hi-po-kon′dre-ak) Region of the abdomen beneath the ribs; having a morbid anxiety about health.

hypodermic Beneath the skin.

hypogastric Pertaining to the lower middle region of the abdomen.

hypoglycemia (hi-po-gli-sēm′e-ah) An excessively low concentration of glucose in the blood.

hyponychium (hi-po-nik′e-um) Cornified epithelium under the free border of a nail.

hypoparathyroidism (hi-po-par″ah-thy′roid-izm) Subnormal secretion of parathyroid hormone.

hypophysectomy (hi″po-fis-ek′to-me) Removal or obliteration of the pituitary gland.

hypophysis (hi-pof′is-is) Pituitary gland.

hyposmotic (hip″os-mot′ik) Producing decreased rate of osmosis.

hypotension Low arterial blood pressure.

hypothalamus (hi-po-thal′ă-mus) Anterior portion of brainstem, which regulates pituitary function, body temperature, and other functions.

hypothermia Below-normal body temperature.

hypothyroidism (hi-po-thi′roid-izm) Subnormal secretion of thyroid hormone.

hypotonic Having less than normal osmotic pressure.

hypovolemic (hi-po-vol-em′ik) **shock** A severe drop in blood pressure due to loss of blood volume.

hypoxia (hīp-ox′e-ah) A deficiency of oxygen.

ICF Intracellular fluid.

ICSH Interstitial-cell-stimulating hormone.

ileum (il′e-um) The lower part of the small intestine.

ilium (il′e-um) A bone of the pelvis.

immune reaction The response of the body to invasion by foreign substances.

immune surveillance theory A theory stating that a seek and destroy mechanism detects and destroys mutated cells before they can produce malignant growth.

immunity (im-u′nit-e) Resistance to disease.

immunoglobulin (im″u-no-glob′u-lin), **Ig** An antibody.

imperforate anus Failure of the tissue closing the embryonic anus to disappear.

impetigo (im-pet-i′go) An inflammatory skin disease characterized by isolated pustules.

implantation The attachment of the embryo to the endometrium of the uterus.

impotence (im′po-tens) Inability to copulate; usually used to refer to males.

impulse A signal conducted along a nerve or muscle fiber; action potential.

inclusion A product or nutrient stored in a cell.

incontinence (in-kon′ten-ens) Inability to control the release of urine from the urinary bladder.

incus Anvil; middle of three bones of the ear.

independent assortment A principle of genetics that two or more inherited traits are inherited independently, provided the alleles for each trait are on different chromosomes.

infarction (in-fark′shun) The formation of necrotic (dying) tissue, especially in the heart as a result of blood vessel blockage.

inferior Below or beneath.

infertility Inability to produce offspring.

inflammatory (in-flam′ma-to″re) **reaction** Localized response to an injury that includes dilation of blood vessels and invasion of leukocytes.

infundibulum (in″fun-dib′u-lum) Funnel-shaped passage or structure.

ingestion (in-jest'shun) The taking of food or fluid into the stomach.

inguinal (in-gwi'nal) Pertaining to the groin.

inhibition Stoppage or suppression of a function.

inhibitory postsynaptic potential, IPSP Excessive polarization of a postsynaptic membrane that causes a neuron to be less easily excited.

innervation Nerve supply.

insertion Attachment of a muscle to a bone at the most movable end.

inspiration Breathing in.

inspiratory reserve Additional air that can be inhaled after a normal inhalation.

insulin (in'su-lin) A hormone from the pancreas that lowers blood sugar.

integral An inseparable part of.

integumentary (in-teg'u-men'ta-re) Pertaining to the skin and its accessory organs.

intercalated (in-ter'kal-āt-ed) **disc** Thin membrane between cells of cardiac muscle.

intercellular Between cells.

intercellular fluid Fluid between cells.

interferon (in-ter-fer'on) A substance produced by virus-infected cells that helps to prevent the infection of other cells.

internal On the inside.

internal environment The environment of cells within the body.

interneuron (in'ter-nu'ron) A neuron that relays signals between a sensory and a motor neuron, typically found in the spinal cord.

interosseous (in-ter-os'se-us) Situated between bones.

interphase (in'ter-fāz) Stage of cell cycle during which the cell is not dividing.

interstitial (in''ter-stish'al) Pertaining to spaces between cells.

interstitial fluid Fluid in spaces between cells.

intracellular Within a cell.

intracellular fluid Fluid contained within a cell.

intrafusal (in''tră-fu'zal) Striated cells within a muscle spindle.

intrapleural (in-tră-plu'ral) Within the pleural cavity.

intrapulmonary (in-tră-pul'mon-a-re) Within the lungs.

intrathoracic (in-tră-tho-ras'ik) Within the chest cavity.

intrauterine (in-tră-u'ter-in) **device, IUD** Object inserted in the uterus as a contraceptive device.

intrinsic (in-trin'sik) Entirely within.

intrinsic factor Substance produced by the gastric mucosa that is necessary for the transport and absorption of vitamin B_{12}.

invagination (in-vaj-in-a'shun) The folding of one part into another.

inversion Turning inward; a rearrangement in the sequence of DNA in a chromosome.

ion (i'on) A charged atom or group of atoms.

ionic (i-on'ik) **bond** A chemical bond through which atoms are held together by the attraction of unlike charges.

ionization The process by which atoms become ions.

ionizing radiation Radioactive emission that causes ionization of atoms within cells.

ipsilateral (ip-se-lat'er-al) On the same side.

IPSP Inhibitory postsynaptic potential.

iris Muscular diaphragm anterior to the lens of the eye that controls the amount of light entering the eye.

irritability Ability to respond to a stimulus.

ischemia (is-ke'me-ah) Reduction in blood flow to an area.

islets of Langerhans Groups of cells in the pancreas that produce hormones.

isometric (i-so-met'rik) Same length.

isosmotic (īs'os-mot''ik) Having the same osmotic pressure.

isotonic (i''so-ton'ik) Having the same tension or pressure.

isotope (i'so-tōp) An atom of an element that has the same number of protons and electrons but a different number of neutrons than other atoms of the same element.

isovolumetric (i-so-vol''u-met'rik) Having the same volume.

isthmus (is'mus) Neck or constriction.

IUD Intrauterine device used for birth control.

jaundice (jawn'dis) Yellowishness of skin and membranes due to bile in the blood.

jejunum (je'ju'num) The middle section of the small intestine.

joint Region of union between two or more bones.

juxtaglomerular (jux''tă-glom-er'u-lar) **apparatus** Cells near the distal tubules and afferent arterioles of the kidneys capable of releasing renin.

juxtamedullary (jux''ta-med-u-lar'e) Near or adjoining the medulla, especially with reference to the kidney.

keratin (ker'ah-tin) An insoluble protein in the outer layer of the skin and in hair and nails.

keratohyaline (ker''ah-to-hi'al-in) A form of hyaline found in the skin.

ketogenic (ke''to-gen'ik) Causing the production of ketone bodies.

ketone (ke'tōn) Molecule having $C = O$ in carbon chain.

ketone bodies Substances produced during excessive metabolism of fat.

ketonuria (ke-to-nu're-ah) Presence of ketone bodies in the urine.

ketosis (ke''to'sis) Accumulation of ketone bodies in blood and urine.

kilocalorie (kil''o-kal'o-re) Amount of heat required to raise 1 kilogram of water 1°C.

kinesthesia (kin-es-the'ze-ah) The sensing of movement.

kinetic (kin-et'ik) Energy of motion.

kinin (ki'nin) One of several substances that cause increased permeability and dilation of blood vessels or movement of neutrophils to injured tissue.

Klinefelter's syndrome A syndrome resulting from the presence of XXY chromosomes and producing a sterile male individual.

Krause corpuscle (kor'pus-el) A sensory end organ that is stimulated by cold or extreme heat.

Krebs cycle Major metabolic pathway by which carbohydrates and most other substances are oxidized; citric acid cycle; tricarboxylic acid cycle.

Kupffer cells   Phagocytic cells in the sinusoids of the liver.

kyphosis (ki-fo'sis)   Excessive concave anterior curvature of the spine.

labia (la'be-ah)   Lip-shaped structures.

labor   Process that leads to the expulsion of a fetus from the uterus.

labyrinth (lab'ĭ-rinth)   A maze.

lacrimal (lak'rĭ-mal)   Pertaining to tears.

lactation (lak-ta'shun)   Milk production and secretion.

lacteal (lak'te-al)   A lymph vessel within a villus of the small intestine.

lactic (lak'tik) **acid**   End product of glycolysis under anaerobic conditions.

lactiferous (lak'tif-er-us)   Producing or conveying milk.

lactogenic (lak''to-jen'ik) **hormone**   Anterior pituitary hormone that stimulates milk secretion by the mammary glands; prolactin.

lactose (lak'tōs)   Sugar found in milk.

lacuna (lah-ku'nah)   Small cavity occupied by one or more cells in bone and cartilage.

lambdoidal (lam-doid'al)   Like the Greek letter lambda—λ; refers to a ridge and suture in the skull.

lamella (lam-el'ah)   Thin layer.

lamina (lam'in-ah)   Thin, flat plate or layer.

lamina propria (lam'in-ah pro'pre-ah)   Connective tissue layer underlying epithelium in mucous membranes.

laryngopharynx (lah-ring''go-far'ingks)   The part of the pharynx that lies behind the larynx and leads to the esophagus.

laryngotracheal (lah-ring''go-tra'ke-al)   Pertaining to the larynx and trachea.

larynx (lar'ingks)   Voicebox; portion of respiratory system between the pharynx and trachea.

latent period   In muscle physiology, the time between the application of a stimulus and the contraction of a muscle.

lateral   On the side.

learning   A permanent change in behavior as a result of experience.

lens   Transparent, biconvex structure behind the iris of the eye that changes shape to focus eye on far and near objects.

Lesch-Nyhan syndrome   A genetic disorder inherited as a recessive characteristic that leads to degeneration of the nervous system and early death.

lesion (le'zhun)   An injury or wound.

leukemia (lu-ke'me-ah)   A malignant increase in the number of leukocytes.

leukocyte (lu'ko-sīt)   A white blood cell, WBC.

leukocytosis (lu''ko-si-to'sis)   Increase in the number of leukocytes in response to an infection.

lever   A simple mechanical device consisting of a rod, fulcrum, weight, and a source of energy applied to some point on the rod.

Leydig cells   Secretory cells of the testes.

LH   Luteinizing hormone.

ligament (lig'ah-ment)   Fibrous connective tissue that attaches bones together.

ligamentum arteriosum (lig-am-en'tum ar-ter''e-o'sum)   Remains of fetal ductus arteriosus.

ligamentum nuchae (nu'sha-e)   Bandlike ligament at the back of the neck.

limbic (lim'bik) **system**   Portion of the brain mainly associated with emotions.

liminal (lim'in-al)   Pertaining to a threshold.

linea alba (lin'e-ah al'bah)   White line; connective tissue along midline of anterior abdominal wall.

linea aspera (lin'e-ah as'per-ah)   A rough longitudinal line on the posterior surface of the shaft of the femur.

lingual (ling'gwal)   Pertaining to the tongue.

lipase (li'pāsz)   An enzyme that digests fat.

lipid (lip'id)   Fats and fatlike substances.

lipogenesis (lip''o-gen'e-sis)   Synthesis of fat.

lipolysis (lip-ol'ĭ-sis)   The digestion of fat.

lipoprotein (lip''o-pro'te-in)   A substance consisting of lipid and protein.

liter (le'ter)   A metric measure of fluid volume.

lobule (lob'ūl)   A small lobe.

locus ceruleus (lo'kus se-ru'le-us)   A nucleus of the reticular formation involved in the regulation of sleep and wakefulness.

longitudinal (lon-jit-u'din-al)   Lengthwise; parallel to the long axis of the body.

loop of Henle   A U-shaped segment of a nephron.

lordosis (lor-do'sis)   Excessive concave posterior curvature of the spine.

lumbar (lum'bar)   Pertaining to the region of the loins.

lumbosacral (lum-bo-sa'kral)   Pertaining to the region of the loins and lower back.

lumen (lu'men)   The space inside a tubular structure.

lunula (lu'nu-lah)   Whitish crescent at the root of a nail.

lutein (lu'te-in)   A yellow pigment.

luteinizing (lu'te-in-iz''ing) **hormone, LH**   Anterior pituitary hormone that stimulates maturation of ovarian follicles in females and secretion of testosterone in males; ICSH.

luteotropic (lu''te-o-trōp'ik)   Stimulating the corpus luteum.

lymph (limf)   Intercellular fluid that has entered a lymphatic vessel.

lymphatic (lim-fat'ik)   Pertaining to lymph; referring to a vessel that carries lymph.

lymph node   Small nodule of lymphatic tissue interposed along the path of a lymphatic vessel.

lymphocyte (lim'fo-sīt)   A leukocyte that participates in the immune response.

lymphoid (lim'foid)   Resembling lymph.

lysosome (li'so-sōm)   Membrane-bound organelle that releases digestive enzymes.

macromolecule (mak''ro-mol'e-kūl)   Large molecule.

macrophage (mak'ro-fāj)   A large phagocytic cell found in connective tissue.

macula (mak'u-lah)   A structure in the inner ear that contains the sensory receptors for static equilibrium.

macula densa (mak'u-lah den'sah) Modified cells of the distal convoluted tubules of the kidneys, associated with the juxtaglomerular apparatus.

macula lutea (mak'u-lah lu'te-ah) A yellowish depression in the retina of the eye that is associated with acute vision.

malignancy (mal-ig'nan-se) A tendency to progress in virulence; a cancerous growth.

malleolus (mal-e'o-lus) Rounded prominence; root meaning, hammer.

malleus (mal'e-us) A bone of the middle ear; root meaning, hammer.

malnutrition (mal"nu-trish'un) Inadequate or faulty nutrition (food intake).

maltose (mawl'tōs) Disaccharide found in milk.

mammary (mam'ar-e) **gland** Gland that produces milk; breast.

mammillary (mam'il-a-re) **body** A nucleus on the inferior surface of the hypothalamus.

manic-depressive psychosis A mental illness characterized by wide mood swings.

manubrium (man-u'bre-um) A handle; upper part of the sternum.

marrow (mar'o) Fatty substance found in the internal cavity of bones.

mast cell Cell of connective tissue believed to release histamine and heparin.

mastication (mas"tĭ-ka'shun) The act of chewing.

mastoid (mas'toid) Nipple-shaped; part of temporal bone behind the ear.

matrix (ma'triks) The substance between the cells of connective tissues.

mean arterial pressure The average of systolic and diastolic pressures in an artery.

meatus (me-a'tus) A canal or passage.

mechanoreceptor (mek-an"o-re-sep'tor) A sensory receptor that responds to pressure, touch, or other mechanical stimulation.

medial (me'de-al) Toward or near the midline.

median (me'de-an) In the middle.

mediastinum (me"de-ah-sti'num) Region of thoracic cavity between the lungs containing the heart, trachea, and part of the esophagus.

medulla (mĕ-dul'lah) Core or inner part of an organ.

megakaryocyte (meg'ah-kar'e-o-sīt) A large bone marrow cell that produces blood platelets.

meiosis (mi-o'sis) A process of cell division by which gametes containing half the normal number of chromosomes are produced.

Meissner's corpuscle (kor'pus-el) A sensory end organ in the skin that responds to touch.

melanin (mel'ah-nin) A dark brown pigment found in hair, skin, and some other structures.

melanocyte (mel'ah-no-sīt) A cell that contains melanin.

melatonin (mel"ah-ton'in) A secretion of the cells of the pineal gland.

membrane A thin sheet of tissue that covers or lines an organ; surface layer of a cell or organelle.

membrane potential The electrical potential difference between the inside and outside of a cell.

memory The power or process of storing and recalling previous experiences.

menarche (mĕ-nar'ke) The onset of the menstrual cycle.

Meniere's disease An inflammatory disease of the semicircular canals that leads to pallor, vertigo, and disturbances of sight and hearing.

meninges (mĕ-nin'jēz) The membranes that enclose the brain and spinal cord.

meniscus (men-is'kus) A crescent-shaped interarticular fibrocartilage, such as that found in the knee joint.

menopause (men'o-pawz) The cessation of the menstrual cycle.

menstrual (men'stru-al) **cycle** A repetitive sequence of events including the sloughing of the uterine lining, the development and release of an ovum, and the replacement of the sloughed uterine lining.

menstruation (men"stroo-a'shun) The periodic discharge of blood and fluid from the uterus.

merocrine (mer'ok-rīn) A gland that produces a water secretion with little or no cytoplasm from the secretory cells; the secretion of such a gland.

mesenchyme (mes'en-kīm) Undifferentiated embryonic cells.

mesentery (mes'en-ter-e) A double layer of peritoneum that suspends organs in the abdominal cavity.

mesoderm (mez'o-derm) The middle of the three embryonic germ layers.

mesonephros (mes-o-nef'ros) A temporary, embryonic kidney.

mesothelium (mes-o-the'le-um) A layer of simple, squamous epithelium that covers the surface of serous membranes.

messenger RNA, mRNA A kind of RNA that carries information in the form of codons from DNA and thereby directs protein synthesis.

metabolic (met-ah-bol'ik) **rate** The rate at which nutrients are oxidized.

metabolic (met-ah-bol'ik) **water** Water derived from the oxidation of nutrients.

metabolism (mĕ-tab'o-lizm) The sum of all chemical processes in the body.

metabolite (mĕ-tab'o-līt) An intermediate or final product of metabolism.

metacarpal (met"ah-kar'pal) One of five bones that form the palm of the hand.

metanephros (met"ah-nef'ros) The embryonic kidney from which the adult functional kidney is derived.

metaphase (met'ah-fāz) A stage of mitosis during which chromosomes align along the middle of the cell.

metarteriole (met-ar-te're-ōl) A vessel containing smooth muscle fibers that connects an arteriole with a capillary bed.

metastasis (met-as'tas-is) The transfer of disease from one organ to another.

metatarsal (met-ah-tar'sal) One of the five bones of the arched part of the foot.

micelle (mis-el') Small fat droplet found in chyme.

microfilaments (mi"kro-fil'ah-mentz) Small, hollow protein fibers found within the cytoplasm of a cell.

microglia (mi-crog'le-ah)   Small phagocytic cells of the central nervous system.

microtubule (mi''kro-tu'būl)   A cylindrical organelle that contributes to the mitotic spindle.

microvilli (mi'kro-vil'e)   Tiny cytoplasmic projections from the surface of intestinal epithelial cells.

micturition (mik''tu-rish'un)   Urination.

mineralocorticoid (min''er-al-o-kor'tĭ-koid)   Adrenocortical hormone that regulates mineral metabolism, especially that of sodium and potassium.

mitochondria (mi''to-kon'dre-ah)   Oval organelles containing many enzymes that carry out various energy-producing processes.

mitosis (mi-to'sis)   A kind of cell division in which two identical cells are produced.

mitral (mi'tral) **valve**   A bicuspid valve between the atrium and ventricle on the left side of the heart.

mixture   A combination of two or more substances in any proportions, in which the substances do not lose their original properties.

modiolus (mo-di'o-lus)   A supporting structure of the cochlea.

mole   A gram molecular weight of a substance.

molecule (mol'ĕ-kūl)   The smallest quantity of a substance that retains its chemical properties.

monoamine oxidase (mon'o-am-in ox'id-ās)   An enzyme containing a single amine group that breaks down neurotransmitters.

monoblast (mon'o-blast)   An immature monocyte.

monocyte (mon'o-sīt)   A large agranular leukocyte with phagocytic properties.

monoglyceride (mon''o-gli'cer-īd)   A fat molecule consisting of one fatty acid and one glycerol.

monosaccharide (mon''o-sak'ah-rid)   A simple sugar.

monosynaptic (mon''o-sin-ap'tik)   Pertaining to a neural pathway having only one synapse.

morula (mor'u-lah)   A solid ball of cells; an early stage in embryonic development.

mossy fiber   A kind of neuron found in the cerebellum.

motility (mo-til'it-e)   The ability to move spontaneously; usually refers to sperm or to contractions of digestive tract muscle.

motor   Pertaining to movement or activity.

motor end plate   The portion of the sacrolemma of a muscle cell that lies beneath nerve endings.

mRNA   Messenger RNA.

mucin (mu'sin)   A glycoprotein found in ground substance and many mucous secretions.

mucociliary escalator (mu''co-sil'e-ar-e es''kah-la'tor)   The mechanism by which cilia and mucus of the respiratory tract move debris toward the pharynx.

mucosa (mu-ko'sah)   Mucous membrane that lines cavities and tubes.

mucous membrane   A membrane that produces a mucous secretion and lines cavities and tubes.

mucus (mu'kus)   Material secreted by a mucous gland.

multiaxial joint   A joint at which motion occurs along more than two axes.

multiple sclerosis (skler-os'is)   A disease of the nervous system that involves hardening of patches of tissue in the brain or spinal cord or both.

murmur   Sound heard from within the body, particularly from the heart valves, lungs, or blood vessels.

muscle spindle   A spindle-shaped structure in skeletal muscle that acts as a proprioceptor or detector of position or movement.

muscular dystrophy (dis'tro-fe)   Progressive atrophy of muscles.

muscularis (mus-ku-la'ris)   (1) A muscular layer in the wall of an organ or tube; (2) a muscular portion of the mucosa of the digestive tract.

mutation (mu-ta'shun)   A change in genetic information in a cell.

myasthenia gravis (mi''as-the'ne-ah gră'vis)   Progressive weakening and paralysis of muscles, especially those of the face, lips, tongue, and throat.

myelin (mi'el-in)   An insulating lipid material deposited in layers around many axons.

myelinated (mi'el-in-a''ted)   Having a sheath of myelin.

myeloblast (mi'el-o-blast)   A cell that gives rise to muscle.

myeloid (mi'el-oid)   Pertaining to or derived from bone marrow.

myenteric (mi-en-ter'ik)   Pertaining to the muscular layer of the intestine.

myocardium (mi-o-kar'de-um)   The muscle of the heart.

myoepithelial (mi''o-ep-ĕ-the'le-al)   Pertaining to epithelial cells that have the ability to contract.

myofibril (mi-o-fi'bril)   Contractile fibril arranged longitudinally in muscle cells.

myoglobin (mi''o-glo'bin)   A pigmented compound found in muscle tissue that stores oxygen.

myometrium (mi''o-me'tre-um)   Muscular portion of the uterus.

myoneural (mi''o-nu'ral) **junction**   The site at which motor neurons terminate at the membrane of a muscle cell.

myopia (mi-o'pe-ah)   Nearsightedness.

myosin (mi'o-sin)   A protein that makes up the thick filaments of a myofibril.

myxedema (mik''sĕ-de'mah)   Hypothyroidism occurring in an adult.

NAD   Nicotinamide adenine dinucleotide.

NADP$^+$ Nicotinamide adenine dinucleotide phosphate; a hydrogen carrier essential for supplying hydrogen in the synthesis of triglycerides.

narcosis (nar-ko'sis)   An unconscious state often produced by a narcotic drug.

nares (na'rēz)   Openings of the nasal cavity; nostrils.

nasal cavity   The mucous membrane–lined cavity of the nose.

nasolacrimal (na''zo-lak'rim-al) **duct**   A tube leading from the lacrimal sac to the nasal cavity.

nasopharynx (na''zo-far'ingks)   The upper portion of the pharynx that connects with the nasal cavity.

neck   A constricted area.

negative feedback   A mechanism by which the output of a system suppresses or inhibits the activity of the system.

Neisseria gonorrhoeae (ni-ser′e-ah gon″o-re′ah-e)   The bacterium that causes gonorrhea.

neocortex (ne-o-kor′tex)   The most recently evolved portion of the cerebrum.

neonate (ne′o-nāt)   A newborn infant.

nephron (nef′ron)   A functional unit of the kidney consisting of a renal corpuscle and its attached tubule.

nerve   A cordlike structure consisting primarily of axons of neurons covered with connective tissue sheaths; conveys signals in the nervous system; may or may not be myelinated.

nerve deafness   Impairment of hearing due to damage to sensory receptors in the cochlea or to nerve fibers leading from those receptors.

neural   Pertaining to the nervous system.

neural crests   Cells derived from the neural tube that give rise to sensory neurons, sympathetic nervous system, and adrenal medulla.

neural tube   A tube formed from the invagination of ectoderm in the embryo that gives rise to the nervous system.

neurilemma (nu-ril-em′ah)   The sheath of Schwann.

neurofibrils (nu-ro-fi′brils)   Small intracellular fibrils found in the cytoplasm of the cell body of a neuron.

neuroglia (nu-rog′le-ah)   Cells of the nervous system that do not participate in conduction signals.

neurohypophysis (nu″ro-hi-pof′is-is)   The posterior, neural portion of the pituitary gland.

neuromuscular (nu-ro-mus′ku-lar)   Pertaining to the association between the nervous and muscular systems.

neuron (nu′ron)   A cell that conveys signals in the nervous system.

neuronal (nu′ro-nal) **pool**   A complex set of synapses, usually in the central nervous system.

neurosecretion (nu″ro-se-kre′shun)   A chemical substance released by an axon that transmits a signal across a synapse; secretion of the neurohypophysis.

neurotransmitter (nu″ro-trans′mit-ter)   A chemical substance that transmits a signal across a synapse.

neurulation (nu″ru-la′shun)   The process by which the neural tube forms in embryonic development.

neutron (nu′tron)   An uncharged particle in the nucleus of an atom.

neutrophil (nu′tro-fil)   A granular leukocyte that does not stain with either acidic or basic dyes.

niacin (ni′a-sin)   One of the B vitamins; nicotinic acid.

nicotinamide adenine dinucleotide (nĭ-ko-tin′am-id ah′den-in di-nu′kle-o-tīd)   A coenzyme that carries hydrogen atoms for oxidation-reduction reactions.

Nissl (nis′l) **body**   RNA-containing granules and associated endoplasmic reticulum found in nerve cell bodies and dendrites.

nitrogen balance   The relationship between the amount of nitrogen ingested and the amount excreted by an organism.

nociceptor (no-sis-ep′tor)   A sensory ending that responds to painful stimuli.

node of Ranvier   A gap in the myelin sheath of an axon.

nodule   A small node; a packed mass of cells.

non-REM sleep   Sleep during which rapid eye movements do not occur.

noradrenaline   Norepinephrine.

norepinephrine (nor′ep-ĭ-nef′rin)   The neurotransmitter released by adrenergic nerve endings; a secretion of the adrenal medulla.

nuchal (nu′kal)   Pertaining to the back of the neck.

nuclear (nu′kle-ar)   Pertaining to the nucleus.

nuclease (nu′kle-ās)   An enzyme that breaks down nucleic acids into nucleotides.

nucleic (nu kle′ik) **acid**   A polymer containing units of sugar, phosphate, and a nitrogenous base; DNA and RNA.

nucleolus (nu-kle′o-lus)   An RNA-containing body within the nucleus.

nucleoplasm (nu′-kle-o-plazm″)   The substance of the nucleus.

nucleosome (nu′kle-o-sōm)   A subunit of a chromosome.

nucleotidase (nu kle-ot′id-ās)   An enzyme that breaks down nucleotides into nucleotides and phosphate groups.

nucleotide (nu′kle-o-tīd″)   A unit composed of a sugar, a nitrogenous base, and a phosphate group found in DNA and RNA.

nucleus (nu′kle-us)   (1) The organelle that controls cellular function; (2) the central portion of an atom; (3) an aggregation of cell bodies in the central nervous system.

nucleus pulposus (pulp-o′sus)   A jellylike material in the center of an intervertebral disc.

nutrition (nu-trish′un)   The act of providing all the substances necessary for maintaining health through the ingestion of food.

nystagmus (nis-tag′mus)   Rapid involuntary rolling movements of the eyeball.

obesity (o-bēs′ĭ-te)   An excessive amount of fat.

obturator (ob′tu-ra-tor)   A structure that closes an opening.

occipital (ok-sip′ĭ-tal)   Pertaining to the back of the head.

occlusion (ok-lu′shun)   The closing of a tube or duct.

odontoid (o-don′toid)   Like a tooth.

olecranon (o-lek′ran-on)   A curved process of the ulna at the elbow.

olfactory (ol-fak′to-re)   Pertaining to the sense of smell.

oligodendrocyte (ol″ĭ-go-den′dro-sīt)   A type of neuroglial cell that forms myelin and connects neurons to blood vessels.

oliguria (ol-ig-u′re-ah)   Reduced daily output of urine.

omentum (o-men′tum)   A double layer of mesentery between certain abdominal organs.

oncotic (ong-kot′ik) **pressure**   Osmotic pressure created by the presence of protein molecules.

oocyte (o′o-sīt)   A cell destined to give rise to an ovum.

oogenesis (o-o-jen′is-is)   The process by which an ovum develops.

ootid (o′o-tid)   One of four cells derived from a primary oocyte.

open reduction   The realignment of the ends of a fractured bone using surgical procedures.

ophthalmic (of-thal′mik)   Pertaining to the eye.

optic (op′tik)   Pertaining to the eye or the properties of light.

optic chiasma (ki-az′ma)   An area anterior to the pituitary gland where some fibers of the optic nerve cross from one side of the body to the other.

optic disc   The region of the retina where fibers of the optic nerve leave the eye; blind spot.

orbit   A spherical bony cavity.

organ   A structure composed of several kinds of tissue capable of carrying out particular functions; a component of a system.

organ of Corti   The structure within the inner ear that detects sound.

organelle (or″gah-nel′)   A tiny organ within a cell.

organic (or-gan′ik)   Pertaining to carbon-containing substances.

orgasm (or′gazm)   The culmination of sexual intercourse.

orifice (or′i-fis)   An opening.

origin   The less movable attachment of a muscle.

oropharynx (o″ro-far′ingks)   The central portion of the pharynx that communicates with the oral cavity.

osmol (oz′mol)   A gram molecular weight of a substance divided by the number of ions each molecule produces when it dissociates.

osmolarity (oz″mo-lar′ĭ-te)   The osmotic concentration of a solution determined by the number of osmotically active particles it contains.

osmoreceptor (oz″mo-re-sep′tor)   Hypothalamic receptors that respond to changes in the osmotic pressure of the blood.

osmosis (oz-mo′sis)   The movement of water across a membrane from the area of lower to the area of higher concentration of the solvent.

osmotic (oz-mot′ik) **pressure**   The pressure produced by osmosis.

ossicles (os′ik-ls)   Small bones of the middle ear.

ossification (os″ĭ-fĭ-ka′shun)   The formation of bone.

osteoarthritis (os″te-o-ar-thri′tis)   Chronic multiple degenerative joint disease.

osteoblast (os′te-o-blast″)   A cell that forms bone matrix.

osteoclast (os′te-o-clast″)   A cell that dissolves bone.

osteocyte (os′te-o-sīt)   A cell occupying a lacuna in bone.

osteomalacia (os″te-o-mal-a′se-ah)   Softening of the bones in adults as a result of vitamin D deficiency.

osteon (os′te-on)   A Haversian system; a central canal and surrounding concentric lamellae in compact bone.

osteoporosis (os″te-o-po-ro′sis)   Abnormal porousness of bone.

otolith (o′to-lith)   A small particle of calcium carbonate associated with the receptors of equilibrium; ear stone.

otosclerosis (o″to-sklĕ-ro′sis)   Abnormal formation of bone within the middle ear that may interfere with the transmission of sound vibrations to the hearing receptors.

oval window   A membrane-covered opening between the middle and inner ear.

ovary (o′var-e)   A female gonad that produces ova and hormones.

oviduct (o′vĭ-dukt)   Tube that transports ova to the uterus; Fallopian tube; uterine tube.

ovulation (o″vu-la′shun)   The release of an ovum from an ovarian follicle.

ovum (o′vum) (plural, **ova**)   A female gamete.

oxidation (ok″si-da′shun)   The loss of an electron, the loss of hydrogen, or the addition of oxygen.

oxidative phosphorylation (ox′ĭ-da′tiv fos-for″ĭ-la′shun)   The production of ATP in association with oxidation.

oxygen debt   The amount of oxygen required to oxidize metabolites produced anaerobically during strenuous activity.

oxyhemoglobin (ok″sĭ-he″mo-glo′bin)   Hemoglobin that is carrying oxygen.

oxytocin (ok″sĭ-to′sin)   A posterior pituitary hormone that causes uterine contractions and release of milk during lactation.

pacemaker   A group of spontaneously discharging cells that excite other cells, especially those of the sinoatrial node of the heart.

Pacinian corpuscle (pă-sin′e-an kor′pus-el)   A receptor that responds to pressure.

palate (pal′at)   A flat plate forming the roof of the mouth.

palmar (pahl′mar)   Pertaining to the palm of the hand.

pancreas (pan′kre-as)   An accessory organ of the digestive tract that produces both digestive secretions and hormones.

pantothenic (pan″to-then′ik) **acid**   A B vitamin that forms part of coenzyme A.

Pap smear   A sample of cells from the cervix for microscopic examination to detect cervical cancer.

papilla (pah-pil′ah)   A nipplelike projection.

papillary (pah-pil′ar-e) **muscles**   Projections of cardiac muscle attached to the chordae tendinae.

paradoxical sleep   Sleep during which rapid eye movements occur and the EEG pattern resembles wakefulness.

paraplegia (par-ah-ple′je-ah)   Paralysis of the legs and lower part of the body.

parasympathetic (par″ah-sim-path-et′ik) **division**   A component of the autonomic nervous system that regulates visceral function in conjunction with the sympathetic division; responsible for returning functions to normal after a stressful situation.

parasympathomimetic (par″ah-sim″path-o-mim-et′ik)   Pertaining to a substance that acts to mimic the action of the parasympathetic nervous system.

parathormone (par″ah thor′mōn)   The hormone produced by the parathyroid glands.

parathyroid (par″ah-thi′roid) **glands**   Endocrine glands imbedded in the surface of the thyroid gland.

parietal (pah-ri′et-al)   Pertaining to the wall of a cavity.

Parkinsonism (park′in-son″izm)   Muscle rigidity and tremor due to lack of dopamine action in an area of the brainstem.

parotid (pah-rot′id) **gland**   A large salivary gland located inferiorly and anteriorly to the ear.

partial pressure   The pressure exerted by one gas in a mixture of gases.

parturition (par″tu-rish′un)   Childbirth.

passive transport   Any process that causes movement of substances without the expenditure of energy.

pathology (pah-thol'o-je)   The study of disease processes.

pectoral (pek'tor-al)   Pertaining to the attachment of the upper appendages to the trunk.

pedicle (ped'ik-el)   A process that connects the lamina and centrum of a vertebra.

pedigree (ped'ĭ grē)   The tracing of a genetic characteristic through several generations.

peduncle (ped'ung-kl)   A stalk or stem.

pelvic (pel'vik)   Pertaining to the attachment of the lower appendages to the trunk.

pelvis (pel'vis)   (1) Bones that attach the lower appendage to the trunk; (2) the cavity enclosed by those bones; (3) a basin.

penis (pēn'is)   The male organ of copulation.

pepsin (pep'sin)   A proteolytic enzyme produced by the gastric mucosa.

peptidase (pep'tĭ-dās)   An enzyme that breaks peptide bonds.

peptide (pep'tīd) **bond**   A chemical bond that links amino acids.

perception   Conscious interpretation of signals from sensory receptors.

perfusion (per-fu'shun)   The passage of blood through vessels to supply cells.

pericardium (per''ĭ kar'de-um)   A fibrous sac that encloses the heart.

perichondrium (per''ĭ kon'dre-um)   A connective tissue membrane that covers cartilage.

perilymph (per'ĭ-limf'')   A clear fluid in the osseous labyrinth that surrounds the membranous labyrinth.

perimysium (per''ĭ-mīs'e-um)   A connective tissue sheath that covers bundles of skeletal muscle fibers.

perineum (per''ĭ-ne'um)   The region of the pelvic outlet.

perineurium (per'ĭ-nu're-um)   A connective tissue sheath that covers bundles of nerve fibers.

periodontal (per''e-o-don'tal)   Situated around a tooth.

periosteum (per''e-os'te-um)   A connective tissue membrane that covers a bone, except at its articular surfaces.

peripheral (pe-rif'er-al)   Outer.

peripheral nervous system   The part of the nervous system outside the brain and spinal cord.

peripheral resistance   Resistance to blood flow in the systemic circulation.

peristalsis (per''ĭ-stal'sis)   Wavelike contractions that propel substances along tubular structures.

peritoneum (per''ĭ-to-ne'um)   A serous membrane that lines the abdominopelvic cavity.

peritonitis (per''it-o-ni'tis)   An inflammation of the peritoneum.

peritubular (per''ĭ-tub'u-lar)   Surrounding a tube, especially the tubule of a nephron.

pernicious (per-nish'us) **anemia**   A kind of anemia caused by a deficiency of vitamin B_{12} or the intrinsic factor that facilitates its absorption.

petrous (pet'rus)   Stony.

Peyer's patches   Elevated areas of lymphoid tissue of the mucosa of the small intestine.

pH   The negative logarithm of the hydrogen ion concentration; a measure of acidity or alkalinity.

phagocytosis (fag''o-si-to'sis)   The engulfment and digestion of particles by a scavenger cell.

phalanx (fa'langks, fa-lan'jes) (plural, **phalanges**)   A bone of a digit.

pharmacology (far''ma-kol'o-je)   The study of drugs.

pharyngitis (far''in-ji'tis)   Inflammation of the pharynx.

pharynx (far'ingks)   The part of the digestive tract between the oral cavity and esophagus, some of which is a common pathway of the respiratory tract.

phenotype (fēn'o-tīp)   The appearance of an individual with regard to an inherited characteristic or all inherited characteristics.

phosphocreatine (fos''fo-kre'ah-tin)   A molecule capable of storing energy in muscle tissue.

phosphogluconate (fos''fo-glu'con-āt) **pathway**   A metabolic pathway through which five-carbon sugars, carbon dioxide, and reduced NADP are formed.

phospholipid (fos''fo-lip'id)   A fatty substance containing phosphoric acid.

phosphorylation (fos-for'ĭ-la'shun)   The addition of a phosphate group to an organic molecule.

photoreceptor (fo''to-re-cep'tor)   A sensory receptor that responds to light.

phrenic (fren'ik)   Pertaining to the diaphragm.

physiology (fis''e-ol'o-ge)   The study of function in living organisms.

pia mater (pi'ah ma'ter)   The delicate, innermost meningis covering the brain and spinal cord; Latin, soft mother.

pineal (pin'e-al) **gland**   A small organ on the dorsal midline of the brain.

pinna (pin'nah)   External flaplike portion of the ear.

pinocytosis (pi-no-si-to'sis)   Cell drinking; process by which cells take in small fluid droplets.

pituitary (pĭ-tu'ĭ-tar''e) **gland**   Master gland of the endocrine system attached to the base of the brain; hypophysis.

pK   The negative logarithm of the dissociation constant of a substance.

placenta (pla-sen'tah)   A round, flat organ present in the uterus during pregnancy that provides for the exchange of substances between the mother and the fetus.

plantar (plan'tar)   Pertaining to the sole of the foot.

plantarflexion   Movement of the foot and toes downward and away from the shin.

plaque (plahk)   Any patch or flat area.

plasma (plaz-mah)   The fluid portion of blood, including the inactive clotting elements.

plasma cell   A cell derived from a B lymphocyte that produces antibodies.

plasma membrane   Cell membrane.

plasmin (plaz'min)   An enzyme that dissolves blood clots.

platelet (plāt'let)   A fragment of a megakaryocyte that circulates in the blood and participates in the blood-clotting mechanism.

pleura (ploo'rah)   A serous membrane that covers the lungs and lines the thoracic cavity.

pleural (ploo'ral) **space**   A potential space between the parietal and visceral pleura.

pleurisy (plu′ris-e) Inflammation of the pleura.

plexus (plek′sus) A network, usually of nerves or blood vessels.

plicae circulares (pli′ke sir-ku-la′rez) Transverse folds in the mucosa of the small intestine.

pneumonia (nu-mo-ne-ah) An inflammation of the lungs.

pneumotaxic (nu″mo-tax′ik) **center** An area of the brain involved in regulating breathing.

pneumothorax (nu-mo-thōr′ax) The presence of air in the pleural space, usually causing collapse of a lung.

podocyte (po′do-sīt) Epithelial cell with footlike processes found in the glomerular capsule, where its processes wrap around capillaries.

point of effort The point at which the contraction of a muscle exerts a force on a bone so as to create movement.

point mutation A modification of a single base in a molecule of DNA.

polar body A cell containing chromosomes and very little cytoplasm, produced during female gametogenesis.

polar compound A molecule that has a charged area.

polarization (po″lar-i-za′shun) The production of different electrical potentials between two points, such as across a cell membrane.

poliomyelitis (po″le-o-mi′ĕ-li″tis) Inflammation of motor cells in the anterior horn of the spinal cord.

pollex (pol′eks) Thumb.

polycythemia (pol″e-si-the′me-ah) An abnormal excess of erythrocytes.

polydipsia (pol-e-dip′se-ah) Frequent drinking.

polymerization (pol″e-mer-iz-a′shun) The union of similar molecules to produce a high molecular weight compound usually consisting of a chain of the units.

polymorphonuclear leukocyte (pol″e-mor-fo-nu′kle-ar lu′ko-sīt) A white blood cell with an irregularly shaped nucleus.

polypeptide (pol-e-pep′tīd) A chain of a number of amino acids.

polysaccharide (pol-e-sak′ar-īd) A long, sometimes branched chain of simple sugars.

polyuria (pol-e-u′re-ah) Excessive production of urine.

pons (ponz) A part of the brainstem associated with the cerebellum.

pontine (pon′ten) Pertaining to the pons.

popliteal (pop″lit′e-al) Pertaining to the posterior surface of the knee.

portal circulation Circulation of blood from the intestinal capillaries to the liver by way of the hepatic portal vein.

portal triad A set of three vessels (branches of the hepatic artery, hepatic portal vein, and bile duct) around the edges of liver lobules.

postabsorptive (post″ab-sorp′tive) **state** The nutritional state following the absorption of food, during which energy is provided by stored nutrients.

posterior Toward their rear; dorsal in humans.

postganglionic (post″gang-le-on′ik) Referring to a neuron encountered after a signal passes through a ganglion; the second neuron in an autonomic pathway.

postsynaptic (post″sin-ap′tik) Referring to the neuron that receives a signal by synaptic transmission.

postural hypotension A lowering of blood pressure on assuming a standing position.

potential A difference in electrical charge between two points, usually across a nerve or muscle cell membrane.

potential energy Energy due to position, as a rock at the top of a hill.

precursor Something that precedes another thing.

preganglionic (pre″gang-le-on′ik) Referring to a neuron that conveys a signal to a ganglion; the first neuron in an autonomic pathway.

pregnancy (preg′nan-cē) Gestation; state of a female carrying a child.

prepuce (pre′pūs) Foreskin; fold of skin covering the glans penis or glans clitoris.

presbyopia (pres-be-o′pe-ah) Elder vision; loss of accommodation ability.

pressor Substance that causes a rise in blood pressure.

pressure Stress due to compression.

presynaptic (pre″sin-ap′tik) Referring to a neuron that conveys a signal to a synapse.

primary bronchus (bronk′us) A main branch from the trachea that carries air to and from a lung.

primary follicle (fol′i-kl) An early stage in the development of an ovarian follicle.

primary germ layers The first layers of cells to differentiate in an embryo; ectoderm, mesoderm, and endoderm.

prime mover A muscle that directly causes a particular movement.

probability A mathematical statement of the likelihood of a particular event occurring among all possible events.

process (1) An extension or outgrowth; (2) a mode of action.

progesterone (pro-jes′tĕ-rōn) A steroid hormone from the corpus luteum and placenta that is important in maintaining pregnancy.

projection fibers Nerve fibers that connect the cerebral cortex with other parts of the central nervous system.

prolactin (pro-lak′tin) Anterior pituitary hormone that stimulates secretion of milk by the mammary glands.

proliferative phase The phase of uterine change in which cells of the endometrium divide and increase in number.

pronation (pro-na′shun) (1) Rotation of the forearm causing the palm of the hand to face backward; (2) facing the abdomen downward, as lying in prone position.

pronephros (pro-nef′rus) The most primitive form of kidney in a vertebrate embryo.

pronucleus (pro-nu′kle-us) Either the male or the female nucleus that combines to form the nucleus of the zygote.

prophase (pro′fāz) The first stage of mitosis, during which the chromosomes become distinct.

proprioceptor (pro″pre-o-sep-tor) A sensory receptor in a muscle, joint, or tendon that detects position or movement.

prostaglandin (pros″tah-glan′din) A substance derived from a fatty acid; may have any of a number of physiological actions.

prostate (pros′tāt) A gland that surrounds the urethra near the

prostate (cont.)
   urinary bladder in a male.
prostatitis (pros-ta-ti′tis)   Inflammation of the prostate gland.
protein (pro′te-in)   Macromolecule consisting of amino acids.
protein turnover   The breakdown and synthesis of protein molecules.
proteinuria (pro″te-in-u′re-ah)   Excretion of protein in the urine.
proteolytic (pro″te-o-lit′ik)   Having the ability to break down protein.
prothrombin (pro-throm′bin)   A plasma protein that, when converted to thrombin, helps to cause clotting of blood.
proton (pro′ton)   A positively charged particle in the nucleus of an atom.
protraction (pro-trak′sun)   Movement of the mandible forward.
proximal (prok′si-mal)   Nearest the body or nearest a point of attachment.
pterygoid (ter′ig-oid)   Winglike; refers to processes on bones.
puberty (pu′ber-te)   A period of time or a sequence of events that lead to maturation of sexual organs.
pudendum (pu-den′dum)   External genitalia, usually referring to the female.
pulmonary (pul′mo-ner″e)   Pertaining to the lungs or pulmonary vessels.
pulmonary ventilation   The quantity of air delivered to the lungs per unit time.
pulp cavity   An inner cavity of a tooth that contains blood vessels and nerves.
pulse   Rhythmic expansion and contraction of an artery caused by the pumping action of the heart.
pulse pressure   Variations in the pressure in an artery due to heart action.
Punnett square   A diagram used to determine the possible genotypes and phenotypes of the offspring of a particular set of parents.
pupil   The circular opening in the center of the iris through which light rays enter the eye.
Purkinje cell   A particular kind of neuron found in the cerebellum that has very large numbers of synapses with other cells.
Purkinje fibers   Terminal ends of fibers of the heart's conduction system.
putamen (pu-ta′men)   Part of the basal nuclei.
pylorus (pi-lo′rus)   The portion of the stomach nearest its attachment to the small intestine.
pyramidal (pir″ĭ-mid′al) **tracts**   Motor nerve fibers that pass through the pyramids of the medulla.
pyridoxine (pir″ĭ-dok′sēn)   A B vitamin essential for fatty acid metabolism.
pyrogen (pi′ro-jen)   A substance that increases body temperature.
pyruvic (pi-roo′vik) **acid**   An intermediate in the metabolism of carbohydrates.

quadrate (kwod′rāt)   Four sided.
quadriplegia (kwad″ra-ple′je-ah)   Paralysis of all four limbs.

radioactivity (ra″de-o-ak-tiv′it-e)   The capacity to emit alpha or beta particles, or gamma rays.
ramus (ra″mus)   A projection from an irregularly shaped bone; root means a branch.
raphe (ra′fe)   A seamlike ridge.
raphe nuclei   A group of cell bodies that form part of the reticular formation and are involved in the regulation of sleep and wakefulness.
rapid-eye-movement sleep, REM   A sleep interval during which the eyeballs move and the EEG resembles wakefulness; paradoxical sleep.
RAS   Reticular activating system.
RBC   Red blood cell, erythrocyte.
reabsorption (re″ab-sorp′shun)   The taking up again of something that has been excreted.
receptor (re-sep′tor)   (1) A sense organ; the peripheral endings of sensory nerves; (2) a specific site or chemical configuration on a cell membrane or inside a cell with which a specific substance (hormone or neurotransmitters) may combine and alter cell function.
recessive (re-ses′iv)   In genetics, a characteristic that appears in the phenotype only when two alleles for the characteristic are present in the genotype.
reciprocal innervation   The neural connections whereby one process is slowed as another is accelerated, such as the contraction of one muscle and the relaxation of its antagonist.
recombinant (re-kom′bin-ant) **DNA**   The union (in the laboratory) of DNA from two different species.
rectum (rek′tum)   The terminal portion of the digestive tract that leads to the anal canal.
rectus (rek′tus)   Straight.
red nucleus   A midbrain nucleus that gives rise to the rubrospinal tract.
red pulp   The portion of the spleen that contains numerous blood sinuses.
reduced hemoglobin   Hemoglobin that is not carrying oxygen.
reduction (re-duk′shun)   (1) The gain of an electron, the gain of hydrogen, or the loss of oxygen; (2) the realignment of a fractured bone.
referred pain   Pain that is perceived to have originated at a site other than its actual origin.
reflex (re′fleks)   An involuntary response to the stimulation of a receptor.
refraction (re-frak′shun)   The bending of light rays as they pass from a medium having one density to a medium having a different density.
refractory (re-frak′to-re) **period**   A period immediately after stimulation, during which a cell cannot respond to another stimulus.
relaxin (re-lax′in)   A hormone from the corpus luteum of pregnancy.
releasing hormones   Secretions from the hypothalamus that stimulate the secretion of anterior pituitary hormones.
REM sleep   Rapid-eye-movement sleep.

remission (re-mish'un) The diminution or abatement of symptoms of a disease; a period during which such diminution occurs.

renal (re'nal) Pertaining to the kidney.

renin (ren'in) A secretion of the kidney that causes a rise in blood pressure by activating angiotensin.

rennin (ren'in) An enzyme from the gastric mucosa that digests milk protein.

replication (rep''lĭ-ka'shun) Duplication.

repolarization (re''po-lar-ĭ-za'shun) The restoring of the resting potential in an excitable cell.

reproduction The process by which an offspring is formed.

residual volume The volume of air remaining in the lungs following a maximal forceful exhalation.

resistance Opposition to flow, as in blood vessels.

respiration Breathing; the exchange of gases between the environment and the blood or between the blood and the cells.

respiratory center A group of neurons in the brainstem that regulate respiration.

respiratory distress syndrome A condition in which respiration is labored and gas exchange is impaired.

respiratory quotient (RQ) The ratio of carbon dioxide produced to oxygen consumed.

response The action elicited by a stimulus.

resting potential Electrical potential difference between the inner and outer surfaces of a membrane in a cell that has not been recently stimulated.

rete (re'te) A net or meshwork of blood vessels or nerves.

reticular (re-tik'u-lar) Pertaining to a net or meshwork.

reticular activating system, RAS A network of fibers in the brainstem that stimulate electrical activity in the cerebral cortex and thus arousal.

reticular formation A network of fibers in the brainstem having numerous connections to other parts of the brain; includes the reticular activating system.

reticuloendothelial (re-tik''u-lo-en-do-the'le-al) **system** A diverse group of macrophages or phagocytic cells that are found in the linings of sinuses in the liver, spleen, and other organs.

retina (ret'ĭ-nah) The innermost layer of the eye, which contains the receptor cells that respond to light.

retinene (ret'ĭ-nēn) A pigment in the eye involved in the response to light.

retraction (re-trak'shun) Movement of the mandible backward.

retroperitoneal (ret''ro-per''ĭ-to-ne'al) Behind the peritoneum.

reverberating (re-ver'ber-āt-ing) **circuit** A neuronal circuit in which collateral signals restimulate the input neuron, thus prolonging neural activity.

Rh factor An antigen found on the red blood cells of Rh-positive individuals.

rheumatoid arthritis (ru''ma-toid' ar-thri'tis) An inflammatory disease of the joints thought to involve autoimmunity.

rhodopsin (ro-dop'sin) A protein of retinal rods that is altered by light.

riboflavin (ri''bo-fla'vin) A B vitamin that forms part of the flavin coenzymes.

ribonucleic (ri''bo-nu-kle'ik) **acid, RNA** A nucleic acid involved in protein synthesis.

ribosomal (ri''bo-som'al) **RNA** Ribonucleic acid that forms part of the structure of a ribosome, the cell organelle responsible for protein synthesis.

ribosome (ri''bo-sōm') An organelle consisting of ribonucleic acid and protein, usually associated with the endoplasmic reticulum and important in protein synthesis.

rickets (rik'etz) A childhood disorder in which the bones fail to harden because of a calcium deficiency.

rigor mortis (ri'gor mor'tis) Rigidity or stiffening of the muscles following death.

RNA Ribonucleic acid.

RNA polymerase (pol-im'er-ās) An enzyme involved in the synthesis of RNA.

rod A receptor in the eye that responds to dim light and is responsible for black-and-white vision.

root Base or foundation.

rotation Movement of a part about its own axis.

round window A membrane-covered opening between the middle and inner ear.

Ruffini corpuscles Sensory receptors in the skin that respond to warm temperatures.

rugae (ru'ge) Creases or folds.

saccule (sak'ūl) A little sac, especially a sac in the vestibule of the inner ear.

sacroiliac (sak'ro-il'e-ak) **joint** The joint between the sacrum and the ilium.

saddle joint A joint having a saddle-shaped articulating surface.

sagittal (saj'i-tal) Pertaining to an antero-posterior direction; referring to a plane that divides left and right sides.

salivary (sal'ĭ-ver-e) Pertaining to saliva or to the glands that produce it.

saltatory (sal'tah-tor-e) Leaping; referring to the jumping of a nerve impulse from one node of Ranvier to the next.

S-A node Sinoatrial node.

saphenous (saf-e'nus) Pertaining to the superficial veins of the leg.

sarcolemma (sar-ko-lem'ah) The cell membrane of a muscle fiber.

sarcomere (sar''ko-mēr) A contractile unit of striated muscle.

sarcoplasm (sar'ko-plazm) The nonfibrillar portion of a muscle cell.

sarcoplasmic reticulum (sar''ko-plaz'mik rĕ-tik'u-lum) A network of tubules and vesicles associated with the myofibrils of striated muscle.

satiety (sat'ĭ-te) **center** A hypothalamic center concerned with the regulation of food intake.

saturated fatty acid A fatty acid having no double bonds in the carbon chain.

scala tympani (ska'lah tim'pan-e) The lower canal of the cochlea.

scala vestibuli (ska'lah ves-tib'u-le)   The upper canal of the cochlea.

schizophrenia (skiz-o-fre'ne-ah)   A mental disorder characterized by a complex set of disturbances in thinking and feeling.

Schwann cell   Cell that insulates the axons of peripheral nerve fibers; neurilemmal cell; myelin-producing cell.

sciatic (si-at'ik)   Pertaining to the hip.

sclera (skle'rah)   The outermost layer of the eyeball.

scoliosis (sko''le-o'sis)   A lateral curvature of the spine.

scotopsin (sko-top'sin)   A protein pigment found in the rods of the retina.

scrotum (skro'tum)   A pouch containing the testes.

sebaceous (se-ba'ce-us)   Pertaining to sebum or the glands that produce it.

sebum (se'bum)   A substance composed of fat and epithelial cell debris.

secretagogue (se-krēt'ag-og)   A substance that stimulates secretion.

secretin (se-kre'tin)   A hormone from the intestinal mucosa that stimulates secretion of pancreatic fluid and bile.

secretion   (1) The product of a gland; the process of releasing a substance from a gland; (2) the active transport of substances from kidney tubule cells to the lumen of the tubule.

secretory (se''kre-to're) **granules**   Small particles within the cytoplasm of cells that produce secretions.

secretory phase   That portion of the menstrual cycle in which the uterine mucosa develops glands.

section   A cut surface or a thin slice.

segmentation (seg''men-ta'shun)   (1) Splitting into segments; (2) alternating contractions of segments of the small intestine.

segmentation contraction   Repetitive contractions of circular muscle in the digestive tract that create a chopping action.

segregation   The separation of chromosomes into gametes.

selectively permeable   The property of allowing some substances to pass through while preventing the passage of other substances; applied to membranes.

sella turcica (sel'ah tur'sik-ah)   A saddle-shaped depression in the sphenoid bone that contains the pituitary gland; root means Turkish saddle.

semen (se'men)   The secretion from the male reproductive tract that contains sperm and a variety of other substances.

semicircular canals   Three mutually perpendicular tubes that contain fluid and receptors for dynamic equilbrium.

semilunar   Shaped like a half-moon.

seminal vesicles   Convoluted saclike structures near the ductus deferens that contribute secretions to the semen.

seminiferous (sem''ĭ-nif'er-us) **tubules**   Coiled tubules of the testes that produce sperm.

sensor   A device that responds to a stimulus.

sensory   Pertaining to sensation.

septum (plural, **septa**) (sep'tum, sep'tah)   A wall or partition.

serosa (se-ro'sah)   A membrane that secretes a watery substance and lines body cavities.

serotonin (sehr''o-to'nin)   A chemical substance secreted by certain cells of the brain and gut; thought to be a neuro-transmitter.

serous (ser'us)   Watery.

serrated (ser'āt-ed)   Saw-toothed.

Sertoli cell   A supporting cell of the seminiferous tubules.

serum (se'rum)   The fluid portion of clotted blood.

sesamoid (ses'a-moid)   Resembling a sesame seed; pertaining to a bone formed in a tendon.

sex-linked inheritance   Transmission of heritable characteristics on the X chromosome.

shaft   Rodlike structure; diaphysis of a long bone.

sheath of Schwann   Membrane containing myelin produced by Schwann cells; neurilemma.

shock   Failure of the blood vessels to deliver blood to the tissues.

sickle cell anemia   A kind of anemia in which erythrocytes assume a sickle shape under low oxygen conditions caused by a hereditary defect in hemoglobin.

SIDS   Sudden infant death syndrome.

sigmoid (sig'moid)   Shaped like the letter S.

signet ring cells   Fat cells, so called because the nucleus is pushed to one side of the cell, giving it a shape in cross section similar to a signet ring.

simple goiter   Enlargement of the thyroid gland due to deficiency of iodine.

sinoatrial (si-no-a'tre-al) **node, S-A node**   An aggregation of spontaneously firing cells that initiate contraction of the heart; pacemaker.

sinus (si'nus)   A recess or cavity.

sinusitis (si''nus-i'tis)   An inflammation of a sinus in a bone.

sinusoid (si'nus-oid)   Blood vessel similar to a capillary but having a larger diameter.

sliding filament theory   An explanation of the mechanism by which muscles contract.

slow-wave sleep   Phase of sleep characterized by slow brain waves and absence of eye movements.

sodium-potassium pump   An active transport system that moves sodium ions out of a cell and potassium ions into a cell against a concentration gradient.

sodium pump   Sodium-potassium pump.

solute   A dissolved substance.

solution   The process of dissolving; a liquid containing two or more substances, the molecules of which are homogeneously dispersed.

solvent   A substance capable of causing certain solutes to dissolve.

soma (so'mah)   Body; a cell body of a neuron.

somatic (so-mat'ik)   Pertaining to the body.

somatic (so-mat'ik) **motor area**   A functional area of the cerebrum from which voluntary actions are initiated.

somatic sensory area   A functional area of the cerebrum in which sensations from the skin and taste buds are perceived.

somatostatin (so-mat'o-stat''in)   Growth hormone–releasing hormone, GH-RH.

somatotropin (so-mat'o-trop-in)   Growth hormone; anterior pituitary hormone that promotes growth and maintains adult size.

somite (so'mīt)   Mesodermal segment of an embryo.

spasm (spazm)   A sudden, violent, involuntary contraction of a muscle or group of muscles.

spastic (spas'tik)   Pertains to increased muscle tone.

spatial summation   Increased excitability of a neuron due to the action of several adjacent excitatory presynaptic potentials.

specific dynamic action, SDA   The increased metabolic rate associated with the ingestion of food, especially protein.

specific gravity   Density; the weight of any substance compared to that of water.

specificity (spec''ĭ-fis'ĭ-te)   The quality of being specific, as an enzyme acting on a particular substrate or an antibody reacting with a particular antigen.

spectrin (spek'trin)   A protein in erythrocytes that contributes to their deformability.

spermatic (sper-mat'ik) **cord**   A cord extending from the scrotum to the inguinal ligament containing the ductus deferens, arteries, veins, lymphatics, and nerves.

spermatids (sper-mah-tids')   Immature spermatozoa.

spermatocytes (sper-mat'o-sīts)   Cells that give rise to spermatozoa.

spermatogenesis (sper''mah-to-jen'e-sis)   The production of spermatozoa.

spermatozoa (sper''mah-to-zo'ah)   Male gametes; sperm.

sphenoid (sfe'noid)   Winglike; refers to a skull bone.

sphincter (sfingk'ter)   A muscle that can close an opening when it contracts.

sphygmomanometer (sfig''mo-mah-nom'e-ter)   An instrument used to measure blood pressure.

spicule (spik'ūl)   A needle-shaped structure.

spinal nerve   One of thirty-one pairs of nerves that branch from the spinal cord.

spinal shock   A condition following spinal injury during which spinal reflexes below the injury are lost.

spinal tap   A procedure in which spinal fluid is withdrawn from the spinal cord.

spine   (1) Vertebral column; (2) a short, sharp process on a bone.

spinous (spi'nus)   Like a spine.

spiral organ   Organ of Corti.

splanchnic (splank'nik)   Pertaining to the viscera.

sprain   A joint injury in which surrounding tissues may be damaged but the joint is not dislocated.

sprue (spru)   A disease in which the lining of the gastrointestinal tract is inflamed and partially destroyed.

squamous (skwa'mus)   Scalelike.

stapes (sta'pez)   Stirrup; one of the ossicles of the middle ear.

starch   A polysaccharide composed of glucose units.

static equilibrium   The maintenance of balance when the head is stationary.

stem cell   An undifferentiated cell that gives rise to blood cells.

stenosis (sten-o'sis)   A narrowing.

sterility   The inability to produce offspring.

steroid (ste'roid)   A substance related to the lipids having a characteristic four-ring structure; cholesterol, adrenocortical, and sex hormones.

stethoscope (steth'o-skōp)   A device for listening to sounds within the body.

stimulus (stim'u-lus)   A change in the environment that in some way modifies the activity of protoplasm.

stomodeum (sto-mo-de'um)   An evagination in the ectoderm from which the mouth and upper pharynx form.

strabismus (stra-biz'mus)   A condition in which the two eyes do not focus together on the same object.

strain   A stretching of tissues around a joint.

stratum (strat'um)   A layer, especially of tissues.

stress   A condition of the body produced by a variety of injurious agents.

stressor (stres'or)   That which produces stress.

stretch receptor   A structure within a lung that responds to stretching as air is inhaled; similar structures in tendons.

stretch reflex   Contraction of a muscle following stimulation of stretch receptors in the muscle or its tendon.

striated   Striped.

stroke volume   The volume of blood pumped per contraction of the heart.

stroma (stro'mah)   Framework; usually connective tissue that supports an organ.

styloid (sti'loid)   A slender process like a stylus.

subarachnoid (sub''ah-rak'noid)   Beneath the arachnoid layer.

subcutaneous (sub''ku-ta'ne-us)   Beneath the skin.

subliminal (sub-lim'in-al)   Pertaining to a stimulus below the level of conscious perception or below the threshold level.

sublingual (sub-ling'gwal)   Beneath the tongue.

submandibular (sub''man-dib'u-lar)   Beneath the mandible.

submucosa   A connective tissue layer beneath a mucous membrane.

subneural (sub-noo'ral) **cleft**   A fold in the sarcolemma that contains receptor sites for a neurotransmitter.

substantia nigra (sub-stan'che-ah ni'grah)   A nucleus of pigmented cells related to the basal nuclei.

substrate   A substance acted on by an enzyme.

subthreshold   Below the threshold level, as a stimulus too weak to cause a response.

sucrose (su-krōs)   A disaccharide composed of glucose and fructose; table sugar.

sugar   A saccharide; a small carbohydrate molecule.

sulcus (sul'kus)   Groove.

summation (sum-ma'shun)   An adding of effects.

superficial   Near the surface.

superior   Above or higher than.

supination (soo''pĭ-na'shun)   Rotation of the forearm so that the palm of the hand faces forward in anatomical position.

supraorbital (soo''prah-or'bit-al)   Above the orbit of the eye.

surfactant (ser-fak'tant)   A substance that reduces surface tension; refers to substance produced in lungs.

suspensory (sus-pen'sor-e)   Serving to hold up a part.

suture (soo'cher)   An immovable fibrous joint.

sympathetic (sim-pa-thet'ik) **division**   A component of the autonomic nervous system that regulates visceral function in conjunction with the parasympathetic division; responsible for stimulating the body to respond to a stressful situation.

sympathomimetic (sim-path″o-mim-et′ik)   Pertaining to a drug that mimics the action of the sympathetic nervous system.

symphysis (sim′fi-sis)   A slightly movable cartilaginous joint.

synapse (sin′aps)   A junction between neurons across which a neurotransmitter diffuses.

synapsis (si-nap′sis)   The coming together of members of a pair of chromosomes.

synaptic (si-nap′tik) **cleft**   The space between neurons of a synapse.

synaptic vesicles   Small membrane-bound particles near the cell membrane of the end-feet of axons.

synarthrosis (sin-ar-thro′sis)   An immovable joint with no intervening tissue between the bones.

synchondrosis (sin-kon-dro′sis)   A slightly movable or immovable joint in which two bones are joined by cartilage.

syncytium (sin-sish′e-um)   A group of cells that have lost the membranes that divided them.

syndesmosis (sin-des-mo′sis)   A joint in which two bones are bound together by fibrous connective tissue.

syndrome (sin′drōm)   A group of signs and symptoms that occur together.

synergist (sin′er-jist)   A muscle that assists a prime mover.

synovial (si-no′ve-al) **joint**   A freely movable joint having a fibrous capsule lined with synovial membrane and filled with synovial fluid.

systemic (sis-tem′ik)   Pertaining to the whole organism.

systole (sis′to-le)   Contraction.

systolic (sis-tol′ik) **pressure**   The highest pressure reached in an artery during heart systole; the pressure during contraction of the ventricles.

T₃, T₄   Tri-iodothyronine and tetra-iodothyronine (thyroxine).

tachycardia (tak″ĕ-kar′de-ah)   An abnormally rapid heartbeat.

tactile (tak′til)   Pertaining to touch.

tardive dyskinesia (tar′dīv dis-kin-e′se-ah)   Involuntary movements that may result from long-term treatment with tranquilizers.

target organ   An organ or tissue acted on by a hormone.

tarsal (tar″sal)   One of seven bones forming the heel and instep.

taste bud   Structure containing receptor cells for taste, located in papillae of the tongue.

T-cell   Cells of the immune system that produce cell-mediated immunity.

tectorial (tek-tor′e-al) **membrane**   A membrane overlying the hair cells of the organ of Corti.

telophase (tel′o-fāz)   The last stage of mitosis, during which the nuclei reform.

temporal (tem′por-al) **lobe**   A functional area of the cerebrum that contains auditory and olfactory areas.

temporal summation   An increased response of a nerve because of increased frequency of excitation.

tendon   A cord of fibrous connective tissue attaching a muscle to a bone.

tendon organ   Sensory receptor in a tendon that responds to stretching.

tendon sheath   A synovial membrane found around certain tendons.

tenia coli (te″ne-ah ko′le)   Any of the three bands of longitudinal muscle fibers in the large intestine.

teratogen (ter-at′o-jen)   An agent that causes defects during embryonic development.

testis (tes′tis)   A male gonad.

testosterone (tes-tos′ter-ōn)   The main hormone of the male gonad.

tetanus (tet′an-us)   (1) A sustained contraction produced by repeated stimulation; (2) lockjaw, a disease produced by a bacterial toxin.

tetany (tet′an-e)   A disorder involving involuntary contraction of skeletal muscles.

tetrad (tet′rad)   (1) A group of four things; (2) duplicated, paired chromosomes.

tetralogy (tet-ral′o-ge) **of Fallot**   A group of four congenital defects in the heart that commonly occur together.

thalamus (thal′am-us)   Gray matter near the anterior end of the brainstem.

theca (the′kah)   Sheath; covering of ovarian follicle.

thermoreceptor   A heat-sensitive receptor.

thiamin   A B vitamin important in several metabolic reactions as a coenzyme.

thirst center   A nucleus in the hypothalamus that responds to osmotic changes in the blood, causing drinking behavior when the osmotic pressure increases.

thoracic (thor-as′ik)   Pertaining to the chest.

thoracic duct   A large lymph vessel extending from the cysterni chyli to the left subclavian vein and draining lymph from the body except for the upper right side.

thoracolumbar (tho-rak-o-lum′bar)   A division of the autonomic nervous system responsible for sympathetic action.

thorax (tho′raks)   The chest.

threshold   (1) The weakest stimulus that will produce a response; (2) the concentration of a substance that can be returned to the blood from the kidney.

threshold stimulus   A stimulus just strong enough to cause a nerve or muscle cell to respond.

thrombin (throm′bin)   An enzyme that converts fibrinogen to fibrin in the blood-clotting reaction.

thrombocyte (throm′bo-sīt)   Platelet.

thromboplastin (throm-bo-plas′tin)   A substance that initiates the extrinsic pathway of the blood-clotting mechanism.

thrombosis (throm-bo′sis)   Formation of a thrombus.

thrombus (throm′bus)   A blood clot adhering to the wall of a blood vessel.

thymine (thi′mēn)   A nitrogenous base in DNA.

thymosin (thi′mo-sin)   A hormone produced by the thymus gland.

thymus (thi′mus)   A lymphoid organ in the upper thoracic cavity that processes and activates T lymphocytes.

thyroid (thi′roid) **gland**   An endocrine gland in the neck that secretes thyroxine and calcitonin.

thyroid-stimulating hormone   A hormone released by the

anterior pituitary gland that causes synthesis and release of thyroid homrones.

thyrotropin (thi-ro'tro-pin) An anterior pituitary hormone that stimulates the thyroid gland to secrete thyroid hormones; thyroid-stimulating hormone.

thyroxine (thi-rok'sin), T_4 Tetra-iodothyronine, the main hormone of the thyroid gland.

tidal volume The volume of air normally moving into and out of the lungs during quiet breathing.

tight junction Intercellular junction in which adjacent cells are fused.

timbre (tahn'br) The musical quality in a tone or sound.

tissue An aggregation of similar cells and the intercellular substances associated with them.

tissue fluid Interstitial fluid; fluid surrounding cells.

T lymphocyte (lim'fo-sīt) Cells associated with cell-mediated immunity.

tone Normal tension maintained in muscle.

tonic Pertaining to continuous activity.

tonsil (ton'sil) An aggregate of lymphatic tissue in the pharynx.

toxemia (tox-em'e-ah) Accumulation of toxins, sometimes occurring in pregnancy.

toxin (tox'in) A poisonous substance.

trabecula (tra-bek'u-lah) A septum; a spicule of spongy bone.

trachea (tra'ke-ah) Passage from the larynx to the bronchi.

tract A bundle of myelinated neurons in the brain or spinal cord.

transamination (trans-am"in-a'shun) The transferral of an amino group from one molecule to another.

transcription (tran-skrip'shun) The process of transferring the genetic code from DNA to mRNA.

transduction The conversion of a signal from a sensory receptor to an electrical signal in a neuron.

transferrin (trans-fer'in) A plasma protein that carries iron.

transfer RNA, tRNA RNA molecules that carry amino acids to ribosomes and align them in the protein according to base-pairing of the tRNA anticodon and the mRNA codon.

translation The process by which information in mRNA codons is used to determine the sequence of amino acids in a protein.

translocation The transfer of a portion of a chromosome from its normal location to a location on another chromosome.

transmission The act of transmitting; refers to the passage of nerve signals across synapses, the passage of genetic characteristics from one generation to the next, and the passage of infectious agents from one individual to another.

transmitter A substance that transmits signals across synapses; neurotransmitter.

transverse Crosswise.

transverse tubules Tubules running crosswise of the myofibrils in skeletal muscle, responsible for conveying an impulse from the sarcolemma to the myofibrils.

trauma (traw'ma) Injury.

Treponema pallidum (tre"po-ne'mah pal'ĭ-dum) A bacterium that causes syphilis.

treppe (trep'eh) A gradual increase in the extent of muscular contraction following rapidly repeated stimulation; root means staircase.

triad Any group of three.

tricarboxylic (tri"kar-box-il'ik) **acid cycle** Krebs cycle.

tricuspid (tri-kus'pid) Having three processes.

triglyceride (tri-glǐ'ser-īd) A molecule consisting of glycerol and three fatty acids; a fat.

trigone (tri'gōn) A triangle; the triangle formed in the urinary bladder by the openings of the ureters and urethra.

tRNA Transfer RNA.

trochanter (tro-kan'ter) Large, rounded bony process.

trochlea (trok'le-ah) Pulley; forms pulleylike attachment for superior oblique eye muscle; process on humerus.

trophoblast (trof'o-blast) Outer layer of a blastocyst, which establishes connection with maternal tissue and gives rise to chorionic villi.

tropomyosin (tor-po-mi'o-sin) A protein of muscle involved in the relaxation of a contracted muscle.

troponin (tro'po-nin) A protein of muscle involved in the relaxation of a contracted muscle.

trypsin (trip'sin) A proteolytic enzyme released from the pancreas.

T-tubule Transverse tubule.

tubercle (tu'ber-kl) Small, rounded protrusion.

tuberculosis (tu-ber-ku-lo'sis) A disease most often affecting the lungs and caused by a bacterium.

tuberosity (tu-ber-os'it-e) Large, rounded protrusion.

tunica (tu'nik-ah) A coat; a layer, as in blood vessels, the eye, and the testes.

Turner's syndrome A condition in which only a single X chromosome (without another X or a Y chromosome) is present; produces a sterile female.

twitch Response of a muscle to a single stimulus.

tympanic (tim-pan'ik) **membrane** Eardrum; membrane dividing external and middle ear.

umbilical (um-bil'ic-al) **cord** A cord connecting the fetus with the placenta and consisting of two umbilical arteries and an umbilical vein.

umbilicus (um-bil-i'kus) Site of attachment of umbilical cord to fetus; navel.

uniaxial joint A joint that moves about only one axis.

unilateral On one side only.

unmyelinated (un-mi'el-in-āt"ed) Lacking myelin.

unsaturated fatty acid Fatty acid having one or more double bonds in its carbon chain.

uracil (ur'ah-sil) A nitrogenous base found in RNA.

urea (u-re'ah) The main nitrogenous waste product found in the urine.

uremia (u-re'me-ah) A disorder caused by the toxic accumulation of urea and other wastes in the blood, usually due to kidney failure.

ureter (u-re'ter) Tube that carries urine from the kidney to the urinary bladder.

urethra (u-re'thrah) Tube that carries urine from the urinary bladder outside the body.

uric (u′rik) **acid** A nitrogenous waste product from the breakdown of purines.

urinalysis (u-rin-al′is-is) Chemical and microscopic study of the constituents of urine.

urinary (u′rin-a″re) **bladder** Stretchable sac where urine is stored.

urine Excretory product of the kidneys.

uterine (u′ter-in) **tube** Fallopian tube; oviduct; tube that carries ova from ovaries to uterus.

uterus (u′ter-us) Hollow, pear-shaped organ in which the fetus develops.

utricle (u′trik-l) Large chamber in the vestibule of the ear that contains receptors for equilibrium.

uvula (u′vu-lah) Soft projection from soft palate.

vagina (fah-ji′nah) Passageway from the uterus to the vestibule.

varicose (var′ik-ōs) Unnaturally swollen.

vasa recta (va′sah rek′tah) Straight vessels, especially capillaries found in the renal pyramids.

vasa vasorum (va′sah vas-o′rum) Blood vessels within the walls of larger blood vessels.

vascular (vas′ku-lar) Pertaining to blood vessels.

vas deferens (vas def′er-enz) Tube from epididymis to the ejaculatory duct; ductus deferens.

vasectomy (vas-ek′to-me) Removal of a segment of the vas deferens, usually for purpose of rendering sterile.

vasoconstriction (va″so-kon-strik′shun) Narrowing of the lumen of a blood vessel.

vasodilation (va″so-di-la′shun) Widening of the lumen of a blood vessel.

vasomotor (va-so-mo′tor) **center** An area in the brainstem that regulates the diameter of blood vessels, especially arterioles.

vasopressin (va-so-pres′in) A posterior pituitary hormone that causes constriction of blood vessels in large doses; antidiuretic hormone, ADH.

vein (vān) A blood vessel carrying blood to the heart.

ventilation (ven-til-a′shun) Exchange of air between the lungs and the atmosphere.

ventral (ven′tral) Pertaining to the belly; anterior in humans.

ventricle (ven′trik-l) A small cavity.

ventricular (ven-trik′ul-ar) Pertaining to a ventricle.

venule (ven′ūl) A small vein connecting capillaries with a larger vein.

vermis (ver′mis) A wormlike structure; a portion of the cerebellum.

vertigo (ver′tig-o) Dizziness.

vesicle (ves′ik-l) A small sac within a cell or within an organ.

vestibule (ves′tib-ūl) A space at the entrance of a tube or canal.

vestigial (ves-tij′e-al) Pertaining to a rudimentary structure.

villikinin (vil″e-kīn′in) A hormone from the small intestine that stimulates movement of the villi.

villus (plural, **villi**) (vill′lus, vil′le) Tiny projection of mucosa into the lumen of the small intestine.

viscera (vis′er-ah) Internal organs.

visceroceptor (vis″er-o-sep′tor) A sensory receptor in a visceral organ.

viscosity (vis-kos′ĭ-te) Tendency of a fluid to resist flowing.

visual area A functional area in the occipital lobe of the cerebrum where impulses from the retina are received and interpreted.

vital capacity The largest volume of air that can be exhaled after a maximal inspiration.

vital center Center in brainstem essential to life.

vitamin (vi′tam-in) An organic substance required for life but not produced in the body.

vitreous (vit′re-us) Glassy.

Volkmann's canals Channels that carry blood vessels through the matrix of bone to the Haversian system.

vulva (vul′vah) Female external genitalia.

Wallerian degeneration The process of disintegration that occurs in the axon of an injured neuron beyond the point of the injury.

water intoxication Entry of water into cells because of reduced osmotic pressure in extracellular fluids.

Wharton's duct The duct of the submaxillary salivary gland.

Wharton's jelly A soft, pulpy connective tissue forming the matrix of the umbilical cord.

white matter Myelinated nerve fibers of the central nervous system.

white pulp Tissue of the spleen consisting of aggregations of lymphocytes.

withdrawal reflex A reflex causing flexion and removal of a limb from a painful stimulus.

Wormian (wer′me-an) **bone** A small accessory bone sometimes found between the larger bones of the skull.

xiphoid (zi′foid) Shaped like a sword; a process of the sternum.

zona fasciculata (zo′nah fas-ik″u-la′ta) Middle layer of adrenal cortex.

zona glomerulosa (zo′nah glo-mer″u-lo′sah) Outer layer of adrenal cortex.

zona pellucida (zo′nah pel-u′sid-ah) Translucent layer surrounding an oocyte while still in the ovarian follicle.

zona reticularis (zo′nah re-tik″u-la′ris) Inner layer of adrenal cortex.

zygomatic (zi-go-mat′ik) Pertaining to the malar (cheek) bone.

zygote (zi′-gōt) Single cell formed by the union of an ovum and a sperm; first cell of a new individual.

INDEX

lamin(a)- layer	**necr-** dead	**pars-** part
lapar- loins	**nephr-** kidney	**partur-** give birth
lat(a)- wide	**neur-** nerve	**patell-** little dish
later- side	**neutr-** neither	**path(o)-** suffering, disease
-lemma sheath	**nom-** name	**pauc-** few
leuco- white	**noxi-** harmful	**ped(i)-** foot
leva- lift	**nuc-** nut	**-pedia** child
levo- left side	**nuch-** nape of neck	**pelv-** basin
liga- tied, bound	**nunci-** messenger	**pent-** five
lipo- fatty	**nutri-** feed, nourish	**pep-** digest
lith- stone	**nyc-** night	**per-** through
lumb- loin	**o-(ov-)** egg	**peri-** around
lut(e)- yellowish	**ob-** against	**peripat-** walking about
lys- loose	**obtur-** stop up	**pernic-** destructive
macer- soften	**oc-** against	**-pes** foot
macr(o)- large	**occip-** back of head	**phag-** eat
macula spot	**occlu-** shut	**phalan-** bone of finger or toe
mal- bad	**ocul-** eye	**phleb-** vein
mast- breast	**odon-** tooth	**phob-** fear
mastic- chew	**olecran-** elbow	**-phragm** fence
meat(us) passage	**olfact-** smell	**pil(i)-** hair
medi- middle	**-ology** science of	**pinn(a)-** wing
medull- marrow	**-oma** tumor	**plant(a)-** sole of foot
melan- black	**omentum** fat skin	**plasm-** something molded
mens- month	**omni-** all	**pleur-** side, rib
ment- mind, chin	**onco-** tumor	**plex-** network
mer(e)- part	**op-** reversed	**pne-** breath, breathe
mes(o)- middle	**-opia** vision	**pneumo-** lungs
met(a)- change	**opt- (opthalm-)** eye	**pod-** foot
micell- little piece	**ora-** mouth	**poly-** many
mill- one thousandth	**orth-** upright	**pons** bridge
mon- one	**os-** bone	**popl-** back of knee
morb- disease	**-ose** full of	**porphyr-** purple
morph- form	**-osis** condition, disease	**post-** behind
morul- mulberry	**-osity** fullness	**pre-** before
mult- many	**osmo-** pushing	**presby-** old
myelo- marrow, spinal cord	**-ostium** small opening	**pro-** in front, before
myo- muscle	**oto-** ear	**proct-** anus, rectum
myop- short-sighted	**-ous** full of	**propri-** one's own
narc- numbness	**oxi-** sharp, acid	**pros-** to, before
nas- nose	**palp-** feel	**proto-** first, original
nebul- mist	**papill-** nipple	**pseudo-** false